EMERGENCY
MEDICAL TECHNICIAN
EMT in Action

Second Edition

Barbara Aehlert, RN

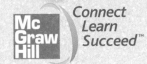

Mc Graw Hill

Connect
Learn
Succeed™

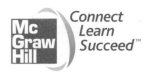

EMERGENCY MEDICAL TECHNICIAN: EMT IN ACTION

Published by McGraw-Hill, a business unit of The McGraw-Hill Companies, Inc., 1221 Avenue of the Americas, New York, NY, 10020. Copyright © 2011 by The McGraw-Hill Companies, Inc. All rights reserved. Previous edition © 2009. No part of this publication may be reproduced or distributed in any form or by any means, or stored in a database or retrieval system, without the prior written consent of The McGraw-Hill Companies, Inc., including, but not limited to, in any network or other electronic storage or transmission, or broadcast for distance learning.

Some ancillaries, including electronic and print components, may not be available to customers outside the United States.

This book is printed on acid-free paper.

2 3 4 5 6 7 8 9 0 RJE/RJE 1 0 9 8 7 6 5 4 3 2 1

ISBN   978-0-07-338289-0
MHID   0-07-338289-2

Vice president/Editor in chief: *Elizabeth Haefele*
Vice president/Director of marketing: *John E. Biernat*
Sponsoring editor: *Barbara Owca*
Director of Development, Business Careers: *Sarah Wood*
Editorial coordinator: *Vincent Bradshaw*
Marketing manager: *Matthew R. McLaughlin*
Lead media producer: *Damian Moshak*
Digital developmental editor: *Kevin White*
Director, Editing/Design/Production: *Jess Ann Kosic*
Lead project manager: *Rick Hecker*
Senior production supervisor: *Janean A. Utley*
Senior designer: *Srdjan Savanovic*
Senior photo research coordinator: *Lori Hancock*
Digital production coordinator: *Brent dela Cruz*
Outside development house: *Laura Horowitz*
Cover and interior design: *Gino Cieslik*
Typeface: *10/12 ITC New Baskerville*
Compositor: *Aptara, Inc.*
Printer: *R. R. Donnelley*
Cover credit: *© Rick Brady*

Go to http://mhhe.com/aehlertemtb2e for Aehlert's updated instructions for cardiopulmonary resuscitation based on the 2010 guidelines on CPR from the American Heart Association.

Library of Congress Cataloging-in-Publication Data

Aehlert, Barbara.
    Emergency medical technician : EMT in action/Barbara Aehlert. – 2nd ed.
        p. cm.
    Includes index.
    ISBN-13: 978-0-07-338289-0 (alk. paper)—ISBN-10: 0-07-338289-2 (alk. paper)
    1. Emergency medicine. 2. Emergency medical technicians. I. Title. [DNLM: 1. Emergency Treatment—methods.
    2. Emergency Medical Services—methods. 3. Emergency Medical Technicians. WB 105 A246e 2011]
RC86.7.A354   2011
616.02'5—dc22   2009039625

www.mhhe.com

Dedication

In memory of my mother, Ronella Su Light Mahoney Grisham

Author and Contributors

About the Author

Barbara Aehlert is the President of Southwest EMS Education, Inc., in Phoenix, Arizona, and Pursley, Texas. She has been a registered nurse for more than 30 years, with clinical experience in medical/surgical and critical care nursing and, for the past 23 years, in prehospital education. Barbara is an active CPR, First Aid, ACLS, and PALS instructor.

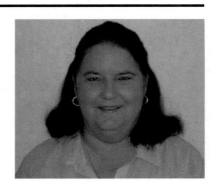

Contributors

Lynn Browne-Wagner, RN, BSN
EMS Program Director
Northland Pioneer College
Holbrook, Arizona

Randy Budd, RRT, CEP
City of Mesa Fire Department
Mesa, AZ

Major Raymond W. Burton (Retired)
Plymouth Academy/Plymouth County Sheriff's Academy
Plymouth, MA

Holly Button, CEP
City of Mesa Fire Department
Mesa, AZ

Suzy Coronel, CEP
Sportsmedicine Fairbanks
Fairbanks, AK

Janet Fitts, RN, EMT-P, Educational Consultant
Prehospital and Emergency Medical Services
Pacific, MO

Paul Honeywell, CEP
Southwest Ambulance
Mesa, AZ

Travis Kidd, EMT-P
Orange County Fire/Rescue
Orlando, FL

Andrea Lowrey, RN
Dallas, TX

Terence Mason, RN
City of Mesa Fire Department
Mesa, AZ

Kim McKenna, RN, EMT-P
Director of Education
St. Charles County Ambulance Service
St. Peters, MO

Sean Newton, CEP
City of Scottsdale Fire Department
Scottsdale, AZ

Gary Smith, MD
Medical Director: Apache Junction, Gilbert, and Mesa
*   Fire Departments*
Apache Junction, Gilbert, and Mesa, AZ

Edith Valladares
Director, Foreign Languages and Academic ESL
Central Piedmont Community College
Charlotte, NC

Reviewers

Leaugeay C. Barnes, BS, NREMT-P, CCEMT-P
Program Director, Emergency Medical Sciences
Oklahoma City Community College
Oklahoma City, OK

Gerria Berryman, EMTP
Emergency Medical Training Professionals
Lexington, KY

Amanda Bowen
Firefighter/Paramedic/Instructor
Memphis Fire Department
Memphis, TN

Debra Cason, RN, MS, EMT-P
Associate Professor and Program Director
Emergency Medicine Education
University of Texas Southwestern Medical Center
Dallas, TX

Mark Chapman
EMS Academy Coordinator
Underwood Memorial Hospital
Woodbury, NJ

Jeff Clayton
EMS
Lanier Technical College
Oakwood, GA

Richard A. Criste, BHS, NREMT-P
EMS Department Chair
Fayetteville Technical Community College
Fayetteville, NC

W. Scott Crowley
EMT Program Director
Phoenix College
Phoenix, AZ

George W. DeTuccio, EMT-P Instructor
Austin Community College
Austin, TX

Martha C. Driscoll, AAS, NREMT-P
Clinical Coordinator, Associate Professor
School of Emergency Services
Daytona State College
Daytona Beach, FL

Christopher Dunn, EMT-P
EMT-B Coordinator
Northwest Community Hospital EMSS
Arlington Heights, IL

Jason Ferguson, BPA, AAS, NREMT-P
EMS Program Head
Central Virginia Community College
Lynchburg, VA

Jeff Fritz, BS, LP, NREMT-P
Chair
EMS Professions
Temple College
Temple, TX

Jonathan Greenwald, BA, EMT-P
Chair, EMS Department
Arapahoe Community College
Littleton, CO

Sheldon Guenther, BS, DC, NREMT-P
Associate Professor
Kansas City Kansas Community College
Kansas City, KS

Darryl J. Haefner
Fire Science Coordinator
College of DuPage
Glen Ellyn, IL

Thomas R. Herron Jr., AAS, EMT-P
EMS Coordinator
Cape Fear Community College
Wilmington, NC

Marvin Hudson, AAS, NREMT-P
Richmond Community College
Hamlet, NC

Craig Jacobus, BA/BS, DC, NREMT-P, EMSI
PHTLS Region 3 Coordinator
EMS Education
Metropolitan Community College
Fremont, NE
FF/PM, Schuyler Fire Department, Schuyler, NE

Charlene Jansen, BS, MM, EMT-P
EMS Programs Coordinator
St. Louis Community College
St. Louis, MO

Shawn Komorn, MA, LP
Director of Initial Education/Assistant Professor
Department of Emergency Health Sciences
University of Texas Health Science Center
San Antonio, TX

Dean C. Meenach, RN, BSN, AAS, CEN, EMT-P
Director of EMS Education
Mineral Area College
Park Hills, MO

Keith A. Monosky, PhD(c), MPM, EMT-P
Associate Professor
Department of Nutrition, Exercise, and Health Sciences
Central Washington University
Ellensburg, WA

Kenneth Moorhouse
Assistant Professor
School of Emergency Services
Daytona State College
Daytona Beach, FL

Kevin O'Hara
Nassau County EMS Academy
East Meadow, NY

Donna Olafson, MA, NREMT-P
Director, EMT/MICT Program
Kansas City, KS

Steve Peterson, CPhT, BS, MEd
Director of Education, Fortis College
Phoenix, AZ

Lorna Ramsey, RN, MSN, NREMT-P
Program Director, Emergency Medical Services
Tidewater Community College
Virginia Beach, VA

Steve Rollin, Paramedic
BLS Program Coordinator
Yavapai College Public Services
Prescott Valley, AZ

Dawn Sgro, NREMTP, BS, EMSI
Program Director
Allied Health and Nursing
Lorain County Community College
Elyria, OH

Kristal Smith
Paramedic Technology
Central Georgia Technical College
Macon, GA

Todd E. R. Strom, JD, MS, NREMT-P
Paramedic Instructor
Hennepin County Medical Center
Minneapolis, MN

Adriana Laura Torrez, LP, AAS
EMS Education Coordinator
Methodist Health Systems of Dallas
Dallas, TX

Karen Urick, EMT, SEI
EMT Program Coordinator
North Seattle Community College
Seattle, WA

Lance Villers, PhD, LP
Assistant Professor and Chair
Department of Emergency Health Sciences
University of Texas Health Science Center
San Antonio, TX

Technical Editors

Lynn Browne-Wagner, RN, BSN
EMS Program Director
Northland Pioneer College
Holbrook, AZ

Thomas Falvo, DO, MBA
Department of Emergency Medicine
York Hospital
York, PA
Medical Director
Newberry Township Fire Department & EMS, Inc.
Etters, PA

Dean C. Meenach, RN, BSN, AAS, CEN, EMT-P
Director of EMS Education
Mineral Area College
Park Hills, MO

Bonnie L. Pastorino, AAS
EMT Department
Northland Pioneer College
Holbrook, AZ

Brief Contents

Module 1

Preparatory 1

▶ CHAPTER 1
EMS Systems and Research 2

▶ CHAPTER 2
Workforce Safety and Wellness 28

▶ CHAPTER 3
Legal and Ethical Issues and Documentation 79

▶ CHAPTER 4
EMS System Communications 109

▶ CHAPTER 5
Medical Terminology 121

Module 2

Function and Development of the Human Body 137

▶ CHAPTER 6
The Human Body 138

▶ CHAPTER 7
Pathophysiology 175

▶ CHAPTER 8
Life Span Development 188

Module 3

Pharmacology 203

▶ CHAPTER 9
Principles of Pharmacology 204

▶ CHAPTER 10
Medication Administration 211

▶ CHAPTER 11
Emergency Medications 218

Module 4

Airway Management, Respiration, Ventilation 241

▶ CHAPTER 12
Airway Management 242

▶ CHAPTER 13
Respiration 259

▶ CHAPTER 14
Artificial Ventilation 279

Module 5

Patient Assessment 293

▶ CHAPTER 15
Therapeutic Communications and History Taking 294

▶ CHAPTER 16
Scene Size-Up 310

▶ CHAPTER 17
Patient Assessment 325

Module 6

Medical Emergencies 368

▶ CHAPTER 18
Medical Overview 371

▶ CHAPTER 19
Neurological Disorders 376

▶ CHAPTER 20
Endocrine Disorders 393

▶ CHAPTER 21
Respiratory Disorders 406

▶ CHAPTER 22
Cardiovascular Disorders 426

► CHAPTER 23
Abdominal and Gastrointestinal Disorders 456

► CHAPTER 24
Genitourinary and Renal Disorders 467

► CHAPTER 25
Gynecologic Disorders 477

► CHAPTER 26
Nontraumatic Musculoskeletal Disorders 486

► CHAPTER 27
Immunology 494

► CHAPTER 28
Toxicology 504

► CHAPTER 29
Psychiatric Disorders 520

► CHAPTER 30
Diseases of the Nose 530

► CHAPTER 31
Hematology 533

Module 7

Shock 538

► CHAPTER 32
Shock 539

Module 8

Trauma 545

► CHAPTER 33
Trauma Overview 547

► CHAPTER 34
Bleeding and Soft Tissue Trauma 554

► CHAPTER 35
Chest Trauma 590

► CHAPTER 36
Abdominal and Genitourinary Trauma 605

► CHAPTER 37
Orthopedic Trauma 612

► CHAPTER 38
Head, Face, Neck, and Spine Trauma 643

► CHAPTER 39
Special Considerations in Trauma 683

► CHAPTER 40
Environmental Emergencies 698

► CHAPTER 41
Multisystem Trauma 728

Module 9

Special Patient Populations 733

► CHAPTER 42
Obstetrics 734

► CHAPTER 43
Neonatal Care 763

► CHAPTER 44
Pediatrics 769

► CHAPTER 45
Older Adults 791

► CHAPTER 46
Patients with Special Challenges 803

Module 10

EMS Operations 813

► CHAPTER 47
Principles of Emergency Response and Transportation 815

► CHAPTER 48
Incident Management 833

► CHAPTER 49
Multiple-Casualty Incidents 838

► CHAPTER 50
Air Medical Transport 844

► CHAPTER 51
Vehicle Extrication 849

► CHAPTER 52
Hazardous Materials Awareness 858

► CHAPTER 53
Terrorism and Disaster Response 866

Appendixes

Appendix A: Cardiopulmonary Resuscitation 875

Appendix B: Rural and Frontier EMS 895

Glossary 899

Credits 925

Index 927

Contents

Foreword   xviii
Preface   xix

Module 1

Preparatory   1

► CHAPTER 1
EMS Systems and Research   2

On the Scene   3
Introduction: The Emergency Medical
   Technician   3
Origins of Emergency Medical Services   4
Overview of the Emergency Medical Services
   System   9
Phases of a Typical EMS Response   17
Characteristics of Professional Behavior   20
Primary Duties as an EMT   22
EMS Research   26
On the Scene: Wrap-Up   27
Sum It Up   27

► CHAPTER 2
Workforce Safety and Wellness   28

On the Scene   30
Introduction   30
Wellness   31
Preventing Disease Transmission   36
Skill Drill 2-1: Removing Gloves   40
Injury Prevention   44
Lifting and Moving Patients   47
Body Mechanics and Lifting Techniques   48
Skill Drill 2-2: Two-Person Power Lift   51
Emergency Moves   53
Urgent Moves (Rapid Extrication)   58
Nonurgent Moves   58
Skill Drill 2-3: Rapid Extrication   59
Transferring a Supine Patient from Bed to Stretcher   60

Skill Drill 2-4: Three-Person Direct Ground
   Lift   61
Skill Drill 2-5: Two-Person Extremity Lift   62
Skill Drill 2-6: Direct Carry   63
Patient Positioning   64
Skill Drill 2-7: Draw Sheet Transfer   65
Equipment   66
Use of Restraints   70
Death and Dying   71
On the Scene: Wrap-Up   76
Sum It Up   76

► CHAPTER 3
**Legal and Ethical Issues
and Documentation**   79

On the Scene   80
Introduction: The Importance of Legal and Ethical
   Care   80
The Legal System   81
Scope of Practice   82
Consent   84
Refusals   85
Advance Directives and Do Not Resuscitate
   Orders   87
Assault and Battery   91
Abandonment   91
Negligence   91
Confidentiality   93
Special Situations   94
Documentation   95
On the Scene: Wrap-Up   106
Sum It Up   106

► CHAPTER 4
EMS System Communications   109

On the Scene   109
Introduction   110
Communications Systems   110

The Call   113
Legal Considerations   119
On the Scene: Wrap-Up   119
Sum It Up   119

▶ CHAPTER 5
Medical Terminology   121
On the Scene   121
Introduction   122
Word Parts   122
Body Positions and Directional Terms   127
Common Medical Abbreviations and
     Acronyms   130
On the Scene: Wrap-Up   135
Sum It Up   136

Module 2

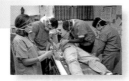

Function and Development of the Human Body   137

▶ CHAPTER 6
The Human Body   138
On the Scene   139
Introduction: Understanding the Structure and Function
     of the Body   140
Structural Organization   140
Homeostasis   140
Body Cavities   142
Body Planes   143
The Musculoskeletal System   144
The Respiratory System   151
The Circulatory System   158
The Nervous System   162
The Integumentary System   165
The Digestive System   165
The Endocrine System   166
The Reproductive System   167
The Urinary System   169
On the Scene: Wrap-Up   169
Sum It Up   169

▶ CHAPTER 7
Pathophysiology   175
On the Scene   176
Introduction: Pathophysiology   176
Cell Function   176
Factors Affecting Cell Function   178
Disease Risk Factors   184
Causes of Disease   184

On the Scene: Wrap-Up   186
Sum It Up   186

▶ CHAPTER 8
Life Span Development   188
On the Scene   188
Introduction: Life Span Development   189
Infants   189
Toddlers   192
Preschoolers   194
School-Age Children   196
Adolescents   197
Early Adulthood   198
Middle Adulthood   199
Late Adulthood   200
On the Scene: Wrap-Up   202
Sum It Up   202

Module 3

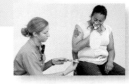

Pharmacology   203

▶ CHAPTER 9
Principles of Pharmacology   204
On the Scene   204
Introduction   205
Drug Legislation and Federal Regulatory Agencies   205
Drug Sources, Names, and References   205
Drug Forms   208
Drug Profile   210
On the Scene: Wrap-Up   210
Sum It Up   210

▶ CHAPTER 10
Medication Administration   211
On the Scene   212
Introduction   212
Drug Administration   212
The Six Rights of Drug Administration   213
Routes of Drug Administration   213
Reassessment and Documentation   215
On the Scene: Wrap-Up   216
Sum It Up   216

▶ CHAPTER 11
Emergency Medications   218
On the Scene   219
Introduction   220
Administered Medications   220

Skill Drill 11-1: Giving Activated Charcoal   222

Skill Drill 11-2: Giving Oral Glucose   225

Assisted Medications   226

Skill Drill 11-3: Administering an Epinephrine Autoinjector   228

Skill Drill 11-4: Assisting a Patient with a Metered-Dose Inhaler   231

Special Situations   233

Skill Drill 11-5: Assisting a Patient with Prescribed Nitroglycerin Tablets   234

Skill Drill 11-6: Assisting a Patient with Prescribed Nitroglycerin Spray   235

On the Scene: Wrap-Up   239

Sum It Up   240

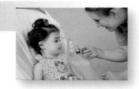

Module 4

Airway Management, Respiration, Ventilation   241

▶ CHAPTER 12

Airway Management   242

On the Scene   243

Introduction: Airway Management   243

The Respiratory System   243

Airway Assessment   246

Inspecting the Airway   248

Airway Obstruction   249

Clearing the Airway   250

Keeping the Airway Open: Airway Adjuncts   253

Skill Drill 12-1: Sizing and Inserting an Oral Airway   254

Skill Drill 12-2: Sizing and Inserting a Nasal Airway   256

On the Scene: Wrap-Up   257

Sum It Up   258

▶ CHAPTER 13

Respiration   259

On the Scene   260

Introduction   261

Physiology of Respiration   261

Pathophysiology of Respiration   262

Assessment of Ventilation   264

Assessment of Oxygenation   267

Supplemental Oxygen   269

Skill Drill 13-1: Setting Up an Oxygen Delivery System   271

Skill Drill 13-2: Discontinuing an Oxygen Delivery System   273

On the Scene: Wrap-Up   277

Sum It Up   277

▶ CHAPTER 14

Artificial Ventilation   279

On the Scene   280

Introduction   280

Is Respiration Adequate or Inadequate?   280

Positive-Pressure Ventilation   280

Skill Drill 14-1: Mouth-to-Mask Ventilation   284

Special Considerations   289

Skill Drill 14-2: Flow-Restricted, Oxygen-Powered Ventilation for a Nonbreathing Patient   290

On the Scene: Wrap-Up   291

Sum It Up   291

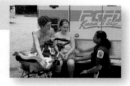

Module 5

Patient Assessment   293

▶ CHAPTER 15

Therapeutic Communications and History Taking   294

On the Scene   295

Introduction   295

The Communication Process   295

Communicating with the Patient   296

Patient History   305

On the Scene: Wrap-Up   308

Sum It Up   309

▶ CHAPTER 16

Scene Size-Up   310

On the Scene   310

Introduction   311

An Overview of Scene Size-Up   311

Standard Precautions Review   312

Scene Safety   312

The Mechanism of Injury or the Nature of the Illness   314

The Number of Patients   322

Additional Resources   322

On the Scene: Wrap-Up   322

Sum It Up   323

▶ CHAPTER 17

Patient Assessment   325

On the Scene   327

Introduction   327

Vital Signs   327

Skill Drill 17-1: Measuring Blood Pressure
   by Auscultation   336
Skill Drill 17-2: Measuring Blood Pressure
   by Palpation   337
Additional Vital Signs   338
An Overview of Patient Assessment   339
Skill Drill 17-3: Performing the Secondary Survey   352
Skill Drill 17-4: Reassessment   363
On the Scene: Wrap-Up   365
Sum It Up   365

Module 6

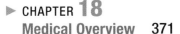

Medical Emergencies   368

▶ CHAPTER 18
Medical Overview   371
On the Scene   371
Introduction   372
The Responsive Medical Patient   372
The Unresponsive Medical Patient   374
On the Scene: Wrap-Up   375
Sum It Up   375

▶ CHAPTER 19
Neurological Disorders   376
On the Scene   377
Introduction   377
Altered Mental Status   377
Seizures   378
Stroke   382
Syncope   385
Headache   387
On the Scene: Wrap-Up   390
Sum It Up   391

▶ CHAPTER 20
Endocrine Disorders   393
On the Scene   394
Introduction   394
Glucose   394
Types of Diabetes Mellitus   395
Complications of Diabetes Mellitus   396
Hypoglycemia   397
Hyperglycemia   398
Patient Assessment   398
Age-Related Considerations   399
Emergency Care   399
Skill Drill 20-1: Performing a Blood Glucose Test
   with a Glucometer   401

On the Scene: Wrap-Up   404
Sum It Up   404

▶ CHAPTER 21
Respiratory Disorders   406
On the Scene   407
Introduction   407
Assessing the Patient with Breathing
   Difficulty   407
Specific Respiratory Disorders   413
Metered-Dose Inhalers   422
On the Scene: Wrap-Up   422
Sum It Up   424

▶ CHAPTER 22
Cardiovascular Disorders   426
On the Scene   427
Introduction   428
Review of Circulatory System Anatomy
   and Physiology   428
Cardiovascular Disease   434
Cardiac Arrest   443
Skill Drill 22-1: Adult Automated External Defibrillator
   Sequence   452
On the Scene: Wrap-Up   453
Sum It Up   453

▶ CHAPTER 23
Abdominal and Gastrointestinal Disorders   456
On the Scene   456
Introduction   457
Review of Digestive System Anatomy
   and Physiology   457
The Acute Abdomen   459
Patient Assessment   462
Emergency Care   463
On the Scene: Wrap-Up   465
Sum It Up   465

▶ CHAPTER 24
Genitourinary and Renal Disorders   467
On the Scene   468
Introduction   468
Review of the Urinary System   468
Renal Disorders   469
Patient Assessment   473
Emergency Care   475
On the Scene: Wrap-Up   475
Sum It Up   475

▶ CHAPTER **25**
Gynecologic Disorders **477**

On the Scene 477
Introduction 478
Review of the Female Reproductive System 478
Assessment of the Gynecologic Patient 479
Emergency Care of the Gynecologic Patient 480
Nontraumatic Gynecologic Conditions 480
Traumatic Gynecologic Emergencies 483
On the Scene: Wrap-Up 484
Sum It Up 484

▶ CHAPTER **26**
Nontraumatic Musculoskeletal Disorders **486**

On the Scene 486
Introduction 487
Review of the Musculoskeletal System 487
Nontraumatic Musculoskeletal Conditions 489
Patient Assessment 491
Emergency Care 492
On the Scene: Wrap-Up 492
Sum It Up 492

▶ CHAPTER **27**
Immunology **494**

On the Scene 494
Introduction 495
Causes of Allergic Reactions 495
What Happens in an Allergic Reaction 497
Patient Assessment 498
Emergency Care 501
Age-Related Considerations 501
On the Scene: Wrap-Up 502
Sum It Up 503

▶ CHAPTER **28**
Toxicology **504**

On the Scene 505
Introduction 505
What Is a Poison? 505
Commonly Misused and Abused Substances 507
Ingested Poisons 514
Inhaled Poisons 515
Injected Poisons 517
Absorbed Poisons 518
On the Scene: Wrap-Up 518
Sum It Up 519

▶ CHAPTER **29**
Psychiatric Disorders **520**

On the Scene 521
Introduction 521
Behavior 521
Behavioral Change 521
Psychological Crises 522
Excited Delirium 526
Assessment and Emergency Care for Patients with Psychiatric Disorders 526
Medical and Legal Considerations 528
On the Scene: Wrap-Up 528
Sum It Up 528

▶ CHAPTER **30**
Diseases of the Nose **530**

On the Scene 530
Introduction 530
Causes of Epistaxis 531
Assessment Findings and Symptoms 531
Emergency Care 531
On the Scene: Wrap-Up 532
Sum It Up 532

▶ CHAPTER **31**
Hematology **533**

On the Scene 533
Introduction 534
Sickle Cell Disease 534
Hemophilia 536
On the Scene: Wrap-Up 536
Sum It Up 536

Module **7**

Shock **538**

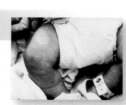

▶ CHAPTER **32**
Shock **539**

On the Scene 539
Introduction 540
Types of Shock 540
The Stages of Shock 541
Shock in Infants and Children 543
Shock in Older Adults 543
Emergency Care of Shock 543
On the Scene: Wrap-Up 544
Sum It Up 544

Module 8

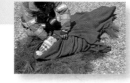

Trauma 545

▶ CHAPTER 33
Trauma Overview 547
On the Scene 547
Introduction 548
Reconsidering the Mechanism of Injury 548
Trauma Patient with Significant Mechanism
    of Injury 550
Trauma Patient with No Significant Mechanism
    of Injury 552
On the Scene: Wrap-Up 552
Sum It Up 553

▶ CHAPTER 34
Bleeding and Soft Tissue Trauma 554
On the Scene 555
Introduction 556
Anatomy Review 556
Bleeding 556
Soft Tissue Injuries 563
Burns 576
Emotional Support 582
Dressing and Bandaging 583
Skill Drill 34-1: Applying a Roller Bandage 586
On the Scene: Wrap-Up 587
Sum It Up 587

▶ CHAPTER 35
Chest Trauma 590
On the Scene 591
Introduction 591
Anatomy of the Chest Cavity 591
Categories of Chest Injuries 591
Closed Chest Injuries 592
Open Chest Injuries 602
On the Scene: Wrap-Up 603
Sum It Up 603

▶ CHAPTER 36
Abdominal and Genitourinary Trauma 605
On the Scene 605
Introduction 606
Abdominal Trauma 606
Genitourinary Trauma 609
Patient Assessment 609
Emergency Care 610

On the Scene: Wrap-Up 610
Sum It Up 610

▶ CHAPTER 37
Orthopedic Trauma 612
On the Scene 613
Introduction 613
The Musculoskeletal System 613
Musculoskeletal Injuries 618
Patient Assessment 622
Emergency Care 623
Splinting 624
Care of Specific Musculoskeletal Injuries 627
Skill Drill 37-1: Immobilizing a Shoulder Injury 627
Skill Drill 37-2: Applying the SEFRS Adaptor 627
Skill Drill 37-3: Applying the Sager SX 405 Unipolar
    Traction Splint 636
Skill Drill 37-4: Applying a Bipolar Traction Splint 638
On the Scene: Wrap-Up 640
Sum It Up 641

▶ CHAPTER 38
Head, Face, Neck, and Spine Trauma 643
On the Scene 644
Introduction 645
Anatomy and Physiology Review 645
Injuries to the Head 647
Injuries to the Face 652
Injuries to the Neck 657
Injuries to the Brain and Spinal Cord 659
Skill Drill 38-1: Applying a Cervical Collar 670
Skill Drill 38-2: Three-Person Logroll 671
Skill Drill 38-3: Spinal Stabilization of a Seated
    Patient 674
Skill Drill 38-4: Spinal Stabilization of a Standing
    Patient 676
Skill Drill 38-5: Helmet Removal 679
On the Scene: Wrap-Up 678
Sum It Up 678

▶ CHAPTER 39
Special Considerations in Trauma 683
On the Scene 684
Introduction 684
Trauma in Pregnancy 684
Pediatric Trauma 688
Trauma in Older Adults 692
Trauma in the Cognitively Impaired Patient 694
On the Scene: Wrap-Up 695
Sum It Up 695

► CHAPTER **40**
Environmental Emergencies 698

On the Scene 698
Introduction 699
Body Temperature 699
Exposure to Cold 701
Exposure to Heat 707
Water-Related Emergencies 709
Bites and Stings 715
On the Scene: Wrap-Up 726
Sum It Up 726

► CHAPTER **41**
Multisystem Trauma 728

On the Scene 728
Introduction 729
Multisystem Trauma 729
Blast Injuries 730
On the Scene: Wrap-Up 731
Sum It Up 731

Module 9

Special Patient Populations 733

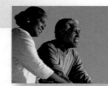

► CHAPTER **42**
Obstetrics 734

On the Scene 735
Introduction 735
Anatomy and Physiology Review 735
Normal Pregnancy 738
Assessing the Pregnant Patient 739
Normal Labor 740
Normal Delivery 742
Pregnancy and Birth—Cultural
  Considerations 748
Complications of Pregnancy 750
High-Risk Pregnancy 756
Complications of Labor 757
Complications of Delivery 757
Postpartum Complications 760
On the Scene: Wrap-Up 760
Sum It Up 761

► CHAPTER **43**
Neonatal Care 763

On the Scene 763
Introduction 764
Caring for the Newborn 764

On the Scene: Wrap-Up 767
Sum It Up 767

► CHAPTER **44**
Pediatrics 769

On the Scene 770
Introduction 770
Anatomical and Physiological Differences
  in Children 771
Assessment of the Infant and Child 775
Common Problems in Infants and
  Children 781
On the Scene: Wrap-Up 788
Sum It Up 789

► CHAPTER **45**
Older Adults 791

On the Scene 791
Introduction 792
Assessment of the Older Adult 792
Common Health Problems in Older Adults 794
On the Scene: Wrap-Up 801
Sum It Up 801

► CHAPTER **46**
Patients with Special Challenges 803

On the Scene 804
Introduction 804
Child Abuse and Neglect 804
Elder Abuse 806
Homelessness 807
Bariatric Patients 808
Patients with Special Healthcare Needs 808
Hospice Care 810
On the Scene: Wrap-Up 811
Sum It Up 811

Module 10

EMS Operations 813

► CHAPTER **47**
**Principles of Emergency Response
and Transportation** 815

On the Scene 816
Introduction 816
Principles of Emergency Response 816
On the Scene: Wrap-Up 831
Sum It Up 831

► CHAPTER **48**

Incident Management   833

On the Scene   833

Introduction   834

Incident Command System   834

On the Scene: Wrap-Up   837

Sum It Up   837

► CHAPTER **49**

Multiple-Casualty Incidents   838

On the Scene   838

Introduction   839

Multiple-Casualty Incidents   839

On the Scene: Wrap-Up   843

Sum It Up   843

► CHAPTER **50**

Air Medical Transport   844

On the Scene   844

Introduction   845

Air Medical Transport Considerations   845

On the Scene: Wrap-Up   847

Sum It Up   848

► CHAPTER **51**

Vehicle Extrication   849

On the Scene   849

Introduction   850

Role of the EMT on an Extrication Scene   850

Equipment   850

Stages of Extrication   850

Additional Scene Hazards   856

On the Scene: Wrap-Up   857

Sum It Up   857

► CHAPTER **52**

Hazardous Materials Awareness   858

On the Scene   858

Introduction   859

Hazardous Materials   859

On the Scene: Wrap-Up   865

Sum It Up   865

► CHAPTER **53**

Terrorism and Disaster Response   866

On the Scene   866

Introduction   867

Types of Weapons of Mass Destruction   867

Weapons of Mass Destruction Incident Response   871

On the Scene: Wrap-Up   873

Sum It Up   873

Appendixes

Appendix A: Cardiopulmonary Resuscitation   875

Skill Drill A-1: One-Rescuer Adult Cardiopulmonary Resuscitation   876

Skill Drill A-2: Two-Rescuer Adult Cardiopulmonary Resuscitation   879

Skill Drill A-3: One-Rescuer Child Cardiopulmonary Resuscitation   882

Skill Drill A-4: One-Rescuer Infant Cardiopulmonary Resuscitation   885

Skill Drill A-5: Adult Automated External Defibrillator Sequence   887

Skill Drill A-6: Clearing a Foreign Body Airway Obstruction in a Conscious Adult   888

Skill Drill A-7: Clearing a Foreign Body Airway Obstruction in an Unconscious Adult   890

Skill Drill A-8: Clearing a Foreign Body Airway Obstruction in a Conscious Child   891

Skill Drill A-9: Clearing a Foreign Body Airway Obstruction in an Unconscious Child   892

Skill Drill A-10: Clearing a Foreign Body Airway Obstruction in a Conscious Infant   893

Skill Drill A-11: Clearing a Foreign Body Airway Obstruction in an Unconscious Infant   894

Appendix B: Rural and Frontier EMS   895

Emergency Response in Rural and Frontier Areas   895

The Challenges of Rural and Frontier EMS   895

Glossary   899

Credits   925

Index   927

Foreword

The world of Emergency Medical Services is rapidly changing. The science of EMS has led to the development of new assessment tools, treatment guidelines, and enhanced communication. These changes have demanded the evolution of pre-hospital professionals who have strong content knowledge, competent practical skills, and effective problem-solving techniques. In 2007 the National Highway Traffic Safety Administration (NHTSA) released the *National EMS Scope of Practice Model,* which confirmed the new label for the second level of Emergency Medical Technician–Basic (EMT-B) as EMT.

The EMS profession, recognizing its role in improving patient outcome, has been an active participant in defining the new 2009 NHTSA *National EMS Education Standards.* This text meets and exceeds the new *National EMS Education Standards.* Barbara Aehlert's approach in this text also successfully incorporates an underlying philosophy shared by many EMS educators: While the EMT must be proficient in basic life support skills, the profession demands that the EMT is ready to function in an advanced life support world.

Barbara Aehlert wrote this text with superior depth and breadth, while maintaining an appreciation for detail. Each chapter begins with an *On the Scene* scenario to capture your interest and to foster clinical decision making. At the conclusion of each objective a *You Should Know* summary is presented to reinforce key content as you read. Detailed illustrations keep your mind active and help make the content real to you. Finally, for easy review, the *Sum It Up* section at the end of each chapter provides a brief summary of key content and EMT care strategies that improve patient outcome.

The emergency medical technician (EMT) provides valuable life-saving basic care and effectively transports and coordinates care with advanced healthcare providers. EMTs are valued members of the healthcare team internationally. Because they are highly skilled, the locations where EMTs may be found are too numerous to count, but include the prehospital and in-hospital settings, industrial areas, casinos, and isolated rural areas. Many EMTs are enthusiastic volunteers in their community. Due to projections in healthcare and an aging population, we will be relying on your continued dedication and commitment to provide EMS service to our communities. We are thankful for your decision to train as an EMT. You will no doubt join us as a proud, skilled, and compassionate member of the EMS profession. Through our shared commitment, the role of the EMT will be recognized and valued within the healthcare community and by all those whom we serve.

Dean C. Meenach, RN, BSN, AAS, CEN, EMT-P
Director of EMS Education
Mineral Area College
Park Hills, Missouri

Preface

This book and the materials that accompany it are designed to teach you how to safely and efficiently provide immediate care to an ill or injured person in accordance with the guidelines established by the Department of Transportation (DOT) *National Emergency Medical Services Education Standards*. Although they may be used alone to increase your awareness about what to do in an emergency situation, these materials are best used in an EMT training program.

This book has been divided into ten modules (divisions) that contain chapters with information relevant to each module. Each chapter begins with a list of knowledge, attitude, and skill objectives that describe what you should be able to do after completing the chapter and related exercises.

Before studying a chapter, first read the knowledge objectives. These objectives will give you an idea of the information you should obtain from reading the material in this book. Next, read the attitude objectives to learn about the behaviors that you are expected to develop as a healthcare professional. Then read the skill objectives to discover the procedures you should be able to perform after reading about, observing, and practicing each skill.

After reviewing the objectives, begin reading the chapter. Each chapter contains illustrations, tables, and other features to help you understand the information presented. For example, most skills discussed in this book are also demonstrated on the DVD that accompanies this text. When you have finished reading the chapter, go through the objectives again to be sure that you have met them.

At the end of each module of the EMT course, time is allowed for skill practice, review, and evaluation. Use the practice questions in the accompanying workbook to help you assess your mastery of the knowledge objectives presented in the course.

Additional information that is related to your role as an EMT is located in the appendixes at the end of this book.

I hope you find this text helpful. If you have comments or suggestions about how I could improve this text, please drop me a line. I would like to hear from you.

Barbara Aehlert, RN
Southwest EMS Education, Inc.
Phoenix, AZ/Pursley, TX

Changes to the Second Edition

The second edition of *Emergency Medical Technician: EMT in Action* has been completely rewritten to conform to the new *National EMS Education Standards*, published by the National Association of EMS Educators (NAEMSE) in January 2009. Specific differences between the first and second editions are outlined below:

- Chapter 1: New coverage on characteristics of professional behavior; additional coverage on primary duties as an EMT.

- Chapter 2: New content on wellness; updated content on injury prevention, lifting and moving patients, body mechanics and lifting techniques, emergency and urgent moves, patient positioning, use of restraints, and death and dying.
- Chapter 3 (from Chapter 11 in the first edition): Updated information on ethics, the legal system, and documentation.
- Chapter 4 (Chapter 10 in first edition): Updated content on EMS system communication.
- Chapter 5 (section of Chapter 11 in first edition): Greatly expanded content on medical terminology, including root words, prefixes, suffixes, combining forms, plural medical terms, body positions, and directional terms (Figures 5-1 and 5-2), and an updated list of common abbreviations and acronyms.
- Chapter 6: Enhanced content on the human body, including three full-page color plates of anatomical figures (Plates A, B, and C).
- Chapter 7: All new content on pathophysiology, including cell function, factors affecting cell function, disease risk factors, and causes of disease.
- Chapter 8: All new content on life span development, covering infants, toddlers, preschoolers, school-age children, adolescents, early adulthood, middle adulthood, and late adulthood.
- Chapter 9 (section of Chapter 12 in first edition).
- Chapter 10 (section of Chapter 12 in first edition): Updated content on medication administration, including six rights of drug administration, reassessment, and documentation.
- Chapter 11: All new content on emergency medications.
- Chapter 12 (section of Chapter 7 in first edition): Updated content on airway management.
- Chapter 13 (section of Chapter 7 in first edition): Expanded coverage of respiration, including physiology and pathophysiology of respiration, and assessment of ventilation and oxygenation.
- Chapter 14: All new content on ventilation.
- Chapter 15 (section of Chapter 5 in first edition): New content on therapeutic communications and updated content on history taking.
- Chapter 16 (Chapter 8 in first edition).
- Chapter 17 (sections of Chapters 5 and 9 in first edition): Updated content on reassessment.
- Chapter 18: All new content on medical overview, the responsive medical patient, and the unresponsive medical patient, including an updated algorithm on assessment of the medical patient (Figure 18-1).
- Chapter 19: All new content on neurological disorders: seizures, stroke, syncope, and headache.
- Chapter 20 (Chapter 15 in first edition): Expanded coverage of endocrine disorders, including new images of the endocrine glands (Figure 20-2), goiter (Figure 20-3), and hyperthyroidism (Figure 20-4).
- Chapter 21 (Chapter 13 in first edition): Expanded coverage of respiratory disorders, including determining the patient's level of respiratory distress, pertussis, cystic fibrosis, spontaneous pneumothorax, and metered-dose inhalers.
- Chapter 22 (Chapter 14 in first edition): New information on cardiogenic shock and the chain of survival.
- Chapter 23: New content on abdominal and gastrointestinal disorders; review of digestive system anatomy and physiology; the acute abdomen; and new images of referred pain (Figure 23-3) and the best position for abdominal examination (Figure 23-4).
- Chapter 24: New content on genitourinary/renal disorders, including review of urinary system, renal disorders, and new images of AV shunts (Figure 24-2) and arteriovenous fistulas (Figure 24-3).

- Chapter 25: New content on gynecologic disorders, including nontraumatic and traumatic gynecological conditions, such as PID, STDs, ovarian cyst, and apparent sexual assault.
- Chapter 26: New content on nontraumatic musculoskeletal disorders, such as arthritis, osteoporosis, and overuse syndromes.
- Chapter 27 (Chapter 16 in first edition): Updated information on immunology, including age-related considerations.
- Chapter 28 (Chapter 17 in first edition): Updated content on toxicology.
- Chapter 29 (Chapter 19 in first edition): Updated content on psychiatric disorders, including new content on excited delirium.
- Chapter 30 (section of Chapter 22 in first edition): Expanded coverage on diseases of the nose, and on epistaxis.
- Chapter 31: New coverage on hematology, including sickle cell disease and hemophilia.
- Chapter 32 (Chapter 21 in first edition): Expanded coverage on shock, including shock in older adults.
- Chapter 33: New coverage on trauma overview, including reconsidering the MOI and trauma patient with significant MOI.
- Chapter 34 (section of Chapter 22 in first edition): Expanded coverage of bleeding and soft tissue trauma.
- Chapter 35 (section of Chapter 25 in first edition): Updated coverage of chest trauma, including new content on commotio cordis.
- Chapter 36 (section of Chapter 25 in first edition): Expanded coverage of abdominal and genitourinary trauma, including closed and open abdominal injuries.
- Chapter 37 (Chapter 23 in first edition): Updated content on orthopedic trauma, including a new Skill Drill 37-2 (Applying the SEFRS Adaptor) and an updated Skill Drill 37-3 (Applying the Sager SX 405 Unipolar Traction Splint).
- Chapter 38 (Chapter 24 in first edition): Expanded coverage, including injuries to the face and injuries to the neck.
- Chapter 39: (sections of Chapters 20 and 26 in first edition) Expanded content on special considerations in trauma, including trauma in pregnancy and pediatric trauma, and new content on trauma in older adults.
- Chapter 40 (Chapter 18 in first edition).
- Chapter 41: New content on multisystem trauma including blast injuries.
- Chapter 42 (Chapter 20 in first edition): Updated coverage of obstetrics, including abuse, substance abuse, and diabetes mellitus as complications of pregnancy; high-risk pregnancy; and postpartum complications.
- Chapter 43 (section of Chapter 20 in first edition): Expanded coverage on neonatal care.
- Chapter 44 (Chapter 26 in first edition): Expanded coverage on pediatrics, including new images of anatomy of children (Figure 44-2), epiphyseal growth plates (Figure 44-3), and using a bulb syringe (Figure 44-9).
- Chapter 45 (Appendix B in first edition): Greatly expanded content on older adults, including common health problems in older adults, such as problems of the cardiovascular and respiratory systems and metabolic and endocrine problems.
- Chapter 46: New content on patients with special challenges, including sections on child abuse and neglect, elder abuse, homelessness, bariatric patients, patients with special healthcare needs, and hospice care.
- Chapter 47 (Chapter 27 in first edition).
- Chapter 48: Expanded content on incident management, including coverage of NIMS components of command and management, preparedness, resource management, communications and information management, supporting technologies, and ongoing management and maintenance.

- Chapter 49 (section of Chapter 29 in first edition): Expanded coverage of multiple-casualty incidents, including algorithms for START and JumpSTART triage systems (Figures 49-2 and 49-4).
- Chapter 50 (section of Chapter 27 in first edition): Expanded coverage of air medical transport, including schematic of a helicopter landing zone (Figure 50-3).
- Chapter 51 (Chapter 28 in first edition): Updated coverage, including new content on hazard control and safety considerations, such as information on alternative fuels and renewable fuels.
- Chapter 52 (section of Chapter 29 in first edition).
- Chapter 53 (Appendix D in first edition).

Supplements

The supplements for the second edition of *Emergency Medical Technician* are designed around the student and are based on the new *National EMS Education Standards* released in January 2009 by the DOT NHTSA Office of EMS.

For the Student

- ***Emergency Medical Technician Workbook*** Includes features to help you study and master the material in each chapter: Reading Assignment, Sum It Up, Tracking Your Progress, Chapter Quiz, and Answer Section.
- **Connect™ Assignments** Web-based assignments that are tied to the *National EMS Education Standards* and the textbook material.
- **Media Rich eBook** Electronic book that incorporates video and animation directly into the pages of the textbook.
- **LearnSmart** An online diagnostic learning system that determines the level of student knowledge, then feeds the student appropriate content. Students take an online pre-test to qualify medical terms they already know, think they know, or don't know at all. Based on a new approach to learning, the system forces students to think about whether they really know the terms, which will generate stronger metacognitive skills.
- **ActivSim** A web-based EMS field simulator that prepares students for certification and enables them to hone their medical skills by using virtual patients with real-life cases and real-time feedback.

For the Instructor

- **Asset Map** Correlates the Aehlert textbook chapters to the NAEMSE *Education Standards* and all available McGraw-Hill resources.
- **Instructor Manual** Contains objectives, class preparation and personnel, key terms, skills, lesson outlines that are linked to the objectives and the PowerPoint slides, and lesson enhancements including chapter quizzes, quiz answers, and activities.
- **McGraw-Hill Connect™** Web-based gradable assignment and assessment platform that helps students connect to their coursework, helps instructors become more efficient, and helps administrators report results. The Connect content is tied to the NAEMSE *Education Standards* and the Aehlert objectives.
- **FISDAP Test Bank** Contains over 2,000 test questions developed by FISDAP to prepare students for National Registry exams. The questions are tied to the textbook and mapped to the *Education Standards* and Bloom's taxonomy.
- **Resource Table** Located on the Connect site, the Resource Table includes files of the textbook assets (art files, videos, animations, and text) for those instructors who prefer to create their own PowerPoint presentations or lectures.

Acknowledgments

No book is published without the assistance of many people. My heartfelt thanks to Laura Horowitz for her assistance with all of the components of this book. You have been a joy to work with. Thanks also to the staff at McGraw-Hill. A special thanks to Rick Hecker, whose attention to detail during the production process was sincerely appreciated.

The contributors for this book and the materials that accompany it were selected because of their experience in EMS. Whether a physician, nurse, or paramedic, they each treat their patients with compassion and respect, and display professionalism every day they are on the job. Their commitment to excellence and professionalism in EMS is evident throughout this book. Thank you to Gary Smith, MD; Lynn Browne-Wagner, RN; Andrea Lowrey, RN; Terence Mason, RN; Suzy Coronel, CEP; Paul Honeywell, CEP; Travis Kidd, EMT-P; Captain Randy Budd, CEP; Captain Holly Button, CEP; Captain Sean Newton, CEP; and Major Raymond Burton. Special thanks to Janet Fitts, RN, and Edith Valladares for their invaluable contributions to the *Spanish Guide to Patient Assessment for the Emergency Medical Technician* featured on the student CD.

Thanks to Kim McKenna, RN, for her suggestions for the first edition of this book. Rick Brady did an outstanding job taking the photos that appear in this book. Thanks to Carin Marter, CEP; the City of Mesa Fire Department, the City of Tempe Fire Department, and AirEvac Services (Phoenix, AZ) for providing additional photos.

Thanks to the many EMS professionals who reviewed this text and the materials that accompany it. Each reviewer provided valuable comments and suggestions that were carefully read and discussed. Modifications have been made where needed based on your comments.

Barbara Aehlert, RN
Southwest EMS Education, Inc.
Phoenix, AZ/Pursley, TX

Guided Tour

Features to Help You Study and Learn

Knowledge, Attitude, and Skill Objectives

Knowledge Objectives alert students to what they should expect as they progress through the chapter. The Knowledge Objectives are tied to the new *National Emergency Medical Services Education Standards.*

The use of knowledge, attitude, and skill objectives is easier for students to grasp.
—Karen Bowlin
Mid-Plains Community College – North Platte

On the Scene and On the Scene: Wrap-Up

Setting the stage with a description of an EMS call, **Think About It** questions give EMT students a feel for scene size-up and the primary survey. At the end of the chapter, the **Wrap-Up** completes the case study by outlining the primary survey and emergency care for the patient.

The On the Scene and Wrap-Up sections provide the students an opportunity to apply the knowledge that they have just gained to real-life situations.
—Dawn Sgro
Lorain County Community College

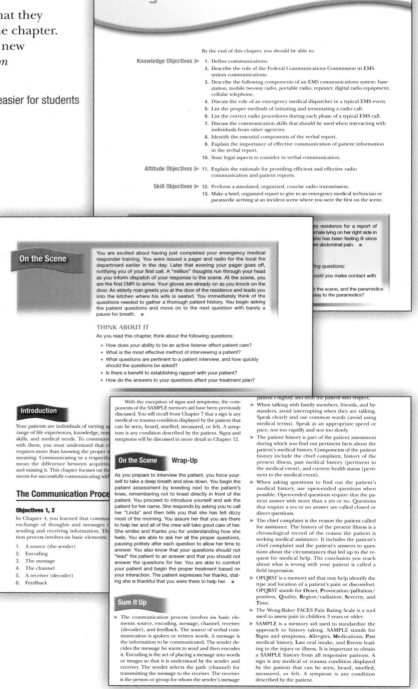

Stop and Think!

Practical advice and safety tips for EMTs.

Very comprehensive text, student friendly.
—Kevin Dobbe
Coconino Community College

Memory Aids

Memory aids are shown in color to help the students find and remember them.

Keeps simple things simple and clarifies difficult concepts.
—Chris Coughlin
Glendale Community College

Remember This

Information that is important for the EMT to remember in the field.

[These boxes] bridge the gap between the "textbook world" and the "real world" very effectively.
—Jason Segner
Blinn College

Stop and Think!

Always practice proper lifting techniques. Learning to lift by using proper body mechanics takes training and practice. When practicing, use "spotters" to alert you when you are performing a technique incorrectly. Practice and practice again until using correct lifting techniques become a habit. One bad lift can damage your back for the rest of your life!

Carrying Patients and Equipment

Objective 33

Guidelines for avoiding injury when carrying patients and equipment:

listen (a
to ident
identify
hol on the patient's breath, body, or clothing. Because it can cause pain, palpation should be performed last. **DCAP-BTLS** is a helpful memory aid to remember what to look and feel for during the physical exam:

DCAP-BTLS
Deformities
Contusions (bruises)
Abrasions (scrapes)
Punctures/penetrations
Burns
Tenderness
Lacerations (cuts)
Swelling

Another memory aid that may be helpful is **DOTS**:

Deformities
Open injuries
Tenderness
Swelling

your care.

Remember This

- Do *not* place a patient with a known or suspected spinal injury in the recovery position, but assess the need for suctioning frequently.
- There is a potential risk for nerve and vessel injury if the patient lies on one arm for a prolonged period in the recovery position. To avoid these types of injuries, it may be necessary to roll the patient to the other side.

Keeping the Airway Open: Airway Adjuncts

You Should Know

Lists the assessment findings and symptoms for the medical and trauma conditions covered in the text.

Provide the student with excellent reinforcement.
—James Norris
Jefferson State Community College

A straightforward presentation of the key information. Easy to read and understand.
—Mike Ditolla
University of Utah

You Should Know
Assessment Findings and Symptoms of Pulmonary Embolism
Common findings and symptoms:
- Sudden onset of dyspnea
- Apprehension, restlessness
- Increased respiratory rate
- Increased heart rate

Possible findings and symptoms:
- Pleuritic chest pain
- Cough
- Blood-tinged sputum
- Hypotension

Emergency Care
Allow the patient to assume a position of comfort unless hypotension is present. If the patient is alert but

You Should Know
Assessment Findings and Symptoms of Acute Pulmonary Edema
- Restlessness, anxiety
- Dyspnea on exertion
- Orthopnea
- Paroxysmal nocturnal dyspnea
- Frothy, blood-tinged sputum
- Cool, moist skin
- Use of accessory muscles
- Jugular venous distention
- Wheezing
- Crackles (rales)
- Rapid, labored breathing
- Increased heart rate
- Increased or decreased blood pressure (depending on severity of edema)

Making a Difference

Highlights how health care professionals can make a difference in the lives of their patients.

Making a Difference

The patient who has an isolated arm injury is often most comfortable in a sitting or semisitting position. If the patient's condition requires that he be positioned on his back, the weight of the patient's arm and splint on his chest and upper abdomen can hamper chest movement. If the patient *must* be positioned on his back and the arm must be immobilized with the elbow bent, try to splint the patient's arm so that the weight of the arm and splint will be supported on the patient's upper legs, rather than on his chest or abdomen. Using a soft pillow under the injured extremity will help alleviate pain and distribute the weight more evenly across the chest and allow better lung expansion if the patient must absolutely be transported flat on his back.

The Sager Emergency Fracture Response System (SEFRS) includes the SX405 compact traction splint and SEFRS Adaptor. The SEFRS compact kit treats any limb fracture in the body without traction and immobilizes

Making a Difference

Taking a medical history is not simply a matter of asking a series of rapid-fire questions in order to complete a report. Obtaining a useful medical history is an art. It requires thoughtful questions, good listening skills, and practice.

Making a Difference
Cultural Considerations

Some healthcare professionals end an interview with a child by patting her on the head. Although this gesture is meant to show friendliness, it may be viewed differently by people of other cultures. For example, this gesture is considered an insult by Southeast Asians. They believe the head is the seat of the soul and the most sacred part of the body. Intentionally touching a child's head without the consent of the parents may make the parents or relatives angry.

When you are caring for patients, a "yes" answer pertaining to an illness or injury indicates a **pertinent positive,** or positive, finding. A "no" indicates a **pertinent negative,** or negative, finding. For example, when you are caring for a patient who has asthma, pertinent positive findings would include shortness of breath and/or a feeling of tightness in the throat or chest. Pertinent neg-

Skill Drills

Present step-by-step procedures for essential skills.

This text goes into great detail and gives good examples.
—Kevin J. O'Hara
Nassau County EMS Academy

Figures

Skill Drill 37-3

Applying the Sager SX 405 Unipolar Traction Splint

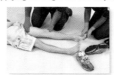
STEP 1 ▲ Expose the fracture site. Ask an assistant to stabilize the patient's leg while you remove the patient's shoe and assess distal pulses, movement, and sensation in the injured leg.

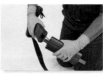
STEP 2 ▲ Remove and unfold the outer shaft assembly.

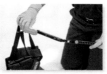
STEP 3 ▲ Remove, unfold, and lock the inner shaft assembly.

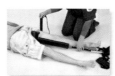
STEP 4 ▲ Insert the inner shaft assembly into the outer shaft assembly. The splint is now ready to be applied.

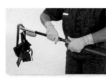
STEP 5 ▲ Position the splint between the patient's legs: Rest the ischial perineal cushion (the saddle) against the ischial tuberosity, with the shortest end of the articulating base toward the ground.

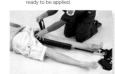
STEP 6 ▲ Press down on the (saddle) cushion while pulling the thigh strap laterally under the thigh to seat the saddle against the ischial tuberosity.

PATIENT ASSESSMENT

Initial Assessment

Scene Size-up

Primary Survey | Secondary Survey

General impression: Appearance (Work of) Breathing Circulation | Vital signs

Airway + Level of responsiveness Cervical spine protection | Focused history (SAMPLE, OPQRST)

Breathing (Ventilation) | Head-to-toe (or focused) physical exam

Circulation (Perfusion)

Disability (Minineurological exam)

Expose

Reassessment

FIGURE 17-12 ▲ Patient assessment.

made safe and you have gained access to the patient (Figure 17-12). It usually requires less than 60 seconds to complete. However, it may take longer if you must provide emergency care to correct an identified problem. Remember to wear appropriate personal protective equipment before approaching the patient.

The primary survey has several parts:
- General impression
- Airway, level of responsiveness, cervical spine protection
- Breathing (ventilation)
- Circulation with bleeding control (perfusion)
- Disability (minineurological exam)
- Expose (for examination)
- Identification of priority patients

General Impression

Objective 29

Whenever you meet someone for the first time, you form a first impression—sometimes without realizing it. You will do the same thing with every patient. A **general**

impression (also called a *first impression*) is an "across-the-room" assessment. As you approach a patient, you will form a general impression of her complaint without her telling you what it is. You can complete it in 60 seconds or less. The purpose of forming a general impression is to decide whether the patient looks "sick" or "not sick." A variation of the sick or not sick approach consists of three questions:

- Does the patient appear stable?
- Does the patient appear stable but is potentially unstable?
- Does the patient appear unstable?

If the patient looks sick (unstable), you must act quickly. As you gain experience, you will develop an instinct for quickly recognizing when a patient is sick.

Remember This

Your patient's condition can change at any time. A patient that initially appears not sick may rapidly worsen and become sick. Reassess your patient often.

Before you speak to your patient and find out what is wrong, stop a short distance from her (Figure 17-13).

Look and listen:
- What things stand out in your mind when you first see her?
- Does the patient look ill (medical patient) or injured (trauma patient)? If the patient looks ill, are there clues around you that suggest the nature of the illness? For example, the presence of an oxygen tank suggests that someone in the home has a chronic medical condition. If the patient is injured, what is the mechanism of injury?

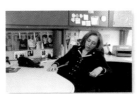
FIGURE 17-13 ▲ Form a general impression by pausing a short distance from the patient.

- Place the patient's right hand under the side of his face.
- Continue to monitor the patient while he is in your care.

Remember This
- Do *not* place a patient with a known or suspected spinal injury in the recovery position, but assess the need for suctioning frequently.
- There is a potential risk for nerve and vessel injury if the patient lies on one arm for a prolonged period in the recovery position. To avoid these types of injuries, it may be necessary to roll the patient to the other side.

Keeping the Airway Open: Airway Adjuncts

Airway adjuncts are devices used to help keep a patient's airway open. When using an airway adjunct, you must first open the patient's airway by using one of the techniques already described. You should then insert the airway adjunct and maintain the proper head position while the device is in place.

Remember This
The use of an airway adjunct does not eliminate the need for maintaining proper head positioning.

Oral Airway

Objective 17

An **oral airway** is a curved device made of rigid plastic. An oral airway is also called an **oropharyngeal airway (OPA)**. An OPA is inserted into the patient's mouth and used to keep the tongue away from the back of the throat. It may be used only in unresponsive patients without a gag reflex.

OPAs are available in a variety of sizes (Figure 12-12). Before inserting an OPA, you must determine the correct size for your patient. To select the correct size, hold the OPA against the side of the patient's face. Select an OPA that extends from the corner of the patient's mouth to the tip of the earlobe, or from the center of the patient's mouth to the angle of the jaw. If you select an airway of the wrong size, you can cause an airway obstruction. An airway that is too long can press the epiglottis against the entrance of the larynx, resulting in a complete airway obstruction (Figure 12-13a). An OPA that is too short may come out of the mouth or it may push the tongue into the back of the throat, causing an airway obstruction

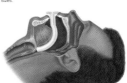
FIGURE 12-12 ▲ Oral airways are available in a variety of sizes.

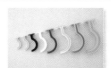
(a)

(b)

FIGURE 12-13 ▲ **(a)** An oral airway that is too long can press the epiglottis against the entrance of the larynx, resulting in a complete airway obstruction. **(b)** An oral airway that is too short may come out of the mouth or it may push the tongue into the back of the throat, causing an airway obstruction.

(Figure 12-13b). A properly sized OPA is one of the best tools for maintaining an open airway (Figure 12-14).

Skill Drill 12-1 shows the steps for sizing and inserting an oral airway.

Tables

This is a modern up-to-date text. It follows the *Education Standards* and the author has expanded further in many of the sections past the minimum standards.
—Gregory Neiman
Virginia Office of EMS

The pictures and tables are excellent resources for the students who are learning the material while trying to work full-time jobs.
—Kristie Skala
Aims Community College

TABLE 17-6 Normal Blood Pressure at Rest			
Life Stage	Age	Systolic Pressure	Diastolic Pressure
Newborn	Birth to 1 month	74 to 100	50 to 68
Infant	1 to 12 months	84 to 106	56 to 70
Toddler	1 to 3 years	98 to 106	50 to 70
Preschooler	4 to 5 years	98 to 112	64 to 70
School-age child	6 to 12 years	104 to 124	64 to 80
Adolescent	13 to 18 years	118 to 132	70 to 82
Adult	19 years and older	100 to 119	60 to 79

Sum It Up

Summarizes all of the chapter's content succinctly.

The Sum It Up section does just that—hits on all of the key points once again.
—Craig Schambow
Gateway Technical College

Sum It Up

► The communication process involves six basic elements: source, encoding, message, channel, receiver (decoder), and feedback. The source of verbal communication is spoken or written words. A message is the information to be communicated. The sender decides the message he wants to send and then encodes it. Encoding is the act of placing a message into words or images so that it is understood by the sender and receiver. The sender selects the path (channel) for transmitting the message to the receiver. The receiver is the person or group for whom the sender's message

Module 1

Preparatory

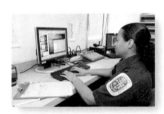

► CHAPTER 1

EMS Systems and Research   2

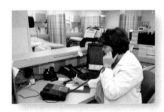

► CHAPTER 2

Workforce Safety and Wellness   28

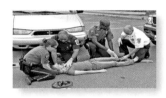

► CHAPTER 3

Legal and Ethical Issues
and Documentation   79

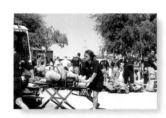

► CHAPTER 4

EMS System Communication   109

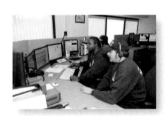

► CHAPTER 5

Medical Terminology   121

EMS Systems and Research

By the end of this chapter, you should be able to:

Knowledge Objectives ▶

1. Define the components of Emergency Medical Services (EMS) systems.
2. Differentiate the roles and responsibilities of the emergency medical technician (EMT) from those of other prehospital care professionals.
3. Define the terms certification, licensure, credentialing, and scope of practice.
4. Describe the benefits of EMT continuing education.
5. Define medical oversight and discuss the emergency medical technician's role in the process.
6. Discuss the types of medical oversight that may affect the medical care given by an EMT.
7. Explain quality management and the EMT's role in the quality management process.
8. Describe the phases of a typical EMS response.
9. Describe examples of professional behaviors in the following areas: integrity, empathy, self-motivation, appearance and personal hygiene, self-confidence, communication, respect, time management, teamwork and diplomacy, patient advocacy, and careful delivery of service.
10. List the primary roles and responsibilities of the EMT.
11. Define the role of the EMT relative to the responsibility for personal safety, the safety of the crew, the patient, and the bystanders.
12. Describe the importance and benefits of research.

Attitude Objectives ▶

13. Characterize the various methods used to access the EMS system in your community.
14. Defend the importance of continuing education and skills retention.
15. Demonstrate professional behaviors in the following areas: integrity, empathy, self-motivation, appearance and personal hygiene, self-confidence, communications, time management, teamwork and diplomacy, respect, patient advocacy, and careful delivery of service.
16. Accept and uphold the responsibilities of an EMT in accordance with the standards of an EMS professional.
17. Assess areas of personal attitude and conduct of the EMT.
18. Explain the rationale for maintaining a professional appearance when on duty or when responding to calls.
19. Describe why it is inappropriate to judge a patient on the basis of a cultural, gender, age, or socioeconomic model, and to vary the standard of care rendered because of that judgment.

20. Value the need to serve as a patient advocate.
21. Assess personal practices relative to the responsibility for personal safety and the safety of the crew, the patient, and the bystanders.
22. Advocate the need for supporting and participating in research efforts aimed at improving EMS systems.

Skill Objectives ▷   No skill objectives are identified for this lesson.

On the Scene

You and your paramedic partner are called to a repair shop for an injured man. When you arrive on the scene, shop workers quickly wave you to the back of the building. A worker has been injured while repairing a gear in a lawn tractor. His hand is stuck in the engine, which still roars loudly. He is writhing in pain and soaked in sweat. Several of his fingers have been cut off. Blood is pooling on his forearm and dripping to the floor. The patient's coworkers gather around, waiting for you to take action. ■

THINK ABOUT IT

As you read this chapter, think about the following questions:

* What is your most important concern as you approach this and all emergency situations?
* What EMT skills might you need in this situation? What others may need to be provided by your paramedic partner?
* What components of the emergency care system is this patient likely to need?

Introduction

The Emergency Medical Technician

An emergency medical technician (EMT) is a member of the Emergency Medical Services (EMS) team who responds to emergency calls, provides efficient emergency care to ill or injured patients, and transports patients to a medical facility. EMTs are an important and essential part of the EMS system. In fact, most prehospital emergency medical care is provided by EMTs. As an EMT, you will be called to respond to many types of emergencies, such as a motor vehicle crash, life-threatening medical situation, or disaster. EMTs may be paid or volunteer as fire department personnel, law enforcement officers, military personnel, members of the ski patrol, teachers, lifeguards, designated industrial/commercial medical response teams, park rangers, coaches, or athletic trainers (Figure 1-1). EMTs may work for public or private agencies. As an EMT, you will be tasked with providing medical assis-

tance and seeking the help of other emergency caregivers as needed.

The emergency medical technician course will help you gain the knowledge, attitude, and skills necessary to be a competent, productive, and valuable member of the healthcare team. The curriculum for this program was developed by representatives of federal and state agencies, professional medical organizations, and education experts.

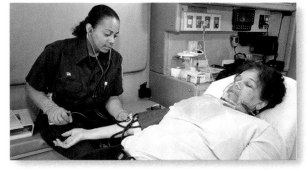

FIGURE 1-1 ▲ An EMT is a member of the EMS team who provides prehospital emergency care.

Origins of Emergency Medical Services

Ancient Times to the 1800s

As an EMT, you will be giving emergency care to ill or injured patients. An **emergency** is an unexpected illness or injury that requires immediate action to avoid risking the life or health of the person being treated. Emergency medical care has been given by one person to another for thousands of years. The Egyptians splinted and dressed wounds. The ill or injured were treated at the site where the emergency happened or were carried to a designated healer or helper. The Good Samaritan stopped to provide care to a man who had been beaten and left lying on the side of the road. He wrapped bandages around the injured man's wounds and then transported him by donkey to the nearest hotel. The Romans and Greeks used chariots to remove injured soldiers from the battlefield.

EMS probably began in 1797 in the Napoleonic Wars during which a system of service was provided to the injured. Baron Dominique-Jean Larrey, a French surgeon general, used light carriages to transport casualties from the field to aid stations. The medical crews operating the carriages were trained to control severe bleeding and splint fractures. The first civilian ambulance services in the United States began as hospital-based services in Cincinnati (in 1865) and New York City (in 1869).

1900 to 1960

The first known air medical transport occurred during the retreat of the Serbian army from Albania in 1915. In 1922, the American College of Surgeons established the Committee on Treatment of Fractures, which later became the Committee on Trauma.

In the mid-1940s, rural communities recognized the need for local fire protection and first aid and began volunteer services to meet the need for these services. In the 1950s, Mobile Army Surgical Hospital (MASH) units used helicopters for evacuation in the Korean War. The rapid evacuation of patients increased survival. In 1958, Dr. Peter Safar demonstrated the importance of mouth-to-mouth ventilation. Cardiopulmonary resuscitation (CPR) was shown to be useful in 1960.

1960 to 1970

In the 1960s, hospital-based mobile coronary care unit ambulances were successfully being used to treat prehospital cardiac patients in Belfast, Ireland. Meanwhile, in the United States, volunteers untrained in emergency care provided minimal stabilization at the scene of an emergency. Transport to the nearest hospital was provided by funeral homes, taxis, and automobile towing companies as an optional service.

This fragmented system of care continued in the United States until the late 1960s. In 1966, the National Academy of Sciences–National Research Council (NAS/NRC) published a paper called *Accidental Death and Disability, The Neglected Disease of Modern Society*. This document is commonly called the "white paper" or "landmark paper." It exposed the gaps in providing emergency care in the United States. Some of the areas identified that needed improvement included the following:

- Improving citizen knowledge of basic first aid
- Improving ambulance design and equipment
- Improving the training of emergency responders (ambulance attendants, police and fire personnel)
- Providing physician oversight (medical direction)
- Improving the care provided by hospital emergency departments
- Improving communications and record keeping
- Increasing local government support to provide the best possible EMS

The Highway Safety Act of 1966 charged the Department of Transportation (DOT) National Highway Traffic Safety Administration (NHTSA) with the responsibility of improving EMS. This act provided funding for the development of highway safety programs to reduce the number of deaths related to highway accidents. The act also established national standards for the training of emergency medical technicians and the minimum equipment required on an ambulance.

You Should Know

Passage of the Highway Safety Act of 1966 was the first national commitment to reducing highway-related injuries and deaths.

The American College of Emergency Physicians (ACEP) was founded in 1968. In the same year, the FCC and AT&T designated 9-1-1 as the universal emergency telephone number, and the American Trauma Society was established. In 1969, the first nationally recognized EMT-Ambulance (EMT-A) curriculum was published.

1970 to 1980

The National Registry of Emergency Medical Technicians (NREMT) was founded in 1970. The NREMT contributes to the development of professional standards. It also verifies the competency of EMS professionals by preparing and conducting examinations. Recognizing a need for an EMS training program for law enforcement personnel, NHTSA developed the *Crash Injury Management for the Law Enforcement Officer* training program in the early 1970s. This 40-hour course later evolved into the First Responder National Standard Curriculum in 1979.

In 1971, the television program *Emergency!* aired, featuring paramedics Johnny Gage and Roy Desoto. This program increased the public's awareness of EMS. The Department of Labor officially recognized EMT-Ambulance as an occupational specialty in 1972. In the same year, demonstration projects were begun in some states to develop model regional EMS systems. The Emergency Medical Services System (EMSS) Act was enacted in 1973. This law mandated that there should be 15 components of EMS systems. The components identified were:

- Manpower
- Training
- Communications
- Transportation
- Facilities
- Critical care units
- Public safety agencies
- Consumer participation
- Access to care
- Patient transfer
- Coordinated patient record keeping
- Public information and education
- Review and evaluation
- Disaster plan
- Mutual aid

By this time, it was clear that patient care could be improved if the components of an EMS system worked together. The EMSS Act provided grant funding to states and communities that developed EMS systems as described in the law.

In 1975, the National Association of Emergency Medical Technicians (NAEMT) was founded. In the same year, a study in Seattle, Washington, showed that the survivability of heart attack victims was improved with early involvement of advanced life support (ALS) personnel. In 1977, national standards were developed for paramedics. In 1979, the American College of Surgeons Committee on Trauma published *Optimal Hospital Resources for Care of the Injured Patient*. To improve hospital capabilities to care for injured patients, this document identified the need for designation of three levels of trauma centers.

1980 to 1990

In 1984, the EMS for Children (EMSC) Program provided funds to improve the EMS system and better serve the needs of infants and children. In 1985, the National Research Council published *Injury in America: A Continuing Public Health Problem*. This document described deficiencies in the progress of addressing the problem of accidental death and disability. In 1986, the Injury Prevention Act (followed by the Injury Control Act of 1990) established the Division of Injury Epidemiology and Control at the Centers for Disease Control and Prevention (changed to the National Center for Injury Prevention and Control in 1992) to provide leadership for a variety of injury-related public health activities. In 1987, the American College of Emergency Physicians published *Guidelines for Trauma Care Systems*. This document identified essential criteria for trauma systems, especially prehospital care components. In 1988, NHTSA began a statewide EMS system Technical Assistance Program (TAP). This program identified 10 essential parts of an EMS system and the methods used to assess these areas. States use the standards set by NHTSA to evaluate the effectiveness of their EMS system.

Components of the NHTSA Technical Assistance Program Assessment Standards

- Regulation and policy
- Resource management
- Human resources and training
- Transportation
- Facilities
- Communications
- Public information and education
- Medical direction
- Trauma systems
- Evaluation

In 1989, *Rescue 911* aired on television. When watching this program, viewers saw reenactments of actual emergency calls. This was significant because previously EMS calls on TV were usually fictionalizations. In this program, viewers saw callers dial "9-1-1" when emergency care was needed. They also saw calls to 9-1-1 being answered by trained personnel who could give lifesaving instructions over the telephone. This program increased awareness of the importance of bystander cardiopulmonary resuscitation (CPR) and resulted in increased training of the community in CPR.

1990s to the Present

Objective 1

In 1990, the Trauma Systems Planning and Development Act created the Division of Trauma and EMS (DTEMS) within the Department of Health and Human Services. To address the needs of injured patients and match them to available resources, this law provided funding to states for the development, implementation, and evaluation of trauma systems. States were responsible for developing a system of specialized care for the triage (sorting) and transfer of trauma patients. DTEMS was disbanded in 1995. Also in 1990, the American College of Surgeons Committee on Trauma published *Resources for Optimal Care of the Injured Patient.* These revised guidelines changed the focus from trauma centers to trauma systems. In 1991, the Commission on Accreditation of Ambulance Services set standards and benchmarks for ambulance services. In 1994, the EMT-Basic National Standard Curriculum was revised. The First Responder National Standard Curriculum was revised in 1995.

In 1996, the National Association of EMS Physicians and the National Association of State EMS Directors created the *EMS Agenda for the Future*. Because it also recommended directions for future EMS development in the United States, this paper is often called a "vision" document. This document reviewed the progress made in EMS over 30 years and proposed continued integration of EMS into the healthcare system.

In 1998, the Paramedic National Standard Curriculum (NSC) was revised followed by revision of the EMT-Intermediate NSC in 1999. In 2000, the *EMS Education Agenda for the Future: A Systems Approach* was released. This document proposed an EMS education system made up of five integrated parts (see Table 1-1).

Following the terrorist attacks on September 11, 2001, the Department of Homeland Security was created with the Homeland Security Act of 2002. In 2003,

---

TABLE 1-1   EMS Education System of the Future—Components

EMS Agenda for the Future	1996 document that created the vision for EMS
EMS Education System of the Future	
1. *National EMS Core Content*	Describes the domain of prehospital care
2. *National EMS Scope of Practice*	• Divides EMS core content into EMS levels of practice • Defines minimum skills and knowledge for each level of EMS professional
3. *National EMS Education Standards*	• Replaces National Standard Curriculum • Defines competencies, clinical behaviors, and judgments that define the performance requirements for each level of student
4. National EMS Education Program Accreditation	EMS education program approval based on universally accepted standards and guidelines
5. National EMS Certification	Standardized testing completed after graduation from an accredited EMS program that leads to state licensure

President George W. Bush directed the Secretary of Homeland Security to develop and administer a National Incident Management System (NIMS). The NIMS provides a consistent nationwide template to enable all government, private sector, and nongovernmental organizations to work together during domestic incidents.

In 2005, the *National EMS Core Content* document was released. This document defines the domain of prehospital care. The *National EMS Scope of Practice* is a document that divides the core content into EMS levels of practice, defining the minimum skills and knowledge for each level of EMS professional. Important dates in the history of EMS are summarized in Table 1-2.

TABLE 1-2   Important Dates in the History of EMS

Year	Event
1797	Napoleonic Wars • Beginning of system of service to the injured. • Light carriages are used for transporting casualties from the field to aid stations. • Medical crews operating the carriages are trained to control severe bleeding and splint fractures.
1860s	First civilian ambulance services in U.S. begin as hospital-based services in Cincinnati and New York City.
1915	First known air medical transport occurs during retreat of the Serbian army from Albania.
1922	American College of Surgeons establishes Committee on Treatment of Fractures (later becomes Committee on Trauma).
Mid-1940s	Rural communities recognize need for local fire protection and first aid and begin volunteer services to meet the need for these services.
1950s	• MASH units use helicopters for evacuation in the Korean War; rapid evacuation of patients increases survival. • American College of Surgeons develops first training program for ambulance attendants. • Dr. Peter Safar demonstrates efficacy of mouth-to-mouth ventilation (1958).
1960	• CPR is shown to be useful. • Ambu introduces bag-valve-mask resuscitator. • Laerdal introduces Resusci Anne.
1965	PhysioControl introduces LifePak 33 heart monitor/defibrillator.
1966	• Beginning of modern EMS. • *Accidental Death and Disability, The Neglected Disease of Modern Society*, published by National Academy of Sciences–National Research Council, identifies injury as a national healthcare problem. • Highway Safety Act of 1966 charges DOT National Highway Traffic Safety Administration (NHTSA) with responsibility of improving EMS, including helping states develop EMS programs; it is the first national commitment to reducing highway-related injuries and deaths.
1967	George Hurst invents Jaws of Life (Hurst Tool).
1968	• 9-1-1 is designated as the universal emergency telephone number. • American Trauma Society is established.
1969	• First nationally recognized EMT-Ambulance (EMT-A) curriculum is published. • Glenn Hare patents the Hare Traction Splint.
1970	National Registry of Emergency Medical Technicians (NREMT) is founded.
1971	*Emergency!* television program airs.

Continued

TABLE 1-2 Important Dates in the History of EMS *Continued*

Year	Event
1972	• Department of Labor officially recognizes EMT-A as an occupational specialty. • Demonstration projects are begun in some states to develop model regional EMS systems.
1973	EMSS Act provides federal guidelines and funding for development of regional EMS systems.
1974	Glenn Hare patents Hare Extrication Collar.
1975	National Association of Emergency Medical Technicians is founded.
1977	National standards are developed for EMT-Paramedics.
1979	• American College of Surgeons Committee on Trauma publishes *Optimal Hospital Resources for Care of the Injured Patient*, which identifies three levels of trauma centers. • Dr. Burt Kaplan and the David Clark Co. patent military antishock trousers.
1981	• Omnibus Budget Reconciliation Act consolidates EMS funding into state preventive block grants; EMSS Act funding is eliminated. • Rick Kendrick invents Kendrick Extrication Device.
1984	EMS for Children program provides funds to improve the EMS system and better serve the needs of infants and children.
1985	• National Research Council publishes *Injury in America: A Continuing Public Health Problem*, which describes the lack of progress in addressing the problem of accidental death and disability. • First Responder, EMT-Ambulance, EMT-Intermediate, and EMT-Paramedic National Standard Curricula are revised by NHTSA.
1986	• Injury Prevention Act (followed by Injury Control Act of 1990) establishes Division of Injury Epidemiology and Control at Centers for Disease Control and Prevention (changed to National Center for Injury Prevention and Control in 1992) to provide leadership for a variety of injury-related public health activities. • Life Support Products develops Automatic Transport Ventilator.
1988	National Highway Traffic Safety Administration establishes EMS Technical Assessment Program; 10 essential components of an EMS system are identified.
1989	*Rescue 911* airs on television.
1990	• Trauma Systems Planning and Development Act creates the DTEMS within the Department of Health and Human Services, provides funding to address needs of injured patients and match them to available resources, and encourages development of trauma systems. • American College of Surgeons Committee on Trauma publishes *Resources for Optimal Care of the Injured Patient*, which changes the focus from trauma centers to trauma systems.
1991	Commission on Accreditation of Ambulance Services sets standards and benchmarks for ambulance services.
1993	Federal Communications Commission approves channels for exclusive Emergency Medical Radio Service (EMRS) use.
1994	EMT-Ambulance National Standard Curriculum is revised and renamed EMT-Basic National Standard Curriculum.
1995	First Responder National Standard Curriculum is revised.

Continued

TABLE 1-2 Important Dates in the History of EMS *Continued*

Year	Event
1996	*EMS Agenda for the Future* is created by the National Association of EMS Physicians and National Association of State EMS Directors, which reviews progress made in EMS over 30 years and proposes continued development of 14 EMS attributes.
1998	Paramedic National Standard Curriculum is revised.
1999	EMT-Intermediate National Standard Curriculum is revised.
2000	• Trauma System Planning and Development Act is reauthorized and funded. • *EMS Education Agenda for the Future: A Systems Approach* is published by NHTSA; it is designed to develop an integrated system of EMS regulation, certification, and licensure.
2002	Homeland Security Act of 2002 creates Department of Homeland Security.
2003	Homeland Security develops and administers the National Incident Management System.
2005	*National EMS Core Content* document is published defining the domain of knowledge of EMS personnel described within the *National EMS Scope of Practice* and universal knowledge and skills of EMS personnel.
2006	*EMS at the Crossroads*, an Institute of Medicine report, is published and contains recommendations related to *EMS Education Agenda*: • State governments should adopt a common scope of practice for EMS personnel, with state licensing reciprocity. • States should require national accreditation of paramedic programs. • States should accept national certification as a prerequisite for state licensure and local credentialing of EMS professionals. *National EMS Scope of Practice* is published by NHTSA: • Divides EMS core content into EMS levels of practice. • Defines practices and minimum competencies for each level of EMS professional. • Guides state legislation. • Promotes reciprocity among states.

Overview of the Emergency Medical Services System

Objective 2

As an EMT, you are a part of the **Emergency Medical Services (EMS) system.** The EMS system is a network of resources that provides emergency care and transportation to victims of sudden illness or injury. An EMS system may be local, regional, statewide, or national. The network of resources includes emergency medical personnel, equipment, and supplies. To be efficient and effective, these resources must function in a coordinated manner.

EMS includes a wide range of emergency care including:

- Recognizing the emergency
- Accessing the EMS system
- Providing emergency care at the scene
- Providing emergency care when indicated during transport to, from, and between healthcare facilities
- Giving medical care to patients during disasters and at mass gatherings, such as a concert or sporting event

An EMS system does not exist by itself. Because EMS professionals provide care to ill or injured members of the public, EMS overlaps with other important areas such as public safety, public health, and the healthcare system. A **healthcare system** is a network of people, facilities, and equipment that is designed to provide for the general medical needs of the population. EMS is a part of the healthcare system.

Legislation and Regulation

To ensure the delivery of quality emergency medical care for adults and children, each state has laws in place that govern its EMS system. Each state must make sure that all ill or injured victims have equal access to appropriate emergency care. This includes making sure there are enough vehicles, equipment, supplies, and trained personnel on hand to meet the needs of local EMS systems. As an EMT, you must know your state and local EMS regulations and policies.

Public Access and Communications

An EMS system must have an effective communications system. The EMS system must provide a means by which a citizen can reliably access the EMS system (usually by dialing 9-1-1). To make sure appropriate personnel, vehicles, and equipment are sent to the scene of an emergency, the communication system must allow contact between different agencies, vehicles, and personnel. For example, there must be a means for:

- Citizen access to the EMS system
- Communication between dispatch center and emergency vehicle
- Communication between emergency vehicles
- Communication to and between emergency personnel
- Communication to and between emergency vehicles and emergency healthcare facilities
- Communication to and between emergency personnel and medical direction
- Communication between emergency healthcare facilities
- Communication between agencies, such as between EMS and law enforcement personnel
- Methods for relaying information to the public

Remember This

The 9-1-1 network is an important part of our nation's emergency response and disaster preparedness system. Because there is no "11" on a telephone pad, 9-1-1 should always be referred to as "nine-one-one," not "nine-eleven." The sequence 9-1-1 is easily remembered, even by young children.

When an emergency occurs in the United States, the person who places a call for help expects a prompt response to the scene of the emergency. For example, law enforcement and fire department personnel are typically dispatched to the scene of a motor vehicle crash after the patient or a bystander calls 9-1-1. Note that 9-1-1 is the official national emergency number in the United States and Canada. When the numbers 9-1-1 are dialed, the caller is quickly connected to a single location called a *Public Safety Answering Point (PSAP)*. The PSAP dispatcher is trained to route the call to local emergency medical, fire, and law enforcement agencies. Although EMS is usually activated by dialing 9-1-1 from a standard telephone, other methods of activating an emergency response include emergency alarm boxes, citizen band radios, amateur radios, local access numbers, and wireless telephones and texting. **Enhanced 9-1-1, or E9-1-1,** is a system that routes an emergency call to the 9-1-1 center closest to the caller and automatically displays the caller's phone number and address. Most 9-1-1 systems that exist today are E9-1-1 systems. The Federal Communications Commission (FCC) has established a program requiring wireless telephone carriers to provide E9-1-1 capability. Wireless E9-1-1 provides the precise location of a 9-1-1 call from a wireless phone, within 50 to 100 meters (164 to 328 feet) in most cases. It is important that you know how the citizens of your community access the EMS system.

Human Resources and Education

An EMS system must have qualified, competent, and compassionate people to provide quality EMS care. Persons working in an EMS system are expected to be trained to a minimum standard. The ***National EMS Scope of Practice*** is a document that defines four levels of EMS professionals: emergency medical responders (EMRs), EMTs, advanced EMTs (AEMTs), and paramedics. This document also defines what each level of EMS professional legally can and cannot do.

For many years, the minimum standard for education of EMS professionals was the DOT National Standard Curriculum (NSC) for each level. The ***National EMS Education Standards*** document is replacing the NSC. This document specifies the objectives that each level of EMS professional must meet when completing his or her education.

EMS education occurs in many different settings, including hospitals, community colleges, universities, technical centers, private institutions, and fire departments. To ensure quality, EMS systems should:

- Monitor educational programs regularly.
- Use qualified instructors.
- Use a standardized curriculum for each level of EMS professional throughout the state.
- Incorporate EMS standards, using an educationally sound curriculum development process.
- Use standardized testing methods.

TABLE 1-3 Levels of EMS Training

Basic Life Support	Emergency Medical Responder (EMR)	An EMR is the first person with medical training who arrives at the scene of an emergency. An EMR provides initial emergency care, including assessing for life-threatening conditions, opening and maintaining an airway, ventilating patients, performing CPR, controlling bleeding, caring for medical emergencies, bandaging wounds, stabilizing the spine and injured limbs, assisting with childbirth, and assisting other EMS professionals.
	Emergency Medical Technician (EMT)	An EMT is more skilled than an EMR and, at the scene of an emergency, continues the care begun by EMRs. EMTs can perform all EMR skills. Additional skills include helping patients with specific prescribed medications and giving oral glucose, aspirin, and other medications when indicated.
Advanced Life Support	Advanced Emergency Medical Technician (AEMT)	An AEMT is more skilled than an EMT. An AEMT can perform all EMT skills and has received additional training in patient assessment, provision of IV fluids and medications, and advanced airway procedures.
	Paramedic	A paramedic has more training than an AEMT and has additional education in pathophysiology, physical examination techniques, assessment of abnormal heart rhythms using a heart monitor, and invasive procedures.

Levels of Prehospital Education

Objective 2

There are four levels of nationally recognized prehospital professionals: emergency medical responder, emergency medical technician, advanced EMT, and paramedic (Table 1-3).

Emergency Medical Responder

An **emergency medical responder (EMR)** is a person who has the basic knowledge and skills necessary to provide lifesaving emergency care while waiting for the arrival of additional EMS resources. EMRs were formerly called *First Responders*. In some states, First Responders were called *Emergency Care Attendants (ECAs)*. Most EMRs have a minimal amount of equipment available with which to assess a patient and provide initial emergency care. An EMR is also trained to assist other EMS professionals.

Emergency Medical Technician

An **emergency medical technician (EMT)** is a member of the EMS team who responds to emergency calls, provides efficient emergency care to ill or injured patients, and transports the patient to a medical facility. An EMT has successfully completed a training program that adheres to the *National EMS Education Standards*. An EMT is trained to perform a more detailed assessment and can perform more skills than an EMR. At the scene of an emergency, EMTs continue the care begun by EMRs, including stabilizing the patient,

assisting a patient with medications, and transporting the patient.

Advanced Emergency Medical Technician

An **advanced EMT (AEMT)** has additional training in skills such as conducting a patient assessment, administering intravenous (IV) fluids and medications, and performing advanced airway procedures.

You Should Know

Advanced EMTs were formerly known as EMT-Intermediates.

Paramedic

A **paramedic** can perform the skills of an AEMT and has had additional instruction in pathophysiology (changes in the body caused by disease), physical examination techniques, assessment of abnormal heart rhythms using a heart monitor, and invasive procedures.

You Should Know

EMRs and EMTs provide basic emergency care. They are referred to as basic life support, or BLS, personnel. Advanced EMTs and paramedics provide more advanced care than EMRs and EMTs. They are often referred to as advanced life support, or ALS, personnel.

Right to Practice

Licensure, Certification, Credentialing

Objective 3

Statutes are laws established by Congress and state legislatures. Every state has statutes that establish an EMS regulatory body, such as a state EMS office. Each state has the authority and responsibility to regulate EMS within its borders and determine how its EMS personnel are certified or licensed. **Certification** is a designation that ensures a person has met predetermined requirements to perform a particular activity. Certification typically involves an examination process that is designed to verify that an individual has achieved minimum competency to ensure safe and effective patient care. **Licensure** is the granting of written permission by the state to perform medical acts and procedures not permitted without the authorization. State laws detail the **scope of practice,** that is, the medical procedures and functions that can be legally performed by certified or licensed healthcare professionals. In other words, scope of practice is a description of what a certified or licensed individual legally can and cannot do. **Credentialing** is a local process by which an individual is permitted by a specific entity (such as a medical director) to practice in a specific setting (such as an EMS agency). Because EMS statutes vary from state to state, ask your instructor about the laws in your area that affect you as an EMT. When working as an EMT, remember that you must also follow your EMS employer's policies and procedures.

EMT Certification

To be certified as an EMT, state agencies require successful completion of an EMT course that follows the DOT EMT National Standard Curriculum (or *National EMS Education Standards*). The NREMT provides examinations for certification and registration that may be required by your state. To be recognized as a nationally registered EMT, you must successfully complete a written and practical skills examination.

Certification as an EMT is good for a limited time, usually two years. Maintenance of current certification and licensure is a personal responsibility and one that you must take seriously. Working as an EMT without current certification and licensure has criminal implications. Participation in continuing education (CE) courses or an EMT Refresher Course is required for recertification.

You Should Know

National Registry of Emergency Medical Technicians

The NREMT helps develop professional standards. It also verifies the skills and knowledge of EMS professionals by preparing and conducting examinations.

Maintaining Knowledge and Skills

Objective 4

Your EMT education does not end with completing the EMT course. As a healthcare professional, you must keep your knowledge and skills current through continuing education and refresher courses. CE and refresher courses are helpful because they assist you in keeping current the skills and knowledge you learned during your initial training. CE and refresher courses also provide information about advances in medicine, skills, and equipment. In addition, they educate you about changes in local protocols and national guidelines that affect EMS.

CE may occur in different forms and includes attending skill labs, lectures, workshops, conferences and seminars; participating in case reviews and/or quality management reviews; reading professional journals; and reviewing DVDs and/or audiotapes.

Transportation

It has been estimated that EMS treats and transports more than 20 million patients per year in the United States. **Emergency transportation** is the process of moving a patient from the scene of an emergency to an appropriate healthcare facility. Healthcare facilities include hospitals, urgent care centers, physicians' offices, and other medical facilities. All patients who need transport must be moved safely in a properly staffed and equipped vehicle. Ground ambulances staffed by qualified emergency medical personnel are used to transport most patients (Figure 1-2). Patients with more serious injuries or illnesses may require transportation by helicopter (Figure 1-3). Boats and fixed-wing aircraft are other forms of transportation that are used in some areas.

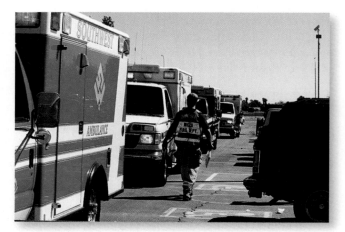

FIGURE 1-2 ▲ Most patients can be moved effectively in a ground ambulance staffed by qualified EMS personnel.

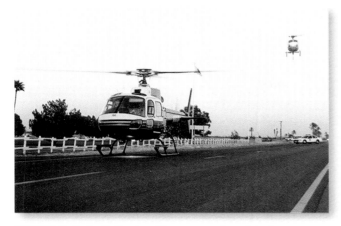

FIGURE 1-3 ▲ Patients with more serious injuries or illnesses may need to be moved rapidly by air medical services.

Medical Oversight

Objectives 5, 6

A physician oversees all aspects of patient care in an EMS system. In the United States, the medical care provided to patients by physicians is closely governed by laws called **medical practice acts.** These laws vary greatly from state to state and may address the ability of physicians to delegate certain skills and tasks to non-physicians, including EMTs, AEMTs, and paramedics.

   Medical oversight is the process by which a physician directs the emergency care provided by EMS personnel to an ill or injured patient. Medical oversight is also referred to as *medical control* or *medical direction.*

Every EMS system *must* have medical oversight. The physician who provides medical oversight is called the **medical director.** The medical director is responsible for making sure that the emergency care provided to ill or injured patients is medically appropriate. The two types of medical oversight are on-line and off-line.

On-Line Medical Direction

On-line medical direction, also called *direct* or *concurrent medical direction,* is direct communication with a physician by radio or telephone—or face-to-face communication at the scene—before EMS personnel perform a skill or administer care (Figure 1-4).

Off-Line Medical Direction

Off-line medical direction, also referred to as *indirect, prospective,* or *retrospective medical direction,* is the medical supervision of EMS personnel by means of policies, treatment protocols, standing orders, education, and quality management reviews.

Prospective Medical Direction

Prospective medical direction refers to activities performed by a physician medical director before an emergency call. Because it is impossible for the medical director to be physically present at every emergency, treatment protocols and standing orders are developed by the medical director, usually with the assistance of a local EMS advisory group. The development of treatment protocols and standing orders are examples of prospective medical direction.

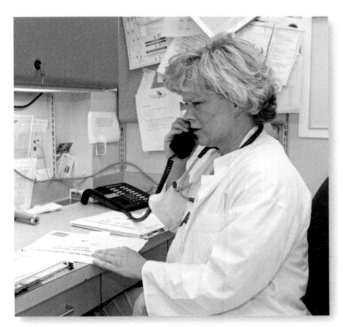

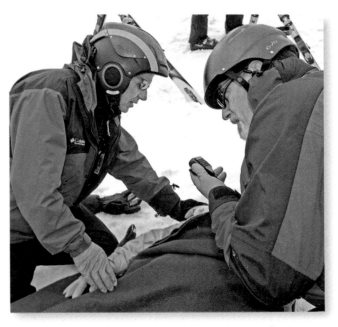

FIGURE 1-4 ▲ On-line medical direction is direct communication with a physician by radio or telephone or by face-to-face communication at the scene.

Treatment Protocols A **treatment protocol** is a list of steps to be followed when EMS personnel are providing emergency care to an ill or injured patient. For example, a patient experiencing a heat-related illness may be treated by using the steps outlined in a Heat-Related Emergencies treatment protocol.

Sample Treatment Protocol: Heat-Related Illness

If the patient has moist pale skin that is normal to cool in temperature, cool the patient by following these steps:

• Remove the patient from the hot environment.
• Administer oxygen.
• Remove as much of the patient's clothing as possible. Loosen clothing that cannot be easily removed.
• Cool the patient by fanning him or her. Do not cool the patient to the point of shivering.
• Place the patient on his or her back or side (if no contraindications exist).
• Consult medical direction for further instructions.

Standing Orders **Standing orders** are written orders that allow EMS personnel to perform certain medical procedures before making direct contact with a physician. Most protocols and standing orders are consistent with state and national standards and regional guidelines.

Standing orders are used in critical situations in which a delay in treatment would most likely result in harm to the patient. They may also be used when technical or logistical problems delay establishing on-line communication. Direct communication with a physician should be made as soon as the patient's condition allows.

Retrospective Medical Direction

Retrospective medical direction refers to activities performed by a physician after an emergency call. The physician (or the designee) may review the documentation related to the call. This review is done as part of an ongoing quality management program to make sure that appropriate medical care was given to the patient.

Facilities

An ill or injured patient receives definitive care in the hospital. Seriously ill or injured patients must be delivered in a timely manner to the closest *appropriate* healthcare facility. Hospital care includes many specialties and patient care resources. When the patient arrives at the hospital by ambulance, healthcare professionals from the hospital's emergency department continue the care

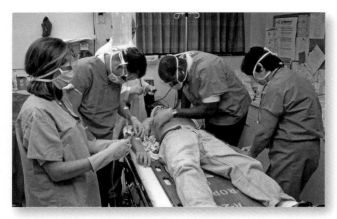

FIGURE 1-5 ▲ When the patient arrives at the hospital by ambulance, healthcare professionals from the hospital's emergency department continue the care begun by prehospital personnel.

begun by prehospital personnel (Figure 1-5). The patient is usually first seen by a nurse, who quickly assesses the severity of the patient's illness or injury, and then by a physician. The patient may be seen by other members of the healthcare team, depending on the patient's illness or injury and the resources of the receiving facility.

Remember This

The healthcare facility closest to the scene of an emergency is not always the most appropriate facility.

Members of the healthcare team who are available at most hospitals include physicians and physician assistants, nurses and nurse practitioners, respiratory therapists, and laboratory and radiology technicians. Additional resources available within the hospital include surgery and intensive care, among many others.

Specialty Centers

Some hospitals provide routine and emergency care but may specialize in the care of certain conditions or emergencies. Specialty centers have resources available, such as trained personnel and equipment, to help provide the best possible care for the patient's illness or injury. A trauma center is one type of specialty center (Figure 1-6). In a trauma center, specially trained personnel and equipment are available 24 hours a day to care for patients with serious injuries. Other types of specialty centers are shown in Table 1-4.

You Should Know

In both urban and rural areas, a patient may be stabilized at a closer hospital and then transferred to a specialty center if the patient requires care beyond that available at the initial receiving facility.

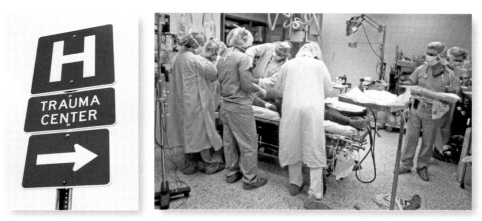

FIGURE 1-6 ▲ A trauma center is a specialty facility with trained personnel and equipment available 24 hours a day to care for seriously injured patients.

TABLE 1-4	Types of Specialty Centers
Burn Centers	Burn centers specialize in the care of patients with burns ranging from relatively mild to life-threatening injuries. Services include helping the patient and family with the emotional stress that often comes with a burn injury and providing daily assistance with exercise, scar control, wound care, splinting, and activities of daily living.
Heart/Cardiovascular Centers	Heart and cardiovascular centers specialize in treating disorders of the heart and blood vessels.
Hyperbaric Centers	Hyperbaric centers specialize in hyperbaric oxygen (HBO) therapy, which uses the administration of 100% oxygen at a controlled pressure (greater than sea level) for a set amount of time. Carbon monoxide poisoning and smoke inhalation are two conditions that may be treated with HBO therapy.
Pediatric Centers	Pediatric centers have trained professionals who recognize the medical, developmental, and emotional needs of children. Children are not just small adults. Their bodies are different, and the illnesses and injuries they experience often produce signs and symptoms that differ from those of an adult.
Perinatal Centers	Perinatal centers specialize in the care of women with high-risk pregnancies and infants with at-risk fetal conditions.
Poison Centers	Poison centers specialize in providing information in the treatment of poisonings and drug interactions. Some poison centers also provide education programs for medical professionals and the public about responding to biological and chemical terrorist incidents, as well as to nonterrorist incidents, such as epidemics and hazardous material incidents.
Spinal Cord Injury Centers	Spinal cord injury centers specialize in the medical, surgical, rehabilitative, and long-term follow-up care of patients with spinal cord injuries.
Stroke Centers	Stroke centers specialize in diagnosing and treating diseases of the blood vessels of the brain. A stroke occurs when blood vessels to a part of the brain suddenly burst or become blocked. The staff at a stroke center work very quickly to determine the cause of the stroke, identify where it is located, and give appropriate care.

Rehabilitation Services

Soon after their condition has been stabilized and they have been moved from the emergency department, some patients will require the services of healthcare professionals who specialize in rehabilitation. These healthcare professionals include rehabilitation nurses, physicians, physical therapists, occupational therapists, and social workers who work with the patient and family to return the ill or injured patient to his previous state of health.

Each state must have a quality management program to review and improve the effectiveness of EMS services provided to adults, infants, and children.

Making a Difference

To be sure that your patient receives the best possible care for an illness or injury, you must be familiar with the capabilities of the healthcare facilities in your area.

Public Health and Injury Prevention

Public health (also called *community health*) is the science and practice of protecting and improving the health of a community as a whole. Public health differs from individual patient care. Public health efforts focus on the prevention of disease and promotion of health, instead of treatment of a patient's specific illness or injury. Examples of public health accomplishments include the following:

- Widespread vaccinations
- Clean drinking water
- Sewage systems
- Declining infectious disease
- Fluoridated water
- Reduction in the use of tobacco products
- Prenatal care

EMS is a public health system and provides a critical public health function. For example, EMS professionals are first-line caregivers and their patient care reports may provide information on epidemics of disease that is important to public health agencies.

EMTs are healthcare professionals who have a responsibility to educate the public. Public education and injury prevention programs often lead to more appropriate use of EMS resources. Community involvement is discussed later in this chapter.

Evaluation

Quality Management

Objective 7

EMS systems use quality management programs to determine the effectiveness of the services the system provides. **Quality management** is a system of internal and external reviews and audits of all aspects of an EMS system. Quality management is used to identify areas of the EMS system needing improvement and to make sure that patients receive the highest quality medical care.

Your Role in the Quality Management Process

Objective 7

Quality management involves the constant monitoring of performance and is an important part of EMS. It includes:

- Obtaining information from the patient, other EMS professionals, and facility personnel about the quality and appropriateness of the medical care you provided
- Reviewing and evaluating your documentation of an emergency call (Figure 1-7)
- Evaluating your ability to properly perform skills
- Evaluating your professionalism during interactions with the patient, EMS professionals, and other healthcare personnel
- Evaluating your ability to follow policies and protocols
- Evaluating your participation in continuing education opportunities

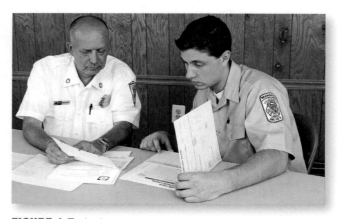

FIGURE 1-7 ▲ Quality management is an important part of EMS. It involves the constant monitoring of performance, including reviewing call documentation.

Phases of a Typical EMS Response

Objective 8

When an emergency occurs, a bystander frequently recognizes the event and activates the EMS system by calling 9-1-1 or another emergency number (Figure 1-8). The EMS dispatcher gathers information and activates an appropriate EMS response based on the information received. The bystander is often given instructions on how to provide basic first aid, including CPR if necessary (Figure 1-9).

On the way to the scene, EMTs prepare for the patient and situation on the basis of the information given by the dispatcher. They consider a number of factors, including:

- Scene safety
- Possible problems in gaining access to the patient
- The number of patients
- Potential complications that could result from the patient's reported illness or injury
- The equipment and supplies that will need to be brought to the patient to begin emergency care

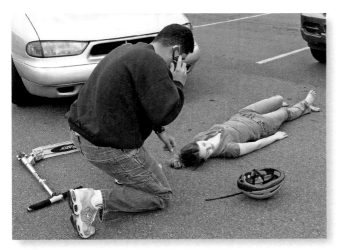

FIGURE 1-8 ▲ When an emergency occurs, a bystander frequently recognizes the event and activates the EMS system.

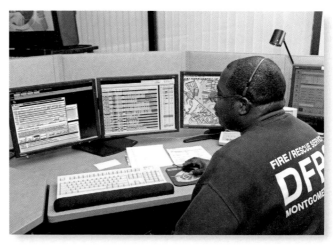

FIGURE 1-9 ▲ While in contact with the EMS dispatcher, the bystander is often provided with instructions regarding how to administer basic first aid.

Upon arriving at the scene, EMTs quickly "size up" the scene to find out if it is safe to enter. A **scene size-up** is done to:

- Find out if the scene is safe.
- Identify the mechanism of injury or the nature of the illness.
- Identify the total number of patients.
- Request additional resources if necessary.

The EMTs look for hazards or potential hazards such as downed electrical lines, possible hazardous materials, traffic hazards, unstable vehicles, signs of violence or potential violence, and weather hazards (Figure 1-10).

The phases of a typical EMS response are listed in Table 1-5 and shown in Figure 1-11.

Stop and Think!

If the scene is not safe and you cannot make it safe, *do not enter*. If a safe scene becomes unsafe, leave. Lives have been lost when a well-meaning rescuer has attempted to assist in an emergency without enough training, assistance, or equipment. Contact the dispatcher for additional equipment and personnel if needed.

After making sure that the scene is safe, EMTs quickly perform a **patient assessment** to find out the seriousness of the patient's condition or the extent of

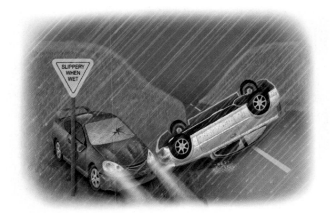

TABLE 1-5 Phases of a Typical EMS Response

- Detection of the emergency
- Reporting of the emergency (the call made for assistance)
- Dispatch/response (medical resources sent to the scene)
- On-scene care
- Care during transport
- Transfer to definitive care

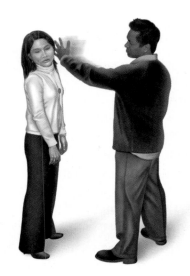

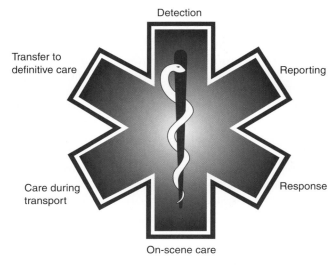

Detection

Transfer to definitive care

Reporting

Care during transport

Response

On-scene care

FIGURE 1-11 ▲ The phases of a typical EMS response.

injuries (Figure 1-12). Assessment is important to determine the emergency medical care the patient requires. EMTs will safely and efficiently provide emergency medical care for life-threatening emergencies at the scene until additional EMS resources arrive.

If more highly trained medical professionals arrive at the scene, EMTs give the arriving personnel a brief description of the emergency and a summary of the care provided before transferring patient care to them (Figure 1-13). If the patient's condition requires further emergency care, EMTs help lift the stretcher and place the patient into an ambulance. During transport, prehospital professionals assess the patient often and give additional emergency care as needed en route to an appropriate receiving facility, such as a hospital, for definitive care (Figure 1-14). EMTs may be required to assist ALS personnel as the patient is transferred to the receiving facility.

On arrival at the receiving facility, EMTs help lift and carry the patient out of the ambulance and into the receiving facility. The EMTs give a brief description

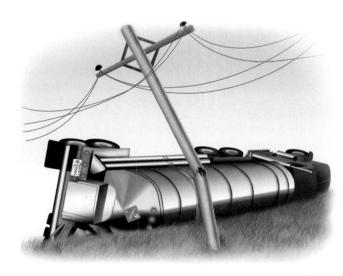

FIGURE 1-10 ▲ Arriving EMTs will quickly evaluate the safety of the scene, looking for hazards or potential hazards.

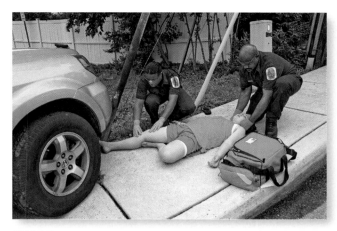

FIGURE 1-12 ▲ After ensuring the scene is safe, EMTs quickly assess the patient to determine the seriousness of the patient's condition or the extent of injuries.

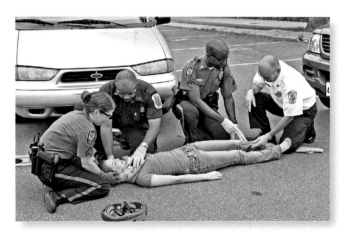

FIGURE 1-13 ▲ If more highly trained medical professionals arrive at the scene, a brief description of the emergency and a summary of the care provided are given before transferring patient care.

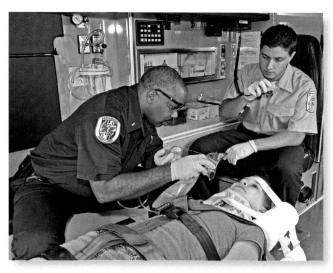

FIGURE 1-14 ▲ If the patient's condition requires further emergency care, the patient is loaded into an ambulance and transported to an appropriate receiving facility, such as a hospital.

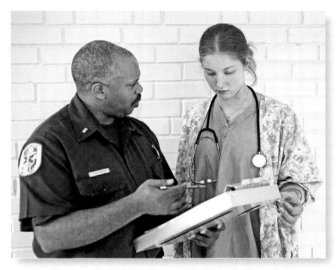

FIGURE 1-15 ▲ On arrival at the receiving facility, a brief description of the emergency and a summary of the care provided are given to a healthcare professional whose level of medical training is the same as or greater than that of the EMT before transferring patient care.

of the emergency and a summary of the care provided to a healthcare professional whose level of medical training is the same as or greater than that of the EMT. Patient care is then transferred (Figure 1-15). After documentation of the call is finished, supplies are restocked. EMTs restock and replace used linens, blankets, and other supplies that were used during the emergency call. They also clean all equipment using appropriate disinfecting procedures. EMTs carefully check all equipment to make sure the vehicle is ready for the next call. They make sure that the emergency vehicle is clean, washed, and kept in neat, orderly condition. The inside of the vehicle is disinfected as needed in accordance with federal, state, or local regulations.

After the call is completed, a review may be held with the other members of the EMS crew to discuss what went well and what could go better in the future.

The review also identifies opportunities for improving patient care at the scene and during transport.

You Should Know

You must know the locations of the healthcare facilities in your area and their capabilities to determine the most appropriate facility to which the patient should be transported.

Characteristics of Professional Behavior

Integrity

The public assumes that EMS professionals have **integrity,** which means honesty, sincerity, and truthfulness. Many consider integrity the single most important quality that an EMS professional can possess. As an EMT, it is important that you display integrity in all actions. Examples of behavior demonstrating integrity include the following:

- Telling the truth
- Providing complete and accurate information and documentation

Empathy

Empathy is the ability to identify with and understand the feelings, situations, and motives of others. You must demonstrate empathy to patients, families, and other healthcare professionals. Examples of behavior demonstrating empathy include the following:

- Showing care and compassion for others
- Demonstrating an understanding of patient and family feelings
- Demonstrating respect for others
- Exhibiting a calm, compassionate, and helpful demeanor toward those in need
- Being supportive and reassuring of others

Self-Motivation

EMS professionals must be self-motivated, which requires enthusiasm and an internal drive for excellence. EMS professionals must also be self-directed, which means that they recognize what needs to be done and set about doing it without having to be told to take action. Examples of behavior demonstrating self-motivation include the following:

- Taking initiative to complete assignments
- Taking initiative to improve and/or correct behavior
- Taking on and following through on tasks without constant supervision
- Showing enthusiasm for learning and improvement
- Demonstrating a commitment to quality management
- Accepting constructive feedback in a positive manner
- Taking advantage of learning opportunities

Appearance and Hygiene

It has been said that you never get a second chance to make a good first impression. As an EMT, you will meet individuals who are experiencing a medical emergency. In 30 seconds or less, they will form an opinion about you based on what they see, hear, and sense. When you approach a patient and prepare to provide needed emergency care, you are expecting the patient to place his or her trust in you. Presenting a neat, clean, and professional appearance invites trust. It also instills confidence, enhances cooperation, and brings a sense of order to an emergency.

Good personal hygiene is essential to presenting a professional appearance. It includes the following:

- Bathing daily
- Using a deodorant or antiperspirant
- Making sure your hair is clean and, if long, restrained so that is will not fall into open wounds or into your working space
- Making sure that your fingernails are clean and neatly trimmed

Good grooming includes making sure that your uniform is clean, is mended, and fits well. Shoes should be clean and comfortable, provide support, and fit properly. You should wear a watch that displays seconds for timing things such as a patient's heart rate, breathing rate, and labor pains.

Appropriate attire is usually defined by the event that is taking place. Your safety is important when selecting appropriate attire when working in EMS. For example, a patient who is confused or combative may pull at dangling jewelry or hair. Dangling jewelry should not be worn, and hair longer than shoulder length should be restrained. Beards and mustaches should be clean and kept short. Because they may be offensive and nauseating to patients, fragrances should not be worn. Tattoos, if present, should be covered by your uniform. Studs, rings, and bars should not be worn in visible body piercings, such as the tongue, nose, and eyebrow.

Making a Difference

The patient, the patient's family, and bystanders often view the attention you pay to your appearance as a reflection of the care you give. If you are courteous and respectful and present a professional appearance, they are reassured that you will provide quality patient care. If you are ill-mannered or your appearance is untidy, they may assume that the care you provide will be of poor quality.

Self-Confidence

Many emergency calls involve minor injuries, and the medical care that is required is straightforward. However, you will come across situations involving life-threatening injuries, as well as patients and family members who are upset. Others will look to you, as an EMT, as the person in control of the situation. Even though you may feel anxious, you must be able to adapt to such situations, remain calm, and display confidence. Self-confidence requires that you honestly assess and maintain awareness of your personal and professional strengths and limitations. Examples of behavior demonstrating self-confidence include the following:

- Demonstrating the ability to trust your personal judgment
- Demonstrating an awareness of your strengths and limitations

Making a Difference

Your contact with the patient, family, bystanders, and other members of the healthcare team must be respectful and professional, even in stressful or chaotic situations.

Communication

Communication is the exchange of thoughts, messages, and information. As an EMS professional, you must be able to convey information to others verbally and in writing. You must also be able to understand and interpret verbal and written messages. Examples of behavior demonstrating good communication skills include the following:

- Speaking clearly
- Writing legibly
- Listening actively
- Adjusting communication strategies to various situations

Respect

Respect is the willingness to feel and show polite regard, consideration, and appreciation for others. Examples of behavior demonstrating respect include being polite to others, not using insulting or demeaning terms, and showing behavior in a manner that brings credit to yourself, your employer and coworkers, and your profession. For instance, when you arrive at the patient's side, begin by introducing yourself: "Hello. My name is _____, and I am an emergency

medical technician. I am here to help you. What is your name?" An older adult should be addressed by his or her last name preceded by, Mr., Mrs., or Ms. Terms such as "hon" or "dear" should not be used because they are disrespectful.

Time Management

EMS professionals work in high stress situations and adverse conditions. You must be able to prioritize tasks, while providing patient care, and work quickly to accomplish those tasks. Examples of behaviors demonstrating good time management include the following:

- Being punctual
- Completing tasks and assignments on time

Teamwork and Diplomacy

Teamwork and diplomacy are two important traits that EMS professionals must possess. **Teamwork** is the ability to work with others to achieve a common goal. **Diplomacy** is the tact and skill in dealing with people. Examples of behavior demonstrating teamwork and diplomacy include the following:

- Placing the success of the team above your own self-interests
- Not undermining the team
- Helping and supporting other team members
- Showing respect for all team members
- Remaining flexible and open to change
- Communicating with coworkers in an effort to resolve problems

As an EMT, you will be working with persons from many other community resources. Examples of community resources include the following:

- Public safety agencies
- Public health departments
- Social service agencies and organizations
- Healthcare networks
- Community health educators

You will often work with public safety personnel, including police officers, firefighters, emergency management personnel, and other EMS professionals. You will be an important link in your community's healthcare system. The information you give members of these organizations about the first few minutes after the emergency will be helpful for providing continuation of patient care following the emergency response. Consider this real-life example: You are called to the home of a 93-year-old man for "difficulty breathing." When you arrive, you find the patient's home in complete disarray. He lives alone with his dog. The animal appears malnourished. The temperature outside is about 27°F, and it is very cold in the patient's home. While you begin caring for the patient, your partner notices that the patient's pantry is bare. The refrigerator contains one item—a carton of milk that was outdated three weeks ago. The patient tells you he has not been feeling well for the past few days and has been too weak to go to the store for food. Because he lives on a fixed income, he does not want to turn the heat on in his home. In situations such as this, it will be important for you to relay what you saw at the scene to the healthcare professionals at the hospital who will provide further patient care. The hospital has access to many resources that can help improve the patient's situation.

Patient Advocacy

One of your responsibilities as an EMT is to serve as the patient's advocate. An **advocate** is a person who supports another. You must protect the patient from further injury and act in the best interests of the patient. At the same time, you must accept the rights of other individuals to differ with you and not impose your beliefs (religious, ethical, political, social, legal) on others. Examples of behavior demonstrating patient advocacy include the following:

- Not allowing personal biases to affect patient care
- Placing the needs of patients above your own interests
- Protecting patient confidentiality

If the patient is unable to speak, you must be the patient's voice and act in the patient's best interests. You must protect the patient's rights, privacy, and dignity. For example, if it is necessary to remove the patient's clothing for assessment, you must make sure that the patient is shielded from the view of others. If bystanders ask you questions about a patient's illness or injury, you must protect the patient's privacy and not give out that information.

Careful Delivery of Service

EMS professionals deliver the highest quality of patient care with careful attention to detail and critically evaluate their performance and attitude. Examples of behavior demonstrating a careful delivery of service include the following:

- Mastering and refreshing skills
- Performing complete equipment checks
- Operating emergency vehicles carefully and safely
- Following policies, procedures, and protocols
- Following orders of superiors

Remember This

Characteristics of Professional Behavior

- Integrity
- Empathy
- Self-motivation
- Appearance and hygiene
- Self-confidence
- Communication
- Respect
- Time management
- Teamwork and diplomacy
- Patient advocacy
- Careful delivery of service

Primary Duties as an EMT

You have many roles and responsibilities as an EMT. When you are dispatched to the scene of an emergency, you are expected to respond promptly and provide competent medical care to the ill and injured.

No matter where they work, EMTs are expected to provide the same standard of care in an emergency. **Standard of care** refers to the minimum level of care expected of similarly trained healthcare professionals. In other words, you are expected to provide the same level of care as that provided by another EMT with similar training and experience in similar circumstances.

You are expected to accept and uphold the responsibilities of an EMT according to the standards of an EMS professional. These responsibilities include preserving life, relieving suffering, promoting health, and doing no harm. You must respect and hold in confidence all information of a confidential nature that was obtained in the course of your work as an EMT, unless you are required by law to report the information.

It is not appropriate to judge a patient or vary the care you provide because of a patient's race, ethnicity, national origin, religion, gender, age, mental or physical disability, sexual orientation, or ability to pay for the care provided. The emergency medical care you provide as an EMT must be based on the patient's needs without regard to any of these factors. Every patient has the right to expect competent, considerate, respectful care from every member of the healthcare team at all times and under all circumstances (Figure 1-16).

Many patient complaints about medical care result from the patient's belief that he or she was not treated

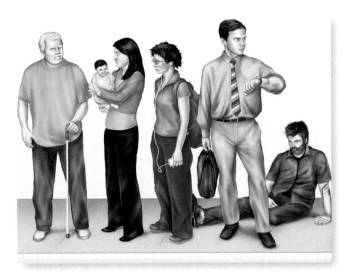

FIGURE 1-16 ▲ Healthcare personnel, including EMTs, must give all patients competent, considerate, and respectful care at all times and under all circumstances.

with respect. As an EMS professional, you have an obligation to do the following:

- Respect each patient as an individual.
- Provide emergency medical care to every patient to the best of your ability.
- Listen attentively to your patients, and take their concerns and complaints seriously.
- Provide clear explanations.
- Provide patients with emotional support to help ease fear and anxiety.
- Preserve each patient's dignity during examinations.

Preparation and Safety

Objectives 10, 11

Preparation for an emergency response includes being physically, mentally, and emotionally ready. Your job as an EMT has physical demands that require stamina and endurance. You will have to walk, stand, and assist in lifting and carrying ill or injured patients who may weigh more than 125 pounds (250 pounds, with assistance). Climbing and balancing may be required to gain access to the patient, such as on stairs or a hillside. You may also have to help transport the patient safely. In some situations, patients may be found in a location where patient assessment is possible only if you stoop, kneel, crouch, or crawl.

To make sure that your well-being, as well as that of the patient and your coworkers, is not at risk in these situations, you must first take care of yourself. Maintain your personal health by exercising regu-

larly. Exercise prepares you to handle the physical demands of the job by improving muscle tone and circulation. Exercise also provides a physical release for stress. Getting enough sleep, rest, and good nutrition is important to staying healthy and doing your job well. You should also keep your immunizations up to date.

Preparation for an emergency response includes having appropriate equipment and supplies ready and keeping your EMS knowledge and skills current to ensure that you deliver the highest quality of care possible to your patients.

Safety must *always* be considered on every call. Although the patient's well-being is an important concern at the scene of an emergency, your personal safety *must* be your primary concern, followed by the safety of your crew, patients, and bystanders.

Stop and Think!

Safety Priorities
1. Personal safety
2. Crew safety
3. Patient safety
4. Bystander safety

Response

When you are notified of an emergency, prepare for the patient and the situation on the basis of the information given to you. If you are responsible for driving an emergency vehicle, drive to the address or location given using the most expeditious route, depending on traffic and weather. Be sure to observe traffic laws and regulations regarding emergency vehicle operation. On arrival at the scene, park the emergency vehicle in a safe location to avoid additional injury.

Scene Size-Up

When you arrive at the scene and before you begin patient care, size up the scene. You should first determine whether the scene is safe. You should then identify the mechanism of the injury or the nature of the illness, identify the total number of patients, and request additional help if necessary. If law enforcement personnel are not present on the scene, create a safe traffic environment. This may require placing safety cones, removing debris, or redirecting traffic to protect the injured and those who are helping with their care. Before approaching the patient, put on appropriate personal protective equipment (PPE). This helps reduce your risk of exposure to potentially infectious body fluid substances or other infectious agents (see Chapter 2).

Remember This

Before approaching the patient, make sure the scene is safe for you to provide care.

Gaining Access to the Patient

You must gain access to the patient in order to perform a patient assessment and provide emergency care. In some situations, you may need additional resources at the scene, such as law enforcement personnel, the fire department, the utility company, or a special rescue team. In these situations, be sure to notify the dispatcher as soon as possible of the need for these resources.

If the patient has been involved in a motor vehicle crash, you must make sure the scene is safe and provide necessary care to the patient before **extrication.** Extrication is the process of removing structural components from around a patient to facilitate patient care and transport. You must also make sure that the patient is removed in a way that minimizes further injury. To accomplish these tasks, you will need to work closely with the rescuers responsible for extrication.

Remember This

Patient care comes before extrication unless a delay in movement would endanger the life of the patient or rescuer.

Patient Assessment

After reaching the patient, you must perform a systematic assessment to determine what is wrong and to quickly identify life-threatening conditions. Your assessment will include obtaining the patient's vital signs. **Vital signs** are measurements of breathing, pulse, skin temperature, pupils, and blood pressure. Gather additional information about the emergency by observing the scene and speaking with the patient and bystanders. Find out who called 9-1-1.

Emergency Care

As an EMT, you will give emergency medical care to adults, children, and infants on the basis of your findings. When providing emergency care, follow your local protocols and contact medical direction as needed.

Depending on the patient's illness or injury, you may need to perform certain skills, including:

- Performing airway management (opening the airway using a head tilt–chin lift or jaw thrust without head tilt, inserting an oral airway, suctioning the upper airway)
- Providing respiratory assistance (giving oxygen when indicated, performing bag-mask ventilation)

- Providing trauma care (manually stabilizing the cervical spine, controlling bleeding, performing emergency moves, manually stabilizing injured limbs, controlling bleeding, performing emergency moves)
- Providing medical care to patients with respiratory, cardiac, diabetic, allergic, behavioral, and environmental emergencies, and suspected poisonings (performing cardiopulmonary resuscitation, operating an automated external defibrillator, or AED, which delivers an electrical shock to the heart)
- Assisting in childbirth
- Assisting patients with prescribed medications, including sublingual nitroglycerin, epinephrine autoinjectors, and handheld aerosol inhalers
- Administering oxygen, oral glucose, and aspirin when indicated

Your help may be needed to lift and move patients when you are providing emergency care. For example, an unresponsive woman who is found on the floor of her home will need to be lifted onto a stretcher and then into an ambulance. To lift and move a patient safely, you must know about body mechanics, lifting and carrying techniques, and principles of moving patients. You must also be familiar with equipment used for lifting and moving. Lifting and moving techniques are discussed in Chapter 2.

Stop and Think!

Back injuries are common among EMS personnel. Remember: Your personal safety comes first. Keep yourself (and your back) safe by learning and using proper lifting and moving techniques.

Once you begin emergency care, you must continue that care until:

- An individual with medical training equal to or greater than your own assumes responsibility for the patient, *or*
- You are physically unable to continue providing care because of exhaustion, *or*
- There is a change in the scene that weakens or endangers your physical well-being, *or*
- An adult patient, of adequate mental capabilities and fully informed of the risks and benefits of treatment, elects to terminate care.

Transport/Transfer of Care

Some patients will require only basic life support (BLS) care. In these situations, you will transport the patient to a healthcare facility. Other patients will require a level of care beyond that which you can give. In these situations, contact dispatch as soon as you recognize the need for advanced level care. Provide what emergency care you can, and prepare the patient for transport.

Quickly decide where you will meet the ALS unit. In some cases, the ALS unit will meet you at the scene of the emergency. However, it is sometimes necessary for you to begin transport to the receiving facility and have the ALS unit meet you at a prearranged location. This is most likely to occur when the arrival of the ALS unit to the scene is estimated to be longer than your transport time to the hospital.

When transferring patient care to a healthcare professional with medical training equal to or greater than your own, be sure to include the following elements in your verbal report:

- Identify yourself as an EMT.
- Report the patient's age, gender, primary problem (chief complaint), and current condition.
- Describe what happened and the position in which the patient was found.
- Describe pertinent assessment findings, including vital signs.
- Report any medical history you obtained from the patient.
- Describe the emergency medical care that you gave.
- Describe the patient's response to the treatment given.
- Report the orders received from medical direction (if applicable).

Remember This

Remember the four Cs when giving a verbal report: Courteous, Clear, Complete, and Concise.

Documentation

Documentation is an important aspect of prehospital care. Information contained in a **prehospital care report (PCR)** is used for many purposes. Your documentation should reflect what you saw and heard at the scene. It should also include the emergency care you gave and the patient's response to that care. Your documentation of an EMS call must be accurate, complete, and concise (see Chapter 3). Other healthcare professionals will use the information contained in your report to note changes in the patient's condition. Changes in the patient's condition are particularly important to healthcare personnel assuming care of the patient.

Some of the information contained in the PCR is used for data collection and research purposes. For example, data such as the time you were dispatched to a call, arrived on the scene, and left the scene en route to the hospital are used for quality management purposes. With this information, the quality management program can determine how long EMS units are taking to respond to calls and how much time is being spent on the scene.

Returning to Service

Your rapid preparation for the next call can be very beneficial to the entire EMS system. It will be your responsibility to clean equipment as needed, restock any disposable equipment that you may have used, and return equipment to its storage area. It is very important that you understand your company's policies and arrangements made with receiving facilities or other agencies regarding restocking of supplies.

Community Involvement

As an EMT, you should be actively involved in educating the public about how and when to call EMS and how to prevent illness and injuries (Figure 1-17). CPR and first aid programs can improve a citizen's ability to recognize an emergency and provide appropriate care until more advanced care arrives. Teaching in the community also enhances the visibility and positive image of EMS professionals.

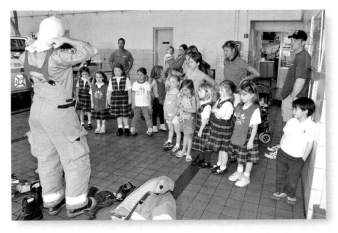

FIGURE 1-17 ▲ EMTs should educate the public about accessing the EMS system and preventing injuries.

Examples of Injury Prevention Programs

- Bicycle safety
- Child passenger safety
- Safe boating
- Poisoning prevention
- Fire-related injury prevention
- Dog bite prevention
- Drowning prevention
- Fireworks injury prevention
- Fall injury prevention for older adults
- Playground injury prevention

Personal Professional Development

Healthcare professionals are responsible for their personal professional development. Examples of ways in which professional development occurs include the following:

- Participating in continuing education activities
- Mentoring individuals who are new to the profession and/or your department
- Getting involved in professional organizations
- Supporting and participating in research activities

EMS Research

Objective 12

Many of the emergency care interventions performed in the prehospital setting were borrowed from hospital emergency departments. In the early years of EMS, assumptions were made that if a treatment worked for a patient in the hospital, it would be similarly useful in the field. As a result, some of the techniques used in the field were not studied to find out if they were actually effective in the prehospital environment. EMS-related research conducted before 1980 usually focused on one disease or operations issue, and was often conducted in only one EMS system. Therefore, the conclusions drawn may not have been valid or applicable in other EMS systems.

Today, scientific evidence through research is the foundation for medical practice decisions and changes in patient management. Research is essential to determine the effectiveness of new procedures, medications, and treatments in improving patient care and outcome. For instance, CPR guidelines change at least every five years on the basis of current research.

Primary Duties of the EMT

- Maintain vehicle and equipment readiness.
- Operate emergency vehicles.
- Perform scene assessment and provide scene leadership.
- Gain access to the patient.
- Perform patient assessment.
- Provide cardiac care.
- Provide respiratory care.
- Provide medical care.
- Provide trauma care.
- Provide obstetrical/gynecological care.
- Provide pediatric care.
- Provide emotional support.
- Resolve an emergency incident.
- Transfer of care.
- Maintain medical legal standards, including documentation.
- Return to service.
- Develop and maintain community relations.
- Provide administrative support.
- Enhance professional development.

Research results cause a chain reaction in EMS education and practice. For example, research findings drive changes in the development of the *National EMS Core Content*, which represents the entire domain of prehospital knowledge and skills. The *National EMS Core Content* drives the *National EMS Scope of Practice*, which names and defines the national levels of EMS practice. The knowledge and skill objectives for each level of practice identified in the *National EMS Scope of Practice* are defined by the *National EMS Education Standards*. Changes in the *National EMS Education Standards* affect medical publishers, EMS instructors, and those participating in EMS-related programs.

As an EMT, you may be asked to participate in EMS research. Your participation might involve using a new piece of equipment or performing a new skill. You may be asked to carefully document scene times, treatment times, or the patient's response to specific interventions as part of a study. You may be asked to participate in focus groups and interviews. No matter how you are asked to participate in research, approach this responsibility seriously and complete the task assigned to the best of your ability. The data obtained from your efforts may help improve the care of patients treated in the future.

After making sure the scene is safe to enter, you quickly turn off the lawn tractor engine and free the patient's hand. You then lay him down in a safe area and control the bleeding. Your paramedic partner assesses the patient and then starts an intravenous line. You check the patient's breathing rate, heart rate, and blood pressure and relay that information to your partner. While the paramedic gives the patient some pain medicine, you locate the severed fingers and package them appropriately. The patient is then transported to a trauma center, where two of his fingers are successfully reattached. He stops in to thank you two weeks later on his way home from a rehabilitation session. ∎

Sum It Up

▶ An EMT is a member of the EMS team who provides prehospital emergency care.

▶ A healthcare system is a network of people, facilities, and equipment designed to provide for the general medical needs of the population. The EMS system is part of the healthcare system.

▶ The *National EMS Scope of Practice* is a document that defines four levels of EMS professionals: EMRs, EMTs, advanced EMTs, and paramedics. This document also defines what each level of EMS professional legally can and cannot do. EMRs and EMTs provide basic life support. AEMTs and paramedics provide advanced life support.

▶ The *National EMS Education Standards* document specifies the objectives that each level of EMS professional must meet when completing his or her education.

▶ Each state has the authority and responsibility to regulate EMS within its borders and determine how its EMS personnel are certified or licensed. Certification is a designation that ensures a person has met predetermined requirements to perform a particular activity. Licensure is the granting of written permission by the state to perform medical acts and procedures not permitted without the authorization. Credentialing is a local process by which an individual is permitted by a specific entity (such as a medical director) to practice in a specific setting (such as an EMS agency).

▶ Every EMS system must have a medical director. A medical director is a physician who provides medical oversight and is responsible for making sure that the emergency care provided to ill or injured patients is medically appropriate.

▶ Medical oversight may be on-line or off-line. On-line medical direction is direct communication with a physician by radio or telephone or face-to-face communication at the scene before a skill is performed or care is given. Off-line medical direction is the medical supervision of EMS personnel by means of policies, treatment protocols, standing orders, education, and quality management review.

▶ A treatment protocol is a list of steps to be followed when EMS personnel are providing emergency care to an ill or injured patient. Standing orders are written orders that allow EMS personnel to perform certain medical procedures before making direct contact with a physician.

▶ Public health is the science and practice of protecting and improving the health of a community as a whole. Public health differs from individual patient care. Public health (also called community health) efforts focus on the prevention of disease and promotion of health, instead of treatment of a patient's specific illness or injury.

▶ Quality management is a system of internal and external reviews and audits of all aspects of an EMS system. Quality management is used to identify areas of the EMS system needing improvement. This system helps to make sure that the patient receives the highest quality medical care.

▶ The phases of a typical EMS response include detection of the emergency, reporting the emergency (the call made for assistance), dispatch/response (medical resources sent to the scene), on-scene care, care during transport, and transfer to definitive care.

▶ Characteristics of professional behavior include integrity, empathy, self-motivation, appearance and hygiene, self-confidence, communication, respect, time management, teamwork and diplomacy, patient advocacy, and careful delivery of service.

▶ Primary duties of the EMT include maintaining vehicle and equipment readiness; operating emergency vehicles; performing scene assessment and providing scene leadership and gaining access to the patient; performing a patient assessment to identify life-threatening conditions; providing cardiac, respiratory, medical, trauma, obstetrical/gynecological, and pediatric care; providing emotional support; resolving an emergency incident; transferring patient care and maintaining medical legal standards, including documenting the emergency per local and state requirements; returning to service; developing and maintaining community relations; providing administrative support; and enhancing professional development.

▶ Research is essential to determine the effectiveness of new procedures, medications, and treatments in improving patient care and outcome. If you are asked to participate in research, approach this responsibility seriously and complete the task assigned to the best of your ability.

CHAPTER

2

Workforce Safety and Wellness

By the end of this chapter, you should be able to:

Knowledge Objectives ▶

1. Discuss the concept of wellness.
2. Define the components of wellness.
3. Discuss the components of wellness associated with physical well-being.
4. Define stress.
5. Discuss the benefits of physical fitness.
6. Discuss the importance of obtaining adequate rest.
7. Define stressor and name common stressors associated with working in Emergency Medical Services.
8. Give examples of stressful situations that may be encountered in EMS.
9. Describe the body's fight-or-flight response.
10. Give examples of physical, behavioral, mental, and emotional signs of stress.
11. State the possible steps that EMS professionals may take to help reduce or alleviate stress.
12. State the possible reactions that members of the EMS professional's family may exhibit due to their outside involvement in EMS.
13. Define traumatic incident and give examples of traumatic incident situations.
14. Recognize the signs and symptoms of traumatic incident stress.
15. Define infection, pathogen, and communicable disease.
16. Describe methods of disease transmission.
17. Define infectious disease exposure.
18. Discuss the classification of communicable diseases.
19. Discuss the importance of standard precautions.
20. Describe the steps EMS professionals should take for personal protection from airborne and bloodborne pathogens.
21. Describe how to document and manage an infectious disease exposure.
22. Distinguish among the terms cleaning, disinfection, and sterilization.
23. Describe how to clean or disinfect items following patient care.
24. Define hazardous material and list the personal protective equipment necessary in a hazardous materials situation.
25. List the personal protective equipment necessary during rescue operations.
26. List the personal protective equipment necessary at a violent scene.
27. List possible warning signs of danger at residences, street scenes, and highway encounters.
28. List methods to avoid disturbing evidence at a crime scene.
29. Describe the indications for an emergency move, urgent move, and non-urgent move.

30. Describe the steps for performing an emergency move, urgent move, and nonurgent move.

31. Define body mechanics.

32. Discuss the guidelines and safety precautions that need to be followed when lifting a patient.

33. Describe the guidelines and safety precautions for carrying patients and/or equipment.

34. Describe correct and safe carrying procedures on stairs.

35. State the guidelines for reaching and their application.

36. Describe correct reaching for logrolls.

37. State the guidelines for pushing and pulling.

38. Discuss positioning patients with different conditions such as unresponsiveness, chest pain/discomfort or difficulty breathing, suspected spine injury, shock (hypoperfusion), and pregnancy.

39. Discuss the various devices associated with moving a patient in the prehospital setting.

40. Describe how to restrain a patient safely.

41. Describe the information that must be documented regarding the use of restraints.

42. Give examples of changes in circumstances that can cause an individual to go through the grieving process.

43. Describe the stages of grief.

44. List signs of obvious death.

45. Discuss the EMS professional's approach to a patient who is dying.

46. Discuss how an EMS professional should convey the news of a death to concerned survivors.

47. Discuss the possible reactions that a patient's family member may exhibit when confronted with death and dying.

Attitude Objectives ▶ 48. Improve personal physical well-being through achieving and maintaining proper body weight, regular exercise, and proper nutrition.

49. Promote and practice stress management techniques.

50. Advocate and practice the use of personal safety precautions in all scene situations.

51. Advocate and serve as a role model for other EMS professionals relative to the use of standard precautions.

52. Explain the rationale for properly lifting and moving patients.

53. Explain the role of EMS professionals regarding patients with do not resuscitate (DNR) orders.

54. Explain the rationale for the needs, benefits, and use of advance directives.

55. Defend the need to respect the emotional needs of dying patients and their families.

56. Communicate with empathy to patients being cared for, as well as with family members, and friends of the patient.

Skill Objectives ▶ 57. Given a scenario with potential infectious exposure, demonstrate the use of appropriate personal protective equipment. At the completion of the scenario, demonstrate proper removal and disposal of the protective garments.

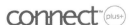

58. Given a scenario in which equipment and supplies have been exposed to body substances, demonstrate proper cleaning, disinfection, and disposal of the items.

59. Demonstrate proper lifting, carrying, and reaching techniques.

60. Given a scenario, determine when an emergency move, urgent move, and nonurgent move is indicated.

61. Working with a partner (when indicated), demonstrate emergency moves, urgent moves, and nonurgent moves.

62. Working with a partner, demonstrate the transfer of a supine patient from a bed to a stretcher using a direct carry.

63. Working with a partner, demonstrate the transfer of a supine patient from a bed to a stretcher using a draw sheet.

64. Demonstrate positioning patients with different conditions: unresponsiveness, chest pain/discomfort or difficulty breathing, suspected spine injury, shock (hypoperfusion), vomiting or nausea, and pregnancy.

65. Working with a partner, prepare each of the following devices for use, transfer a patient to the device, properly position the patient on the device, move the device to the ambulance, and load the patient into the ambulance: wheeled stretcher, bariatric stretcher, portable stretcher, stair chair, scoop stretcher, long spine board, basket stretcher, and flexible stretcher.

66. Working with a partner, demonstrate techniques for the transfer of a patient from an ambulance stretcher to a hospital stretcher.

67. Demonstrate safe techniques for managing and restraining a patient.

On the Scene

It is 3:30 a.m. Your spouse looks frustrated as the familiar beep of your volunteer fire department pager gets progressively louder. "Not again," she groans as you grab your gear and move quickly to your truck. I have to go, you think, noting the address is that of a close friend. You radio your response status and hear other members of your department notify the dispatcher that they are en route. As you walk into your friend's living room and past his wife, you see him. He is slumped forward at the kitchen table. He is not aware of your approach. You can feel your heart racing. Your hand trembles as you reach toward the carotid artery. You cannot feel a pulse and note that the patient's skin is cold to your touch. His wife looks on as other members of your department help you quickly move the patient to the floor. You note that his limbs are rigid and cold. His wife tells you that she got up to see why her husband had not come to bed and she found him in this position at the table. ■

THINK ABOUT IT

As you read this chapter, think about the following questions:

- How might you respond emotionally to this call?
- How will you approach the patient's wife?
- What methods will you use to determine whether you should begin resuscitation?
- What personal protective equipment will you need in this situation?

Introduction

To effectively care for others, you must first take care of yourself. Before working in healthcare, it is a good idea to have a physical examination to determine your baseline health status.

In this chapter you will learn about wellness and injury prevention. You will learn how to manage stress through changes in your lifestyle and work environment, how to prevent the spread of disease, how to lift and move patients safely, how to safely apply restraints, and how to assist the dying patient and the patient's family.

Wellness

Objectives 1, 2

Wellness is a state of health and happiness (well-being) that involves lifestyle choices in pursuit of an optimal state of health. Physical well-being and mental well-being are components of wellness.

Physical Well-Being

Objectives 3, 4, 5

Physical well-being includes keeping physically fit, maintaining adequate nutrition and proper body fat, obtaining adequate rest, and preventing disease and injury. Infectious disease prevention and injury prevention are discussed later in this chapter.

Regular exercise is important to keeping physically and mentally fit. It helps you meet the physical requirements of your responsibilities. **Stress** is a chemical, physical, or emotional factor that causes bodily or mental tension. Sustained aerobic activity causes the body to release endorphins. These natural chemicals can relieve stress and bring about a sense of well-being. Exercise also allows you to "burn off" pent-up emotions. Benefits of physical fitness include the following:

- Improved personal appearance and self-image
- Decreased resting heart rate and blood pressure
- Increased oxygen-carrying capacity
- Increased muscle mass and metabolism

Maintaining adequate nutrition and developing good dietary habits are important to your physical well-being. An excess of substances such as caffeine, sugar, fatty foods, and alcohol can exaggerate your body's response to stress. These substances can also influence your behavior. Good dietary habits include the following:

- Limiting the amount of fat, saturated fat, and cholesterol you eat
- Reducing or avoiding the intake of sugar, caffeine, and alcohol
- Eating a variety of foods each day, such as fruits and vegetables, whole grain breads and cereals, and lean meats
- Limiting the amount of salt you eat by cooking with only small amounts, avoiding salty snacks, and using less salt at the table

Objective 6

According to 2001 data from the Bureau of Labor Statistics, almost 15 million Americans work evening shifts, night shifts, rotating shifts, or other employer-arranged irregular schedules. Both shift work and long work hours have been associated with health and safety risks. Disturbances in the amount, quality, and consistency of sleep can result in sleep deprivation. Signs of sleep deprivation are shown in the following *You Should Know* box. Although it is sometimes difficult for EMS personnel because of the shifts and hours worked, obtaining adequate rest is necessary to restore energy, maintain a healthy immune system, handle stress, and function at your best.

You Should Know

Signs of Sleep Deprivation

- Decreased ability to concentrate
- Slower reaction times
- Decreased reasoning ability (judgment)
- Lack of memory, confusion
- Excessive sleepiness
- Suspiciousness
- Speaking at a slower pace than usual
- Slurred speech
- Blurred vision, itchy eyes, headache
- Tremors
- Extremes of emotion

Mental Well-Being

As an EMS professional, you will experience personal stress and will encounter patients and bystanders in severe stress (Figure 2-1). You will rarely

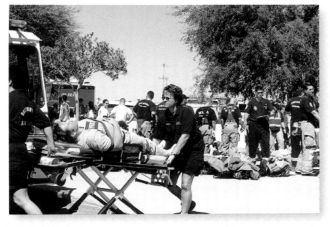

FIGURE 2-1 ▲ EMTs respond to many different types of stressful situations.

witness the actual mishap or violent act that occurred. However, you will be repeatedly exposed to the human suffering and tragedies that result from them. When you are dealing with an ill or injured person, the patient, the patient's family and friends, and bystanders will expect you to provide excellent medical care. They will also depend on you for emotional support.

You may feel emotions such as joy, pride, and contentment when you are able to make a positive difference in a patient's life (Figure 2-2). You may experience emotions such as anger, anxiety, frustration, fear, grief, and feelings of helplessness when you are unable to relieve a patient's suffering or when a patient dies despite your best efforts at resuscitation. You may feel sick at the sight of a severe injury. You may feel sad or anxious when dealing with a dying patient. These emotions are common and expected. You should not feel embarrassed or ashamed when these situations affect you. As you gain experience, you will learn to recognize and control these feelings while caring for patients. Despite the situation, you must act professionally. You must also be able to work quickly and confidently, think clearly, and make appropriate decisions about your patient's care.

Remember This

The delivery of emergency medical care has an emotional impact on the patient, the patient's family, bystanders, and you.

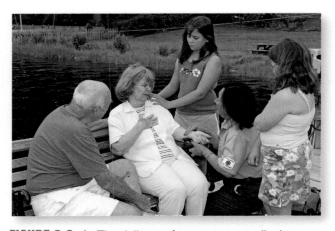

FIGURE 2-2 ▲ The delivery of emergency medical care has an emotional impact on the patient, the patient's family, bystanders, and you.

Objectives 7, 8, 9

A **stressor** is any event or condition that has the potential to cause bodily or mental tension. Because each of us responds differently to an emergency, it is important that you learn how to anticipate and recognize signs and symptoms of stress in yourself and others, and learn how to manage them when they occur. Common stressors associated with working in EMS are shown in Table 2-1. Examples of stressful situations are listed in Table 2-2.

When you encounter a stressor, your brain tells the rest of your body how to adjust to it. The part of your body that is first aware of the stressor, such as your eyes or nose, sends a message along your nerves to your brain. Your brain receives the message and tells specific body organs to release chemicals. These

TABLE 2-1 Common Stressors Associated with Working in EMS		
Environmental Stressors	**Psychosocial Stressors**	**Personal Stressors**
• Lights, siren, alarm noise	• Family relationships	• Life-and-death decision making
• Long hours and shifts	• Conflicts with supervisors or coworkers	• Personal expectations
• Absence of challenge between calls	• Agitated, combative, or abusive patients	• Feelings of guilt and anxiety
• Weather conditions and temperature extremes	• Dealing with critically ill and injured or dying patients	• Dealing with death and dying
• Confined work spaces	• Patients under the influence of drugs or alcohol	
• Emergency driving and rapid scene response	• Incompatibility with partner(s)	
• Demanding physical labor	• Getting used to new shift or assignment	
• Multiple role responsibilities		
• Dangerous situations		

TABLE 2-2 Stressful Situations and Additional Factors That May Cause Stress

Examples of Stressful Situations	Additional Factors That May Cause Stress
• Mass-casualty incidents	• Dangerous situations
• Infant and child trauma	• Challenging locations and terrain
• Death, terminal illness	• Weather conditions
• Amputations	• Severe time pressures
• Violence	• Media attention
• Death of a child	
• Infant, child, elder, or spousal abuse	
• Death or injury of a coworker or other public safety personnel	
• Emergency response to illness or injury of a friend or family member	

chemicals activate the body's *fight-or-flight response* (Figure 2-3). The fight-or-flight response prepares the body to protect itself.

When the stressor is removed, the body should return to its normal state. If the stress does not stop, the brain keeps the body in a state of high alert and the body becomes exhausted. Over time, this state takes its toll on the body. Stress-induced illnesses result. Examples of stress-induced illnesses include the following:

- Headaches
- Upset stomach
- Rashes
- Insomnia
- Ulcers
- High blood pressure
- Heart disease
- Stroke

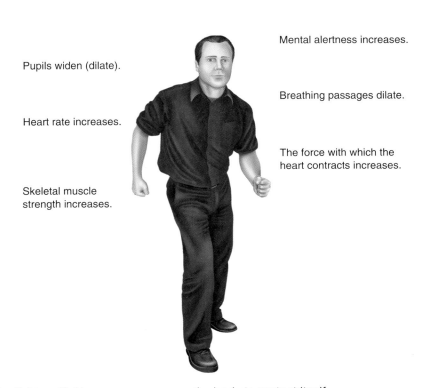

Pupils widen (dilate).

Mental alertness increases.

Heart rate increases.

Breathing passages dilate.

Skeletal muscle strength increases.

The force with which the heart contracts increases.

FIGURE 2-3 ▲ The fight-or-flight response prepares the body to protect itself.

TABLE 2-3 Signs of Stress

Physical Signs	Behavioral Signs	Mental Signs	Emotional Signs
• Increased heart rate • Pounding/racing heart • Elevated blood pressure • Sweaty palms • Tightness of the chest, neck, jaw, and back muscles • Headache • Diarrhea, constipation • Trembling, twitching • Stuttering and other speech difficulties • Nausea, vomiting • Sleep disturbances • Fatigue • Dryness of the mouth or throat • Susceptibility to minor illness	• Crying spells • Hyperactivity or under-activity • Changes in eating habits • Increased substance use or abuse, including smoking, alcohol consumption, medications, and illegal substances • Excessive humor or silence • Violence, aggressive behavior (such as driving aggressively) • Withdrawal • Hostility • Being prone to accidents • Impatience	• Inability to make decisions • Forgetfulness • Reduced creativity • Lack of concentration • Diminished productivity • Lack of attention to detail • Disorganized thoughts • Lack of control or a need for too much control	• Irritability • Angry outbursts • Hostility • Depression • Jealousy • Restlessness • Withdrawal • Anxiousness • Diminished initiative • Feelings of unreality or overalertness • Reduction of personal involvement with others • Tendency to cry • Being critical of others • Nightmares • Impatience • Reduced self-esteem

Recognizing Warning Signs of Stress

Objective 10

Stress can affect your mental well-being and the way in which you interact with your patients and family. Signs of stress may be physical, behavioral, mental, or emotional (Table 2-3). Become aware of your stressors and your responses to them. Recognizing the warning signs and sources of stress will help you develop a plan about what to do to avoid its occurrence or decrease its impact.

You Should Know

Common Signs and Symptoms of Stress

- Irritability toward coworkers, family, or friends
- Inability to concentrate
- Difficulty sleeping or nightmares
- Anxiety
- Indecisiveness
- Guilt
- Loss of appetite
- Loss of interest in sexual activities
- Isolation
- Loss of interest in work

Cumulative stress is common in EMS. It results from repeated exposure to smaller stressors that build up over time. In EMS, cumulative stress is often referred to as *burnout*. Causes of cumulative stress may include not getting enough sleep for several days in a row, job-related problems, or family and relationship issues.

You Should Know

Signs of Cumulative Stress

- Physical and emotional exhaustion
- A negative attitude toward others
- A disrespectful attitude toward patients
- Increased absences
- Emotional outbursts
- Decreased work performance

Managing Stress

The key to managing stress is prevention. Leading authorities in stress management recommend two important approaches to managing stress. First, ensure that your personal needs for food, drink, warmth, and companionship are met. Second, develop personal and departmental stress management strategies.

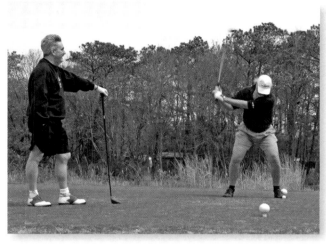

FIGURE 2-4 ▲ Learning to create balance in your life will allow you to manage the stress associated with EMS work.

Lifestyle Changes

Objective 11

There are several things you can do to manage stress in a healthy way. These steps include developing good dietary habits and exercising. Relaxation techniques such as meditation, deep-breathing exercises, yoga, reading, listening to music, and visual imagery can help reduce stress. Effectively managing the stress associated with caring for ill or injured people also requires learning to balance work, family and friends, fitness, and recreation (Figure 2-4). Consider the following suggestions to help maintain balance in your life:

- Develop a recreational outlet or hobby.
- Get away so you can "recharge" your emotional reserves.
- Learn to say no when you need time for yourself.
- Make sure you get adequate sleep. Be as consistent with your sleep schedule as possible.
- Develop mutually supportive friendships and relationships.

Family and Friends

Objectives 11, 12

Your role as an EMS professional can take a toll on those close to you. Family and friends may not understand the stressors that are a part of EMS work. After a particularly difficult call, you may arrive home too emotionally drained to take part in family activities. Family and friends may not understand the closeness and trust that develops among EMS professionals. Those who are close to you may become frustrated when you do the following:

- Eat, breathe, and sleep EMS.
- Work long hours.
- Sleep away from home.
- Are on call when you are at home.
- Agree to work yet another shift.
- Miss important family events because of your shift schedule.

The spouses of many EMS professionals frequently feel that they are of secondary importance, that "the job comes first."

EMS professionals may find it hard to discuss feelings about their work with loved ones. Some EMTs want to protect their loved ones from the horrors of the job. They may also need to protect confidential information. In addition, EMS professionals may be unwilling to expose themselves as being vulnerable. Family and friends become frustrated because they sense something is wrong and want to share your pain, but you refuse to let them do so. They may feel ignored and fear separation when you withdraw from them. These feelings often worsen if you prefer to talk with your coworkers about your feelings or spend your free time with your coworkers instead of with your family.

You Should Know

Responses to Stress by the Family and Friends of EMS Workers

- Lack of understanding of prehospital care
- Fear of separation or being ignored
- Frustration caused by the on-call nature of the job and the inability to plan activities
- Frustration caused by wanting to share

Because your family and friends are a base of support for you, communication of stressors can be helpful and positive in certain circumstances, helping you cope with the stressors associated with EMS work (Figure 2-5). *Do not assume they will not understand.* They can appreciate your feelings about a good or difficult call without knowing the details. Consider the following examples:

- "I had a tough call today. A 2-year-old drowned in a backyard pool."
- "You won't believe what happened today! I performed abdominal thrusts on a person who was choking. The patient coughed up a piece of chicken and is going to be fine."

Make it a point to talk about your day with your loved ones. Actively listen to what they have to say when

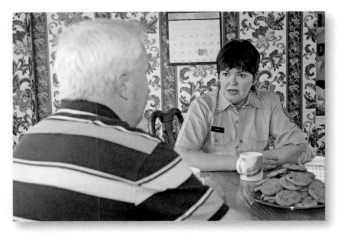

FIGURE 2-5 ▲ Your family and friends are a base of support and can help you cope with the stressors associated with caring for ill or injured people.

they tell you about theirs. Plan time for your family and friends. Say no to work when a request would require that you alter family plans.

Work Environment Changes

Objective 11

To help balance work and family, request work shifts that allow you more time for relaxation with family and friends. If you recognize the warning signs of stress, consider asking for a temporary rotation to a less stressful assignment.

Professional Help

Objective 11

When you need help coping with stress, seek assistance from a coworker, mental health professional, social worker, or member of the clergy. Many organizations have employee assistance programs. These programs offer confidential counseling to prehospital professionals. These resources can help you understand and effectively deal with stress.

Traumatic Incident Stress

Objectives 13, 14

A **traumatic incident** is a situation that causes a healthcare provider to experience unusually strong emotions. This type of incident may interfere with the provider's mental ability to cope and function either immediately or later. Examples of traumatic incidents include the following:

- Line-of-duty death or serious injury
- Mass-casualty incident

Making a Difference

EMS professionals often create their own methods of dealing with stress. After a particularly difficult call, some individuals prefer to be quiet and reflect on the events that occurred. Some individuals prefer to talk with their coworkers about different aspects of the call. Some of these conversations are serious, while others may be done in a joking manner. During these conversations, feelings are generally not directly discussed. Instead, phrases are substituted for the word "feelings." For example, "What went through your mind when . . . ?" or "What did you think about . . . ?" The companionship among EMS professionals often plays an important role in stress management.

- The suicide of a coworker
- Serious injury or death of a child
- Dead bodies or body parts
- Events with excessive media interest or criticism
- Victims who are known to you
- Any event that has an unusual impact on personnel
- Any disaster

Traumatic incident stress is a normal stress response to abnormal circumstances. Traumatic incident stress can affect all levels of EMS personnel. It can also affect bystanders, law enforcement officers, dispatchers, nurses, physicians, and other healthcare workers.

One symptom of traumatic incident stress is exhaustion, which often results from disturbing elements, such as the sounds, smells, or sights that occurred at the incident. When awake, a person may have flashbacks of the disturbing elements. Nightmares may occur during sleep. Other signs and symptoms include anxiety, depression, irritability, an inability to concentrate, indecisiveness, and either hyperactivity or underactivity. If you experience traumatic incident stress, seek mental health support if your symptoms or distress continues for several weeks or interferes with your daily activities.

Preventing Disease Transmission

Objective 15

As an EMT, you will provide emergency care to persons who are ill or injured. When you are providing care, one of the most serious risks to which you will be exposed is infection. An **infection** results when the body is invaded by **pathogens** (germs capable of producing disease), such as bacteria and viruses. A **communicable** (contagious) **disease** is an infection that can be spread from one person to another. The germs multiply and cause tissue damage, which may result in illness and disease. Signs of illness or disease may or may not be obvious.

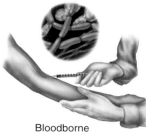
Airborne

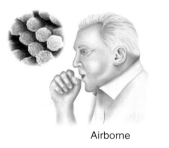
Bloodborne

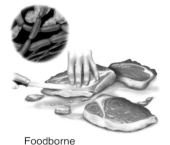
Foodborne

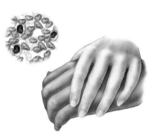
Sexually transmitted

FIGURE 2-6 ▲ Communicable diseases may be classified as airborne, bloodborne, foodborne, or sexually transmitted.

You Should Know

Factors That Increase Susceptibility to Infection

- Age (the very young and the elderly)
- Poor nutrition
- Excessive stress or fatigue
- Chronic illness
- Poor hygiene
- Alcoholism
- Body damage resulting from trauma
- Crowded or unsanitary living conditions
- The use of drugs that decrease the body's ability to fight infection

Methods of Disease Transmission

Objective 16

Communicable diseases can be spread in different ways. Contact with drainage from an open sore is an example of *direct* contact. Germs can also be spread through *indirect* contact with contaminated materials or objects, such as needles, toys, drinking glasses, eating utensils, and bandages. Wearing gloves can help prevent the spread of disease from direct and indirect contact. Germs can also be transmitted in droplets suspended in the air through coughing, talking, and sneezing. Wearing a mask can help prevent the spread of infection from droplets. Wearing a mask that shields the eyes offers even better protection.

Classification of Communicable Diseases

Objective 17

Communicable diseases may be classified as airborne, bloodborne, foodborne, or sexually transmitted (Figure 2-6):

- **Airborne diseases** are spread by droplets produced by coughing or sneezing. Examples include tuberculosis, measles, meningitis, rubella, smallpox, and chickenpox (varicella).
- **Bloodborne diseases** are spread by contact with the blood or body fluids of an infected person. Exam-

ples include hepatitis B virus (HBV), hepatitis C, human immunodeficiency virus (HIV), and syphilis.
- **Foodborne diseases** are spread by the improper handling of food or by poor personal hygiene. Examples include salmonella (food poisoning) and hepatitis A.
- **Sexually transmitted diseases (STDs)** are spread by either blood or sexual contact. Examples include chlamydia, gonorrhea, and HIV.

You Should Know

HBV can survive up to 1 week outside the human body. HIV can survive only a short time (hours) outside the body.

Infection Control

Objective 18

An **exposure** is direct or indirect contact with infected blood, body fluids, tissues, or airborne droplets. An accidental exposure to infectious material can occur when your skin is pricked or cut, allowing the entry of germs. Germs can also enter your body through nicks or scrapes on your skin or through mucous membranes (such as your eyes, nose, or mouth). An exposure to a communicable disease does not automatically result in infection.

Preventing Disease Transmission ◄ **37**

Objective 19

Standard precautions have been developed by the **Centers for Disease Control and Prevention (CDC)** to reduce the risk of exposure to infection. These standards have been adopted by the **Occupational Safety and Health Administration (OSHA)**, which is a branch of the federal government responsible for safety in the workplace. **Standard precautions** refer to self-protection against all body fluids and substances. These fluids and substances include blood, urine, semen, feces, vaginal secretions, tears, and saliva. Standard precautions include handwashing and using personal protective equipment. They also include the proper cleaning, disinfecting, and disposing of soiled materials and equipment.

Stop and Think!

When caring for patients, assume that all human blood and body fluids are infectious. For your safety, use appropriate standard precautions during *every* patient contact.

Remember This

Standard Precautions

Standard precautions include the following:

- Handwashing
- Using personal protective equipment
- Cleaning, disinfecting, and disposing of soiled materials and equipment

Handwashing

Objective 20

Handwashing is the single most important method you can use to prevent the spread of communicable disease (Figure 2-7). Frequent handwashing removes germs picked up from other people or from contaminated surfaces. Wash your hands before and after contact with a patient (even if gloves were worn), after removing your gloves, and between patients.

Remember This

Soap combined with scrubbing action is what helps dislodge and remove germs.

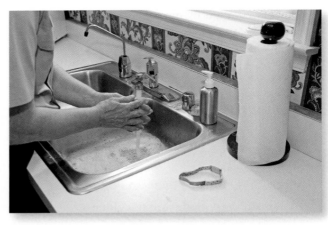

FIGURE 2-7 ▲ Handwashing is the single most important method you can use to prevent the spread of disease.

Proper handwashing begins with removing all jewelry from your hands and arms. If your hands are visibly dirty or soiled with blood or other body fluids, wash your hands with soap and water. Avoid using hot water because repeated exposure to hot water may increase the risk of skin irritation. If no visible soil or blood is noted after removing gloves, an alcohol-based hand gel is recommended. Wet your hands first with water and then apply soap (or hand gel). Briskly rub your hands together for at least 15 seconds, washing the palm and back surface of each hand, your wrists, and exposed forearms. Scrub under and around your fingernails with a brush. With your fingers pointing downward, rinse your wrists, hands, and fingers with running water. Use a paper towel to dry them. Also use a paper towel to turn off the faucet. Avoid touching any part of the sink once your hands are clean, and use the paper towel to open the door so that you do not touch the doorknob with clean hands.

Stop and Think!

Handwashing

- Wearing gloves does *not* eliminate the need for handwashing after each patient contact.
- Wash your hands immediately after exposure to blood and/or body fluids and after removing disposable gloves.
- Spend more time washing your hands after providing care to a patient at high risk for infection.

A waterless hand-cleansing solution can be used initially on the scene if you do not have access to soap and running water. Follow with a complete handwashing as soon as possible after completing patient care.

Personal Protective Equipment

Objective 20

Personal protective equipment and standard precautions are a part of scene safety. PPE includes eye protection and protective gloves, gowns, and masks. These items provide a barrier between you and infectious material. The infectious condition of a patient is usually unknown. Therefore, you *must* wear PPE when an exposure to blood or other potentially infectious material may be likely, especially since this type of exposure can occur when it is not expected. Make it a habit to put on appropriate PPE before providing any patient care.

Eye Protection

Eye protection should be worn when body fluids may be splashed into your face or eyes. This splashing can occur during childbirth, in suctioning an airway, or with a coughing or spitting patient. Available eyewear includes goggles and face shields (Figure 2-8). If you wear prescription eyeglasses, removable side shields should be applied to them or form-fitting goggles should be placed over them. To prevent the transfer of germs, remove protective eyewear without touching your face.

Gloves

You should put on disposable gloves before physical contact with *every* patient. When providing patient care, use gloves made of vinyl, latex, or another type of synthetic material. If you have a latex allergy, wear gloves made of a nonlatex material such as nitrile. If you have a cut on your hand or wrist, apply a bandage to the cut before putting on gloves. Check the condition of the gloves before putting them on. Do not use them if they have small holes or tears in them.

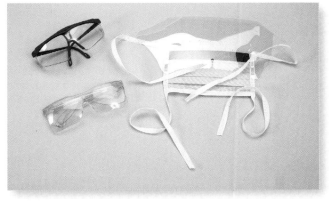

FIGURE 2-8 ▲ Goggles and face shields are types of protective eyewear.

Change your gloves between contacts with different patients. If a glove tears while providing patient care, remove it as soon as you can and replace it with a new one. Consider changing gloves often. For instance, upon entering the ambulance from the patient's residence or scene, before touching a second patient, and before applying a dressing to a nonlife-threatening wound. Throw away contaminated gloves and other PPE in clearly labeled biohazard bags or containers.

When removing gloves, keep in mind that the outer surface of the gloves is considered contaminated. Do not let the outside surface of the gloves come in contact with your skin. Be careful not to let the gloves snap when taking them off. If the gloves snap, germs may become airborne and contact your eyes, mouth, or skin or that of a coworker or patient. The proper technique for removing gloves is shown in Skill Drill 2-1.

Stop and Think!

Using Gloves in Patient Care

- *Always* put on disposable gloves before physical contact with every patient.
- *Always* change gloves before caring for another patient.
- *Always* dispose of gloves properly.
- *Always* wash your hands after removing your gloves.
- *Never* reuse disposable gloves.

Gowns

Disposable, fluid-resistant gowns should be used in situations in which large splashes of blood or body fluids might occur. Examples of such situations include childbirth, vomiting, and massive bleeding. After patient care activities are complete, properly dispose the gown. If a gown is not available and you were exposed to the patient's body fluids when providing care, change your clothes and take a shower as soon as possible after contact with the patient, washing your entire body with soap for 2 minutes. Wash your clothes in hot soapy water for at least 25 minutes. Launder your clothes at work, if possible. If you have to take them home, wash them in a separate load.

Masks

Wear a surgical-type face mask to protect against the possible splatter of blood or other body fluids (Figure 2-9). If you know or suspect that your patient has an airborne disease, such as tuberculosis, wear an **N95** or a **high-efficiency particulate air (HEPA) mask** (Figure 2-10). The mask should be changed if it becomes moist.

Removing Gloves

STEP 1 ▶
- Using your index finger and thumb on one hand, pull the bottom (cuff) of the glove away from your other hand.
- Peel the glove off your hand, being careful not to touch the skin of your wrist or hand with the outside surface of the glove. As you begin to remove the glove, it will turn inside out. This action helps prevent exposure to blood or other possibly infectious fluids on the gloves.

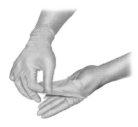

STEP 2 ▶ Place your fingers inside the bottom (cuff) of the other glove. Pull the glove off by turning it inside out.

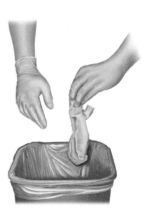

STEP 3 ▶ Dispose the gloves in an appropriate container. Wash your hands thoroughly.

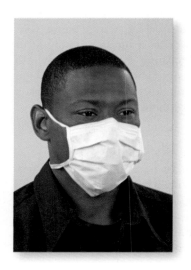

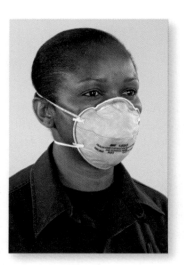

FIGURE 2-9 ◀ A surgical-type mask should cover your mouth, nose, and chin. To keep the mask from slipping, pinch the metal band at the top of the mask. This causes the mask to conform to the shape of your nose.

FIGURE 2-10 ◀ Wear an N95 mask (shown here) or a high-efficiency particulate air (HEPA) mask if you know or suspect that your patient has an air-borne disease, such as tuberculosis.

TABLE 2-4   Guidelines for Using Personal Protective Equipment

PPE	Guidelines for Use
Gloves	Any situation in which the potential for contacting blood or other body fluids exists
Gloves and chin-length plastic face shield (or mask and protective eyewear)	Any situation in which the splashing or spattering of blood or other body fluids is likely (such as suctioning, or a coughing or spitting patient)
Gloves, chin-length plastic face shield (or mask and protective eyewear), and gown	Any situation in which the splashing or spattering of blood or other body fluids is likely and clothing is likely to be soiled (such as childbirth and arterial bleeding)

Remember This

Personal Protective Equipment

PPE includes the following:

- Eye protection
- Gloves
- Gowns
- Masks

Refer to Table 2-4 for guidelines on using PPE.

Immunizations

An infection can cause serious medical problems. Immunizations help your body fight infection. It is important to keep your immunizations current:

- Tetanus prevention (booster every 10 years)
- Hepatitis B vaccine
- Influenza vaccine (yearly)
- Measles, mumps, and rubella (MMR) vaccine (if needed)

Tetanus

Tetanus (lockjaw) is a serious disease caused by bacteria found in the soil, dust, and feces of many household and farm animals such as horses, sheep, cattle, dogs, cats, rats, guinea pigs, and chickens. The bacteria can survive for many years and enter the body through a burn, cut, frostbite, crush injury, or puncture wound (such as that caused by an insect bite, splinter, nail, or intravenous drug use). Tetanus causes serious, painful spasms of all muscles. It can lead to "locking" of the jaw so the patient cannot open his or her mouth or swallow. The tetanus vaccine can prevent tetanus. This vaccine is usually given beginning at the age of 2 months. After receiving three doses of the vaccine (usually during childhood), a booster shot is needed every 10 years.

You Should Know

The Centers for Disease Control and Prevention recommends a diphtheria vaccination every 10 years for healthcare professionals—given with the tetanus vaccine.

Hepatitis B

Hepatitis B is a serious disease caused by HBV. This virus is spread through contact with the blood and body fluids of an infected person. A person can be infected in several ways, including:

- Having unprotected sex with an infected person
- Sharing needles
- Being stuck with a used needle while treating an infected patient
- Having blood splashed into your eyes, mouth, or onto a skin wound
- During birth, when the virus passes from an infected mother to her baby

HBV can cause a loss of appetite, diarrhea and vomiting, tiredness, jaundice (yellow skin or eyes), stomach pain, and pain in muscles and joints. HBV can also cause long-term illness that leads to liver damage (cirrhosis), liver cancer, and death.

The hepatitis B vaccine can prevent hepatitis B. Everyone 18 years of age and younger and adults over

18 who are at risk should receive the hepatitis B vaccine. Adults at risk for HBV infection include:

- Healthcare workers and public safety workers who might be exposed to infected blood or body fluids
- People who have more than one sex partner in 6 months
- Men who have sex with other men
- People who have sexual contact with infected individuals
- People who inject illegal drugs
- People who have household contact with individuals who have chronic HBV infection
- Hemodialysis patients

Many hepatitis B vaccines are available. They are usually given in a series of three immunizations, but some are given in two or four doses.

Influenza

Influenza ("flu") is caused by a virus that spreads from infected persons to the nose or throat of others. Influenza can cause fever, sore throat, chills, cough, headache, and muscle aches. Most people are ill for only a few days. However, some people get much sicker and may need to be hospitalized. According to the CDC, influenza causes an average of 36,000 deaths each year in the United States, mostly among the elderly.

All healthcare workers who breathe the same air as a person at high risk for complications of influenza and do not have a contraindication to the flu vaccine should receive an influenza vaccination every year. The flu season usually peaks from January through March. Therefore, the best time to get the flu vaccine is in October or November.

Measles, Mumps, and Rubella

Measles, mumps, and rubella are serious diseases that are spread from person to person through the air. The measles virus causes a rash, cough, runny nose, eye irritation, and fever. The mumps virus causes fever, headache, and swollen glands. Rubella (German measles) is caused by the rubella virus. It causes a rash and mild fever. If a woman gets rubella while she is pregnant, she could have a miscarriage or her baby could be born with serious birth defects (see Table 2-5).

The MMR vaccine can prevent these diseases. Generally, individuals 18 years of age or older who were born after 1956 should get at least one dose of the MMR vaccine unless they can show that they have had either the vaccine or the diseases.

Chickenpox (Varicella)

Chickenpox (varicella) is a common childhood disease that is usually mild. However, this disease can be serious, especially in young infants and adults. Chickenpox is

TABLE 2-5	The Signs, Symptoms, and Complications of Some Airborne Diseases	
Disease	**Signs and Symptoms**	**Complications**
Measles	Rash Cough Runny nose Eye irritation Fever	Ear infection Pneumonia Seizures Brain damage Death
Mumps	Fever Headache Swollen glands	Deafness Meningitis (infection of the brain and spinal cord covering) Painful swelling of the testicles or ovaries Death (rare)
Rubella (German measles)	Rash Mild fever	Possible serious birth defects
Chickenpox (varicella)	Rash Itching Fever Tiredness	Severe skin infection Scars Pneumonia Brain damage Death

caused by a virus that is spread from person to person through the air or by contact with fluid from chickenpox blisters. The virus causes a rash, itching, fever, and tiredness.

Most people who get the varicella vaccine will not get chickenpox. However, if someone who has been vaccinated does get chickenpox, it is usually very mild. All healthcare workers should be immune to varicella, as a result of either having had chickenpox or receiving two doses of the varicella vaccine. ProQuad is a vaccine recently approved by the U.S. Food and Drug Administration. This vaccine is an MMR vaccine that also contains a vaccine for chickenpox.

Tuberculosis

Tuberculosis (TB) is a disease caused by bacteria that usually attack the lungs. It is spread through the air when a person with TB coughs or sneezes. You may become infected with TB if you breathe in these bacteria. To determine if you have been exposed to TB, you should have a tuberculin skin test at least yearly.

Documenting and Managing an Exposure

Objective 21

If you are exposed to blood or body fluids, immediately wash the affected area with soap and water. If the eyes are exposed, flush them with water. Notify your designated infection control officer, medical director, or other designated individual as soon as possible. Get a medical evaluation and proper immunizations if necessary.

Make sure to document the following:
* The date and time of the exposure
* The circumstances surrounding the exposure
* The type, source, and amount of body fluid to which you were exposed
* The actions you took to reduce the chances of infection

Know your local protocols about when and how soon to have a medical follow-up after an exposure incident. As a rule, exposure follow-up should be done immediately after the exposure. If the patient has HIV or hepatitis B, preventive care is most effective when given quickly.

Cleaning Equipment

Stop and Think!

Do not reuse disposable equipment.

Objectives 22, 23

Germs can be killed or inactivated by cleaning, disinfecting, or sterilizing. Different chemicals or combinations of chemicals kill or inactivate different germs. When providing patient care, use disposable equipment whenever possible. Reusable equipment used in the care of a patient with intact skin usually requires only cleaning or disinfecting.

When dealing with contaminated materials, place them in appropriately labeled leak proof containers or bags. Double-bag disposable items if the patient is known to have a communicable disease.

Cleaning

Cleaning is the process of washing a contaminated object with soap and water. An item must be cleaned before it is disinfected or sterilized. To clean equipment, begin by rinsing the item with cold water to remove obvious body fluid or tissue. Then wash the item with hot, soapy water. If the item has grooves or narrow spaces, use a stiff-bristled brush to clean it. Rinse it well with moderately hot water and then dry it. The item is now considered clean.

Remember This

Physically removing germs by scrubbing is as important as the effect of the agent you use for cleaning or disinfecting.

Disinfecting

Disinfecting is cleaning with chemical solutions such as alcohol or chlorine. These agents destroy some types of germs that may be left after washing. Depending on the type and degree of contamination, items such as stethoscopes, blood pressure cuffs, backboards, and splints usually need only cleaning followed by disinfection. Isopropyl (rubbing) alcohol is often used to disinfect surfaces. However, rubbing alcohol may discolor, swell, harden, and crack rubber and certain plastics after prolonged and repeated use. When chlorine bleach is used as a disinfectant, it must be diluted. A solution of 1 part bleach and 10 parts water or 1 part bleach and 100 parts water may be used. The solution used depends on the amount of material (such as blood, mucus, or urine) present on the surface to be cleaned and disinfected. These disinfectants are not tuberculocidal. If a patient known to have TB is transported, equipment and surfaces should be cleaned with a disinfectant solution that is tuberculocidal (the label will state that).

Many commercial disinfectants are available. Follow the manufacturer's instructions to disinfect equipment.

Sterilizing

Sterilizing is a process that uses boiling water, radiation, gas, chemicals, or superheated steam to destroy all the germs on an object. Reusable equipment that is inserted into a patient's body should always be sterilized.

Stop and Think!

Chemical solutions can be harmful. Always protect yourself by wearing gloves and goggles.

Injury Prevention

Hazardous Materials Scenes

Objective 24

You may be required to respond to situations involving hazardous materials. The National Fire Protection Association (NFPA) defines a **hazardous material** as "a substance (solid, liquid, or gas) that, when released, is capable of creating harm to people, the environment, and property." A hazardous materials scene may involve liquids, solids, or gases that are toxic. To prevent further injury, you must be able to recognize that a hazardous materials situation exists.

Use binoculars to identify possible hazards before approaching the scene. Look for signs or placards that provide information about the contents of containers or vehicles. A placard is a four-sided, diamond-shaped sign. It is displayed on trucks, railroad cars, and large containers that carry hazardous materials (Figure 2-11). The placard will contain a four-digit identification number to guide you to reference information found in the *Emergency Response Guidebook*, which is published by the U.S. Department of Transportation (Figure 2-12). The *Guidebook* provides information to help identify the type of hazardous material involved. In addition, it outlines basic initial actions to take at the scene. The placard will also contain a class or division number that indicates whether the material is flammable, radioactive, explosive, or poisonous.

Stop and Think!

Learn how to contact your local hazardous materials team.

If you are the first person on the scene of an incident involving a hazardous material, *do not enter the scene.* Contact law enforcement and your local hazardous materials response team immediately. Stay upwind and on higher ground than the incident site. Keep unnecessary people away from the area.

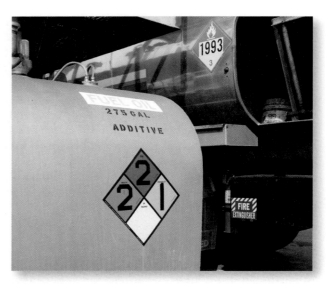

FIGURE 2-11 ▲ A placard is a diamond-shaped sign that is displayed on trucks, railroad cars, and large containers carrying hazardous materials.

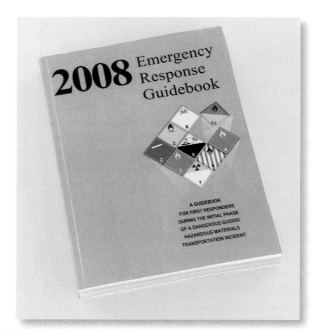

FIGURE 2-12 ▲ The four-digit identification number on a hazardous materials placard can be used to find information about the material in the *Emergency Response Guidebook*.

Hazardous materials incidents require specialized protective equipment that is not commonly available to EMTs. In general, protective clothing for a hazardous materials scene includes a hazardous materials suit and a self-contained breathing apparatus (SCBA) (Figure 2-13). Do not enter the scene unless you are trained to handle hazardous materials, are fully protected with the proper equipment, and know how to use that equipment. Provide emergency care only after the scene is safe and the patient is decontaminated.

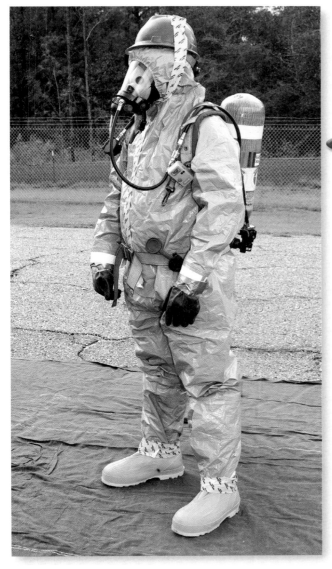

FIGURE 2-13 ▲ Protective clothing for a hazardous materials scene generally includes a hazardous materials suit and a self-contained breathing apparatus (SCBA).

Motor Vehicle Crashes and Rescue Scenes

Stop and Think!

Remember: Your personal safety is your number one priority. *Think* before entering a scene.

The scene of a motor vehicle crash may involve potential threats to your safety. It may also threaten the safety of your crew, the patient, and bystanders. Study the scene before entering, and determine if it is safe to approach the patient. Determine the number and type of vehicles and the extent of damage. Also note the approximate number of persons injured, and look for hazards (see the following *You Should Know* box). Assess the need for additional resources, such as a hazardous materials team or extrication equipment.

You Should Know

Potential Hazards at a Motor Vehicle Crash Scene

- Traffic
- Blood
- Gasoline spills
- Hazardous materials
- Sharp edges and fragments
- Exposed or downed electrical wires
- Fire or potential for fire
- Explosive materials
- Unstable vehicle or structure
- High-voltage batteries in hybrid vehicles
- Environmental conditions (such as heavy rain, heavy snowfall, and flash floods)

Traffic

Traffic is a common danger at a crash scene. If you arrive at a crash scene in a vehicle, be very careful when preparing to exit, especially if your door will open into traffic. Put on appropriate reflective gear, if available. Make sure that the vehicle is in park or that the brake is set. Check your rearview mirror for traffic, and open the door slowly. Request the help of law enforcement personnel to investigate and assist with traffic control. If the fire department responds to the scene, its large trucks are often positioned in a specific way. This positioning is done to shield the collision site and to provide protection while you care for the patient.

Power Lines

Look for downed or exposed power lines, which are a potential source of electrocution. You *must* assume that any downed wire is dangerous. Contact the power company and fire department immediately. Do not attempt to move the downed wire, and make sure not to touch any metal object or water in contact with it. Wait for the power company to shut off the power to the downed line before approaching the patient. If a downed wire is in contact with the vehicle, tell those inside the vehicle to remain inside until additional help arrives. Who makes the call to the utility company varies in EMS systems. In some systems, the call is made by dispatch. In others, it is made by the senior fire officer, first engine on the scene, or the EMS unit. Follow your local protocol regarding utility company contact.

Fire Hazards

Look for fire or potential fire hazards, such as leaking fuel. Do not approach a burning vehicle unless you are trained to handle such situations and are fully protected with proper equipment.

Objective 25

Entrapped Victims

Look for entrapped victims. Request special rescue teams when an extensive or complex rescue is needed. Protective clothing for a rescue scene typically includes turnout gear, puncture-proof gloves, a helmet, eye protection (safety glasses or goggles), and boots with steel toes (Figure 2-14). In cold weather, consider wearing long underwear, a warm head covering, and gloves. In wet weather, you may want to wear waterproof boots and slip-resistant gloves.

Violent Scenes

Remember This

Violence may occur even when police are present on the scene.

Objectives 26, 27, 28

Scenes involving armed or potentially hostile persons are among the most dangerous for emergency care providers and law enforcement personnel. EMS personnel may be mistaken for law enforcement officials because of their uniform or badge. The scene should *always* be secured by law enforcement before you provide patient care. However, a scene that has been declared safe does not mean that it will *continue* to be safe. Reassess scene safety often. Notify law enforcement personnel on the scene if a condition concerning scene safety comes to your attention. Table 2-6 lists some of the warning signs of danger.

Some EMS professionals wear body armor (bulletproof vests). Body armor does not cover the entire body. The areas of the body that are not covered are still vulnerable to injury. Body armor protects covered areas from most handgun bullets and most knives. It does not offer protection from high-velocity (rifle) bullets or from thin or dual-edged weapons (such as an ice pick), nor can it protect when it is not worn. Body armor provides reduced protection when wet.

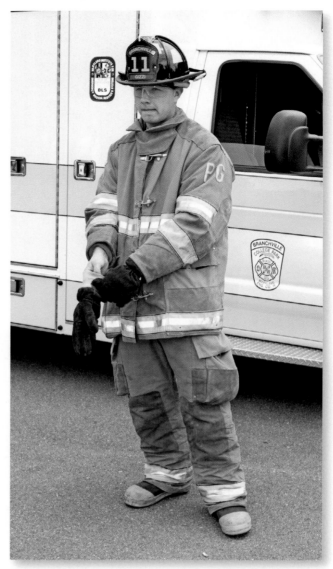

FIGURE 2-14 ▲ Protective clothing for a rescue scene typically includes turnout gear, puncture-proof gloves, a helmet, eye protection (such as safety glasses or goggles), and boots with steel toes.

Stop and Think!

Never enter a potential crime scene or a scene involving a family dispute, a fight, an attempted suicide, drugs, alcohol, or weapons until law enforcement personnel have secured the scene and declared it safe for you to enter and provide patient care.

At a crime scene, law enforcement personnel are responsible for gathering evidence that is needed for investigation and prosecution. EMS personnel are responsible for patient care. Do not disturb the scene

TABLE 2-6 Warning Signs of Danger

Residences	Street Scenes	Highway Encounters
• Unusual silence or a darkened residence • Past history of problems or violence • Known drug or gang area • Loud noises or items breaking • The sight or sound of acts of violence • The presence of alcohol or other drug use • Evidence of dangerous animals (pets, nonpets, infestations)	• Crowds (Groups of people may quickly become large and unpredictable.) • Voices becoming louder • Pushing, shoving • Hostility toward others at the scene (perpetrator, police, victim) • A rapid increase in crowd size • Inability of law enforcement to control crowds	• Disabled vehicles; calls for "man slumped over wheel"; motor vehicle crashes • Suspicious movements within a vehicle • The grabbing or hiding of items • Arguments or fights between passengers • Lack of activity where activity is likely • Signs of alcohol or drug use • Open or unlatched trunks (may hide people)

unless absolutely necessary for medical care. Evidence includes fingerprints, footprints, blood, body fluid, hair, and carpet and clothing fibers.

Avoid disturbing evidence by:
- Being observant
- Touching only what is required for patient care
  —If it is necessary to touch something, remember what you touched and tell the police.
- Wearing gloves
  —Wearing gloves helps provide infection control and prevents leaving your fingerprints at the scene. However, it will not prevent you from smudging other fingerprints.
- Taking the same path into and out of the scene
- Avoiding stepping on bloodstains or splatter
- Disturbing the victim and the victim's clothing as little as possible
- Avoiding cuts to the victim's clothing that may have been caused by a knife, bullet, or other penetrating weapon
- Saving the victim's clothing and personal items in a paper bag

Stop and Think!

Scene Safety in Violent Scenes
- Communicate with dispatch and law enforcement.
- Know an alternate way out of the scene.
- Have a prearranged panic code with dispatch and your partner(s).

Lifting and Moving Patients

Many EMS professionals are injured every year because they attempt to lift or move patients improperly. In fact, surveys show that almost one in two (47%) EMS personnel have sustained a back injury while performing EMS duties. Improper lifting and moving techniques can result in muscle strains and tears, ligament sprains, joint and tendon inflammation, pinched nerves, and related conditions. These conditions may develop gradually or may result from a specific event, such as a single, heavy lift. Pain, loss of work, and disability may result. In most cases, these injuries are preventable. More EMS professionals leave the profession because of disability and complications resulting from a back injury than because of any other reason.

There is no one best way to move all patients. Many circumstances will affect the method you choose to use. The key is to take a brief moment to analyze the situation and think of all your options. Then choose the method that is safest for you, your coworkers, and the patient.

The Role of the Emergency Medical Technician

You will most often provide initial emergency care to patients in the position in which they are found. Your responsibility is to distinguish an emergency from a nonemergency situation. Your role will also include:

- Positioning patients to prevent further injury
- Recognizing when to call for more help
- Assisting other EMS professionals in lifting and moving patients

Principles of Moving Patients

Objectives 29, 30

The big decision: What is an emergency that requires immediately moving a patient from the area? In general, a patient should be moved *immediately* (an **emergency move**) when one of the following situations exists:

1. *The presence of scene hazards.* The patient may need to be moved if you are unable to protect the patient from hazards in the area and there is an immediate danger to you or the patient if he is not moved. Examples of possible scene hazards include:
   - Fire or the danger of fire
   - Uncontrolled traffic
   - Explosives or the danger of an explosion
   - Electrical hazards
   - Rising flood water
   - Toxic gases
   - Radiation
   - Structural collapse or the threat of a structural collapse
   - Potentially violent scenes (such as a shooting or domestic violence)

2. *The inability to reach other patients who need lifesaving care.* For example, if there are multiple patients in a vehicle, you may need to move a patient to reach another who is more seriously injured.

3. *The inability to provide immediate, lifesaving care because of the patient's location or position.* For example, a patient in cardiac arrest who is sitting in a chair or lying on a bed must be moved to the floor in order to provide effective cardiopulmonary resuscitation (CPR).

All these situations put you at great risk. Always consider your safety first, and then make the decision whether to attempt an emergency move or wait for additional resources.

The greatest danger in moving a patient quickly is the possibility of aggravating a spinal injury. Always drag the patient in the direction of the length (the long axis) of the body. This action will provide as much protection as possible to the patient's spine. Never push, pull, or drag a patient sideways. In the rare event that you need to perform an emergency move, realize that you will be putting yourself at risk for injury as well as possibly complicating the patient's injury. Using an emergency move to remove a patient from a vehicle makes it impossible to provide the same level of spine protection that would be accomplished with spine stabilization devices. *Think before you act!* Remember that in most cases—except in the situations listed above—a patient is better off being treated in place until additional help arrives.

Remember This

If no immediate threat to life exists, when ready for transport, move the patient using a **nonurgent move.** Nonurgent moves are the types of moves you will perform most often. They will be done with the help of other EMS professionals. It is important to communicate with each other and the patient before, during, and after the lift. Work as a team for success.

Body Mechanics and Lifting Techniques

Safety Precautions and Preparation

Objective 31

Body mechanics refers to the way we move our bodies when lifting and moving. Body mechanics includes body alignment, balance, and coordinated body movement. Proper body alignment is synonymous with good posture and is an important part of body mechanics (Figure 2-15). Good posture means that the spine is in a neutral position when standing, sitting, or lying. This position recognizes that the spine has four natural curves. These curves are in the areas of the cervical, thoracic, lumbar, and sacral vertebrae (Figure 2-16). When you use good posture, there is minimal strain on your muscles, ligaments, bones, joints, and nerves. By maintaining proper body alignment, you reduce strain on your spine as well as on the muscles and ligaments that support it.

You also improve your balance when you use good posture. Balance can be further improved by:

- Separating your feet to a comfortable distance
- Bending your knees
- Flexing your hips to reach a squatting position

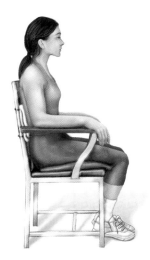

FIGURE 2-15 ▲ Good body mechanics includes good posture.

These actions broaden your base of support and help reduce your risk of injury. To protect yourself and the patient, you should prepare and plan *before* you actually move a patient. Important factors to consider include:

- The patient's weight
- The patient's condition
- The presence of hazards or potential hazards at the scene
- The terrain
- The distance the patient must be moved
- Your physical abilities and any limitations
- The availability of any equipment or personnel to assist with the move

In some cases, a patient may be in an awkward position or a tight space. The patient's position or location may require that you bend or move out of balance. In these situations, it is best to call for additional help before moving the patient. In some situations, the *patient* may be able to tell you the best technique for moving. In all cases, it is very important to communicate clearly and frequently with your partner and the patient throughout the process. Work as a team and remind each other to use proper lifting techniques.

The Power Grip

When you are lifting, your arms and hands are strongest when positioned with your palms up. Use the **power grip (underhand grip)** when lifting an object to take full advantage of the strength of your hands, forearms, and biceps. With your palms up, grasp the object you are preparing to lift. Position your hands a comfortable distance apart, usually about 10 inches. Your palms and fingers should be in complete contact with the object, with all fingers bent at the same angle (Figure 2-17).

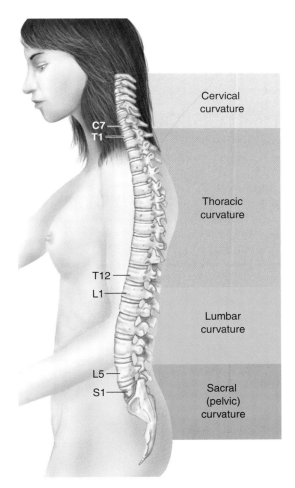

FIGURE 2-16 ▲ The adult spine has four natural curves in the areas of the cervical, thoracic, lumbar, and sacral vertebrae.

Cervical curvature

C7
T1

Thoracic curvature

T12
L1

Lumbar curvature

L5
S1

Sacral (pelvic) curvature

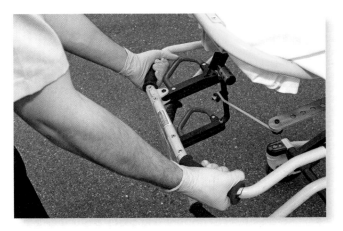

FIGURE 2-17 ▲ The power grip.

Guidelines for Safe Lifting of Cots and Stretchers

Objective 32

Safe lifting means keeping your back aligned as vertically as possible, using your leg strength, and maintaining your center of balance while lifting.

Important rules for preventing injury when lifting:

- Know or find out the weight to be lifted. Consider the weight of the patient, the weight of the equipment being used, and the need for additional help. Know or find out the weight limitations of the equipment being used. Know what to do with patients who exceed the weight limitations of the equipment.
- Know your physical ability and limitations.
- Plan how and where you will move the patient. It is often helpful to mentally picture the patient's final position and work backward to the patient's current position. Working in this way helps prevent arms from getting crossed and bodies from becoming twisted during the actual move. It also prevents you from being stuck in a position in which you are unable to complete the move safely.
- Make sure your path is clear of obstructions.
- Make sure that enough help is available. Use at least two people to lift. If possible, always use an even number of people to lift to maintain balance. Determine in advance who will direct the move. *One* person (usually the person at the patient's head) must assume responsibility for directing the actions of the others. "On my count, lift on three: one, two, three." "On my count, turn on three: one, two, three." Agree in advance that if anyone involved in the move says no, the move will immediately be stopped. The person stopping the move must state what needs to be done in order to complete the move. Sometimes, it's just stopping to turn a corner and get a better grip.
- Position your feet a comfortable distance apart (usually a shoulder's width) on a firm surface. Wear proper footwear to protect your feet and maintain a firm footing.
- Tense the muscles of your abdomen and buttocks before lifting. This tensing helps relieve the stress on your back muscles.
- Bend at your knees and hips, not your waist, and keep your back straight. All movement in the lift comes from your *legs*.
- Use your legs to lift, not your back. Your legs are much stronger than your back.
- Lift using a smooth, continuous motion. *Do not jerk or twist* when lifting. Jerking or twisting increases your risk of injury.
- Keep the patient's weight as close to you as possible. "Hug the load." Doing so moves your center of gravity closer to the patient, helps maintain balance, and reduces muscle strain.
- When possible, move forward rather than backward.
- Walk slowly, using short steps.
- Look where you are going.
- Move slowly, communicating clearly and frequently with other EMS personnel and the patient throughout the move.

Remember This

You must think about these guidelines before *every* lift.

The **power lift** is a way to lift heavy objects, using the proper body mechanics just described. Skill Drill 2-2 shows a two-person power lift being used to lift a wheeled stretcher.

Stop and Think!

Always practice proper lifting techniques. Learning to lift by using proper body mechanics takes training and practice. When practicing, use "spotters" to alert you when you are performing a technique incorrectly. Practice and practice again until using correct lifting techniques become a habit. One bad lift can damage your back for the rest of your life!

Carrying Patients and Equipment

Objective 33

Guidelines for avoiding injury when carrying patients and equipment:

- Whenever possible, transport patients on devices that can be rolled.
- Know or find out the weight to be lifted.
- Know your physical abilities and limitations and those of your crew.
- Work in a coordinated manner and communicate frequently with your partner and the patient.
- Keep the weight as close to the body as possible.

Two-Person Power Lift

STEP 1 ▶ Position your feet shoulder's width apart on a firm surface. Wear proper footwear to protect your feet and maintain a firm footing.

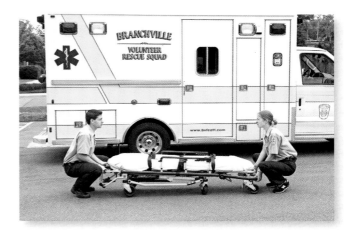

STEP 2 ▶ Use the power grip to grasp the stretcher. Tense the muscles of your abdomen and buttocks. Bend at your knees and hips, not at your waist, and keep your back straight.

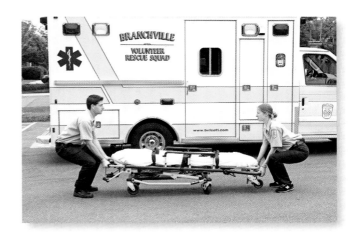

STEP 3 ▶ Communicating with other EMS personnel and the patient, lift at the same time with your legs, not your back. Use a smooth, continuous motion.

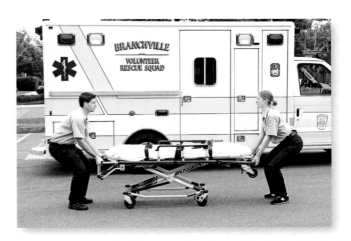

- Keep your back in a locked-in position and avoid twisting.
- Flex at the hips, not at the waist, and bend at the knees.
- Do not hyperextend the back (do not lean back from the waist).
- Whenever possible, you and your partner should be of similar height and strength.
- When carrying a stretcher or backboard with only two crew members, face each other from either the sides or ends of the stretcher.

When using a one-handed carrying technique, pick up and carry with the back in a locked-in position. Avoid leaning to either side to compensate for the imbalance.

Carrying Procedure on Stairs

Objective 34

Guidelines for carrying patients and equipment on stairs:
- When possible, use a commercially made stair chair instead of furniture or a stretcher when transporting patients down stairs.
- Make sure that the stairway is free of obstructions.
- Have another rescuer act as a guide or "spotter," especially if going down the stairs. This person can alert you to the number of steps, changes in footing surfaces, or any potential hazards.
- Make sure that the patient is secured to the stair chair before lifting.
- Carry patients head-first up the stairs and feet-first down the stairs.
- Keep your back in a locked-in position.
- Flex at the hips, not at the waist, and bend at the knees.
- Keep the weight and your arms as close to your body as possible.
- Always communicate with your partner during the move.

Guidelines for Safe Reaching

Objective 35

Important rules for avoiding injury when reaching:
- Keep your back straight.
- Avoid stretching or leaning back from your waist (hyperextending) when reaching overhead. Lean from your hips.
- Avoid twisting while reaching.

- Avoid reaching more than 15–20 inches in front of your body to grasp an object.
- Avoid situations in which prolonged strenuous effort (more than a minute) is needed.

Objective 36

A **logroll** is a technique used to move a patient from a facedown to a face-up position while keeping the head and neck in line with the rest of the body. This technique is also used to place a patient with a suspected spinal injury on a backboard.

Guidelines for correct reaching for logrolls:
- Keep your back straight while leaning over the patient.
- Lean from the hips.
- Use your shoulder muscles to help with the roll.

Guidelines for Safe Pushing and Pulling

Objective 37

Guidelines for avoiding injury when pushing and pulling:
- Push, rather than pull, whenever possible.
- Keep your back straight.
- Avoid twisting or jerking when pushing or pulling an object.
- Push at a level between your waist and shoulders.
- When the patient or object is below your waist, kneel to push or pull.
- When pulling, avoid reaching more than 15–20 inches in front of your body. Change your position (move back another 15–20 inches) when your hands have reached the front of your body.
- Keep the line of the pull through the center of your body by bending your knees.
- Keep the weight close to your body.
- Keep your elbows bent and your arms close to your sides.
- If possible, avoid pushing or pulling from an overhead position.

Remember This

When you are called to the scene of an emergency, it is the patient's emergency. Treat the patient to the best of your ability until you can *safely* move the person. If you are injured in the process of lifting and moving, you have done nothing but caused an additional problem.

Emergency Moves

Drags

Drags are a good way to move patients already on the ground. Dragging or pulling is more difficult than pushing. You will be surprised by how tired you become in a short time. Stabilize the patient's head and neck as much as possible before beginning the move. The clothes drag and blanket drag may be used when the patient must be moved quickly and an injury to the head or spine is suspected. Although it is not ideal material for stabilizing the spine, the patient's clothing or a blanket provides material against which the patient's head and neck are cradled during the move. The patient's clothing or a blanket is used not as a pillow, but as a stabilizer around the sides of the head to prevent rolling.

When dragging a patient, always pull along the length of the spine from either the patient's shoulders or the patient's feet and legs. The surface should be smooth to prevent bobbing of the patient's head over uneven terrain. *Never* pull the patient's head away from the person's neck and shoulders. Broaden your base of support by moving your rear leg back (if you are facing the patient) or by moving your front foot forward (if you are facing away from the patient).

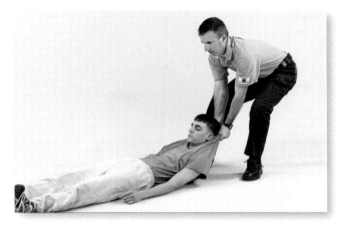

FIGURE 2-18 ▲ The clothes drag.

Stop and Think!

Before performing an emergency move, make sure your path is clear of obstructions. Doing so will protect the patient from being dragged through broken glass, metal fragments, or other sharp objects that can cause additional injury.

Clothes Drag

To perform a **clothes drag** (also called the *clothing pull* or *shirt drag*), position yourself at the patient's head (Figure 2-18). To prevent the patient's arms from being pulled upward during the move, consider securing the patient's wrists together or tucking his hands into his waistband. Gather the shoulders of the patient's shirt and pull him toward you so that a cradle is formed for the patient's head and neck. Make sure you have a firm grasp on the patient's clothing and begin pulling the patient to safety. When using this move, check often to make sure you are not choking the patient as his clothes slide up around his neck.

Blanket Drag

To perform a **blanket drag**, lay a blanket, sleeping bag, tarp, bed sheet, bedspread, or similar material lengthwise beside the patient. Make sure there is approximately 2 feet of the blanket above the patient's head. The uppermost section of the blanket will provide a cradle for the patient's head. It will also be used as the handle with which you will drag the patient. Kneel on the opposite side of the patient and roll him toward you (Figure 2-19a). Grasp the blanket and tuck half the blanket under the patient. Leave the remainder of the blanket lying flat (Figure 2–19b). Quickly but gently, roll the patient onto his back. Pull the tucked portion of the blanket out from under the patient. Wrap the corners of the blanket securely around the patient (Figure 2–19c). Using the blanket "handle" that you created above the patient's head, keep the pull as straight and as in-line as possible and drag the patient to safety. Remember to use your legs, not your back, and keep your back as straight as possible (Figure 2–19d).

Remember This

Always use the part of the blanket under the patient's head as a handle. Doing so will keep the person's head and shoulders slightly raised so that the patient's head will not strike the ground.

Shoulder Drag

A **shoulder drag** is an emergency move that is often used because it does not require any additional materials. To perform a shoulder drag, position yourself behind the patient and prop her up into a sitting position. From your position behind the patient, slide your hands under her armpits and drag her to safety (Figure 2-20). The shoulder drag should be used with caution in older adults because cases of joint damage have been reported after its use.

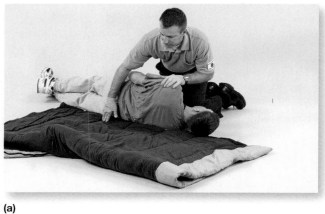

(a)

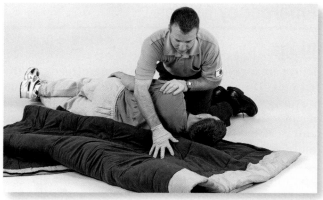

(b)

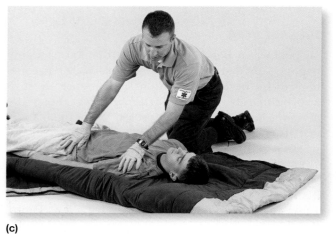

(c)

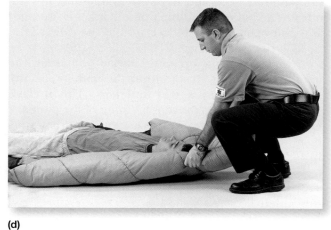

(d)

FIGURE 2-19 ▲ The blanket drag.

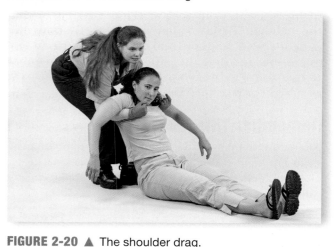

FIGURE 2-20 ▲ The shoulder drag.

FIGURE 2-21 ▲ The forearm drag.

Forearm Drag

To perform a **forearm drag** (also called the *bent-arm drag*), position yourself as you would in a shoulder drag. After sliding your hands under the patient's armpits, grasp her forearms and drag her to safety (Figure 2-21). Note that the forearm drag or shoulder drag provide *no* protection for the patient's spine.

Ankle Drag

To perform an **ankle drag,** grasp the patient's ankles or pant cuffs (Figure 2-22). This emergency move is not recommended because the patient's head is not supported and it may bounce if the patient is not pulled over a smooth surface. However, it is presented here because it is possible that you will encounter a

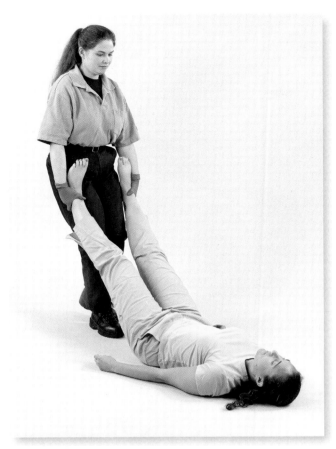

FIGURE 2-22 ▲ The ankle drag.

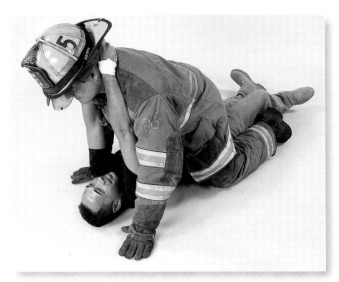

FIGURE 2-23 ▲ The firefighter's drag.

situation in which you have no other means to move the patient.

Firefighter's Drag

The **firefighter's drag** is particularly useful when you must crawl underneath a low structure for a short distance or move a patient from a smoke-filled area. To perform a firefighter's drag, place the patient on his back (Figure 2-23). Cross his wrists and secure them together with gauze, a triangular bandage, or a necktie. Straddle the patient, and lift his arms over your head so that his wrists are behind your neck. As you crawl forward, be sure to raise your shoulders high enough so that the patient's head does not hit the ground.

Remember This

Dragging Tips

- Always drag the patient along the length (long axis) of the spine.
- Never push, pull, or drag a patient sideways.
- Never pull the patient's head away from his or her neck and shoulders.

Carries

Firefighter's Carry

The **firefighter's carry** can be used to quickly move a patient. The patient's abdomen bears the weight with this move. To perform the firefighter's carry, position yourself toe to toe with the patient. Crouch down, grasp the patient's wrists, and pull the patient to a sitting position (Figure 2-24a). Step on the patient's toes with the tip of your shoes. While grasping the patient's wrists, pull the patient to a standing position (Figure 2–24b). Remove your shoes from the patient's toes. Quickly place your shoulder into the patient's abdomen and pull the patient lengthwise across your shoulders (Figure 2–24c). Place one arm through the patient's legs. Use your other hand to grasp one of the patient's arms, secure the patient in position on your shoulders, and then stand up (Figure 2–24d). Remember to lift with your legs and not your back.

Cradle Carry

The **cradle carry** (also called the *one-person arm carry*) may be used if the patient is a child or a small adult. To perform a cradle carry, kneel next to the patient. Place one hand under the patient's shoulders and the other under her knees, and then stand up, using the strength of your legs (Figure 2-25).

Pack-Strap Carry

The **pack-strap carry** requires no equipment. It is best used with a conscious patient unless someone is available to help you position the patient. To perform

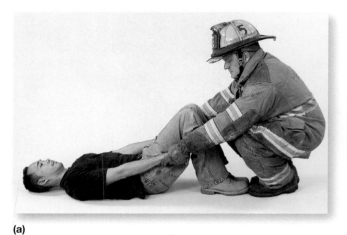

(a)

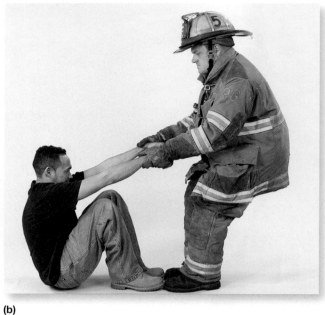

(b)

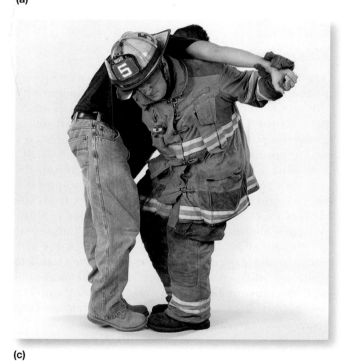

(c)

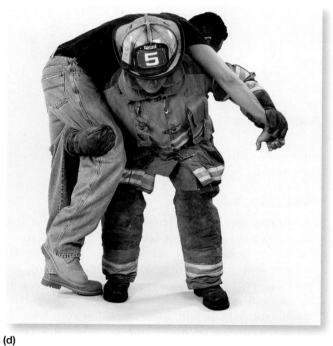

(d)

FIGURE 2-24 ▲ The firefighter's carry.

the pack-strap carry, kneel in front of a seated patient with your back to her. Have the patient place her arms over your shoulders so that they cross your chest. Be sure the patient's armpits are over your shoulders. Cross the patient's wrists in front of you and grasp them. While holding the patient's wrists, lean forward, rise up on your knees, and pull the patient up onto your back. Hold both of the patient's wrists close to your chest as you stand up (Figure 2-26). If the patient

is small, it may be possible to grasp both of her wrists with one hand. This action leaves your other hand free to open doors and move obstructions.

Piggyback Carry

The **piggyback carry** is used when the patient cannot walk but can use her arms to hold onto you. To perform this move, kneel in front of a seated patient

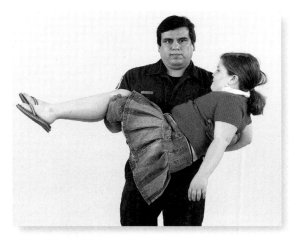

FIGURE 2-25 ▲ The cradle carry.

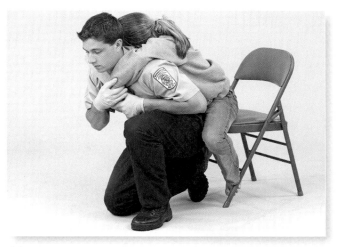

(a)

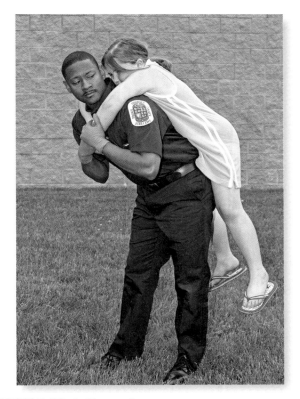

FIGURE 2-26 ▲ The pack-strap carry.

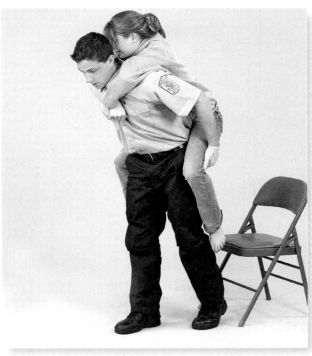

(b)

FIGURE 2-27 ▲ The piggyback carry.

with your back to her. Have the patient place her arms over your shoulders so that they cross your chest. Cross the patient's wrists in front of you and grasp her wrists. While holding her wrists, lean forward, rise up on your knees, and pull the patient up onto your back. Hold both of the patient's wrists close to your chest as you stand up (Figure 2-27a). As you prepare to reposition your arms and hands, instruct the patient to hold onto you with her arms. Position your forearms under the patient's knees and grasp her thighs (Figure 2–27b).

Two-Person Carry

If the patient is unable to walk, two people can make a "seat" for the patient. It is best to have two rescuers of about the same height and size perform this move. To perform the **two-person carry** (also called the *two-person seat carry*), place one arm under the patient's

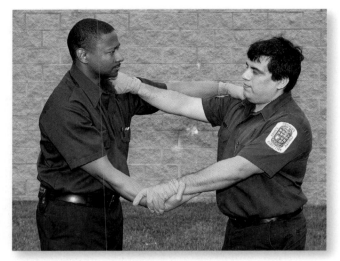

(a)

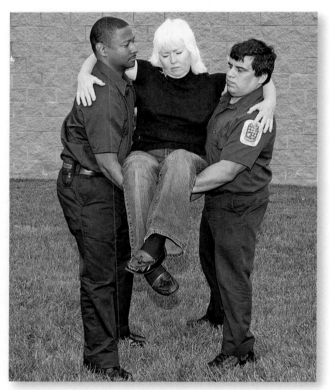

(b)

FIGURE 2-28 ▲ The two-person carry.

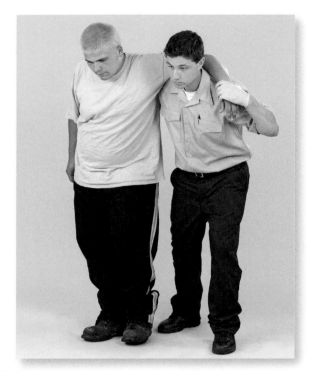

FIGURE 2-29 ▲ The human crutch move.

acting as a crutch. One or two rescuers may be used for this move. To perform the **human crutch move** (also called the *rescuer assist* or *walking assist*), place the patient's arm across your shoulders and hold his wrist with one hand. Place your other hand around his waist and help him to safety (Figure 2-29).

Urgent Moves (Rapid Extrication)

A patient should be moved quickly (**urgent move**) when there is an immediate threat to life, such as in the following situations:

- Altered mental status
- Inadequate breathing
- Shock (hypoperfusion)

Rapid extrication must be accomplished quickly, without compromise or injury to the spine. Skill Drill 2-3 shows the steps for rapid extrication.

Nonurgent Moves

If no threat to life exists, the patient should be moved when ready for transportation (a nonurgent move).

thighs and the other across the patient's back. Grasp the arms of the other rescuer and lock them in position at the elbows, forming a "seat." Both rescuers then rise slowly to a standing position (Figure 2-28).

Human Crutch Move

In some situations, the patient may be able to walk but requires assistance. You can assist him to safety by

Rapid Extrication

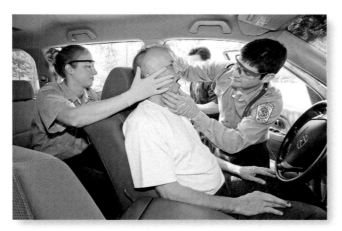

STEP 1 ▲ One EMT positions himself behind the patient. This EMT then places his hands on either side of the patient's head, bringing the cervical spine into a neutral in-line position and providing manual stabilization. At the same time, the EMT begins assessment of the patient's airway.

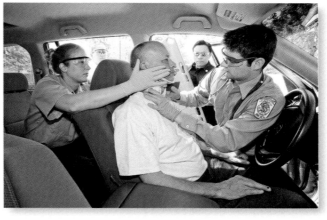

STEP 2 ▲ • A second EMT performs a primary survey and applies a cervical immobilization device.
• At the same time, a third EMT places a long backboard near the door.

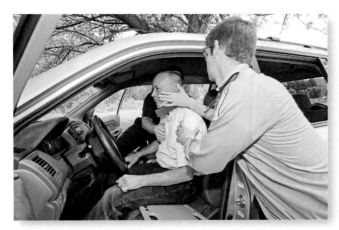

STEP 3 ▲ The second EMT supports the patient's chest and back as the third EMT moves to the passenger seat and frees the patient's legs from the pedals and floor panels.

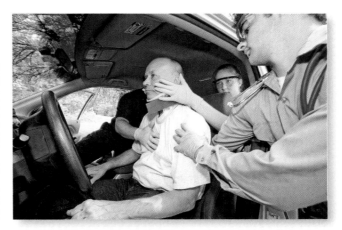

STEP 4 ▲ At the direction of the EMT at the patient's head, the patient is rotated in several short, coordinated moves until the patient's back is in the open doorway and his feet are on the passenger seat.

Continued

Rapid Extrication *Continued*

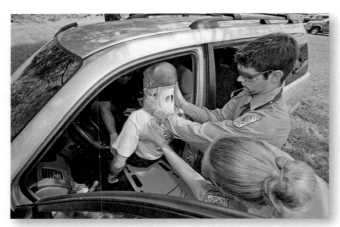

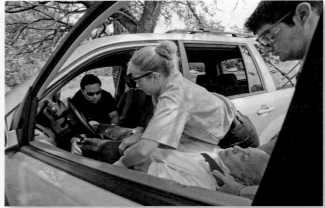

STEP 5 ▲ Because the first EMT cannot usually support the patient's head any longer, another available EMT or emergency worker supports the patient's head as the first EMT gets out of the vehicle and takes support of the head outside the vehicle. The end of the long backboard is placed on the seat next to the patient's buttocks.

STEP 6 ▲
- Assistants support the other end of the board as the first EMT and the second EMT lower the patient onto it.
- The second and third EMTs slide the patient into proper position on the board in short, coordinated moves.

Direct Ground Lift

The **direct ground lift** is used to lift and carry a patient with no suspected spinal injury from the ground to a bed or a stretcher. If the patient is going to be transferred to a stretcher, place the stretcher as close to the patient as possible. Although this lift can be performed with two rescuers, doing it with three is the safest method. A lot of communication and teamwork is necessary to lift and move patients safely. Skill Drill 2-4 shows the steps for a direct ground lift.

Remember This

Do *not* perform a direct ground lift or an extremity lift if trauma to the patient's head, neck, or back is suspected because the head is not stabilized during these moves. The extremity lift must also be avoided if an extremity is injured.

Extremity Lift

The extremity lift is used to lift a patient onto a carrying device, such as a stretcher. Two rescuers are needed to perform an extremity lift. This lift should *not* be used on a patient with a suspected head, neck, back, or extremity injury. Skill Drill 2-5 shows a two-person extremity lift.

Transferring a Supine Patient from Bed to Stretcher

There are two common methods used to transfer a supine patient from a bed to a stretcher. (In the supine position, a patient is lying flat on the back and face-up.) The first method is the direct carry. It is used when you are required to move a patient to a stretcher that cannot be placed parallel to the bed. The second, the draw sheet method, is by far the most common. This method requires that the stretcher be

Direct Ground Lift

STEP 1 ▶
- Three rescuers line up on the same side of a supine patient. Position one at the patient's head, the second at the patient's waist, and the third at the patient's knees.
- To maintain balance throughout the move, all rescuers should kneel on one knee. The same knee should be used by all rescuers. If possible, place the patient's arms across her chest.
- If only two rescuers are available, position one at the patient's chest and the other at the patient's thighs.

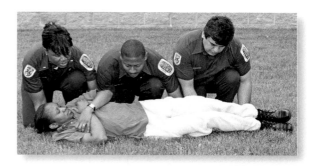

STEP 2 ▶
- The rescuer at the head places one arm under the patient's neck and shoulders, cradling the patient's head. The first rescuer's other arm is placed under the patient's lower back. The second rescuer places one arm above and one arm below the patient's waist. The third rescuer places one arm under the patient's knees and the other under the patient's ankles.
- If only two rescuers are available, the first rescuer places one arm under the patient's head and neck and cradles the patient's head. She places the other hand under the patient's shoulders. The second rescuer places his arms under the patient's lower back and buttocks.

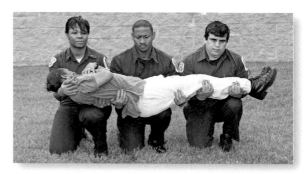

STEP 3 ▶
- On the command of the rescuer at the patient's head, all the rescuers should lift the patient to their knees.
- Once everyone is balanced, the patient is rolled toward the rescuers' chests. This action keeps the weight of the patient close to a rescuer's body, reducing the risk of back injury to the rescuer.

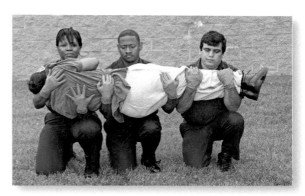

STEP 4 ▶
- On the command of the rescuer at the patient's head, all rescuers should stand and move the patient to the desired location.
- To lower the patient, simply reverse the steps.

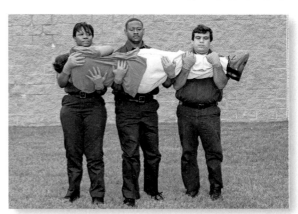

Two-Person Extremity Lift

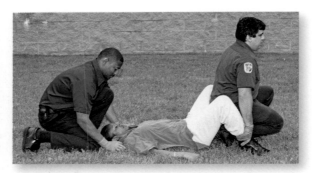

STEP 1 ▲ One rescuer kneels at the patient's head. The second rescuer kneels between the patient's bent knees with his back to the patient.

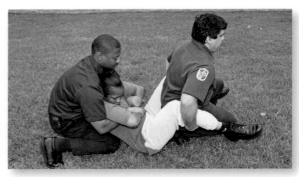

STEP 2 ▲ The rescuer at the patient's head places one hand under each of the patient's armpits and grasps the patient's wrists. The second rescuer slips his hands behind the patient's knees.

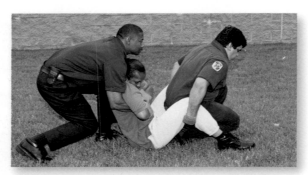

STEP 3 ▲ On a signal from the rescuer at the patient's head, both rescuers move up to a crouching position.

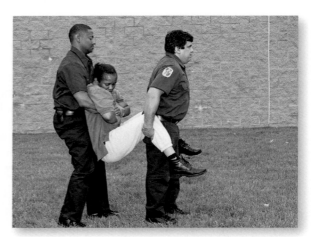

STEP 4 ▲ On a signal from the rescuer at the patient's head, both rescuers stand at the same time and move with the patient.

placed parallel to the patient's bed. In both cases, you will be assisting hospital personnel or another EMS professional. As with previous moves, teamwork and coordination are essential.

Direct Carry

The *direct carry* is used to move a patient with no suspected spinal injury from a bed to a stretcher. Skill Drill 2-6 illustrates a direct carry.

Stop and Think!

Use the following tips when performing a direct carry:

- Some older stretchers do not have brakes. If there is no brake, ask someone to stabilize the stretcher for you.
- Remember to lift with your legs.
- Be careful not to jerk or twist when lifting the patient.

Direct Carry

STEP 1 ▶
- Place the stretcher at a 90-degree angle to the bed, with the head end of the stretcher at the foot of the bed. Prepare the stretcher by unbuckling the straps, adjusting the height of the stretcher so that it is even with the bed, and lowering the side rails. Set the brakes on the stretcher (if so equipped) to the ON position.
- Both rescuers should stand between the bed and the stretcher and face the patient.

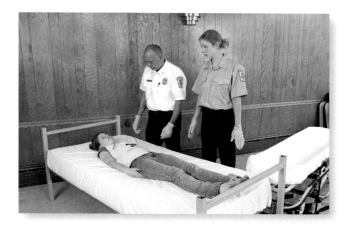

STEP 2 ▶
- Both rescuers kneel. The rescuer at the head slides one arm under the patient's neck, cupping the patient's far shoulder with his hand and cradling the patient's head. The rescuer then slides his other arm under the patient's lower back.
- The second rescuer slides one hand under the patient's hip and lifts slightly. She then places her other arm under the patient's hips and calves.

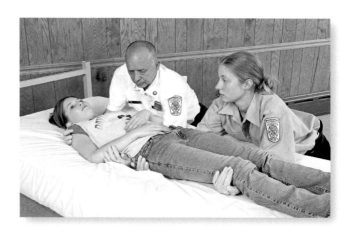

STEP 3 ▶ On a signal from the rescuer at the patient's head, both rescuers slide the patient toward them to the edge of the bed. Both rescuers should lift with their legs.

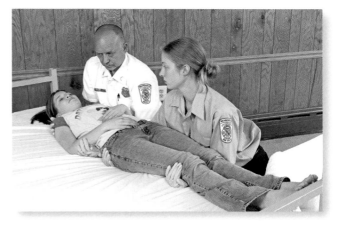

Continued

Direct Carry *Continued*

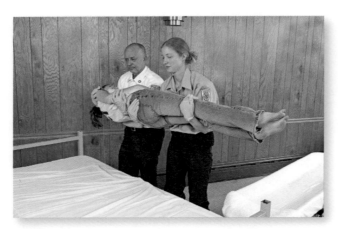

STEP 4 ▲ On a signal from the rescuer at the patient's head, the patient is lifted and curled toward the rescuers' chests. Both rescuers should be careful not to jerk or twist.

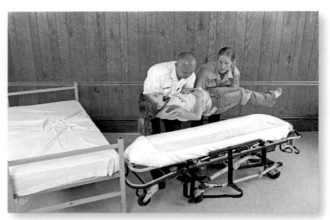

STEP 5 ▲ On a signal from the rescuer at the patient's head, both rescuers then rotate together, lining up with the stretcher, and, reversing the previous steps, gently place the patient onto the stretcher.

Draw Sheet Transfer

A **draw sheet** is a narrow sheet placed crosswise on a bed under the patient. It is used to assist in moving a patient or changing soiled bed sheets. The draw sheet transfer requires a minimum of two people to be performed; however, the use of four rescuers is preferred. To move a patient by using a draw sheet, follow the steps outlined in Skill Drill 2-7.

Patient Positioning

Objective 38

Although patient positioning is often overlooked, it is an essential part of your patient care. In some cases, simply changing the patient's position can improve the person's condition. Consider the following situations:

- Your patient was golfing when he suddenly felt hot and lightheaded. He sat down in the grass to rest. As you approach, he lies down. Your patient is now unresponsive without a possible head, neck, or back injury. He is breathing and a pulse is present. This patient should be placed in the **recovery position** (Figure 2-30). To place a patient

in the recovery position, raise the patient's left arm above his head so that his head will rest on his arm once he is logrolled onto his left side. Kneel on the left side of the supine patient. Grasp the patient's leg and shoulder and roll him toward you, onto his left side. This positioning allows the patient's head to rest on his raised left arm with his face in a slightly downward position. It also helps secretions drain from the patient's nose and

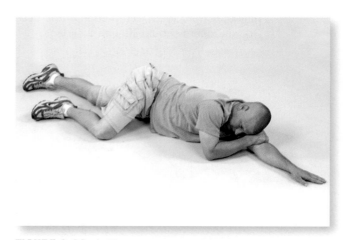

FIGURE 2-30 ▲ The recovery position.

Draw Sheet Transfer

STEP 1 ▶
- Loosen the draw sheet on the bed, and form a long roll to grasp.
- Prepare the stretcher by unbuckling the straps, adjusting the height of the stretcher so that it is even with the bed, and lowering the side rails.
- Set the brakes on the stretcher (if so equipped) to the ON position.
- Position the stretcher next to and touching the patient's bed.

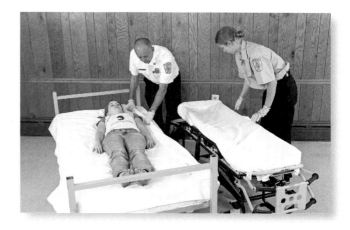

STEP 2 ▶ Both rescuers should stand on the same side of the stretcher and then reach across it to grasp the draw sheet firmly at the patient's head and hips.

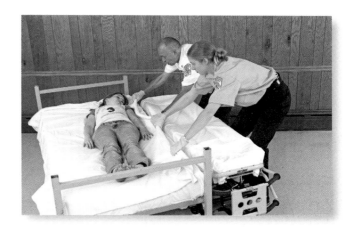

STEP 3 ▶ On a signal from the rescuer at the patient's head, both rescuers gently slide the patient from the bed to the stretcher.

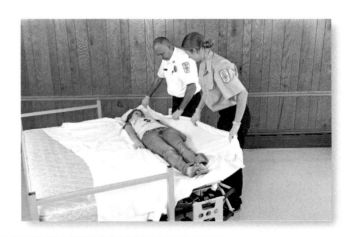

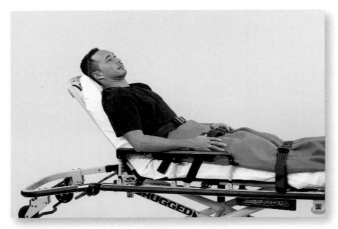

FIGURE 2-31 ▲ The Fowler's position.

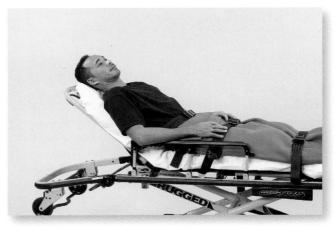

FIGURE 2-32 ▲ The semi-Fowler's position.

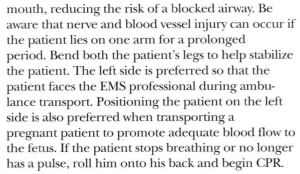

FIGURE 2-33 ▲ The high-Fowler's position.

mouth, reducing the risk of a blocked airway. Be aware that nerve and blood vessel injury can occur if the patient lies on one arm for a prolonged period. Bend both the patient's legs to help stabilize the patient. The left side is preferred so that the patient faces the EMS professional during ambulance transport. Positioning the patient on the left side is also preferred when transporting a pregnant patient to promote adequate blood flow to the fetus. If the patient stops breathing or no longer has a pulse, roll him onto his back and begin CPR.

- Your patient has fallen from a ladder while trimming tree branches. You suspect a head, neck, or back injury. This patient should *not* be moved until additional personnel are on the scene to help you assess the patient and stabilize her spine before moving her to a stretcher. Be sure to have suction readily available should vomiting occur.

- Your patient was running at the track and is now experiencing difficulty breathing. This patient should be allowed to assume a position of comfort. Most often, this will be a seated position. In a **Fowler's position,** the patient is lying on his back with his upper body elevated at a 45- to 60-degree angle (Figure 2-31). In a **semi-Fowler's position,** the patient is sitting up with his head at a 45-degree angle and his legs out straight (Figure 2-32). In a **high-Fowler's position,** the patient is sitting upright at a 90-degree angle (Figure 2-33).

- Your patient is experiencing a sudden onset of severe abdominal pain or nontraumatic back pain. Patients with this complaint are often most comfortable on their back or side with their knees slightly bent.

- Your patient is vomiting. She is awake and alert with a strong pulse. There is no history or evidence of trauma. This patient should be allowed to assume a

position of comfort. Be prepared to manage her airway and place her in the recovery position if her level of consciousness decreases.

- Your patient is complaining of weakness. He has had flu symptoms for three days. He is confused. His skin is pale, cool, and moist, and his heart rate is fast. A patient with signs and symptoms of shock should be placed flat on his back.

Remember This

- Any patient with a suspected spinal injury should be fully stabilized on a long backboard.

- Do not place a patient in the recovery position if you suspect the patient has experienced an injury to the head, neck, or spine.

- *Do not permit a patient complaining of chest pain or difficulty breathing to walk to the stretcher or ambulance.*

- If the stretcher will not fit into a particular area, it may be necessary to place the patient in a chair and then move the patient in the chair to the stretcher.

Equipment

You will encounter many different types of equipment that are used to assist in stabilizing and moving your patients. Most equipment works under the same basic principle with slight design and cosmetic variations. It is important to become familiar with the equipment used in your area. Below are descriptions of commonly used equipment.

Wheeled Stretcher

A wheeled stretcher is a rolling bed that is commonly found in the back of an ambulance (Figure 2-34a). It is used more often than any other patient transfer device. There are many different manufacturers, but all wheeled stretchers have certain characteristics that make them compatible with the need to transfer and maneuver patients from the scene to the transport vehicle. The main bed (patient platform) is about 76 inches in length and about 23 inches wide. It is typically padded with a comfort mattress that will need to be covered with a sheet. It should also include a cover that will stop fluids from penetrating into the mattress. The head of the stretcher can be adjusted to several different angles. Most patients will be more comfortable with their head and body inclined at a slight angle. Cardiac and respiratory patients will generally be unable to lie flat. The platform can incline to a semisitting position.

All patient transport devices must have an effective method of securing the patient to the device. This is generally accomplished with a restraint system. Current recommendations are for restraint devices that incorporate an "over the shoulder" system. This can protect the patient during rapid deceleration. In addition, patient transport equipment must have the ability to be securely fastened to the floor to prevent movement during a rollover type of accident. The actual movement of the patient on the stretcher will be influenced by many factors, such as the size and weight of the patient and the terrain over which you are traveling. Many newer stretchers have large, inflatable tires that allow movement over uneven ground.

Wheeled stretchers have handles for lifting and rolling. If you are lifting a wheeled stretcher with someone who does not operate it often, take the control end so that you can make sure the wheels will drop properly. Be sure you know the weight limitations of the stretcher you are using. Exceeding it could cause injury to the atient, the crew, or both.

Newer types of lifting devices (such as pneumatic or electronic stretchers) are available that offer some type of "power" assist to help reduce your risk of back

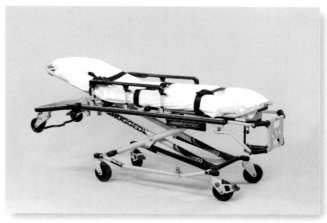

(a)

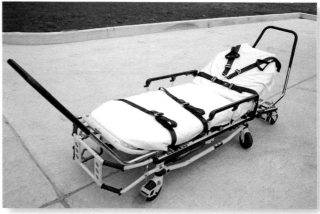

(b)

FIGURE 2-34 ▲ **(a)** A wheeled stretcher; **(b)** a bariatric stretcher.

strain or injury. A bariatric stretcher is designed to hold larger or heavier patients (Figure 2-34b). It may have an ability to be moved into the transport vehicle on a ramp by using a pulley or winch system. Request additional resources if this equipment is unavailable and the patient is large. Lifting a heavy or large patient not only puts your back at risk but also creates a greater possibility of dropping the patient.

Remember This

Keep the stretcher in the lowest, most comfortable position during patient moves. This will keep the patient's center of gravity lower, and the stretcher will be less likely to tip over.

Portable Stretcher

A portable stretcher usually folds or collapses when it is not in use. It is often made of heavy canvas or heavy

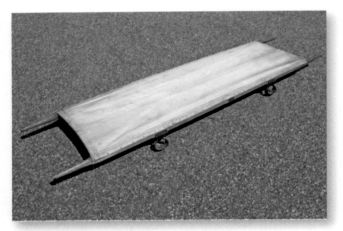

FIGURE 2-35 ▲ A portable stretcher.

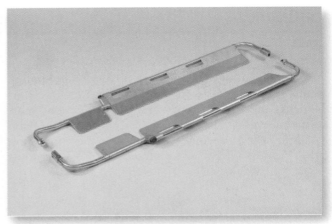
(a)

plastic (Figure 2-35). It may be used in the following situations:

- To carry patients down stairs, down a hill, or over rough terrain
- To remove patients from spaces too confined or narrow for a wheeled stretcher
- To quickly transfer a large number of people from one place to another

Scoop Stretcher

A **scoop (orthopedic) stretcher** is unique in that it is hinged and opens at the head and feet to fit around and under the patient (Figure 2-36). The scoop stretcher is also called a *split litter*. To use this device, you must have access to both sides of the patient. The two halves of the stretcher are adjusted to the patient's length. Each piece is then slid under the patient and reconnected, effectively scooping the patient onto the device. The scoop stretcher may be used to carry a supine patient up or down stairs. However, a scoop stretcher does not adequately stabilize the spine. If a spinal injury is suspected, the patient and scoop stretcher should be secured to a long backboard for stabilization.

Basket Stretcher

A **basket stretcher** (Figure 2-37) is shaped like a long basket and can hold a scoop stretcher or a long backboard. A basket stretcher is also called a *basket litter* or *Stokes basket*. Some basket stretchers are too narrow to hold all widths of backboards. If you will be using a basket stretcher, be sure to check how wide it is to make certain your backboard will fit. There is a military version of basket stretcher that has a leg divider. This device will not accept a long backboard, no matter the width.

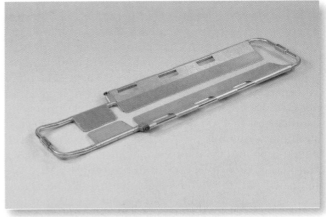
(b)

FIGURE 2-36 ▲ A scoop (orthopedic) stretcher. **(a)** Sides separated; **(b)** sides together.

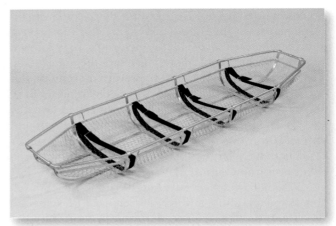

FIGURE 2-37 ▲ A basket stretcher.

The basket is made of fiberglass-plastic composites, plastic with an aluminum frame, or a steel frame with wire or plastic mesh. Some basket stretchers have holes in the bottom of the stretcher to allow water drainage. A basket stretcher is used for moving patients over

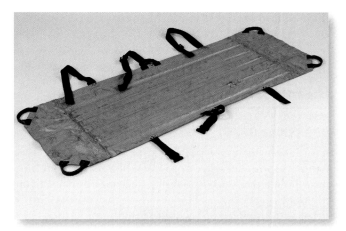

FIGURE 2-38 ▲ A flexible stretcher.

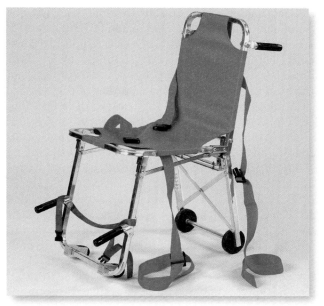

FIGURE 2-39 ▲ A stair chair.

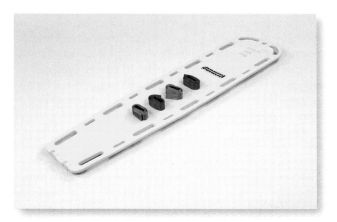

FIGURE 2-40 ▲ A long backboard.

rough terrain, in water rescues, or in high-angle rescues. A basket stretcher that has a solid bottom can also be pulled over snow and ice (and other terrain), much like a sled.

Flexible Stretcher

A **flexible stretcher** can be rolled up for easy storage and carrying but forms a more rigid surface that conforms to the sides of the patient when in use. Examples of flexible stretchers include the Reeves stretcher (Figure 2-38), SKED, and Navy stretcher. Flexible stretchers are made of canvas or flexible, synthetic material with carrying handles. Straps are used to secure the patient. This type of stretcher is particularly useful when space is limited for accessing the patient. It can be used in narrow hallways, stairs, cramped corners, high-angle rescues, and hazardous materials situations. Because the flexible stretcher conforms around the patient, it may not be possible to access all areas of the patient when giving emergency care. Flexible stretchers do not provide the kind of impact protection for the patient that is provided by many basket stretchers. You will need to have greater concern about spinal precautions and exercise greater care when moving your patient in a flexible stretcher. Patients carried in a flexible stretcher should be carried in a supine position to prevent accidental suffocation.

Stair Chair

A **stair chair** is used to transfer patients up or down stairways, through narrow hallways and doorways, into small elevators, or in narrow aisles in aircraft or buses (Figure 2-39). At least two rescuers are required to move the patient in a stair chair. It is a very helpful device when a patient does not need to lie flat. The stair chair has belts and straps with which to secure the patient. It also has handles for lifting.

Backboards

Backboards (also called *spine boards*) come in many different shapes, sizes, and colors. The **long backboard** has holes spaced along the head and foot ends as well as the sides of the board (Figure 2-40). These holes are used as handholds and as places to insert straps. A long backboard is relatively inexpensive, easy to store, and very versatile. The long backboard is used in the following situations:

- Securing a patient who is either lying or standing and needs to be immobilized to prevent worsening a potential spinal injury
- Lifting and moving patients
- Providing secondary support when a short backboard or scoop stretcher is used
- Providing a firm surface on which to perform CPR

Securing a patient properly to a long backboard is essential in order to minimize spinal movement. This is particularly important if it is necessary to tilt the backboard. Tilting the backboard may be necessary if an immobilized patient vomits or if you are transporting a woman in her second or third trimester of pregnancy.

Although the use of a long backboard helps stabilize a patient's spine, it is uncomfortable for the patient. While most prehospital patient encounters are relatively short, the patient may remain on the board for hours after arrival in an emergency department. Patients can develop pressure injuries at body contact points along the board. In some cases, the backboard itself can cause pain and lead to unnecessary tests (such as x-rays) at the hospital to identify the source of the pain. The three most common areas for pressure pain are the back of the head, lower back, and sacrum. Padding at points of contact between the bones in these areas and the backboard can help reduce the patient's discomfort without compromising spinal stabilization.

Vacuum mattresses are being used with increasing frequency in the field. A vacuum mattress can provide spinal stabilization, as does a backboard, and is much more comfortable for the patient than a backboard. A vacuum mattress is particularly helpful for long transports where a hard backboard will cause the patient great discomfort and pain (and possible minor injury). Another benefit of using a vacuum mattress is that it is easier to position a patient who has been immobilized on the side when it is necessary to clear the patient's airway. One drawback of using a vacuum mattress is that access to the posterior aspect of the patient may be difficult. A vacuum mattress is also susceptible to punctures and tears. Carrying a patient in a vacuum mattress requires the assistance of more than two people. The mattress will collapse if it is supported solely at each end, with potentially disastrous results.

The **short backboard** is used to secure the head, neck, and back of a stable patient found in a seated position (Figure 2-41). Once secured, the patient can then be transferred to a long backboard for full stabilization that includes the hips and legs. A vest-type device can be used in place of a short backboard.

Use of Restraints

Objectives 40, 41

Avoid restraining a patient unless the patient is a danger to you, herself, or others. When using restraints, have police present, if possible, and get approval from medical direction. If you must use restraints, apply them with the help of law enforcement and other EMS personnel.

Remember This

Be aware that after a period of combativeness and aggression, some apparently calm patients may cause unexpected and sudden injury to you, themselves, or others.

Avoid the use of unreasonable force. **Reasonable force** is the amount of force necessary to keep a patient from injuring you, himself, or others. Use only the force necessary for restraint. You can determine what is reasonable by looking at all the circumstances involved. These circumstances include the following:

- The patient's size and strength
- The type of abnormal behavior
- The patient's body build and mental state
- The method of restraint

Making a Difference

Avoid acts of physical force that may cause injury to the patient.

When applying restraints, make certain you have enough assistance. You will need at least four healthcare or law enforcement personnel (one for each extremity) (Figure 2-42). Have a plan. Decide who will do what before attempting to restrain the patient. It is extremely important that there be no confusion while you are applying restraints, as confusion will give the patient an opportunity to escape the restraints. Be sure to take standard precautions for protection against body fluids.

Estimate the range of motion of the patient's arms and legs. Stay beyond that range until you are ready to restrain the patient. Once the decision has been made to restrain, act quickly.

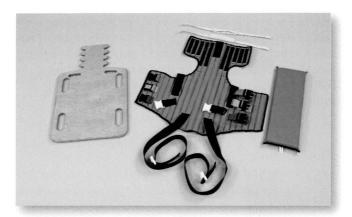

FIGURE 2-41 ▲ A short backboard and vest-type device.

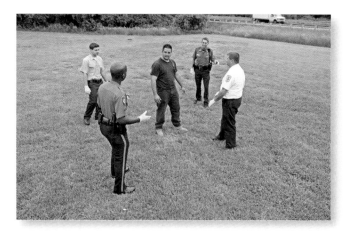

FIGURE 2-42 ▲ Once the decision has been made to restrain a patient, act quickly. One EMS professional should talk to the patient throughout the procedure. At least four persons should approach the patient, one assigned to each of the patient's extremities. Restrain on cue to gain rapid control of the patient.

One EMS professional should talk to the patient throughout the procedure. Tell the patient you are restraining him for his safety and for the safety of those around him. Secure the patient's extremities with restraints approved by medical direction, such as soft leather or cloth. Secure the patient on his back to the stretcher with chest, waist, and thigh straps (Figure 2-43). If the patient is spitting, cover the patient's face with a disposable surgical mask. Reassess the patient's airway, breathing, and circulation frequently (see Chapter 17). Suction as necessary. Chest straps should not hinder the patient's breathing. Reassess distal pulses in each extremity to make sure circulation is not impaired by the restraints.

When using restraints:
- Do not inflict unnecessary pain.
- Do not use unreasonable force.
- Do not leave a restrained patient unattended.
- Do not remove the restraints once they have been applied.

You Should Know

Acceptable Restraints

- Soft leather straps
- Padded cloth straps
- Nylon restraints
- Velcro straps

Stop and Think!

A restrained patient must *never* be left alone. You must constantly reassess the patient who is in your care.

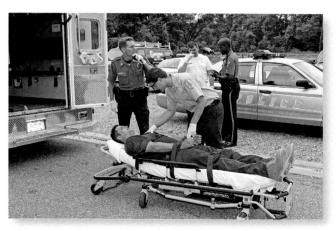

FIGURE 2-43 ▲ Secure the patient on his back to the stretcher with chest, waist, and thigh straps. Reassess the patient's airway, breathing, and circulation frequently.

It is important to document the use of restraints. Make sure to document your findings each time you reassess the patient while the person is in restraints and in your care.

Remember This

Documenting the Use of Restraints

When Caring for a Patient in Restraints, Document the Following Information

- The reason for the restraints
- The number of personnel used to restrain the patient
- The type of restraints used
- The time the restraints were placed on the patient
- The status of the patient's airway, breathing, circulation (ABCs), and distal pulses before and after the restraints were applied
- Reassessment of the patient's ABCs and distal pulses

Death and Dying

The Stages of Grief

Objectives 42, 43

Grief is a normal response that helps people cope with the loss of someone or something that had great meaning to them. Whereas grief is most often associated with death, *any* change of circumstance can cause

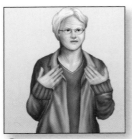 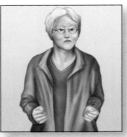 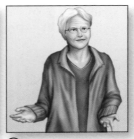 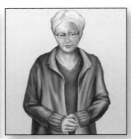 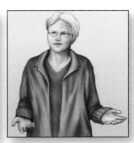

① Denial: "Not me." ② Anger: "Why me?" ③ Bargaining: "OK, but first let me…" ④ Depression: "I don't care anymore." ⑤ Acceptance: "OK, I am not afraid."

FIGURE 2-44 ▲ *Any* change of circumstance can initiate the process of grief.

a person to go through this process (Figure 2-44). How deeply a person feels grief and for how long depends on how important the person believes the loss is. Critically ill or injured patients may experience grief. They may not recognize that they are reacting to the loss of something that was important to them. Knowing about the stages of grief will help you provide appropriate care.

You Should Know

Changes in Circumstances That Contribute to Grief

- Loss or change in status or environment (for example, retirement or relocation)
- Loss of personal possessions (such as a home destroyed by fire)
- Change in a relationship (separation, divorce, death)
- Loss of a significant other (partner, child, parent, close friend, pet)
- Loss of or change in health (including body part or function, physical or mental capacity)
- Loss of or change in security (financial, social, occupational, cultural)

Grief is a very personal and individual process. It is a natural and inevitable part of our journey through life. Elizabeth Kübler-Ross, a world-famous authority on death and dying, developed a model of the stages of grief that a person typically experiences. Although five stages of grief are presented here, a person may move back and forth between stages (see the following *You Should Know* box). An individual may also skip a stage,

go through two or three stages at the same time, go through each stage more than once, or stay in one stage of the process for minutes, hours, days, or longer. Cultural differences will also affect how a person experiences grief.

You Should Know

The Five Stages of Grief

1. Denial
2. Anger
3. Bargaining
4. Depression
5. Acceptance

Denial

"Not me."

Denial is the first phase of the grieving process. Denial is a defense mechanism. It is used to create a buffer against the shock of dying or dealing with an illness or injury. During this stage of the grief process, the person is unable or refuses to believe the reality of what has happened. The patient may try to ignore or deny the seriousness of the illness or injury. The patient may dismiss the symptoms with words such as "only" or "a little." During the denial stage, common reactions from the patient or family include "Not me" or "This can't be happening." During this stage, the patient or family member often does not grasp the information you provide about the illness or injury.

When dealing with a patient in this stage of the grief process, try to find a family member or close friend who can give you more information about the patient's illness or injury. The information you receive can help you make appropriate decisions regarding the patient's care.

Anger

> "Why me?"

Anger is the second stage of the grief process. The ill or injured person's anger comes from several sources. It can be related to discomfort, a limitation of activity, or an inability to control the situation. Family, friends, and medical professionals are common targets for blame. The person often experiences guilt and blames herself for either taking or failing to take specific actions ("If only I had. . .").

In the anger stage, common reactions from the person (or family) include, "Why is this happening to me?" The person's anger may be marked by the following:

- Abusive language
- Criticism of anyone who offers help
- Resentment (particularly of those who are healthy)
- Irritability
- Demanding or impatient manner
- Physical agitation

Stop and Think!

When dealing with an angry person, remember that your safety is your priority. If the scene is not safe and you cannot make it safe, *do not enter.*

When dealing with an angry person, do not take anger or insults personally. Also, do not become defensive. Be tolerant and empathetic, and use good listening and communication skills. Speak to the person in a calm, controlled tone. It is not necessary to agree with the person, but do not challenge how he is feeling. Briefly and honestly explain what the patient can expect from you as well as what you expect from him.

Bargaining

> "Okay, but first let me…"

Bargaining is the third stage of the grief process. During this stage, the person is willing to do anything to change what is happening to her. The person may bargain with herself, her family, God, or medical professionals. Bargaining reflects the person's need for time to accept the situation. Bargaining is marked by statements such as the following:

- "I promise I'll be a better person if…"
- "If I could live to…"
- "Okay, but first let me…"

Depression

> "I don't care anymore."

Depression is the fourth stage of the grief process. Depression is a normal response to the loss of a significant other or the loss of some bodily function. Depression may also result from feeling a loss of control over one's destiny.

A depressed person has the following characteristics:

- Is sad and usually silent
- Appears withdrawn and indifferent
- May take a long time to perform routine activities
- May have difficulty concentrating and following instructions
- May reject your attempts to help
- May accept your help and then fail to react to your interventions
- Shows a lack of interest

Depression is marked by statements such as, "I don't care anymore." You may feel confused, annoyed, defensive, frustrated, or even angry because of the patient's behavior. It is important to recognize these feelings. However, do not communicate them while caring for your patient. Be supportive and nonjudgmental. Provide whatever care is needed.

Acceptance

> "Okay, I am not afraid."

The fifth stage of the grief process is acceptance. The person has come to terms with the loss or change in circumstances and is learning to live with it. If dying, the patient realizes his fate and understands that death is certain. Acceptance does not mean that the patient is happy about dying. Instead, the patient believes that he has done all that is possible in preparing to die. For example, the patient has said what needed to be said and has completed any unfinished business. Acceptance is marked by statements such as, "I am ready for whatever comes," "I know I can't change this," and "Okay, I am not afraid." Friends or family members may need more support during this stage than the patient.

Death

Dealing with death and dying patients is part of the work of an EMS professional. It is important to understand that dying is a process. Death is an event. A person's attitude about dying and death is influenced by culture, experiences, religion, and age. Your reaction to a situation involving the death of a patient will also depend on the circumstances surrounding the event. It is important to look at your own fears, attitudes, and beliefs about death and dying so that you will be prepared when faced with the situation. Doing so can help you understand the needs of the dying patient and his or her family.

You will encounter situations in which you must determine whether a patient is dead or requires emergency medical care. Dying is a process that may take minutes, hours, days, weeks, or months. As a patient is dying, changes occur in the patient's level of responsiveness, breathing, and circulation.

Death occurs when the patient's organs stop functioning. When the patient's heart stops (cardiac arrest), brain death will occur unless circulation is rapidly restored. For this reason, cardiopulmonary resuscitation (CPR) is most effective when started immediately after a cardiac arrest occurs. When you arrive at the scene of a cardiac arrest, CPR should be started immediately if the person is unresponsive, is breathless, and has no pulse (heartbeat). CPR should not be started if a valid do not resuscitate (DNR) order (see the following section) is present or if death is obvious. CPR is discussed in detail in Appendix A.

You Should Know

In some Latin-American and Asian-Pacific cultures, a patient may not be told he has a terminal illness. It is believed that telling this would upset the patient's inner harmony and could hasten the progression of disease or death.

Advance Directives and Do Not Resuscitate Orders

Some patients, such as those who have been diagnosed with a terminal illness, may not want aggressive efforts aimed at reviving them when they are dying. These patients may have an advance directive or a DNR order. An **advance directive** is a legal document that details a person's healthcare wishes when the person becomes unable to make decisions for himself or herself. A **do not resuscitate (DNR) order** is an order written by a physician. It instructs medical professionals not to provide medical care to a patient who has experienced a cardiac arrest.

If you arrive on the scene of a cardiac arrest, begin CPR if:
- A DNR order is not present.
- There are no signs of obvious death.
- A DNR order is present, but the DNR documentation is unclear.
- A DNR order is present, but you are not sure the order is valid.

If you arrive on the scene of a cardiac arrest and a DNR order is present:
- Make sure the form clearly identifies the person to whom the DNR applies.
- Make sure the patient is the person referred to in the DNR document.
- Make sure the document is the correct type, approved by your state and local authorities.

If the patient requires resuscitation, advanced life support (ALS) should be called to the scene. If a DNR exists but you are unsure about the validity of the order, begin CPR immediately. It is possible to stop CPR more easily than it is to begin resuscitation measures when it is too late. If you determine the DNR order is valid, follow the instructions outlined in the document. This may include stopping resuscitation if it has already been started. If required by your local protocol, call advanced life support personnel to the scene to confirm that the patient is dead and/or contact medical direction.

Signs of Obvious Death

Objective 44

In some situations, it will be clear that a person has been dead for some time. An obvious sign of death includes decapitation (beheading). Other signs include putrefaction, dependent lividity, and rigor mortis, which are described in the following sections.

You Should Know

Be sure to let the police know about your observations.

If a person shows signs of obvious death, do not disturb the body or scene. The police or medical examiner will need to authorize removal of the body. It will be important for you to observe and document the following:

- The position of the patient/victim
- The patient's injuries
- The conditions at the scene
- Statements of persons at the scene
- Statements of the patient/victim before death

Putrefaction

Putrefaction is the decomposition of organic matter, such as body tissues.

Dependent Lividity

Dependent lividity refers to the settling of blood in dependent areas of the body. Dependent areas are those areas on which the body has been resting. Dependent lividity is considered an obvious sign of death only when there are widespread areas of discolored skin (reddish-purple skin) in dependent areas of an unresponsive, breathless, and pulseless person. In some EMS systems, both lividity and rigor mortis must be present to be considered signs of obvious death. Lividity is harder to detect on a person with dark skin pigmentation. In addition, lividity may be absent if there was major blood loss before death.

Rigor Mortis

Rigor mortis is the stiffening of body muscles that occurs after death. This stiffening occurs because of chemical changes in muscle tissue. After death, the muscles of the body will normally be relaxed for about 3 hours. They stiffen between 3 hours and 36 hours and then become relaxed again. The condition of the body, the environmental temperature, and the amount of work the muscles performed just before death affect how quickly rigor mortis occurs. The onset of rigor mortis is usually delayed in a cold environment and sped up in a hot one. A high level of muscle activity increases acid production. The presence of acid speeds up the onset of rigor mortis.

Rigor mortis begins in the muscles of the face. It then spreads downward to other parts of the body. Rigor may be more difficult to detect in obese individuals. The state of rigor usually lasts about 24–36 hours or until muscle decay occurs.

You Should Know

Signs of Obvious Death

- Decapitation or other obvious mortal injury
- Putrefaction (decomposition)
- Extreme dependent lividity
- Rigor mortis

Helping the Dying Patient

Objective 45

As an EMT, you may arrive to find that a patient has died or is dying. A dying patient may ask to talk with her family. If the family is not at the scene, it is appro-

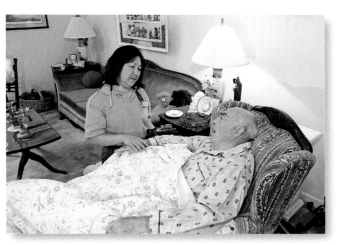

FIGURE 2-45 ▲ The dying patient may want to express feelings and concerns to you.

priate to offer to pass on important messages. Write down the information. Be sure to follow through with the patient's request.

A dying patient may want to express feelings and concerns to you (Figure 2-45). Just being there and listening is often all that the patient wants from you. Remember to preserve the patient's dignity and treat the patient with respect.

Making a Difference

Dealing with the Dying Patient and Family Members

- Be aware that the patient's needs include dignity, respect, sharing, communication, privacy, and control.
- Allow family members to express their feelings.
- Listen empathetically.
- Do not falsely reassure.
- Use a gentle tone of voice.
- Let the patient know that everything that can be done to help will be done.
- Use a reassuring touch, if appropriate.
- Comfort the family.

Helping the Dying Patient's Family

Objectives 46, 47

When conveying news about a patient's death, speak slowly and in a quiet, calm voice. You might begin by saying, "This is hard to tell you, but . . . " and then tactfully explain that the patient is dead. Use the words "death," "dying," or "dead" instead of phrases such as "passed on," "no longer with us," or "has gone to a better place." An empathic response such as, "You have my (our) sincere sympathy," may be used to express your feelings.

The patient's family will go through the grief process. If the patient had a prolonged illness, family members may have had an opportunity to share important messages. They may also have been able to resolve conflict before the patient died. When a person dies suddenly, family members and friends may experience intense grief and guilt. This may be particularly true if messages were left unsaid or harsh words were spoken before death.

The reactions of family members to a loved one's death may include anger, rage, withdrawal, disbelief, extreme agitation, guilt, or sorrow. In some cases, there may be no visible response, or the response may seem inappropriate. Be sensitive to the needs of those who have suffered a loss by acknowledging their grief. They have a right to these feelings.

After a death, members of the family and close friends will often try to make sense of what happened to their loved one. Many will want to learn the details surrounding the death. They may want to talk to those who were present at the time of death. They may also want to view the body. At a possible crime scene, do not disturb the body or the scene.

Some EMS agencies have arrangements with counselors, who can be called to the scene to provide grief support for the family (Figure 2-46). Remain with the family until law enforcement personnel or the medical examiner assumes responsibility for the body. In addition, if grief support services are available in your area, stay with the family members until grief support personnel are on the scene to assist them. If counselors or grief support personnel are not available, give the family members information packets or crisis intervention contact information so that they can seek help from mental health professionals.

Taking caring of ill or injured people is emotionally demanding. Make sure to assess your own physical and emotional response to the situation when the call is over. It may be helpful for you to talk with other EMS professionals afterward. You may find it helpful to discuss your feelings if the call involved death or dying.

On the Scene   Wrap-Up

Your neighbor has no pulse. His jaw and limbs are rigid and cold, and you decide not to resuscitate him. Paramedics arrive moments later and confirm that he is dead. You sit down next to his wife and quietly tell her that her husband is dead. She screams and pushes you away angrily, asking why you didn't do anything to save him. Moments later she moans and says that she shouldn't have gone to bed, that she knew he'd been feeling ill all day.

You go back to the station after the call and tearfully explain to the crew about your lifelong friendship with the patient. Later that week a debriefing is held. Because of your ongoing dreams about the event, you visit a counselor to help you cope with the strong emotions you are feeling. ■

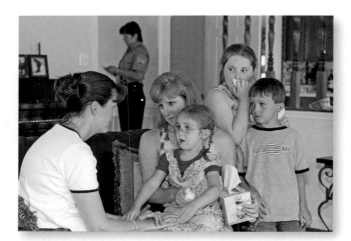

FIGURE 2-46 ▲ Many EMS agencies have arrangements with counselors who can provide grief support for a family on the scene.

Sum It Up

▶ Wellness is a state of health and happiness (well-being) that involves lifestyle choices in pursuit of an optimal state of health. Physical well-being and mental well-being are components of wellness.

▶ As an EMT, you will encounter many stressful situations. A stressor is any event or condition that has the potential to cause bodily or mental tension. To be an effective EMT, you must learn to recognize the physical, behavioral, mental, or emotional signs of stress.

- You should manage stress through lifestyle changes. These changes include developing good dietary habits, exercising, and practicing relaxation techniques. You should also seek to create balance in your life, including time with family and friends.

- Professional help may be needed to help you cope with stress. Many organizations have employee assistance programs that offer confidential counseling to prehospital professionals.

- An EMT is responsible for ensuring the safety of the crew, the patient, and bystanders. However, an EMT's first priority is ensuring his or her own safety at all scenes. This responsibility includes protecting oneself against disease transmission, which includes using personal protective equipment and having the proper vaccinations. It also involves safety at hazardous materials scenes, motor vehicle crashes and rescue scenes, and violent scenes.

- As an EMT, you will most often give initial emergency care to a patient in the position in which the patient is found. You will need to be able to distinguish an emergency from a nonemergency situation. Your role will also include positioning patients to prevent further injury and assisting other EMS professionals in lifting and moving patients.

- Body mechanics is the way we move our bodies when lifting and moving. Body mechanics includes body alignment, balance, and coordinated body movement. Good posture is key to proper body alignment.

- To lift safely, you should use the power grip (underhand grip). To perform this grip, you should position your hands a comfortable distance apart (about 10 inches). With your palms up, grasp the object you are preparing to lift. The power grip allows you to take full advantage of the strength of your hands, forearms, and biceps.

- Safely lifting patients requires that you use good posture and good body mechanics. You should consider the weight of the patient and call for additional help if needed. Plan how and where you will move the patient. It is also important to remember to lift with your legs and not your back. When you are lifting with other EMS professionals, communication and planning are key.

- An emergency move is used when there is an immediate danger to you or the patient. Such dangers include scene hazards, the inability to reach patients who need lifesaving care, and a patient location or position that prevents you from giving immediate and lifesaving care.

- Drags are one type of emergency move. When dragging a patient, remember to stabilize the patient's head and neck as much as possible before beginning the move. Also, always remember to pull along the length of the spine. *Never* pull the patient's head away from his neck and shoulders. You should also never drag a patient sideways. Carries are the second major type of emergency move. As an EMT, you should become familiar with the different types of carries.

- An urgent move is used to move a patient when there is an immediate threat to life, such as in the following situations: altered mental status, inadequate breathing, or shock. Rapid extrication is an example of an urgent move. It must be accomplished quickly, without compromise or injury to the spine.

- Nonurgent moves are used to move, lift, or carry patients with no known or suspected injury to the head, neck, spine, or extremities. The direct ground lift and the extremity lift are the two main types of nonurgent moves.

- The direct carry and the draw sheet method are the two primary methods used to transfer a supine patient to a bed or stretcher. In both transfer types, you will be assisting hospital personnel or another EMS professional. Therefore, teamwork and coordination are essential.

- Patient positioning is an important part of the patient care you provide. In some cases, simply changing a patient's position can improve her condition. As an EMT, you should become familiar with the different types of positions and when to use them.

- Many different types of equipment are used to assist in stabilizing and moving patients. In your role as an emergency care provider, it is important to become familiar with the equipment used in your area. Commonly used equipment includes various types of stretchers and backboards as well as the stair chair.

- Avoid restraining a patient unless the patient is a danger to you, himself, or others. When using restraints, have police present, if possible, and get approval from medical direction. If you must use restraints, apply them with the help of law enforcement and other EMS personnel.

- Critically ill or injured patients may experience grief, which is a normal response to a loss of any kind. The five stages of grief are denial, anger, bargaining, depression, and acceptance. Remember that a person going through grief may skip a stage, go through more than one stage at the same time, or go through each stage more than once. Cultural factors will influence how a person experiences grief.

- Patients may experience any number of emotions in response to their illness or injury. As an EMT, you must be respectful of each patient. Listen with empathy to the patient's concerns but do not give the patient false hope or false reassurance. In dealing with the patient's family or friends or with bystanders, you may need to use many of the same approaches you use in dealing with patients.

▶ Some patients may not want aggressive efforts aimed at reviving them when they are dying. These patients may have an advance directive or a DNR order. An advance directive is a legal document that details a person's healthcare wishes when she becomes unable to make decisions for herself. A DNR order is written by a physician. It instructs medical professionals not to provide medical care to a patient who has experienced a cardiac arrest.

▶ The signs of obvious death include decapitation (beheading), putrefaction (decomposition), dependent lividity, and rigor mortis. If a person shows signs of obvious death, do not disturb the body or scene. The police or medical examiner will need to authorize removing the body. You should document the victim's position and injuries. You should also document the conditions at the scene as well as statements of persons at the scene.

CHAPTER

3

Legal and Ethical Issues and Documentation

By the end of this chapter, you should be able to:

Knowledge Objectives ▶

1. Describe the basic structure of the legal system in the United States.
2. Define the terms plaintiff, defendant, statute of limitations, criminal law, civil law, and tort.
3. Differentiate between criminal and civil law.
4. Discuss the steps in a lawsuit.
5. Differentiate between the scope of practice and the standard of care for emergency medical technician practice.
6. Discuss the concept of medical oversight, including off-line medical direction and on-line medical direction, and its relationship to the EMT.
7. Define ethics.
8. Describe the ethical responsibilities of the EMT.
9. Describe a three-part test used for determining a patient's competence.
10. Define consent and discuss the methods of obtaining consent.
11. Differentiate between expressed and implied consent.
12. Explain the role of consent of minors in providing care.
13. Discuss the implications for the emergency medical technician in patient refusal of transport.
14. Explain the purpose of advance directives relative to patient care and how the EMT should care for a patient who is covered by an advance directive.
15. Define and give examples of comfort care.
16. Differentiate between assault and battery, and describe how to avoid each.
17. Describe what constitutes abandonment.
18. Define negligence, and describe the four elements that must be present in order to prove negligence.
19. State the conditions necessary for the emergency medical technician to have a duty to act.
20. Explain the importance, necessity, and legality of patient confidentiality.
21. List the actions that an emergency medical technician should take to assist in the preservation of a crime scene.
22. State the conditions that require an emergency medical technician to notify local law enforcement officials.
23. Discuss the responsibilities of the EMT relative to emergency care for patients who are potential organ donors.
24. Describe the legal implications associated with the written report.
25. Identify the various sections of the written report.

26. Describe what information is required in each section of the prehospital care report and how it should be entered.

Attitude Objectives ▶ 27. Explain the rationale for the needs, benefits, and usage of advance directives.

28. Explain the rationale for patient care documentation.

Skill Objectives ▶ 29. Given a scenario in which an EMT has a conscious patient in need of care, demonstrate the process used to obtain consent.

30. Demonstrate appropriate patient management and care techniques in a refusal of care situation.

31. Given a scenario in which a patient is injured while an EMT is providing care, determine whether the four components of negligence are present.

32. Complete a prehospital care report.

33. Complete a patient refusal report.

On the Scene

"The scene is safe. Proceed in," the dispatcher calls over the radio. An adult male has evidently shot himself while cleaning his gun. You find the patient sitting in a chair in the living room. He is awake, alert, and oriented, but he looks very pale. He is holding his upper leg, where you can see a small hole in his jeans. You carefully avoid touching the small handgun that is sitting on the table near the patient. The upholstery on the chair under him is soaked with blood. You introduce yourself and prepare to care for the patient, but he says, "No, don't touch me. I'm okay." You recognize that he is a reporter for the local news station. You carefully explain the danger of developing shock and dying if he refuses care. He insists that no care be given, so you call for backup and contact your medical director. ■

THINK ABOUT IT

As you read this chapter, think about the following questions:

- Can the patient refuse to allow you to care for him?
- What can you be accused of if you try to care for him without his consent?
- Is it okay to talk about his case to other coworkers because he is a reporter?
- Could you be accused of negligence in this situation?

Introduction

The Importance of Legal and Ethical Care

As an EMS professional, you will face many situations involving medical, legal, and ethical questions. Consider the following examples.

- You have completed your EMT training and are heading home after a busy day at work. While driving through town, you come upon an automobile crash that apparently happened moments ago. You can see a middle-aged man slumped over the steering wheel. Should you stop and provide emergency care to this person—even though you are off duty?

- You are on shift as an EMT and receive a call from an attorney. The attorney is representing a patient who was involved in a fall while at work. You provided emergency care for the patient about 2 months ago. Should you release patient information to the attorney on the telephone?

- You are on shift as an EMT and are called to a local park where a 7-year-old child fell off a piece of playground equipment. Her arm appears to be broken. The next-door neighbor, an adult, is present on the scene. The child's parents cannot be reached. Can you provide emergency care for this child?

You will face situations like these and other legal and ethical questions every day. You must know how to make correct decisions when these questions arise.

The first and most basic principle for any healthcare professional is to *do no harm*. As an EMT, you have certain legal and ethical duties to your patients, the medical director, and the public. Your patients, the medical director, and the public also have certain expectations of you. If you act in good faith and to an appropriate standard of care, you should be able to satisfy these duties and obligations. In this chapter we will explore common legal definitions and the expectations of your career and practice as an EMT. We will also discuss how proper documentation is vital when facing legal and ethical challenges.

The Legal System

Sources of Law

Objectives 1, 2, 3

The U.S. government is made up of three branches: legislative, executive, and judicial. Each branch is the source of a different type of law. The legislative branch of government is made up of Congress and government agencies such as state legislatures, city councils, district boards, and general assemblies. Law made by this branch of government is called *statutory* or *legislative law.*

The president of the United States is the head of the executive branch. The vice president, cabinet members, state governors, and state and federal administrative agencies that make rules and regulations are also part of the executive branch. An **administrative agency** is a governmental body responsible for implementing and enforcing a particular law passed by the legislative branch of government. These agencies generally have the power to develop rules and regulations and to decide disputes. The rules and regulations made by the executive branch of government are called **administrative law.**

The court system is the judicial branch of government. Courts hear cases that challenge or require explanation of the laws passed by the legislative branch of government and approved by the executive branch. The federal government and each of the state governments have their own court systems.

In the United States, there are generally three levels of courts. Cases are first heard in trial courts, and a decision is made by a judge or jury. In some states, trial courts are called *circuit* or *district courts.* After the trial court has reached a decision, an attorney may request a higher court to hear the case to reverse the trial court's decision. This is called an **appeal.** Most appeals are first heard by an intermediate court, called an *appellate court.* Further appeals may be heard by supreme courts, which have final authority in most of the cases they hear.

In a lawsuit, the **plaintiff** (also called the *complainant*) is the party that files a formal complaint with the court. The **defendant** is the party being sued or accused. The maximum period within which a plaintiff must begin a lawsuit (in civil cases), or a prosecutor must bring charges (in criminal cases), or lose the right to file the suit is called the **statute of limitations.** The length of the statute of limitations varies by state and may differ for cases involving adults and children.

Criminal law is the area of law in which the federal, state, or local government prosecutes individuals on behalf of society for violating laws designed to safeguard society. Criminal laws are punishable by fine, imprisonment, or both. In criminal cases, the plaintiff is a federal, state, or local government agency. **Civil law** is a branch of law that deals with complaints by individuals or organizations against a defendant for an illegal act or wrongdoing **(tort).** Examples of civil cases include personal injury claims, divorce, and contract disputes. In a civil case, the plaintiff asks the court to provide a remedy in the form of an award for damages.

Steps in a Lawsuit

Objective 4

A lawsuit begins when an incident occurs and an individual or organization finds that the problems resulting from the incident require the involvement of the courts. In some states it is necessary to make a formal demand by means of a "lawyer's letter" before a suit can be filed. In this case, the party who has the complaint (the plaintiff) meets with an attorney to discuss the incident and the remedy sought from the other party (the defendant). The plaintiff's attorney gathers available facts concerning the claim and then sends a letter to the defendant. If the issue is not resolved, both parties and their attorneys may meet to discuss the claim and reach a fair resolution.

If this attempt fails, the formal action of filing a lawsuit generally begins. If a lawyer's letter is not required by the state before a suit is filed, the plaintiff's attorney begins by gathering pertinent facts, which may include interviewing witnesses and taking statements from them. The attorney then prepares documents and files a written statement (the complaint) with the court. The complaint explains the plaintiff's claim and the remedy sought from the court. After the complaint is filed, copies of the court documents and a summons (notice) are delivered (served) to the defendant (or the defendant's attorney), notifying him that a lawsuit has been filed against him. In many areas, the summons is served by a deputy sheriff or special process server. In other areas, it is served by mail. Once served, the defendant has a specific period within which to answer the complaint. If the defendant does not file an answer to the complaint within the time specified, the court can enter a default judgment against the defendant. The defendant's attorney prepares a response to the complaint and files it with the court. A copy of the defendant's answer is sent to the plaintiff's attorney.

After a lawsuit is filed, the process of **discovery** begins. The purpose of discovery is to enable each side to learn the facts necessary to prepare its case and narrow the issues to be decided by the jury at trial. To find out more details about the claim, one party may send written questions (interrogatories) to the other party. Either party can also submit a list of facts that must be admitted or denied in writing or request the other party to turn over documents that are relevant to the case. Depositions may be taken by either party during discovery, which means asking individuals oral questions while they are under oath. The questions and answers obtained in a deposition are recorded by a court reporter. A transcript of the deposition is made a part of the case record.

After discovery is completed, the judge will hold a pretrial conference with the attorneys to even further narrow the issues to be decided during the trial. The judge will also attempt to persuade the attorneys to settle their case before the trial. Most cases are settled during this period. If no settlement is reached, the judge sets a date for the trial and the trial is conducted. After the trial is finished, a decision is handed down by a judge or jury. The decision determines guilt or liability and the damages and award, if any, to the plaintiff. The judge then enters a judgment, which means that the decision is filed in public records. Either side may appeal the decision to a higher court if the party believes there were errors in law made by the court during the initial trial.

Scope of Practice

Legal Duties

Objectives 5, 6

As an EMT, you have a legal duty to your patients, medical director, and the public. You must provide for the well-being of your patients by providing necessary medical care outlined in the scope of practice. The scope of practice includes the emergency care and skills an EMT is legally allowed and expected to perform when necessary. These duties are set by state laws and regulations. They are also based on generally accepted standards. States often use the U.S. Department of Transportation (DOT) Emergency Medical Technician Curriculum and/or the National EMS Education Standards to define the EMT's scope of practice. Some states have adopted the *National EMS Scope of Practice* model to define the scope of practice in their state. Some states modify an EMS professional's scope of practice to fit the needs or desires of the state. As a result, what is accepted EMS practice in one state may not be so in another. A medical director and/or your local, regional, or state EMS community may modify an EMT's scope of practice by using standing orders and **protocols**. *Standing orders* are written instructions that authorize EMS personnel to perform certain medical interventions before establishing direct communication with a physician. *Protocols* are written instructions to provide emergency care for specific health-related conditions.

You Should Know

Make sure to check your state rules and regulations to find out the specific skills you are allowed by law to perform.

Regardless of your primary occupation, as an EMT you are expected to provide the same standard of care in an emergency as another EMT with similar training and experience in similar circumstances. Standard of care means the minimum level of care expected of similarly trained healthcare professionals, based on education, experience, laws, and protocols. As an EMT, the laws of the state in which you practice define your scope of practice. Common skills that are within the EMT's scope of practice include:

- Patient assessment
- Inserting oral and nasal airways
- Upper airway suctioning
- Bag-mask ventilation
- Supplemental oxygen therapy
- Cardiopulmonary resuscitation (CPR)
- Automated external defibrillation (AED)
- Rapid extrication
- Pulse oximetry
- Using an automatic transport ventilator
- Obtaining manual and automatic blood pressure readings
- Mechanical patient restraint
- Assisting in lifting and moving patients
- Splinting (cervical spine, spinal stabilization, extremity splinting, traction splinting)
- Assisting patients in taking their own prescribed medications
- Giving specific over-the-counter medications with appropriate medical oversight
- External hemorrhage control
- Bandaging wounds
- Using a tourniquet
- Assisting in childbirth

Your legal right to function as an EMT depends on medical oversight. This means that, for you to practice as an EMT, a physician must oversee your training and practice. A physician acting as medical oversight may allow you to carry out certain medical treatments in specific situations without first making direct contact with a person of higher medical authority (off-line medical direction). Alternatively, the physician may not allow you to provide emergency care without first making telephone or radio contact with a person of higher medical authority (such as a paramedic, nurse, or physician) than you (on-line medical direction). When you practice under medical oversight, you are, in effect, practicing under the physician's license.

Making a Difference

Legal Duties of the Emergency Medical Technician

- Provide for the well-being of the patient by giving emergency medical care as outlined in the scope of practice.
- Provide the same standard of care as another EMT with similar training and experience in similar circumstances.
- Before providing emergency care, make telephone or radio contact with your medical oversight authority (if required to do so).
- Follow standing orders and protocols approved by medical oversight or the local EMS system.
- Follow instructions received from medical oversight.

Ethical Responsibilities

Objectives 7, 8

Ethics are principles of right and wrong, good and bad. Ethics affect our actions and lead to consequences. Ethics are what a person *should* do. As a healthcare professional, you have an ethical responsibility to make the physical and emotional needs of your patient a priority. While you are in contact with a patient, your patient must be your primary concern. Your patient may be a person from a different ethnic or social background or a criminal. None of these circumstances should interfere with the care you give.

Remember This

Value judgments about a patient's character have no place at any level of medical care.

You must treat all patients with respect. Give each patient the best care you are capable of giving. To do this, you have an ethical responsibility to practice and master your skills. This includes taking advantage of continuing education and refresher programs. After a call, review how you did and look for areas in which you can improve. For example, look for ways to improve response times, patient outcomes, and communication skills.

You must be honest and accurate in your written and verbal communications. You must also respect your patient's right to privacy. Much of the information you will get from your patients is considered **protected health information (PHI).** Federal laws exist that forbid sharing patient information that you receive in the course of your work as an EMT without the patient's consent. These laws are discussed in more detail later in this chapter.

As a healthcare professional, you also have a responsibility to work cooperatively with other emergency care professionals. This includes other EMS professionals, law enforcement personnel, fire department and ambulance personnel, and members of the hospital staff. Make sure that your communications and actions with others are professional and respectful.

You Should Know

Ethical Responsibilities of the Emergency Medical Technician

- Responding with respect to the physical and emotional needs of every patient
- Maintaining mastery of skills
- Participating in continuing education and refresher programs
- Critically reviewing your performance and seeking improvement
- Reporting (in written and verbal form) honestly and accurately
- Respecting confidentiality
- Having respect for and working cooperatively with other emergency care professionals

Making a Difference

Treat any patient with the same care and respect you would want a member of your family to receive.

Competence

Objective 9

Before a patient can accept or refuse the care you wish to provide, you must determine whether the patient is capable (competent) of making the decision. **Competence** is the ability of patients to understand the questions you ask. It also means that patients can understand the result of the decisions they make about their care. Patients are considered **incompetent** if they do not have the ability to understand the questions you ask. They are also considered incompetent if they do not understand the possible outcome of the decisions they make about their care.

You Should Know

Because state laws vary, check with your instructor to find out the requirements for legal competence in your state.

How do you determine whether a patient is competent? Well-known EMS attorneys have suggested a three-part test for determining a patient's competence:

1. *Legal competence.* Determine if the patient is legally competent. In most states, this means that your patient is at least 18 years of age, is a minor who is married or pregnant, is economically independent, or is a member of the armed forces.

2. *Mental competence.* Determine if the patient is alert and oriented by asking specific questions. Assess the patient's orientation to the following:
   - *Person:* The patient can tell you her name.
   - *Place:* The patient can tell you where she is.
   - *Time:* The patient can tell you the day, date, or time.
   - *Event:* The patient can tell you what happened.
   Find out if the patient has a mental condition such as Alzheimer's disease, mental retardation, or autism that could affect his or her ability to make an informed decision.

3. *Medical/situational competence.* Some illnesses or injuries can temporarily affect patients' ability to make informed decisions about their care. For example, head trauma, low blood sugar (hypoglycemia), shock, or low blood oxygen (hypoxia) can affect the ability to think clearly.

   In some situations, it may be difficult or impossible to determine whether your patient is competent. An adult is generally considered incompetent if he:
   - Has an altered mental status.
   - Is under the influence of drugs or alcohol.
   - Has a serious illness or injury that affects his ability to make an informed decision about his care.
   - Has been declared legally incompetent related to a known mental disorder.

A patient who has an **altered mental status** is often referred to as *altered.* An altered patient may be "under the influence of drugs," which include legal or prescription drugs. Medical conditions such as diabetes or epilepsy can also alter a patient's mental status. Serious injuries, such as head injuries or injuries that can lead to shock, can cause a change in the patient's mental status or level of responsiveness.

It is generally believed that any amount of alcohol or drugs can affect a patient's judgment. In most cases, a patient who is under the influence of drugs or alcohol is considered incompetent. However, determining competence can be tricky. Is a person who has had one drink or two beers intoxicated or incompetent? The person may not meet the legal definition of intoxicated by blood alcohol content. Your own state laws and medical oversight authority can help you determine the definitions of intoxicated and altered.

Some patients may be judged by the courts to be mentally incompetent. Someone who is truly mentally incompetent or legally mentally incompetent will rarely be alone. A legal guardian who is able to allow or refuse care for the patient will usually be present.

Consent

Objective 10

When patients allow you to provide emergency care, they are giving you permission, or **consent.** You must have consent before assessing or treating patients. Any competent patient has the right to decide about his or her care. The patient's consent is based on the information you give the patient about his or her condition. It is also based on the treatment you will provide and the patient's understanding of that information.

Expressed Consent

Objective 11

Consent may be expressed or implied. You must obtain expressed consent from *every* mentally competent adult before you provide any medical care. Expressed consent is given by a patient who is of legal age and competent to give consent. **Expressed consent** is a type of consent in which a patient gives specific permission for care and transport to be provided. Expressed consent may be given verbally, in writing, or nonverbally. Examples of nonverbal expressed consent include allowing care to be given or a gesture such as a nod or walking to the ambulance.

Expressed consent must be **informed consent.** This means that you must give the patient enough information to make an informed decision; otherwise, the patient's expressed consent may be not considered valid. You must tell the patient what you are going to do, how you will do it, the possible risks, and the possible outcome of what is to be done. To obtain expressed consent:

- Identify yourself and your level of medical training.
- Explain all treatments and procedures to the patient.
- Identify the benefits of each treatment or procedure.
- Identify the risks of each treatment or procedure.

You must give the patient explanations using words and phrases that the patient can understand. Do not use confusing medical terms. If the patient speaks a language different from your own, you must make every attempt to find someone who can translate for you. Remember: In order for expressed consent to be valid, the patient must understand what you are saying. You must also understand what the patient is saying to you.

Remember This

A competent adult can withdraw consent at any time during care and transport.

A competent adult may agree to some medical treatments but not to others. For example, a patient with a cut on his leg may allow you to look at his injury and bandage it but refuse transport for further care. If this situation should occur, follow your local protocol. Your local protocol may require you to contact medical direction and/or call advanced life support (ALS) personnel to the scene to assess the patient and the situation.

Implied Consent

Implied consent is consent assumed from a patient requiring emergency care who is mentally, physically, or emotionally unable to provide expressed consent. Implied consent is sometimes called the *doctrine of implied consent*. Implied consent is based on the assumption that the patient would consent to lifesaving treatment if able to do so. It is effective only until the patient no longer requires emergency care or regains competence to make decisions. For example, an unresponsive diabetic patient with low blood sugar may be treated under implied consent. It is assumed that a patient with low blood sugar would want someone to give her sugar if she was unable to do this for herself. Implied consent does not allow you to treat a competent adult for a condition that is not life threatening.

Special Situations

Objective 12

Children and mentally incompetent adults must have a parent or legal guardian give consent for treatment. Each state has its own laws about when a minor attains legal age to consent to his or her own treatment. In most states, a **minor** refers to a child younger than the age of 18. State laws also address emancipated minors. An **emancipated minor** is a person who is younger than the legal age of consent but who, because of special circumstances, is given the rights of adults. In general, the courts deem an emancipated minor to be one who is married, is economically independent (living independently and is self-supporting), or is in the armed forces. Mental incompetence is also determined by state laws and sometimes involves court hearings and judgments. You must be familiar with your own state laws.

In some situations, a parent may grant permission to another person or agency to allow medical care for his or her child in an emergency. For example, many parents sign a form allowing their child's school, coach, or daycare provider to authorize care in an emergency. A life-threatening emergency may exist for a child or a mentally incompetent adult when no parent or guardian is present. In such cases, you may treat the patient under implied consent.

Remember This

Even if there is written parental consent to treat a child, make every attempt to contact the child's parents or legal guardian as soon as possible.

Refusals

Objective 13

All competent adults have the right to refuse emergency care. If your patient is a child or mentally incompetent adult, only a parent or legal guardian can refuse care on behalf of the patient. A patient's refusal of care may not always be in his or her best interest, but you cannot and should not force any competent patient to accept your care.

You Should Know

Most EMS systems in the United States require phone or radio contact with a base hospital or physician for field refusals. Research, understand, and follow your local protocol.

Examples of High-Risk Refusals

Some examples of high-risk refusals involve the following:

- Abdominal pain
- Chest pain
- Electrical shock
- Foreign body ingestion
- Poisoning
- Pregnancy-related complaints
- Water-related incidents
- Falls >20 feet
- Head injury
- Vehicle rollovers
- High-speed auto crashes
- Auto-pedestrian or auto-bicycle injury with major impact (>5 mph)
- Pedestrian thrown or run over
- Motorcycle crash >20 mph or with the separation of the rider from the bike
- Pediatric patient with a vague medical complaint

If a patient refuses treatment or transport, call advanced medical personnel to the scene as soon as possible to evaluate the patient or contact medical direction. Document any telephone or radio advice given by medical direction. In some instances, a patient who is refusing transport may allow you to perform an assessment. If so, perform an assessment, and document your findings and the patient's refusal of transport as discussed below.

Remember This

If the patient refuses to allow vital signs to be taken or will not answer your questions, make sure to document this in your report.

A refusal of care does not release you from liability if you know that the patient's condition will worsen without care and you do not attempt to inform your patient of the risks of refusing care. Make multiple attempts to try to convince the patient to accept care. You must make sure that the patient fully understands your explanation and the consequences of refusing treatment or transport. Remember to use words and phrases the patient can understand. The patient's

refusal may stem from a lack of understanding because of the effects of illness or injury, pain, or drugs or alcohol. If you have doubts about the competence of your patient, contact medical direction unless the situation is life-threatening and you have begun treatment under implied consent.

Some refusals of care carry a higher risk of legal liability than others. A patient may stumble, fall on the grass, and then refuse care because the patient is certain she is not injured. Considering the nature of the fall, the surface the patient fell on, and the lack of signs of trauma, you may agree that the patient is competent and uninjured. In situations like this, know your EMS system's policy regarding a patient's refusal of care. You may be required to contact medical direction and/or call ALS personnel to the scene to assess the patient. If the patient continues to refuse care, document the refusal.

A patient involved in a high-speed motor vehicle crash may also claim he or she has no injuries. As a trained EMT, you know that even though there are no visible injuries or signs of trauma, there may be hidden internal injuries that require transport and a physician's evaluation. If this patient chooses to refuse emergency care, it would be considered a high-risk refusal because it is likely that the patient has experienced an injury. Document the patient's refusal of care as discussed in the next *You Should Know* box.

Most EMS systems require EMTs to contact their medical oversight authority for high-risk refusals. Some systems require this contact for *any* situation in which a patient refuses treatment or transport. When contacting your medical direction authority, make sure that you clearly describe the events, your assessment, and the information you have given to the patient. This will help medical direction determine whether the patient has enough information to make an informed refusal. If so, medical direction may allow the patient to refuse care. On the basis of the information you relay, if medical direction feels the patient can refuse care but does not yet have enough information to make an informed refusal, medical direction can give you more information to share with the patient.

In some cases, such as those involving drugs or alcohol, medical direction may instruct you to treat and transport the patient against his or her wishes. In these situations, ask law enforcement personnel to help you. In some cases, law enforcement will need to ride with the patient in the ambulance. It is important that you clearly explain to law enforcement what medical direction is requesting. This will help law enforcement decide whether or not to place the patient in custody.

If a patient refuses treatment or transport and medical direction agrees that the patient can be

Documentation of a patient's refusal should include the following:

- Patient name and age
- Date of birth
- Medical history
- Two complete sets of vital signs
- Chief complaint
- Mental status exam findings (speech, gait, appropriate behavior, level of cooperation, ability to follow instructions/commands, etc.)
- Physical exam findings
- Reason for refusal
- Signed refusal form
- Advice given
- Acknowledgment that patient understands risks of refusal
- Acknowledgment that patient understands possible outcome if advice is not followed
- Any telephone or radio advice given by medical direction

allowed to refuse care, you must inform the patient of the following:

- The nature of the illness or injury
- The treatment that needs to be performed
- The benefits of that treatment
- The risks of not providing that treatment
- Any alternatives to treatment
- The dangers of refusing treatment (including transport)

If you are unable to persuade the patient (or the patient's parent or legal guardian) to allow care, you must carefully document the patient's refusal of care. In those instances in which the patient is adamantly refusing, you should ask the patient to read, understand, and sign your agency's refusal form. A sample refusal form is shown in Figure 3-1. Your chart should reflect the fact that you tried to reason with and informed your patient of the risks of not receiving care. Your documentation should also include the patient's name, age, chief complaint, medical history, and two complete sets of vital signs. You should also document details about the patient's mental status. These details include appropriate behavior, cooperation, and the patient's ability to follow instructions or commands. Document your physical examination findings and the patient's reason for refusing treatment and/or transport. Inform the patient of (and document) your willingness to

return should his condition change or should the patient change his mind (Figure 3-2).

The patient's signature should be obtained on a refusal form that notes the advice the patient was given, the patient's understanding of the risks of refusal, and the patient's understanding of the possible outcome if the advice given is not followed. The patient's signature should be witnessed by a law enforcement officer, family member, or friend. If the patient refuses to sign the refusal form, document this and then attempt to have a family member sign as a witness that the patient would not sign the form. You may also have law enforcement personnel or other healthcare professionals at the scene act as witnesses that the patient would not sign the refusal.

Advance Directives and Do Not Resuscitate Orders

Objectives 14, 15

An advance directive is a legal document that details healthcare wishes when people become unable to make decisions for themselves. Any competent patient can refuse resuscitation. What about a patient who is unresponsive? Should all unresponsive patients be treated under implied consent regardless of the circumstances?

Some patients who have been diagnosed with a terminal illness may not want further medical care, even if it could prolong their life. A patient may argue that instead of prolonging her life, you are, in fact, prolonging her death. Continued pain and suffering, a loss of dignity, and artificial life support are some of the reasons a competent patient may not want treatment or resuscitation. Whatever the reason, if it is properly documented and the documentation is available to you, you must honor the patient's request. In such cases, the legal documents are called *advance directives* or *do not resuscitate (DNR)* orders. A DNR order is a type of advance directive that is used when patients wish to outline their care for when they are terminally ill. Patients often fill out advance directive forms or ask their physicians to write DNR orders. In some cases, the patient's next of kin or legal guardian will begin this process for an unresponsive or mentally incompetent patient. When this occurs, it is generally based on what the patient would want if she was able to do this for herself.

Some patients who have a DNR do not have a terminal illness.

All 50 states have laws or protocols that address advance directives and DNR orders. A situation may

REFUSAL OF SERVICES AGAINST MEDICAL ADVICE – RELEASE OF RESPONSIBILITY

CALL NUMBER

☐☐☐☐☐☐

REFUSAL CRITERIA

The patient meets all of the following: (check all that apply)

☐ Is an adult (18 or over), or if under 18, is being released to a parent, guardian, responsible party, or law enforcement personnel.

☐ Is oriented to person, place, time, and event.

☐ Exhibits no evidence of: ☐ Altered level of consciousness ☐ Alcohol or drug ingestion that impairs judgment

☐ Understands the nature of his/her medical condition, as well as the risks and consequences of refusing care.

PATIENT/ GUARDIAN/ POWER OF ATTORNEY HAS BEEN ADVISED: (check all that apply)

☐ That it is the preference of the attending EMT/Paramedic to arrange for transport to the closest appropriate medical facility for further evaluation and treatment.

☐ That an ambulance is available for transportation to the closest appropriate medical facility for treatment.

☐ That transport by means other than by ambulance could be hazardous and is not recommended based upon current condition/complaint, specific injury, or medical illness.

☐ That significant risk(s) could be involved with refusal of EMS treatment and/or transportation, related from, but not limited to; exacerbation of present complaint / condition / injuries, or the possibility of significant disability and/or death occurring from refusal of emergent medical care or transportation.

☐ Patient has been informed of their right to refuse prehospital treatment and/or offer of transport to an appropriate medical facility (after being advised of potential complications) and understands the consequences of his/her decision.

☐ Should the patient change his/her mind or if his/her condition changes, he/she has been advised to contact the healthcare provider of his/her choice (9-1-1, personal physician, emergency department, or urgent care center in his/her area) to address his/her medical needs.

The following section must be signed by the patient, nearest relative, legal guardian, or responsible party/authority in the case of a minor or when the patient is physically or mentally incompetent.

It is my choice and at my own insistence, I _____ elect not to receive ☐ Assessment ☐ Treatment ☐ Transportation against the advice of the attending EMT/Paramedic(s) and the _____ (EMS Agency) and, when applicable, the base hospital physician. The potential risks associated with my refusal have been explained to me before my signature on this document, which includes risk of serious illness, injury, and death. I hereby release the attending Emergency Medical Technician/Paramedic, _____ (EMS Agency) and its employees, officials, agents, volunteers, and when applicable, the base hospital and the base hospital physician from further responsibility for my well-being. I understand there may be injuries or complications not known to EMS personnel at this time, but which may result in further illness, injury, permanent disability, or death. I further deny being physically or mentally impaired by the use of drugs or alcohol. If I change my mind or if my condition changes, I have been advised to contact the healthcare provider of my choice (9-1-1, personal physician, emergency department or urgent care center in my area) to address my medical needs. I also acknowledge that I have been provided with a copy of the _____ (EMS Agency) Notice of Privacy Practices that describes how my health information is used and shared.

I have received and read the above information and am voluntarily signing this release without undue stress, duress, and without pressure.

_____
Patient / Responsible Party Signature
Firma del Paciente / Persona Responsable

_____
Witness
Testigo

_____
Witness
Testigo

Relationship: ☐ Self ☐ _____

If released in care of custody of relative or friend: _____
Name

_____
Relationship

If released in custody of law enforcement agency: _____
Officer's Signature

_____
Agency

FIGURE 3-1 ▲ Sample EMS refusal form.

TIME	PULSE (RATE/QUALITY)	BP	RESP RATE	BREATH SOUNDS / RESP EFFORT		PUPILS	SKIN	SPO2
								☐RA ☐O2
PT REFUSED ALL VITAL SIGNS X3 ATTEMPTS				1.CLEAR ☑ NONLABORED 2.CRACKLES ☐ LABORED 3.RHONCHI ☐ RETRACTIONS 4.WHEEZES ☐ NASAL FLARING 5.DIMINISHED ☐ GRUNTING				☐RA ☐O2 ☐RA ☐O2
								☐RA ☐O2
								☐RA ☐O2

LOC U/A ☑ AWAKE ☑ ALERT ORIENTED: ☑ PERSON ☑ PLACE ☑ TIME ☑ EVENT ☐ VERBAL ☐ PAIN ☐ UNRESP

LOSS OF CONSCIOUSNESS ☐ YES ☑ NO ☐ UNK   **PEDS** AGE–APPROPRIATE? ☐ YES ☐ NO CAP REFILL:

CHIEF COMPLAINT MOTOR VEHICLE CRASH

U/A PT found standing outside vehicle in street next to a 2-car MVC with moderate damage. Pt stated no need for ambulance. Pt states husband was driving when car pulled in front of them making a U-turn and they broadsided a 4-door car. Estimated speed 25-35 mph. Pt was restrained passenger. Airbag deployed. Pt denies alcohol or drugs. Pt states in no physical distress. Pt states she has soreness in both knees and lower back. Denies head, neck, upper back, abdominal, or pelvic pain/soreness. Denies headache, dizziness, loss of consciousness, SOB, CP, and n/v. Pt ambulatory w/o assistance. Pt repeatedly refused assessment including vital signs on scene.

Head / Face / Airway	Pt advised that amlulance on scene and transport for	
Neck	evaluation recommended. Pt declined stating that if pain she would go to MD later. Pt told to go to	
Chest	MD or call 9-1-1 if sudden increase in pain in areas of complaint or sudden onset of pain in	O
	any area. Contacted G Smith MD @ 2210. Orders: Review refusal form with pt.	P
Abd	Ok to refuse treatment/transport. Refusal form	Q
Pelvis	reviewed with pt. Pt verbalized understanding of risks of refusal. Pt and witness signatures obtained.	R
Back		S
Ext		T

FIGURE 3-2 ▲ Sample of an actual EMS refusal narrative for a patient involved in a motor vehicle crash.

occur in which you have doubts about the legality of the order or it does not fit within the protocols of your agency. In this case, it is best to err on the side of caution and begin resuscitation. If the patient or family members on the scene request resuscitation efforts despite the presence of an advance directive, you should immediately begin resuscitation and contact medical direction.

If you arrive on the scene to find that a patient is not breathing, has no pulse, and an advance directive is present:

- Make sure the form clearly identifies the person to whom the DNR applies.
- Make sure the patient is the person referred to in the document.
- Make sure the document you are viewing is the correct type approved by your state and local authorities.

If you determine that the document is valid, follow the instructions outlined in the document.

You Should Know

You must know your local protocol regarding advance directives before you are faced with a situation involving one. In situations involving a patient's death, your local protocol may require contacting medical direction and/or calling ALS personnel to the scene (if available in your area) to confirm that the patient is dead.

Different types of DNR orders exist. In some states, a DNR order may specify that the patient does not want CPR or a shock to the heart if it stops beating. However, the patient may want (and expect) oxygen to be given. The patient may also want medications (given by ALS personnel). Alternatively, a DNR order may specifically state that the patient does not want any resuscitative measures, including CPR, heart shocks, and medications.

Some states recognize only a specific form of advance directive for EMS personnel, regardless of similar forms issued by private physicians or hospitals. Figure 3-3 is an example of the Prehospital Medical Care Directive form currently used in Arizona. This form is considered valid if it is printed on an orange background and includes specific wording on the form. Arizona EMS personnel are not required to accept or interpret medical care directives that do not meet these specific requirements. A person who has a valid Prehospital Medical Care Directive may wear an identifying bracelet on either the wrist or the ankle. In Arizona, the bracelet must be on an orange background and state three specific pieces of information: (1) Do not resuscitate, (2) the patient's name, and (3) the patient's physician. You must be familiar with the laws of your own state and the protocols of your agency and medical direction authority.

What should you do if you are called to a scene where a patient is seriously ill or injured and has a valid

PREHOSPITAL MEDICAL CARE DIRECTIVE

IN THE EVENT OF CARDIAC OR RESPIRATORY ARREST, I REFUSE ANY RESUSCITATION MEASURES INCLUDING CARDIAC COMPRESSION, ENDOTRACHEAL INTUBATION AND OTHER ADVANCED AIRWAY MANAGEMENT, ARTIFICIAL VENTILATION, DEFIBRILLATION, ADMINISTRATION OF ADVANCED CARDIAC LIFE SUPPORT DRUGS AND RELATED EMERGENCY MEDICAL PROCEDURES.

Patient: _____ Date: _____
                  (Signature or mark)

Attach recent photograph here or provide all of the following information below:

Date of Birth _____

Sex _____ Race _____

Eye Color _____

Hair Color _____

(Attach photo here)

Hospice Program (if any) _____

Name and telephone number of patient's physician _____

_____

I have explained this form and its consequences to the signer and obtained assurance that the signer understands that death may result from any refused care listed above.

_____ Date: _____
          (Licensed health care provider)

I was present when this was signed (or marked). The patient then appeared to be of sound mind and free from duress.

_____ Date: _____
          (Witness)

FIGURE 3-3 ▲ Sample Prehospital Medical Care Directive form.

DNR order, but is not in full cardiac or respiratory arrest? Because some EMS personnel interpret the existence of a DNR order as "do not treat," confusion may exist in situations like this. As previously stated, you must be familiar with your state laws and the protocols of your agency and medical direction authority. Unless specified otherwise by your state laws or protocols, if the patient's heartbeat and breathing are adequate, treat within your scope of practice and transport as appropriate. If the patient has a valid DNR order and is not in full respiratory or cardiac arrest, but his or her heartbeat or breathing is inadequate, provide treatment within the scope of your practice and transport as appropriate. Providing **comfort care** means giving care to ease the symptoms of an illness or injury. Comfort care is also called *palliative care* or *supportive care*. Unless specified otherwise by your state laws or protocols, comfort care includes providing emotional support, suctioning the airway, giving oxygen, controlling bleeding, splinting, and positioning the patient for comfort.

Physician Orders for Life-Sustaining Treatment (POLST), which is also called *Medical Orders for Life-Sustaining Treatment (MOLST),* programs exist in some states and are in development in others. The program is recommended for individuals with an advanced chronic progressive illness or terminal illness or patients interested in further defining their end-of-life care wishes. After an extensive discussion with the patient, a physician uses a POLST form to document do not resuscitate orders, do not intubate (DNI) orders, and/or other life-sustaining treatments such as the use of antibiotics, artificially administered fluids, and nutrition. Although the POLST form summarizes advance directives, it does not replace an advance directive. An advance directive applies when an individual loses decision-making capability about healthcare wishes. Use of the POLST form is not conditional on losing decision-making capacity. The color of the POLST form may be bright pink or lime green depending on the state in which the form is used. The form transfers with the patient from one care setting to another (such as home, emergency department, and long-term care facility). Check with your instructor to find out if a POLST program exists in your state.

Remember This

Although a patient may have an advance directive, you must obtain consent for medical treatment from the patient as long as the patient is able to make decisions about healthcare.

Remember This

When looking for an advance directive or POLST form in a patient's home, be sure to look on the refrigerator, behind the patient's bedroom door, and on or in bedside tables and the medicine cabinet.

Assault and Battery

Objective 16

When you hear the words "assault and battery," you may be thinking of some form of physical aggression or attack by one person on another. In medicine, assault and battery are not necessarily defined as attacking or physically striking a patient. Touching a competent adult patient without his or her consent can be considered assault or battery.

There are no universal definitions of assault and battery. Each state has its own laws and definitions. In most states, **assault** is considered to be threatening, attempting, or causing a fear of offensive physical contact with a patient or another person. **Battery** is the unlawful touching of another person without consent. Check your local protocols and definitions concerning these terms. To protect yourself from possible legal action, clearly explain your intentions to your patients and obtain their consent before beginning patient care.

Abandonment

Objective 17

Abandonment is terminating patient care without making sure that care will continue at the same level or higher. You can be charged with abandonment if you turn the patient over to another healthcare professional who has less medical training than you have. You can also be charged with abandonment if you stop patient care when the patient still needs and desires additional care.

Stop and Think!

If a scene is unsafe, it is not abandonment if you leave the scene for your safety with the intention of returning as soon as the scene is made safe. Your safety comes first.

Once you have begun patient care, you must complete it to the best of your ability. Patient care may be transferred to another healthcare professional if that person accepts the patient and has medical qualifications equal to or greater than yours.

Remember This

Once you have begun patient care, you must continue to provide care until it is no longer needed or patient care is transferred to another healthcare professional whose medical qualifications are equal to or greater than yours.

Negligence

Objective 18

Negligence is a deviation from the accepted standard of care, resulting in further injury to the patient. A healthcare professional is negligent if he or she fails to act as a reasonable, careful, similarly trained person would act under similar circumstances. Negligence is the cause of most lawsuits filed against EMS personnel. Four elements must be present to prove negligence: (1) There was a legal duty to act, (2) the healthcare professional breached that duty, (3) injury and/or damages (physical or psychological) were inflicted, and (4) the actions or inactions of the healthcare professional caused the injury and/or damage (proximate cause). A successful negligence lawsuit can result in loss of the healthcare professional's certification or licensure and financial penalties.

You Should Know

Components of Negligence
1. You had a legal duty to act.
2. You breached that duty.
3. Injury and/or damages were inflicted.
4. Your actions or lack of actions caused the injury and/or damage.

Duty to Act

Objective 19

The first element that must be proved in a negligence lawsuit is a **duty to act**. The duty to act may be either a formal, contractual duty or an implied duty. A formal duty occurs when an EMS service has a written contract to provide services. For example, an EMS service may have a formal contract with a community that requires a response to 9-1-1 calls. An ambulance service may have a formal contract with a long-term care facility. Written contracts usually contain clauses that state when service to a patient must be provided or may be refused.

An implied duty occurs, for example, when a patient calls 9-1-1 and the dispatcher confirms that an EMT will be sent. If you are the EMT sent to the scene, you have an implied legal obligation (duty) to care for the patient. When you begin patient care, you have established an implied contract with the patient.

A legal duty to act may not exist. In some states, off-duty EMTs have no legal duty to act if they observe or come upon an emergency. In other states, off-duty healthcare professionals are required to stop and provide care. In some states, any citizen must stop. Check your state laws and EMS agency's policies and procedures regarding your obligation to provide care if you are off duty. Although a legal duty to act may not exist, a moral or ethical duty to act may exist. You must decide if you are morally or ethically bound to provide care in emergency situations.

Making a Difference

Whether you provide patient care on or off duty, the care you provide must be the same as the care another reasonable, prudent (sensible), similarly trained person would provide under similar circumstances.

Breach of Duty

The second element that must be proved in a negligence lawsuit is that a **breach of duty** occurred. A breach of duty occurs when the standard of care that applies in a given situation is violated. Healthcare professionals can perform skills and provide treatment only within their scope of practice. Performing skills or treatments outside your scope of practice can lead to a breach of duty.

A breach of duty may be proved if you failed to act or you acted inappropriately. If you are dispatched to a scene to assist a patient and choose not to respond to the call, you are failing to act. If you respond to the call and act outside your scope of practice or do not complete an assessment or perform all treatments indicated, you are failing to act appropriately.

Remember This

Whatever the situation, you must act as a similarly trained EMT would in a similar situation.

Damages

The third element that must be proved in a negligence case is injury or damage done to the patient. Damages occur if the patient is injured, either physically or psychologically, by your breach of duty.

Proximate Cause

Proximate cause is established when:

- Your action or inaction was either the cause of or contributed to the patient's injury.
- You could reasonably foresee that your action or inaction would result in the damage.

Attorneys usually use statements (testimony) from expert witnesses to prove that an EMT either failed to act or acted inappropriately and that these actions or inactions were the cause of the patient's injury. Expert witnesses can include other EMTs, paramedics, nurses, and doctors.

You can protect yourself against negligence claims by:
- Maintaining your professional attitude and conduct
- Providing care and treatment within your scope of practice

- Maintaining mastery of your skills
- Participating in continuing education and refresher programs
- Following instructions provided by your medical oversight authority
- Following your standing orders or protocols
- Providing your patients with a consistently high standard of care
- Making sure your documentation is thorough and accurate

Confidentiality

Objective 20

Health Insurance Portability and Accountability Act

The **Health Insurance Portability and Accountability Act (HIPAA)** went into effect in 2003. This law was passed by Congress in 1996 to ensure the confidentiality of a patient's health information. HIPAA does the following:

- Provides patients with control over their health information
- Sets boundaries on the use and release of medical records
- Ensures the security of personal health information
- Establishes accountability for the use and release of medical records

Individuals who disobey HIPAA privacy rules face criminal and civil penalties. Some important points about HIPAA include the following:

- Patients have the right to review and copy their medical records. Patients can also request amendments and corrections to these records.
- Healthcare providers (and insurance plans) must tell patients with whom they are sharing their information and how it is being used.

The effects of HIPAA are widespread in medicine. As an EMT, you must protect and keep confidential any health-related information about your patients. You must keep confidential any medical history given to you in a patient interview. You must also keep private any findings you may discover during your patient assessment and any care that you provide. Releasing patient information without proper permission may lead to charges of libel or slander. **Libel** is injuring a person's character, name, or reputation by false and malicious writings. **Slander** is injuring a person's character, name, or reputation by false and malicious spoken words.

Stop and Think!

The HIPAA privacy rules are very complex. A breach of a person's health privacy can have a major impact beyond the physical health of that person. This breach can result in the loss of a job, the alienation of family and friends, the loss of health insurance, and public humiliation. Be sure to check with your EMS agency about its policies regarding patient confidentiality.

Protected Health Information (PHI)

PHI is information that:

- Relates to a person's physical or mental health, treatment, or payment
- Identifies the person or gives a reason to believe that the individual can be identified
- Is transmitted or maintained in *any* format, including oral statements, electronic information, written material, and photographic material

You may use and disclose the patient's PHI for three purposes without any written consent, authorization, or other approvals from the patient. These purposes are treatment, payment, and healthcare operations. Before the patient's PHI is used or disclosed for any reason other than treatment, payment, or healthcare operations, a signed authorization form must usually be obtained from the patient or the patient's authorized representative.

In some situations, you can disclose specific PHI without the patient's authorization. These situations require an opportunity for the patient to verbally agree or object to the disclosure of information. These situations include:

- Disclosures to the patient's next of kin or to another person (designated by the patient) involved in the patient's healthcare
- Notification of a family member (or the patient's personal representative) of the patient's location, general condition, or death
- Disaster situations

Remember This

Be sure to follow your agency's policies when disclosing any PHI. If you are in doubt, contact your supervisor or ask the patient's permission before you release any information.

Persons involved in the patient's care and other contact persons might include blood relatives, spouses, roommates, boyfriends and girlfriends, domestic partners, neighbors, and colleagues. In these situations, disclose only the minimum information necessary. The information you share should be directly related to the person's involvement with the patient's healthcare.

If the patient is injured or in cases of an emergency, you may use your professional judgment to decide if sharing PHI is in the patient's best interest. For example, you may tell your patient's relatives or others involved in the patient's care that he may have experienced a heart attack. You may also provide updates on the patient's condition. In such situations, reveal only the PHI that is directly relevant to the person's involvement with the patient's healthcare.

The patient's consent, authorization, or opportunity to agree or object to the release of PHI is not required in some situations. Examples of these situations include the following:

- When you are required by law to provide this information
- Due to public health activities, such as injury/disease control and prevention
- When the patient is a victim of abuse, neglect, or domestic violence
- For judicial and administrative proceedings
- For specific law enforcement purposes
- To avoid a serious threat to health or safety

You may accidentally reveal PHI when you are caring for a patient. Accidental disclosures usually occur during a radio or face-to-face conversation between healthcare professionals. You may freely discuss all aspects of your patient's medical condition, the treatment you gave, and any of the patient's health information you have with others involved in the patient's medical care. However, when discussing patient information with another healthcare professional, take a moment to look around you. Be sensitive to your level of voice. Make sure that persons who do not need to know this information are not able to hear what is said.

An accidental disclosure may also occur when information about a patient is left out in the open for others to access or see. For example, a prehospital care report may be left on a desk or may be visible on a computer screen when you leave to respond to another call. You must maintain the confidence and security of all material you create or use that contains patient care information. Prehospital care reports should not be left in open bins, on desktops, or on other surfaces. Store them in safe and secure areas. When using a computer, be aware of those who may be able to view the monitor screen. Take simple steps to shield the screen from unauthorized persons.

Special Situations

Medical Identification Devices

You may respond to a call and find the patient wearing medical identification. The identification device may be in the form of a bracelet, a necklace, or an identification card. Medical identification is used to alert healthcare personnel to a patient's particular medical condition. For example, the patient may have diabetes, epilepsy, a heart condition, or a specific allergy. You must consider this information while performing your assessment and patient interview.

Remember This

Even if a patient is wearing a medical identification device, you must always perform a thorough patient assessment. The reason you were called may be completely different from the condition described by the medical identification device the patient is wearing or carrying.

Crime Scenes

Objective 21

During your career as an EMT, you may be dispatched to a crime scene. A crime scene is the responsibility of law enforcement personnel. As an EMT, you are responsible for ensuring your own safety and then providing care for the patient. Your dispatcher should notify you of the potential crime scene at the time you are sent to the call. You may be required to stage (remain at a safe distance) and wait for an "all clear" from law enforcement personnel before entering the scene and providing patient care. Even after law enforcement personnel have declared the scene is safe to enter, you must always assess the scene yourself and ensure your safety. After you are certain the scene is safe, your first priority will be patient care.

Making a Difference

It is important to understand your obligations in providing patient care and balancing your other responsibilities on the scene. For example, a law enforcement officer may need to delay your treatment of patients until a crime scene has been secured.

Crime scenes demand certain actions and responsibilities from medical personnel. For example, you should protect potential evidence by leaving intact any holes in clothing from bullets or stab wounds. Do not disturb any item at the scene unless emergency care requires that you do so. You should always be alert and observe and document anything unusual on a call. These actions are especially important at a crime scene. You may be called to testify in court about what you observed at the scene.

Consider talking with law enforcement personnel on the scene to discuss various crime scene issues:

- Possible victim and suspect statements
- Evidence you observed
- Collection of shoe prints from EMTs for comparison
- The names of all personnel on the scene, including EMTs and fire personnel

Special Reporting Requirements

Objective 22

State or local laws and regulations or agency protocols require that you report certain situations or conditions that you know or suspect have occurred. For example, you are required to report known or suspected abuse of a child or an elderly person and, in some locations, a spouse. You must also report injuries that may have occurred during the commission of a crime, such as gunshot and knife wounds. EMS agencies require that you report exposure to an infectious disease. Because state and local reporting requirements vary, you must learn the requirements for your area and act accordingly.

You Should Know

Generally, you will report special situations such as those mentioned here to law enforcement or the emergency department staff.

Multiple-Casualty Incidents

Multiple-casualty incidents (MCIs) are events that place a great demand on resources—equipment, personnel, or both (such as an airplane crash) and will be covered in detail in Chapter 51. In an MCI, comprehensive documentation must often wait until after the casualties are triaged and transported. You must know and follow local procedures for documentation in these situations. The local MCI plan should include a means of temporarily recording patient information (such as using triage tags, shown in Figure 3-4) that can be used later to complete the prehospital care report (PCR).

Organ Donation

Objective 23

An organ donor is a person who has signed a legal document to donate his organs in the event of his death. This document may be an organ donor card that the patient carries in his wallet. Alternatively, the patient may have indicated his intent to be a donor on his driver's license.

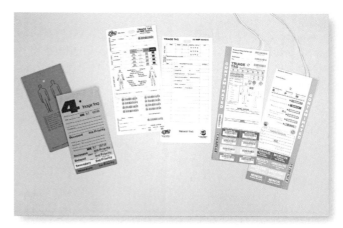

FIGURE 3-4 ▲ In a multiple-casualty incident, triage tags are often used to record patient information.

Family members may also tell you that the patient is an organ donor. A patient who is a potential organ donor should not be treated differently from any other patient who requires your care. Your responsibilities include:

- Providing any necessary emergency care
- Notifying EMS or hospital personnel that the patient is a potential organ donor when you transfer patient care

Documentation

A prehospital care report is known by many names (see the next *You Should Know* box). No matter its name in your area, a PCR is a legal record that documents the patient care delivered in the field. Healthcare professionals use the information in the PCR to begin appropriate treatment after the patient arrives at the receiving facility. Inaccurate, illegible, or incomplete information on the prehospital care report regarding the patient's condition, assessment, and care can have grave consequences. Every emergency medical technician must learn to document accurately, legibly, and completely (Figure 3-5).

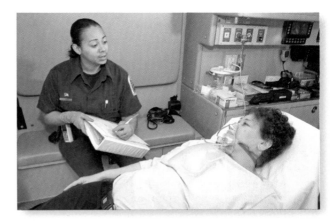

FIGURE 3-5 ▲ An EMT must document accurately, legibly, and completely.

The prehospital care report may also be called the:

- Patient care report
- Run report
- Encounter form
- EMS form
- Run sheet
- Trip sheet
- Incident report
- Ambulance report

The Uses of a Prehospital Care Report

Objective 24

Medical Uses

One of the most important necessities of giving prehospital medical care is the thorough, honest, and complete documentation of that care. Your accurate observation and documentation of the patient's vital signs, medical history, mental status, medications, allergies, and related patient information is very important to the paramedics, physicians, and nurses who will assume the care of your patient. Thus, the PCR is important in helping ensure continued patient care. The PCR may be the only source of information that hospital personnel can refer to later. This report may include important information about the scene, the patient's condition on arrival at the scene, the emergency medical care provided or attempted, and any changes in the patient's condition.

Legal Uses

The PCR is an official record of the care given by EMS. When you transfer patient care to another healthcare professional, you are expected to give a verbal report of what occurred while the patient was in your care. You are also expected to provide that individual with a completed PCR. Your completed PCR becomes part of the patient's medical record.

Because a PCR is a legal document, it must accurately reflect the events that occurred and the time they occurred. When skills are performed, accurately document who performed them and the time they were done. For example, if oxygen was given, document the device used, the time it was applied, who applied it, the liter flow used, and the patient's response to the care given. At a minimum, the patient's response should include a description of mental status, skin color, and oxygen saturation level (if available).

Remember This

Pay attention to time intervals when documenting.

A patient's attorney will often request a copy of a PCR when researching a patient's complaint about care. A poorly documented PCR is more likely to cause a jury to find liability against an EMT than a well-documented report. PCRs that contain "red flags" cause individuals who read the report to question the facts about the emergency care given to a patient. Examples of documentation red flags that must be avoided are shown in the following *Remember This* box.

Remember This

Documentation Red Flags

- It is incomplete.
- It is vague.
- Opinions are included.
- Labeling is used.
- It is late.
- It is inaccurate.
- It is illegible.
- It has been altered.
- The report is missing.

Administrative Uses

A PCR not only provides an accurate record of the circumstances of the patient encounter but also enables the billing department to honestly and accurately bill the appropriate agency or individual for your services. The PCR may also be used to collect agency or service statistics. Examples of statistics that are often assessed in an EMS system include response times, number of calls in which a lights-and-siren response was used, number of interfacility transports, and the number of calls to 9-1-1 for which the patient subsequently refused transport.

Monitoring and evaluating data allow administrative staff to measure the agency's performance, determine whether additional resources are required, and compare performance with similar agencies. Careful analysis of response times may show that your agency needs additional staffing and units at certain times of day and in specific locations. This makes the use of accurate and synchronous clocks very important to the appropriate and timely response to calls for help.

Failing to obtain a signature from the patient at the time of service is a common reason for billing errors. If you are unable to obtain a signature from the patient, be sure to document why the patient was unable to sign. If another person signs the form instead of the patient, document the identity of the signer and the relationship of the signer to the patient.

Educational and Research Uses

PCRs may also be used for educational purposes to show proper documentation and how to handle unusual or uncommon calls. A patient's refusal of treatment and/or transport is an example of a situation that requires careful documentation. EMS agencies often hold continuing education sessions with their personnel to discuss patient refusals and show examples of proper documentation in these situations.

Data obtained from the PCR may be collected and used for research. The medical information that you gather about your patient is intended to help you give the most appropriate care possible. In many instances the protocols or treatments that you use have been developed with information from the research of similar types of calls. Careful study of your patient's response to currently recommended care may reveal a better way to treat this type of problem. Your careful documentation may assist with the care of more than just the patients you treat.

The PCR may also be used to determine the frequency with which an EMT performs specific patient care procedures and determine continuing education needs. For instance, the training officer in your EMS agency may notice that the EMS unit to which you are assigned responds to many trauma calls but not to many pediatric calls. The training officer may schedule a continuing education session for you and your partner to review pediatric assessment and vital signs to make sure that you remain competent in performing these skills.

Quality Management

The information contained in your PCR can and will be used to assess the quality of emergency medical care given to the patient. Most EMS agencies have developed standards for documentation that they expect you to use when completing your report. Completed reports are typically evaluated for:

- Adequacy of documentation
- Compliance with local rules and regulations
- Compliance with agency documentation standards
- Appropriateness of medical care

Making a Difference

Imagine for a moment that you have just finished an EMS call and put the "final touches" on the PCR. If your local newspaper or television news station obtained a copy of that report tomorrow and printed it or aired it for all to see, would you be proud of what you wrote? Would the report reflect the EMS professional that you are? Or would it paint a different picture of you?

The Uses of a Prehospital Care Report

- Medical use (to ensure continued patient care)
- Legal record
- Administrative use (billing as well as agency/service statistics)
- Education
- Research (data collection)
- Quality management

Elements of the Prehospital Care Report

Objective 25

The National Highway Traffic Safety Administration (NHTSA), the Trauma/EMS Systems program of the Health Resources and Services Administration (HRSA), and the National Association of State EMS Directors have been working together to develop a national EMS database. The National Emergency Medical Services Information System (NEMSIS) is the database that will be used to store EMS data from every state in the nation (see the next *You Should Know* box).

The information collected will be useful in the following:

- Developing nationwide EMS training curricula
- Evaluating patient and EMS system outcomes
- Facilitating research efforts
- Determining national fee schedules and reimbursement rates
- Addressing resources for disaster and domestic preparedness
- Providing valuable information on other issues or areas of need related to EMS care

Components of the National EMS Information System

- Dispatch data
- Incident data
- Patient data
  - —Demographics
  - —Medical history
  - —Assessment
  - —Medical device data
  - —Treatment/medications
  - —Procedures
  - —Disposition
- Injury/trauma data
- Cardiac arrest data
- Financial data
- EMS system demographic data
- EMS personnel demographic data
- Quality management indicators
- Outcome indicators
- Domestic terrorism data
- Linkage data

The recommended minimum information that should be included in a PCR is called the **minimum data set** (see the following *Remember This* box).

Remember This

Minimum Data for a Prehospital Care Report

Administrative Information

- Time incident reported to 9-1-1
- Time unit notified
- Time of arrival at patient
- Time unit left scene
- Time of arrival at destination
- Time of transfer of care

Patient Information

- Chief complaint
- Mechanism of injury or nature of illness
- Level of consciousness
- Breathing rate and effort
- Heart rate
- Skin perfusion (capillary refill) for patients younger than 6 years of age
- Skin color and temperature
- Systolic blood pressure for patients older than 3 years of age

Administrative or Dispatch Information Section

Objectives 25, 26

Statistical information pertaining to an EMS call is known by many names (see the following *You Should Know* box).

The statistical portion of a PCR may also be called:

- Run data
- Alarm information
- Alarm history
- Call information
- Dispatch information
- Administrative information
- Statistical data
- Incident information

Examples of additional statistical information that may be required by some EMS agencies is shown in the following *You Should Know* box. Table 3-1 gives examples of how to complete the administrative section of the PCR. The administrative section of a sample PCR is shown in Figure 3-6 on p.100.

Additional Statistical Information

- Shift
- Type of incident
- Time unit en route to hospital
- Arrival at hospital
- Hospital destination
- Time unit available for service
- Total number of patients
- Extrication time
- Additional EMS units on the scene
- Transport type (ground ambulance, air ambulance)
- Transport mode (with or without lights and siren)
- Mileage to the scene, to the hospital, and total mileage
- Employee numbers of the responding EMS unit

When mileage is recorded for billing purposes, it must include four digits and must be accurate to the tenth of a mile. Your agency must establish the appropriate guidelines for this information per federal requirements. Inappropriate documentation or falsification of this information has severe consequences.

TABLE 3-1 Completing the Administrative Section of a Prehospital Care Report

Form Field	Explanation	Example
Alarm number	All calls should have a unique number for tracking purposes. In most cases, this number will be provided by your dispatch center.	2009-12857
Alarm date	Enter the date the call was received, using the date format MM/DD/YY (unless specified otherwise by your EMS agency). If the call *originated* 12 minutes before midnight on 01/01/09 but was completed at 0043 on 01/02/09, the date entered as the *dispatch* date would be 01/01/09.	01/01/09
Unit number or name	Enter your unit's designated radio call sign or unit descriptor.	Medic 51
Alarm time	This is the time that the dispatch center received the call. All times are generally entered as military time. Note: All times should be recorded from accurate and synchronous clocks.	2348
Dispatch time	This is the time that your unit is notified of the call by the dispatch center.	2349
Unit en route	This is the time that your unit begins travel to the scene.	2350
Arrival time	This entry is the time that your unit arrives at or on the scene.	2354
Patient contact	This entry is the time that you make contact with the patient. In some cases, the arrival time and patient contact time may be the same if the patient is waiting for EMS arrival. But in many cases, the arrival time and patient contact time differ. This is because the EMS crew must park the vehicle and then make entry into the patient's home or other location. Additional delays may occur if the scene is not safe to enter and the EMS crew must stage (wait at a safe distance) for law enforcement personnel to secure the scene.	2357
Time unit left scene	If the patient is not transported (or if the patient is transported but your EMS unit is not the transport vehicle), this is the time that your unit leaves the scene. If the patient is transported in your unit, this is the time your unit leaves with the patient toward the destination. (It is not when the patient is placed in the back of the ambulance.)	0015
Time of arrival at destination	This is the time your unit arrives on the grounds of the receiving facility or helicopter landing zone.	0025
Time of transfer of care	This is the time that you transfer care to the receiving facility.	0038
Time unit available	This is the time that your unit is back in service and available for another call.	0043

CALL NUMBER							ALARM DATE				ALARM TIME				DISPATCH TIME				UNIT RPT				ARRIVAL TIME				PT CONTACT		
0	9	1	2	8	5	7	0	1	0	9	2	3	4	8	2	3	4	9	M	5	1		2	3	5	4	2	3	5	7

PT#		TOTAL PTS		LEFT SCENE				DEST ARRIVAL				TRANSFER CARE				AVAILABLE			
0	1	0	1	0	0	1	5	0	0	2	5	0	0	3	8	0	0	4	3

BLOCK NUMBER			DIR		STREET NAME								CITY							ZIP					
1	2	3		W	M	A	I	N		S	T			A	N	Y	T	O	W	N	7	6	1	2	3	

FIGURE 3-6 ▲ The administrative section of a sample PCR.

Patient and Scene Information

Objectives 25, 26

The patient and scene information section of the PCR requires the entry of patient information, including the patient's name, age, address, gender, and weight (Figure 3-7). If the patient is stable, this information is usually obtained while taking the patient's medical history. If the patient is unstable, the minimum information necessary is obtained (such as name and age) on the scene. The rest is obtained on arrival at the receiving facility. This information should be collected from each patient, even if your agency does not perform any billing for EMS. Table 3-2 gives examples of how to complete the patient and scene information portion of a PCR.

TABLE 3-2	**Completing the Patient Information Section of a Prehospital Care Report**	
Form Field	**Explanation**	**Example**
Scene location	This is the location of the patient or scene. This address may differ from the patient's address information. Include street address, city, state, and zip code.	123 W Main Street Anytown, TX 76123
Number of patients	This number is typically noted as 1 of *x*. The first number represents the patient for whom you are filling out the form, and the second number represents the total number of patients at the scene (such as 1 of 3). Each patient will require an additional report completed in its entirety. You may not list multiple patients on the same report.	1 of 3
Patient name	Print the patient's complete first name, middle initial, and last name. Do not use nicknames or abbreviations. It is very important to confirm spelling and include *Sr., Jr.,* or *II* after the last name, if appropriate.	Thomas R. Nixon
Patient gender	Mark whether the patient is male or female.	Male
Patient mailing address	This is the patient's mailing address and may differ from the scene location information. Include street address, city, state, and zip code.	123 W Main Street Anytown, TX 76123
Patient weight (in kilograms)	Enter the patient's current weight in kilograms. If you do not calculate the weight in kilograms, then enter the patient's weight in pounds (lb) and note it on your chart.	80 kg
Patient age	Enter the patient's date of birth, and calculate the patient's age. Use months or days as needed for patients younger than 2 years of age.	75 years
Social Security number	If needed for billing purposes, enter the patient's Social Security number. You may need to inform the patient that all information gathered as part of the care is confidential and may be released only to other healthcare providers.	123-45-6789
Patient phone number	Enter the patient's phone number, including the area code.	(123) 456-7890

NAME	FIRST	MIDDLE	LAST	**AGE**		75	**GENDER**		**WEIGHT**		80	MEDS SENT WITH PATIENT? ✓
	Thomas	R	NIXON	(YRS) MOS WKS DAYS			(M) F		LBS (KG)			

ADDRESS–SAA ☑		**ALLERGIES**	☐ NONE ☐ UNK ☑ PENICILLIN,	**TRIAGE DECISION**
CITY STATE ZIP		DEMEROL, CODEINE		☐ CLOSEST APPROPRIATE FACILITY
Rx ☐ DENIES ☐ UNK		**DR / GROUP**	☐NONE ☐UNK ☑ G SMITH MD	☑ PT/FAMILY REQUEST
METOPROLOL, FUROSEMIDE,		**PMH**	☐DENIES ☐UNK ☐ALZHEIMER'S ☐ASTHMA	☐ TRAUMA TRIAGE
LISINOPRIL, ATROVENT, ASPIRIN		☐CA ☑CARDIAC ☐CONTAGIOUS ☐COPD ☑CVA/TIA ☐DIABETES		☐ MEDICAL DIRECTION ORDER
		☐DRUGS/ETOH ☐GERD ☐HEAD INJURY ☑HTN ☐PACER/ICD		☐
		☐PREGNANCY G P DUE DATE LMP		
		☐PSYCH ☐SEIZURES ☐GALLBLADDER REMOVED 2002		

FIGURE 3-7 ▲ The patient information section of a sample PCR.

Patient Assessment Section

Objectives 25, 26

The patient assessment section of the PCR is also called the *narrative section* of the form (Figure 3-8). Some EMS forms (both paper and electronic) consist of check boxes to record patient assessment information. Other EMS forms have a combination of boxes and blank lines on which you are expected to write a short story (narrative), using information gathered from the patient interview and your assessment findings. Some EMS systems, such as those in Maryland and North Carolina, use web-based electronic reporting (Figure 3-9). Some electronic systems will ask you to check boxes and then will create a short narrative based on your entries. When documenting using check boxes, be sure to fill in the box completely and avoid stray marks. No matter the form of documentation you use, it is your responsibility as an EMS professional to be sure that all documentation is accurate and complete.

TIME	PULSE (RATE/QUALITY)	BP	RESP RATE	BREATH SOUNDS / RESP EFFORT			PUPILS	SKIN		SPO2	
2359	92, S/R	178/94	24	| | |	1.CLEAR 2.CRACKLES 3.RHONCHI 4.WHEEZES 5.DIMINISHED	☑ NONLABORED ☐ LABORED ☐ RETRACTIONS ☐ NASAL FLARING ☐ GRUNTING	PERL	W/P/D	96	☑RA ☐O2
0004	88, S/R	170/90	20				PERL	W/P/D	99	☐RA ☑O2
0009	84, S/R	166/84	18	| | |			PERL	W/P/D	99	☐RA ☑O2
										☐RA ☐O2

LOC U/A ☑AWAKE ☑ALERT ORIENTED: ☑PERSON ☑PLACE ☑TIME ☑EVENT ☐VERBAL ☐PAIN ☐UNRESP
LOSS OF CONSCIOUSNESS ☐YES ☑NO ☐UNK   **PEDS** AGE–APPROPRIATE? ☐YES ☐NO CAP REFILL:
CHIEF COMPLAINT CHEST PRESSURE/WEAKNESS

U/A crew found pt standing lying on couch. Pt appears anxious. States watching TV when suddenly felt weak and	
had a "pressure-type" feeling in the center of his chest. Denies nausea, vomiting. Pt states he feels "a little" short	
of breath, but speaks in complete sentences. Describes pressure as constant. Hx of heart failure and HTN, but	
denies prior episodes of chest discomfort. Took daily aspirin dose with dinner.	
Head / Face / Airway | Airway open; nose & ears clear; no trauma or STI	
Neck Trachea midline, no JVD, no trauma, deformity, or STI	
Chest Lungs clear bilat; chest intact with no trauma, deformity, STI, or pain on palp;	O 2-3 HRS.
equal chest rise & fall; good tidal volume	P AT REST
Abd SNT; no masses or pain on palp; old surgical scar from gallbladder surg	Q "PRESSURE"
Pelvis No trauma, deformity, STI, or pain on palp	R LEFT ARM
Back No trauma, deformity, STI, or pain on palp	S 6/10
Ext Moves all on command; left grip weaker than right due to CVA n 1996; strong and = pulses;	T NO PRIOR HX
no trauma or STI; moderate swelling of feet and ankles bilat	

FIGURE 3-8 ▲ The patient assessment section of the PCR is also called the narrative section of the form.

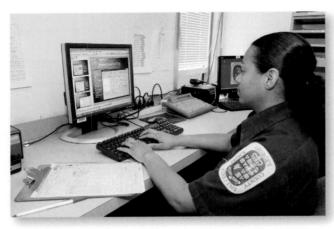

FIGURE 3-9 ▲ Some EMS systems use web-based electronic reporting.

Characteristics of Good Documentation

An EMT is a healthcare professional. A healthcare professional's documentation is a reflection of professionalism and credibility. Just as you must practice to become skilled at assessing a patient, writing a good report is also a skill that requires practice. Characteristics of good documentation are shown in the following *Making a Difference* box.

Making a Difference
Characteristics of Good Documentation

- Complete
- Clear
- Concise
- Objective
- Timely
- Accurate (including spelling)
- Legible

Accurate and complete documentation tells a story about what happened while the patient was in your care. This includes the patient's condition on your arrival at the scene, your assessment findings, the emergency care performed, and the patient's response to the care given. When documenting, describe—don't conclude. Your documentation should contain facts that are supported by what you see, hear, feel, and smell. It should not contain jargon, slang, bias, opinions, or impressions. Do not use phrases like "I felt" or "I thought." Subjective information that can be documented includes what the patient says that pertains to the current illness or complaint.

Remember This

When completing a PCR, *never* "label" a patient. Examples of labeling include using words such as "rude," "confrontational," or "frequent flyer." Words such as these can give the impression that the care you provide to these patients differs from the care you provide to patients who are friendlier or whom you see less often.

When completing a paper report, use a ballpoint pen with black or blue waterproof ink. Since paper PCRs usually consist of multiple pages, you will need to press firmly to make sure the information you write appears on the last page of the form. Use a strong card or separator to ensure that you are not writing through to the next set of report forms. Write neatly and in a manner that is easy to read. Print if necessary. Spelling is important. Many medical terms are spelled similarly but have completely different meanings. If you do not know how to spell a specific word, either look it up or use a different phrase. If you find medical terms confusing, it is generally better to use common words to describe or explain something in your report than to use medical terms incorrectly.

The story that you write in the PCR about a call should be clear and to the point. It is not necessary to write a novel to describe what happened. However, you must include enough detail to enable you to recall events that occurred 2 weeks previously and even 5 years previously. In addition, the story should be clearly written so that the healthcare professionals who assume responsibility for your patient will be able to read the report and know what happened on the basis of what you wrote.

Remember This

Two guidelines you should remember about documentation are:

- If it is not written down, it was not done;

and

- If it was not done, do not write it down.

Although EMS calls are usually very busy scenes, you must make it a habit to document the care you give in a timely manner. Since your ability to recall details will usually begin to fade with time, it is a good idea to make notes throughout a call and then use them to write a complete report when the call is over. Some EMS professionals use preprinted pocket-sized forms to jot down notes while they are interviewing a

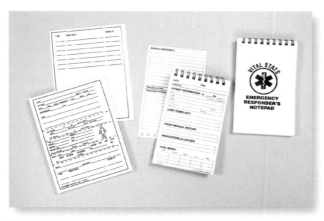

FIGURE 3-10 ▲ You may find it convenient to use a pre-printed pocket-sized form to jot down notes while you are interviewing a patient. This information can then be used for writing a complete report when the call is over.

patient (Figure 3-10). You will need to develop a system that works for you and then use it consistently.

Making a Difference

In most instances it will be the EMT who assesses and documents a patient's vital signs. Your honest reporting of this information to the paramedic *will* make a difference in the care that the patient receives.

Advances in technology have led to the availability and use of mobile and pen-based reporting systems. Electronic prehospital care reports are called *ePCRs*. Some electronic systems can interface with EMS equipment, such as an automated external defibrillator (AED). This allows data recorded from the AED to be sent to the electronic reporting system. Some electronic systems provide anatomical templates that allow EMS personnel to easily document medical or trauma body system findings by patient gender and age. Although this technology will affect the manner in which you complete your prehospital care reports, you are still expected to document the same basic information.

Documentation—General Guidelines

Some important points to keep in mind when writing a PCR include the following:

- Document important observations about the scene such as the presence of empty pill bottles, a suicide note, or weapons.
- Document the events of a call in chronological order.
- Document pertinent positives and negatives. A yes pertaining to an illness or injury is considered a **pertinent positive** or positive finding. A

pertinent negative is a finding expected to accompany the patient's chief complaint but not found during the patient assessment. For example, a patient with asthma pertinent positive findings would have shortness of breath and/or a feeling of tightness in throat or chest. Pertinent negative findings would include no history of a recent cold, bronchitis, pneumonia, or other infection.

- Use abbreviations only if they are standard and approved by your EMS system. A list of common abbreviations is provided in Chapter 5, "Medical Terminology."
- When documenting information of a sensitive nature (such as a communicable disease), note the source of that information, such as the patient, family member, or bystander. For example, if a patient's wife tells you that her husband has "infectious hepatitis" but the patient does not relay this information, you would document, "Patient's wife states patient has infectious hepatitis."
- Document the emergency care delivered.
- Document the time of each intervention, who performed it, and the patient's response to the intervention.
- Document any orders received from medical direction and the results of carrying out the orders.
- Document changes in the patient's condition throughout the call.
- Do not intentionally leave spaces blank; use "NA" if information does not apply.

Confidentiality

The PCR and the information on it are considered confidential. Do not show the form or discuss the information contained on it with unauthorized persons. Violation of patient confidentiality laws can lead to serious consequences. Your report and the information it contains can be distributed only to other healthcare providers who will provide care for your patient and to members of your agency who perform billing or quality management functions.

Local and state protocols and procedures will determine where the different copies of the PCR should be distributed. Know your state laws and local protocols.

Falsification

Falsification of information on the PCR may lead to suspension or revocation of the EMT's certification and/or license and other legal action. Falsifying information may harm the patient because false information may mislead other healthcare professionals about the patient's condition, assessment, and care. Specific areas of difficulty in EMS documentation include vital signs and treatments given. Never attempt to make up vital signs that were not taken or document care that was not given. For example, if an intervention such as oxygen was overlooked, do not chart that the patient was given oxygen.

Error Correction

As previously noted, the PCR is considered a legal document and may be used as evidence in a court proceeding. In most instances, your reports will be written in a very busy and hectic atmosphere. The potential for errors is quite high. Mistakes can and do occur. Your response to a mistake should be honest and very straightforward.

If an error is discovered while the report form is being written, draw a single horizontal line through the error, initial it, and write the correct information beside it (Figure 3-11). Do not erase or try to obliterate the error. Erasures may be interpreted as an attempt to cover up a mistake.

If an error is discovered after the report form is submitted, draw a single line through the error, initial and date it, and add a note with the correct information. If information was omitted, or if additional information comes to your attention after you have written the original report, add a supplemental narrative (called an *addendum* or *amendment*) on a separate report form with the correct information, the date, and your initials and attach it to the original. When documenting the date, record the date and time of the addendum you are writing first and then add the date and time of the event.

When an error pertaining to patient care occurs, document what did or did not happen and what steps were taken (if any) to correct the situation. In addition, your EMS employer is likely to require that you complete a field incident report (or similar reporting form) to document the situation for internal administrative and quality management use.

Most electronic reporting systems have an "error check" feature. The computer program quickly checks your entries for errors, enabling you to correct entries where needed, before closing the report. After a report is closed, the patient record is locked to prevent unauthorized access by another individual. If you discover an error after completing an electronic report, it is necessary to complete an addendum to the original report. Upon completion of the addendum, it is time- and date-stamped and can be electronically retrieved with the original report.

Documentation Formats

Effective documentation requires an organized approach. Although there are several formats to choose from, three of the more commonly used are discussed here. You will need to determine which method works for you, modify it if needed, and then use it consistently to ensure that no important information is omitted when documenting patient care.

TIME	PULSE (RATE/QUALITY)	BP	RESP RATE	BREATH SOUNDS / RESP EFFORT		PUPILS	SKIN	SPO2
2359	92, S/R	178/94	24		1.CLEAR ☑ NONLABORED	PERL	W/P/D	96 ☑RA ☐O2
0004	88, S/R	170/90	20		2.CRACKLES ☐ LABORED 3.RHONCHI ☐ RETRACTIONS	PERL	W/P/D	99 ☐RA ☑O2
0009	84, S/R	166/84	18		4.WHEEZES ☐ NASAL FLARING 5.DIMINISHED ☐ GRUNTING	PERL	W/P/D	99 ☐RA ☑O2
								☐RA ☐O2

LOC U/A ☑AWAKE ☑ALERT ORIENTED: ☑PERSON ☑PLACE ☑TIME ☑EVENT ☐VERBAL ☐PAIN ☐UNRESP

LOSS OF CONSCIOUSNESS ☐YES ☑NO ☐UNK   **PEDS** AGE–APPROPRIATE? ☐YES ☐NO CAP REFILL:

CHIEF COMPLAINT CHEST PRESSURE/WEAKNESS

U/A crew found pt standing lying on couch. Pt appears anxious. States watching TV when suddenly felt weak and
had a "pressure-type" feeling in the center of his chest. Denies nausea, vomiting. Pt states he feels "a little" short
of breath, but speaks in complete sentences. Describes pressure as constant. Hx of heart failure and HTN, but
denies prior episodes of chest discomfort. Took daily aspirin dose with dinner.

Head / Face / Airway	Airway open; nose & ears clear; no trauma or STI	
Neck	Trachea midline, no JVD, no trauma, deformity, or STI	
Chest	Lungs clear bilat; chest intact with no trauma, deformity, STI, or pain on palp;	O 2-3 HRS.
	equal chest rise & fall; good tidal volume	P AT REST
Abd	SNT; no masses or pain on palp; old surgical scar from gallbladder surg	Q "PRESSURE"
Pelvis	No trauma, deformity, STI, or pain on palp	R LEFT ARM
Back	No trauma, deformity, STI, or pain on palp	S 6/10 ~~PA~~ 8/10
Ext	Moves all on command; left grip weaker than right due to CVA n 1996; strong and = pulses;	T NO PRIOR HX
	no trauma or STI; moderate swelling of feet and ankles bilat	

FIGURE 3-11 ▲ If you make an error while writing a report, draw a single horizontal line through the error, initial it, and write the correct information beside it.

SOAP

The **SOAP** method of documentation is one of the most commonly used. SOAP is a memory aid that stands for **S**ubjective findings, **O**bjective findings, **A**ssessment, and **P**lan.

- **Subjective findings.** Subjective findings include information told to you by the patient, family members, or bystanders. Examples include the patient's chief complaint, history of the present illness, related symptoms, and SAMPLE and OPQRST history.
- **Objective findings.** Objective findings include information that can be seen, heard, smelled, measured, or felt. Information contained in this portion of your report includes your primary and secondary survey findings and the patient's vital signs (if they are not recorded elsewhere on the report).
- **Assessment.** The information that should be documented here is your field impression of the patient's illness or injury based on the subjective and objective findings found during your interaction with the patient.
- **Plan.** Document the emergency care given, patient's response to each intervention, mode of patient transport, transportation destination, and ongoing assessment findings.

The following is an example of documentation using the SOAP format.

S Chief complaint: 44-year-old woman complaining of pain in hip and lower back.

SAMPLE: Allergies: hydrocodone. Takes no medications, no pertinent PMH. Breakfast at 0700. Patient was climbing stairs in bank building because elevator wasn't working. Slipped and fell about 6 steps. Rates hip and lower back pain 6 on 0 to 10 scale.

O Fall injury. Patient found between floor 7 and 8 in stairwell of bank building.

Head/face/airway: Awake, alert, and oriented to person, place, time, event. Denies hitting head during fall or loss of consciousness. DCAP-BTLS negative; denies pain on palpation. PERL. No drainage from ears or nose.

Neck: DCAP-BTLS negative, trachea midline.

Chest: DCAP-BTLS negative, breath sounds clear/equal bilaterally.

Abdomen: Soft, nontender; DCAP-BTLS.

Pelvis: Complains of left hip pain on palpation, femoral pulses strong and equal.

Back: Complains of lumbar pain on palpation.

Extremities: DCAP-BTLS negative; equal pulses, movement, sensation.

A Fall injury with hip and lower back trauma.

P Oxygen by nonrebreather mask at 15 L/min. Patient refused spinal stabilization (cervical collar, spider straps, head blocks, backboard). Transported down remaining stairs on backboard and then placed in position of comfort on stretcher. Transported code 2 by ground ambulance to XYZ hospital.

CHART

CHART is another commonly used documentation format. CHART stands for **C**hief complaint, **H**istory, **A**ssessment, **R**x (treatment), and **T**ransport. The main difference between the SOAP and CHART formats is that the subjective information in SOAP is separated into two parts in CHART (chief complaint and history).

- **Chief complaint.** The chief complaint is the patient's description of illness or injury. If the patient is unresponsive or has an altered mental status, this information is usually obtained from family members, bystanders, or your evaluation of the scene.
- **History.** Document the patient's history of the present illness (including OPQRST if appropriate) and SAMPLE history.
- **Assessment.** Document objective findings from your primary and secondary surveys that can be seen, heard, smelled, measured, or felt. Include vital signs if they are not recorded elsewhere on the report.
- **Rx (treatment).** Document any treatment the patient received before your arrival, as well as the emergency care you provided. Document the patient's response to each intervention.
- **Transport.** Document the mode of patient transport, transportation destination, ongoing assessment findings, any treatment provided en route, and the patient's response to the treatment given.

The following is an example of documentation using the CHART format.

C **Chief complaint.** 44-year-old woman complaining of pain in hip and lower back.

H **History.** Fall injury. Patient found between floor 7 and 8 in stairwell of bank building. Patient was climbing stairs in bank building because elevator wasn't working. Slipped and fell about 6 steps. Rates hip and lower back pain 6 on 0 to 10 scale. Allergies: hydrocodone. Takes no medications, no pertinent PMH. Breakfast at 0700.

A **Assessment.** Head/face/airway: Awake, alert, and oriented to person, place, time, event. Denies hitting head during fall or loss of consciousness.

DCAP-BTLS negative; denies pain on palpation. PERL. No drainage from ears or nose.

Neck: DCAP-BTLS negative, trachea midline.

Chest: DCAP-BTLS negative, breath sounds clear/equal bilaterally.

Abdomen: Soft, nontender; DCAP-BTLS.

Pelvis: Complains of left hip pain on palpation, femoral pulses strong and equal.

Back: Complains of lumbar pain on palpation.

Extremities: DCAP-BTLS negative; equal pulses, movement, sensation.

R   Rx. Oxygen by nonrebreather mask at 15 L/min. Patient refused spinal stabilization (cervical collar, spider straps, head blocks, backboard). Transported down remaining stairs on backboard and then placed in position of comfort on stretcher.

T   Transport. Transported code 2 by ground ambulance to XYZ hospital.

Narrative

The narrative documentation format is like writing a short story about the events of the call. Documentation includes assessment findings, pertinent historical information, treatment, patient responses, and transport data in chronological order. Although this method of documentation is easy to learn, locating specific information is often difficult.

The following is an example of documentation using the narrative format. Please note that explanations for some abbreviations are provided in parentheses for clarity. This would not be done in an actual report because it would defeat the purpose of using the abbreviations.

R/T (respond to) fall injury. 44-year-old woman found between floor 7 and 8 in stairwell of bank building. Patient was climbing stairs in bank building because elevator wasn't working. Slipped and fell about 6 steps. C/O (complains of) hip and lower back pain; rates pain 6 on 0 to 10 scale. Allergies: hydrocodone. Takes no medications, no pertinent PMH. Breakfast at 0700.

Head/face/airway: Awake, alert, and oriented to person, place, time, event. Denies hitting head during fall or loss of consciousness. DCAP-BTLS negative; denies pain on palpation. PERL. No drainage from ears or nose.

Neck: DCAP-BTLS negative, trachea midline.

Chest: DCAP-BTLS negative, breath sounds clear/equal bilaterally.

Abdomen: soft, nontender; DCAP-BTLS.

Pelvis: Complains of left hip pain on palpation, femoral pulses strong and equal.

Back: Complains of lumbar pain on palpation.

Extremities: DCAP-BTLS negative; equal pulses, movement, sensation.

Rx: Oxygen by nonrebreather mask at 15 L/min. Patient refused spinal stabilization (cervical collar, spider straps, head blocks, backboard). Transported down remaining stairs on backboard and then placed in position of comfort on stretcher. Transported code 2 by ground ambulance to XYZ hospital.

On the Scene   Wrap-Up

As paramedics arrive on the scene, the patient vomits and then says, "I don't feel so good; maybe I should go to the hospital." You quickly cut away his jeans, being careful to avoid the area the bullet penetrated. As you are controlling the bleeding, he admits that his girlfriend shot him during an argument.

A few hours later, a reporter from the local news station calls to check on the patient and find out what happened. You politely tell the reporter that you are not able to share any information about the patient's care because of privacy laws. The reporter is not happy with your answer and says she will call the hospital and try to get the information she wants. ■

Sum It Up

▶ The U.S. government is made up of three branches: legislative, executive, and judicial. Law made by the legislative branch of government is called statutory or legislative law. The rules and regulations made by the executive branch of government are called administrative law. The court system makes up the judicial branch of government. Courts hear cases that challenge or require explanation of the laws passed by the legislative branch of government and approved by the executive branch.

▶ In a lawsuit, the plaintiff (also called the complainant) is the party that files a formal complaint with the court. The defendant is the party being sued or accused.

▶ The maximum period within which a plaintiff must begin a lawsuit (in civil cases) or a prosecutor must bring charges (in criminal cases) or lose the right to file the suit is called the statute of limitations.

▶ Criminal law is the area of law in which the federal, state, or local government prosecutes individuals on behalf of society for violating laws designed to safeguard society.

- Civil law is a branch of law that deals with complaints by individuals or organizations against a defendant for an illegal act or wrongdoing (tort).

- A lawsuit begins when an incident occurs and an individual or organization find that the problems resulting from the incident require the involvement of the courts. The plaintiff's attorney gathers pertinent facts, prepares documents, and files a written statement (the complaint) with the court. After the complaint is filed, copies of the court documents and a summons (notice) are delivered (served) to the defendant (or the defendant's attorney) notifying her that a lawsuit has been filed against her. The defendant's attorney prepares a response to the complaint and files it with the court. A copy of the defendant's answer is sent to the plaintiff's attorney. After a lawsuit is filed, discovery begins. To find out more details about the claim, one party may send written questions (interrogatories) to the other party. Depositions may be taken by either party during discovery, which means asking individuals oral questions while they are under oath. After discovery is completed, the judge will hold a pretrial conference with the attorneys to even further narrow the issues to be decided during the trial even further. After the trial is finished, a decision is handed down by a judge or jury. The decision determines guilt or liability and the damages and award, if any, to the plaintiff.

- The scope of practice includes the emergency care and skills an EMT is legally allowed and expected to perform. These duties are set by state laws and regulations. As an EMT, your ethical responsibilities include treating all patients with respect and giving each patient the best care you are capable of giving. You must also determine if patients are competent (that is, if they can understand the questions you ask and the consequences of the decisions they make about their care).

- A competent patient must give you consent (permission) before you can provide emergency care. Expressed consent is one in which a patient gives specific permission for care and transport to be provided. Expressed consent may be given verbally, in writing, or nonverbally. Implied consent is consent assumed from a patient requiring emergency care who is mentally, physically, or emotionally unable to provide expressed consent.

- Mentally competent adults have the right to refuse care and transport. As an EMT, you must make sure that the patient fully understands your explanation and the consequences of refusing treatment or transport. In high-risk situations in which the patient's injuries may not be obvious, you must contact medical direction or call ALS personnel to the scene to assess the patient.

- An advance directive is a form filled out by the patient. It outlines the patient's wishes for care if the patient is not able to express any wishes. A do not resuscitate order is written by a physician and details the patient's wishes for care when terminally ill.

- Assault is considered threatening, attempting, or causing a fear of offensive physical contact with a patient or other person. Battery is the unlawful touching of another person without consent. Because each state has its own definitions of assault and battery, you should check your local protocols concerning these terms.

- Abandonment is terminating patient care without making sure that care will continue at the same level or higher. You can also be charged with abandonment if you stop patient care when the patient still needs and desires additional care.

- A healthcare professional is negligent if failing to act as a reasonable, careful, similarly trained person would act under similar circumstances. Negligence includes the following four elements: (1) the duty to act, (2) a breach of that duty, (3) injury or damages (physical or psychological) that result, and (4) proximate cause (the actions or inactions of the healthcare professional that caused the injury or damages).

- A medical identification device is used to alert healthcare personnel to a patient's particular medical condition. This identification device may be in the form of a bracelet, a necklace, or an identification card.

- If you are sent to a crime scene, you must wait for law enforcement personnel to declare that the scene is safe to enter. After you are certain the scene is safe and you ensure your safety, your first priority will be patient care. You should be alert and document anything unusual on the call.

- An organ donor is a person who has a signed legal document to donate his organs in the event of death. The patient may have an organ donor card or may have indicated the intent to be a donor on a driver's license.

- Good documentation is complete, clear, concise, objective, timely, accurate, and legible.

- A PCR has many important functions.
  - *Continuity of care.* The PCR may be used by receiving facility staff to help determine the direction of treatment following the EMS treatments given.
  - *Legal document.* Good documentation reflects the emergency medical care provided, status of the patient on arrival at the scene, and any changes upon arrival at the receiving facility.
  - *Education and research.* The PCR can be used to show proper documentation and how to handle

unusual or uncommon situations, as well as identify training needs for the EMS providers.

- *Administrative.* The PCR is used for billing and EMS service statistics.
- *Quality management.* Completed reports are typically evaluated for adequacy of documentation, compliance with local rules and regulations, compliance with agency documentation standards, and appropriateness of medical care.

▶ A PCR generally consists of an administrative section, patient and scene information section, and patient assessment (narrative) section.

- The administrative section includes data pertaining to the EMS call, such as the date, times, service, unit, and crew information.
- The patient and scene information section includes data such as the patient's name, age, gender, weight, address, date of birth, and insurance information.
- The patient assessment section includes the patient's chief complaint, mechanism of injury/ nature of illness, location of the patient, treatment given before arrival of EMS, patient signs and symptoms, care given, vital signs, medical history, and changes in condition.

▶ The PCR form and the information on it are considered confidential. Local and state protocols and procedures determine where the different copies of the PCR should be distributed.

▶ When documenting information of a sensitive nature (such as a communicable disease), note the source of that information, such as the patient, family member, or bystander.

▶ Falsification of information on the PCR may lead not only to suspension or revocation of the EMT's certification/license but also to poor patient care because other healthcare professionals have a false impression of which assessment findings were discovered or which treatment was given.

▶ When a documentation error occurs, do not try to cover it up. Instead, document what did or did not happen; include the time and date; and initial your change.

EMS System Communications

By the end of this chapter, you should be able to:

Knowledge Objectives ▶
1. Define communications.
2. Describe the role of the Federal Communications Commission in EMS system communications.
3. Describe the following components of an EMS communications system: base station, mobile two-way radio, portable radio, repeater, digital radio equipment, cellular telephone.
4. Discuss the role of an emergency medical dispatcher in a typical EMS event.
5. List the proper methods of initiating and terminating a radio call.
6. List the correct radio procedures during each phase of a typical EMS call.
7. Discuss the communication skills that should be used when interacting with individuals from other agencies.
8. Identify the essential components of the verbal report.
9. Explain the importance of effective communication of patient information in the verbal report.
10. State legal aspects to consider in verbal communication.

Attitude Objectives ▶
11. Explain the rationale for providing efficient and effective radio communication and patient reports.

Skill Objectives ▶
12. Perform a simulated, organized, concise radio transmission.
13. Make a brief, organized report to give to an emergency medical technician or paramedic arriving at an incident scene where you were the first on the scene.

On the Scene

You and your EMT partner respond to a private residence for a report of abdominal pain. You arrive to find a 17-year-old female lying on her right side in her bed. The patient is awake and reports that she has been feeling ill since yesterday. She is complaining of a fever and severe abdominal pain. ■

THINK ABOUT IT

As you read this chapter, think about the following questions:

* After being dispatched to the call, when should you make contact with the dispatcher?
* You summon an advanced life support unit to the scene, and the paramedics arrive quickly. What information should you relay to the paramedics?

One of the most amazing abilities we possess is the capacity for communication. We can express fear, describe symptoms, ask questions, inform crew members, give a radio report, relay information to hospital staff, and even offer condolences when needed. This special ability is an important component of prehospital care. As an emergency medical technician, you must be able to communicate effectively with crew members, emergency dispatchers, medical direction, and other healthcare professionals; law enforcement personnel and other public safety workers; the patient; and the patient's family. Communication with medical direction may be necessary when a patient refuses care or when you encounter difficult patient management situations. As an EMT, you must learn to communicate patient information to other healthcare professionals in a concise, organized manner. This chapter focuses on the basic requirements for successfully communicating with your dispatch center, your partner, your patients, and other healthcare professionals.

Communications Systems

Objective 1

Communication is the exchange of thoughts and messages that occurs by sending and receiving information. This interaction may occur on a radio or cell phone with dispatch personnel, between crew members, with a patient's family, or with the staff of the receiving facility. Effective communication requires that we send and receive this information using an understandable and commonly recognized language. This "language" requirement is not just as simple as speaking English or Spanish. Using terminology that is too technical or too advanced may create confusion. Information that is misunderstood can lead to inappropriate treatment or care. To alleviate this potential problem, most Emergency Medical Services (EMS) systems in the United States require the use of clear text or speech to relay data from one point to another. To understand its importance, we must consider the history, terminology, and basic concepts of communication.

History

Modern EMS communication began with the use of telephones to contact local rescue squads or personnel. This usually required calling a specific local number or the local operator, who then contacted EMS personnel. In many towns across the United States, this contact may have initiated the sounding of a bell or siren located on a tower near the station that housed the ambulance. Sounding the bell notified local volunteers to assemble for a call. You can imagine the time that may have elapsed from the original call to arrival at the scene.

Communication Centers

Communication capabilities and equipment have changed significantly in just the last two decades. Cellular phones that used to be the size of a toaster are now small enough to fit in your pocket. This has helped reduce the overall time needed to find a telephone to report a medical problem. Despite all the advances in technology, we still rely heavily on the ability of all the people connected with the EMS system to verbally communicate with each other.

Regulation

Objective 2

The **Federal Communications Commission (FCC)** is the U.S. government agency responsible for regulation of interstate and international communications by radio, television, wire, satellite, and cable. The FCC is charged with the development and enforcement of rules and regulations pertaining to radio transmissions. In addition, the FCC is mandated to do the following:

- Control licenses and allocate frequencies.
- Establish technical standards for radio equipment.
- Monitor frequencies for appropriate usage.
- Spot-check for licenses and records.

Remember This

Always speak in a professional manner during radio communication. Inappropriate language or use of radio frequencies may lead to enforcement action by the FCC. Keep in mind that many people have scanners in their homes and may hear all communications shared back and forth.

Radio Frequencies and Ranges

Objective 3

In the United States, the FCC regulates the use of nongovernmental radio frequencies. The **Interagency Radio Advisory Committee (IRAC)** is responsible for coordinating radio use by agencies of the federal government. The **Emergency Medical Radio Service (EMRS)** is a group of frequencies designated by the FCC exclusively for use by EMS providers. EMRS includes many frequencies in the **VHF** (very high frequency) and **UHF** (ultrahigh frequency) bands (a *band* is a group of radio frequencies close together).

Very High Frequency

VHF radio frequencies can be subdivided into low band and high band. Low-band frequencies generally have a greater range than high-band VHF frequencies.

Radio waves in the low-band frequency range bend and follow the curvature of the Earth, allowing radio transmission over long distances. These radio waves are subject to interference by atmospheric conditions, including weather disturbances, and electrical equipment. These waves do not penetrate solid structures (such as buildings) well, making VHF low band less effective for use in metropolitan areas.

Radio waves in the high-band frequency range travel in a straight line. This straight-line quality means that the radio wave is easily blocked by topography such as a hill, mountain, or large building. Although less interference occurs in this band than in VHF low band, its susceptibility to interference by solid structures may result in gaps or "holes" in radio coverage. This band is generally better for use in metropolitan areas than is VHF low band.

Ultrahigh Frequency

Radio waves in the UHF frequency travel in a straight line but do have an ability to reflect off or bounce around buildings. This band has a shorter range than VHF high or low bands. This type of frequency has a greater ability to enter buildings or structures through openings or mediums that are radio frequency permeable. UHF frequently requires the use of repeaters because of its short range. A **repeater** is a device that receives a transmission from a low-power portable or mobile radio on one frequency and then retransmits it at a higher power on another frequency so that it can be received at a distant location.

You Should Know

Line-of-sight and straight-line radio coverage problems are generally overcome with the use of repeaters placed on high ground or on top of a large structure or tower.

800-Megahertz Frequencies

The 800-megahertz (MHz) frequencies are UHF radio signals that use computer technology to make transmissions more secure than the other types of radio transmissions. These frequencies allow clear communication with minimal interference. They also use a trunk system that allows routing of a transmission to the first available frequency. Many channels are available to choose from. Although 800-MHz frequencies generally have a limited range and are very straight line, these problems are overcome by using multiple repeaters. This makes 800-MHz frequencies very effective for use in urban areas.

Remember This

Knowing the capabilities of your equipment may mean the difference in communicating effectively with a distant site.

Equipment

Base Station

A **base station** is a transmitter/receiver at a stationary site such as a hospital, mountaintop, or public safety agency (Figure 4-1). At a minimum, a base station is made up of a transmitter, a receiver, a transmission line, and an antenna. A **transmitter** is a device that sends out data on a given radio frequency. A radio signal generated by the base station may be sent directly to a receiving unit or to a repeater as needed.

Mobile Two-Way Radio

A **mobile two-way radio** is a vehicular-mounted communication device (Figure 4-2). It usually transmits at a lower power than do base stations (typically 20–50 watts). The typical transmission range is 10–15 miles over average terrain. Transmission over flat land or water increases range. Urban areas, mountains, and dense foliage decrease transmission range.

Portable Radio

A **portable radio** is a handheld communication device (Figure 4-3). Typical power output is 1–5 watts, which limits its range. Portable radios are used for radio communication away from the emergency vehicle. They may have a single channel or multiple channels. A portable radio is often used in conjunction with repeaters to increase transmission range.

Repeater

A repeater is designed to receive a lower-powered transmission and then boost the signal for retransmittal. This may allow greater geographic coverage and can assist with the transmission of portable signals to other units in the system. Repeaters can be fixed or mobile. For portable communications, repeaters may be located in the vehicle or on radio towers. Mobile communications use repeaters on radio towers. Repeater signals can be retransmitted by radio waves, microwaves, or telephone landlines.

Digital Radio Equipment

Digital pagers are used in many EMS systems. An audible signal and/or text message can be transmitted quickly by the dispatch center to alert EMS personnel to respond to a call.

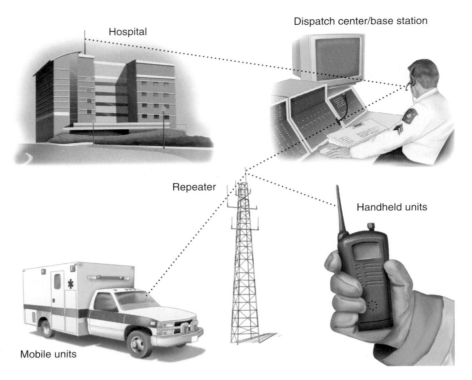

FIGURE 4-1 ▲ Example of an EMS communication system.

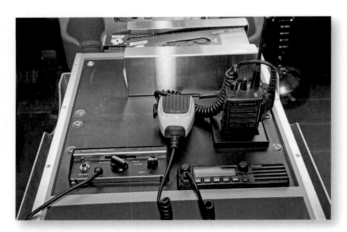

FIGURE 4-2 ▲ A mobile radio.

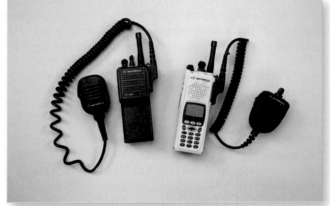

FIGURE 4-3 ▲ Portable (handheld) radios.

Some EMS systems use **mobile data computers (MDCs)** (also called *mobile data terminals,* or *MDTs*). An MDC is a computer that is mounted in an emergency vehicle (Figure 4-4). The computer displays information pertaining to the calls for which EMS personnel are dispatched. Examples of information displayed include text from dispatch pertaining to the call, the address of the incident, and a local map pointing directly to the incident. The computer is used to log response times and indicate the status of the EMS crew and vehicle (in service and available for calls, on the scene, responding to a call, en route to the hospital, etc.). The computer is also used to send and receive text messages between the EMS crew and the dispatch center.

Many EMS vehicles are equipped with an **Automatic Vehicle Locator (AVL)**. An AVL is a device that uses the **Global Positioning System (GPS)** to track a vehicle's location. GPS uses a system of satellites and receiving devices to compute the receiver's geographic position on the Earth. If the MDC is equipped with the necessary software, EMS vehicles equipped with an AVL appear on the local map that is displayed on the computer terminal.

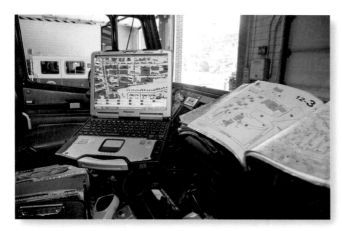

FIGURE 4-4 ▲ Mobile data computers display information pertaining to the calls for which EMS personnel are dispatched.

Cellular Telephones

Geographic areas are divided into "cells." Each cell has a base station to transmit and receive signals. Cellular communication systems can track a mobile unit's movements from cell to cell and transfer the unit's radio activity to the appropriate cell base station.

Transmission Modes

Four transmission modes are generally used in an EMS communication system: one way, simplex, duplex, and multiplex. A one-way transmission mode is generally used for paging systems. In one-way mode, a signal is sent to any unit monitoring the appropriate frequency, but the receiving unit has no ability to transmit a message.

A **simplex system** uses a single frequency to transmit and receive messages. As a result, only one signal may be transmitted or received at a time. Simultaneous radio transmissions will block a message from being received. An advantage of this type of system is that it allows the speaker to relay a message without interruption. However, communication using a simplex system takes away the ability to have a discussion regarding a patient or situation.

A **duplex system** is a mode of radio transmission that uses two frequencies to transmit and receive messages, allowing simultaneous two-way communication. An advantage of using this system for radio transmission is that either party can interrupt as necessary. Two-way communication aids discussion regarding a patient or situation. A disadvantage of this type of system is that the user at each end has a tendency to interrupt the other.

A **multiplex system** is a mode of radio transmission that permits simultaneous transmission of voice and other data, using one frequency. Advantages of using

this system for radio transmission are that either party can interrupt as necessary and two-way communication aids discussion regarding a patient or situation. Disadvantages of this type of system are that voice signals can interfere with data transmission.

The Call

An EMS communications network must provide a means by which a citizen can reliably access the EMS system (usually by dialing 9-1-1). To ensure adequate EMS system response and coordination, there must also be a means for dispatch center to emergency vehicle communication, communication between emergency vehicles, communication from the emergency vehicle to the hospital, hospital-to-hospital communication, and communication between agencies, such as between EMS and law enforcement personnel.

The sequence 9-1-1 is the official national emergency number in the United States and Canada. When the numbers 9-1-1 are dialed, the caller is quickly connected to a single location called a **Public Safety Answering Point (PSAP).** A PSAP is a facility equipped and staffed to receive and control 9-1-1 access calls. A dispatch center, alarm room, and police department are examples of facilities that may host the PSAP. Information coming into the PSAP may be processed at the PSAP, or the PSAP may route the call to an appropriate agency for processing. The PSAP dispatcher is trained to route the call to the appropriate local emergency medical, fire, and law enforcement agencies. Although EMS is usually activated by dialing 9-1-1 from a standard telephone, other means of activating an emergency response include emergency alarm boxes, citizen band radios, and wireless telephones.

Enhanced 9-1-1, or E9-1-1, is a system that routes an emergency call to the 9-1-1 center closest to the caller and automatically displays the caller's phone number and address. E9-1-1 speeds up the transfer of information from the caller to the call taker and helps decrease the number of false alarms. It also assists in callbacks to obtain more complete information. Most 9-1-1 systems that exist today are E9-1-1 systems.

The FCC has established a program that requires wireless telephone carriers to provide E9-1-1 services. Wireless E9-1-1 provides the precise location of a 9-1-1 call from a wireless phone, within 50–100 meters in most cases. Wireless E9-1-1 is not yet available in all areas.

Voice over Internet Protocol (VoIP), also known as *Internet Voice,* is technology that allows users to make telephone calls by means of a broadband Internet connection instead of a regular telephone line. Companies offering this service provide different features. Some services allow you to call only other people using the same service. Others allow you to call anyone who has a telephone number. Some services do not work during power outages and may not offer backup power. Some services offer E9-1-1 support as an optional service. Subscribers register and pay a fee for E9-1-1. With their subscription, an emergency call is automatically routed to the PSAP that handles 9-1-1 emergencies. If the subscriber is unable to speak, the PSAP operator will know the subscriber's location and be able to dispatch emergency personnel. If the user declines E9-1-1 service, the person does not have direct access to emergency personnel via Internet Voice.

You Should Know

If a 9-1-1 caller does not speak English, the 9-1-1 call taker can add an interpreter from an outside service to the line. Communications centers that answer 9-1-1 calls also have special telephones for responding to 9-1-1 calls from deaf or hearing- or speech-impaired callers.

Dispatch

When an emergency occurs, a bystander frequently recognizes the event and activates the EMS system by calling 9-1-1 or another emergency number. The emergency medical dispatcher (Figure 4-5) gathers information and activates ("tones out") an appropriate EMS response based on the information received.

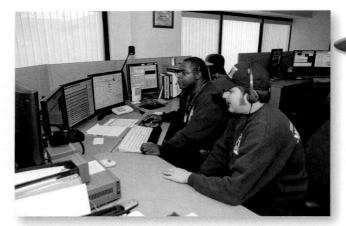

FIGURE 4-5 ▲ Example of an EMS dispatch center. Emergency medical dispatchers are trained to provide prearrival instructions to the caller by phone when necessary. How to provide cardiopulmonary resuscitation, emergency care for choking, and bleeding control techniques are among the most common prearrival instructions provided by EMDs.

You Should Know

Telephone conversations with the caller and telephone and radio transmissions between the dispatch center and police, fire, and EMS personnel are recorded. Courts have forced dispatch centers to release tapes of 9-1-1 calls in response to lawsuits by the media, attorneys, or other involved parties. The 9-1-1 tapes may subsequently be heard on radio and television news. With this in mind, *always* be professional when communicating with others in the workplace and on an emergency call.

Emergency Medical Dispatchers

Objective 4

Formal emergency medical dispatch protocols and training began in the 1980s. Before this time, medical dispatchers averaged less than 1 hour of medical training. The Emergency Medical Dispatch program has been developed to certify personnel as **emergency medical dispatchers (EMDs).** An EMD is knowledgeable about the geography of the area, the EMS system's capabilities, and the activities of other public service agencies. An EMD is responsible for:

- Verifying the address of the incident
- Asking questions of the caller
- Assigning technicians to the incident
- Alerting and activating personnel to the incident
- Providing prearrival instructions to the caller
- Communicating with technicians
- Recording incident times

You Should Know

Emergency medical dispatchers are trained to provide prearrival instructions to the caller by phone when necessary. The cardiopulmonary resuscitation (CPR) procedure, emergency care for choking, and bleeding control techniques are among the most common prearrival instructions provided by EMDs.

Computer-aided dispatch (CAD) is used in many EMS systems (Figure 4-6). When a call comes into a PSAP that uses CAD, the address and phone number of the caller are automatically entered into the CAD system. The dispatcher types a description of the emergency into the computer and then assigns a priority level to the call. As a result, an "event" is created and many activities related to it can be tracked, retrieved, and evaluated. The software used by the CAD system can

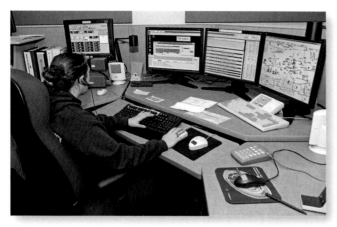

FIGURE 4-6 ▲ Computer-aided dispatch is used in many EMS systems.

connect dispatchers with local, state, and national computer database systems. Important times pertaining to an emergency call that are tracked and evaluated in most EMS systems include the following:

- Call received
- EMS crew dispatched
- EMS crew vehicle en route
- EMS crew on the scene
- EMS crew making patient contact
- EMS crew en route to receiving facility
- EMS crew arrival with patient at receiving facility
- EMS crew returning from the hospital
- EMS crew available for service
- EMS crew arrival at the station or quarters

Objective 5

When the dispatcher has enough information about an EMS call to determine the type of response needed and the proper unit to send, a signal is sent to begin the activation process. The crew may receive a signal by pager, radio, or cell phone. General guidelines to ensure effective radio communication during the activation and response phase of a typical EMS call are listed in the following *Making a Difference* box.

Making a Difference

Guidelines for Effective Radio Communication

- Make sure that you have checked that your equipment is available and in good working order at the start of your shift.
- Before speaking into the radio:
  —Make sure the radio is on and the volume is properly adjusted.
  —Reduce background noise as much as possible.
  —Listen to the frequency that you will be transmitting on to make sure that it is clear before speaking.
  —Hold the radio's microphone about 2–3 inches away from your mouth.
  —Locate and press the "push to talk" (PTT) button. To make sure your first words are not cut off, pause (with the PTT button depressed) for about 1–2 seconds before speaking.
- Using a normal tone of voice, address the unit being called by its name and number. Then identify the name of your unit (and number, if appropriate) as determined by your local protocols.
- Wait for the unit being called to signal you to begin your transmission by saying, "Go ahead," or some other term standard in your area. A response of "Stand by" means, "Wait until further notice."
- When the unit being called has acknowledged your call (and has stopped speaking), relay your message. Speak clearly, keeping your transmissions brief.
- At the end of your message, the unit being called may repeat the pertinent information from your message to make sure that the unit has received the information correctly. If the information is verified as correct, acknowledge the unit's transmission and announce that you are clear.
- Use plain English in your radio communications. Avoid the use of "ten codes" and slang.
- Avoid meaningless phrases, such as "Be advised."
- Do not use profanity on the air. (The FCC may impose substantial fines.)
- Avoid words that are hard to hear like "yes" and "no"; use "affirmative" and "negative."
- Courtesy is assumed; there is no need to say "please," "thank you," and "you're welcome."
- When transmitting a number that might be confused with another, give the individual digits. For example, do not say "fifty-one." Instead, say "five one."
- Develop a working field impression, recognizing that it may change during your assessment of the patient's chief complaint and mechanism of injury or nature of the illness. Remain objective and impartial in describing patients.

En Route to the Call

Objective 6

The format for your radio report may be determined by local or state protocols. The following script may help you understand a typical call. The script below begins with the electronic or tone activation of a radio or pager. We will use "Medic 51" to indicate your communication with dispatch.

Dispatch Center:	"Medic 51 (five, one), respond code 3 to 4321 (four, three, two, one) East Main Street for a report of difficulty breathing. Call number 987 (nine, eight, seven). Time out 1402 (fourteen, zero, two)."
Medic 51:	Dispatch, Medic 51 (five, one) received. Responding to report of difficulty breathing at four, three, two, one East Main Street."
Dispatch Center:	"Medic 51 (five, one), Dispatch received; you are responding. Caller reports your patient is 70-year-old female in the kitchen of this address. The door will be unlocked. 1403 (fourteen, zero, three)."
Medic 51:	"Dispatch, Medic 51 (five, one), received. 70-year-old female in the kitchen, and the door will be unlocked."

Arrival at the Scene

Objective 6

Additional radio contact with the dispatch center will be needed on your arrival at the scene.

Medic 51:	"Dispatch, Medic 51 (five, one). We are on scene."
Dispatch Center:	"Medic 51 (five, one), received, on scene at 1406 (fourteen, zero, six)."

Communicating with the Patient

When communicating with a patient, begin by identifying yourself and establishing your role. Respectfully explain that you are there to provide assistance. Methods of patient communication are discussed in detail in Chapter 15, "Therapeutic Communications and History Taking."

Communicating with Individuals from Other Agencies

Objectives 7, 8

Communications with individuals from other agencies should be organized, concise, thorough, and accurate. When receiving a report from others at the scene (such as bystanders or emergency medical responders), listen carefully to their report (Figure 4-7). Ask questions

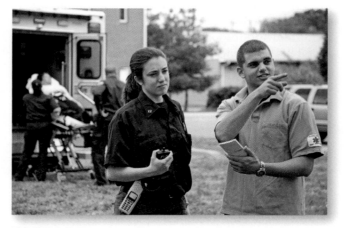

FIGURE 4-7 ▲ When receiving a report from others at the scene (such as an EMR), listen carefully to the report.

if any information is unclear. Be professional and thank them for their efforts.

You must give a verbal report to EMS professionals arriving on the scene where you have been providing care. Keeping your report brief and pertinent, you will need to relay the following information:

- Identify yourself as an EMT.
- Report the patient's name (if known), age, gender, primary problem (chief complaint), and current condition.
- Describe what happened and the position in which the patient was found.
- Describe pertinent assessment findings, including vital signs.
- Report any medical history you obtained from the patient.
- Describe the emergency medical care that you gave.
- Describe the patient's response to the treatment given.
- Report orders received from medical direction (if applicable).

Communicating with Medical Direction

You may need to contact medical direction for advice, if a patient refuses care, during difficult patient management situations, or to obtain orders to give medications. When you are communicating with medical direction, it is very important that your radio or telephone communication be professional, organized, concise, and pertinent (Figure 4-8). The information that you give to the physician must be accurate because the physician will use this information to determine whether to order medications and procedures.

After receiving an order (or a denial of a request), use the "echo" procedure. This means that you must repeat the order back to the physician, word for word.

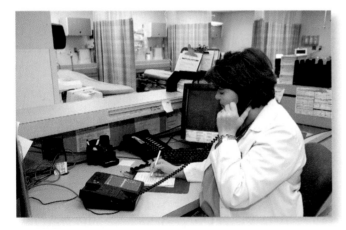

FIGURE 4-8 ▲ When you are communicating with medical direction, it is very important that your radio or telephone communication be professional, organized, concise, and pertinent.

Be sure to document any orders received and question any orders that are unclear.

En Route to the Receiving Facility

Objectives 6, 9

Contact your dispatch center as you begin patient transport to the receiving facility.

Medic 51:	"Medic 51 (five, one) to Dispatch."
Dispatch Center:	"Dispatch. Medic 51 (five, one)—go ahead."
Medic 51:	"Dispatch, Medic 51 (five, one) is transporting one patient to Anytown Medical Center—nonemergent."
Dispatch Center:	"Received, Medic 51 (five, one). Transporting one patient to Anytown Medical Center—nonemergent. Time: 1426 (fourteen, two, six)."

In most EMS systems, EMS personnel are required to notify any receiving facility of the condition of the patient they are transporting to that facility. The essential elements of this type of report and the order in which they should occur are as follows:

- Identity of the unit and the level of the care provider (such as BLS, ALS)
- Estimated time of arrival at facility
- Patient's age and gender
- Chief complaint
- Brief, pertinent history of present illness or problem
- Major past illnesses
- Mental status
- Vital signs
- Pertinent physical exam findings
- Emergency medical care given
- Response to emergency medical care

Your ability to communicate effectively with the receiving facility directly affects the care that the patient receives. This report is your chance to paint a very clear picture in the minds of the receiving facility staff. The clearer you paint the picture, the better prepared they will be for your arrival and the subsequent treatment of your patient. If you do not use the standard reporting format, you run the risk of omitting essential information, and patient care may be delayed while the hospital attempts to get the information it needs. This could negatively affect your patient's health.

A sample radio report simulating communication with a receiving facility is shown below. You will need to practice a radio report like this one many times to become proficient.

Medic 51:	"Anytown Medical Center, Medic 51 (five, one)."
Anytown Medical Center:	"Anytown Medical Center. Go ahead Medic 51 (five, one)."
Medic 51:	"Anytown Medical Center, EMT Smith on Medic 51 (five, one). We are en route to your facility. Expected arrival time: 10 minutes. The patient is a 70-year-old woman with a chief complaint of difficulty breathing that started yesterday. Patient denies any past medical history or medications. Patient is awake and oriented to person, place, time, and event. Baseline vital signs follow: respirations 20, pulse 80, blood pressure 130/78 (one thirty over seventy-eight). Exam reveals swelling of both of the patient's legs to the level of her calves. We have placed the patient in a semi-Fowler's position and put her on oxygen by nonrebreather mask at 15 L/min (fifteen liters per minute). The patient reports feeling 'a little better.' Any questions or orders?"
Anytown Medical Center:	"Medic 51 (five, one), Anytown Medical Center report received [your report may be repeated to ensure accuracy]. No orders or questions. Contact us if there is any change in patient condition before arrival. Anytown Medical Center clear."
Medic 51:	"Medic 51 (five, one) clear."

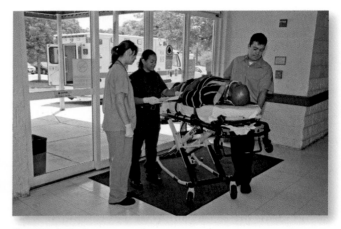

FIGURE 4-9 ▲ Give a verbal report to the receiving facility staff in a polite and respectful manner.

professional of equal or higher medical skills. Begin the verbal report by introducing the patient by name (if known). Summarize the information already provided by radio or telephone to the receiving facility:

- Patient's chief complaint
- Pertinent patient history that was not previously given
- Emergency medical care given en route and the patient's response to the treatment given
- Vital signs taken en route
- Any additional information collected en route but not transmitted to the receiving facility

Give your verbal report in a polite and respectful manner (Figure 4-9). The receiving facility staff may ask you questions to clarify information or may have additional questions about the patient or your observations at the scene. Effective communication with the receiving facility staff is important. It can make the difference between prompt, efficient care for the patient's injury or illness and problems and confusion that may delay patient care.

Arrival at the Receiving Facility

Objectives 6, 8

Notify dispatch as soon as you arrive at the receiving facility.

| Medic 51: | "Dispatch, Medic 51 (five, one). Arrival at Anytown Medical Center." |
| Dispatch Center: | "Received, Medic 51 (five, one). Arrival at Anytown Medical Center at 1448 (fourteen, four, eight)." |

On arrival at the receiving facility, the staff expects a verbal report that follows a specific format. The verbal report (sometimes called a *hand-off report*) is essentially a summary of the information that you gave over the radio. Give your verbal report to a healthcare

En Route to the Station

Objective 6

Notify dispatch when you are leaving the receiving facility and are en route to the station.

Medic 51:	"Medic 51 (five, one) to Dispatch."
Dispatch Center:	"Dispatch. Go ahead Medic 51 (five, one)."
Medic 51:	"Dispatch, Medic 51 (five, one) is leaving Anytown Medical Center en route to our station."
Dispatch Center:	"Received, Medic 51 (five, one). En route to your station. Time: 1510 (fifteen, ten)."

Contact dispatch again on arrival at the station or earlier, when you enter your service area, per your agency's guidelines.

Medic 51:	"Medic 51 (five, one) to Dispatch."
Dispatch Center:	"Dispatch. Medic 51 (five, one), go ahead."
Medic 51:	"Dispatch, Medic 51(five, one) is back at our station and in service."
Dispatch Center:	"Received, Medic 51 (five, one). In station and available for service. Time: 1518 (fifteen, eighteen)."

Legal Considerations

Objective 10

Your interaction with a patient should always be direct, polite, and honest. There are legal limits to the information that you may share with others about your patient. These legal limitations are found in the Health Insurance Portability and Accountability Act (HIPAA) (see Chapter 3). Generally, you may share medical information about your patient only with those healthcare professionals who will have direct contact with your patient. These legal limitations extend to the radio report given to the receiving facility. Do not use any patient "identifiers" beyond the age and gender of your patient over the radio. Individuals who disobey HIPAA privacy rules face criminal and civil penalties.

On the Scene   Wrap-Up

Communication with dispatch is important. You should notify dispatch when acknowledging notification of the call, responding to the call, and arriving at the scene. If you are responsible for patient transport, notify dispatch when leaving the scene for the receiving facility, arriving at the receiving facility, and leaving the hospital for the station. Contact dispatch again on arrival at the station or earlier, when you enter your service area, per your agency's guidelines.

Before transferring patient care to the paramedics, identify yourself as an EMT and give them a brief report. Introduce the patient by name, indicating that she is 17 years old and complaining of a fever and severe abdominal pain that began yesterday. Explain that you found her lying in bed, and relay pertinent assessment findings, including vital signs. Report any medical history you obtained from the patient, the emergency medical care that you gave, and the patient's response to the treatment given. If you contacted medical direction before the paramedic's arrival, relay this information and any orders received. ∎

Sum It Up

▶ Communication is the process of sending and receiving information. As an EMT, you must be able to communicate effectively with crew members, emergency dispatchers, medical direction, and other healthcare professionals; law enforcement personnel and other public safety workers; the patient; and the patient's family.

▶ The Federal Communications Commission is the U.S. government agency responsible for the development and enforcement of rules and regulations pertaining to radio transmissions.

▶ Very high frequency radio frequencies can be subdivided into low band and high band. Low-band frequencies generally have a greater range than high-band VHF frequencies. Radio waves in the low-band frequency range bend and follow the curvature of the Earth, allowing radio transmission over long distances. Radio waves in the high-band frequency range travel in a straight line. This straight-line quality means that the radio wave is easily blocked by topography such as a hill, mountain, or large building.

▶ Ultrahigh frequency radio waves travel in a straight line but do have an ability to reflect off or bounce around buildings. The 800-megahertz frequencies are UHF radio signals that use computer technology to make transmissions more secure than the other types of radio transmission.

▶ A base station is a transmitter/receiver at a stationary site such as a hospital, mountaintop, or public safety agency. A radio signal generated by the base station may be sent directly to a receiving unit or to a repeater as needed. A mobile two-way radio is a vehicular-mounted communication device. A portable radio is a handheld communication device. A repeater is a device that receives a transmission from a low-power portable or mobile radio on one frequency and then retransmits it at a higher power on another frequency so that it can be received at a distant location.

▶ Mobile data computers (also called mobile data terminals) are computers mounted in emergency vehicles that display information pertaining to the calls for which EMS personnel are dispatched. The computer is also used to send and receive text messages between the EMS crew and the dispatch center.

▶ An EMS communications network must provide a means by which a citizen can reliably access the EMS system (usually by dialing 9-1-1). To ensure adequate EMS system response and coordination, there must also be a means for dispatch center to emergency vehicle communication, communication between emergency vehicles, communication from the emergency vehicle to the hospital, hospital-to-hospital communication, and communication between agencies, such as between EMS and law enforcement personnel.

▶ The sequence 9-1-1 is the official national emergency number in the United States and Canada. When the numbers 9-1-1 are dialed, the caller is quickly connected to a single location called a Public Safety Answering Point. Although EMS is usually activated by dialing 9-1-1 from a standard telephone, other methods of activating an emergency response include emergency alarm boxes, citizen band radios, and wireless telephones. Enhanced 9-1-1, or E9-1-1, is a system that routes an emergency call to the 9-1-1 center closest to the caller and automatically displays the caller's phone number and address. Voice over Internet Protocol (also known as Internet Voice) is technology that allows users to make telephone calls by means of a broadband Internet connection instead of a regular telephone line.

▶ Emergency medical dispatchers are trained professionals who are responsible for verifying the address of the incident, asking questions of the caller, assigning technicians to the incident, alerting/activating technicians to the incident, providing prearrival instructions to the caller, communicating with technicians, and recording incident times.

▶ After being dispatched to the call, dispatch should be notified when the EMS crew is receiving the call, responding to the call, arriving at the scene, leaving the scene for the receiving facility, arriving at the receiving facility, leaving the hospital for the station, returning to service, and arriving at the station.

▶ When communicating with individuals from other agencies, be organized, concise, thorough, and accurate.

▶ It may be necessary to contact medical direction for advice or receive other orders. The information given to the physician must be accurate. Repeat orders back to the physician, word for word.

▶ Use a standardized reporting format when relaying a verbal report to medical direction or to the staff of the receiving facility.

▶ The Health Insurance Portability and Accountability Act limits the medical information that may be shared about an individual.

CHAPTER

Medical Terminology

By the end of this chapter, you should be able to:

Knowledge Objectives ▶
1. Identify and define the main parts of a medical term.
2. Identify and define a combining vowel and combining form.
3. Describe standard anatomical position.
4. Identify and define terms that describe directions and positions of the body.
5. Identify and define commonly used medical abbreviations and acronyms.

Attitude Objectives ▶
6. Explain the rationale for using medical terminology correctly.
7. Show appreciation for proper terminology when describing a patient or patient condition.

Skill Objectives ▶
There are no skill objectives identified for this lesson.

On the Scene

You and your EMT partner are called to a local grocery store for an "ill man." As you enter the store, you are quickly directed to the patient's location. You find a 30-year-old man lying prone on the floor with several people kneeling next to him. As you get closer to the man on the floor, one of the women kneeling near the patient says, "This is my husband. He has diabetes and hypertension. I think he may be hypoglycemic. He took his insulin this morning but may not have eaten as much as he was supposed to." Fire department paramedics are en route to the scene. ■

THINK ABOUT IT

As you read this chapter, think about the following questions:

- How does your knowledge of medical terminology and anatomical terms assist you with understanding the scene and the potential for a life-threatening medical emergency?
- What terminology may be used to help determine what is possibly wrong with this patient?
- Why is it important to be able to understand the terminology associated with the patient's prior medical history?
- How does your understanding of simple medical and anatomical terms influence or alter your care?
- What type of terminology will you use to relay scene and patient information to the responding medical crew?

An EMT is a healthcare professional. Healthcare professionals use medical terms to communicate information about a patient's illness or injury. To correctly relay what you are seeing and what the patient is saying in your written and verbal reports, you must know medical terms and their meanings. You must also spell medical terms correctly because a spelling error may completely alter the meaning of the word and result in incorrect information being conveyed to other healthcare professionals.

Word Parts

Objective 1

Many medical terms originate from Greek and Latin words. Although it is not necessary to know these languages to learn and use medical terminology, an understanding of common medical terms is important. Medical terms are made up of three main parts: a root word, prefix, and suffix. When learning medical terms, slashes are often used to differentiate the parts of a term. Each word part is discussed below. Medical terms for body positions, directional terms,

and common medical abbreviations, which are used to save time when documenting, are discussed later in this chapter.

Root Words

All medical terms have a root word (also called the *stem*). A *root word* is the main part of a word and conveys the body system, part, disease, or condition being discussed. Although some root words are complete words by themselves, many are combined with a prefix, suffix, and/or another root word to form a more descriptive word.

Prefixes

A prefix is a syllable placed at the beginning of a root word to modify its meaning. Many medical terms do not have a prefix. When a prefix is written alone, a hyphen follows it. For example, the prefix *a-* or *an-* means "without or absence of." The root word *algesia* means "sensitivity to pain." The hyphen that follows *an-* indicates that another word part follows the prefix to form a complete word. Combining the prefix and root word results in the medical term *analgesia*, which means "without or absence of pain." Common prefixes are shown in Table 5-1. Prefixes pertaining to color are shown in Table 5-2.

TABLE 5-1 Common Prefixes

Prefix	Meaning	Prefix	Meaning
a-, an-	without, from, absence of	de-	down, lack of
ab-	away from	derma-	skin
ad-	toward, near	dia-	through, completely
aden-	pertaining to gland	dys-	difficult, bad, painful, abnormal
ana-	up, toward, apart		
ante-	before	ec-, ecto-, ex-, exo-, extra-	out, outside, without
anti-	against, opposing		
auto-	self	edem-	swelling
bi-	two	en-, end-	inside, within
brady-	slow	endo-	within, inner
circum-	around, about	ep-, epi-	upon, on, over
contra-	opposite, against	eu-	good, normal

Continued

TABLE 5-1 Common Prefixes *Continued*

Prefix	Meaning	Prefix	Meaning
hemi-	half	peri-	around
hyper-	excessive, high, above	poly-	many, much, excessive
hypo-	too little, low, beneath, under	post-	after, behind
infra-	beneath, under	pre-	before, in front of
inter-	between	pseudo-	false
intra-	within	quadri-	four
macro-	great, abnormal largeness	retro-	behind, backward
mal-	bad	semi-	half
mega-	large, great	sub-	under, beneath
megalo-	large, great	super-	above, beyond
micro-	small	supra-	above, beyond
mid-	middle	sym-	joined, together, with
multi-	many, much	syn-	joined, together, with
my-	pertaining to muscle	tachy-	fast
oligo-	little, scanty	trans-	across
para-	near, beside, abnormal	tri-	three
per-	through, by, excessive	uni-	one, single

Suffixes

A *suffix* is a syllable placed at the end of a root word to modify its meaning. When a suffix is written alone, a hyphen precedes it. For example, the suffix *-itis* means "inflammation." The root word *gastr* means "stomach." The hyphen that precedes *-itis* indicates that another word part precedes the suffix to form a complete word. Combining the root word and suffix results in the medical term *gastritis*, which means "inflammation of the stomach." Common suffixes are shown in Table 5-3.

Combining Forms

Objective 2

A vowel is often added between a root word and suffix or between two word roots to make the new term easier to pronounce. The vowel used is called a *combining vowel*. The root word plus the combining vowel is called

TABLE 5-2 Prefixes Pertaining to Color

Prefix	Meaning
alb-	white
chlor-, chloro-	green
cyan-, cyano-	blue
eryth-, erythro-	red
leuk-, leuko-	white
melan-, melano-	dark, black
xanth-, xantho-	yellow

a *combining form*. Although the most common combining vowel used is *o*, the vowels *a*, *e*, *i*, *u*, and *y* are sometimes used as well. A combining vowel is not used to connect a prefix and word root.

TABLE 5-3   Common Suffixes

Suffix	Meaning	Suffix	Meaning
-able, -ible	capable of, able to	-megaly	enlargement
-ac, -iac	pertaining to	-oid	resembling
-al, -an	pertaining to	-ole	little, small
-algia	pain	-oma	tumor, swelling
-ar, -ary	pertaining to	-opia	vision
-ase	enzyme	-opsy	to view
-centesis	surgical puncture to remove fluid	-ose	sugar
		-osis	condition of
-cidal	killing	-ostomy	creation of an opening
-cyte	cell	-ous	pertaining to or characterized by
-dipsia	thirst		
-eal	pertaining to	-para	a woman who has given birth
-ectomy	surgical removal or cutting out	-paresis	weakness
-edema	swelling	-partum	birth, labor
-emesis	vomiting	-pathy	disease condition
-emia	blood condition	-phagia	eating
-esthesia	sensation, perception	-phasia	speech
-eum, -ium	membrane	-phobia	fear
-genic	causing, produced by	-plasty	surgical repair/reshaping
-gram	record	-plegia	paralysis
-graph	recording	-pnea	breathing
-graphy	process of recording	-rhythmia	rhythm
-ia, -iasis, -ism	condition	-rrhagia, -rrhage	rapid flow or discharge
-iac	one who suffers	-rrhea	flow, discharge
-ic, -ical	pertaining to	-sclerosis	hardening
-ictal	seizure, attack	-scope	instrument for visual examination
-itis	inflammation	-scopy	insertion of a lighted instrument to view inner areas of the body
-ive	pertaining to		
-lexia	words, phrases	-sepsis	infection
-lith	stone or calculus	-spasm	sudden, involuntary muscle contraction
-logy	science, study of		

Continued

TABLE 5-3 Common Suffixes *Continued*

Suffix	Meaning	Suffix	Meaning
-stalsis	contraction	-tomy	incision, cut into
-stomy	formation of an opening (stoma)	-tripsy	surgical crushing
		-trophy	development
-therapy	treatment	-ule	little, small
-tic	pertaining to	-uria	urine, urination

To better understand combining forms, consider this example. When the term *hematology* is broken down into its parts, the root word is *hemat*, which means "blood." The suffix, *-logy*, means "study of." The combining vowel is the letter *o*. *Hemat* and the combining vowel *o* (*hemato*) make up a combining form. When all the parts are combined, *hematology* means "the study of blood."

A combining vowel is dropped when it is added to a word that begins with a vowel. For example, the combining form *neur/o* means "nerve" and the suffix *algia* means "pain." When the word parts are joined, the combining vowel (*o*) is dropped. The term *neuralgia* means "pain along a nerve." Common root words and combining forms are shown in Table 5-4.

Plural Medical Terms

In the English language, the plural form of a noun is often made by adding *-s* or *-es* to the root word. Medical terms derived from Greek or Latin words have different rules that must be applied when forming the plural form of the root word. Use the examples provided in Table 5-5 to learn how to create the plural forms of most medical terms.

TABLE 5-4 Common Root Words

Root Word/ Combining Form	Meaning	Root Word/ Combining Form	Meaning
abdomin/o	abdomen	col/o	colon (large intestine)
algesia	sensitivity to pain	cost/o	rib
angi/o	vessel	cutane/o	skin
arter/o, arteri/o	artery	encephal/o	brain
arthr/o	joint	enter/o	intestine
axill/o	armpit	gastr/o	stomach
brachi/o	arm	gluc/o	sugar
bronch/o	bronchi (lungs)	glyc/o	sugar
carcin/o	cancer	gravid/o	pregnancy
cardi/o	heart	hem/a, hem/o	blood
carp/o	wrist	hemat/o	blood
cephal/o	head	hepat/o	liver
chondr/o	cartilage	hydr/o	water, fluid
chron/o	time	immune/o	protection

Continued

TABLE 5-4 Common Root Words *Continued*

Root Word/ Combining Form	Meaning	Root Word/ Combining Form	Meaning
laryng/o	larynx (voice box)	physi/o	nature
lingu/o	tongue	pneumon/o	lungs
lith/o	stone	pulmon/o	lungs
mamm/o	breast	py/o	pus
mast/o	breast	pyr/o	fever, heat
my/o	muscle	ren/o	kidney
naso	nose	rhin/o	nose
nephr/o	kidney	splen/o	spleen
neur/o	nerve	therm/o	heat
ophthalm/o	eye	thorac/o	chest
oro	mouth	thromb/o	clot
oste/o	bone	thyr/o	shield, thyroid
ot/o	ear	tox/o, toxic/o	poison
path/o	disease	trache/o	trachea (windpipe)
ped/o	child, foot	vas/o, vascul/o	vessel
pharyng/o	throat	ven/o	vein
phleb/o	vein		

TABLE 5-5 Plural Word Forms

Singular Ending	Plural Ending	Example
-a	-ae	Singular: vertebra Plural: vertebrae
-ax	-aces	Singular: pneumothorax Plural: pneumothoraces
-en	-ina	Singular: lumen Plural: lumina
-ex	-ices	Singular: cortex Plural: cortices
-is	-es	Singular: psychosis Plural: psychoses
-itis	-ides	Singular: arthritis Plural: arthritides

Continued

TABLE 5-5 Plural Word Forms *Continued*

Singular Ending	Plural Ending	Example
-ix	-ices	Singular: appendix Plural: appendices
-ma	-s or mata	Singular: carcinoma Plural: carcinomas or carcinomata
-nx	-nges	Singular: phalanx Plural: phalanges
-on	-a	Singular: protozoon Plural: protozoa
-um	-a	Singular: atrium Plural: atria
-us	-i	Singular: alveolus Plural: alveoli
-y (preceded by a vowel)	-s	Singular: survey Plural: surveys
-y (preceded by a consonant)	-ies	Singular: artery Plural: arteries
-yx	-yces	Singular: calyx Plural: calyces

Body Positions and Directional Terms

Objectives 3, 4

Medical terms are used to convey to others the location of a patient's injury or symptoms so that further care can be given. Directions refer to the body when it is in the **anatomical position.** In the anatomical position, a person is standing, arms to the sides with the palms turned forward, feet close together and pointed forward, the head pointed forward, and the eyes open (Figure 5-1). Definitions and examples of common directional terms are given in Table 5-6 and Figure 5-2.

- *Superior/inferior.* **Superior** means above or in a higher position than another portion of the body. The head is the most superior part of the body. The neck is superior to the chest because it is closer to the head. **Inferior** means in a position lower than another. The soles of the feet are the most inferior part of the body. The knees are inferior to the pelvis because they are closer to the feet.

- *Anterior/posterior.* **Anterior**, or *ventral*, represents the front portion of the body or body part. The heart is anterior to the spine. **Posterior**, or *dorsal*, is the back side of the body or body part. The spine is posterior to the heart.

- *Proximal/distal.* These terms are most often used when referring to an extremity (arm or leg). **Proximal** means closer to the midline or center area of the body. When this term is used to reference an extremity, it means nearer to the point of attachment to the body. The knees are proximal to the toes. **Distal** means farther from the midline or center area of the body. With reference to an extremity, it means farthest from the point of attachment to the body. The elbow is distal to the shoulder.

- *Midline.* The **midline** is an imaginary line down the center of the body that divides the body into right and left sides. Using the midline as a reference point will assist in describing whether an injury is **lateral** (toward the side) or **medial** (toward the midline). The **sternum** (breastbone) is medial to the left nipple. The **axilla** (armpit) is lateral to the sternum. The word **bilateral** means pertaining to both sides. **Contralateral** means

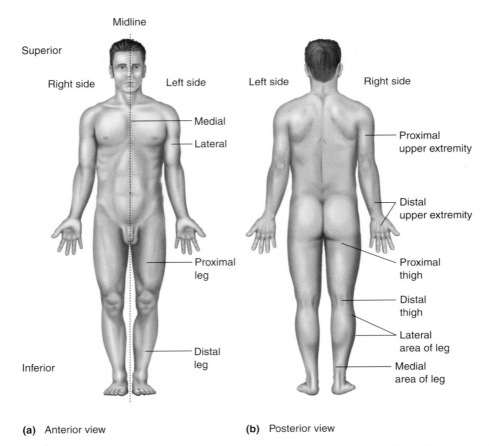

(a) Anterior view   (b) Posterior view

FIGURE 5-1 ▲ The anatomical position and directional terms. **(a)** Front (anterior) view; **(b)** back (posterior) view.

TABLE 5-6	Common Directional Terms	
Term	**Definition**	**Example**
Superior	Above or in a higher position than another portion of the body	The head is the most superior part of the body. The neck is superior to the chest because it is closer to the head.
Inferior	In a position lower than another	The soles of the feet are the most inferior part of the body. The knees are inferior to the pelvis because they are closer to the feet.
Anterior, ventral	The front portion of the body or body part	The heart is anterior to the spine.
Posterior, dorsal	The back side of the body or body part	The spine is posterior to the heart.
Proximal	Closer to the midline or center area of the body; most often used when referring to an extremity, meaning nearer to the point of attachment to the body.	The knees are proximal to the toes.

Continued

TABLE 5-6 Common Directional Terms *Continued*

Term	Definition	Example
Distal	Farther from the midline or center area of the body; with reference to an extremity, it means farthest from the point of attachment to the body	The elbow is distal to the shoulder.
Midline	An imaginary line down the center of the body that divides the body into right and left sides; used to assist in describing whether an injury is lateral (toward the side) or medial (toward the midline)	
Lateral	Toward the side	The *axilla* (armpit) is lateral to the sternum.
Medial	Toward the midline	The *sternum* (breastbone) is medial to the left nipple.
Bilateral	Pertaining to both sides	
Contralateral	On the opposite side	
Ipsilateral	On the same side	
Midaxillary line	An imaginary vertical line drawn from the middle of the patient's armpits (axillae), parallel to the midline; it divides the body into anterior and posterior sections	
Midclavicular line	An imaginary vertical line drawn through the middle portion of the collarbone (clavicle) and nipple, parallel to the midline	

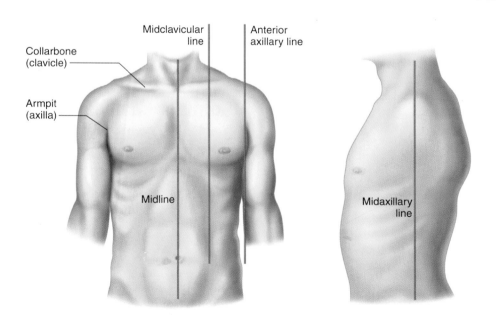

FIGURE 5-2 ▲ The midaxillary line is an imaginary vertical line drawn from the middle of the patient's armpits (axillae), parallel to the midline. The midclavicular line is an imaginary vertical line drawn through the middle portion of the collarbone (clavicle) and nipple, parallel to the midline.

TABLE 5-7 Position Terminology

Term	Definition
Erect	A person standing up
Supine	A person lying flat on the back, face up
Prone	A person lying facedown and flat
Lateral recumbent	A person lying on his side
Left lateral recumbent	A person lying on her left side
Right lateral recumbent	A person lying on his right side

on the opposite side. **Ipsilateral** means on the same side.

- *Midaxillary line.* The **midaxillary line** refers to an imaginary vertical line drawn from the middle of the patient's armpits (axillae), parallel to the midline. It divides the body into anterior and posterior sections.
- *Midclavicular line.* The **midclavicular line** refers to an imaginary vertical line drawn through the middle portion of the collarbone (clavicle) and nipple, parallel to the midline (Figure 5-2).

Remember This

- When you look at a patient in the anatomical position, describe the patient's injuries from the patient's perspective. In other words, right and left always refers to the *patient's* right and left.
- If you forget the proper medical term for something, use a plain, understandable description instead. For example, if you forget that the back is posterior, then refer to the "back of the patient." Do not make up or guess at terms—it could be embarrassing. It could also lead to misinterpretation by others.

Ill and injured patients are found in many positions. Table 5-7 has terminology for positions. A person standing upright is said to be **erect**. A person lying flat on the back (face up) is said to be in a **supine** position. A person lying facedown and flat is in a **prone** position. If a person is found on her side, she is in a **lateral recumbent position.** If he is found

on his left side, he is in a left lateral recumbent position. If she is on her right side, she is in a right lateral recumbent position.

Remember This

It is important to use body position and directional terms properly so that you can describe the position in which the patient is found and transported.

As an EMT, you may choose to place a patient in a specific position based on the patient's condition. For example, Fowler's position is lying on the back with the upper body elevated at a 45- to 60-degree angle. In a semi-Fowler's position, the patient is sitting up with the head at a 45-degree angle and legs out straight. In a high-Fowler's position, the patient is sitting upright at a 90-degree angle. A patient who is short of breath is often placed in one of these positions.

Common Medical Abbreviations and Acronyms

Objective 5

Abbreviations and acronyms are used to save time and space when documenting. An abbreviation is a shortened form of a word or name, such as *abd* for "abdominal." An acronym is a word formed from the first letter or letters of several words, such as *CHF* for "congestive heart failure." Use abbreviations and acronyms only if they are standard and approved by your EMS system. Common abbreviations and acronyms are shown in Table 5-8. Common units of measure are listed in Table 5-9.

TABLE 5-8 Common Abbreviations and Acronyms

Abbreviation/Acronym	Meaning	Abbreviation/Acronym	Meaning
<	less than	ARDS	adult respiratory distress syndrome
>	more than	ASA	aspirin
=	equal	ASHD	atherosclerotic heart disease
~	approximately, about	AV	arteriovenous, atrioventricular
↑	increased		
↓	decreased	BBO_2	blow-by oxygen
→	going to or leading to	BCP	birth control pills
△	change	Bilat	bilateral
♀ or F	female	Bld	blood
♂ or M	male	BLS	basic life support
ā	before	BM	bowel movement, bag-mask
AAA	abdominal aortic aneurysm	BOW	bag of waters
A&O	alert and oriented	BP	blood pressure
A&O×4	alert and oriented to person, place, time, and event	bpm	beats per minute
A&P	anterior and posterior; anatomy and physiology	BS	breath sounds, blood sugar
		BSA	body surface area
ABD, abd	abdomen	BW	birth weight
ABG	arterial blood gas	c̄	with
AC	antecubital (vein)	c/m	cool and moist
ACE	angiotensin converting enzyme	C/O	complains of
ACS	acute coronary syndrome	CA, Ca, ca	cancer, carcinoma
AFib	atrial fibrillation	CABG	coronary artery bypass graft
AIDS	acquired immunodeficiency syndrome	CAD	coronary artery disease
ALS	advanced life support	caps	capsules
AMA	against medical advice	CC, C.C.	chief complaint
AMI	acute myocardial infarction	CCU	coronary care unit
Amt	amount	CHF	congestive heart failure
Ant	anterior	Clr	clear

Continued

TABLE 5-8 Common Abbreviations and Acronyms *Continued*

Abbreviation/Acronym	Meaning	Abbreviation/Acronym	Meaning
CMS	circulation, motor, sensory	DOE	dyspnea on exertion
CN	courtesy notification	DPT	diphtheria, pertussis, and tetanus
CNS	central nervous system	DX, Dx, dx	diagnosis
CO	carbon monoxide, cardiac output	ECG	electrocardiogram
CO_2	carbon dioxide	ED	emergency department
Conc	conscious	EDC	expected date of confinement (due date)
Cond	condition	ENT	ear, nose, and throat
COPD	chronic obstructive pulmonary disease	Epi	epinephrine
CP	chest pain	ETA	estimated time of arrival
CPh	cellular phone	ETOH	ethyl alcohol
CPR	cardiopulmonary resuscitation	Exam	examination
C-spine	cervical spine	Ext	extremities
CSF	cerebrospinal fluid	F/U	follow-up
CT	computed tomography	FDA	Food and Drug Administration
CVA	cerebrovascular accident	FSI	full spinal immobilization
D/C	discontinue	FUO	fever of undetermined origin
D/T	dispatched to	Fx	fracture
DCAP-BTLS	*d*eformities, *c*ontusions, *a*brasions, *p*unctures, *b*urns, *t*enderness, *l*acerations, *s*welling	GB	gallbladder
		GI	gastrointestinal
		GLF	ground level fall
Defib	defibrillation	GSW	gunshot wound
D50	50% dextrose	GU	genitourinary
D5W	5% dextrose in water	GYN, gyn	gynecology
DKA	diabetic ketoacidosis	H/A	headache
DM	diabetes mellitus	h/d	hot/dry
DNP	did not patch	h/m	hot/moist
DO	doctor of osteopathy	HEENT	*h*ead, *e*yes, *e*ars, *n*ose, *t*hroat
DOA	dead on arrival		

Continued

TABLE 5-8 Common Abbreviations and Acronyms *Continued*

Abbreviation/Acronym	Meaning	Abbreviation/Acronym	Meaning
Hgb	hemoglobin	MD	medical doctor, muscular dystrophy
HIV	human immunodeficiency virus	MDI	metered dose inhaler
HPI	history of present illness	MI	myocardial infarction
HR	heart rate	MOI	mechanism of injury
HTN	hypertension	MRI	magnetic resonance imaging
Hx	history		
ICS	intercostal space	MS	multiple sclerosis, morphine sulfate
ICU	intensive care unit	MVA	motor vehicle accident
inf	inferior	MVC	motor vehicle crash, motor vehicle collision
inj	injection		
IUD	intrauterine device	N/C	nasal cannula, no charge
IV	intravenous	n/v	nausea/vomiting
JVD	jugular vein distention	n/v/d	nausea/vomiting/diarrhea
K+	potassium	NA	not applicable
kg	kilogram	Na+	sodium
KO	keep open	NaCl	sodium chloride
KVO	keep vein open	NFO	no further orders
LAD	left anterior descending (coronary artery)	NG, N/G	nasogastric
lat	lateral	NKA	no known allergies
LMP	last menstrual period	NKDA	no known drug allergies
LOC	loss of consciousness, level of consciousness	No △	no change
		NPA	nasal airway, nasopharyngeal airway
LR	Lactated Ringer's		
lt	left	NPO	nothing by mouth
LUQ	left upper quadrant	NS	normal saline
LV	left ventricle	NTG	nitroglycerin
MAE	moves all extremities	OB	obstetrics

Continued

TABLE 5-8 Common Abbreviations and Acronyms *Continued*

Abbreviation/Acronym	Meaning	Abbreviation/Acronym	Meaning
OB/GYN	obstetrics and gynecology	PVC	premature ventricular complex
OPA	oral airway, oropharyngeal airway	q	*quodque* (Latin for "each, every")
OTC	over-the-counter	q.h.	*quaque hora* (Latin for "every hour")
$\overline{p}$	after		
P	pulse	R	respirations
PCN	penicillin	R/O	rule out
Peds	pediatrics	R/T	respond to
PERL	pupils equal, round, reactive to light	RBC	red blood cell
		RLQ	right lower quadrant
PERLA	pupils equal, round, reactive to light and accommodation	RN	registered nurse
		ROM	range of motion
pH	hydrogen ion concentration	ROS	rate of speed
PI	present illness	RP	reporting or responsible party
PID	pelvic inflammatory disease	RUQ	right upper quadrant
PMH	past medical history	Rx	prescription, treatment
PMS	premenstrual syndrome; *pulses, movement* (motion), *sensation*	$\overline{s}$	without
		S&S, S/S	signs and symptoms
P.O.	*per os* (Latin for "by mouth")	SCBA	self-contained breathing apparatus
		sec	second
POC	products of conception	SIDS	sudden infant death syndrome
POV	privately owned vehicle		
p.r.n.	*pro re nata* (Latin for "as needed, as necessary")	SNT	soft, nontender
		SO	standing order
PSVT	paroxysmal supraventricular tachycardia	SOB	shortness of breath
PT	physical therapy	stat	immediately
PTA	prior to arrival	STD	sexually transmitted disease
PTCA	percutaneous transluminal coronary angioplasty	Subcut	subcutaneous
		SVN	small volume nebulizer

Continued

TABLE 5-8 Common Abbreviations and Acronyms *Continued*

Abbreviation/Acronym	Meaning	Abbreviation/Acronym	Meaning
Sx	symptom	UA	urinalysis
Sz	seizure	URI	upper respiratory infection
T	temperature	UTI	urinary tract infection
Tabs	tablets	VF	ventricular fibrillation
TB	tuberculosis	VS	vital signs
temp.	temperature	VT	ventricular tachycardia
TIA	transient ischemic attack	w/d	warm/dry
TKO	to keep open	w/d/p	warm/dry/pink
TMJ	temporomandibular joint	w/m	warm/moist
TPR	temperature, pulse, respirations	W/O	without
TRX, x-port	transport	WBC	white blood cell
TV	tidal volume	x-fer	transfer
Tx	treatment	y.o./YO	year old
U/A	upon arrival		

TABLE 5-9 Abbreviations for Common Units of Measure

cm	centimeter	mEq	milliequivalent
ft	foot, feet	mg	milligram
g, gm	gram	ml, mL	milliliter
hr	hour	mm	millimeter
l, L	liter	oz	ounce
lb	pound	ppm	parts per million
m	meter	tsp	teaspoon
mcg	microgram		

On the Scene Wrap-Up

Your training helps you understand that this patient has diabetes and may also have heart problems. As you kneel next to him, you ask the patient's wife if the patient fell or was assisted to the ground. She tells you that she helped him lie down after he complained of feeling dizzy and weak. You know that laying facedown (prone) may compromise your patient's airway. As you move him to his back and assess him, the patient responds to you saying that he still feels dizzy.

As you assess the patient's blood glucose level, the local fire department arrives. You are able to give a good hand-off report to the fire department paramedic using proper medical terminology. You explain that the patient is hypoglycemic (low blood sugar) and has a history of hypertension (high blood pressure). The fire department paramedic thanks you for your assistance and assumes care of the patient. Minutes later the patient is loaded into the back of the ambulance, accompanied by the fire department paramedic. ■

Sum It Up

► Healthcare professionals use medical terms to communicate information about a patient's illness or injury. To correctly relay what you are seeing and what the patient is saying in your written and verbal reports, you must know medical terms and their meanings. You must also spell medical terms correctly because a spelling error may completely alter the meaning of the word.

► Medical terms are made up of three main parts: a root word, prefix, and suffix. A root word is the main part of a word and conveys the body system, part, disease, or condition being discussed. A prefix is a syllable placed at the beginning of a root word to modify its meaning. A suffix is a syllable placed at the end of a root word to modify its meaning.

► A vowel is often added between a root word and suffix or between two word roots to make the new term easier to pronounce. The vowel used is called a combining vowel. The root word plus the combining vowel is called a combining form.

► In your role as an EMT, it is important to know the terms used to describe body positions and directions. You must be able to use these terms correctly so that you can describe the position in which a patient is found and transported. You will also need to know body positions so that you can place a patient in a specific position based on the patient's condition.

► Abbreviations and acronyms are used to save time and space when documenting. Use abbreviations and acronyms only if they are standard and approved by your EMS system.

Module 2

Function and Development of the Human Body

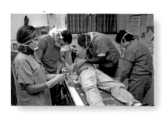

▶ CHAPTER 6

The Human Body   138

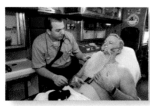

▶ CHAPTER 7

Pathophysiology   175

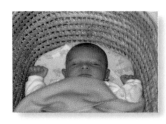

▶ CHAPTER 8

Life Span Development   188

CHAPTER

6

The Human Body

By the end of this chapter, you should be able to:

Knowledge Objectives ▶

1. Define anatomy and physiology.
2. Describe the structure and function of a typical cell.
3. Name and describe the levels of organization of the body.
4. Name the organ systems of the body.
5. Define homeostasis, and give an example of a typical homeostatic mechanism.
6. Define cell metabolism, aerobic metabolism, and anaerobic metabolism.
7. Explain the importance of water to the function of the body.
8. Define intracellular and extracellular fluid.
9. Name the body cavities and some organs within each cavity.
10. Explain the four quadrants of the abdomen, and name the organs in those areas.
11. Describe the sagittal, midsagittal, transverse, and frontal planes.
12. List the functions of the musculoskeletal system.
13. Identify the two major subdivisions of the skeleton, and list the bones in each area.
14. Explain how bones are classified, and give an example of each.
15. Name the bones of the skull and face.
16. Describe the structure of the vertebral column and thoracic cage.
17. Explain the purpose of muscles and the basic differences between skeletal, smooth, and cardiac muscles.
18. Explain the purpose of tendons and ligaments.
19. State the general function of the respiratory system.
20. Describe the anatomy and function of each of the structures in the upper and lower airway.
21. Define tidal volume, anatomic dead space, and minute volume.
22. Describe the changes in air pressure within the chest cavity during ventilation.
23. Differentiate between ventilation and respiration.
24. Differentiate between internal and external respiration.
25. Discuss alveolar-capillary gas exchange and cell-capillary gas exchange.
26. Describe the components and functions of the circulatory system.
27. Name the chambers of the heart and their function.
28. Trace the flow of blood through the heart's chambers and valves.
29. Describe the primary functions of blood.
30. List the formed elements of blood, and state the primary functions of each.
31. Describe the structure and function of each of the blood vessels: arteries, arterioles, capillaries, venules, and veins.

32. Name the major arteries, and describe their location and the parts of the body they nourish.
33. Name the major veins, and describe their location and the parts of the body they drain of blood.
34. Define pulse, and differentiate between a central and a peripheral pulse, giving examples of each.
35. Define blood pressure, systolic blood pressure, and diastolic blood pressure.
36. Name the divisions of the nervous system, and state the general functions of each.
37. Describe the location and function of the meninges and cerebrospinal fluid.
38. State the functions of the parts of the brain, and locate each part on a diagram.
39. Compare the function of the sympathetic and parasympathetic divisions of the autonomic nervous system.
40. State the functions of the integumentary system.
41. Describe the layers of the skin and, where applicable, the structures contained within them.
42. Describe the functions and components of the digestive system.
43. Describe the functions and components of the endocrine system.
44. Describe the functions and components of the male and female reproductive systems.
45. Describe the functions and components of the urinary system.

Attitude Objectives ▶   There are no attitude objectives identified for this lesson.

Skill Objectives ▶   There are no skill objectives identified for this lesson.

On the Scene

It has already been a tough assignment for your unit on this security detail. Then, just after lunch, while patrolling the perimeter of your area, you hear a blast and the sound of glass breaking. An initial team goes to investigate, and then you are sent in to check out the one officer injured by the explosion. Your patient is lying on the ground, awake and moaning. He was struck by flying debris and thrown approximately 12 feet from an armored carrier during the blast.

A member of the initial team maintains the officer's spine position while you quickly perform your initial assessment. The patient has strong radial and carotid pulses, and you find no immediate life threats. As you wait for the EVAC unit, you continue your head-to-toe assessment. He has several open cuts superior to his right eyebrow. His face is tender over the mandible area, and he is having trouble speaking because of the pain. There is tenderness to the cervical spine area. You note bruising on his chest lateral to his right nipple, and his ribs are tender. He jumps with pain when you palpate over his sternum but says he is not having any difficulty breathing. When you palpate the left upper quadrant of his abdomen, the patient pushes your hand away. There is deformity in the area of his femur. Luckily, you can feel a strong dorsalis pedis pulse in both feet, and normal movement and sensation is present distal to the injury. ■

As you read this chapter, think about the following questions:

- On the basis of your physical exam, what underlying structures may be injured?
- Which injuries could lead to trouble with breathing or circulation?
- Where are the mandible, the cervical spine, the sternum, and the femur located?
- Where are the carotid, radial, and dorsalis pedis pulses found?

Introduction

Understanding the Structure and Function of the Body

Objective 1

Anatomy is the study of the structure of an organism, such as the human body. **Physiology** is the study of the normal functions of an organism, such as the human body. As an emergency medical technician, you must be familiar with the structure and function of the human body so that you can better assess an injured or ill patient. For example, if a patient was stabbed in the right upper area of the **abdomen** and you had an understanding of anatomy and physiology, you would then know which organs might be affected. You would understand their function in the body and could anticipate possible complications. The knife blade may have injured the liver, gallbladder, intestines, blood vessels, diaphragm, lungs, and kidneys, depending on the length of the blade and the direction of the stab (for example, whether it was upward, straight, or downward). Your understanding of the human body is essential in order to give proper emergency care.

Structural Organization

Objectives 2, 3, 4

The human body is made up of billions of **cells**, the basic building blocks of the body. Cells vary in size, shape, and function. For example, some nerve cells are very long and threadlike, enabling them to quickly transmit messages from one part of the body to another. Red blood cells are small, circular, and flexible, allowing them to squeeze through blood vessels. The components of a typical cell are shown in Figure 6-1 and described in Table 6-1.

Cells that cluster together to perform a specialized function are called **tissues**. For example, nervous tissue is specialized to receive and conduct electrical signals over long distances in the body. Muscle tissue is com-

posed of similar cells that can contract, usually in response to an electrical signal from a nerve. An **organ** is made up of at least two different types of tissue that work together to perform a particular function. Examples of organs include the brain, stomach, and liver. **Vital organs** are organs such as the brain, heart, and lungs that are essential for life. An **organ system** (also called a body system) is made up of tissues and organs that work together to provide a common function. The human body consists of 10 major organ systems:

- Skeletal
- Muscular
- Respiratory
- Circulatory
- Nervous
- Integumentary
- Digestive
- Endocrine
- Reproductive
- Urinary

Homeostasis

Objectives 5, 6, 7, 8

Organ systems rely on each other to maintain a constant internal environment (**homeostasis**) and perform the required functions of the entire body. Homeostasis is also called a *steady state.*

Thousands of chemical reactions occur within every cell in the body every second. **Cell metabolism** is the sum of the chemical reactions that occur within cells, enabling them to maintain a living state. **Aerobic metabolism** is cell metabolism that occurs in the presence of oxygen. When cells are deprived of oxygen, cell metabolism can continue but much less efficiently. Cell metabolism that does not require the presence of oxygen is called **anaerobic metabolism**. Aerobic metabolism yields considerably more energy for use by the cells than anaerobic metabolism. The process of cell metabolism is discussed in more detail in Chapter 7.

All body systems need nutrients, oxygen, water, and appropriate temperature to survive. To function at their best, cells need a continuous supply of oxygen and glucose. To accomplish this, the respiratory and cardiovascular systems work hand in hand. The blood and blood vessels provide the transport mechanism for

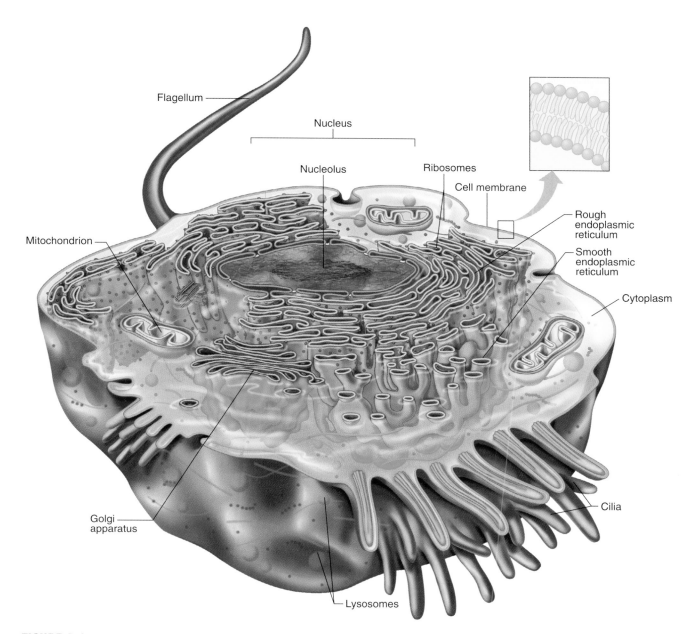

FIGURE 6-1 ▲ A typical cell and its parts.

Labels: Flagellum, Nucleus, Nucleolus, Ribosomes, Cell membrane, Rough endoplasmic reticulum, Smooth endoplasmic reticulum, Cytoplasm, Mitochondrion, Golgi apparatus, Lysosomes, Cilia

moving nutrients such as oxygen, carbohydrates, proteins, and fats to the cells of the body.

Body fluids contain water, electrolytes (such as sodium and potassium), proteins, and other substances. Water is the most abundant component of body fluid, providing the fluid base necessary for chemical reactions, body secretions, and excretions. Body fluids are housed in two main compartments. The **intracellular fluid (ICF)** compartment is actually many small compartments because it is made up of the fluid contained within the walls of the billions of body cells. Intracellular fluid accounts for about two-thirds of body water. The remaining one-third or so of body water is found in the **extracellular fluid (ECF)** compartment, which is

the fluid outside the body cells. Extracellular fluid includes the fluid within the blood vessels (intravascular fluid, or plasma) and the fluid within the tissues (interstitial fluid). The cell membrane is the division between the intracellular and extracellular compartments. To maintain homeostasis, water and the substances dissolved or suspended within it are exchanged between the intracellular and extracellular compartments.

The human body has various "checks and balances" systems to maintain homeostasis. For example, the body's organ systems require a relatively constant temperature for essential chemical reactions to occur normally. If the body's temperature is too low, the muscles shiver to produce heat. If the body's temperature is too high, blood

TABLE 6-1 Cell Structure and Function

Cell Structure	Function
Cell membrane	Forms the outer boundary of the cell; controls the movement of substances into and out of the cell
Cytoplasm	A gelatinous, semitransparent fluid that surrounds the nucleus and is itself encircled by the cell membrane
Nucleus	Control center that contains genetic information (DNA); directs the activities of the cell
Nucleolus	Small, dense body of protein and ribonucleic acid where ribosome production occurs
Mitochondria	"Power plants" of the cell; contain enzymes that release energy from glucose and other nutrients to transform it into a readily useable form (adenosine triphosphate)
Golgi apparatus	Processes and packages proteins
Ribosomes	Sites for protein production
Lysosomes	"Garbage disposals"; contain digestive enzymes that destroy debris and worn-out cell parts
Endoplasmic reticulum (ER)	Tubular communication system for transport of protein and other components through the cytoplasm; ER that lacks ribosomes is called smooth ER and contains enzymes important in fat absorption and the breakdown of alcohol and drugs; rough ER contains ribosomes and is found in cells that manufacture proteins
Cilia	Tiny, hairlike structures that produce a wavelike sweeping motion to move fluid, such as mucus, across the surface of the cilia
Flagellum	Long, taillike structure found on sperm cells that enable the sperm to swim

vessels near the skin's surface **dilate** (expand). This dilation brings more blood to the body surface and allows heat to be passed off into the environment. Sweating is another means of cooling the body through evaporation.

When an organ system does not function properly because of illness or injury, other body functions are affected. For example, the circulatory and respiratory systems need the kidneys to perform their function in order for the body to maintain its balanced environment. If the kidneys fail to produce urine, the circulatory system will retain too much fluid within the bloodstream. This will cause a backup of fluid into the lungs and affect the patient's breathing, disrupting the body's internal balance.

Body Cavities

Objectives 9, 10

A **body cavity** is a hollow space in the body that contains internal organs (Figure 6-2). The **cranial cavity** is located in the head. It contains the brain and is protected by the skull. The **spinal cavity** extends from the bottom of the skull to the lower back. It contains the spinal cord and is protected by the vertebral (spinal) column. The brain and spinal cord make up the **central nervous system**

(CNS). This system allows the body to carry electrical signals from the body's organ systems to the brain and spinal cord as well as to the various organ systems of the body.

The **thoracic (chest) cavity** is located below the neck and above the diaphragm and is protected by the rib cage. The thoracic cavity contains the heart, major blood vessels, and the lungs. The heart is surrounded by another cavity, the **pericardial cavity.** The lungs are surrounded by the **pleural cavities.** The right lung is located in the right pleural cavity; the left lung is located in the left pleural cavity.

The abdominal and pelvic cavities are often called the abdominopelvic cavity. The **abdominal cavity** is located below the diaphragm and above the pelvis (see Plates A, B, and C at the end of this chapter). The abdominal cavity contains the stomach, intestines, liver, gallbladder, pancreas, and spleen. The **peritoneal cavity** is a potential space between two membranes that line the abdominal cavity, separating the abdominal organs from the abdominal wall. Although not separated by any kind of wall, the area below the abdominal cavity is called the **pelvic cavity.** The pelvic cavity contains the urinary bladder, part of the large intestine, and the reproductive organs.

To make it easier to identify the abdominal organs and the location of pain or injury, the abdominal

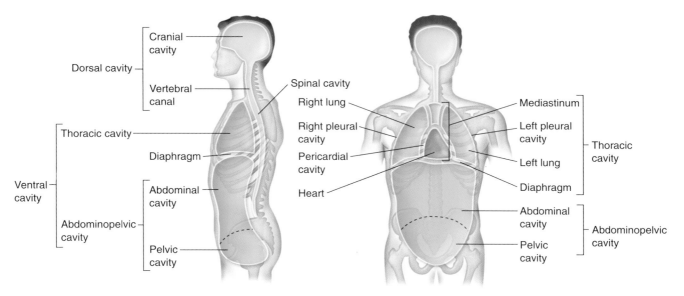

FIGURE 6-2 ▲ Body cavities.

cavity is divided into four quadrants (Figure 6-3). These quadrants are created by drawing two imaginary lines that intersect with the midline through the **navel (umbilicus)**. The **right upper quadrant (RUQ)** contains the liver, the gallbladder, portions of the stomach, and the major blood vessels. The **left upper quadrant (LUQ)** contains the stomach, spleen, and pancreas. The **right lower quadrant (RLQ)** contains the appendix. The **left lower quadrant (LLQ),** along with the other three quadrants, contains the intestines. In females, the right and left lower quadrants contain the ovaries and fallopian tubes. The uterus is in the midline superior to (above) the pelvis and just posterior to (behind) the bladder. Knowing the organs found within each of the four quadrants will help you describe the location of an injury or the symptoms of a sick or injured patient.

Body Planes

Objective 11

The human body is often discussed in terms of sections (cuts) along a plane, which is a flat surface. Planes consist of imaginary lines that are drawn through an upright body (Figure 6-4).

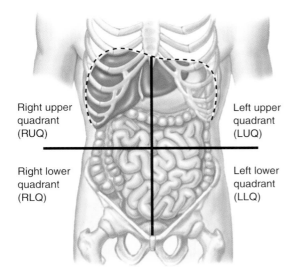

FIGURE 6-3 ▲ The abdominal area is divided into four quadrants.

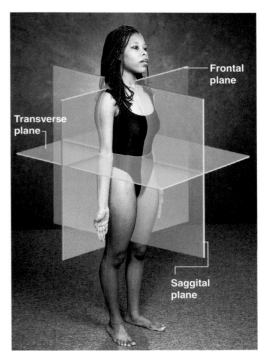

FIGURE 6-4 ▲ Body planes.

The **frontal plane** is the vertical (lengthwise) field that passes through the body from side to side, dividing the body (or any of its parts) into anterior (ventral) and posterior (dorsal) parts. The frontal plane is also called the *coronal plane.*

The **sagittal plane** is the vertical field that passes through the body from front to back, dividing the body (or any of its parts) into right and left sections. The sagittal plane is also called the *lateral plane.* In a sagittal cut, the right and left sides do not have to be equal. The midsagittal plane is the sagittal field that divides the body into two equal halves.

The **transverse plane** is the crosswise field that divides the body (or any of its parts) into superior (upper) and inferior (lower) sections. The transverse plane is also called the *horizontal* or *axial plane.* A cut in the transverse plane may also be called a *cross section.*

The Musculoskeletal System

Objective 12

The musculoskeletal system gives the human body its shape and ability to move and protects the major organs of the body. It consists of the skeletal system (bones) and the muscular system (muscles).

The Skeletal System

Objectives 13, 14

The **skeletal system** consists of 206 bones of varying types. Bones store minerals for the body, such as calcium and phosphorus. Many bones have a hollow cavity that contains a substance called *bone marrow.* Bone marrow produces the body's blood cells—the red blood cells, white blood cells, and platelets.

The skeletal system is divided into two groups of bones. The **axial skeleton** is the part of the skeleton that includes the skull, spinal column, sternum, and ribs (Figures 6-5 and 6-6). The **appendicular skeleton** is made up of the upper and lower extremities (arms and legs), the shoulder girdles, and the pelvic girdle. The **shoulder girdle** is the bony arch formed by the collarbones (clavicles) and shoulder blades (scapulae). The **pelvic girdle** is made up of bones that enclose and protect the organs of the pelvic cavity. It provides a point of attachment for the lower extremities and the major muscles of the trunk. It also supports the weight of the upper body.

Bones are classified by their shape and size—long, short, flat, and irregular (Figure 6-7 on p. 147). Long bones are the relatively cylindrical bones of the upper and lower extremities, such as the humerus of the upper arm. Short bones can be found in the carpal bones of the hand and the tarsal bones of the feet. The

shoulder blade (scapula) is an example of a flat bone. The vertebrae are examples of irregular bones.

The Skull

Objective 15

The **skull** is the bony skeleton of the head that protects the brain from injury and gives the head its shape. It is made up of two main groups of bones, the bones of the cranium and the bones of the face (Figure 6-8 on p. 147). The **cranium** contains eight bones that house and protect the brain:

- Frontal (forehead) bone
- Two parietal (top sides of cranium) bones
- Two temporal (lower sides of cranium) bones
- Occipital (back of skull) bone
- Sphenoid (central part of floor of cranium) bone
- Ethmoid (floor of cranium, nasal septum) bone

The skull is supported by the neck, which receives its strength from the vertebrae. Attached to the skull are many facial bones. Muscles attached to these bones allow eye movements and facial expressions. These muscles also allow the tongue to be held in position so that the airway remains open. Without these important mouth muscles, a person would not be able to swallow food or fluids without gagging and choking. The face contains the following bones:

- Orbits (eye sockets)
- Nasal bones (upper bridge of nose)
- Maxilla (upper jaw)
- Mandible (lower jaw)
- Zygomatic bones (cheek bones)
- Auditory ossicles (bones within the ear)

The mandible is the largest and strongest bone of the face. It is the only movable bone of the face. The ear contains six bones, which are located in the middle ear and are called the *auditory ossicles.* The tongue is anchored to

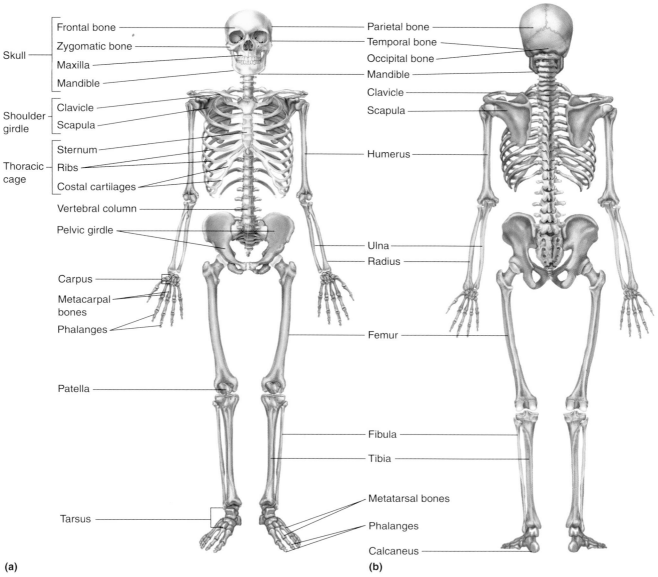

FIGURE 6-5 ▲ The adult skeleton. **(a)** Anterior view; **(b)** posterior view. The appendicular skeleton is colored blue and the rest is axial skeleton.

the hyoid bone. The hyoid bone is the only bone in the body that does not connect to another bone.

The Spine

Objective 16

The **spine (vertebral column)** is made up of 32–33 vertebrae that are arranged in regions (Figure 6-9 and Table 6-2 on p. 147). The vertebrae of each region have a distinctive shape. The vertebral column is made up of 7 cervical (neck) vertebrae, 12 thoracic vertebrae, 5 lumbar vertebrae, 5 fused vertebrae that form the sacrum, and 3–4 fused vertebrae that form the coccyx (tailbone). The vertebral column provides rigidity to the body while allowing movement. It also encloses and

protects the spinal cord. It extends from the base of the skull to the coccyx.

The seven cervical vertebrae of the neck, the **cervical spine**, hold up the head and allow it to rotate left and right as well as move backward, forward, and side to side. On the scene of an emergency, rescuers often refer to the cervical spine as the *c-spine*. The first cervical vertebra, the atlas, supports the skull. The second cervical vertebra is called the *axis*. The 12 thoracic vertebrae form the upper back and the posterior portion of the thorax. Below the thoracic vertebrae are five lumbar vertebrae. The lumbar vertebrae are the largest and strongest of the vertebrae because they carry the bulk of the body's weight. Below the lumbar vertebrae are five fused vertebrae that form the sacrum (the back wall of the pelvis) and eventually attach to three to four

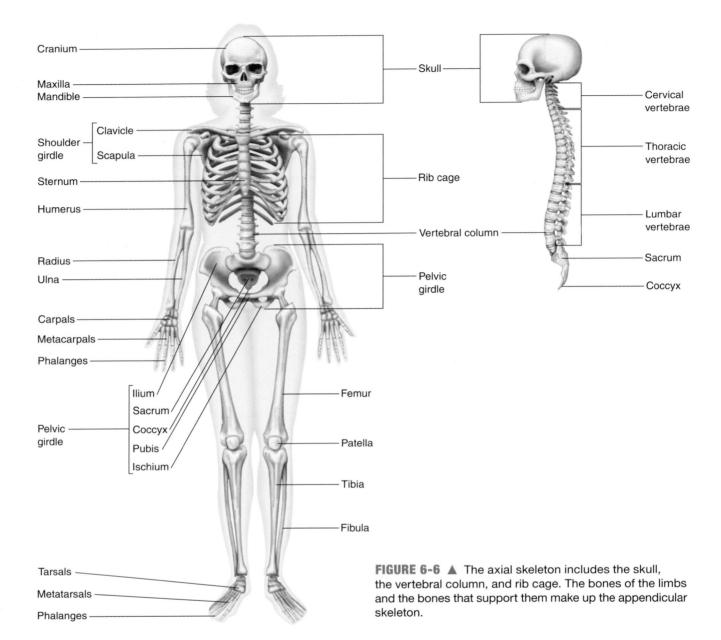

Cranium

Maxilla
Mandible

Shoulder girdle — Clavicle

Scapula

Sternum

Humerus

Radius

Ulna

Carpals

Metacarpals

Phalanges

Ilium

Sacrum

Pelvic girdle — Coccyx

Pubis

Ischium

Tarsals

Metatarsals

Phalanges

Skull

Rib cage

Vertebral column

Pelvic girdle

Femur

Patella

Tibia

Fibula

Cervical vertebrae

Thoracic vertebrae

Lumbar vertebrae

Sacrum

Coccyx

FIGURE 6-6 ▲ The axial skeleton includes the skull, the vertebral column, and rib cage. The bones of the limbs and the bones that support them make up the appendicular skeleton.

fused vertebrae that form the coccyx. The fused sacral vertebrae are connected to the pelvis, which attaches the lower appendicular skeleton to the axial skeleton.

You Should Know

The adult spinal cord is about 16–18 inches in length and about .75 inch in diameter in the midthorax. The length of the spinal cord is shorter than the length of the bony vertebral column. The spinal cord extends down to only about the second lumbar vertebra. In the cervical and thoracic areas of the vertebral column, the spinal cord lies very close to the walls of the vertebrae. The spinal cord is at risk of injury in these areas.

Between every two vertebrae is a disk. Each disk is a tiny pad that is made up mainly of water (Figure 6-10 on p. 148). These disks help protect the spinal nerves. The disks between the vertebrae are soft and rubbery, cushioning each of the vertebrae and acting as shock absorbers. The spinal nerves exit the spinal cord at openings between the vertebrae. They send signals to the body's muscles and organs (Figure 6-11 on p. 148).

The Chest

Objective 16

The **chest (thorax)** is made up of the 12 thoracic vertebrae, 12 pairs of ribs, and the breastbone (sternum) (see Figure 6-12 on p. 148, and Plate A at the end of

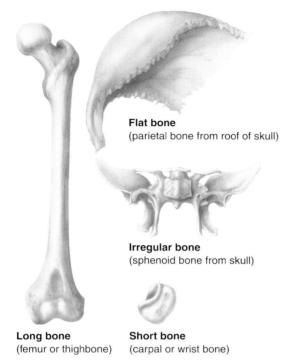

Flat bone
(parietal bone from roof of skull)

Irregular bone
(sphenoid bone from skull)

Long bone
(femur or thighbone)

Short bone
(carpal or wrist bone)

FIGURE 6-7 ▲ Bones are classified by their shape and size.

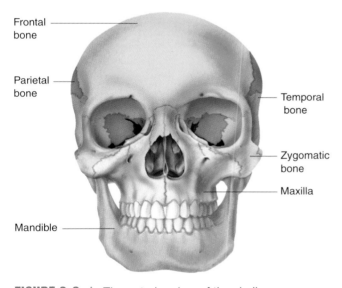

Frontal bone

Parietal bone

Temporal bone

Zygomatic bone

Maxilla

Mandible

FIGURE 6-8 ▲ The anterior view of the skull.

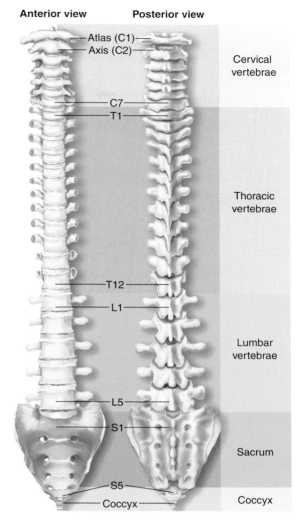

Anterior view Posterior view

Atlas (C1)
Axis (C2)

Cervical vertebrae

C7
T1

Thoracic vertebrae

T12

L1

Lumbar vertebrae

L5

S1

Sacrum

S5

Coccyx

Coccyx

FIGURE 6-9 ▲ The vertebral column (spine), anterior and posterior views.

TABLE 6-2	Regions of the Spinal Column
Region	**Number of Vertebrae**
Cervical spine (neck)	7
Thoracic spine (chest, upper back)	12
Lumbar spine (lower back)	5
Sacrum	5 (fused)
Coccyx	3 to 4 (fused)

the chapter). These structures form the thoracic cage, serving to protect the organs within the thoracic cavity, such as the heart, lungs, and major blood vessels. The sternum is attached to the ribs and collarbones (clavicles). All the ribs are attached posteriorly to the thoracic vertebrae by ligaments. Pairs 1 through 10 are attached to the front of the sternum. Pairs 1 through 7 are attached to the front of the sternum by cartilage and are called **true ribs**. Rib pairs 8 through 10 are attached to the cartilage of the seventh ribs. These ribs are called **false ribs**. Pairs 11 and 12 are not attached to the front of the sternum; these ribs are called **floating ribs**.

The **sternum (breastbone)** consists of three sections. The **manubrium** is the superior (uppermost)

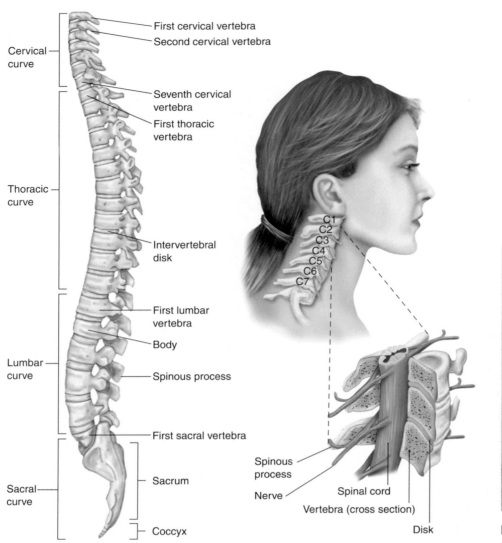

Cervical curve

First cervical vertebra

Second cervical vertebra

Seventh cervical vertebra

First thoracic vertebra

Thoracic curve

Intervertebral disk

Lumbar curve

First lumbar vertebra

Body

Spinous process

First sacral vertebra

Sacral curve

Sacrum

Coccyx

C1
C2
C3
C4
C5
C6
C7

Spinous process

Nerve

Spinal cord

Vertebra (cross section)

Disk

FIGURE 6-10 ▲ The vertebral column.

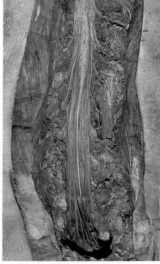

FIGURE 6-11 ▲ A dissected spinal cord and roots of the spinal nerves.

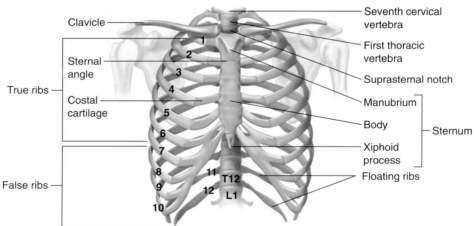

Clavicle

Sternal angle

True ribs

Costal cartilage

False ribs

1
2
3
4
5
6
7
8
9
10
11
12
T12
L1

Seventh cervical vertebra

First thoracic vertebra

Suprasternal notch

Manubrium

Body

Xiphoid process

Floating ribs

Sternum

FIGURE 6-12 ▲ The thoracic cage (anterior view). The thoracic cage includes 12 pairs of ribs and the 12 thoracic vertebrae with which they join. The thoracic cage also includes the breastbone (sternum).

portion; it connects with the clavicle and first rib. The body is the middle portion, and the **xiphoid process** is the inferior portion. This landmark is important when determining the proper hand position for chest compressions in cardiopulmonary resuscitation (CPR). The superior portion of the sternum is attached to the clavicles, which join the axial skeleton to the appendicular skeleton.

The Upper Extremities

The **upper extremities** are made up of the bones of the shoulder girdle, the arms, the forearms, and the hands (Figure 6-13). The **humerus** is the upper arm bone to which the biceps and triceps muscles are attached, allowing the shoulder to rotate, flex, and extend. The humerus is the largest bone of the upper extremity and is the second-longest bone in the body. The clavicles (collarbones) and the scapulae (shoulder blades) form the capsule into which the proximal portion of the humerus inserts to form the shoulder joint. The forearm contains two bones, the **radius** (lateral, thumb side) and **ulna** (medial side). The ulna is the longer of the two bones. The **olecranon** (elbow) is the joint where the humerus connects with the radius and the ulna. The forearm is connected to the **carpals** (wrist) and then to the **metacarpals** (hand) and the **phalanges** (fingers). There are multiple bones and joints within the wrist and hand, allowing humans to have a great deal of flexibility, movement, and use.

The Lower Extremities

The **lower extremities** are made up of the bones of the pelvis, upper legs, lower legs, and feet (Figure 6-14). In general, the bones of the lower extremities are thicker, heavier, and longer than the upper extremity bones. The bones of the lower extremities support the body and are essential for standing, walking, and running. The **pelvis** is a bony ring formed by three separate bones that fuse to become one by adulthood. The lower extremities are attached to the pelvis at the hip joint. The hip joint is formed by the socket of the **acetabulum** (hip bone) and the head of the **femur** (thigh bone). The femur is the longest, heaviest, and strongest bone of the body. The **greater trochanter** is the large, bony prominence on the lateral shaft of the femur to which the buttock muscles are attached. The head of the femur is the upper end of the bone and is shaped like a ball.

The knee is the largest joint in the body. It is a hinge joint that allows the distal leg to move in flexion and extension. The knee is protected anteriorly by the **patella** (kneecap). It attaches the femur to the two lower leg bones, the **tibia** (shinbone) and **fibula.** The tibia is the larger of the two bones of the lower leg. The lower leg attaches to the foot by the ankle, which is similar to the wrist of the upper extremities. Like the hand, the foot contains several smaller bones and joints, allowing free movement of the foot at the ankle. The **tarsal** bones

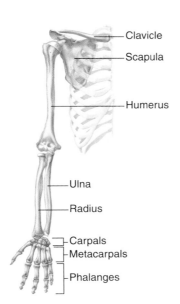

FIGURE 6-13 ▲ The shoulder girdle and upper extremity bones.

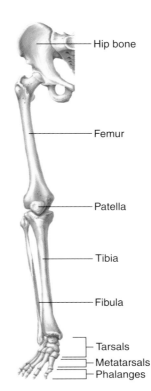

FIGURE 6-14 ▲ Lower extremity bones.

make up the back part of the foot and heel. The **metatarsal** bones make up the main part of the foot. The toes (**phalanges**) are the foot's equivalent to the fingers.

The Muscular System

Objectives 17, 18

The muscular system provides several functions for the body:

- Gives the body shape
- Protects internal organs
- Provides for movement of the body
- Maintains posture
- Helps stabilize joints
- Produces body heat

Muscles allow you to smile, open your mouth, breathe, speak, blink, walk, talk, and move food through your digestive system. The heart is a muscle that pumps blood through the body.

Muscles are classified according to their structure and function: skeletal (voluntary) muscle, smooth (involuntary) muscle, and cardiac muscle.

Skeletal Muscles

Skeletal muscles move the skeleton, produce the heat that helps maintain a constant body temperature, and maintain posture. Skeletal muscles are *voluntary* because you can determine how they move. Most skeletal muscles are attached to bones by means of tendons. **Tendons** are strong cords of connective tissue that firmly attach the end of a muscle to a bone. The tendons of many muscles cross over joints, and this helps stabilize the joint. **Ligaments** are tough groups of connective tissue that attach bones to bones and bones to cartilages. They provide support and strength to joints and restrain excessive joint movement. Rupture or tearing of a ligament can lead to pain and/or impaired function of the joint. Skeletal muscles produce rapid, forceful contractions but do not contract unless they are stimulated by a nerve. When a skeletal muscle contracts, it shortens, pulling on the structure next to it to cause movement. Although the contractions produced are forceful, skeletal muscle tires easily and must rest after short periods of activity. Regular exercise maintains or increases the size and strength of skeletal muscles. When contraction occurs, the bones work together with muscles to produce body movement. For example, when the forearm bends or straightens at the elbow, the bones and muscles function as a lever (Figure 6-15).

Even when you are not moving, your muscles are in a state of partial contraction. This state is referred to as **muscle tone**. Because of electrical signals sent from nerve cells, some muscle fibers are continuously contracted at any given time. This state of constant tension keeps your head in an upright position, your back straight, and the muscles of your body prepared for action.

Smooth Muscle

Smooth (involuntary) muscle is found within the walls of tubular structures of the gastrointestinal tract and urinary systems, blood vessels, the eye, and the bronchi of the respiratory system. Smooth muscle is *involuntary* because you cannot control its movement. Smooth muscle contractions are strong and slow. They respond to stimuli such as stretching, heat, and cold. In the iris of the eye, smooth muscle regulates pupil size. The contraction of the smooth muscle that surrounds the intestines causes food and feces to move along the digestive tract. In blood vessels, smooth muscle helps maintain blood pressure. In the bronchi, the constriction of smooth muscle may result in breathing problems.

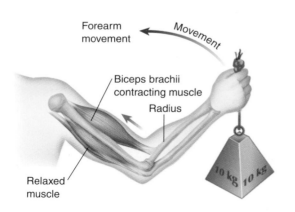
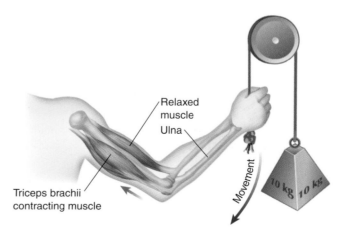

FIGURE 6-15 ▲ When the forearm bends or straightens at the elbow, the bones and muscles function as a lever.

TABLE 6-3 Comparison of Muscle Types

	Location	Function	Type of Control
Skeletal	Attached to bone	• Move the skeleton. • Produce heat that helps maintain a constant body temperature. • Maintain posture.	Voluntary
Smooth	Walls of the esophagus, stomach, intestines, bronchi, uterus, blood vessels, glands	• Move food through the digestive tract. • Adjust the size of blood vessels to control blood flow.	Involuntary
Cardiac	Walls of the heart	• Contract and relax the heart. • Move blood through the body.	Involuntary

A person has no voluntary control over smooth muscle. The contraction and relaxation of smooth muscle is controlled by the body's needs. For example, when a person eats, he does not think about the digestive process. The food is broken down in the stomach and moved forward to the intestinal tract. Nutrients are absorbed and waste is excreted. This process occurs involuntarily (without thought) and with each meal eaten.

Cardiac Muscle

Cardiac muscle, found in the walls of the heart, produces the heart's contractions and pumps blood. Cardiac muscle is found *only* in the heart and has its own supply of blood through the coronary arteries. It can tolerate an interruption of its blood supply for only very short periods. Normal cardiac muscle contractions are strong and rhythmic.

Like smooth muscle, cardiac muscle is involuntary. The heart has the ability to change its rate, rhythm, and strength of contraction according to the needs of the other muscles and organ systems within the body. The heart is the body's hardest working muscle. It beats about 100,000 times every day, without rest, year after year, to move blood through the body.

A comparison of the different muscle types is presented in Table 6-3.

The Respiratory System

Objectives 19, 20

The body's cells need a continuous supply of oxygen to sustain life. The air that we breathe in is made up of a mixture of gases. At sea level, this gas mixture consists of about 78% nitrogen, 21% oxygen, 0.9% argon, and 0.03% carbon dioxide. The percentage of oxygen in the air inhaled is called the **fraction of inspired oxygen** (FiO_2). The FiO_2 ranges from 21% (the percentage of oxygen in room air) to 100% (pure oxygen).

Working with the circulatory system, the respiratory system supplies oxygen from the air we breathe to the body's cells. It also transports carbon dioxide (a waste product of the body's cells) to the lungs. Carbon dioxide is removed from the body in the air that we exhale.

The respiratory system is divided into the upper and lower airways (Figure 6-16). The upper airway is made up of structures outside the chest cavity. These structures include the nose, the **pharynx** (throat), and the **larynx** (voice box). The lower airway consists of parts found almost entirely within the chest cavity, such as the **trachea** (windpipe) and the lungs.

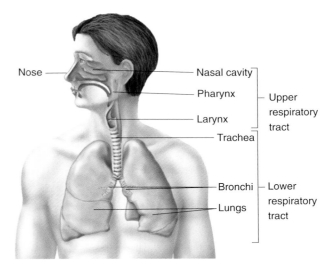

FIGURE 6-16 ▲ The upper and lower respiratory tract.

Air enters the body through the nose or the mouth (Figure 6-17). The nostrils are also called the **external nares.** The nostrils open into the nasal cavity. Air is warmed, moistened, and filtered as it moves over the damp, sticky lining (mucous membrane) of the nose. The nasal septum (a wall, or partition, that separates two cavities) divides the nasal cavity into right and left portions. The floor of the nasal cavity is bony and is called the **hard palate.** The **soft palate** is fleshy and extends behind the hard palate. It marks the boundary between the nasopharynx and the rest of the pharynx.

Four nasal **sinuses** (spaces or cavities inside some cranial bones) drain into the nose. Sinuses produce mucus and trap bacteria; they can become infected when bacteria become entrapped in the sinus tissues. Because they are filled with air, sinuses lighten the weight of the bones that make up the skull. They provide additional surface area to nasal passages for warming and humidifying air. Each side of the nose has several **turbinates** (shelflike projections that protrude into the nasal cavity). As air moves within the turbinates, it is warmed, humidified, and filtered. The turbinates protect structures of the lower airway from foreign body contamination.

Air then travels down the throat through the larynx and the trachea. The pharynx is a muscular tube about 5 inches long. It is used by both the respiratory and the digestive systems. It serves as a passageway for food, liquids, and air. The pharynx is made up of three parts.

- **Nasopharynx.** The nasopharynx is located directly behind the nasal cavity. It serves as a passageway for air only. The tissues of the nasopharynx are extremely delicate and bleed easily.

- **Oropharynx.** The oropharynx is the middle part of the throat. It opens into the mouth and serves as a passageway for both food and air. It is separated from the nasopharynx by the soft palate. The **uvula** is the small piece of tissue that looks like a miniature punching bag and hangs down in the back of the throat.

- **Laryngopharynx.** The laryngopharynx is the lowermost part of the throat. It surrounds the openings of the esophagus and larynx. It opens in the front into the larynx and in the back into the esophagus. It serves as a passageway for both food and air.

The larynx connects the pharynx with the trachea. It functions in voice production; the length and tension of the vocal cords determine voice pitch. The larynx provides a passageway for air to enter and exit the lungs. It is made up of nine cartilages connected to each other by muscles and ligaments. The **thyroid cartilage** (Adam's apple) is the largest cartilage of the larynx and is shaped like a shield. It can be felt on the front surface of the neck. The hyoid bone is a U-shaped bone that sits above the larynx. It helps move the larynx upward during swallowing. The epiglottis is the uppermost cartilage and is shaped like a leaf. It is attached along the interior anterior border of the thyroid cartilage in a hingelike fashion. You cannot swallow and breathe at the same time because the **epiglottis,** a special flap of cartilage, covers the trachea when you are eating or drinking so that food or liquids do not enter the lungs (Figure 6-18). The

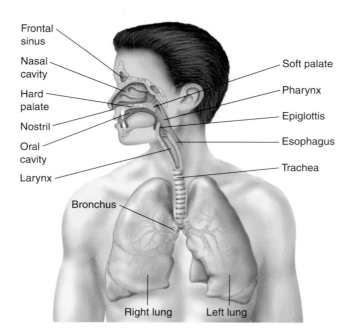

FIGURE 6-17 ▲ Structures of the respiratory system.

Frontal sinus
Nasal cavity
Hard palate
Nostril
Oral cavity
Larynx
Bronchus
Right lung   Left lung
Soft palate
Pharynx
Epiglottis
Esophagus
Trachea

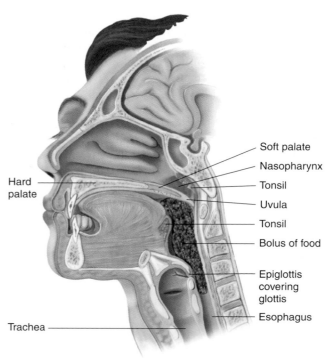

FIGURE 6-18 ▲ The structures involved in swallowing.

Hard palate
Trachea
Soft palate
Nasopharynx
Tonsil
Uvula
Tonsil
Bolus of food
Epiglottis covering glottis
Esophagus

cricoid cartilage is the lowermost cartilage of the larynx. It is the only complete ring of cartilage in the larynx. The cricoid cartilage forms the base of the larynx on which the other cartilages rest. The vocal cords stretch across the inside of the larynx. The space between the vocal cords is called the **glottis.**

You Should Know

Cricoid pressure (also called the *Sellick maneuver*) is a technique used for unresponsive patients. When pressure is applied to the cricoid cartilage, the trachea is pushed backward and the esophagus is compressed (closed) against the cervical vertebrae. This compression helps decrease the amount of air entering the stomach during artificial ventilation.

The trachea is located in the front of the neck. It is kept permanently open by C-shaped cartilages. The **esophagus,** which is part of the digestive system, is a muscular tube located behind the trachea. It serves as a passageway for food. The open part of each C-shaped cartilage faces the esophagus. This allows the esophagus to expand slightly into the trachea during swallowing.

The trachea continues into the chest, where it branches into large airway tubes called the *right primary bronchus* and *left primary bronchus* (Figure 6-19). The right primary bronchus is shorter, wider, and straighter than the left. Each **bronchus** is joined to a lung, so one tube leads to the right lung and the other leads to the left lung. The inside walls of the bronchi are covered with mucus, which traps dirt and germs that get into the lungs. Small, hairlike structures (cilia) work like brooms to get rid of the debris caught in the mucus. The primary bronchi branch into smaller and smaller tubes called **bronchioles.** Bronchioles end in microscopic tubes called *alveolar ducts.* Each alveolar duct ends in several alveolar sacs. At the end of each alveolar duct, the collections of air sacs **(alveoli)** look like a cluster of grapes. The wall of an alveolus consists of a single layer of cells. A thin film of **surfactant** coats each alveolus and prevents the alveoli from collapsing.

You Should Know

The bronchi and bronchioles serve as passageways for air to enter and exit the alveoli. The point at which the trachea divides into two primary bronchi forms an internal ridge called the **carina.** The mucous membrane of the carina is one of the most sensitive areas of the respiratory system and is associated with the cough reflex.

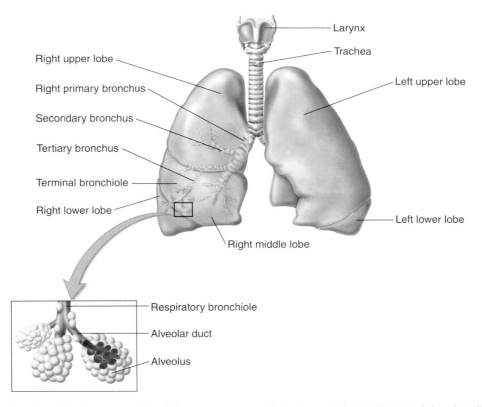

Larynx
Trachea
Right upper lobe
Right primary bronchus
Secondary bronchus
Tertiary bronchus
Terminal bronchiole
Right lower lobe
Right middle lobe
Left upper lobe
Left lower lobe

Respiratory bronchiole
Alveolar duct
Alveolus

FIGURE 6-19 ▲ The bronchial tree consists of the passageways that connect the trachea and the alveoli.

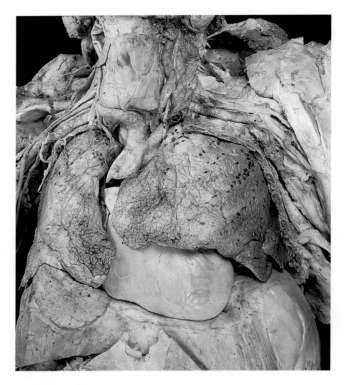

FIGURE 6-20 ▲ Anterior view of the chest.

The **lungs** are spongy, air-filled organs. They are bound superiorly by the clavicles and inferiorly by the diaphragm (see Figure 6-20, and Plate A at the end of the chapter). The primary function of the lungs is gas exchange—bringing air into contact with the blood so that oxygen and carbon dioxide can be exchanged in the alveoli. The apex of the lung is the uppermost portion of the lung; it reaches above the first rib. The base of the lung is the portion of the lung resting on the diaphragm. The **mediastinum** is part of the space in the middle of the chest, between the lungs. The mediastinum extends from the sternum (breastbone) to the spine. It contains all the organs of the thorax—the heart, major blood vessels, the esophagus, the trachea, and nerves—except the lungs.

The lungs are divided into lobes. The right lung has three lobes. It is shorter than the left lung because the diaphragm is higher on the right to make room for the liver that lies below it. The left lung has two lobes. Because two-thirds of the heart lies to the left of the midline of the body, the left lung contains a notch to make room for the heart (see Plates A and B at the end of the chapter).

The lungs "float" within separate pleural cavities. They are separated from the chest wall by a space containing pleural fluid. The **pleurae** are the serous (oily) double-walled membranes that enclose each lung (Figure 6-21). The **parietal pleura** is the outer lining and lines the wall of the chest cavity (the rib cage, diaphragm, and mediastinum). The **visceral pleura** is the inner layer and covers the surface of the lungs. The **pleural space** is a space between the visceral and parietal pleura filled with a small amount of oily fluid. Pleural fluid allows the lungs to glide easily against each other as the lungs fill and empty during breathing. Certain illnesses or injuries can cause air, blood, or both to fill the pleural space. This can cause a collapse of the lung on the affected side.

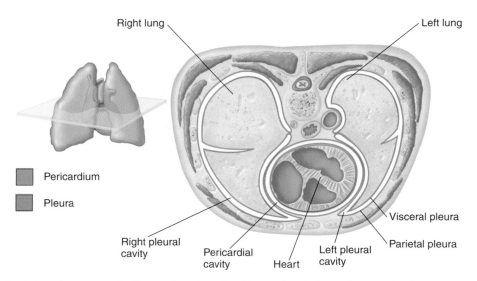

Right lung

Left lung

Pericardium

Pleura

Right pleural cavity

Pericardial cavity

Heart

Left pleural cavity

Parietal pleura

Visceral pleura

FIGURE 6-21 ▲ Each lung is surrounded by a pleural cavity. The parietal pleura lines each pleural cavity, and the visceral pleura covers the surface of the lungs. The potential spaces between the pleural membranes (the left and right pleural cavities) are shown here as actual spaces.

The respiratory system can be divided into two divisions based on their function. The conducting (ventilating) division consists of the areas of the respiratory system that are involved in the transport of gases to and from the alveoli. This division includes the oral and nasal cavities, pharynx, larynx, trachea, and bronchi, ending at the terminal bronchioles, which are the smallest airway passages outside the alveoli. The respiratory division consists of the areas of the respiratory system that are involved in the exchange of gases between the air and blood. It includes the alveolar ducts, alveolar sacs, and alveoli.

Ventilation

Objectives 21, 22, 23

Breathing (also called *pulmonary ventilation*) is the mechanical process of moving air into and out of the lungs. **Inspiration** (inhalation) is the process of breathing in and moving air into the lungs. **Expiration** (exhalation) is the process of breathing out and moving air out of the lungs.

Respiration is the exchange of gases between a living organism and its environment. A single respiration consists of one inspiration and one expiration. Normal respiratory rates depend on age. **Tidal volume** is the amount of air moved into or out of the lungs during a normal breath. You can indirectly assess tidal volume by watching the rise and fall of the patient's chest and abdomen. The tidal volume of a healthy adult at rest is about 500 mL. Of the 500 mL, only about 350 mL reaches the alveoli for gas exchange with the red blood cells. About 150 mL remains in the **anatomic dead space**, which is the volume of air contained in the conducting airways, where gas exchange does not take place. **Minute volume** is the amount of air moved in and out of the lungs in 1 minute. Minute volume is determined by multiplying the tidal volume by the respiratory rate. An inadequate tidal volume *or* respiratory rate can result in inadequate ventilation.

The rate and depth of breathing are controlled by the brain. Sensory receptors called **chemoreceptors** monitor the levels of oxygen and carbon dioxide in the body. **Central chemoreceptors** are located in the medulla oblongata in the brainstem. These chemoreceptors are sensitive to changes in the carbon dioxide content of the blood. In most people, a rise in the level of carbon dioxide in the bloodstream is the stimulus that triggers the respiratory center in the brain. When the level of carbon dioxide in the blood is increased, a person breathes faster and deeper to get rid of the carbon dioxide and bring in more oxygen, which is necessary for cell function. **Peripheral chemoreceptors**, located in the carotid arteries and arch of the aorta, monitor changes in carbon dioxide and oxygen levels. However, their most important role is in monitoring the level of oxygen in the blood. Peripheral chemoreceptors exert little control over ventilation until the level of oxygen in the blood has dropped very low.

Chronic respiratory diseases may alter the normal respiratory drive over time. Instead of an increase in carbon dioxide levels stimulating breathing, low levels of oxygen in the blood become the breathing stimulus. This kind of breathing stimulus is called **hypoxic drive**.

When the brain senses a rise in the carbon dioxide level in the bloodstream, it sends a signal to the diaphragm and **intercostal muscles** (muscles between the ribs), causing them to contract. The **diaphragm** is the dome-shaped muscle below the lungs. It separates the chest cavity from the abdominal cavity and is the main muscle of respiration. The right and left phrenic nerves conduct motor impulses to the muscle fibers of the diaphragm, causing it to contract. Stimulation of the diaphragm via the phrenic nerves allows it to descend on inspiration, increasing lung volume. Injury to the phrenic nerve will result in paralysis of the portion of the diaphragm that it stimulates. The external intercostal muscles are located between the ribs. The internal intercostal muscles, muscles above the collarbones, and abdominal muscles are called **accessory muscles for breathing**. These muscles may be used for breathing during periods of respiratory distress. A patient who is having trouble breathing will often sit up and lean forward. This position lets the respiratory muscles expand to help the patient breathe.

Breathing and gas exchange in the lungs depend on appropriate atmospheric pressure. **Atmospheric pressure** is the force exerted by air on the body surface. Air moves from the environment into the body and through the respiratory system to the alveoli because of pressure differences within the system. When the diaphragm and external intercostal muscles contract, the chest cavity enlarges and fills with air. This causes the pressure within the lungs to decrease as compared to the air pressure outside the body. Air begins to rush in from the area of higher pressure (outside the body) to the area of lower pressure (the lungs), normally entering the body through the mouth and nose. This process is called *inspiration*. Inspiration is considered an active process because it requires muscle contraction.

Inspiration stops when the respiratory muscles stop contracting and air pressures inside the chest cavity and outside the body equalize. Oxygen and carbon dioxide are then exchanged in the lungs. The exchange of oxygen and carbon dioxide is discussed in more detail below. Stretch receptors that respond to changes in pressure are located in the smooth muscle of the bronchi and bronchioles and in the visceral pleurae. When the lungs are inflated, the stretch receptors are stimulated. They quickly send impulses by means of vagus nerves to the medulla in the brain to stop inspiration and allow expiration to occur. This is called the *inflation* or *Hering-Breuer reflex*. Stretch receptors play an important role in adjusting respiratory rate and tidal volume in response to changes in the elasticity of the lungs and resistance to air flow.

When the diaphragm and external intercostal muscles relax, the chest cavity becomes smaller, the lungs are compressed, and the stretch receptors become quiet. As a result, the pressure within the chest cavity is higher than that outside the body, and air is forced out the mouth and nose. This process is called *expiration*. Expiration is normally a passive process because the lungs recoil as a result of their elasticity (Figure 6-22). Expiration becomes an active process when the respiratory passages become narrowed due to spasms of the bronchioles (as in asthma) or become filled with secretions, such as mucus or fluid (as in pneumonia).

You Should Know

Structures in the Chest Wall That Support Ventilation

- Pleurae
- Diaphragm
- Intercostal muscles
- Phrenic nerves
- Pulmonary capillaries

Respiration

Objectives 24, 25

You will recall that respiration is the exchange of gases between a living organism and its environment. There are two types of respiration: internal and external. Internal respiration (also called *cellular respiration*) is the process whereby energy is released from molecules such as glucose and made available for use by the cells and tissues of the body. The carbon dioxide produced in the cell during this process is absorbed by the blood and transported to the lungs. External respiration is the exchange of gases between the lungs and the blood cells in the pulmonary capillaries.

Oxygen is the component of air that is an essential "fuel" needed by all body cells for survival. Most cells begin to die if their oxygen supply is interrupted for even a few minutes. Alveoli are the sites where

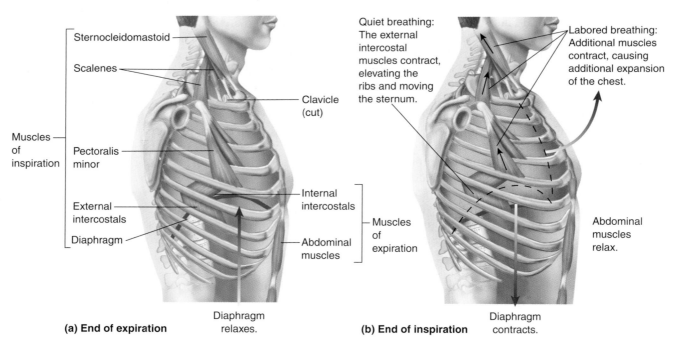

(a) End of expiration

Muscles of inspiration
- Sternocleidomastoid
- Scalenes
- Clavicle (cut)
- Pectoralis minor
- External intercostals
- Diaphragm
- Internal intercostals
- Abdominal muscles

Diaphragm relaxes.

(b) End of inspiration

Quiet breathing: The external intercostal muscles contract, elevating the ribs and moving the sternum.

Labored breathing: Additional muscles contract, causing additional expansion of the chest.

Muscles of expiration

Abdominal muscles relax.

Diaphragm contracts.

FIGURE 6-22 ▲ **(a)** Muscles of respiration at the end of expiration; **(b)** muscles of respiration at the end of inspiration. During inhalation, the diaphragm and external intercostal muscles between the ribs contract causing the volume of the chest cavity to increase. During a normal exhalation these muscles relax and the chest volume returns to normal.

gases—oxygen and carbon dioxide—are exchanged between the air and the blood. **Erythrocytes** (red blood cells) contain hemoglobin. **Hemoglobin** is an iron-containing protein that chemically bonds with oxygen. About 97% of the oxygen in the body is bound to hemoglobin molecules. The remaining 3% of the body's oxygen is dissolved in the liquid portion of the blood called plasma. Each red blood cell has about 250 million hemoglobin molecules. Each hemoglobin molecule can carry up to four oxygen molecules. Thus, hemoglobin is the part of the red blood cell that picks up oxygen in the lungs and transports it to the body's cells. If a hemoglobin molecule carries four of the four possible oxygen molecules, it is 100% saturated with oxygen. If the hemoglobin molecule carries only two of the four possible oxygen molecules, it is 50% saturated, and so forth.

Carbon dioxide (CO_2) is a waste product produced by the body's cells. It is transported in the blood in three forms. Most of the body's carbon dioxide is transported in the blood as bicarbonate, which is created when carbon dioxide combines with water. Some of the body's carbon dioxide is transported on the hemoglobin molecule. Hemoglobin can transport oxygen and CO_2 at the same time. This is possible because oxygen attaches to the iron portion of the hemoglobin molecule and CO_2 attaches to the globin, or protein portion, of the hemoglobin. A small amount of CO_2 is carried in the plasma as a dissolved gas.

Each alveolus is surrounded by a network of pulmonary capillaries (Figure 6-23). Each time you breathe in, oxygen-rich air enters the alveoli. Oxygen is then passed from the alveoli into the pulmonary capillaries to enrich the blood low in oxygen. This is called *alveolar-capillary gas exchange*. As they expand, the alveoli become thinner, making the exchange of oxygen or carbon dioxide easier. The oxygen-rich blood is distributed to the cells of the body where the oxygen is passed

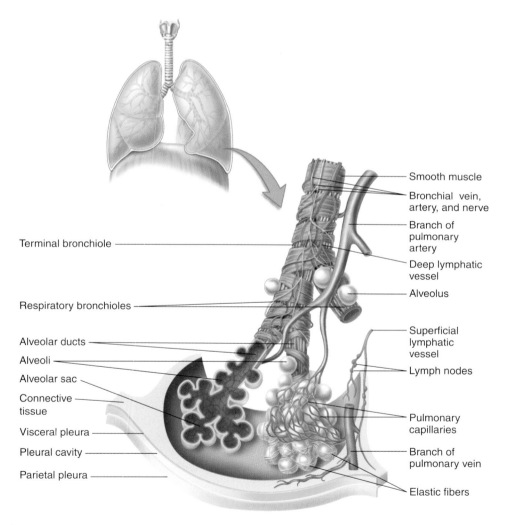

Terminal bronchiole

Respiratory bronchioles

Alveolar ducts

Alveoli

Alveolar sac

Connective tissue

Visceral pleura

Pleural cavity

Parietal pleura

Smooth muscle

Bronchial vein, artery, and nerve

Branch of pulmonary artery

Deep lymphatic vessel

Alveolus

Superficial lymphatic vessel

Lymph nodes

Pulmonary capillaries

Branch of pulmonary vein

Elastic fibers

FIGURE 6-23 ▲ The primary bronchi branch into smaller and smaller tubes called bronchioles. At the ends of the bronchioles are tiny sacs that look like clusters of grapes. These tiny sacs are called the alveoli. Alveoli are the sites of gas exchange between the air and blood.

from the capillaries to the cells of the body. Red blood cells in the capillaries gather the waste carbon dioxide from the cells and transport it to the lungs, where the carbon dioxide is passed from the capillaries to the alveoli and exhaled from the body. This process is called *cell-capillary gas exchange.*

The Circulatory System

Objective 26

The **circulatory system** is made up of the cardiovascular and lymphatic systems. The **cardiovascular system** is made up of three main parts: a pump (the heart), fluid (blood), and a container (the blood vessels). The **lymphatic system** consists of lymph, lymph nodes, lymph vessels, tonsils, the spleen, and the thymus gland. The spleen and liver are also associated with the circulatory system because they form and store blood.

The functions of the circulatory system are the following:

- Deliver oxygen-rich blood and nutrients to body tissues.
- Help maintain body temperature.
- Protect the body against infection.
- Control bleeding (hemostasis).
- Remove waste and by-products of metabolism from the body tissues.
- Transport hormones and other chemical messengers to targeted tissues of the body.

The Heart

Objectives 27, 28

The **heart** is located slightly to the left of the center of the chest (see Plate B at the end of the chapter). It is attached to the chest through the **great vessels** (pulmonary arteries and veins, the aorta, and the superior and inferior vena cavae). With its thick walls of cardiac muscle, the heart functions to pump blood through the vessels of the body (Figure 6-24).

The heart has four hollow chambers. The two upper chambers are the right and left **atria.** The job of the atria is to receive blood from the body and lungs. The two lower chambers of the heart are the right and left **ventricles.** The ventricles are larger and have thicker walls than the atria because their job is to pump blood to the lungs and body.

The right atrium receives blood that is low in oxygen from the body by means of veins. Blood flows from the right atrium through a one-way valve, the tricuspid valve. The tricuspid valve forces the blood to always

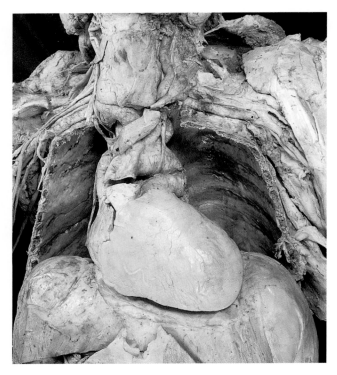

FIGURE 6-24 ▲ Anterior view of the human heart in the chest (without the lungs).

move in the correct direction, into the right ventricle. When the right ventricle contracts, blood is pumped through another one-way valve, the pulmonic valve, into the pulmonary arteries. Blood flows from the pulmonary arteries to the lungs, where it receives a fresh supply of oxygen. From the lungs, the oxygen-rich blood flows along the pulmonary veins to the left upper chamber of the heart, the left atrium. The left atrium pumps the blood through the mitral (bicuspid) valve to the left ventricle. The left ventricle is about three times thicker than the right ventricle because it has to produce enough pressure to push the blood out of the heart, through the aortic valve, and into the aorta, the body's largest artery (Figure 6-25). The aorta and its branches distribute the oxygen-rich blood throughout the body.

The normal heartbeat begins as an electrical signal in a small area of specialized tissue in the upper right atrium of the heart. The impulse spreads through a system of pathways called the *conduction system.* A disruption of these pathways can cause the heart to malfunction. For example, a heart attack disrupts the flow of oxygen and nutrients to the heart's cells. This disruption can cause the heart to beat too quickly or too slowly. It can also affect the heart's ability to contract and pump blood to the rest of the body.

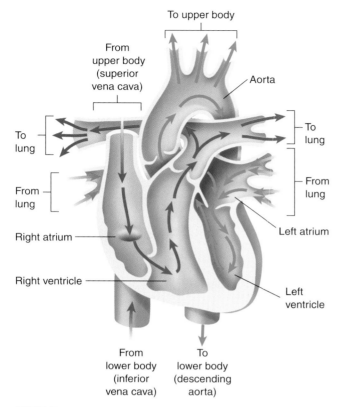

FIGURE 6-25 ▲ Blood flow through the heart and lungs.

Blood

Objectives 29, 30

Blood is a type of transport system. It is the means by which oxygen, food, hormones, minerals, and other essential substances are carried to all parts of the body. An adult has about 5–6 liters of blood flowing through the circulatory system. Blood carries carbon dioxide and other waste material from the body's cells

to the lungs, kidneys, or skin for removal. To help maintain body temperature, blood vessels constrict (narrow) and dilate (widen) as needed to keep or lose heat at the skin's surface. The blood and lymphatic system work together to protect the body against infection.

Blood is made up of liquid and formed elements (Figure 6-26). The liquid portion of the blood is called **plasma**. Plasma carries oxygen, blood cells, vitamins, proteins, glucose, and many other substances throughout the body. The formed elements of the blood include erythrocytes, leukocytes, and thrombocytes. Erythrocytes (red blood cells) have two main functions: (1) to pick up oxygen from the lungs and transport it to tissues throughout the body and (2) to pick up carbon dioxide from body tissues and transport it to the lungs. Erythrocytes contain hemoglobin. Hemoglobin is red and therefore gives blood its red color.

Leukocytes (white blood cells) attack and destroy germs that enter the body. **Thrombocytes (platelets)** are irregularly shaped blood cells that have a sticky surface. When a blood vessel is damaged and starts to bleed, platelets gather at the site of injury. The platelets begin sticking to the opening of the damaged vessel and seal it, stopping the flow of blood.

Blood Vessels

Objective 31

Blood vessels that carry blood away from the heart to the rest of the body are called **arteries** (Figure 6-27). Blood is forced into the arteries when the heart contracts. Arteries have thick walls because they transport blood under high pressure. Arteries normally carry oxygen-rich blood. However, the pulmonary artery and its two branches, the left and right pulmonary arteries, carry oxygen-poor blood.

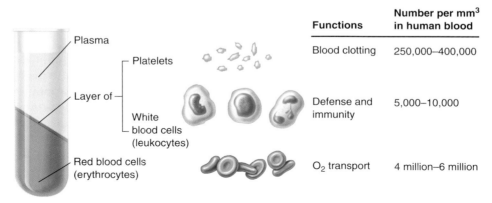

	Functions	Number per mm³ in human blood
Platelets	Blood clotting	250,000–400,000
White blood cells (leukocytes)	Defense and immunity	5,000–10,000
Red blood cells (erythrocytes)	O₂ transport	4 million–6 million

FIGURE 6-26 ▲ Blood is made up of liquid (plasma) and formed elements (red blood cells, white blood cells, and platelets).

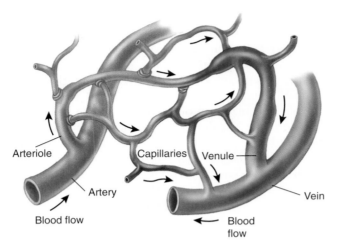

FIGURE 6-27 ▲ Blood flow from the heart through the body moves through the following vessels: Arteries → arterioles → capillaries → venules → veins.

Arterioles are the smallest branches of arteries. They connect arteries to capillaries. **Capillaries** are the smallest and most numerous blood vessels. They are very thin (thinner than a human hair) and connect arterioles and venules. The exchange of oxygen, nutrients, and waste products between blood and body cells occurs through the walls of capillaries. **Venules** are the smallest branches of veins. They connect capillaries and veins. **Veins** are vessels that return blood to the heart. Veins normally carry oxygen-poor blood. However, the pulmonary vein and its two branches (the left and right pulmonary veins) carry oxygen-rich blood. (There are four pulmonary veins, two from each lung). The walls of veins are thinner than those of arteries. Because the pressure in the veins is low, most veins contain one-way valves that help keep the blood flowing toward the heart (Figure 6-28).

Remember This

Arteries = Away. In illustrations of the circulatory system, *arteries* are usually drawn in *red* to show that the blood in them is filled with hemoglobin on its way to the body. *Veins* are usually shown in *blue* to indicate they are carrying oxygen-poor blood back to the heart.

Major Arteries

Objective 32

Blood flows from the **aorta**, the largest artery in the body, to all parts of the body. The aorta lies in front of the spine in the thoracic and abdominal cavities (Figure 6-29). Because the heart must have a constant blood supply, it supplies itself with oxygenated blood

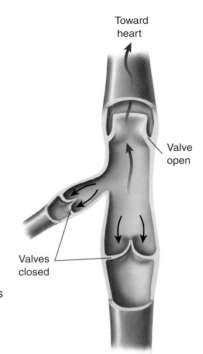

FIGURE 6-28 ▶ Veins contain one-way valves that help keep blood flowing toward the heart.

first through the coronary arteries. The coronary arteries are the first blood vessels that branch off the aorta. When the heart relaxes, the coronary arteries fill with blood in between beats and supply the heart muscle with the oxygen it needs.

Branches of the aorta form the carotid and subclavian arteries. The left and right carotid arteries are the major arteries of the neck, supplying the head and neck with blood. A carotid pulse can be felt on either side of the neck. The subclavian arteries run under the clavicles and supply blood to the upper extremities. The subclavian arteries branch into the axillary and brachial arteries in the upper arm. A brachial pulse can be felt on the inside of the arm between the elbow and the shoulder. This artery is used when determining a blood pressure (BP) with a BP cuff and stethoscope. The brachial arteries branch into the radial and ulnar arteries. These arteries supply the forearm with blood. The radial artery is the major artery of the lower arm. A radial pulse can be felt on the side of the wrist below the thumb.

The femoral arteries are the major arteries of the thigh, supplying the lower extremities with blood. A femoral pulse can be felt in the groin area (the crease between the abdomen and the thigh). Behind the knees, the femoral arteries become the popliteal arteries. The popliteal arteries supply blood to the lower legs. Slightly below the knee, the popliteal arteries become the tibial arteries. The posterior tibial pulse is located just behind the inner ankle bone. At the ankle, one of the tibial arteries becomes the dorsalis pedis artery, which supplies blood to the foot. A dorsalis pedis pulse (often called a *pedal pulse*) can be felt on the top of the foot.

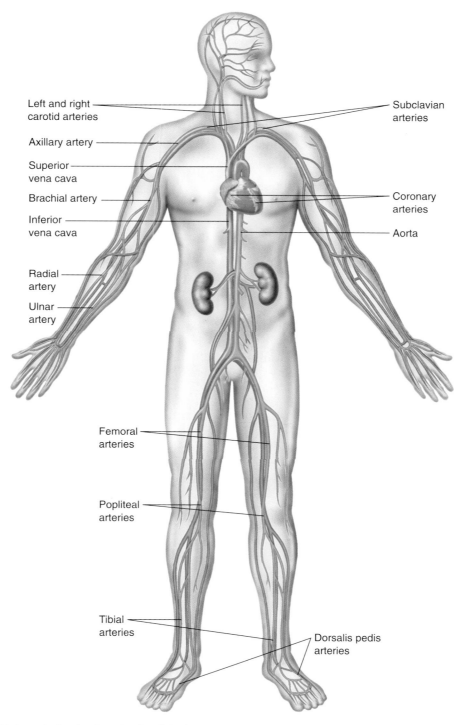

Left and right carotid arteries

Axillary artery

Superior vena cava

Brachial artery

Inferior vena cava

Radial artery

Ulnar artery

Femoral arteries

Popliteal arteries

Tibial arteries

Subclavian arteries

Coronary arteries

Aorta

Dorsalis pedis arteries

FIGURE 6-29 ▲ Major arteries (red) and veins (blue).

Major Veins

Objective 33

The two largest veins in the human body are the inferior vena cava and the superior vena cava. These two veins empty oxygen-poor blood into the heart's right atrium. The superior vena cava returns blood from the head, chest, and upper extremities to the heart. The inferior vena cava returns blood from the abdomen and lower extremities to the heart.

The Physiology of Circulation

Pulse

Objective 34

When the left ventricle contracts, a wave of blood is sent through the arteries, causing the arteries to expand and recoil. A **pulse** is the regular expansion and recoil of an artery caused by the movement of blood from the heart as it contracts. A pulse can be felt anywhere an artery passes near the skin surface and over a bone. Central pulses are located close to the heart, such as the carotid and femoral pulses. Peripheral pulses are located farther from the heart, such as the radial, brachial, posterior tibial, and dorsalis pedis pulses.

Blood Pressure

Objective 35

Blood pressure is the force exerted by the blood on the inner walls of the heart and arteries. The **systolic blood pressure** is the pressure in an artery when the heart is pumping blood (systole). The **diastolic blood pressure** is the pressure in an artery when the heart is at rest (diastole). A blood pressure measurement is made up of both the systolic and the diastolic pressures. It is measured in millimeters of mercury (mm Hg). Blood pressure is written as a fraction (for example, 115/78), with the systolic number first. In an adult, a normal systolic blood pressure ranges from 100 to 120 mm Hg. A normal diastolic blood pressure ranges from 60 to 80 mm Hg. Blood pressure is dependent on the contraction of the heart, blood volume, and the condition of the blood vessels. A slow or fast heart rate, a loss of blood, or changes in the elasticity of the blood vessels may lead to changes in the blood pressure. Methods used to measure blood pressure are discussed in Chapter 17, "Patient Assessment."

The Nervous System

Objective 36

The **nervous system** is a collection of specialized cells that conduct information to and from the brain. The functions of the nervous system are to:

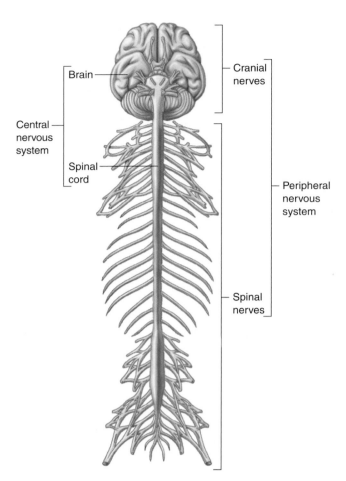

FIGURE 6-30 ▲ The central nervous system (CNS) consists of the brain and spinal cord. The peripheral nervous system (PNS) consists of cranial nerves, which arise from the brain and spinal nerves, which arise from the spinal cord. The nerves actually extend throughout the body.

- Control the voluntary (conscious) and involuntary (unconscious) activities of the body.
- Provide for mental activity (such as thought, emotion, learning, and memory).

The nervous system has two divisions: the central nervous system (CNS) and the peripheral nervous system (PNS) (Figure 6-30).

The Central Nervous System

Objectives 37, 38

The central nervous system consists of the brain and the spinal cord. The brain is made up of many nerve cells (**neurons**) that are involved in higher mental function. These higher functions include the ability to think, to perform unconscious motor functions such as breathing and controlling blood vessel diameter, and to experience and express emotion.

The brain is located in the cranium, where it is protected. The spinal cord is protected in the spinal canal where it travels through the **foramen magnum**, which is the opening in the base of the skull, and down the vertebral column. The central nervous system is also protected by the **meninges**, a covering over the brain and spinal cord, and **cerebrospinal fluid (CSF)**, a clear liquid that is circulated continuously. CSF acts as a shock absorber for the central nervous system. It also provides a means for the exchange of nutrients and wastes between the blood, the brain, and the spinal cord.

You Should Know

Meninges (literally, "membranes") are three layers of connective tissue coverings that surround the brain and spinal cord. The **pia mater** (literally, "gentle mother") forms the delicate inner layer that clings gently to the brain and spinal cord. It contains many blood vessels that supply the nervous tissue. The **arachnoid** (literally, "resembling a spider's web") layer is the middle layer with delicate fibers resembling a spider's web; it contains few blood vessels. The **dura mater** (literally, "hard" or "tough mother") is the tough, outermost layer that sticks to the inner surface of the skull. **Meningitis** is an inflammation of the tissue coverings of the brain and spinal cord.

The **cerebrum** is the largest part of the human brain (Figure 6-31). It consists of two cerebral hemispheres. The **corpus callosum**, a very thick bundle of nerve fibers, joins the two hemispheres. The outer layer of the cerebrum is called the **cerebral cortex**. Although no area of the brain functions alone, each cerebral hemisphere is divided into four lobes named for the bones that lie over them:

1. *Frontal.* The frontal lobes control goal-oriented behavior, personality, short-term memory, elaboration of thought, inhibition of emotions, and the programming and integrating of motor activity, including speech.
2. *Parietal.* The parietal lobes receive and process information about touch, taste, pressure, pain, heat, and cold.
3. *Occipital.* The occipital lobes receive and interpret visual information.
4. *Temporal.* The temporal lobes receive auditory signals and interpret language. They are also involved in personality, behavior, emotion, long-term memory, taste, and smell, and they have some influence on balance.

You Should Know

Think of the CNS as a computer system. The right and left hemispheres of the brain are two computers in the network. The corpus callosum is the cable that connects (networks) the two computers.

The **cerebellum** is the second-largest part of the human brain. It is responsible for the precise control of muscle movements as well as maintaining posture and balance. The **diencephalon** is the part of the brain between the cerebrum and the brainstem. It contains the thalamus and hypothalamus. The **thalamus** functions as a relay station for impulses going to and from the cerebrum. The **hypothalamus** plays an important role in the control of thirst, hunger, and body temperature. It also serves as a link between the nervous and endocrine systems.

The **brainstem** is made up of the midbrain, the pons, and the medulla oblongata. The midbrain connects the pons and cerebellum with the cerebrum. It acts as a relay for auditory and visual signals. The pons, which means "bridge," connects parts of the brain with one another by means of tracts. It influences respiration. The medulla oblongata is the lowest part of the brainstem. It joins the brainstem to the spinal cord. The medulla contains nerves that pass from the spinal cord to the brain and nerves that pass from the brain to the spinal cord. The medulla is involved in controlling blood vessel diameter, respiration, and centers that control reflexes such as coughing, swallowing, sneezing, and vomiting.

The **reticular formation** is a complex network of nerve fibers located throughout the medulla, pons, and midbrain that connect with nerve fibers of other structures, including the hypothalamus, cerebellum, and cerebrum. A portion of the reticular formation, the reticular activating system (RAS), is responsible

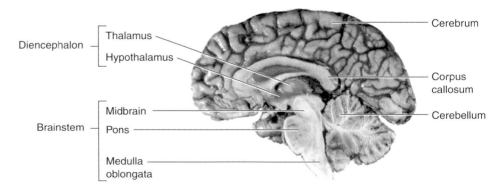

FIGURE 6-31 ▶ The areas of the brain.

for states of consciousness, such as alertness and sleep, and filtering incoming sensory information. The cerebral cortex is constantly bombarded with sensory information. As a filter for the cerebral cortex, the RAS determines if sensory information received is important. For example, while reading this page, you may be sitting in a room in which conversations are taking place among other individuals, a clock may be ticking, a bird may be chirping outside a window, and traffic may be passing by on the street outside the building. These stimuli are largely ignored by the cerebral cortex because they are filtered by the RAS and deemed unimportant. However, if someone calls your name, the RAS recognizes the stimulus as an important one and activates the cerebral cortex into a state of wakefulness, thus bringing the stimulus to your conscious attention. Visual and auditory stimuli and mental activity can stimulate the RAS to maintain attention and alertness. Sleep centers in the hypothalamus and other areas of the brain inhibit the activity of the RAS, inducing drowsiness or sleep. The activity of the RAS may also be suppressed by alcohol, tranquilizers, and general anesthetics. Severe injury to the RAS can result in permanent unconsciousness (irreversible coma).

The **spinal cord** is continuous with the medulla and is the center for many reflex activities of the body. It relays electrical signals to and from the brain and peripheral nerves (see Figure 6-30).

The Peripheral Nervous System

Objective 39

The **peripheral nervous system (PNS)** is made up of nerves that connect the brain and spinal cord to the rest of the body. Twelve pairs of **cranial nerves** are linked directly to the brain. Even though the cranial nerves exit from the brain, they are still considered a part of the peripheral nervous system. The cranial nerves are involved in special senses such as vision, hearing, smell, and taste. They are also involved in eye, face, and tongue movements. Cranial nerves relay signals to and from the brain.

Spinal nerves are any of 31 pairs of nerves that relay impulses to and from the spinal cord. There are three types of spinal nerves: sensory, motor, and mixed nerves. Sensory nerve cells receive information from the body. They send electrical signals *to* the brain and spinal cord, allowing the body to respond to sensory input. The brain and spinal cord's response is sent along motor nerve cells. Motor nerves send electrical signals *from* the brain and spinal cord. For example, when a person touches hot water, the sensory nerve signal travels up to the brain and then back down via motor nerve cells to the muscles of the involved extremity, causing movement away from the hot water.

The PNS has two divisions. The **somatic** (voluntary) **division** has receptors and nerves concerned with the external environment. It influences the activity of the musculoskeletal system. The **autonomic** (involuntary) **division** has receptors and nerves concerned with the internal environment. It controls the involuntary system of glands and smooth muscle and functions to maintain a steady state in the body.

The autonomic division is further divided into the sympathetic division and parasympathetic division. The **sympathetic division** mobilizes energy, particularly in stressful situations. This is called the *fight-or-flight response*. Its effects are widespread throughout the body. The **parasympathetic division** conserves and restores energy ("rest and digest"); its effects are localized in the body (Table 6-4).

TABLE 6-4   Effects of Stimulation of the Autonomic Nervous System

Effects of Sympathetic Stimulation: "Fight or Flight"	Effects of Parasympathetic Stimulation: "Rest and Digest"
• Heart rate increases.	• Heart rate decreases.
• Heart's force of contraction increases.	• Heart's force of contraction decreases.
• Pupils widen.	• Pupils narrow.
• Digestion decreases.	• Digestion increases.
• Mouth and nose secretions decrease.	• Mouth and nose secretions increase.
• Bronchial muscles relax.	• Bronchial muscles constrict.
• Urine secretion decreases.	• Urine secretion increases.

The Integumentary System

Objectives 40, 41

The **integumentary system** is made up of the skin, hair, nails, sweat glands, and sebaceous (oil) glands (Figure 6-32). The skin protects the body from the environment, bacteria, and other organisms, as well as keeping the fluids inside the body. Blood vessels and the sweat glands in the skin help control and maintain body temperature. The skin acts as a sense organ, detecting sensations such as heat, cold, touch, pressure, and pain. The skin relays this information to the brain and spinal cord.

The skin has multiple layers, including the epidermis, dermis, and subcutaneous tissue, which lie over muscle and bone. Each layer contains different structures. The **epidermis** is the outer portion of the skin. It does not contain blood vessels and is thickest on the palms of the hands and the soles of the feet. The **dermis** is the thick layer of skin below the epidermis. The dermis contains hair follicles, sweat and oil glands, small nerve endings, and blood vessels. The **subcutaneous layer** is thick and lies below the dermis. It contains fat and insulates the body from changes in temperature. This layer is loosely attached to the muscles and bones of the musculoskeletal system.

The Digestive System

Objective 42

Function

The digestive system performs the following functions:

- **Ingestion.** The digestive system brings nutrients, water, and electrolytes into the body.
- **Digestion.** It chemically breaks down food into small parts so that absorption can occur.
- **Absorption.** It moves nutrients, water, and electrolytes into the circulatory system so that they can be used by body cells.
- **Defecation.** It eliminates unabsorbed waste.

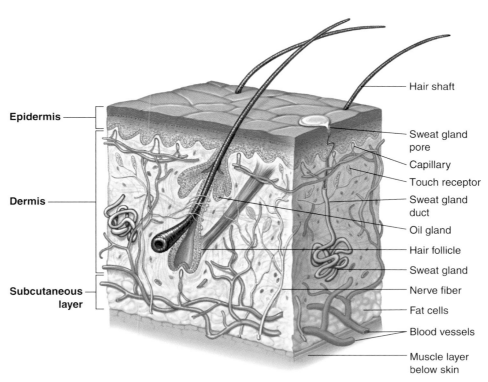

Epidermis

Dermis

Subcutaneous layer

Hair shaft

Sweat gland pore

Capillary

Touch receptor

Sweat gland duct

Oil gland

Hair follicle

Sweat gland

Nerve fiber

Fat cells

Blood vessels

Muscle layer below skin

FIGURE 6-32 ▲ Human skin consists of the epidermis and dermis. The subcutaneous layer is beneath the dermis. Associated structures include hair follicles, sweat glands, and sebaceous (oil) glands.

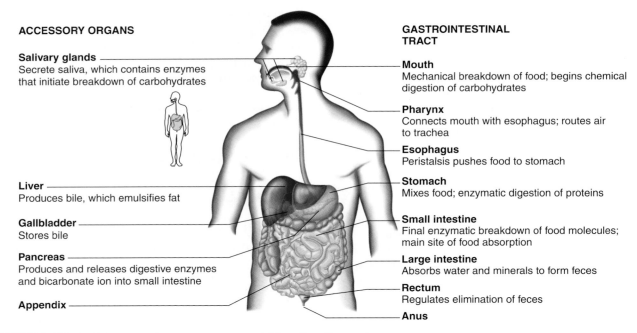

ACCESSORY ORGANS

Salivary glands —
Secrete saliva, which contains enzymes
that initiate breakdown of carbohydrates

Liver —
Produces bile, which emulsifies fat

Gallbladder —
Stores bile

Pancreas —
Produces and releases digestive enzymes
and bicarbonate ion into small intestine

Appendix —

**GASTROINTESTINAL
TRACT**

Mouth
Mechanical breakdown of food; begins chemical
digestion of carbohydrates

Pharynx
Connects mouth with esophagus; routes air
to trachea

Esophagus
Peristalsis pushes food to stomach

Stomach
Mixes food; enzymatic digestion of proteins

Small intestine
Final enzymatic breakdown of food molecules;
main site of food absorption

Large intestine
Absorbs water and minerals to form feces

Rectum
Regulates elimination of feces

Anus

FIGURE 6-33 ▲ Primary and accessory organs of the digestive system.

Components

The primary organs of the digestive system are the mouth, pharynx, esophagus, stomach, small intestine, large intestine, rectum, and anal canal (Figure 6-33). The **accessory organs of digestion** are the teeth and tongue, salivary glands, liver, gallbladder, pancreas, and appendix. **Peristalsis** is the involuntary wavelike contraction of smooth muscle that moves material through the digestive tract.

The mouth, teeth, and salivary glands begin the process of digestion. The tongue manipulates food for chewing and swallowing. Chemicals (enzymes) in the salivary glands begin the breakdown of food. The salivary glands also moisten and lubricate food so that it can be swallowed. The teeth mince food into small pieces so that it can be swallowed when mixed with saliva.

Swallowing moves food from the pharynx into the esophagus. The esophagus transports food from the pharynx to the stomach by peristalsis. The stomach stores food. It mixes food with gastric juices and breaks it down into chyme. The **chyme** (partially digested food) is moved into the small intestine by peristalsis.

The **small intestine** is about 20 feet (6 meters) long (see Plate B at the end of the chapter). It is smaller in diameter than the large intestine. It receives food from the stomach and secretions from the pancreas and liver. It completes the digestion of food that began in the mouth and stomach. Most digestion and absorption occurs here. The small intestine selectively absorbs nutrients that can be used by the body. It is composed of three sections (listed in the order in which food passes through them): **duodenum, jejunum,** and **ileum.**

The **large intestine (colon)** is about 5 feet (1.5 meters) in length (see Plate B). It absorbs water and electrolytes from the remaining chyme and changes it from a fluid to a semisolid mass. It excretes waste as feces. The large intestine is subdivided into the following sections (listed in the order in which food passes through them): **cecum, ascending colon, transverse colon, descending colon, sigmoid colon, rectum,** and **anal canal.**

The **liver** is the largest internal organ of the body (Plate A at the end of the chapter). It produces bile, which breaks up (emulsifies) fats. It stimulates the gallbladder to secrete stored bile into the small intestine. It stores minerals and fat-soluble vitamins (A, D, E, and K). It also stores blood. The **gallbladder** stores bile until it is needed by the small intestine (Plates A and B at the end of the chapter). The **pancreas** secretes juices that contain enzymes for protein, carbohydrate, and fat digestion into the small intestine (Plate C at the end of the chapter).

The Endocrine System

Objective 43

Function

The **endocrine system** is a system of glands that secrete chemicals (hormones) directly into the circulatory system (Figure 6-34). The chemicals released into the bloodstream trigger a response in specific body cells. As a result, the endocrine system influences body activities and functions. The endocrine system works closely with the nervous system to maintain homeostasis.

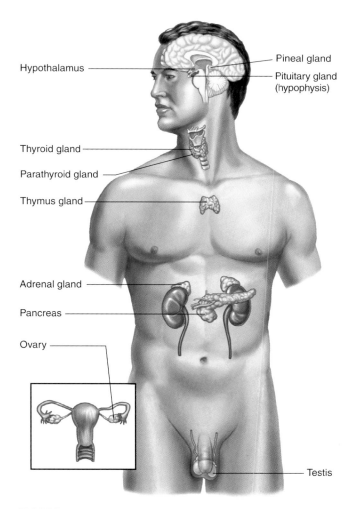

Hypothalamus

Pineal gland

Pituitary gland
(hypophysis)

Thyroid gland

Parathyroid gland

Thymus gland

Adrenal gland

Pancreas

Ovary

Testis

FIGURE 6-34 ▲ The endocrine system.

Components

The **thyroid gland** lies in the neck, just below the larynx. Its shape resembles that of a butterfly. The thyroid gland produces hormones that stimulate body heat production and bone growth. It also controls the body's metabolic rate. The **parathyroid glands** are located behind the thyroid gland. They secrete a hormone that maintains the calcium level in the blood. **Adrenal glands** are located on top of each kidney. The outer tissue of an adrenal gland is called the *cortex*. The inner tissue of an adrenal gland is called the *medulla*. The adrenal medulla releases epinephrine and norepinephrine. Epinephrine and norepinephrine help prepare the body for its fight-or-flight response.

The **pituitary gland** is buried deep in the cranial cavity at the base of the brain. In an adult, it is about the size and shape of a garbanzo bean. The pituitary gland is the "master gland" of the body. It regulates growth and controls other endocrine glands. The hypothalamus produces or controls hormones released by the pituitary. It controls the part of the nervous

system that controls involuntary body functions, hormones, and functions such as regulating sleep and stimulating appetite. The **pineal gland** is located near the center of the brain. It is responsible for producing **melatonin,** which has a role in regulating daily rhythms, such as sleep. Levels of melatonin increase at night and are low or undetectable during the day.

The **islets of Langerhans** are located in the pancreas. Alpha cells secrete glucagon, which increases blood glucose concentration. Beta cells secrete **insulin,** which decreases blood glucose concentration.

Other glands of the endocrine system include the **thymus gland, ovaries,** and **testes.** The thymus gland plays a role in the body's immune system. The ovaries secrete estrogens, which are female sex hormones. The testes secrete testosterone and other male hormones.

The Reproductive System

Objective 44

Function

The **reproductive system** makes cells (sperm, eggs) that allow continuation of the human species.

Components

Male

The testes produce sperm and the hormone testosterone (Figure 6-35). Reproductive ducts allow passage of sperm. Ducts include:

- Epididymis
- Ductus (vas) deferens
- Ejaculatory duct
- Urethra

Seminal vesicles secrete fluid that nourishes and protects sperm. The **prostate gland** secretes fluid that increases sperm movement and neutralizes the acidity of the vagina during intercourse. The **penis** serves as the outlet for sperm and urine. The **scrotum** is the loose sac of skin that houses the testes (Plate A).

Female

The ovaries are a pair of almond-shaped organs that produce eggs (ova) (see Figure 6-36 and Plate C). They are located on either side of the uterus in the pelvic cavity. The ovaries produce the hormones estrogen and progesterone. **Fallopian tubes (oviducts)** receive the ovum and transport it to the uterus after ovulation. The **uterus** is a hollow, muscular organ in which a fertilized ovum implants and receives nourishment until birth. The **vagina (birth canal)** receives the penis during

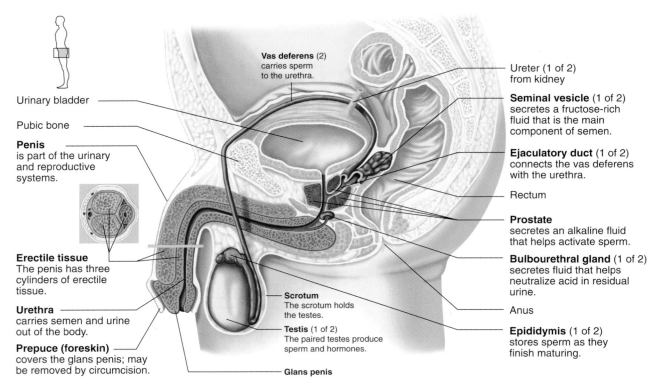

Vas deferens (2) carries sperm to the urethra.

Urinary bladder

Pubic bone

Penis
is part of the urinary and reproductive systems.

Erectile tissue
The penis has three cylinders of erectile tissue.

Urethra
carries semen and urine out of the body.

Prepuce (foreskin)
covers the glans penis; may be removed by circumcision.

Ureter (1 of 2) from kidney

Seminal vesicle (1 of 2) secretes a fructose-rich fluid that is the main component of semen.

Ejaculatory duct (1 of 2) connects the vas deferens with the urethra.

Rectum

Prostate
secretes an alkaline fluid that helps activate sperm.

Bulbourethral gland (1 of 2) secretes fluid that helps neutralize acid in residual urine.

Anus

Epididymis (1 of 2) stores sperm as they finish maturing.

Scrotum
The scrotum holds the testes.

Testis (1 of 2)
The paired testes produce sperm and hormones.

Glans penis

FIGURE 6-35 ▲ The male reproductive system.

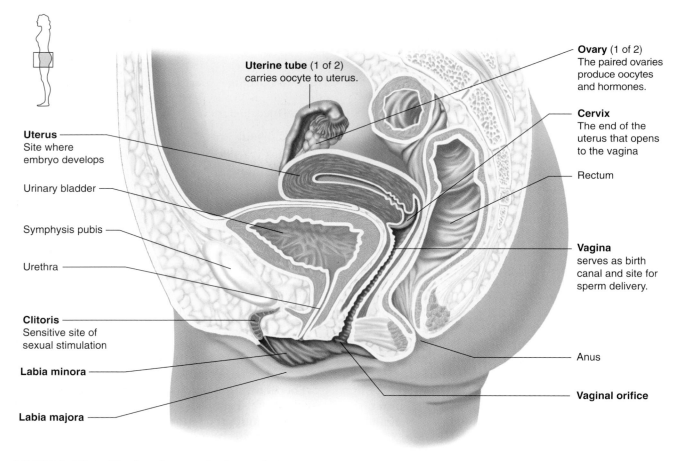

Uterine tube (1 of 2)
carries oocyte to uterus.

Uterus
Site where embryo develops

Urinary bladder

Symphysis pubis

Urethra

Clitoris
Sensitive site of sexual stimulation

Labia minora

Labia majora

Ovary (1 of 2)
The paired ovaries produce oocytes and hormones.

Cervix
The end of the uterus that opens to the vagina

Rectum

Vagina
serves as birth canal and site for sperm delivery.

Anus

Vaginal orifice

FIGURE 6-36 ▲ The female reproductive system.

intercourse and serves as a passageway for menstrual flow and delivery of an infant. Accessory organs include the **mammary glands (breasts)**, which function in milk production after delivery of an infant.

The external genitalia include the mons pubis, clitoris, urethral opening, Bartholin's gland, vagina, labia minora, labia majora, and hymen. The **perineum** is the area between the vaginal opening and the anus.

The Urinary System

Objective 45
Function

The urinary system is responsible for removing body wastes, assisting in regulating blood pressure, and helping to control the amount and composition of water and other substances in the body.

Components

The **kidneys** are located at the back of the abdominal cavity on each side of the spinal column (Plate C). They produce urine, maintain water balance, aid in regulation of blood pressure, and regulate levels of many chemicals in the blood. The **ureters** are tubes that drain urine from the kidneys to the urinary bladder. The **urinary bladder** serves as a temporary storage site for urine. The **urethra** is a canal that passes urine from the urinary bladder to the outside of the body (Figure 6-37). In males, the urethra also transports semen from the body. The male urethra is longer than that of females.

A summary of the organ systems discussed in this chapter is shown in Table 6-5 on p. 170.

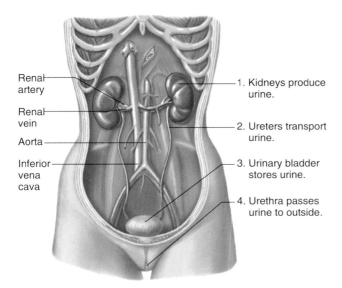

Renal artery
Renal vein
Aorta
Inferior vena cava

1. Kidneys produce urine.
2. Ureters transport urine.
3. Urinary bladder stores urine.
4. Urethra passes urine to outside.

FIGURE 6-37 ▲ The urinary system.

Sum It Up

▶ The body's most basic building block is a cell. The human body contains billions of cells. Cell metabolism is the sum of the chemical reactions that occur within cells, enabling them to maintain a living state. Aerobic metabolism is cell metabolism that occurs in the presence of oxygen. Cell metabolism that does not require the presence of oxygen is called anaerobic metabolism.

▶ Clusters of cells form tissues. Specialized types of tissues form organs such as the brain and the liver. An organ system (also called a body system) consists of tissues and organs that work together to provide a specialized function. The circulatory and respiratory systems are examples of organ systems.

▶ Organ systems work together to maintain a state of homeostasis (balance). These systems need a constant internal environment to perform the required functions of the body.

▶ A body cavity is a hollow space in the body that contains internal organs. Knowing the body cavities and the organs found within each cavity will help you describe the location of the injury or symptoms of a sick or injured patient.

▶ The human body is often discussed in terms of sections (cuts) along a plane, which is a flat surface. The frontal plane is the vertical (lengthwise) field that passes through the body from side to side, dividing the body (or any of its parts) into anterior (ventral) and posterior (dorsal) parts. The sagittal plane is the vertical field that passes through the body from front to back, dividing the body (or any of its parts) into right and left sections. The midsagittal plane is the sagittal field that divides the body into two equal halves. The transverse plane is the crosswise field that divides the body (or any of its parts) into superior (upper) and inferior (lower) sections.

TABLE 6-5 Organ Systems

System	Components	Function
Skeletal	Ligaments, cartilage, and bones	Gives the body shape; protects vital internal organs
Muscular	Skeletal muscle, smooth muscle, and cardiac muscle	Gives the body shape; protects internal organs; movement of parts of the skeleton
Respiratory	Air passages (mouth, nose, trachea, larynx, bronchi, and bronchioles) and lungs	Brings oxygen into the body; removes carbon dioxide from the body
Circulatory	Heart, blood, blood vessels, lymph, and lymph vessels	Delivers oxygen and nutrients to the tissues; removes waste products from the tissues
Nervous	Brain, spinal cord, and nerves	Controls the voluntary and involuntary activity of the body; provides for higher mental function (thought, emotion)
Integumentary	Skin, hair, fingernails, toenails, sweat glands, and sebaceous glands	Protects the body from the environment, bacteria, and other organisms; helps regulate the temperature of the body; senses heat, cold, touch, pressure, and pain
Digestive	Mouth, esophagus, stomach, liver, pancreas, and intestines	Performs ingestion and digestion of food, which is absorbed into the body through the membranes of the intestines
Endocrine	Pituitary gland, thyroid gland, parathyroid glands, adrenal glands, thymus gland, ovaries, testes, pineal gland, and the islets of Langerhans in the pancreas	Interacts with the nervous system to regulate many body activities; secretes chemicals (hormones) to stimulate many body functions
Reproductive	Female: ovaries, uterus, vagina, and mammary glands Male: testes and penis	Manufactures cells (eggs, sperm) that allow continuation of the species
Urinary	Kidneys, urinary bladder, ureters, and urethra	Removes body wastes; assists in regulating blood pressure; helps control the amount and composition of water and other substances in the body

▶ The musculoskeletal system gives the human body its shape and ability to move and protects the major organs of the body. It consists of the skeletal system (bones) and the muscular system (muscles).

▶ The respiratory system supplies oxygen from the air we breathe to the body's cells. It also removes carbon dioxide (a waste product of the body's cells) from the lungs when we breathe out. This system is made up of an upper and a lower airway. The upper airway includes the nose, the pharynx (throat), and the larynx (voice box). The lower airway consists of structures found mostly within the chest cavity, such as the trachea (windpipe) and the lungs.

▶ Breathing (also called pulmonary ventilation) is the mechanical process of moving air into and out of the lungs. Inspiration (inhalation) is the process of breathing in and moving air into the lungs. Expiration (exhalation) is the process of breathing out and moving air out of the lungs. Respiration is the exchange of gases between a living organism and its environment. A single respiration consists of one inspiration and one expiration.

▶ The circulatory system is made up of the cardiovascular and lymphatic systems. This system has three main functions: (1) to deliver oxygen-rich blood and nutrients to body tissues, (2) to help maintain body temperature, and (3) to protect the body against infection. The cardiovascular system consists of the heart, blood, and blood vessels. The lymphatic system consists of lymph, lymph nodes, lymph vessels, tonsils, the spleen, and the thymus gland.

▶ Red blood cells (erythrocytes) contain hemoglobin. Hemoglobin chemically bonds with oxygen and transports it to the body's cells.

- A pulse is the regular expansion and recoil of an artery caused by the movement of blood from the heart as it contracts. Central pulses are located close to the heart, such as the carotid and femoral pulses. Peripheral pulses are located farther from the heart, such as the radial pulse.

- Blood pressure is the force exerted by the blood on the inner walls of the heart and arteries. The systolic blood pressure is the pressure in an artery when the heart is pumping blood (systole). The diastolic blood pressure is the pressure in an artery when the heart is at rest (diastole). A blood pressure measurement is made up of both the systolic and the diastolic pressures.

- The nervous system is a collection of specialized cells that transfer information to and from the brain. The two main functions of the nervous system are to control the voluntary (conscious) and involuntary (unconscious) activities of the body and to provide for higher mental function (such as thought and emotion). The nervous system has two divisions: (1) the CNS and (2) the PNS. The PNS has two divisions. The somatic (voluntary) division has receptors and nerves concerned with the external environment. It influences the activity of the musculoskeletal system. The autonomic (involuntary) division has receptors and nerves concerned with the internal environment. It controls the involuntary system of glands and smooth muscle and functions to maintain a steady state in the body. The autonomic division is divided into the sympathetic division and parasympathetic divisions. The sympathetic division mobilizes energy, particularly in stressful situations. This is called the fight-or-flight response. Its effects are widespread throughout the body. The parasympathetic division conserves and restores energy; its effects are localized in the body

- The integumentary system is made up of the skin, hair, nails, sweat glands, and oil (sebaceous) glands. The skin is the largest organ of the body. It protects the body from the environment, bacteria, and other organisms and plays an important role in temperature regulation.

- The digestive system brings nutrients, water, and electrolytes into the body (ingestion). It chemically breaks down food into small parts so absorption can occur (digestion). It moves nutrients, water, and electrolytes into the circulatory system so they can be used by body cells (absorption). It also eliminates undigested waste (defecation). The primary organs of the digestive system are the mouth, pharynx, esophagus, stomach, small intestine, large intestine, rectum, and anal canal. The accessory organs are the teeth and tongue, salivary glands, liver, gallbladder, and pancreas.

- The endocrine system is a system of glands that secrete chemicals (hormones) directly into the circulatory system. It influences body activities and functions. The endocrine system works closely with the nervous system to maintain homeostasis.

- The reproductive system makes cells (sperm, eggs) that allow continuation of the human species. The urinary system is responsible for removing body wastes, assisting in regulating blood pressure, and helping to control the amount and composition of water and other substances in the body.

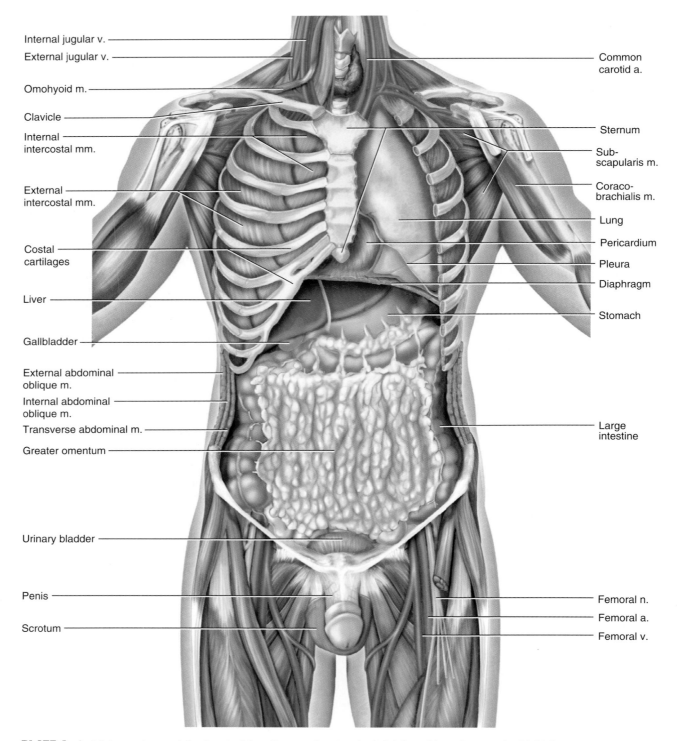

Internal jugular v.

External jugular v.

Omohyoid m.

Clavicle

Internal intercostal mm.

External intercostal mm.

Costal cartilages

Liver

Gallbladder

External abdominal oblique m.

Internal abdominal oblique m.

Transverse abdominal m.

Greater omentum

Urinary bladder

Penis

Scrotum

Common carotid a.

Sternum

Sub-scapularis m.

Coraco-brachialis m.

Lung

Pericardium

Pleura

Diaphragm

Stomach

Large intestine

Femoral n.

Femoral a.

Femoral v.

PLATE A ▲ Male anatomy at the level of the rib cage (anatomical right) and lung (anatomical left) (a. = artery; v. = vein; m. = muscle; mm. = muscles; n. = nerve).

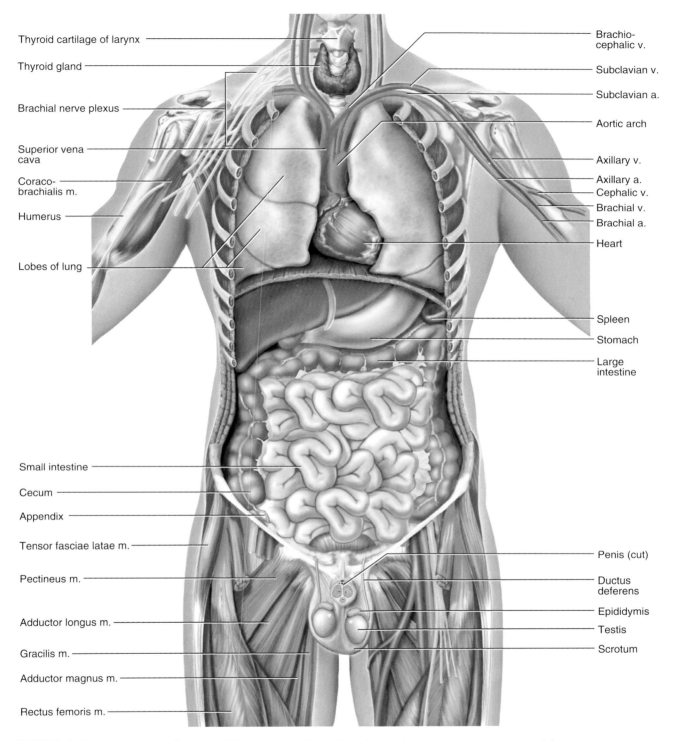

Thyroid cartilage of larynx

Thyroid gland

Brachial nerve plexus

Superior vena cava

Coraco-brachialis m.

Humerus

Lobes of lung

Small intestine

Cecum

Appendix

Tensor fasciae latae m.

Pectineus m.

Adductor longus m.

Gracilis m.

Adductor magnus m.

Rectus femoris m.

Brachio-cephalic v.

Subclavian v.

Subclavian a.

Aortic arch

Axillary v.

Axillary a.

Cephalic v.

Brachial v.

Brachial a.

Heart

Spleen

Stomach

Large intestine

Penis (cut)

Ductus deferens

Epididymis

Testis

Scrotum

PLATE B ▲ Male anatomy at the level of the lungs and intestines (a. = artery; v. = vein; m. = muscle).

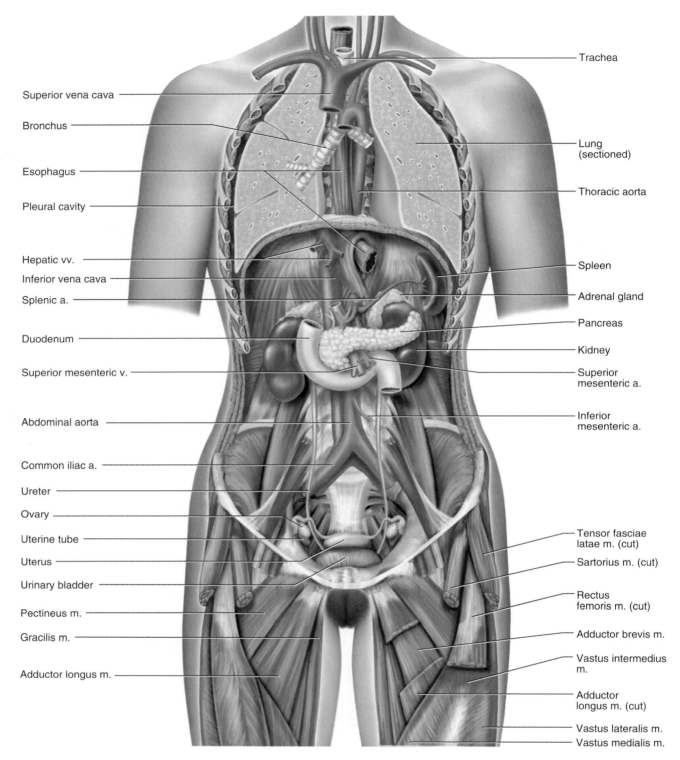

Superior vena cava

Bronchus

Esophagus

Pleural cavity

Hepatic vv.

Inferior vena cava

Splenic a.

Duodenum

Superior mesenteric v.

Abdominal aorta

Common iliac a.

Ureter

Ovary

Uterine tube

Uterus

Urinary bladder

Pectineus m.

Gracilis m.

Adductor longus m.

Trachea

Lung
(sectioned)

Thoracic aorta

Spleen

Adrenal gland

Pancreas

Kidney

Superior
mesenteric a.

Inferior
mesenteric a.

Tensor fasciae
latae m. (cut)

Sartorius m. (cut)

Rectus
femoris m. (cut)

Adductor brevis m.

Vastus intermedius
m.

Adductor
longus m. (cut)

Vastus lateralis m.

Vastus medialis m.

PLATE C ▲ Female anatomy at the level of the retroperitoneal viscera. The heart is removed, the lungs are sectioned frontally, and the viscera of the peritoneal itself are removed (a. = artery; v. = vein; vv. = veins; m. = muscle).

Pathophysiology

By the end of this chapter, you should be able to:

Knowledge Objectives ▶

1. Define disease, pathology, and pathophysiology.
2. Define anabolism and catabolism.
3. Discuss cellular respiration.
4. Discuss glycolysis and aerobic and anaerobic metabolism.
5. Discuss cell reproduction.
6. Discuss benign and malignant tumors.
7. Define metastasis.
8. Discuss free radicals and their effects on the body.
9. Define hypoxia and ischemia, and explain their effects on the body.
10. Explain how an inadequate rate or depth of breathing affects cellular respiration.
11. Define perfusion, cardiac output, and stroke volume.
12. Define venous return, and explain the effect of decreased venous return on cardiac output.
13. Discuss the effect of heart rate on cardiac output.
14. Describe the structure of blood vessel walls.
15. Describe the function of large- and medium-sized arteries, arterioles, capillaries, venules, and veins.
16. Explain peripheral vascular resistance.
17. Explain the relationship between blood pressure, cardiac output, and peripheral vascular resistance.
18. Discuss shock (hypoperfusion).
19. Discuss the major categories of shock: hypovolemic, cardiogenic, obstructive, and distributive.
20. Describe factors that increase the risk of disease.
21. Define pathogenesis, etiology, and idiopathic.
22. Define sign, symptom, and syndrome, and then differentiate between a sign and a symptom.
23. Describe the causes of disease.
24. Define antigen, antibody, allergen, and anaphylaxis.

Attitude Objective ▶ 25. Advocate the need to understand and apply the knowledge of pathophysiology to patient assessment and treatment.

Skill Objectives ▶ There are no skill objectives identified for this lesson.

You and your partner are called to a private residence for an 85-year-old woman who "doesn't feel well." You arrive to find her sitting in a chair with her legs resting on an ottoman. She says that she has "not been feeling right" for a couple of weeks, but today she noticed swelling in her legs that concerns her. She has a history of rheumatoid arthritis. As you examine her, you note that her skin is flushed, very warm, and dry. Swelling is present in both legs from her calves to her feet. Her right foot is warm and red. You note that her respiratory rate is 36 breaths per minute, heart rate is 120 beats per minute, and her blood pressure is 148/84. While you continue your assessment, your partner contacts dispatch and requests that a paramedic unit to be sent to the scene. ■

THINK ABOUT IT

As you read this chapter, think about the following questions:

- Based on your assessment of the patient's skin, do you think her peripheral vascular resistance is increased or decreased? Why?
- The patient's right foot is showing signs of inflammation. What is a sign? What are the classic signs of inflammation?
- The patient's history of rheumatoid arthritis is an example of what type of immune disorder?

Introduction

Pathophysiology

Objective 1

As you learned in Chapter 6, anatomy and physiology involve the study of the body's normal structure and function. **Disease** is an abnormal condition in which the body's steady state (homeostasis) is threatened or cannot be maintained. **Pathology** is the study of disease. **Pathophysiology** is the study of the physical, chemical, and mechanical processes that cause or are caused by disease or injury, producing changes in the structure and function of the body. In this chapter we discuss the basic concept of disease processes. By understanding disease processes, you will better understand the patient's illness or injury, anticipate the patient's needs and potential complications of the illness or injury, and provide appropriate care.

Cell Function

Cell Metabolism

Objectives 2, 3, 4

As discussed in Chapter 6, cell metabolism is the sum of the chemical reactions that occur within cells, enabling them to maintain a living state. There are two types of **cell metabolism.** In **anabolism,** a cell uses energy to make larger molecules from smaller ones. For example, substances such as amino acids are combined to form enzymes. In **catabolism,** the cell breaks down large molecules into small ones, releasing energy. For example, carbohydrates, fats, and proteins can be broken down into smaller substances.

You will recall from Chapter 6 that cellular respiration is the process whereby energy is released from molecules such as glucose and made available for use by the cells and tissues of the body. The energy that is released is eventually converted into adenosine triphosphate (ATP), which is used by cells throughout the body.

The breakdown (catabolism) of glucose into a usable energy form by the cells is called **glycolysis.** During the first step of this process, one molecule of glucose is converted into two molecules of pyruvate (an acid), which is then converted into two molecules of ATP (Figure 7-1). This step does not require oxygen. What happens next to the pyruvate depends on whether or not oxygen is available.

Cell metabolism that does not require the presence of oxygen is called **anaerobic metabolism.** Anaerobic metabolism occurs in the cytoplasm of the cell. If oxygen is not available for the next step, pyruvic acid is converted to lactic acid, which produces no additional ATP. If oxygen is still not available, lactic acid builds up in body cells and fluids and eventually inhibits glycolysis and ATP production. Lactic acid is toxic, and oxygen is needed to break it down. If oxygen becomes available, the liver converts the lactic acid that has

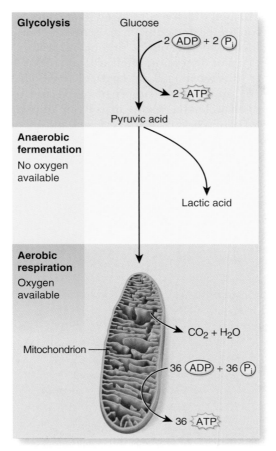

Glycolysis	Glucose
Anaerobic fermentation No oxygen available	Pyruvic acid → Lactic acid
Aerobic respiration Oxygen available	Mitochondrion → $CO_2 + H_2O$

$2\ ADP + 2\ P_i$
$2\ ATP$

$36\ ADP + 36\ P_i$
$36\ ATP$

FIGURE 7-1 ▲ Glycolysis produces pyruvic acid and two molecules of adenosine triphosphate (ATP). If oxygen is not available, pyruvic acid is converted to lactic acid, which produces no additional ATP. In the presence of oxygen, aerobic metabolism occurs in the mitochondria and produces a much greater amount of ATP.

moved into the blood back to pyruvic acid, and the process of aerobic metabolism can begin.

Aerobic metabolism is cell metabolism that occurs in the presence of oxygen. If an ample amount of oxygen is available, the pyruvic acid produced by glycolysis moves into the power plants (mitochondria) of the cell. Here pyruvic acid is broken down into carbon dioxide and water. In the presence of oxygen, each molecule of pyruvate is converted into 18 molecules of ATP. You will recall that at the start of the process, one molecule of glucose was converted into two molecules of pyruvate. Therefore, in the presence of oxygen, 1 glucose molecule will yield a total of 36 molecules of ATP, plus the 2 ATP molecules from the first step in the process, for a total of 38 ATP molecules. As you can see, aerobic metabolism is much more efficient than anaerobic metabolism and yields considerably more energy (ATP) for use by the cells.

After a meal, some of the glucose absorbed from the digestive system is used immediately by cells as fuel for energy. However, most of the glucose is stored as glycogen in muscle and the liver or stored as fat and converted to fuel for energy later. Because glucose is a large molecule, it cannot easily enter the body's cells where it is needed. Insulin, a hormone released from the pancreas, helps transport glucose from the blood into cells, including muscle, liver, and fat cells, to be used for energy.

Cell Reproduction

Objectives 5, 6, 7

Cell reproduction, also called *cell division,* is necessary for body growth, wound healing, and replacement of old, injured, or dead cells. During reproduction, cells begin to differentiate (specialize) in one type of function or act with other cells to perform a more complex task. For example, some cells become skin cells, blood-forming cells, cells that line the intestine, or bone cells. Although most cells reproduce as quickly as they die, some cells, such as those in the pancreas, and certain nerve cells in the brain and spinal cord, do not reproduce.

Cell reproduction that occurs too often or in a disorderly fashion results in a **tumor** (also called a *neoplasm*). A tumor is a growth of cells that multiply without a purpose. A **benign tumor** is noncancerous. It usually develops slowly, remains in place (localized) like a lump, and may eventually interfere with the function of healthy tissue by compressing nearby tissue or obstructing an organ. A **malignant tumor** is cancerous (Figure 7-2). The original tumor is called

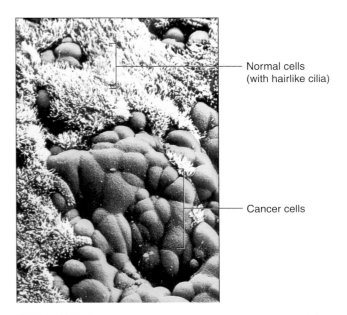

Normal cells (with hairlike cilia)

Cancer cells

FIGURE 7-2 ▲ A cancer cell is rounder and less specialized than surrounding healthy cells. It secretes substances that invade nearby tissue and stimulate formation of blood vessels that foster the tumor's growth.

the *primary cancer* or *primary tumor* and is usually named for the part of the body or the type of cell in which it begins. As it multiplies, the tumor can invade and extend into surrounding tissue. If not stopped by surgery, radiation, or chemicals, the cancerous cells will eventually reach the circulatory system and be transported by the blood and lymph to one or more areas of the body. **Metastasis** is a word used to describe the spread of cancerous cells from their site of origin to sites elsewhere in the body. Some cancers tend to spread to certain parts of the body. For example, lung cancer often spreads to the brain or bones, colon cancer frequently spreads to the liver, and breast cancer often spreads to the bones, lungs, liver, or brain.

Cell Injury and Death

Objectives 8, 9

Cells have the ability to adapt to their environment to protect themselves from injury. But cellular injury can occur if the cell is changed or damaged to the extent that normal function is negatively affected or permanently impaired. Most diseases start with an injury to the cells. There are many causes of cellular injury including free radicals, hypoxia, trauma, bacteria, toxins, viruses, drugs, and chemical agents. Free radicals and hypoxia are discussed below. The others are discussed later in this chapter as causes of disease.

Free radicals are highly reactive molecules that are a by-product of many normal cellular reactions within the body such as inflammatory processes and the breakdown of fats and proteins. Oxygen atoms are the most common source of free radicals. An excessive number of free radicals can damage cells and impair the body's ability to fight illness. Stress and exposure to cigarette smoke, pesticides, air pollution, and ultraviolet light are examples of conditions that can cause an overproduction of free radicals. Antioxidants, such as vitamins C and E and beta-carotene (a precursor to vitamin A), block the production of free radicals, inactivate them, or transform them into nondamaging substances.

Hypoxia, which is a lack of oxygen available to the tissues, is the most common cause of cellular injury. Cells within the brain, heart, and kidney are the most rapidly affected by hypoxia because of their high demand for oxygen. Hypoxia deprives the cell of oxygen and interferes with energy (ATP) production. It may result from decreased amounts of oxygen in the air, loss of hemoglobin or hemoglobin function, decreased production of red blood cells, poisoning of substances within the cells, or diseases of the respiratory or cardiovascular systems.

Ischemia, which is a reduced blood supply, is the most common cause of hypoxia. Ischemia often affects blood flow to specific vessels, producing localized tissue injury. Pain or discomfort often accompanies ischemia, serving as a warning that a part of the body is not receiving an adequate supply of blood and oxygen. Prolonged ischemia results in cellular injury. If the cause of the ischemia is not reversed and blood flow restored to the affected area, ischemia may lead to cellular injury and, ultimately, cell death. Injured cells have been cut off from or have experienced a severe reduction in their blood and oxygen supply. Death of tissue due to ischemia is called an **infarct.**

A common cause of ischemia is narrowing of arteries and blockage of the vessel by plaque or a blood clot (thrombus). For example, ischemia of the heart muscle can occur if a coronary artery is blocked. If the vessel is partially blocked, medications such as nitroglycerin may be used to dilate the affected vessel, allowing blood flow to resume and oxygenation to be restored. If the vessel is completely blocked, ischemia can lead to cell and tissue death, which is called *necrosis*. The process of the heart muscle dying is called a **myocardial infarction** or heart attack. An infarct in the brain is called a **cerebrovascular accident (CVA)** or stroke.

Factors Affecting Cell Function

The balanced state that the body requires to function properly is very sensitive to changes caused by illness or injury. Disease or injury affecting the respiratory or cardiovascular systems can affect the delivery of oxygen and nutrients to the cell and the removal of waste products from the cell, thus disrupting homeostasis. Interruption of the body's oxygen supply and/or removal of carbon dioxide can lead to shock. Unless adequate blood flow is quickly restored, death may soon follow.

Oxygenation and Ventilation

Objective 10

The respiratory system delivers oxygen from the atmosphere to the blood where it gets distributed to body cells and removes carbon dioxide produced by the body cells to the atmosphere. Your patient must have an open airway in order for these essential processes to occur. In addition, adequate oxygenation requires that sufficient oxygen must be present in the surrounding air. Adequate movement of gases into and out of the lungs (ventilation) is dependent on an open airway and an adequate rate and depth of movement of the thoracic cage by the respiratory muscles.

Perfusion

Objectives 10, 11

Perfusion is the circulation of blood through an organ or a part of the body. A balance between ventilation and perfusion must exist to ensure adequate gas exchange. Illnesses and injuries can affect ventilation and/or perfusion, disrupting homeostasis. For example, alveoli may be ventilated but not perfused or, conversely, alveoli may be perfused but not ventilated.

A blocked airway, or an injury or disease that affects oxygenation or ventilation, can lead to hypoxia (a lack of oxygen) and/or **hypercarbia** (an increase in carbon dioxide). Possible causes of a blocked airway include the presence of a foreign body, the tongue blocking the airway in an unconscious patient, blood or secretions, swelling, and trauma to the neck.

Even if the patient's airway is open, cell metabolism can be disrupted if there is inadequate oxygen in the air that is breathed in. Possible causes include a low oxygen environment, toxic gases, lung infection, infection or disease that narrows the airway and causes wheezing, excess fluid in the lungs, excess fluid between the lungs and blood vessels, and poor circulation. **Wheezing** is a high- or low-pitched whistling sound that is usually heard on exhalation. Wheezing suggests that the lower airways are partially blocked with fluid or mucus.

If a patient's rate or depth of breathing is not adequate, an insufficient volume of air will be moved into and out of the lungs. An inadequate tidal volume *or* respiratory rate can result in inadequate ventilation. This, in turn, affects oxygenation and elimination of carbon dioxide, resulting in decreased ATP production. Possible causes of an inadequate rate or depth of breathing include disease, poisoning or overdose, chest injury, unconsciousness, or altered mental status (a change in a patient's level of awareness).

Cardiac Output

Objectives 11, 12, 13

Perfusion depends on cardiac output (CO), peripheral vascular resistance (PVR), and the transport of oxygen. **Cardiac output** is the amount of blood the heart pumps each minute. Cardiac output is determined by multiplying stroke volume (SV) by heart rate (HR). **Stroke volume** is the amount of blood ejected by the ventricles of the heart with each contraction. An average adult man has a normal blood volume of about 5 to 6 L (5,000 to 6,000 mL). In a healthy person, stroke volume is usually about 60 to 100 mL per contraction. In an adult, the heart rate is usually 60 to 100 beats per minute at rest. Therefore, a patient who has a stroke volume of 80 mL per contraction and a heart rate of 70 beats per minute has a cardiac output of 5,600 mL per minute.

$$80 \text{ SV} \times 70 \text{ HR} = 5,600 \text{ CO}$$

A change in either stroke volume *or* heart rate can affect cardiac output. The amount of blood returning to the ventricles is called **venous return.** In a healthy heart, an increase in the volume of blood in the ventricles causes the fibers in the heart muscle to stretch, resulting in a more forceful contraction. This principle is called the **Frank-Starling law of the heart.** For example, the amount of blood that enters the heart from the veins increases during exercise. The muscle fibers in the ventricles stretch to adjust to the increased volume, and the next contraction is stronger than normal, increasing stroke volume and cardiac output. A decrease in the amount of blood returning to the heart and entering the ventricles causes less muscle fiber stretch, decreased force of contraction, and decreased stroke volume. **Hemorrhage** (also called *major bleeding*), an extreme loss of blood from a blood vessel, is one cause of decreased venous return.

Certain hormones, medications, and stimulation of the heart by sympathetic nerves can also cause an increase in the strength of contraction. However, if the heart's muscle fibers are continuously stretched, this responsiveness is lost and the heart contracts less forcefully than normal. When this occurs, cardiac output will no longer be increased by an increased stroke volume. A decrease in the force of the heart's contractions can be caused by heart disease and medications, among other causes.

Heart rate also affects cardiac output. If the patient's heart rate is too fast, the ventricles will have less time to refill before the next contraction. As a result, the stroke volume and, subsequently, cardiac output will decrease. In healthy individuals, a slow heart rate may reflect good physical condition. However, in many individuals a heart rate below 50 beats per minute will result in decreased cardiac output and reduced perfusion of vital body organs.

You Should Know

Signs and Symptoms of Decreased Cardiac Output

- Restlessness
- Changes in mental status
- Fatigue
- Cold, clammy skin
- Skin color changes
- Difficulty breathing, shortness of breath
- Changes in blood pressure
- Abnormal heart rhythms

Blood Vessel Walls

Objective 14

The walls of arteries and veins are made up of three layers (tunics) of tissue (Figure 7-3). The innermost layer (tunica intima) is normally smooth, enabling blood to flow easily along its surface. Conditions such as high blood pressure, high cholesterol, smoking, and diabetes can damage this inner layer. The middle layer of an artery and vein (tunica media) is usually the thickest. It is made up of smooth muscle and, sometimes, elastic tissue. The amount of smooth muscle and elastic tissue varies depending on the vessel's function. For example, the large arteries have a lot of elastic tissue, enabling them to stretch in response to the pumping action of the heart. The presence of smooth muscle allows the vessel to constrict (narrow) and dilate (widen), changing the vessel's diameter. This characteristic plays an important role in regulating blood pressure and blood flow to various organs.

The outermost layer (called the *tunica externa* or *tunica adventitia*) is often continuous with neighboring blood vessels, nerves, or other organs. This layer is made of tough tissue that protects the vessel, gives it strength to withstand high blood pressure, and provides a passageway for small nerves, smaller blood vessels, and lymphatic vessels.

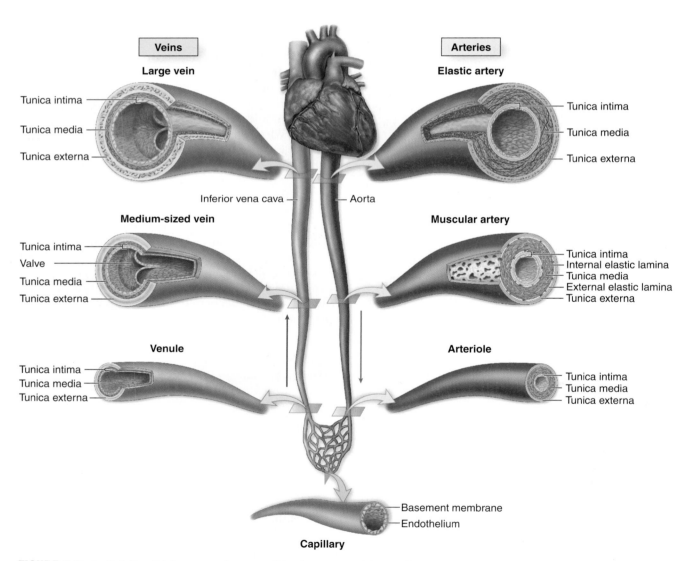

FIGURE 7-3 ▲ Relative thickness and composition in comparable arteries and veins.

Blood Vessel Function

Objective 15

Large arteries are called *conductance vessels* because their main purpose is to carry blood away from the heart through smaller arteries and capillaries to other body systems. The aorta, carotid arteries, and pulmonary arteries are examples of large arteries. The walls of large arteries are thick and elastic, allowing them to expand and recoil. When ventricular contraction occurs, blood pressure rises and the walls of the large arteries expand. Blood pressure falls with ventricular relaxation and the arterial walls recoil. The elasticity of the large arteries reduces the variation in pressure exerted on the smaller arteries.

Large arteries divide into progressively smaller arteries. Medium-sized arteries, such as the brachial and femoral arteries, are called *distributing vessels* because they are farther away from the heart than are the large arteries and they deliver blood to specific organs. Medium-sized arteries are primarily made up of smooth muscle. Because they have less elasticity than larger arteries, the diameter of medium-sized arteries remains relatively constant with changes in blood pressure. A medium-sized artery provides a greater resistance to blood flow than a large artery because its lumen (interior space) is narrower.

The smallest arteries, arterioles, are made up of smooth muscle. They provide the greatest resistance to blood flow through the arterial circulation because the lumen of an arteriole is narrower than that of medium and large arteries. For this reason, arterioles are called *resistance vessels*. Arterioles have a rich supply of fibers of the sympathetic division of the autonomic nervous system and are the primary sites at which the body controls the amounts of blood sent to various organs. In most areas of the body, blood from arterioles enters capillaries. Some arterioles connect directly to venules, and this enables blood to bypass the capillary networks. These connections are called *arteriovenous shunts*.

Capillaries (exchange vessels) are considered the functional units of the circulatory system because it is through them that the exchange of oxygen, nutrients, and waste products between blood and body cells occurs. Capillaries are the most numerous blood vessels and are very thin, consisting of just one cell layer, enabling exchanges between the blood and tissue fluid. Capillaries form extensive networks so that few cells in the body are more than a fraction of a millimeter away from any capillary. Exceptions include tendons and ligaments, which contain few capillaries. Cartilage and the cornea and lens of the eye contain no capillaries. A *precapillary sphincter* is a band of smooth muscle that is present at the opening of each capillary network (Figure 7-4). The

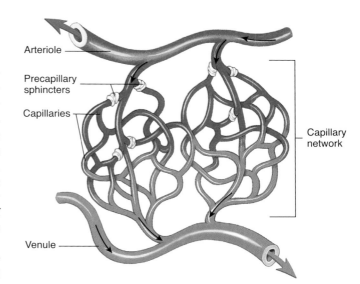

FIGURE 7-4 ▲ Precapillary sphincters are present at the openings of capillary networks.

amount of blood entering a capillary network and flowing to an organ is controlled by precapillary sphincters and the arterioles in the organ.

Capillaries connect to venules, which are the smallest branches of veins. Blood is delivered from venules into progressively larger vessels that empty into the large veins. Examples of large veins include the superior and inferior vena cavae. Veins and venules are called *capacitance vessels* because they function as reservoirs, stretching as they receive blood and returning it to the heart. Some veins are located between groups of skeletal muscles. Because the pressure in the veins is low, contraction of the skeletal muscles provides a massaging action that squeezes the veins and moves blood through one-way valves (located within the veins) toward the heart. Inactivity, such as sitting for long periods or being bedridden, decreases the rate at which blood is returned to the heart. Conversely, vigorous exercise increases the rate of venous return.

You Should Know
Blood Vessel Function

- Large arteries are conductance vessels.
- Medium arteries are distributing vessels.
- Arterioles are resistance vessels.
- Capillaries are exchange vessels.
- Veins and venules are capacitance vessels.

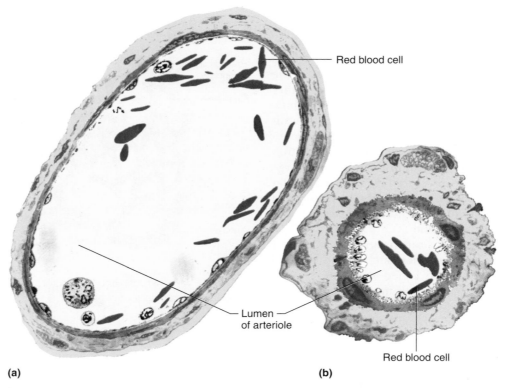

FIGURE 7-5 ▲ Vasodilation and vasoconstriction. **(a)** Relaxation of smooth muscle in the arteriole wall produces dilation; **(b)** contraction of the smooth muscle causes constriction.

Peripheral Vascular Resistance

Objective 16

Peripheral vascular resistance (PVR) (also called *systemic vascular resistance*, or *SVR*) is the opposition that blood encounters in the blood vessels as it travels away from the heart. Because the resistance to flow in the venous circulation is very low, peripheral vascular resistance generally refers to the opposition to flow encountered in the arterial circulation. As previously discussed, the arterioles, because of their small diameter, are the vessels in the arterial circulation that have the greatest resistance to blood flow. However, changing the diameter of the arterioles alters their resistance to blood flow. For example, if arterioles widen, peripheral resistance is decreased, which means there is less resistance to blood flow. Widening of a vessel is called **vasodilation.** If arterioles narrow, peripheral resistance is increased and there is increased resistance to blood flow. Narrowing of a vessel is called **vasoconstriction** (Figure 7-5).

Remember This

Narrowing of a vessel (vasoconstriction) increases peripheral resistance. Widening of a vessel (vasodilation) decreases peripheral resistance.

Blood Pressure

Objective 17

Pressure, provided by the circulatory system, is required to move the blood that carries oxygen and other nutrients to the cells of the body. Blood pressure is the force exerted by the blood on the inner walls of the heart and arteries. It is affected by cardiac output (heart) and peripheral vascular resistance (blood vessels) and can be expressed as the following equation:

$$\text{Blood pressure} = \text{cardiac output} \times \text{peripheral vascular resistance}$$

Therefore, a change in cardiac output *or* peripheral vascular resistance will also affect blood pressure (Figure 7-6).

Pressure receptors in the body continuously send electrical signals to the medulla oblongata. Similarly, electrical signals are continuously sent from the medulla by means of sympathetic nerves to the smooth muscles in the walls of the arterioles. The walls of the arterioles are usually kept in a state of continuous contraction to maintain the peripheral vascular resistance associated with normal blood pressure. If blood pressure falls (such as a systolic blood pressure of less than 80 mm Hg), the pressure receptors send a

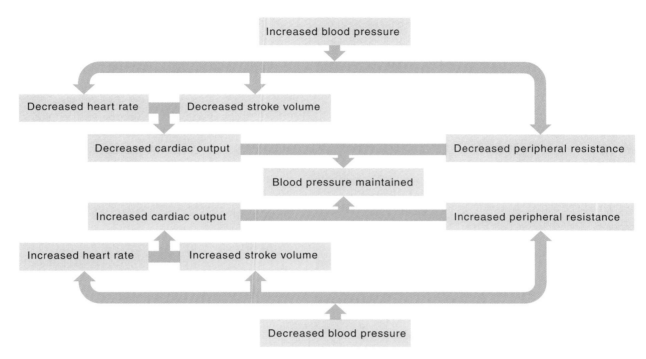

FIGURE 7-6 ▲ Cardiac output and peripheral resistance regulates blood pressure.

message to the medulla, which responds by sending signals to the sympathetic nerves. The arterioles respond to sympathetic stimulation by narrowing, increasing peripheral vascular resistance. In the heart, sympathetic stimulation causes an increase in heart rate and force of contraction. Together, increased peripheral vascular resistance, increased heart rate, and increased contractility help restore blood pressure to normal. As the blood pressure improves, perfusion to the heart, lungs, and brain improves. Conversely, if blood pressure rises excessively, signals are sent to the parasympathetic division of the autonomic nervous system to decrease heart rate and cardiac output. Signals are also sent to reduce the degree of arteriolar narrowing. The decrease in heart rate, cardiac output, and vascular resistance combine to reduce the blood pressure.

Shock

Objectives 18, 19

Maintenance of normal perfusion requires a functioning heart, adequate blood volume, and intact blood vessels that are able to respond to changes in blood pressure. Inadequate perfusion can result if any of these components is disrupted, decreasing cell oxygenation and energy (ATP) production.

Shock is the inadequate circulation of blood through an organ or a part of the body. Shock is also called *hypo-*

perfusion. Because the presence of shock affects the body's ability to oxygenate and perfuse cells, shock can lead to death if it is not corrected. Disruptions in circulatory function that can cause shock include the following:

- **Hypovolemic shock** is a condition in which there is a loss of blood, plasma, or water from the body resulting in an inadequate volume of fluid in the circulatory system to maintain adequate perfusion. This type of shock may occur because of bleeding, vomiting, diarrhea, or burns, among other causes.

- **Cardiogenic shock** is a condition in which the heart fails to function effectively as a pump. As a result, the heart does not pump enough blood to maintain adequate perfusion. This type of shock may be due to disease of or injury to the conduction system, abnormal heart rhythms, or damage to cardiac muscle.

- **Obstructive shock** occurs when blood flow is slowed or stopped by a mechanical or physical obstruction. This type of shock may occur when blood collects in the sac surrounding the heart, preventing efficient cardiac contraction or when air is present in the chest due to a lung injury, putting pressure on the great vessels in the chest and limiting blood flow.

- **Distributive shock** refers to conditions that cause massive dilation of the blood vessels, redistributing the fluid volume within the circulatory system. This type of shock may occur because of a massive infection

(septic shock), severe allergic reaction (anaphylaxis), a loss of nervous system control **(neurogenic shock),** or psychological causes **(psychogenic shock).**

Shock is discussed in more detail in Chapter 32, "Shock."

Disease Risk Factors

Objective 20

Conditions that may increase a person's chance of developing a disease are called **risk factors** or *predisposing factors.* While some risk factors can be changed, others cannot. Examples of risk factors include age, gender, lifestyle, environment, and heredity.

- *Age.* Age is an important risk factor associated with the onset and progression of some diseases. For example, the newly born are at risk of disease because their immune systems are not fully developed and able to fight off infection. As we age, our risk of developing conditions such as Alzheimer's disease, Parkinson's disease, cancer, stroke, heart disease, and arthritis increases.
- *Gender.* Some diseases are more common in one gender than in the other. For example, osteoporosis, multiple sclerosis, breast cancer, and rheumatoid arthritis are more common in women. Lung cancer, gout, and Parkinson's disease are more common in men.
- *Lifestyle.* An individual's personal habits and lifestyle can increase the risk of disease. Constant stress, smoking, excessive alcohol intake, lack of exercise, and poor nutrition are examples of behaviors that can be modified to improve health and decrease the risk of disease.
- *Environment.* Some of the most hazardous occupations in our country include logging, mining, farming, fishing, and hunting. The risk of disease or injury in these occupations may be due to a combination of factors, including exposure to pesticides or other chemicals and safety concerns around machinery. Studies have demonstrated an association between environmental exposure and certain diseases or other health problems. Examples include the following:
  —Radon and lung cancer
  —Arsenic and cancer in several organs
  —Lead and nervous system disorders
  —Contaminated meat and water containing *E. coli* and gastrointestinal illness and death
- *Heredity.* Heredity is an important risk factor for some diseases. For example, a family history of heart disease combined with an inactive lifestyle

and poor personal habits can greatly increase one's risk of a heart attack.

Causes of Disease

Objectives 21, 22

Pathogenesis refers to the mechanism by which a disease develops. Examples of pathogenesis include infection, inflammation, tumors, and tissue breakdown. **Etiology** means the study of cause. The etiology (cause) of many diseases is known. For example, we know that croup, a common childhood respiratory infection, is caused by a virus. The phrase "unknown etiology" or **"idiopathic"** is used when the cause of a disease is unknown.

Some diseases develop in stages. For instance, a disease (such as measles) may have an incubation period, followed by a period during which signs and symptoms are evident, and then a convalescent (recovery) period. The **incubation period** is the interval between the exposure to a disease-causing agent and the appearance of signs and symptoms. A **sign** is a medical or trauma condition of the patient that can be seen, heard, smelled, measured, or felt by the examiner. Examples of signs include a rash, unusual chest movement, bleeding, swelling, pale skin, and a fast pulse. Because signs can be seen, heard, smelled, measured, or felt, they are considered **objective findings.** Some of the ways signs (also called *clinical findings*) can be determined include physical or psychological examination, laboratory tests, and imaging studies (such as x-rays). A **symptom** is a condition described by the patient. Shortness of breath, nausea, abdominal pain, chills, chest pain, and dizziness are examples of symptoms. Symptoms are **subjective findings** because they are dependent on (subject to) the patient's interpretation and description of the complaint. A **syndrome** is a group of signs and symptoms that together are characteristic of a specific disease or disorder.

Remember This

Signs (objective findings, clinical findings)	Medical or trauma conditions of the patient that can be seen, heard, smelled, measured, or felt by the examiner	*Examples:* Rash, unusual chest movement, bleeding, swelling, pale skin, fast pulse
Symptoms (subjective findings)	Conditions described by the patient	*Examples:* Shortness of breath, nausea, abdominal pain, chills, chest pain, dizziness

Physical Agents

Objective 23

Damage to cells and the subsequent development of disease or injury can be caused by physical agents such as mechanical forces, extremes of temperature, electrical forces, and radiation exposure. Injury due to mechanical forces occurs when the body impacts another object, as in a motor vehicle crash, fall, or physical abuse. These types of injuries can cause mechanical damage such as tearing of tissue, breaking of bones, and injuring of blood vessels. Impaired blood flow because of injury to the cells will affect cell metabolism.

Extremes of temperature can cause cellular injury. Exposure to cold causes vasoconstriction and decrease in blood flow. Depending on the degree and duration of cold exposure, this may lead to tissue hypoxia and, possibly, tissue and organ death. Exposure to heat can result in burns, depending on the nature, intensity, and extent of the heat source. Excessive heat causes cell injury by disrupting cell membranes, injuring vessels, and altering cell metabolism.

The extent of tissue damage that results from an electrical injury depends on voltage, type of current (direct or alternating), amperage, tissue resistance, the pathway of the current, and the duration of exposure. In addition to causing tissue damage, electrical injuries can disrupt the conduction of impulses in the heart and nervous system.

Exposure to radiation can cause cell damage. Non-ionizing radiation, which includes infrared light, ultrasound, microwaves, and laser energy, can cause thermal injury. Ionizing radiation, which includes x-rays and radiation therapy used in cancer treatment, can damage cells by interfering with their blood supply or directly altering the structure of DNA within the cell.

Chemical Agents

Objective 23

Chemical agents or irritants can injure the cell membrane and other cell structures or produce free radicals that continue to damage cell components. Examples of chemical agents include poisons, air and water pollutants, heavy metals (such as lead), carbon monoxide, ethanol, preservatives, and social or street drugs (such as marijuana, cocaine, and heroin).

Inflammation and Infection

Objective 23

Inflammation is a tissue reaction to disease, injury, irritation, or infection. It is characterized by pain, heat, redness, swelling, and sometimes a loss of function. You will recall from Chapter 2 that an infection results when the body is invaded by pathogens (germs capable of producing disease), such as bacteria and viruses. When a pathogen grows and multiplies in the body, its ability to cause disease depends on its ability to invade and destroy cells and produce substances that are toxic to the body. Inflammation may be present without an infection, as in a sunburn. However, an infection is usually accompanied by signs of inflammation.

Immune Disorders

Objectives 23, 24

The body's **immune system** consists of specialized cells, tissues, and organs that protect the body against disease by distinguishing the body's healthy cells from pathogens and then killing the foreign invaders. Immune system disorders include allergies, autoimmune disorders, and immunodeficiency.

An **antigen** is any substance that is foreign to an individual and causes antibody production. When the body's immune system detects an antigen, white blood cells respond by producing antibodies specific to that antigen. An **antibody** is a substance that defends the body against bacteria, viruses, or other antigens. When an antigen causes signs and symptoms of an allergic reaction, the antigen is called an **allergen.** Some allergic reactions are mild, causing symptoms that are annoying but not life-threatening. For example, inhaling an antigen such as plant pollen can result in irritation of the eyes, nose, and respiratory tract. Signs and symptoms often include red, watery eyes; sneezing and a runny nose; and coughing. When an allergic reaction is severe and affects multiple body systems, it is called **anaphylaxis.** Anaphylaxis is a life-threatening emergency.

Autoimmune disorders result when a hyperactive immune system attacks its own normal tissues as if they were foreign organisms. Rheumatoid arthritis is an example of a common autoimmune disease.

Immunodeficiency disorders occur when the immune system is unable to defend the body against disease because of a decrease or absence of white blood cells. Patients who have an immunodeficiency disorder usually have recurring infections. Immunodeficiency may be caused by a genetic disease, medications, chemotherapy, radiation, or an infection, such as acquired immune deficiency syndrome (AIDS) that is caused by the human immunodeficiency virus (HIV).

Hereditary Factors

Objective 23

Heredity plays a role in some diseases. A congenital disease or condition is one that is present at birth. Some congenital conditions are obvious at the time of birth, whereas others may not show signs and symptoms until later in life.

Examples of congenital conditions include dwarfism, epilepsy, muscular dystrophy, sickle cell anemia, and Down syndrome. Some congenital conditions, although present at birth, are not inherited. Cerebral palsy, a condition associated with a difficult delivery, is one example.

Nutritional Imbalances

Objective 23

Proper nutrition is essential to good health. A diet lacking essential nutrients can affect the body's ability to break down, absorb, or use food. Being overweight or obese increases the risk of many diseases and health conditions including hypertension (high blood pressure), diabetes, osteoarthritis (a degeneration of cartilage and its underlying bone within a joint), heart disease, stroke, gallbladder disease, respiratory problems, and some cancers (such as breast and colon).

On the Scene   Wrap-Up

You and your partner administer oxygen and remain with the patient until the arrival of the paramedic unit. The patient's skin is flushed, very warm, and dry. The presence of flushed skin suggests that her arterioles have widened (resulting in vasodilation), and blood flow to the skin is increased. If arterioles widen, peripheral resistance is decreased, which means there is less resistance to blood flow. The patient's right foot is showing signs of inflammation. A sign is a medical or trauma condition of the patient that can be seen, heard, smelled, measured, or felt by the examiner. The classic signs of inflammation are redness, heat, swelling, pain, and a possible loss of function. You recall that rheumatoid arthritis is an autoimmune disorder, a result of a hyperactive immune system that attacks its own normal tissues as if they were foreign organisms. When they arrive, the paramedics listen to your report, assess the patient, and start an intravenous line. A few hours later, they call you with patient follow-up information, indicating that she was diagnosed with sepsis (a massive infection). She will remain in the hospital for a few days undergoing treatment with IV antibiotics. ∎

Sum It Up

▶ Disease is an abnormal condition in which the body's steady state (homeostasis) is threatened or cannot be maintained. Pathology is the study of disease. Pathophysiology is the study of the physical, chemical, and mechanical processes that cause or are caused by disease or injury, producing changes in the structure and function of the body.

▶ The basic building block of the human body is the cell. Cell metabolism is the sum of the chemical reactions that occur within cells, enabling them to maintain a living state. There are two types of cell metabolism. In anabolism, a cell uses energy to make larger molecules from smaller ones. In catabolism, the cell breaks down large molecules into small ones, releasing energy.

▶ To function at their best, cells need a continuous supply of oxygen and glucose. The breakdown (catabolism) of glucose into a usable energy form by the cells is called glycolysis. Cell metabolism that does not require the presence of oxygen is called anaerobic metabolism. Aerobic metabolism is cell metabolism that occurs in the presence of oxygen. Aerobic metabolism is much more efficient than anaerobic metabolism and yields considerably more energy (ATP) for use by the cells.

▶ Cell reproduction, also called cell division, is necessary for body growth, wound healing, and replacement of old, injured, or dead cells. Cell reproduction that occurs too often or in a disorderly fashion results in a tumor (also called a neoplasm).

▶ Most diseases start with an injury to the cell. Although cells have the ability to adapt to their environment to protect themselves from injury, cellular injury can occur if the cell is changed or damaged to the point that normal function is negatively affected or permanently impaired.

▶ Hypoxia, which is a lack of oxygen available to the tissues, is the most common cause of cellular injury. Hypoxia deprives the cell of oxygen and interferes with energy (ATP) production. Ischemia, which is a reduced blood supply, is the most common cause of hypoxia. Death of tissue due to ischemia is called an infarct.

▶ Disease or injury affecting the respiratory or cardiovascular systems can affect the delivery of oxygen and nutrients to the cell and the removal of waste products from the cell, thus disrupting homeostasis. Your patient must have an open airway in order for these essential processes to occur. In addition, adequate oxygenation requires that sufficient oxygen must be present in the surrounding air. Adequate movement of gases into and out of the lungs (ventilation) is dependent on an open airway and an adequate rate and depth of movement of the thoracic cage by the respiratory muscles. Perfusion is the circulation of blood through an organ or a part of the body. A balance between ventilation and perfusion must exist to ensure adequate gas exchange.

▶ Perfusion depends on cardiac output, peripheral vascular resistance, and the transport of oxygen. Cardiac output is the amount of blood the heart pumps each minute. Cardiac output is determined by multiplying stroke volume by heart rate. Stroke volume is the amount of blood ejected by the ventricles of the heart with each contraction.

► The amount of blood returning to the ventricles is called venous return. In a healthy heart, an increase in the volume of blood in the ventricles causes the fibers in the heart muscle to stretch, resulting in a more forceful contraction. This principle is called the Frank-Starling law of the heart. Hemorrhage (also called major bleeding), an extreme loss of blood from a blood vessel, is one cause of decreased venous return.

► Peripheral vascular resistance (also called systemic vascular resistance) is the opposition that blood encounters in the blood vessels as it travels away from the heart. The smallest arteries, arterioles, are made up of smooth muscle. They provide the greatest resistance to blood flow through the arterial circulation because the lumen of an arteriole is narrower than that of medium and large arteries. Narrowing of a vessel (vasoconstriction) increases peripheral resistance. Widening of a vessel (vasodilation) decreases peripheral resistance.

► Blood pressure is the force exerted by the blood on the inner walls of the heart and arteries. It is affected by cardiac output (heart) and peripheral vascular resistance (blood vessels).

► Shock is the inadequate circulation of blood through an organ or a part of the body. Shock is also called hypoperfusion. Because the presence of shock affects the body's ability to oxygenate and perfuse cells, shock can lead to death if it is not corrected.

► Conditions that may increase a person's chance of developing a disease are called risk factors or predisposing factors. Examples of risk factors include age, gender, lifestyle, environment, and heredity.

► Pathogenesis refers to the mechanism by which a disease develops. The etiology (cause) of many diseases is known. The phrase "unknown etiology" or "idiopathic" is used when the cause of a disease is unknown.

► Some diseases develop in stages. The incubation period is the interval between the exposure to a disease-causing agent and the appearance of signs and symptoms. A sign is a medical or trauma condition of the patient that can be seen, heard, smelled, measured, or felt by the examiner. A symptom is a condition described by the patient. Symptoms are subjective findings because they are dependent on (subject to) the patient's interpretation and description of the complaint. A syndrome is a group of signs and symptoms that together are characteristic of a specific disease or disorder.

Life Span Development

By the end of this chapter, you should be able to:

Knowledge Objectives ▶

1. Discuss the physiologic, cognitive, and psychosocial characteristics of an infant.
2. Discuss the physiologic, cognitive, and psychosocial characteristics of a toddler.
3. Discuss the physiologic, cognitive, and psychosocial characteristics of a preschool child.
4. Discuss the physiologic, cognitive, and psychosocial characteristics of a school-age child.
5. Discuss the physiologic, cognitive, and psychosocial characteristics of an adolescent.
6. Discuss the physiologic, cognitive, and psychosocial characteristics of an early adult.
7. Discuss the physiologic, cognitive, and psychosocial characteristics of a middle-aged adult.
8. Discuss the physiologic, cognitive, and psychosocial characteristics of an older adult.

Attitude Objective ▶

9. Value the uniqueness of infant, toddler, preschool, school-age, adolescent, early adulthood, middle-aged, and late adulthood physiologic, cognitive, and psychosocial characteristics.

Skill Objectives ▶

There are no skill objectives identified for this lesson.

On the Scene

You and your EMT partner are called to a local daycare facility for an ill child. As you enter the building, you are approached by a woman who asks you to "take a look at one of the children." She directs you to one of the rooms that are set aside for the 3- to 5-year-old children. Upon entering, you see a child seated on the edge of a chair in the corner of the room. She looks to be about 3 years old. You immediately notice that the muscles in her neck stand out with each attempt to breathe. As you approach the child, she turns her head toward you. You try to count her breaths, and she appears to be breathing about 40 times per minute. Her skin is pale. ■

Introduction

Life Span Development

Life span refers to the period during which something is functional. For example, the life span of a battery means the amount of time the battery will last. In humans, life span is the period from birth to death. Human development is the process of growing to maturity. The stages of human development discussed in this chapter are listed in the *You Should Know* box below.

Each stage of human development is accompanied by physiologic, cognitive, and psychosocial milestones. Physiologic milestones pertain to growth, body system changes, and changes in vital signs. Vital signs are measurements of breathing, pulse, skin temperature, pupils, and blood pressure. Cognitive milestones pertain to mental processes such as reasoning, imagining, and problem solving. Psychosocial milestones pertain to personality, emotions, social interactions and expectations. By knowing the milestones for each stage of development, you will be able to recognize what is typical and what is unusual as you begin patient care.

You Should Know

Stages of Human Development

Infancy	birth to 12 months
Toddler	12 to 36 months
Preschooler	3 to 5 years
School-age	6 to 12 years
Adolescence	13 to 19 years
Early adulthood	20 to 40 years
Middle adulthood	41 to 60 years
Late adulthood	61 years and older

Infants

Physiologic Changes

Objective 1

A North American infant usually weighs about 7 pounds (3.2 kilograms) at birth, doubles the birth weight by 3 to 4 months of age, and triples it by the end of the first year. An infant is usually about 19 to 20 inches long (48 to 51 centimeters) at birth, reaching about 29 to 30 inches (74 to 76 centimeters) at 12 months. Infants will usually sleep 16 to 18 hours per day with sleep and wakefulness evenly distributed over a 24-hour period (Figure 8-1). Sleep requirements gradually decrease to 14 to 16 hours per day, with 9 to 10 hours of sleep time occurring at night. Most infants sleep through the night at 2 to 4 months. An infant is usually easily arousable from sleep. The inability to arouse a baby should be considered an emergency.

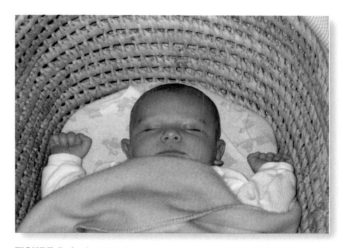

FIGURE 8-1 ▲ Infants will usually sleep 16–18 hours per day.

The head and trunk of an infant and young child are large in proportion to the rest of the body, giving the child a "top heavy" appearance. The chest circumference of an infant is usually less than the head circumference. By about 9 or 10 months, the circumference of the head and that of the chest are about the same. After 1 year of age, the chest circumference is larger. Growth of the hips, legs, and feet catches up in later childhood.

At birth, the heads of many newborns are misshapen because of the molding of the head that occurs during vaginal deliveries. Molding is possible because of small diamond-shaped openings called fontanels (soft spots) that are present on both the top and back of the head. **Fontanels** are "gaps" in the bones of the head of an infant that allow flexibility during delivery and growth of the brain. These areas will not completely close until about 6 months of age for the rear fontanel and 18 months for the top one.

Newborns possess a number of reflexes, which are involuntary responses to a stimulus. Touching a baby's cheek stimulates a feeding reflex called the *rooting reflex*, which causes the baby to turn its mouth toward the side that was touched and start to suck. This reflex usually disappears after 4 months. The sucking reflex, another feeding reflex, causes a newborn to suck when its lips are touched (such as with a nipple, fingers, or toes). This reflex is present throughout infancy. If the newborn's hearing is intact, the baby will react with a startle to a loud noise (the Moro reflex). In contrast, the rhythmic, soothing sound of a lullaby or heartbeat will put an infant to sleep. The palmar grasp reflex, which disappears after 3 months, occurs when a small object is placed against the palm of the newborn's hand, causing the fingers to curl around it.

At birth, the most developed of the senses is hearing and the least developed is sight. Within days, an infant will recognize the sound of the mother's voice and turn toward it. Newborns are able to smell, and some quickly recognize the smell and handling of their caregiver. They are also sensitive to pain and extremes of temperature. Most newborns respond positively when touched, held, and cuddled. An infant's response to pain is similar to that of an older child.

The heart rate of the newly born is usually between 100 and 160 beats per minute during the first 30 minutes of life, and then slows to about 120 beats per minute. In the first year of life, an infant's heart rate is usually between 80 and 140 beats per minute (Figure 8-2). The respiratory rate of the newly born is usually between 40 and 60 breaths per minute, dropping to about 30 to 40 breaths per minute after the first few minutes of life, and slowing to 20 to 30 breaths per minute by 1 year.

The respiratory anatomy of infants and young children differs from that of older children and adults. In general, all structures are smaller. Because they are smaller, they are more easily blocked than is

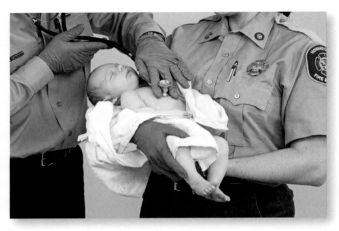

FIGURE 8-2 ▲ An infant's heart rate is usually between 80 and 140 beats per minute.

the case in adults. The nasal passages are soft and narrow and have little supporting cartilage. It is important to keep the nasal passages clear in infants under 6 months of age because they breathe mostly through their noses, not their mouths. If the nasal passages are blocked as a result of tissue swelling or a buildup of mucus, difficulty in breathing and problems with feeding can result.

The tongue takes up proportionally more space in the mouth of a child than in that of an adult. The tracheal rings are softer and more flexible in infants and children. This puts the airway at risk of compression if the neck is not positioned properly.

The chest wall of infants and young children is softer and more elastic than that of older children and adults. This is because it is made of more cartilage than bone. Children also have fewer and smaller alveoli. Thus, the potential area for exchanging oxygen and carbon dioxide is smaller. Because the chest wall is soft and flexible, rib and sternum fractures are less common in children than in adults. However, the force of the injury is more easily transmitted to the delicate tissues of the underlying lung. This results in bruising of the lung and bleeding in the alveoli, which reduces the number of alveoli available for gas exchange. This type of injury is potentially life-threatening.

Infants and young children depend more heavily on the diaphragm for breathing than do adults. Air can build up in the stomach during rescue breathing or improperly performed CPR. As a result, the stomach swells with air, movement of the diaphragm is limited, and effective breathing is reduced.

You Should Know

The main cause of cardiac arrest in infants and children is an uncorrected respiratory problem.

TABLE 8-1 Motor and Social Development in Infants

Age	Motor and Social Development	Age	Motor and Social Development
Newly born	Can follow large moving objects Blinks in response to bright light and sound	7 months	Is fearful of strangers Imitates simple acts and sounds Quickly changes from crying to laughing
2 months	Recognizes familiar faces May be soothed by rocking Has control of eye muscles Lifts head when on stomach	8 months	Sits alone without support Responds to "no" Feeds self with fingers Plays peek-a-boo Cries when scolded
3 months	Coos and babbles; laughs aloud Moves objects to mouth with hands Shows primary emotions with distinct facial expressions	9 months	Responds to adult anger Waves "bye-bye" Can pull up to a standing position Grasps rattle and can transfer it from hand to hand Explores objects by mouthing, sucking, chewing, and biting
4 months	Drools without swallowing Sits with support Rolls over Grasps objects with both hands Reaches out to people	10 months	Is responsive to own name Looks under an object for toy Crawls well Pulls self to sitting position
5 months	Sleeps throughout the night without food Grasps object and moves it to mouth Can tell the difference between family and strangers	11 months	Attempts to walk without assistance Reacts with frustration to restrictions
6 months	Sits upright in a highchair Grasps dangling objects Makes one-syllable sounds such as "ba" and "da"	12 months	Walks with some assistance Knows own name Can put objects into a container Helps dress self

An infant's nervous system undergoes significant growth during the first year of life. Neurons (nerve cells) grow and form increasingly dense connections, enabling faster and more efficient message transmission. As the nervous system develops, motor skills progress from simple reflexes to increasingly complex activities such as grasping, reaching, crawling, standing, and walking.

Teething begins at about 6 months of age, with eruption of the lower central incisors occurring between 6 and 8 months of age. By 12 months, an infant typically has 6 to 8 teeth.

Infants and young children are susceptible to changes in temperature. Children have a large body surface area (BSA) compared with their weight. The larger the BSA that is exposed, the greater the area of heat loss.

An infant's skin is thin with few fat deposits under it. This condition contributes to an infant's sensitivity to extremes of heat and cold. Infants also have poorly developed temperature-regulating mechanisms. For example, newborns are unable to shiver in cold temperatures, and their sweating mechanism is immature in warm temperatures. Because infants and children are at risk of **hypothermia** and **hyperthermia,** it is very important to keep their temperature regulated.

Typical motor and social development of infants is shown in Table 8-1.

Cognitive Changes

Infants 2 to 6 months of age are increasingly aware of their surroundings and begin to explore their bodies. By 6 months, an infant should make eye contact. Lack of eye contact in an infant could be a sign of significant illness or depressed mental status. Between 6 and 12 months of age, an infant begins looking for things not in sight, such as a toy hidden under a pillow. Infants begin babbling at about 6 months of age. By 12 months many infants speak their first understandable words.

Psychosocial Changes

Crying is an infant's method of communication. In fact, newborns spend about 1 to 4 hours each day crying. Babies cry for many reasons such as having a wet or soiled diaper, or being hungry, tired, bored, lonely, hot or cold, or in pain. Crying may be preceded by signals such as anxious facial expressions, flailing arms, and excited breathing. Parents and researchers have identified three unique types of cries: the basic cry, the angry cry, and the pain cry. The basic cry begins softly and gradually increases in intensity, usually signaling that the infant is hungry or tired. The angry cry is more intense than the basic cry. The pain cry begins suddenly with a long burst of crying, followed by a long pause and gasping. When obvious reasons for crying have been addressed, persistent crying can be a sign of illness.

Implications for the Healthcare Professional

Infants are completely dependent on others for their needs (Figure 8-3). Young infants (birth to 6 months of age) are unafraid of strangers and have no modesty. Older infants (6 months to 1 year of age) do not like to be separated from their caregiver (separation anxiety). They may be threatened by direct eye contact with strangers.

When providing care for an infant, watch the baby from a distance before making contact (see Chapters 15 and 17). If possible, assess the baby on the caregiver's lap. Avoid loud noises; bright lights; and quick, jerky movements. Smile and use a calm, soothing voice. Allow the baby to suck on a pacifier for comfort, if appropriate. Be sure to handle an infant gently but firmly, always supporting the head and neck if the baby is not on a solid surface.

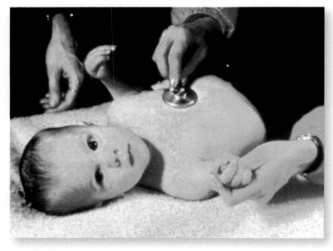

FIGURE 8-3 ▲ Infants are completely dependent on others for their needs.

An infant must be kept warm and covered as much as possible, particularly the head. The head has the largest BSA in infants and young children. Heat loss from this area significantly cools the rest of the body. Make sure your hands and stethoscope are warmed before touching an infant.

Stop and Think!

An increased risk of a foreign body airway obstruction begins at about 6 months of age, when a child is able to grasp objects. Be careful not to leave small objects within an infant's reach.

You Should Know

Shaken baby syndrome is a severe form of head injury. It occurs when an infant or child is shaken by the arms, legs, or shoulders with enough force to cause the baby's brain to bounce against the skull. This shaking can cause bruising, swelling, and bleeding of the brain. It can lead to severe brain damage or death.

Just 2 to 3 seconds of shaking can cause bleeding in and around the brain. *Never shake or jiggle an infant or child.*

Toddlers

Objective 2

Physiologic Changes

A typical toddler looks chubby with relatively short legs and a large head. A typical 2-year-old measures between 32 and 36 inches (81 to 91 centimeters), which is about half of the adult height. A toddler's heart rate is usually between 80 and 130 beats per minute, and the respiratory rate is about 20 to 30 breaths per minute.

A toddler's body systems continue to grow and are relatively mature by the end of the toddler years. The terminal airways of the respiratory system continue to branch, and the alveoli increase in number. In the musculoskeletal system, muscle mass and the bone thickness increase. Continued development of the nervous system allows effortless walking and other basic motor skills. Gross and fine motor skills are developing, such as throwing a ball and scribbling. A toddler can eat most food without help and drink from a cup. By age 3, a toddler can walk, run, climb, jump, and ride

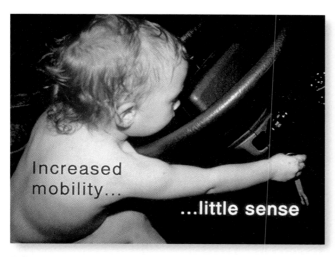

FIGURE 8-4 ▲ Toddlers are always on the move. As a result, they are prone to injury.

a tricycle. The brain has achieved 80% to 90% of its ultimate weight at 3 years of age.

A toddler is always on the move. As a result, toddlers are prone to injury (Figure 8-4). Remember that infants and toddlers are "top-heavy"; the head is larger and heavier relative to the rest of the body. The skull of an infant or a child is thin and flexible. When an infant or a child suffers trauma to the head, force is more likely to be transferred to the brain instead of fracturing the skull. In infants and young children, the ligaments of the neck are underdeveloped, and the muscles of the neck are relatively weak. In addition, young children have less muscle mass and more fat and cartilage than older children.

Injuries to the spinal cord and spinal column are uncommon in infants and young children. When they do occur, children younger than 8 years of age tend to sustain injury to the uppermost area of the cervical spine.

A toddler is more susceptible to minor respiratory and gastrointestinal infections because the immunity that he had from his mother is lost. At this stage, immunity to common pathogens develops as exposure occurs. Many toddlers (and preschoolers) develop colds and minor infections because of their exposure to pathogens in group settings, such as daycare.

The digestive system continues to develop, and the stomach's capacity increases, allowing for the typical schedule of three meals per day. A toddler may not be able to grind up food before swallowing due to a lack of molars, thus increasing the risk of choking on food. An important development in the digestive and urinary systems is the voluntary control of elimination. A child is physiologically capable of toilet training by 12 to 15 months and psychologically ready between 18 and 30 months. The average age for completion is about 28 months.

Cognitive Changes

At 12 to 18 months, a toddler imitates older children and parents, knows major body parts, and knows four to six words. By 18 to 24 months, the child begins to understand cause and effect, can identify objects, and can talk in short sentences. By 24 months, a toddler knows about 100 words.

Psychosocial Changes

A toddler responds appropriately to an angry or friendly voice. When separated from their primary caregivers, most toddlers experience strong separation anxiety. Toddlers are easily frustrated and may have temper tantrums in an attempt to control others. Persistent crying or irritability can be a symptom of serious illness.

A toddler can answer simple questions and follow simple directions. However, you cannot reason with a toddler. Toddlers are likely to be more cooperative if given a comfort object like a blanket, stuffed animal, or toy. They are afraid of being left alone, of monsters, of interruptions in their usual routine, and of getting hurt (such as a fall or cut).

Implications for the Healthcare Professional

Toddlers understand "soon," "bye-bye, "all gone," and "uh-oh." A toddler's favorite words are "no" and "mine," so avoid asking questions that can be answered with a yes or no. If you ask questions that begin with "May I," "Can I," or "Would you like to," a toddler will probably say no. If you then do whatever you asked anyway, you will immediately lose the toddler's trust and cooperation. You are more likely to have cooperation if you state clearly what you are going to do in simple terms, rather than asking for permission from the child (see Chapter 15).

Toddlers view illness and injury as punishment. They are distrustful of strangers. Toddlers are likely to resist examination and treatment. When touched, they may scream, cry, or kick. Toddlers do not like having their clothing removed and do not like anything on their face.

Encourage the child's trust by gaining the cooperation of the caregiver. When the child sees you talking with the caregiver first and understands that the adult is not threatened, the child may be more at ease. When possible, allow the child to remain on the caregiver's lap. If this is not possible, try to keep the caregiver within the child's line of vision. Approach the child slowly and address her by name. Talk to her at eye level, using simple words and short phrases. Speak to her in a calm, reassuring tone of voice.

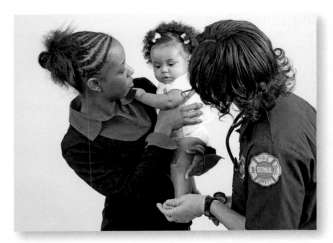

FIGURE 8-5 ▲ Talk to toddlers at eye level and use a calm reassuring voice.

Although the child may not understand your words, she will respond to your tone. Try a game such as counting toes or fingers to enlist the child's cooperation (Figure 8-5).

Assess the child's head last. Start with either her trunk or feet and move upward. Respect the child's modesty by keeping her covered. When it is time to remove an item of clothing, ask the child's caregiver to do so, if possible. Replace clothing promptly after assessing each body area. Be sure to praise the child for cooperative behavior.

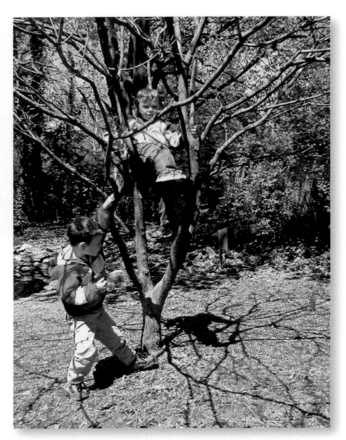

FIGURE 8-6 ▲ Preschoolers can climb, hop, swing, and run and may be able to skip.

Remember This

Do not tell children that they cannot cry or they need to be strong. Instead, reassure the child that it is okay to cry, be angry or frightened, and express emotion. However, you can remind the child that hitting, kicking, or biting is not allowed.

Preschoolers

Objective 3

Physiologic Changes

A preschooler appears taller and thinner than a toddler, and this may be mistaken for weight loss by the child's caregiver. The heart rate of a preschooler is usually between 80 and 120 beats per minute, and the respiratory rate about 20 to 30 breaths per minute. A preschooler can stand on one foot for 10 seconds or longer; can hop, swing, and climb; and may be able to skip (Figure 8-6). Preschoolers begin to skate and swim by age 5. Most preschoolers can dress themselves and brush their own teeth. By this age, left- or right-handedness has been established.

Cognitive Changes

Preschoolers have a better understanding of the concept of time and can count 10 or more objects. Their attention span increases, and they have a vocabulary of about 1,500 words. Sentences now consist of six to eight words. Preschoolers can correctly name at least four colors and can say their name and address. They understand a three-part request such as, "Find your teddy bear," "Pick it up," and "Bring it to me." Their speech is clearly understood by strangers.

Psychosocial Changes

A child of preschool age likes to sing, dance, and act and wants to be like her friends. Preschoolers are certain that they know everything and may be rude when you ask them to do something they do not want to do. Preschoolers are able to play more independently and may be able to spend more time apart from their caregivers without becoming too upset. Preschoolers explore their bodies and find playing "doctor" an interesting activity.

Implications for the Healthcare Professional

Preschoolers are afraid of the unknown, the dark, being left alone, and adults who look or act mean. They may think their illness or injury is punishment for bad behavior or thoughts (Figure 8-7). Approach the child slowly and talk to him at eye level. Use simple words and phrases and a reassuring tone of voice. Assure the child that he was not bad and is not being punished.

A preschooler may feel vulnerable and out of control when lying down. Assess and treat the child in an upright position when possible. Preschoolers are modest. They do not like being touched or having their clothing removed. When assessing a child, keep in mind that she has probably been told not to let a stranger touch her. Remove clothing, assess the child, and then quickly replace clothing. Allow the caregiver to remain with the child whenever possible.

Preschoolers are curious and like to "help." Encourage the child to participate. Tell the child how things will feel and what is to be done just before doing it. For example, a preschooler may fear being suffocated by an oxygen mask. It may be helpful to use a doll or a stuffed animal to explain the procedure. The child may want to hold or look at the equipment first (Figure 8-8). Avoid procedures on the child's dominant hand or arm.

Preschoolers are highly imaginative. When talking with a preschooler, choose your words carefully. Avoid baby talk and frightening or misleading terms. For example, avoid words such as "take," "cut," "shot," "deaden," or "germs." Instead of saying, "I'm going to take your pulse," you might say, "I'm going to see how fast your heart is beating." Instead of saying, "I'm going to take your blood pressure," you might say, "I'm going to hug your arm" or "I'm going to see how strong your muscles are." Because preschoolers are afraid of blood, dress and bandage wounds right away.

Depending on the child's age, you may find that distracting the child is helpful. Remember that children are self-centered—they imagine that the world revolves around them. Paying attention to their world and needs will improve your ability to assess and care for your pediatric patients.

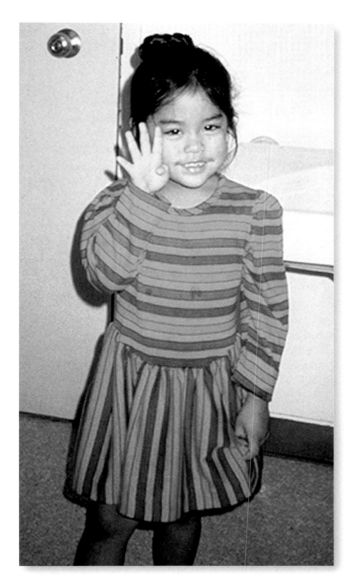

FIGURE 8-7 ▲ Preschoolers are highly imaginative and may think their illness or injury is punishment for bad behavior or thoughts.

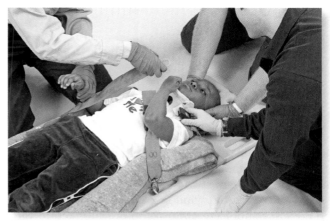

FIGURE 8-8 ▲ Calling the straps "seat belts" helped this preschooler feel more comfortable.

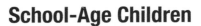
Distractions

- Ask a child about favorite foods, games, cartoon characters, movies, or computer games.
- Ask the child to visually locate an item in the area.
- Ask the child to sing a song or tell you about school.
- Use a flashlight as a distraction or a stuffed animal as a distraction or comfort item.

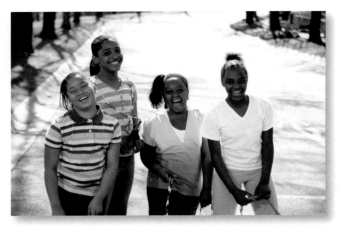

FIGURE 8-9 ▲ School-age children form friendship groups based on gender, interests, and the same race or ethnic group.

School-Age Children

Objective 4

Physiologic Changes

The heart rate of a school-age child is usually 70 to 110 beats per minute, the respiratory rate is 20 to 30 breaths per minute, and the systolic blood pressure is 80 to 120 mm Hg. Growth in height and weight continues to occur in the school-age child, but at a slower pace as compared with earlier years. Growth spurts, occurring in girls at age 10 and in boys at age 12, begins before the onset of puberty.

Function increases in both hemispheres of the brain. The school-age child can run, ride a bicycle, climb, jump, hop, and skip. Fine motor skills continue to develop such as writing, drawing, working on puzzles, typing, playing the piano, and building model cars. During the school-age years, the baby teeth are lost and permanent teeth come in, giving an appearance of teeth that are too large for the child's face.

Cognitive Changes

The school-age child thinks logically and is able to see things from another's point of view. An important skill, the ability to read, is acquired.

Psychosocial Changes

School, school-related activities, popularity, and peer groups are important to school-age children. Friendships are most common between children of the same age, gender, interests, and race or ethnic group (Figure 8-9). The school-age child has more interaction with adults and other children, begins comparing himself

with others, develops self-esteem, and takes pride in learning new skills. At age 6 and 7, the child prefers playing with others of the same gender. By age 8 and 9, the child is interested in relationships with the opposite gender but will not admit it. Around age 10 to 12, the child begins developing relationships with the opposite gender.

Body image is also important to the school-age child. Children with a chronic illness or disability are very self-conscious. Physical differences, such as having a bumpy nose, needing glasses, being overweight, or wearing a hearing aid often result in taunts from other children, and can have lasting effects.

The school-age child begins to understand that death is permanent and that it eventually happens to everyone. However, the child may feel responsible and guilty for a loved one's death. Help the child understand that he or she did not cause the death. Phrases such as, "Grandma is only sleeping," should be avoided because they may be taken literally, causing confusion. A child's grief reaction to death varies and may include denial, anger, the hope that the deceased will return, physical ailments, and problems at school.

Implications for the Healthcare Professional

School-age children are less dependent on their caregivers than are younger children. They are usually cooperative (Figure 8-10). They fear pain, permanent injury, and disfigurement. They are also afraid of blood and prolonged separation from their caregivers. A school-age child is very modest and does not like his body exposed to strangers. A child of this age may still view

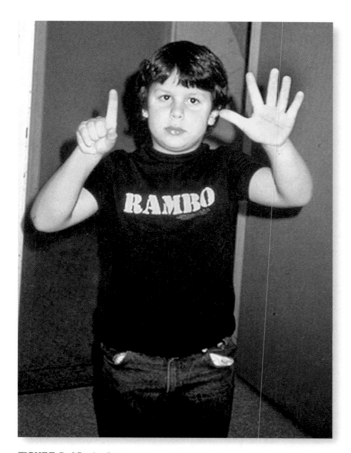

FIGURE 8-10 ▲ School-age children are usually cooperative.

illness or injury as punishment. Reassure the child that what is happening is not related to being punished.

When caring for a school-age child, approach her in a friendly manner and introduce yourself. Talk directly to the child about what happened, even if you also obtain a history from the caregiver. Explain procedures before carrying them out. Because school-age children often view things in concrete terms, choose your words carefully. For example, the phrase "I am going to take your pulse" will concern a school-age child. She will wonder why you are taking it away and when she will get it back. Allow the child to see and touch equipment that may be used in her care.

Honesty is very important when interacting with school-age children. If you are going to do something to the child that may cause pain, warn the child just before you do it. Give a simple explanation, just before the procedure, of what will take place so that the child does not have long to think about it. For example, if a child has a possible broken leg and you must move the leg to apply a splint, warn the child just before you move the leg. Do not threaten an uncooperative child.

Adolescents

Objective 5

Physiologic Changes

During adolescence, the size and strength of the heart increases, blood volume increases, systolic blood pressure increases, and heart rate decreases. An adolescent's heart rate is usually 55 to 105 beats per minute, respiratory rate is 12 to 20 breaths per minute, and systolic blood pressure is 100 to 120 mm Hg. Muscle size and strength increase, and bone growth is nearly complete. Most adolescents experience a rapid 2- to 3-year growth spurt that begins distally with enlargement of the feet and hands, followed by enlargement of the arms and legs. Enlargement of the chest and trunk occurs in the final stage. Physical maturity occurs at different times beginning at age 10 and ending about age 16 in girls and beginning at age 12 and ending about age 18 in boys.

Primary and secondary sexual development occurs during adolescence. Primary sexual development refers to changes in the internal and external organs responsible for reproduction, such as the ovaries, uterus, breasts, and penis. Secondary sexual development refers to body changes that are the result of hormonal change, such as voice changes and the development of facial and genital hair.

Menarche is the onset of menstruation during puberty. In the United States the average age of menarche is 12.5 years. **Menstruation,** which is the periodic discharge of blood and tissue from the uterus, occurs about every 28 days. Each occurrence of menstruation is called a period. The onset of menarche and subsequent sexual activity increase the risk of teen pregnancy and sexually transmitted disease (STD).

Cognitive Changes

Adolescents have the ability to reason and think beyond the present. They are concerned about the opinions of others. Adolescents develop morals, questioning adults who say one thing but do another.

Psychosocial Changes

An adolescent wants to be treated like an adult, yet conflicts between an adolescent and his or her parents are common. While the adolescent is developing an identity, the parent wants to protect the teen from harm or something the teen may later regret.

During adolescence, self-consciousness increases, peer pressure increases, and interest in the opposite sex increases. Antisocial behavior peaks around eighth or ninth grade. Hormone surges cause wide mood swings.

Peer groups are important to an adolescent, and school is typically the focus of social life. Body image is of great concern at this age. Adolescents continuously compare themselves with their peers and determine if they are "normal" on the basis of what they observe. Some adolescents do not adjust well to the demands and responsibilities of adolescence. For example, although many adolescent girls accept menstruation and changes in their bodies as a matter of course, others are distressed and frightened. Teens often experience an increase in weight and fat distribution during their growth spurt. Eating disorders are common because the adolescent desires the "perfect" body, or at least a slimmer one. Some teens respond to the stressors of adolescent life in unhealthy ways, such as experimentation with tobacco, alcohol, and illicit drugs. Depression and suicide are more common in adolescents than any other age group.

Between 15 and 17 years of age, the teen cautiously establishes relationships. An adolescent usually knows by this time if he or she is homosexual or heterosexual. Around the age of 18, adolescents begin to understand who they are and start to feel comfortable with that. An attachment to another person develops and stable relationships form.

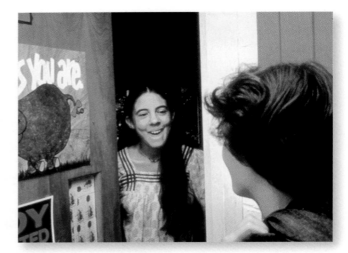

FIGURE 8-11 ▲ Adolescents expect to be treated as adults.

You Should Know

Adolescence is a time of hormonal surges, emotions, and peer pressure with an increased risk for substance abuse, self-endangerment, pregnancy, and dangerous sexual practices.

Implications for the Healthcare Professional

Adolescents often show inconsistent and unpredictable behavior, although they expect to be treated as adults (Figure 8-11). Talk to an adolescent in a respectful, friendly manner, as if speaking to an adult. If possible, obtain a history from the patient instead of a caregiver. Expect an adolescent to have many questions and to want detailed explanations about what you are planning to do or what is happening to her. Explain things clearly and honestly. Be honest about procedures that will cause discomfort. Allow time for questions. Give the patient choices when appropriate, but do not bargain with an

adolescent in order to do what you need to do. Recognize the tendency for adolescents to overreact. Do not become angry with an emotional or hysterical adolescent.

Adolescents fear pain, permanent damage to their bodies that results in a change in appearance or scarring, and death. They may go back and forth between being very modest and openly displaying their bodies. Respect the patient's modesty and cover him after the physical examination is complete. Address concerns and fears about the lasting effects of any injuries (especially cosmetic), and, if appropriate, provide reassurance. Try to have an adult of the same gender as the child present while you examine the patient. Allow the caregiver to be present during your assessment if the patient wishes. However, some adolescents may prefer to be assessed privately, away from their caregivers.

Peers are a major influence in the life of an adolescent. When you are providing care, an adolescent may prefer to have a peer close by for reassurance. When caring for an adolescent, do not tease or embarrass her—particularly in front of peers.

Early Adulthood

Objective 6

Physiologic Changes

Peak physical conditioning occurs between 19 and 26 years of age, and adults develop lifelong habits and routines during this time. All body systems function at optimal performance. The heart rate of an early adult averages 70 beats per minute, the respiratory rate averages 16 to 20 breaths per minute, and the blood pressure averages 120/80 mm Hg. Doctor visits during early adulthood are usually related to pregnancy or injuries. Accidents are a leading cause of death in this age group.

You Should Know

Early adulthood is considered the prime of life in terms of peak physical condition.

Cognitive Changes

The thought process of adolescents is closely related to logic. As a result, they often feel that the only solution (or solutions) to a problem is a logical one. Young adults recognize that, in some situations, there is no single correct solution. In fact, the solution may vary from situation to situation. This type of thought process is practical, flexible, and involves emotion and logic.

Psychosocial Changes

During early adulthood, individuals typically become independent of their parents, complete their education, and establish a career. High levels of job stress are experienced during this time. The young adult usually establishes an intimate relationship with a significant other and decides whether to have children. Childbirth occurs more often in this age group than in any other. A new family provides the young adult with new challenges and stress.

Friendships are important, particularly if a young adult is single. Friendships between men typically involve outdoor activities and talk about work, sports, politics, and cars (Figure 8-12). In contrast, friendships between women usually involve conversations about their personal weaknesses, secrets about their past, personal health issues, or problems with their significant other or family.

Young adults demonstrate reckless behavior (such as driving at a high rate of speed) less often than adolescents do. Young adults are more likely to abuse alcohol and use illicit drugs and have more serious emotional difficulties (such as major depression and rage) than older adults. Eating disorders are more common in this age group than at other ages.

Implications for the Healthcare Professional

Talk to a young adult in a respectful, friendly manner. Obtain a history from the patient. Explain what you are planning to do and why it needs to be done. Allow time for questions. Provide clear and honest explanations.

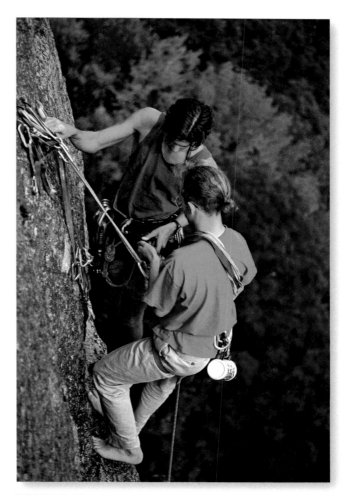

FIGURE 8-12 ▲ Friendships between young adult men often involve outdoor activities.

Middle Adulthood

Objective 7

Physiologic Changes

The heart rate of a middle adult averages 70 beats per minute, the respiratory rate averages 16 to 20 breaths per minute, and the blood pressure averages 120/80 mm Hg. In an adult's early 40s, his body is still functioning as effectively as it did in his 20s.

However, as the years go by, many physical changes take place. Near vision declines by the late 40s. Taste sensations diminish, and the ability to hear high-frequency sounds decreases, particularly in men. Metabolism slows, making weight control more difficult. Cardiovascular health becomes a concern as blood vessels lose elasticity and become thicker. Cholesterol levels increase and cardiac output decreases throughout this period. Hormonal changes occur in both women and men. In women, **menopause** (cessation of menstruation) occurs in the late 40s or early 50s. In men, testosterone levels gradually decline and sperm production decreases. The hair begins to thin and turn gray. The skin's elasticity and moisture decrease and wrinkling occurs. Cancer often strikes in this age group.

Cognitive Changes

The middle adult's memory, perception, learning, problem solving, and creativity change very little. Reaction time may diminish toward the later part of middle adulthood. In the workplace, the middle adults' experience and expertise allows them to surpass younger workers in their problem-solving abilities.

Psychosocial Changes

Middle adults approach problems more as challenges than threats. They are typically in the center of the family, between aging parents, adult children, and grandchildren. Some may be burdened by financial commitments for them.

Middle adults may experience empty nest syndrome, which is a feeling of sadness and loneliness when one or more of their children leaves home. However, after the children have left home, most middle adult couples find that their relationship strengthens as they have more time for each other and can pursue mutual interests and activities. It has been estimated that about half the young adults in the United States return to their parents' home at least once after moving out.

Implications for the Healthcare Professional

Talk to the patient in a respectful, friendly manner. Obtain a history from the patient, listening carefully to the patient's answers to your questions. Explain what you are planning to do and why it needs to be done. Allow time for the patient to ask you questions. Provide clear and honest explanations.

Late Adulthood

Objective 8

Physiologic Changes

Maximum life expectancy is the oldest age to which any person lives. At present, maximum life expectancy for humans is about 120 years. Average life expectancy is the age at which half the people born in a particular year will die. A baby born in 2004 in the United States would have an average life expectancy of 77.9 years (Figure 8-13).

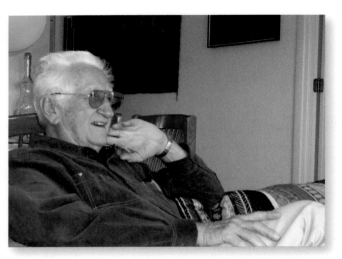

FIGURE 8-13 ▲ At 81 years of age, this man still lives in his own home, travels, gardens, cooks, and cleans.

An older adult's heart rate, respiratory rate, and blood pressure depend on the person's physical health. Cardiovascular system changes associated with aging include thickening of the blood vessels, decreased vessel elasticity, and increased peripheral vascular resistance, all of which contribute to reduced blood flow to organs. There is often a marked increase in the systolic blood pressure and a slight increase in the diastolic blood pressure because of increased peripheral vascular resistance. The heart's valves become hard and thick, affecting the heart's ability to adequately fill and empty. Normally, heart rate (and cardiac output) increases with exercise. In older adults, the heart is less responsive to exercise. When a rapid heart rate occurs, it is not well tolerated and is slow to return to normal.

Changes in the respiratory system include diminished elasticity of the diaphragm and weakening of the chest wall muscles. Coughing is often ineffective because of weakened expiratory muscles. Damage or loss of the elastic fibers in the small airways and thickening of the alveoli result in a decreased number of alveoli that participate in gas exchange. The activity of the cilia in the lungs is decreased, and this results in an increased collection of mucous in the respiratory tract and an increased susceptibility to infection.

Sensory changes that occur in older adults include a loss of taste buds, loss of hearing, and a diminished sense of smell, vision, perception of pain, and reaction time.

Older adults have less subcutaneous tissue, inefficient blood vessel constriction, diminished shivering and sweating, diminished perception of temperature, and diminished thirst perception. These factors increase an older adult's likelihood of experiencing a heat- or cold-related emergency.

Older adults experience a loss of muscle strength and a decrease in the number of muscle cells. Regular exercise can help slow this process. Older adults also experience a loss of bone mass. Bone loss is greater in women, particularly after the onset of menopause. Falls are common in older adults. They occur because of vision and/or balance problems, physical weakness, environmental hazards (such as poor lighting and throw rugs), urinary problems, and the effects of taking multiple medications.

In the urinary system of some older adults, blood flow to the kidneys is reduced because of thickening of the blood vessels and subsequent narrowing of the renal arteries. The amount of urine the bladder holds decreases with age and the need to urinate becomes more frequent. As a result, older adults often arise during the night to urinate.

Many changes occur in the older adult's gastrointestinal (GI) system. Some older adults have no teeth and depend on dentures. Many have dentures but do not wear them. Others cannot afford to purchase them. The amount of saliva normally present in the mouth declines with age. Loss of smooth muscle in the stomach causes a delayed emptying time. GI secretions are decreased. Liver blood flow is decreased, resulting in less efficient breakdown of protein. A decrease in pancreatic secretions results in less efficient breakdown of fats. Impaired absorption of B vitamins, calcium, and iron can cause vitamin and mineral deficiencies.

In the nervous system, there is a loss of nerve cells, which can result in memory impairment. Older adults are able to learn new material, but they may have difficulty retrieving information. Balance and coordination are decreased. Sleep disorders are common in older adults. Most older adults feel drowsy more often in the daytime, take more naps, take longer to fall asleep, spend less time in deep sleep, and wake up more often.

Cognitive Changes

Some cognitive abilities decline with aging, while others remain stable or improve. Short-term memory, which is what a person has in mind at a given moment (such as remembering a phone number long enough to dial it), is relatively unaffected in older adults. Age-related changes in memory most often occur in recent memory. Recent memory is that which is used every day, such as information pertaining to current events or a recently read article. Long-term memory, such as memories of childhood friends and events, is essentially unaffected by the aging process.

Psychosocial Changes

In addition to adjusting to decreasing physical strength and health, older adults face many psychosocial changes, including the following:

- Making personal choices to find the meaning of life
- Evaluating one's self-worth

- Adjusting to retirement
- Adjusting to reduced income
- Establishing satisfactory living arrangements
- Adjusting to the death of a spouse or companion
- Maintaining contact with friends and family
- Meeting social and civic obligations, such as through volunteering and political activities

Implications for the Healthcare Professional

When communicating with an older adult, obtain a history from the patient, speaking to him or her in a respectful, friendly manner. "Elder speak" should be avoided. **Elder speak,** often unknowingly used by young adults when speaking to an older adult, is a style of speech that resembles baby talk and contains the following features:

- A slower rate of speaking
- A patronizing tone
- High pitch
- Increased volume
- Increased repetition
- Simpler vocabulary and grammar than in normal adult speech
- Statements that sound like questions
- Exaggeration of words

Elder speak does not communicate appropriate respect. Its use implies that the older adult is dependent and incompetent, lacking the ability to understand and respond. The use of elder speak when talking with an older adult can cause confusion and decrease comprehension. For example, speaking too slowly can affect an older adult's ability to focus on the main point you are trying to make. It is also hard to understand a statement that sounds like a question. Exaggerating words can cause confusion. Slow speech, shortened sentences, and using simple vocabulary sounds like baby talk and is perceived by most older adults as demeaning. An older adult will better understand you if you repeat and reword what you are saying. It is important to note that there is a difference between elder speak and speaking so that you can be understood by a patient who does not hear well. If an older adult does not hear well, it is okay to speak up to be sure that your patient can hear you. This can easily be accomplished while simultaneously avoiding the use of elder speak.

Remember This

When speaking with a patient, using terms of endearment like "hon," "dear," "sweetie," "grandma," or "good girl" is inappropriate and disrespectful.

Recognizing that the child is about 3 years of age, you recall that children of this age can answer simple questions, follow simple directions, and are likely to be more cooperative if given a comfort object. You remember that it is best to avoid asking questions that can be answered with a yes or no. Because most 3-year-olds are distrustful of strangers, this child is likely to resist examination and treatment. To help ease the child's anxiety, begin by talking with the child's caregiver and allow the child to remain on the caregiver's lap if possible. Talk to the child at eye level while addressing her by name. Examine her trunk or feet first and her head last. Replace clothing promptly after assessing each body area.

During your initial approach to the patient, you rapidly compare her general appearance, work of breathing, and skin color to what you have been trained to expect from a healthy child of the same age and level of development. You expect the child to be relaxed and breathing without difficulty at a rate of about 20 to 30 breaths per minute. Instead, you find this patient is struggling to breathe and breathing too fast for her age. From your calm demeanor and tone of voice, the child understands that you are there to help her. As you continue to talk to her, her rate of breathing slows a little to about 36 breaths per minute. The child's parents arrive, and you give them a brief report while administering supplemental oxygen to the patient. All agree that you and your partner will transport the child to the closest appropriate hospital for additional care. ∎

Sum It Up

▶ Life span refers to the period during which something is functional. In humans, life span is the period from birth to death.

▶ Human development is the process of growing to maturity. Stages of human development include the following:

- Infancy: birth to 12 months
- Toddler: 12 to 36 months
- Preschooler: 3 to 5 years
- School-age: 6 to 12 years
- Adolescence: 13 to 19 years
- Early adulthood: 20 to 40 years
- Middle adulthood: 41 to 60 years
- Late adulthood: 61 years and older

▶ Each stage of human development is accompanied by physiologic, cognitive, and psychosocial milestones. Physiologic milestones pertain to growth, body system changes, and changes in vital signs. Vital signs are measurements of breathing, pulse, skin temperature, pupils, and blood pressure. Cognitive changes pertain to mental processes such as reasoning, imagining, and problem solving. Psychosocial milestones pertain to personality, emotions, social interactions, and expectations.

▶ Maximum life expectancy is the oldest age to which any person lives. At present, maximum life expectancy for humans is about 120 years. Average life expectancy is the age at which half the people born in a particular year will have died. A baby born in 2004 in the United States would have an average life expectancy of 77.9 years.

Module 3

Pharmacology

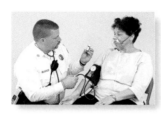

► CHAPTER 9

Principles of Pharmacology 204

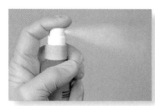

► CHAPTER 10

Medication Administration 211

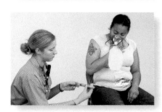

► CHAPTER 11

Emergency Medications 218

Principles of Pharmacology

By the end of this chapter, you should be able to:

Knowledge Objectives ▶

1. Define pharmacology and pharmacodynamics.
2. Discuss drug legislation in the United States.
3. List the main sources of medications.
4. Differentiate among the chemical, generic, and trade names of a drug.
5. Give examples of reputable sources of drug information.
6. Discuss the forms in which medications may be found.
7. Differentiate between local and systemic effects of medications.
8. Describe the components of a drug profile, including actions, indications, contraindications, adverse effects, dose, and route of administration for the medications an EMT can administer or assist with administering.

Attitude Objectives ▶

There are no attitude objectives identified for this lesson.

Skill Objectives ▶

There are no skill objectives identified for this lesson.

On the Scene

You are dispatched for an "unknown medical problem." The address is one that you recognize as a home healthcare facility. On arrival, you find a man sitting upright in a chair. He looks to be about 60 years of age. You quickly note that he is responsive, but his voice sounds weak. He is complaining of chest discomfort and pain in his left arm and jaw. His symptoms began about 30 minutes after eating lunch. He has a history of pulmonary hypertension, for which he takes Revatio. ■

THINK ABOUT IT

As you read this chapter, think about the following questions:

- What is the definition of *pharmacology* and *pharmacodynamics?*
- What is the difference between a drug's generic name and trade name, and how does this affect your care?
- How does understanding the pharmacodynamics about this patient's medication affect the care you deliver?

Introduction

Objective 1

Pharmacology is the study of drugs or medications and their effect on living systems. **Pharmacodynamics** is the study of the effects of drugs and their mechanisms of action at target sites in the body. This chapter introduces you to the principles of pharmacology. You must be familiar with medications carried on the EMS unit and physician-prescribed medications that medical direction will authorize you to assist patients in taking. Although drugs may be lifesaving when properly given, they may be fatal if improperly administered. This chapter includes information about the very important responsibilities that you will have to your patients when giving a medication.

Drug Legislation and Federal Regulatory Agencies

Objective 2

From the very earliest recorded history, humankind has used herbs, plants, and minerals to ease pain and treat diseases. The realization that these plants, herbs, and minerals had an effect on the body was the beginning of the science of pharmacology. This science continues to advance every day with the use of chemical compounds that help in the fight against illnesses and disease. The medications that we consider as a part of everyday life have developed with time. In addition, the safety and regulation of the medications that we use has also changed.

Drug Legislation in the United States

Drug legislation in the United States has been put in place to protect the public from contaminated or mislabeled drugs. Important events and laws pertaining to the purchasing, distribution, dispensing, and giving of drugs are shown in Table 9-1. Controlled substances are listed in Table 9-2.

Federal Regulatory Agencies and Services

The Drug Enforcement Agency (DEA) is a division of the Justice Department. It became the sole legal drug enforcement agency in July 1973 and replaced the Bureau of Narcotics and Dangerous Drugs (BNDD).

The Food and Drug Administration (FDA) is a part of the U.S. Department of Health and Human Services.

It enforces the Federal Food, Drug, and Cosmetic Act by means of seizure and criminal prosecution as necessary.

Drug Sources, Names, and References

Drug Sources

Objective 3

Drugs can be obtained from many sources. Morphine, a commonly used drug for pain relief, is an example of a drug obtained from a plant. Some drugs are obtained from minerals or mineral products, such as iron. Advances in technology have enabled drug companies to make many drugs in the laboratory that were formerly obtained from animals and humans (such as insulin and some vaccines). Drugs that are made in a laboratory are called **synthetic drugs. Semisynthetic drugs** are naturally occurring substances that have been chemically altered, such as antibiotics.

Drug Names

Objective 4

Chemical Name

A drug's **chemical name** is a description of its composition and molecular structure. For example, the chemical name for epinephrine is (+)-3,4-dihydroxy-alpha-((methylamino) methyl) benzyl alcohol. This name is useful for determining the effects of a drug on the body.

Generic Name

The **generic name** (also called the *nonproprietary name*) is the name given to a drug by the company that first manufactures it. It is often a simplified version of the drug's chemical name or structure. Generic names are printed in lowercase letters, such as epinephrine.

Trade Name

A drug's **trade name** is also known as its *brand name* or *proprietary name*. Trade names are capitalized, such as EpiPen. When a company makes a new drug, the manufacturer patents the drug and its trade name. The patent usually lasts 20 years. During that time, the drug company that holds the patent has the sole right to make, market, and sell the drug. When the patent expires, other drug companies can make and sell generic versions of the drug, but they cannot use the drug's original trade name. As a result, a drug may have several different trade names if it is made and sold by different manufacturers (see Table 9-3 on p. 208).

TABLE 9-1   Landmarks in Food and Drug Legislation in the United States

Year	Legislation/Event	Notes
1848	Drug Importation Act	Required U.S. Customs Service inspectors to stop entry of contaminated drugs from overseas
1862	President Lincoln appointed a chemist to serve in the new Department of Agriculture	Beginning of the Bureau of Chemistry, the predecessor of the Food and Drug Administration
1902	Biologics Control Act	Passed to ensure purity and safety of serums, vaccines, and similar products used to prevent or treat diseases in humans
1906	Pure Food and Drug Act	Prohibited interstate commerce in misbranded and impure foods, drinks, and drugs
1912	Shirley Amendment	Prohibited labeling medicines with false therapeutic claims intended to defraud the purchaser
1914	Harrison Narcotic Act	• Established the word "narcotic" • Required prescriptions for products exceeding the allowable limit of narcotics • Required increased record keeping for physicians and pharmacists who dispense narcotics
1927	Bureau of Chemistry reorganized into two separate entities	• Regulatory functions located in the Food, Drug, and Insecticide Administration • Nonregulatory research located in the Bureau of Chemistry and Soils
1930	Name of the Food, Drug, and Insecticide Administration shortened to Food and Drug Administration (FDA)	Name shortened as a result of an agricultural appropriations act
1937	Death of 107 persons, many of whom were children, due to Elixir of Sulfanilamide	Emphasized the need to establish drug safety before marketing (Elixir of Sulfanilamide was a liquid that contained a poison)
1938	Federal Food, Drug, and Cosmetic (FDC) Act of 1938	• Required that new drugs be shown to be safe before marketing • Established the FDA's responsibility for supervising and regulating drug safety • Authorized factory inspections • Required that drugs contain a label listing all of the ingredients and directions for use
1951	Durham-Humphrey Amendment	Required that prescription drugs (also called *legend drugs*) must carry the following label: "Caution: Federal law prohibits dispensing without a prescription."
1962	Kefauver-Harris Drug Amendments	• Thalidomide, a sleeping pill, found to have caused birth defects in thousands of babies born in western Europe • 1962 drug amendments passed to ensure drug effectiveness and greater drug safety • Drug manufacturers required to prove to FDA the effectiveness of their products before marketing them

Continued

TABLE 9-1 Landmarks in Food and Drug Legislation in the United States *Continued*

Year	Legislation/Event	Notes
1970	Comprehensive Drug Abuse Prevention and Control Act (Controlled Substances Act)	• Consolidated over 50 federal narcotic, marijuana, and dangerous drug laws into one law • Designed to regulate the manufacture, importation, possession, and distribution of certain drugs in the United States • Established five schedules (classifications) of drugs based on their accepted medical use in the United States, abuse potential, and potential for addiction
1983	Orphan Drug Act	Enabled FDA to promote research and marketing of drugs needed for treating rare diseases
1988	Food and Drug Administration Act of 1988	Officially established FDA as an agency of the Department of Health and Human Services
1990	Anabolic Steroid Act	Identified anabolic steroids as a class of drugs and specified over two dozen items as controlled substances

TABLE 9-2 Schedule of Controlled Substances

Schedule	Description
I	• No acceptable medical use in United States • Used for research, analysis, or instruction only • High abuse potential • May lead to severe dependence • Examples: heroin, peyote, marijuana (cannabis), lysergic acid diethylamide (LSD), Ecstasy, XTC
II	• Acceptable medical use in United States • High abuse potential • May lead to severe physical and/or psychological dependence • Examples: morphine, meperidine (Demerol), codeine, oxycodone (OxyContin, Percocet, Tylox, Roxicodone, Roxicet), methadone, propoxyphene (Darvon), amphetamines, cocaine, opium
III	• Acceptable medical use in United States • Less abuse potential than drugs in Schedules I and II • May lead to moderate/low physical or high psychological dependence • Examples: anabolic steroids ("body-building" drugs); preparations containing limited narcotic quantities, or combined with one or more active ingredients that are noncontrolled substances, such as acetaminophen with codeine (Tylenol 3), or acetaminophen with hydrocodone (Vicodin)
IV	• Acceptable medical use in United States • Lower abuse potential compared with drugs in Schedule III • May lead to limited physical or psychological dependence • Examples: alprazolam (Xanax), diazepam (Valium), lorazepam (Ativan), midazolam (Versed), phenobarbital
V	• Acceptable medical use in United States • Low abuse potential compared with drugs in Schedule IV • May lead to limited physical or psychologic dependence • Examples: narcotic-containing preparations to suppress cough (Robitussin A-C) or control diarrhea (Lomotil)

TABLE 9-3 Additional Examples of Drug Names

Generic Name	Trade Name	Chemical Name
albuterol	Proventil, Ventolin	2-(hydroxymethyl)-4-[1-hydroxy-2-(tert-butylamino) ethyl]phenol
ibuprofen	Motrin, Advil	(±)-2-(p-isobutylphenyl) propionic acid
sildenafil citrate	Viagra, Revatio	1-[[3-(6,7-dihydro-1-methyl-7-oxo-3-propyl-1H-pyrazolo [4,3-d] pyrimidin-5-yl)-4-ethoxyphenyl]sulfonyl]-4-methylpiperazine citrate

Making a Difference

In the field, the generic and trade names are the names most often used to identify a drug or medication. An informed emergency medical technician is able to recognize both these names.

Sources of Drug Information

Objective 5

Before giving *any* medication, you have a responsibility to the patient to know as much as you can about the drug you will be giving or assisting the patient in taking. There are many sources of drug information available to help you find out more about a drug.

The *United States Pharmacopeia–National Formulary* is an official publication that contains information about drugs marketed in the United States. It lists approved drugs and gives directions for their general use.

The *American Hospital Formulary Service (AHFS) Drug Information* is an electronic database published by the American Society of Hospital Pharmacists. It is available in hospital pharmacies and most emergency departments. It contains information about drugs for Food and Drug Administration–approved uses as well as some investigational uses of medications.

The *Physician's Desk Reference* (PDR) is well known to healthcare professionals. This publication contains a collection of packaged inserts provided by drug manufacturers. The information includes the accepted uses, dosages, and adverse effects of commercially available drugs. It lists specific drugs for FDA-approved uses. The PDR also contains a product identification guide showing actual sizes and color pictures of commonly prescribed drugs.

Patient packaged inserts are published by drug companies. They are required by law, and their content is approved by the FDA. Other sources of information include pharmacists, poison centers, and drug references produced by medical publishers.

Drug Forms

Objectives 6, 7

Every drug is supplied in a specific form by the drug's manufacturer. This is done to allow properly controlled concentrations of the drug to enter the bloodstream where the drug has an effect on the target body system.

A drug's effects may be local or systemic. A **local effect** of a drug usually occurs only in a limited part of the body (usually at the site of drug application). For instance, if you apply calamine lotion to a rash on your arm or leg, the effects of the drug are limited to the extremity to which the drug was applied.

Drugs with **systemic effects** are absorbed into the bloodstream and distributed throughout the body. For example, when you go to a dentist to have a cavity fixed, the dentist may give you an injection in the mouth where the dental work will be done. The drug used is often a combination of lidocaine and epinephrine. Lidocaine numbs the area (a local effect). Epinephrine constricts the blood vessels in the area to limit bleeding (a local effect). However, another effect of epinephrine is an increase in heart rate (a systemic effect).

Gas Forms

Drugs that are in a gas form are breathed in and absorbed through the respiratory tract. Oxygen is an example of a drug that you will be giving in gas form.

Liquid Drugs

Liquid drugs contain medication that is ground into a powder and mixed with a substance, such as water. Table 9-4 shows examples of different types of liquid drug forms.

TABLE 9-4 Liquid Drug Forms

Liquid Drug Form	Description	Example
Elixir	Clear liquid made with alcohol, water, flavors, or sweeteners	Terpin hydrate, NyQuil
Emulsion	Mixture of two liquids, one distributed throughout the other in small globules	Cold cream
Gel	Clear or transparent semisolid substance that liquefies when applied to the skin or a mucous membrane	Glucose
Lotion	Preparation applied to protect the skin or treat a skin disorder	Calamine lotion
Solution	Liquid preparation of one or more chemical substances, usually dissolved in water	5% dextrose in water, 0.9% normal saline
Spirit	Volatile substance dissolved in alcohol	Spirit of ammonia
Suspension	Drug particle mixed with, but not dissolved in, a liquid	Oral antibiotics (amoxicillin), activated charcoal
Syrup	Drug suspended in sugar and water	Cough syrup
Tincture	Alcohol solution prepared from an animal or vegetable drug or chemical substance	Tincture of iodine

TABLE 9-5 Solid Drug Forms

Solid Drug Form	Description	Example
Caplet	Oval-shaped tablet that has a film-coated covering	Tylenol caplets
Capsule	Small gelatin container containing a medication dose in powder or granule form	Actifed
Enteric-coated tablet	Tablet that has a special coating so that it breaks down in the intestines instead of the stomach	Aspirin
Gelcap	Small gelatin container containing a liquid medication dose	DayQuil gelcaps
Powder	Drug ground into fine particles	Calcium carbonate
Suppository	Drug mixed in a firm base such as cocoa butter that, when placed into a body opening, melts at body temperature	Glycerin, aspirin
Tablet	Powdered drug, molded or compressed into a small form	Nitroglycerin

Solid Drugs

A drug that is in solid form is usually swallowed. In some cases (such as when a patient takes aspirin for chest pain), the drug is chewed first and then swallowed. Although solid drugs are generally easy to administer, the patient must be responsive and cooperative and have an intact gag reflex. Table 9-5 shows examples of different types of solid drug forms.

Drug Profile

Objective 8

You must be knowledgeable about the characteristics of each drug that you administer. A **drug profile** is a description of a drug's characteristics. Common elements of a drug profile include the following:

- **Name:** Generic and trade names of the drug
- **Mechanism of action:** How the drug exerts its effect on body cells and tissues
- **Indications:** The condition(s) for which the drug has documented usefulness
- **Dose:** The amount of the drug that should be given to the patient at one time
- **Route of administration:** The route and form in which the drug should be given to the patient
- **Contraindications:** Condition(s) for which a drug should not be used because it may cause harm to the patient or offer no improvement of the patient's condition or illness
- **Adverse effects:** An undesired effect of a drug
- **Special considerations:** Factors to consider when giving the drug, such as the impact of age and weight on medication administration (children, older adults, pregnant patients); tips for administration of the drug

Drug profiles for medications frequently administered by EMTs appear in Chapter 11.

Stop and Think!

Emergency medical technicians are responsible for their own actions when giving drugs. Although drugs may be lifesaving when given properly, they may cause death if they are improperly given.

On the Scene   Wrap-Up

After careful assessment of the patient, you believe that his pain is due to a possible cardiac problem. The patient's blood pressure is 116/74, pulse 88, and respiratory rate 16. Routine emergency care generally includes administering supplemental oxygen and sublingual nitroglycerin, if no contraindications exist.

You recognize that the generic name of the medication the patient is taking is sildenafil and that a trade name for this medication is Viagra. You recall that sildenafil may cause problems (such as hypotension) if the patient receives nitroglycerin. On arrival at the receiving facility, you relay this important information during your hand-off report to the nurse. She thanks you for the "heads up." ■

Sum It Up

▶ Pharmacology is the study of drugs or medications and their effect on living systems. Pharmacodynamics is the study of the effects of drugs and their mechanisms of action at target sites in the body.

▶ Drug legislation in the United States has been put in place to protect the public from contaminated or mislabeled drugs.

▶ The Drug Enforcement Agency became the sole legal drug enforcement agency in July 1973 and replaced the Bureau of Narcotics and Dangerous Drugs. The Food and Drug Administration enforces the Federal Food, Drug, and Cosmetic Act by means of seizure and criminal prosecution as necessary.

▶ A drug's chemical name is a description of its composition and molecular structure. The generic name (also called the nonproprietary name) is the name given to a drug by the company that first manufactures it. A drug's trade name is also known as its brand name or proprietary name.

▶ A local effect of a drug usually occurs only in a limited part of the body (usually at the site of drug application). Drugs with systemic effects are absorbed into the bloodstream and distributed throughout the body.

▶ Each drug is in a specific medication form to allow properly controlled concentrations of the drug to enter the bloodstream where the drug has an effect on the target body system.

▶ You must be knowledgeable about the characteristics of each drug that you administer. A drug profile is a description of a drug's characteristics. Common elements of a drug profile include the following:

- The drug's mechanism of action: The desired effects the drug should have on the patient
- Indications for the drug's use, including the most common uses of the drug in treating a specific illness
- Contraindications: Situations in which the drug should not be used because it may cause harm to the patient or offer no possibility of improving the patient's condition or illness
- Correct dose (amount) of the drug to be given
- The proper route by which the drug is given
- Adverse effects: Undesired effects of a drug
- Special considerations: Factors to consider when giving the drug, such as the impact of age and weight on medication administration (children, older adults, pregnant patients); tips for administration of the drug

Medication Administration

By the end of this chapter, you should be able to:

Knowledge Objectives ▶
1. Describe the conditions that must exist for an EMT to give, or assist a patient in taking, medications.
2. List and explain the six rights of medication administration.
3. List and differentiate routes of drug administration, including the enteral and parenteral routes.
4. Discuss the use of standard precautions and personal protective equipment when administering a medication.
5. Discuss the advantages, disadvantages, and techniques for each route of drug administration.

Attitude Objectives ▶
6. Explain the rationale for using the six rights of medication administration when giving a drug.
7. Comply with EMT standards of medication administration.
8. Comply with standard precautions during medication administration.

Skill Objectives ▶
9. Demonstrate use of standard precautions during medication administration.
10. Read the labels and inspect each type of medication.
11. Demonstrate general steps for assisting the patient with self-administration of oral medications.
12. Demonstrate general steps for assisting the patient with self-administration of medications by the inhalation route.
13. Demonstrate preparation and general steps for administration of autoinjected medications.
14. Demonstrate proper disposal of contaminated items and sharps.

You are dispatched to a report of chest pain at a local business address. You arrive to find a 58-year-old man complaining of severe pain in the center of his chest. He states his discomfort began about 1 hour ago. Your partner applies an oxygen delivery device to the patient as you check his vital signs. The patient denies any allergies. He has a history of angina pectoris, for which he takes nitroglycerin spray when needed. He has this prescribed medication with him at his desk. His vital signs are as follows: blood pressure 154/78, pulse 82, respirations 16. ■

THINK ABOUT IT

As you read this chapter, think about the following questions:

- What questions will you ask before assisting the patient in taking his medication?
- How is this medication administered?
- How do the buccal and sublingual routes of medication administration differ?

Introduction

This chapter introduces you to the rights and routes of drug administration. Knowing the rights of drug administration helps ensure safe and effective administration of a drug. The route of drug administration is one of the most important factors influencing the effects of a drug and the rate at which the onset of drug action occurs. Although some drugs can be used both locally and systemically, most drugs are given via a single route of administration.

Drug Administration

General Guidelines

Objective 1

An EMT can give, or assist a patient in taking, medications only by the order of a licensed physician. The physician's order may be a written protocol (standing order) or a verbal order.

Before giving any drug, you must assess the patient (see Chapter 17). The extent of the physical examination you perform will depend on the patient's illness or present condition. The physical exam provides baseline information by which you will be able to evaluate the effectiveness of the medications given.

Obtain a medication history from the patient including the following:

- Prescribed medications (name, strength, daily dosage)
- Over-the-counter medications
- Allergies to medications

Stop and Think!

Many patients use herbal and nontraditional medications. Always ask your patients for information about any herbs and herbal remedies that they may have used (or routinely take) before giving any medication. In these situations, you must consider the possibility of a negative interaction between the drug you are about to give and the substances the patient has already taken. If the patient has taken any herbal or nontraditional medications, consult medical direction before giving any medication.

You will recall from Chapter 9 that you must be knowledgeable about each drug you give, knowing the drug's mechanism of action, indications, dose, route of administration, contraindications, and adverse effects. You must also be aware of any special considerations pertaining to the drug, such as the impact of the patient's age and weight on medication administration.

Before giving a medication, consult with medical direction. When speaking with medical direction, be sure to relay relevant information about the patient, including the following:

- Patient's age
- Chief complaint
- Vital signs
- Signs and symptoms
- Allergies
- Current medications
- Pertinent past medical history

The physician's order will include the name, dose, and route of administration of the drug to be given. Make sure you clearly understand the orders received from medical direction. Repeat the orders back to the physician, including the name of the drug, dose, and route of administration. If an order received from medical direction is unclear or seems incorrect, ask the physician to repeat the order.

The Six Rights of Drug Administration

Objective 2

The six "rights" of drug administration before giving a drug:

1. *Right patient.* If assisting a patient who is taking medication, make sure that the medication is prescribed for *that* patient.
2. *Right drug.* Select the right medication. Use only medications that are in a clearly labeled container. If the label is unclear or blurred, do not give the drug. Carefully read the label and check it three times before administering: (1) when removing the drug from the drug box (or other medication storage device), (2) when preparing the drug for administration, and (3) before actually giving the drug to the patient. Check the drug's expiration date.
3. *Right dose.* Check and recheck the dose ordered against the dose to be given.
4. *Right route.* You must know the route(s) by which a drug is to be given.
5. *Right time (frequency).* Although many drugs are ordered for one-time administration, some may be repeated. Determine from medical direction the frequency with which a drug may be given.
6. *Right documentation.* After giving a drug, document the time you gave it, document the patient's response to the drug, monitor the patient for possible adverse (harmful) effects, as well as expected results, and reassess and record the patient's vital signs.

Routes of Drug Administration

Objective 3

Enteral and parenteral are two primary categories of drug administration. The **enteral** route of administration involves passage of the medication through any portion of the digestive tract. Routes of administration that fall into the enteral category include the oral, buccal, and sublingual routes. A drug that is given by a **parenteral** route does not pass through the digestive tract. Drugs given by a parenteral route are injected, inhaled, or infused. Routes of administration that fall into the parenteral category include the subcutaneous and intramuscular routes.

Enteral Routes
Oral

Objectives 4, 5

The oral route of drug administration is the most frequently used route in the hospital and home settings, but it is used infrequently in the prehospital setting. Commonly used oral dosage forms include liquids, tablets, and capsules. Drugs administered orally require a responsive, cooperative patient. Aspirin (see Chapter 22) and activated charcoal (see Chapter 28) may be given by this route (Figure 10-1).

The oral medication route is painless, convenient, and readily available because of the accessibility of the oral cavity. Drugs given orally are easy to administer and generally easy to store. Oral medications are absorbed in

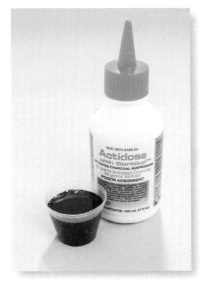

FIGURE 10-1 ▲ Activated charcoal is a suspension. It contains drug particles that are mixed with, but not dissolved in, a liquid.

the gastrointestinal tract, primarily in the small intestine. Disadvantages of the oral route of drug administration include slow or erratic absorption of the drug. For example, the presence of food in the stomach or a digestive system disorder will affect the rate of absorption and flow of the medicine through the gastrointestinal tract. Digestive enzymes present in the stomach can also destroy certain drugs if given orally, making them ineffective. Irritation of the gastrointestinal tract by some drugs, such as aspirin, may produce adverse effects such as nausea and vomiting. Possible complications of oral medication administration can also include airway obstruction and aspiration pneumonia. Inflammation of the esophagus due to oral tablet or capsule administration is called *pill esophagitis*. A relatively uncommon condition, pill esophagitis is primarily the result of a chemical reaction between the released contents of a tablet or capsule and the lining of the esophagus. The midesophagus is the most commonly affected site. To minimize the risk of this condition, the patient should drink an adequate amount (usually 4–6 ounces) of fluid with the medication and remain upright for 10–15 minutes after drug administration.

Giving oral medications usually does not involve exposure to a patient's blood or other body fluids. However, wearing appropriate personal protective equipment (such as gloves) is a common practice to minimize the chances of communicable disease exposure. The inside of the medicine container, its contents, and the inside of the container's cap are considered clean. When giving a medication, be careful not to touch these areas.

When administering a tablet, open the container and pour the correct number into the inside cap of the container. Transfer the tablets by pouring them into the patient's hand, making sure not to contaminate the inside cap of the container, and then carefully recap the container.

Stop and Think!

Patients who are unresponsive, uncooperative, have no gag reflex, or are vomiting should *not* be given drugs orally.

Buccal

Objectives 4, 5

Drugs administered buccally are absorbed through the mucous membranes of the mouth. **Buccal** means, "pertaining to the cheek." To give a drug by this route, the drug is placed in the mouth against the mucous membranes of the cheek until the drug is dissolved. The drug may act locally on the mucous membranes of the mouth or systemically when swallowed in the saliva. Oral glucose may be given by this route (see Chapter 20).

The amount of drug absorbed by the buccal route depends on many factors, including the concentration of the drug and the length of time it is in contact with the mucosal surface. The rate of drug absorption is affected by the amount of saliva present. Salivation and swallowing remove the drug from the absorptive mucosal surface. The presence of an insufficient amount of saliva will hinder dissolution of the drug at the desired rate.

One of the advantages of the buccal administration route is the ease of drug administration because of the accessibility of the oral cavity. Buccal drug administration is painless. The surfaces of most mucous membranes have a rich blood supply, enabling drugs that penetrate the mucous membrane to be delivered directly into the bloodstream. Disadvantages include a smaller absorptive surface area in comparison to the absorptive surface area of the small intestines and a risk of choking if the patient does not have a gag reflex. The number of medications that can be administered buccally is limited.

When administering a drug buccally, use appropriate personal protective equipment. Place the medication against the mucous membrane of the cheek until it dissolves.

Remember This

Use caution when working near a patient's mouth because it is possible a patient may clench his teeth onto your hand.

Sublingual

Objectives 4, 5

Sublingual drugs are given under the tongue. The drug must remain under the tongue until it is dissolved and absorbed. An EMT may assist a patient in taking prescribed nitroglycerin (NTG) sublingual tablets or spray (see Chapter 22).

Drugs given sublingually are easy to administer, and the drug is rapidly absorbed into the bloodstream because of the rich blood supply under the tongue. Administration of sublingual tablets and sprays is painless. A disadvantage of the sublingual route is the limited number of medications that can be administered sublingually. When giving a nitroglycerin tablet, the presence of an insufficient amount of saliva will hinder dissolution of the drug at the desired rate. If the patient's mouth is very dry, ask the patient to rinse her mouth with water and then place the tablet under her tongue.

When administering a drug sublingually, use appropriate personal protective equipment. When giving NTG, it is particularly important to wear gloves so that the drug is not absorbed through your skin. The patient should not swallow the drug or take it with water. If swallowed, the drug may be inactivated by gastric juice in the stomach. Because hypotension is a common and significant adverse effect of NTG administration, vital signs should be obtained before and after administration of this drug.

Parenteral Routes
Inhalation
Objectives 4, 5

Drugs given by the **inhalation** route have a rapid onset of action because of the large surface area and blood supply of the lungs. To make sure that normal gas exchange of oxygen and carbon dioxide is continuous in the lungs, drugs given by inhalation must be in the form of a gas (such as oxygen) or fine mist (such as an aerosol). Oxygen is given for its systemic effects. A metered-dose inhaler (MDI) such as albuterol is given for its localized effect on the lungs.

Administration of drugs by the inhalation route is easy and painless. Inhaled drugs are rapidly absorbed into the bloodstream. However, the amount of medication absorbed is affected by airway size and the degree of obstruction within the airways due to mucous plugs, bronchoconstriction, and inflammation. Oxygen administration is discussed in Chapter 11. Medications contained in a MDI are usually beta-2 agonists. This means that the drug stimulates beta-2 receptor sites in the lungs. When these receptor sites are stimulated in the bronchioles, the smooth muscle tissue relaxes (dilates), reducing airway resistance. This makes it easier for the patient to move air in and out. Inhaled steroids are another type of medication that may be given by means of an MDI. Inhaled steroids help decrease inflammation in the airways. Assisting a patient with the use of a prescribed MDI is discussed in Chapter 21.

In some states, EMTs are permitted to give naloxone in cases of narcotic overdose. With an order from medical direction, the EMT gives naloxone to the patient by means of an atomizer that is connected to a syringe. The atomizer is placed a short distance (about 1.5 cm) into the patient's nose. When the EMT pushes the plunger on the syringe, the atomizer disperses a mistlike spray onto the inner surface of the patient's nostril, where the drug is quickly absorbed. Contraindications to the use of an atomizer include nasal trauma or congestion or the presence of blood or mucous in the nose.

Subcutaneous
Objectives 4, 5

Drugs given by the **subcutaneous route** are given by means of a needle inserted underneath the skin into the subcutaneous tissue. The subcutaneous route is readily available and allows delivery of a variety of medications. The onset of drug action via the subcutaneous route is faster than that by the oral route but slower than that by the intramuscular route. Disadvantages of the subcutaneous route include delayed drug absorption in circulatory collapse, such as shock. A subcutaneous injection is painful and requires technical skill to perform. Improper technique can cause local tissue injury and nerve damage. Only a small volume of drug can be given by this route.

Intramuscular
Objectives 4, 5

When a drug is given by the **intramuscular (IM) route**, a medication in a liquid form is injected into a large mass of skeletal muscle (Figure 10-2). Sites commonly used in prehospital care include the arm (deltoid muscle) and midlateral thigh (vastus lateralis muscle). The injection is usually made with a longer needle than that used with a subcutaneous injection. Epinephrine is an example of a drug that may be given by this route.

The IM route is readily available and allows delivery of a variety of medications. Larger volumes can be given by the intramuscular route than by the subcutaneous route. The onset of action is faster than that by the subcutaneous route because of the muscle's blood supply and large absorbing surface. An IM injection is painful and requires technical skill to perform. Improper technique can cause local tissue injury and nerve damage.

Reassessment and Documentation

After giving a drug, document the reason the drug was given, the medication administered, and the time you gave it. When giving an injectable drug, be sure to document the site where the drug was administered. Reassess the patient and document the patient's vital signs and response to the drug. Continue to monitor the patient for possible adverse effects, as well as expected results.

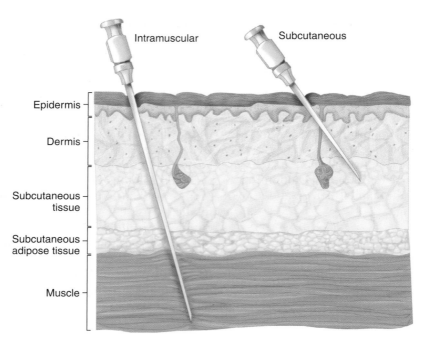

Intramuscular   Subcutaneous

Epidermis

Dermis

Subcutaneous
tissue

Subcutaneous
adipose tissue

Muscle

FIGURE 10-2 ▲ Intramuscular and subcutaneous injections.

On the Scene   Wrap-Up

Your patient rates his chest discomfort an 8 on a 0 to 10 scale. You recall that you can assist this patient in taking his prescribed nitroglycerin spray only by the order of a licensed physician. The physician's order may be a written protocol (standing order) or a verbal order. Before giving any drug, you must assess the patient, including assessment of his vital signs. You must also obtain a medication history from the patient. Based on your assessment findings and the patient's symptoms, you assist the patient in taking his medication and move him into the ambulance. Five minutes after administration of the drug, you reassess his vital signs and find that they are as follows: blood pressure 148/74, pulse 86, respirations 16. The patient states his discomfort is still an 8 on a 0 to 10 scale. Based on this information, you prepare to assist the patient in taking a second dose of his medication. ■

Sum It Up

▶ An EMT can give, or assist a patient in taking, medications only by the order of a licensed physician. The physician's order may be a written protocol (standing order) or a verbal order.

▶ Before giving any drug, you must assess the patient and obtain a medication history from the patient.

Then consult with medical direction. When speaking with medical direction, be sure to relay relevant information about the patient, including the patient's age, chief complaint, vital signs, signs and symptoms, allergies, current medications, and pertinent past medical history. The physician's order will include the name, dose, and route of the drug to be given. Repeat the orders back to the physician including the name of the drug, the dose, and the route of administration.

▶ Before giving a drug, use the six "rights" of drug administration: Right patient, right drug, right dose, right route, right time (frequency), and right documentation. After giving a drug, document the time you gave the drug, document the patient's response to the drug, monitor the patient for possible adverse (harmful) effects, and reassess and record the patient's vital signs.

▶ The enteral route of drug administration involves passage of the medication through any portion of the digestive tract. Routes of administration that fall into the enteral category include the oral, buccal, and sublingual routes.

▶ A drug that is given by a parenteral route does not pass through the digestive tract. Drugs given by a parenteral route are injected, inhaled, or infused. Routes of administration that fall into the parenteral category include the subcutaneous and intramuscular routes.

▶ The oral route is painless, convenient, and readily available because of the accessibility of the oral cavity.

Oral medications are easy to administer and generally easy to store. Disadvantages of the oral route of drug administration include slow or erratic absorption of the drug.

▶ Drugs administered buccally are absorbed through the mucous membranes of the mouth. Advantages of the buccal route include ease of drug administration because of the accessibility of the oral cavity, painlessness, and delivery of the drug directly into the bloodstream. However, there is a smaller absorptive surface area in comparison to the absorptive surface area of the small intestines (as with oral drug administration). There is also a risk of choking if the patient does not have a gag reflex. Few medications can be administered buccally.

▶ Sublingual drugs are given under the tongue. The drug must remain under the tongue until it is dissolved and absorbed. Sublingual drugs are easy to administer and painless. They are rapidly absorbed into the bloodstream because of the rich blood supply under the tongue. However, few medications can be administered sublingually.

▶ Drugs given by the inhalation route have a rapid onset of action because of the large surface area and blood supply of the lungs. Drugs given by inhalation must be in the form of a gas (such as oxygen) or fine mist (such as an aerosol). The inhalation route is painless. Inhaled drugs are easy to administer and have a rapid onset of action. However, the amount of medication absorbed is affected by airway size and the degree of obstruction within the airways due to mucous plugs, bronchoconstriction, and inflammation.

▶ Drugs given by the subcutaneous route are given by means of a needle inserted underneath the skin into the subcutaneous tissue. This route is readily available and allows delivery of a variety of medications. The onset of action of subcutaneous drugs is faster than the oral route but slower than the intramuscular route. Drug absorption is delayed in circulatory collapse, such as shock. The subcutaneous route is painful and requires technical skill to perform. Only a small volume of drug can be given by this route.

▶ When a drug is given by the IM route, a medication in a liquid form is injected into a large mass of skeletal muscle. The IM route is readily available and allows delivery of a variety of medications. Larger volumes can be given by the IM route than the subcutaneous route, and the onset of action is faster than the subcutaneous route. The IM route is painful and requires technical skill to perform.

Emergency Medications

By the end of this chapter, you should be able to:

Knowledge Objectives ▶

1. State the generic and trade names, action, indications, contraindications, adverse effects, dose, medication form, and administration for activated charcoal.

2. State the generic and trade names, action, indications, contraindications, adverse effects, dose, medication form, and administration for aspirin.

3. State the generic and trade names, action, indications, contraindications, adverse effects, dose, medication form, and administration for oral glucose.

4. State the action, indications, contraindications, adverse effects, dose, medication form, and administration for oxygen.

5. State the generic and trade names, action, indications, contraindications, adverse effects, dose, medication form, and administration for the epinephrine autoinjector.

6. Give examples of generic and trade names, action, indications, contraindications, adverse effects, dose, medication form, and administration for inhaled bronchodilators.

7. State the generic and trade names, action, indications, contraindications, adverse effects, dose, medication form, and administration for nitroglycerin (NTG).

8. Explain what a nerve agent is and give examples.

9. Define antidote.

10. Describe the signs and symptoms of nerve agent exposure.

11. Identify the medications contained in the Mark I and DuoDote autoinjectors.

12. State the generic and trade names, action, indications, contraindications, adverse effects, dose, medication form, and administration for the medications contained in the Mark I and DuoDote autoinjectors.

13. State the generic and trade names, action, indications, contraindications, adverse effects, dose, medication form, and administration for the diazepam autoinjector.

Attitude Objectives ▶

14. Explain the rationale for administering activated charcoal.

15. Explain the rationale for administering aspirin.

16. Explain the rationale for administering oral glucose.

17. Explain the rationale for administering oxygen.

18. Explain the rationale for administering epinephrine using an autoinjector.

19. Explain the rationale for administering inhaled bronchodilators.

20. Explain the rationale for administering NTG.

21. Explain the rationale for the administration of the Mark I or DuoDote kits.

22. Explain the rationale for administering diazepam using an autoinjector.

Skill Objectives ▶ 23. Demonstrate the steps in the administration of activated charcoal.

24. Demonstrate the assessment and documentation of patient response to activated charcoal.

25. Demonstrate the steps in the administration of aspirin.

26. Demonstrate the assessment and documentation of patient response to aspirin.

27. Demonstrate the steps in the administration of oral glucose.

28. Demonstrate the assessment and documentation of patient response to oral glucose.

29. Demonstrate the use of an epinephrine autoinjector.

30. Demonstrate the assessment and documentation of patient response to an epinephrine injection.

31. Perform the steps in facilitating the use of inhaled bronchodilators.

32. Demonstrate the assessment and documentation of patient response to inhaled bronchodilators.

33. Perform the steps in facilitating the use of NTG for chest pain or discomfort.

34. Demonstrate the assessment and documentation of patient response to NTG.

35. Demonstrate the steps for self-administration of a nerve agent antidote by means of an autoinjector.

36. Demonstrate the steps for administration of a nerve agent antidote by means of an autoinjector to a peer.

On the Scene

While performing a standby at a local grade school soccer game, you notice one of the players slap at her leg and cry out in pain. The player runs to the sidelines and starts talking with the coach. A parent runs from the sidelines to be with the player. Her parent helps her lie down on the ground as other parents huddle around her. You and your partner are flagged over. As you approach, you notice that the patient seems to be having trouble breathing. As you kneel at the patient's side, the child's mother introduces herself. She tells you that her daughter has just been stung by a bee and is allergic to bees. In addition, she says that she is unable to find her daughter's "sting kit." ■

THINK ABOUT IT

As you read this chapter, think about the following questions:

- What do you need to know about this scene?
- What questions will you ask?
- Is there any danger to you or your partner?
- How will you get additional help if it is needed?
- What pharmacological intervention is needed to help this patient?
- Do you have the training, knowledge, and ability to help?
- What information will need to be relayed to the hospital if you transport this patient?

Introduction

This chapter introduces the emergency medications you are most likely to give, or assist a patient in taking, while working as an emergency medical technician. The procedure for administering these medications is also discussed.

Administered Medications

The medications that are most commonly found in EMS units include activated charcoal, aspirin, oral glucose, and oxygen. This list may vary from state to state and even from EMS system to EMS system. The expiration date for medications carried on the EMS unit should be checked daily.

Activated Charcoal

Objective 1

In some EMS systems, activated charcoal is administered in specific situations involving ingested poisons (Figure 11-1). **Activated charcoal** binds with many toxic substances in the gastrointestinal (GI) tract to prevent them from being absorbed and then carries them out of the GI tract. If the patient is alert and cooperative, medical direction may instruct you to give the patient this medication. To reduce or prevent absorption of ingested poisons, activated charcoal should ideally be given within the first hour of the ingestion.

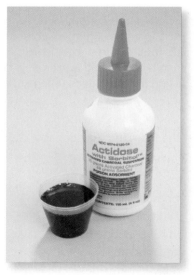

FIGURE 11-1 ▲ Activated charcoal is a suspension. It contains drug particles that are mixed with, but not dissolved in, a liquid.

Action

Activated charcoal binds (adsorbs) with many (but not all) chemicals, slowing down or blocking absorption of the chemical in the GI tract.

Activated charcoal is produced by heating wood pulp to high temperatures and then "activating" it with steam or strong acids. This process creates tiny pores on each particle of charcoal that increase its surface area. With this large surface area, activated charcoal will bind to many ingested toxins. However, charcoal can only bind to a drug that is *not yet absorbed* from the GI tract.

Activated charcoal does not bind well to such substances as some pesticides (malathion), cyanide, strong caustics (acids and alkalis), iron, mercury, ethanol, methanol, and petroleum products (such as gasoline, turpentine, and kerosene).

Indications

If ordered by medical direction (and approved by your state and local EMS system), you may give activated charcoal for some ingested poisons.

Contraindications

Contraindications for activated charcoal administration include the following:

- The patient has an altered mental status.
- The patient is unable to swallow.
- Medical direction does not give authorization.
- The patient has ingested acids or alkalis. Examples of acids include rust removers, phenol, and battery acid. Examples of alkalis include ammonia, household bleach, and drain cleaner.

Adverse Effects

Adverse effects of activated charcoal include abdominal cramping, constipation, and black stools. Some patients, particularly those who have ingested poisons that cause nausea, may vomit. If the patient vomits, consider repeating the dose once (check with medical direction).

Dosage

The dosage of activated charcoal for adults and children is 1 gram of activated charcoal per kilogram of body weight. The usual adult dose is 25 to 50 grams. The usual dose for an infant or child is 12.5 to 25 grams. If the activated charcoal is not premixed, mix the appropriate dosage in a glass of water (8 ounces) to produce a thick slurry.

You Should Know

Activated charcoal is given in doses according to the patient's body weight. The recommended dose is 1 gram (g) of activated charcoal per kilogram (kg) of the patient's body weight. One kg is equal to 2.2 pounds (lb). An *estimate* of the patient's weight in kg can be made by dividing by the patient's weight in pounds by 2 and then subtracting 10%. For example,

$$Patient\ weight = 200\ lb$$
$$200/2 = 100$$
$$100 \times 10\% = 10$$
$$100 - 10 = 90\ kg$$

In this example, a 200-lb patient weighs about 90 kg. The patient would receive about 90 g of activated charcoal. This is not an acceptable conversion method for a pediatric patient. For children, the preferred method is the actual calculation of the conversion in most cases. When obtaining authorization to give the medication from medical direction, request a dose amount from the physician (be prepared to give the patient's weight).

Route

Activated charcoal is administered orally.

Special Considerations

- Obtain an order from medical direction either on-line or off-line to give the medication.
- Before giving any medication, use appropriate personal protective equipment and make sure you have the right patient, right drug, right dose, right route, and right time. After giving the medication, document the patient's response to the medication.
- Activated charcoal can be harmful or fatal if the patient accidentally inhales it. Before giving this drug, you must make sure that the patient is awake, cooperative, has an open airway, and can swallow.

- Activated charcoal looks like mud. It is often helpful to put the medication in a cup, cover it with a lid, and have the patient drink the mixture through a straw.
- Do not give activated charcoal with ice cream, sherbet, milk, or other drinks. Because charcoal binds with whatever it is mixed with, flavoring with drinks impairs charcoal's capacity to bind with other substances.
- After giving charcoal, reassess the patient's airway, breathing, and circulatory status. Be prepared for the patient to vomit or for the patient's condition to worsen. Signs of worsening patient condition include decreasing mental status, increasing breathing difficulty, and decreasing blood pressure. If the patient's condition improves, give supportive care. Reassess the patient every 5 minutes. Transport promptly to the closest appropriate medical facility.

Administration Procedure

Skill Drill 11-1 shows the procedure for giving a patient activated charcoal.

Remember This

- Before giving activated charcoal, you must determine if your patient can follow directions and swallow safely.
- Activated charcoal looks like tar, stains any material with which it comes in contact, and does not taste good. Be prepared for the patient to spit out the medication.

Aspirin

Objective 2

Aspirin is a drug that has been used for many years. It is a nonnarcotic pain reliever, fever reducer, and anti-inflammatory medication.

Action

At low doses, aspirin inhibits platelet clumping, thus interfering with blood clotting. In prehospital care, aspirin is used for this purpose. In somewhat higher doses, it reduces fever and relieves aches and pains. In relatively large doses, aspirin reduces pain and inflammation in rheumatoid arthritis and several related diseases.

Giving Activated Charcoal

STEP 1 ▶ Put on appropriate personal protective equipment. Because charcoal will stain any clothing it contacts, take additional precautions as necessary. Obtain an order from medical direction either on-line or off-line. Make sure that the patient is awake, cooperative, has an open airway, and can swallow.

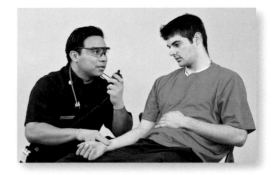

STEP 2 ▶ Make sure that the activated charcoal is not expired. Grasp the container in your hand and shake thoroughly.

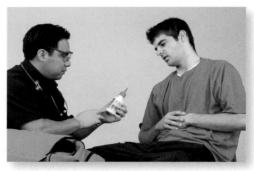

STEP 3 ▶ Cover the patient's lap or chest with old towels and have a large basin available should the patient vomit. Because charcoal looks like black mud, the patient may need to be persuaded to drink it. Place a straw in the container, or pour the activated charcoal into a covered opaque container, and ask the patient to drink it. If the patient does not drink all the medication in the first drink, shake the container before the second dose because the activated charcoal will settle to the bottom of the container or glass. Some patients, particularly those who have ingested poisons that cause nausea, may vomit. Vomiting may also occur when charcoal is drunk either too slowly or too rapidly. If the patient vomits, consider repeating the dose once (check with medical direction).

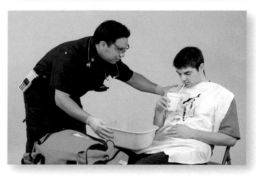

STEP 4 ▶ Document the patient's name, drug name and dose given, time of administration, and the patient's response to the drug. If an on-line order was received by medical direction, document the name of the physician giving the order. The patient will need to be transported for additional care. Reassess the patient every 5 minutes.

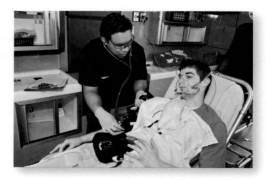

Indications

Aspirin is indicated for chest pain or other signs/symptoms suspected to be of cardiac origin, unless the patient is hypersensitive to aspirin. If ordered by medical direction, aspirin should be given as soon as possible after the patient's onset of chest discomfort.

Contraindications

Aspirin is contraindicated in the following situations:

- Known allergy or sensitivity to aspirin or other nonsteroidal anti-inflammatory medications (NSAIDs)
- Bleeding ulcer or bleeding disorders
- Children and adolescents

Adverse Effects

Adverse effects of aspirin administration may include the following:

- Rapid pulse
- Flushing
- Wheezing
- Nausea, vomiting
- Gastrointestinal bleeding
- Diarrhea
- Heartburn
- Loss of appetite
- Ringing in the ears (tinnitus)
- Rash
- Hives
- Bruising

Dosage

The adult dose of aspirin is two to four 81-mg tablets (pediatric aspirin), chewed and swallowed. Prehospital personnel should not administer aspirin to children and adolescents.

Route

Aspirin is administered orally. The patient must be awake, cooperative, have an open airway, and able to swallow.

Special Considerations

- Obtain an order from medical direction either on-line or off-line to give the medication.
- If ordered by medical direction, aspirin should be given as soon as possible after the patient's onset of chest discomfort.
- Use appropriate personal protective equipment.

- Practice the six rights of drug administration.
- Use with caution in patients with a history of asthma, nasal polyps, or nasal allergies. Severe allergic reactions in sensitive patients have occurred.

Administration Procedure

When administering aspirin, remember that the inside of the medicine container, its contents, and the inside of the container's cap are considered clean. Be careful not to touch these areas. Open the container, and pour the correct number into the inside cap of the container. Transfer the tablets by pouring them into the patient's hand, making sure not to contaminate the inside cap of the container, and then carefully recap the container.

You Should Know

In most EMS systems, an EMS dispatcher will ask a few precautionary screening questions and then instruct a patient who is experiencing a possible heart attack to take aspirin (if there are no contraindications).

Oral Glucose

Objective 3

Glucose, a sugar, is the basic fuel for body cells. If approved by medical direction (and your state and local EMS system), you may give **oral glucose** to a patient who has an altered mental status and a history of diabetes controlled by medication and is able to swallow (Figure 11-2). Oral glucose given to a patient with an altered mental status and a known history of diabetes can make a difference between development of coma (unconsciousness) and ability to maintain consciousness.

Before giving any medication, you must make sure that the medication to be given is indicated for the patient and that the patient does not have any allergies to

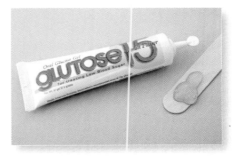

FIGURE 11-2 ▲ Oral glucose.

the medication. Even though you are giving glucose, it is possible that the patient may have an allergy to the way the drug is packaged or manufactured. If a drug contains any preservatives, the patient may have an adverse reaction to the preservative in the medication. Next, you must make sure that the patient is responsive, has an open airway, and can swallow. Because any patient who has an altered mental status has the potential to become unresponsive without warning, it is essential to make sure the patient has (and maintains) an open airway. If all these criteria are met and medical direction has given the order to administer the drug, oral glucose can be given.

Action

When administered, oral glucose increases the amount of sugar available for use as energy by the body.

Indications

Oral glucose is indicated for patients with an altered mental status who have a known history of diabetes controlled by medication and can swallow.

Remember This

Measurement of a patient's glucose level is an important part of the assessment of any patient who has an altered mental status. A patient's glucose level is measured by means of a glucometer. Use of a glucometer is not within an EMT's scope of practice in all states. Ask your instructor about the use of glucometers by EMTs in your area.

Contraindications

Oral glucose should not be given in the following situations:

- Medical direction does not give permission.
- The patient is unresponsive.
- The patient is unable to swallow.
- The patient has a known allergy to the glucose preparation.

Adverse Effects

Oral glucose may cause nausea. The drug may be aspirated by the patient without a gag reflex.

Dosage

The usual dose of glucose is one tube of oral glucose gel.

Route

Oral glucose is administered buccally.

Special Considerations

Ensure that the patient has signs and symptoms of altered mental status with a known history of diabetes. Make sure the patient is responsive, can swallow, and can protect her airway. Obtain an order from medical direction to give the medication. Before giving any medication, use appropriate personal protective equipment. Practice the six rights of drug administration.

Administration Procedure

Skill Drill 11-2 shows the procedure for giving a patient oral glucose.

Oxygen

Objective 4

Oxygen is a molecule that is needed for body metabolism. It is an odorless, colorless, and tasteless gas normally present in the atmosphere. When administered to a patient, oxygen is considered a medication and is the most common medication that you will administer. An oxygen delivery system is used to deliver oxygen from an oxygen cylinder to the patient (Figure 11-3). Oxygen administration is explained in more detail in Chapter 13, "Respiration."

Action

Giving oxygen increases the amount available in the bloodstream for use by the body's cells.

Indications

Oxygen is used in cardiac or respiratory arrest and any suspected cardiopulmonary emergency, especially complaints of shortness of breath or chest pain. Oxygen is

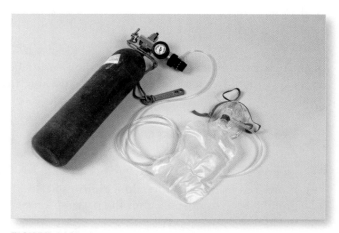

FIGURE 11-3 ▲ An oxygen delivery system.

Giving Oral Glucose

STEP 1 ▶
- Put on appropriate personal protective equipment.
- Obtain an order from medical direction either on-line or off-line.
- Confirm that the patient has an altered mental status, has a history of diabetes controlled by medication, and is able to swallow and protect his airway.

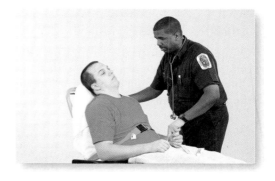

STEP 2 ▶ Squeeze the glucose from the tube onto a tongue depressor.

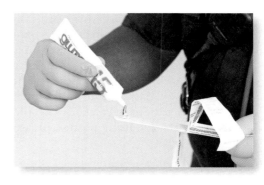

STEP 3 ▶
- Place the tongue depressor between the patient's cheek and gum.
- Remove the tongue depressor from the patient's mouth once the gel is dissolved or if the patient loses consciousness or seizes.

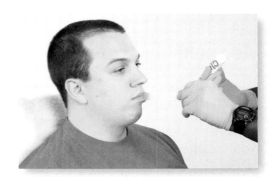

STEP 4 ▶
- Document the patient's name, drug name and dose given, time of administration, and response to the drug.
- If an on-line order was received by medical direction, document the name of the physician giving the order.
- Reassess every 5 minutes, continuously monitoring the patient's airway and breathing.

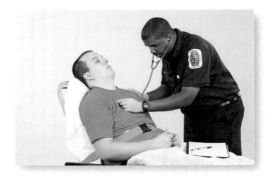

also indicated in cases of suspected low oxygen levels (hypoxia) from any cause. There are many causes of hypoxia. Examples include shock, heart failure, drowning, burns, seizures, diabetic emergency, altered mental status, trauma, pneumonia, hemorrhage, heart attack, head injury, or toxic inhalation.

Adverse Effects

Oxygen may reduce the respiratory drive in some patients with chronic obstructive pulmonary disease (see Chapter 21). Oxygen administration causes drying of the mucous membranes.

Dosage

Several oxygen delivery devices are used to administer oxygen. A nasal cannula and nonrebreather mask are used to deliver oxygen to a spontaneously breathing patient. Positive-pressure ventilation is used to deliver oxygen to a nonbreathing patient. The dosage of oxygen is determined by the patient's condition and the oxygen delivery device used. A nasal cannula is used with a liter flow of 1 to 6 L/min. A nonrebreather mask is used with a liter flow of 10 to 15 L/min. A patient in cardiac or respiratory arrest is given 100% oxygen using positive-pressure ventilation (see Chapter 14).

Route

Oxygen is administered as an inhaled gas.

Assisted Medications

After consulting with medical direction, some medications can be given to patients who fit established criteria. An EMT can assist a patient in taking the following physician-prescribed medications when authorized by medical direction:

- Epinephrine autoinjector
- Inhaled bronchodilators
- Nitroglycerin

Epinephrine

Objective 5

An epinephrine autoinjector is used to treat the patient experiencing a severe allergic reaction. An EMT may assist a patient with using an epinephrine autoinjector at the discretion of the EMT's program medical director. In some states, EMTs now carry epinephrine autoinjectors (EpiPens) on their EMS units and are not limited to administering the medication to patients who have been prescribed one.

An **autoinjector** is a drug delivery system that is designed to work through clothing. Applying firm, even pressure to the injector propels a spring-driven needle into the patient's skin (usually the thigh) and then injects the drug into the muscle. Physician authorization to administer the medication can be given either online or by standing orders at the discretion of the medical director.

Action

Epinephrine works by relaxing the bronchial passages of the airway and constricting the blood vessels. The opening of the airway allows the patient to move more air into and out of the lungs, and this will increase the amount of oxygen in the bloodstream. Constriction of the blood vessels slows the leakage of fluid from the blood vessels into the space around the cells of the body.

Indications

As an EMT, you can give epinephrine by means of an autoinjector if all the following criteria are met:

- The patient exhibits signs and symptoms of a severe allergic reaction, including respiratory distress and/or signs and symptoms of shock (see Chapter 32).
- The medication is prescribed for the patient, or your EMS system authorizes EMTs to carry the medication.
- Medical direction has authorized use for the patient.

Contraindications

There are no contraindications when an epinephrine autoinjector is used in a life-threatening situation.

Adverse Effects

Adverse effects of epinephrine include the following:

- Rapid heart rate
- Anxiety
- Excitability
- Nausea, vomiting
- Chest pain or discomfort
- Headache
- Dizziness

Dosage

EpiPens are available in two strengths (Figure 11-4). The EpiPen autoinjector (0.3 mg) is used for individuals weighing 66 pounds or more. The EpiPen Jr autoinjector (0.15 mg) is for individuals weighing between 33 and 66 pounds. Both strengths deliver a single dose.

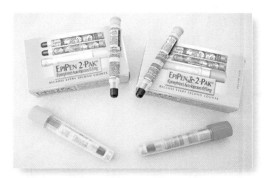

FIGURE 11-4 ▲ Epinephrine autoinjectors are available for adults and children.

Route

Epinephrine is administered intramuscularly by means of an autoinjector.

Special considerations:

- Use appropriate personal protective equipment.
- Practice the six rights of medication administration.
- Place the patient on a pulse oximeter, and give oxygen by nonrebreather mask. Monitor the patient's breath sounds, heart rate, and blood pressure closely before and after administration.
- Assess the patient's lung sounds before administration of epinephrine to establish a baseline (see Chapter 17). Assess lung sounds again after administration of epinephrine, and compare your findings.
- The effects of the injected epinephrine last about 10 to 20 minutes.
- Because a single dose of epinephrine may not completely reverse the effects of an anaphylactic reaction (even when the proper dose is given), the patient's physician may prescribe more than one autoinjector.
- Look closely at the autoinjector container. Make sure that the epinephrine is not expired (Figure 11-5). Look into the clear window of

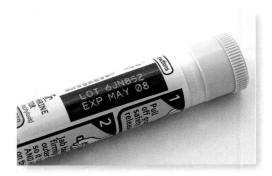

FIGURE 11-5 ▲ Look at the autoinjector container, and make sure that the epinephrine is not expired.

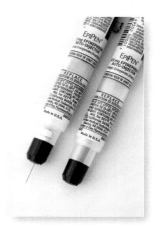

FIGURE 11-6 ▲ Look into the clear window of the EpiPen container. If a red flag is present in the window of the autoinjector, the epinephrine has already been injected.

the EpiPen container. The solution should be clear. If the solution is discolored or contains solid particles (precipitate), do not use the medication. If a red flag is present in the window of the autoinjector, the epinephrine has already been injected (Figure 11-6). Find out if the patient has already taken any doses before your arrival today or if the patient used the autoinjector in the past and forgot to get a new EpiPen.

You Should Know

- A physician may prescribe a child an EpiPen Jr, then change the child's prescription to the EpiPen because the recommended dose increases with age.
- Sometimes a child will not use the prescribed EpiPen due to fear of a potentially painful needlestick.

Administration Procedure

Skill Drill 11-3 shows the procedure for using an epinephrine autoinjector.

Inhaled Bronchodilators

Objective 6

A **metered-dose inhaler (MDI)** is used to deliver **bronchodilators** (inhaled respiratory medications) (Figure 11-7). A patient who has a prescribed MDI typically has reversible constriction of the airways. An MDI is small and consists of two parts, the medication canister and a plastic dispenser with a mouthpiece. Because some patients find it hard to coordinate breathing

Skill Drill 11-3

Administering an Epinephrine Autoinjector

STEP 1 ▶ Put on appropriate personal protective equipment. Confirm that the patient has signs or symptoms of a severe allergic reaction. Confirm that the patient has a physician-prescribed epinephrine autoinjector (or state/local protocols permit an EMT to carry and administer an autoinjector). Obtain an order from medical direction either on-line or off-line. Make sure that the epinephrine is not expired. Look into the clear window of the EpiPen container. The solution should be clear.

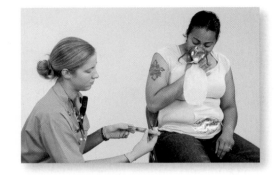

STEP 2 ▶ Remove (or assist the patient in removing) the EpiPen from its container by unscrewing the cap off of the EpiPen carrying case and removing the EpiPen from its storage tube.

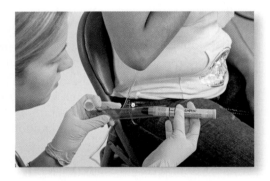

STEP 3 ▶ Grasp (or assist the patient in grasping) the EpiPen with the black tip pointing downward.

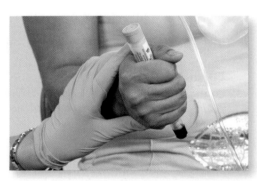

STEP 4 ▶ Form a fist (or have the patient do so) around the EpiPen (black tip down). With the other hand, pull off the "safety" cap from the other end of the autoinjector

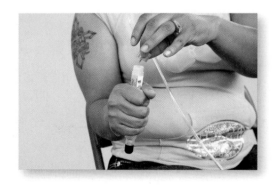

STEP 5 ▶ Press the autoinjector against the outside portion of one thigh (or assist the patient in doing so) for about 10 seconds until you hear it release. Hold the EpiPen perpendicular (at a 90-degree angle) to the thigh. It is designed to work through clothing but make sure pockets (if present) at the injection site are empty. The autoinjector will propel a spring-driven needle into the patient's thigh and then inject the drug into the muscle of the outer thigh. This will cause pain, and the patient may move very suddenly.

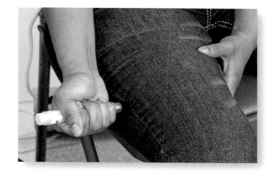

STEP 6 ▶ After the drug has been delivered, the window on the autoinjector will show red. Remove the EpiPen from the patient's thigh (or have the patient do so), and massage the injection area for 10 seconds. Carefully reinsert the EpiPen (without replacing the safety cap) needle-first into the storage tube. Document the patient's name, drug name and dose given, time of administration, and the patient's response to the drug. If an on-line order was received by medical direction, document the name of the physician giving the order. The patient will need to be transported for additional care. Reassess the patient every 5 minutes, continuously monitoring the patient's airway and breathing.

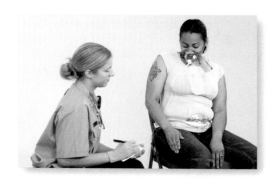

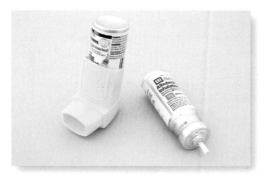

FIGURE 11-7 ▲ A metered-dose inhaler.

in and pressing the inhaler at the same time, a physician will often prescribe a "spacer" to be used with the MDI. The spacer increases the amount of medication delivered into the respiratory tract. The patient squeezes the MDI into a plastic holding chamber, then inhales the medication from the chamber. The use of spacers is very common in children and older adults.

Action

Medications contained in an MDI are usually beta-2 agonists. This means that the drug stimulates beta-2 receptor sites in the lungs. When these receptor sites are stimulated in the bronchioles, the smooth muscle tissue relaxes (dilates), reducing airway resistance. This makes it easier for the patient to move air in and out. Examples of inhaled bronchodilators include the following:

- albuterol (Proventil, Ventolin)
- isoetharine (Bronkosol)
- metaproterenol (Alupent, Metaprel)
- terbutaline (Bricanyl)
- formoterol fumarate (Foradil)
- pirbuterol (Maxair)
- salmeterol (Serevent)
- terbutaline (Brethine, Bricanyl)
- ipratropium bromide (Atrovent) (Note: Atrovent is not a beta-2 agonist)

Indications

As an EMT, you can assist a patient in using a prescribed inhaler if *all* the following criteria are met:

- The patient has signs and symptoms of a respiratory emergency.
- The patient has a physician-prescribed handheld inhaler.
- There are no contraindications to giving the medication.
- You have specific authorization by medical direction.

Contraindications

Assisting a patient with the use of an MDI is contraindicated if any of the following conditions exists:

- The patient is unable to use the device (this may be a result of the level of the patient's respiratory distress).
- The inhaler is not prescribed for the patient.
- Permission is not received from medical direction.
- The patient has already met the maximum prescribed dose before your arrival.

Adverse Effects

Adverse effects of inhaled bronchodilators include the following:

- Increased heart rate
- Shaking or tremors
- Restlessness
- Nervousness
- Nausea
- Headache
- Dizziness

Dosage

An MDI automatically delivers a specific dose of medication each time it is activated. The usual dosage is two puffs every 3 to 4 hours as needed for shortness of breath, associated with asthma and chronic obstructive pulmonary disease. The number of inhalations is based on medical direction's order or the patient's physician order.

Route

Although bronchodilators are available in many forms, the EMT may assist a patient in using a prescribed bronchodilator packaged in a metered-dose inhaler.

Special Considerations

- Use appropriate personal protective equipment.
- Practice the six rights of medication administration.
- Assist the patient in finding the MDI if it is not readily available.
- Assess the patient's vital signs, lung sounds, and oxygen saturation before administration of an MDI to establish a baseline. Assess vital signs, lung sounds, and oxygen saturation again after administration of the MDI, and compare your findings.
- Wait at least 3 minutes before assisting with another dose from the MDI.
- Reassess vital signs and the patient's degree of breathing difficulty.

Administration Procedure

Skill Drill 11-4 shows the procedure for assisting a patient with the prescribed MDI.

Nitroglycerin

Objective 7

Nitroglycerin (NTG) is used to treat chest discomfort that is believed to be cardiac in origin.

Action

NTG causes dilation (expansion) of the smooth muscle of blood vessel walls. Relaxation of the veins results in pooling of blood in the dependent portions of the body as a result of gravity. This effect reduces the amount of blood returning to the heart, decreasing the heart's workload. NTG causes some relaxation of the walls of arteries, including the coronary arteries. This helps reduce the resistance the heart must overcome to pump blood throughout the body, thus decreasing the heart's workload.

Indications

As an EMT, you can assist a patient in taking prescribed NTG if all the following criteria are met:

- The patient has signs and symptoms of chest pain or discomfort.
- The patient has physician-prescribed NTG.
- There are no contraindications to giving the medication.
- You have specific authorization by medical direction (off-line or on-line).

Assisting a Patient with a Metered-Dose Inhaler

STEP 1 ▶
- Contact medical direction for an order to assist with giving this medication.
- Make sure that you have the right medication, right patient, right route of administration, and that the patient is alert enough to use the medication.
- Check the expiration date of the inhaler.
- Check to see when the last dose was taken by the patient.
- Make sure the inhaler is at room temperature or warmer.
- Shake the inhaler, vigorously, several times.
- If the patient is wearing an oxygen mask, remove it now.

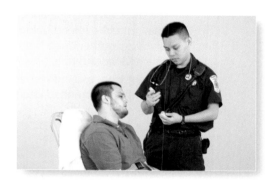

STEP 2 ▶ Invert the inhaler as shown. Have the patient exhale deeply, and then have him put his lips around the mouthpiece of the inhaler.

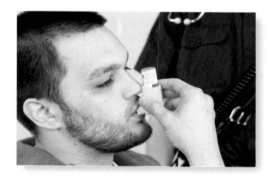

STEP 3 ▶ If the patient has a spacer device for use with the inhaler, it should be used. If a spacer is used, have the patient depress the inhaler to inject the dose into the chamber of the spacer. This is done before placing the mouthpiece of the spacer in the mouth.

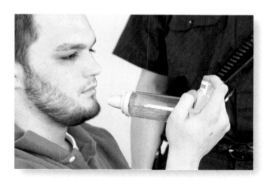

STEP 4 ▶
- Have the patient depress the MDI as he begins to inhale deeply. Help the patient direct the spray into his mouth as he attempts to take a breath.
- Instruct the patient to hold his breath as long as he comfortably can. (This helps with medication absorption.)

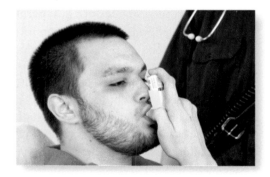

Continued

Assisting a Patient with a Metered-Dose Inhaler *Continued*

STEP 5 ▶
- If the patient is using a spacer, have him depress the inhaler, breathe in and hold his breath, breathe out, and then take another deep breath through the mouthpiece of the spacer and hold his breath.
- A patient who is using a spacer should try to take two deep breaths from the spacer and hold them for each puff from his inhaler.

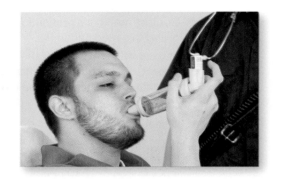

STEP 6 ▶
- Replace the previously removed oxygen mask. Recheck the patient's lung sounds, vital signs, oxygen saturation, and degree of breathing difficulty.
- Repeat the dose after 1–3 minutes per instructions from medical direction.
- When finished with the inhaler, wipe off the mouthpiece with an alcohol swab and replace the cap.
- After using an MDI, have the patient rinse his mouth out with water. This will decrease the possibility of adverse effects from the medication.

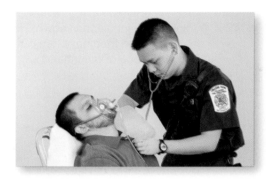

Contraindications

Assisting a patient in taking prescribed nitroglycerin is contraindicated if *any* of the following conditions exists:

- Medical direction does not give permission.
- The medication is not prescribed for the patient.
- The patient has already taken the maximum prescribed dose before the EMT's arrival.
- The patient has hypotension (systolic blood pressure below 100 mm Hg).
- The patient has a heart rate less than 50 beats/minute or more than 100 beats/minute.
- The patient has had a head injury (recent) or stroke (recent).
- The patient is an infant or child.
- The patient has taken a medication for erectile dysfunction within the last 24 to 48 hours.

Adverse Effects

Hypotension is a common and significant adverse effect. Other adverse effects include tachycardia, bradycardia, headache, palpitations, and fainting.

Dosage

The dosage is one tablet or one spray under the tongue. This dose may be repeated in 3 to 5 minutes (maximum of three doses) if:

- The patient experiences no relief.
- The patient's systolic blood pressure remains above 100 mm Hg.
- The patient's heart rate remains between 50 and 100 beats/minute.
- There are no other contraindications.
- The EMT is authorized by medical direction to give another dose of the medication.

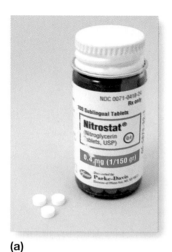
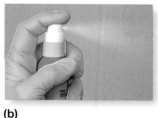

(a)   **(b)**

FIGURE 11-8 ▲ Sublingual nitroglycerin is available in **(a)** tablet and **(b)** spray form.

Route

NTG is available in many forms. An EMT may assist a patient in taking prescribed sublingual NTG tablets or spray (Figure 11-8).

Special Considerations

- Wear appropriate personal protective equipment.
- Practice the six rights of drug administration.
- NTG works quickly. Relief of chest pain or discomfort may occur within 1 to 2 minutes of administration. Its effects last about 5 to 7 minutes.
- If authorized by medical direction, NTG can be repeated every 5 minutes for up to three tablets or sprays (provided the patient's vital signs remain stable). Ask the patient to rate the discomfort after each dose so you can detect any changes in the patient's condition.
- Monitor the patient's heart rate and blood pressure closely before and after administration. Compare the patient's blood pressure after each dose of NTG with the baseline blood pressure.
- Do not give another dose of NTG if the patient's blood pressure drops below 100 mm Hg systolic or is 30 mm Hg or more below the patient's baseline systolic blood pressure. If the blood pressure is below 100 mm Hg systolic, place the patient in a supine position and reassess the blood pressure.

Remember This

- NTG is a frequently "shared" medication. Make sure that the medication belongs to the patient and that you have contacted medical direction before giving it.

- You will need to ask the patient if he or she has taken any drugs for sexual enhancement, such as Viagra or Cialis. Although once thought to be used only by men for erectile problems, these medications are also used by women. Giving NTG to a patient who has taken these drugs within 24 to 48 hours may lead to irreversible hypotension and death.

Administration Procedure

Skill Drills 11-5 and 11-6 show the procedure for assisting a patient with prescribed NTG.

Special Situations

Nerve Agent Antidotes

Objectives 8, 9, 10, 11, 12

Nerve agents are chemical weapons that interrupt nerve signals, causing a loss of consciousness within seconds and death within minutes of exposure. Examples include tabun, sarin, soman, VX or organophosphate (Lorsban, Cygon, Delnav, Malathion, Supracide, Parathion, Carbopenthion), or carbamate (Sevin) pesticides. Routes of exposure to nerve agents include inhalation as a gas, absorption through the skin, or ingestion of a liquid or food.

An **antidote** is a substance that neutralizes a poison. Nerve agent antidotes are used for individuals experiencing symptoms after suspected exposure to these substances. Signs and symptoms of exposure are listed in Table 11-1 on p. 236.

Atropine sulfate and pralidoxime chloride (nerve agent antidotes) are the initial medications used in treating individuals who have symptoms of a nerve agent exposure. These medications are conveniently packaged in autoinjectors known as Mark I kits. In the event of a mass exposure to a nerve agent, these kits are designed for self-treatment and treatment of other members of the initial emergency response team. Administer a nerve agent autoinjector kit if you or a peer has serious signs or symptoms that indicate the presence of nerve agent poisoning and you are authorized to do so by medical direction. Do not administer the nerve agent autoinjector kit if mild signs and symptoms, such as tearing or runny nose, are the only signs of nerve agent poisoning present.

Nerve agent antidotes are available in two types. The Mark I kit contains two separate autoinjectors—one for atropine and one for pralidoxime chloride (Figure 11-9 on p. 236). The Mark I kit is also called

Assisting a Patient with Prescribed Nitroglycerin Tablets

STEP 1 ▶
- Put on appropriate personal protective equipment.
- Confirm that the patient has signs or symptoms of chest pain/discomfort. Place the patient on a pulse oximeter, and give oxygen by nonrebreather mask.

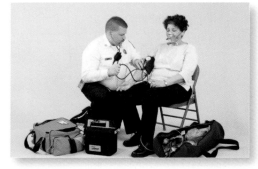

STEP 2 ▶
- Confirm that the patient has physician-prescribed nitroglycerin. Make sure that the nitroglycerin is not expired and that the patient is alert.
- Determine if the patient has already taken any doses. If so, find out the time of the last dose and the effects of the medication.
- Assess the patient's vital signs to make sure that the patient's systolic blood pressure is 100 mm Hg or greater and her heart rate is between 50 beats/minute and 100 beats/minute.
- If there are no contraindications, obtain an order from medical direction (either on-line or off-line) to assist the patient in taking the medication.

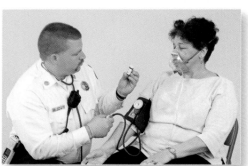

STEP 3 ▶
- Remove the oxygen mask from the patient.
- Pour one nitroglycerin tablet into the bottle cap. Ask the patient to lift her tongue while you place the tablet under the tongue (while wearing gloves), or have the patient place the tablet under the tongue.
- Have the patient keep her mouth closed with the tablet under the tongue (without swallowing) until it is dissolved and absorbed.

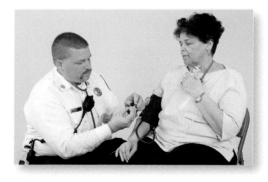

STEP 4 ▶
- Replace the oxygen mask on the patient.
- Recheck the patient's vital signs within 2 minutes. Reassess the patient's degree of discomfort.
- Document the patient's name, drug name and dose given, time of administration, and the patient's response to the drug.
- If an on-line order was received by medical direction, document the name of the physician giving the order.
- Reassess every 5 minutes, continuously monitoring the patient's airway and breathing.

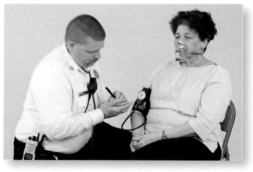

Assisting a Patient with Prescribed Nitroglycerin Spray

STEP 1 ▶
- Put on appropriate personal protective equipment.
- Confirm that the patient has signs or symptoms of chest pain/discomfort.

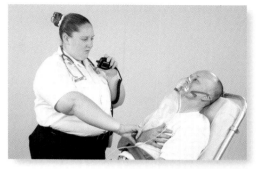

STEP 2 ▶
- Confirm that the patient has physician-prescribed nitroglycerin. Make sure that the nitroglycerin is not expired and that the patient is alert.
- Determine if the patient has already taken any doses. If so, find out the time of the last dose and the effects of the medication.
- Assess the patient's vital signs to make sure that the patient's systolic blood pressure is 100 mm Hg or greater and his heart rate is between 50 beats/minute and 100 beats/minute.
- If there are no contraindications, obtain an order from medical direction (either on-line or off-line) to assist the patient in taking the medication.

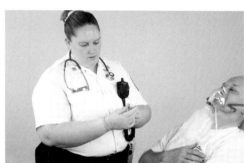

STEP 3 ▶
- Remove the oxygen mask from the patient.
- Ask the patient to lift his tongue while you spray the medication under his tongue (while wearing gloves), or have the patient self-administer the drug under his tongue.
- Have the patient keep his mouth closed (without swallowing) until the drug is absorbed.

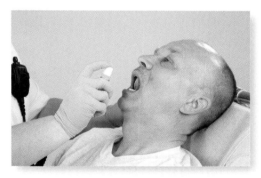

STEP 4 ▶
- Replace the oxygen mask on the patient.
- Recheck the patient's vital signs within 2 minutes. Reassess the patient's degree of discomfort.
- Document the patient's name, drug name and dose given, time of administration, and the patient's response to the drug.
- If an on-line order was received by medical direction, document the name of the physician giving the order.
- Reassess every 5 minutes, continuously monitoring the patient's airway and breathing.

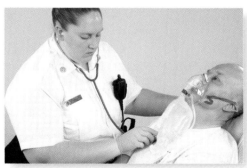

TABLE 11-1 Signs and Symptoms of Nerve Agent Exposure

Mild signs/symptoms	Tearing Unexplained runny nose
Moderate signs/symptoms	Drooling Excessive sweating Nausea and/or vomiting Abdominal cramps Diarrhea Tightness in chest Muscle twitching at site of exposure Pinpoint pupils resulting in blurred vision Difficulty breathing, shortness of breath, wheezing
Severe signs/symptoms	Strange or confused behavior Severe difficulty breathing or severe secretions from the airway Muscle twitching, jerking, staggering Drowsiness General weakness Headache Involuntary urination Involuntary defecation (bowel movement) Seizures Apnea Unconsciousness

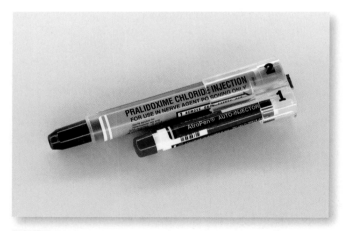

FIGURE 11-9 ▲ The Mark I kit contains two separate autoinjectors—one for atropine and one for pralidoxime chloride.

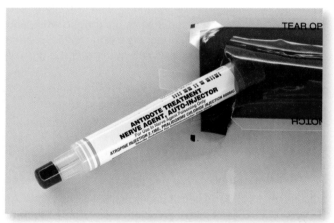

FIGURE 11-10 ▲ The DuoDote, approved by the FDA in 2007, is a prefilled autoinjector that delivers atropine and pralidoxime chloride in one intramuscular injection.

Nerve Agent Antidote Kit, or NAAK. DuoDote, approved by the FDA in 2007, is a prefilled autoinjector that delivers atropine and pralidoxime chloride in one intramuscular injection (Figure 11-10). Nerve agents are discussed in more detail in Chapters 28 and 53.

Atropine

Action

Atropine reverses some effects of nerve agent poisoning. It increases heart rate, relaxes bronchioles, dries secretions, and decreases gastric motility. Atropine also dilates pupils.

Indications

An EMT can self-administer an atropine autoinjector or can administer it to a peer if *all* the following criteria are met:

- The EMT or a peer has signs and symptoms consistent with nerve agent exposure.
- The EMT has specific authorization by medical direction.

Contraindications

In the face of life-threatening poisoning by chemical nerve agents, there are no absolute contraindications for the use of atropine.

Adverse Effects

Adverse effects of atropine administration may include the following:

- Mild to moderate pain possible at the site of injection
- Dryness of the mouth
- Blurred vision
- Confusion
- Headache
- Dizziness
- Tachycardia
- Palpitations
- Flushing
- Urinary hesitance or retention
- Constipation
- Nausea, vomiting

Dosage

One adult autoinjector contains about 2 mg of atropine in 0.7 mL.

Route

Atropine is administered intramuscularly by means of an autoinjector.

Special Considerations

More than one dose of atropine may be necessary initially, especially when exposure is massive or symptoms are severe. However, no more than three doses should be administered unless under the supervision of trained medical personnel. High doses of atropine may be required for many hours following high-dose exposure. Generally, one Mark I or DuoDote kit is used to treat moderate symptoms, and three kits are used for severe symptoms.

Atropine needs to be kept at room temperature. It should not be refrigerated or exposed to extreme heat, such as in the glove compartment of an emergency vehicle during the summer. Do not expose the atropine autoinjector to direct sunlight; light and heat can cause atropine to degrade.

When transferring care to receiving facility personnel, relay (and document) the following information:

- The substance (nerve agent) the patient was exposed to
- How long ago the exposure occurred
- The signs and symptoms the patient experienced (difficulty breathing, secretions, pinpoint pupils, etc.) before the atropine was administered
- The time and dose of the atropine administered
- Any change(s) in the patient's condition after the atropine was administered

Administration Procedure

Put on appropriate personal protective equipment. Reassure the patient and administer oxygen. If the patient is confused, disoriented, or unconscious, place the patient in a supine position. If the patient has a weak, rapid pulse and/or cool, clammy skin, place the patient in a supine position.

Confirm that the patient has signs or symptoms of nerve agent exposure and that atropine administration is warranted. Obtain an order from medical direction either on-line or off-line. Make sure that the atropine is not expired and that the solution in the window of the autoinjector is clear.

Remove the atropine autoinjector (AtroPen™) from its container by unscrewing the cap of the AtroPen carrying case and removing the AtroPen from its storage tube. Grasp the AtroPen with the tip pointing downward. Form a fist around the AtroPen (tip down). With the other hand, pull off the safety cap from the other end of the autoinjector. Do not place your fingers over the tip of the autoinjector when removing the safety cap or after the safety cap has been removed.

Press the autoinjector against the outside portion of one thigh for about 10 seconds until you hear it release. Hold the AtroPen perpendicular (at a 90-degree angle) to the thigh. The AtroPen can be injected through clothing but make sure pockets (if present) at the injection site are empty. Remove the autoinjector from the thigh, and massage the injection site for several seconds. Record the time of the injection. Properly dispose of the AtroPen after it has been activated. The manufacturer recommends showing used AtroPens to the next medical person you encounter to allow them to see the number and dose of AtroPens administered. Check your agency's policy regarding this practice.

Document the patient's name, drug name and dose given, time of administration, and the patient's response to the drug. If an on-line order was received by medical direction, document the name of the physician giving the order. The patient will need to be transported for additional care. Reassess the patient every 5 minutes, continuously monitoring the patient's airway and breathing.

Pralidoxime Chloride

Pralidoxime chloride (2-PAM) is given in conjunction with atropine in cases of nerve agent poisoning. Its trade name is 2-PAM chloride.

Action

Pralidoxime chloride reverses some effects of nerve agent poisoning, such as muscle twitching and difficulty breathing.

Indications

An EMT can self-administer a 2-PAM autoinjector or can administer it to a peer if all the following criteria are met:

- The EMT or a peer has signs and symptoms consistent with nerve agent exposure.
- The EMT has specific authorization by medical direction.

Contraindications

In the face of life-threatening poisoning by chemical nerve agents, there are no absolute contraindications for the use of pralidoxime chloride.

Adverse Effects

Adverse effects of pralidoxime chloride may include the following:

- Mild to moderate pain experienced at the site of injection 40 to 60 minutes after intramuscular injection
- Tachycardia
- Hypertension
- Muscle weakness
- Nausea
- Blurred or double vision
- Dizziness
- Increased blood pressure
- Loss of coordination
- Headache
- Drowsiness

Dosage

One adult autoinjector contains 600 mg of pralidoxime chloride in 2 mL.

Route

Pralidoxime chloride is administered intramuscularly by means of an autoinjector.

Special Considerations

Generally, one 2-PAM kit is used to treat moderate symptoms, and three kits are used for severe symptoms. When transferring care to receiving facility personnel, relay (and document) the following information:

- The substance (nerve agent) the patient was exposed to
- How long ago the exposure occurred
- The signs and symptoms the patient experienced (difficulty breathing, secretions, pinpoint pupils, etc.) before the 2-PAM was administered
- The time and dose of the 2-PAM administered
- Any change(s) in the patient's condition after the 2-PAM was administered

Administration Procedure

Put on appropriate personal protective equipment. Reassure the patient and administer oxygen. If the patient is confused, disoriented, or unconscious, place the patient in a supine position. If the patient has a weak, rapid pulse and/or cool, clammy skin, place the patient in a supine position.

Confirm that the patient has signs or symptoms of nerve agent exposure and that 2-PAM administration is warranted. Obtain an order from medical direction either on-line or off-line. Make sure that the drug is not expired and that the solution in the window of the autoinjector is clear.

Remove the 2-PAM autoinjector from its container by unscrewing the cap of the autoinjector carrying case and removing the autoinjector from its storage tube. Grasp the 2-PAM autoinjector with the tip pointing downward. Form a fist around the 2-PAM autoinjector (tip down). With the other hand, pull off the safety cap from the other end of the autoinjector. Do not place your fingers over the tip of the autoinjector when removing the safety cap or after the safety cap has been removed.

Press the autoinjector against the outside portion of one thigh for about 10 seconds until you hear it release. Hold the 2-PAM autoinjector perpendicular (at a 90-degree angle) to the thigh. The 2-PAM autoinjector can be injected through clothing but make sure pockets (if present) at the injection site are empty. Remove the autoinjector from the thigh and massage the injection site. Record the time of the injection. Properly dispose of the autoinjector after it has been activated. When using a DuoDote autoinjector, the manufacturer recommends leaving used DuoDote autoinjectors with the patient to allow other medical personnel to see the number of DuoDote autoinjectors administered. Check your agency's policy regarding this practice.

Document the patient's name, drug name and dose given, time of administration, and the patient's response to the drug. If an on-line order was received by medical direction, document the name of the physician giving the order. The patient will need to be transported for additional care. Reassess the patient every 5 minutes, continuously monitoring the patient's airway and breathing.

Diazepam

Objective 13

Diazepam (Valium) is used to control seizures following severe exposure to nerve agents (and similar toxins). Diazepam may be carried in a single autoinjector called *convulsant antidote for nerve agent (CANA)* (Figure 11-11).

Action

Diazepam relaxes skeletal muscle and controls seizures.

Indications

Seizures that occur because of nerve agent exposure often respond to atropine and pralidoxime chloride. Therefore, diazepam is generally recommended only if seizures persist after three Mark I (or DuoDote) kits have been given and the EMT has specific authorization by medical direction.

Contraindications

Use of a diazepam autoinjector is contraindicated if the patient is sensitive to any component of the product.

Adverse Effects

Mild to moderate pain may be experienced at the site of injection 40 to 60 minutes after intramuscular injection. Diazepam administration may result in dizziness, drowsiness, confusion, and respiratory depression.

Dosage

One autoinjector contains 10 mg of diazepam.

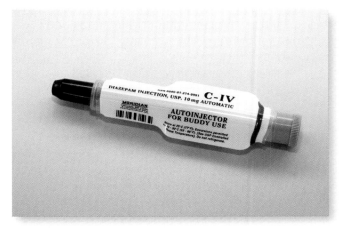

FIGURE 11-11 ▲ Diazepam is used to control seizures following severe exposure to nerve agents (and similar toxins).

Route

Diazepam is administered intramuscularly by means of an autoinjector.

Special Considerations

Diazepam is a relatively short-acting drug. Seizure activity may recur. When administered intramuscularly, the onset of action of diazepam is about 15 to 30 minutes. Monitor blood pressure, pulse, and respiratory rate every 5 minutes.

Administration Procedure

Put on appropriate personal protective equipment. Place the patient in a supine position and administer oxygen, if possible. Obtain an order from medical direction either on-line or off-line. Make sure that the diazepam is not expired and that the solution in the window of the autoinjector is clear.

Remove the diazepam autoinjector from its container by unscrewing the cap of the carrying case and removing the autoinjector from its storage tube. Grasp the autoinjector with the tip pointing downward. Form a fist around the autoinjector (tip down). With the other hand, pull off the safety cap from the other end of the autoinjector. Do not place your fingers over the tip of the autoinjector when removing the safety cap or after the safety cap has been removed.

Press the autoinjector against the outside portion of one thigh for about 10 seconds until you hear it release. Hold the autoinjector perpendicular (at a 90-degree angle) to the thigh. The autoinjector can be injected through clothing but make sure pockets (if present) at the injection site are empty. Remove the autoinjector from the thigh. Record the time of the injection. Properly dispose of the autoinjector after it has been activated.

Document the patient's name, drug name and dose given, time of administration, and the patient's response to the drug. If an on-line order was received by medical direction, document the name of the physician giving the order. The patient will need to be transported for additional care. Reassess the patient every 5 minutes, continuously monitoring the patient's airway and breathing.

On the Scene   Wrap-Up

Because you work in an area that allows EMTs to carry and give an EpiPen autoinjector, you are able to assist the patient with the use of this lifesaving drug. Your knowledge of the indications, contraindications, adverse effects, and appropriate dose of the medications discussed in this chapter can and will help you save lives. ■

▶ The medications that are most commonly found in EMS units include activated charcoal, aspirin, oral glucose, and oxygen.

▶ In some EMS systems, activated charcoal is administered in specific situations involving ingested poisons. Activated charcoal binds with many toxic substances in the GI tract to prevent them from being absorbed and then carries them out of the GI tract.

▶ Aspirin is a nonnarcotic pain reliever, fever reducer, and anti-inflammatory medication. At low doses, aspirin inhibits platelet clumping, thus interfering with blood clotting. In prehospital care, aspirin is used for this purpose. Aspirin is indicated for chest pain or other signs/symptoms suspected to be of cardiac origin, unless the patient is hypersensitive to aspirin.

▶ Glucose, a sugar, is the basic fuel for body cells. If approved by medical direction (and your state and local EMS system), you may give oral glucose to a patient who has an altered mental status and a history of diabetes controlled by medication and is able to swallow.

▶ Oxygen is a molecule that is needed for body metabolism. It is an odorless, colorless, and tasteless gas normally present in the atmosphere. When administered to a patient, oxygen is considered a medication and is the most common medication that you will administer. An oxygen delivery system is used to deliver oxygen from an oxygen cylinder to the patient.

▶ After consulting with medical direction, some medications can be given to patients who fit established criteria. An EMT can assist a patient in taking the following physician-prescribed medications when authorized by medical direction: epinephrine autoinjector, inhaled bronchodilators, and nitroglycerin.

▶ An epinephrine autoinjector is used to treat the patient experiencing a severe allergic reaction. An EMT may assist a patient with using an epinephrine autoinjector at the discretion of the program medical director. In some states, EMTs now carry EpiPens on their EMS units and are not limited to administering the medication to patients who have been prescribed one.

▶ A metered-dose inhaler is used to deliver inhaled respiratory medications. A patient who has a prescribed MDI typically has reversible constriction of the airways. Medications contained in an MDI are usually beta-2 agonists. This means that the drug stimulates beta-2 receptor sites in the lungs. When these receptor sites are stimulated in the bronchioles, the smooth muscle tissue relaxes (dilates), reducing airway resistance. This makes it easier for the patient to move air in and out.

▶ Nitroglycerin is used to treat chest discomfort that is believed to be cardiac in origin. NTG causes relaxation (dilation) of the smooth muscle of blood vessel walls. Relaxation of the veins results in pooling of blood in the dependent portions of the body as a result of gravity. This effect reduces the amount of blood returning to the heart, decreasing the heart's workload. NTG causes some relaxation of the walls of arteries, including the coronary arteries. This helps reduce the resistance the heart must overcome to pump blood out to the body, thus decreasing the heart's workload.

▶ Nerve agents are chemical weapons that interrupt nerve signals, causing a loss of consciousness within seconds and death within minutes of exposure. Routes of exposure to nerve agents include inhalation as a gas, absorption through the skin, or ingestion of a liquid or food. An antidote is a substance that neutralizes a poison. Nerve agent antidotes are used for individuals experiencing symptoms after suspected exposure to these substances.

▶ Atropine sulfate and pralidoxime chloride (nerve agent antidotes) are the initial medications used in treating individuals with symptoms of nerve agent exposure. Diazepam (Valium) is used to control seizures following severe exposure to nerve agents (and similar toxins).

Module 4

Airway Management, Respiration, Ventilation

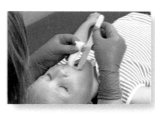

► CHAPTER 12

Airway Management   242

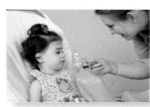

► CHAPTER 13

Respiration   259

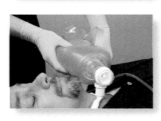

► CHAPTER 14

Artificial Ventilation   279

12

Airway Management

By the end of this chapter, you should be able to:

Knowledge Objectives ▶

1. Name and describe the locations and functions of the organs of the respiratory system.
2. Discuss the mechanics of breathing.
3. Discuss how the respiratory system anatomy of infants and young children differs from that of older children and adults.
4. Discuss how the respiratory system anatomy of older adults differs from that of younger adults.
5. List the signs of an adequate airway.
6. List the signs of an inadequate airway.
7. Describe the purpose, indications, contraindications, complications, and procedure for performing the head tilt–chin lift.
8. Relate mechanism of injury to opening the airway.
9. Describe the purpose, indications, contraindications, complications, and procedure for performing the modified jaw thrust maneuver.
10. Describe assessment findings and symptoms of a foreign body airway obstruction.
11. Describe the manual techniques used to relieve a foreign body airway obstruction.
12. State the importance of having a suction unit ready for immediate use when providing emergency medical care.
13. Discuss the advantages and disadvantages of mechanically powered suction devices.
14. Discuss the advantages and disadvantages of hand-powered suction devices.
15. Describe the purpose, indications, contraindications, complications, and procedure for suctioning the upper airway.
16. Describe the purpose of the recovery position and the steps for placing a patient in this position.
17. Describe the purpose, indications, contraindications, complications, and procedure for using an oral airway.
18. Describe the purpose, indications, contraindications, complications, and procedure for using a nasal airway.

Attitude Objectives ▶

19. Explain why airway protective skills take priority over most other basic life support skills.
20. Demonstrate a caring attitude toward patients with airway problems who request medical assistance.
21. Place the interests of the patient with airway problems as the foremost consideration when making patient care decisions.

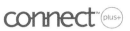
22. Communicate with empathy to patients with airway problems, as well as with family members and friends of the patient.
23. Demonstrate the steps in performing the head tilt–chin lift.
24. Demonstrate the steps in performing the modified jaw thrust maneuver.
25. Demonstrate the techniques of suctioning.
26. Demonstrate how to insert an oral airway.
27. Demonstrate how to insert a nasal airway.

On the Scene

You and your partner pull up to a house for "an unconscious person." After donning gloves and grabbing your emergency kit, you approach the door where a tearful woman directs you to the bathroom. She tells you, "It's my brother—I can't wake him up." An elderly man is seated limply on the toilet with his chin on his chest. You can see that his skin is gray and his chest is slowly rising and falling. You hear a harsh, high-pitched sound when he inhales. ■

THINK ABOUT IT

As you read this chapter, think about the following questions:

* How does your knowledge of airway anatomy and physiology help you identify the patient's medical problem?
* What findings suggest that he has an inadequate airway?
* What resources or equipment will be needed to properly care for this patient?
* What is the most appropriate method to open his airway?

Introduction

Airway Management

All living cells of the body require oxygen and produce carbon dioxide. Oxygen is particularly important to cells of the nervous system because, without it, brain cells begin to die within 4 to 6 minutes. The most stressful and chaotic scene usually involves a difficult airway. A nonbreathing patient or a patient with difficulty breathing is experiencing a true emergency. To prevent death, you must be able to recognize early signs of breathing difficulty and know what to do.

The Respiratory System

The Functions of the Respiratory System

One of the major functions of the respiratory system is to deliver oxygen from the atmosphere to the bloodstream (Figure 12-1). Another major function is to remove carbon dioxide produced by the body cells from the bloodstream and release it in the atmosphere. As an emergency medical technician, you must make sure these functions happen by maintaining an open airway and ensuring that the patient is breathing adequately. Maintaining an open airway allows a free flow of air into and out of the lungs.

Anatomy Review

The upper airway is made up of structures outside the chest cavity. These structures include the nose, the pharynx, and the larynx. The lower airway consists of parts found almost entirely within the chest cavity, such as the trachea and the lungs.

The Upper Airway

Objective 1

The nose warms, humidifies, and filters the air before it enters the lungs. A wall of tissue called the **septum** separates the right and left nostrils. A bent nasal septum is called a **deviated septum.** The nasal septum may

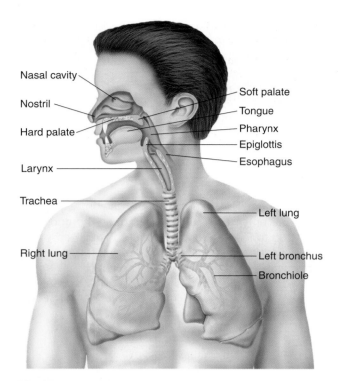

Nasal cavity
Nostril
Soft palate
Hard palate
Tongue
Pharynx
Epiglottis
Larynx
Esophagus
Trachea
Left lung
Right lung
Left bronchus
Bronchiole

FIGURE 12-1 ▲ The anatomy of the respiratory system.

bend because of trauma, such as during birth or a blow to the nose. A deviated septum can obstruct the nasal cavity, making breathing difficult.

The nose is lined with a mucous membrane that is fragile. When the nose is subjected to trauma, it is prone to bleed and become inflamed, and this can cause an airway obstruction. The nose is susceptible to trauma because of its location on the face. The nasal cavity is separated from the cranium by a thin bone that can become fractured as a result of head trauma. The nasal cavity is separated from the oral cavity by the hard palate.

The mouth, also call the *oral cavity,* is formed by the cheeks, lips, hard palate, and soft palate. Air enters the body through the mouth or nose and passes down the pharynx (throat), past the epiglottis, down the trachea, and into the lungs. Air entering the mouth is not filtered or warmed as efficiently as air entering the nostrils.

The **pharynx** is a funnel-shaped muscular tube that serves as a passageway for food, liquids, and air. The uppermost part of the pharynx, the **nasopharynx,** is located directly behind the nasal cavity and serves as a passageway for air only. The **oropharynx** opens into the mouth and serves as a passageway for both food and air. It is separated from the nasopharynx by the soft palate. The lowermost part of the throat, the **laryngopharynx,** surrounds the openings of the esophagus and larynx. It opens in the front into the larynx and in the

back into the esophagus. It serves as a passageway for both food and air.

The **larynx** contains the vocal cords. This area is the narrowest part of an adult's airway. The vocal cords are responsible for sound production. The space between the vocal cords is called the *glottis.* The largest cartilage of the larynx is the thyroid cartilage, also called the *Adam's apple.* The **cricoid cartilage** is the most inferior (lowest) of the cartilages of the larynx. The narrowest part of a child's airway is at the level of the cricoid cartilage. The **epiglottis** is a piece of cartilage that protects the lower airway from **aspiration.** When we swallow, the epiglottis helps in closing the glottic opening, preventing food and liquid from entering the trachea. Choking may result if the epiglottis fails to close.

The upper airway is the most common place for an airway obstruction to occur. When a patient becomes unresponsive, the tongue falls back into the posterior oropharynx (the back of the mouth). This can cause a complete airway obstruction. Other common causes of upper airway obstruction are dislodged teeth or dentures, blood, body secretions, and foreign objects. An airway obstruction at or below the vocal cords will affect the ability to produce sound. You must be able to recognize signs of an airway obstruction and act quickly to remove the object in order for the patient to survive.

You Should Know

The jobs of the upper airway are to warm, filter, and humidify air. Upper airway problems often begin suddenly. Patients with upper airway problems must be watched closely because they may quickly worsen while you are providing care.

The job of the lower airway is the exchange of oxygen and carbon dioxide. Lower airway problems usually take longer to develop than upper airway problems. Although patients must be watched closely, lower airway problems are less likely to cause sudden changes in a patient's condition while you are providing care.

The Lower Airway

Objective 1

The **trachea,** or windpipe, connects the larynx to the main bronchi. It extends to the level of the upper and middle portion of the breastbone (sternum). The trachea is protected and supported by C-shaped rings of cartilage. This allows for some expansion during breathing and coughing. At about the middle of the breastbone, the trachea divides into two main branches. One branch, the right primary bronchus, allows air in and out of the right lung. The other, the left primary bronchus, allows air in and out of the left lung. The junction where the trachea splits to form the right and left primary bronchi is reinforced by a ridge of cartilage called the **carina.** The primary bronchi branch into smaller and smaller tubes called **bronchioles.** Microscopic tubes called terminal bronchioles connect to respiratory bronchioles that lead to alveolar ducts. Each alveolar duct ends in several alveolar sacs. Alveolar sacs are clusters of alveoli. The alveoli are surrounded by capillaries and are the location where oxygen and carbon dioxide are exchanged. When an adequate blood volume and blood pressure are present, the capillaries return oxygenated blood to the heart.

The lungs are very elastic and are made up of many tiny air sacs (alveoli). The lungs are divided into three separate lobes on the right and two lobes on the left. Even a tiny blockage in the lower airways can completely collapse a segment of the lung, making breathing much more difficult. This situation can also occur because of a penetrating injury to the lung, such as a stab or gunshot wound. If an opening occurs between the outside atmosphere and the lung, the lung will collapse and require emergency treatment.

The Mechanics of Breathing

Objective 2

Below the lungs is the diaphragm, the primary muscle of breathing. The dome-shaped diaphragm divides the chest cavity from the abdominal cavity. It works in concert with the external intercostal muscles, which are located between the ribs. The external intercostal muscles assist with **inhalation.** The internal intercostal muscles and abdominal muscles may be used during forceful **exhalation.**

As the diaphragm moves down and in, the external intercostal muscles move the ribs up and out and the chest expands, increasing the volume of the chest cavity. The pressure within the lungs decreases to allow for inspiration. After inhalation, tiny air sacs (alveoli) are inflated while oxygen and carbon dioxide cross their membranes. Oxygen enters the circulation, while carbon dioxide enters the alveoli. Carbon dioxide is exhaled into the atmosphere as the diaphragm returns to its resting state, reducing the volume of the chest cavity and pushing air from the lungs.

Special Patient Populations
Infant and Child Anatomy

Objective 3

The respiratory anatomy of infants and young children differs from that of older children and adults. The epiglottis is large and floppy. The teeth are either absent or very delicate. Infants less than 6 months of age breathe primarily through the nose, not the mouth. The airway is much smaller, allowing a greater opportunity for obstruction. One such obstruction is the tongue, which is large in size compared to the size of the mouth.

The trachea is softer and more flexible in infants and children. The supporting cartilage of a child's trachea is less developed than that of an adult's, making it prone to compression with improper neck positioning. Be sure to place an infant's head in a neutral position, which may require slight elevation of the infant's shoulders. This can be done by placing padding under the shoulders to compensate for the proportionately larger head.

The narrowest part of a child's airway is at the cricoid cartilage, which is lower in the child's airway than it is in an adult's. A small change in airway size (because of conditions such as swelling or inflammation) can result in significant breathing problems. These differences allow for easier airway obstruction in an infant or child.

The chest wall of the infant and young child is flexible because it is composed of more cartilage than bone. Because of the flexibility of the ribs, children are more resistant to rib fractures than adults. The force of the injury, however, is easily transmitted to the lungs. Chest injury may result in bruising of the lungs (pulmonary contusion) or more serious injury.

Infants and children depend more heavily on the diaphragm for breathing. Gastric distention (swelling) is common in the ventilation of infants and children. If enough air builds up in the child's stomach to push on the lungs and diaphragm, effective breathing can be compromised. When assisting the breathing of an infant or child, avoid using too much volume. Use only enough volume to cause a gentle chest rise.

Older Adult Anatomy

Objective 4

The respiratory system undergoes many changes with age. Cartilage between the sternum and ribs calcifies and stiffens. Over time, the thoracic cage assumes a shape resembling that of a barrel. This physical finding is described as a "barrel chest." The diaphragm becomes less elastic, and the muscles of the chest wall, including the accessory muscles for breathing, weaken. Weakened ventilatory muscles tire easily and can result in symptoms such as difficulty breathing.

The protective reflexes involved in coughing, gagging, and swallowing diminish with age. The activity of the cilia in the lungs decreases and mucus thickens, making the patient vulnerable to infection. Damage or loss of the elastic fibers in the small airways makes them prone to collapse.

Blood volume does not significantly change with age, but the amount of blood present in the pulmonary circulation at any given time does decrease. The anatomic dead space, the volume of air contained in the conducting airways where gas exchange does not take place, increases with age. In addition, thickening of the alveoli results in a decreased number of alveoli that participate in gas exchange. When the older adult's body demands additional oxygen, such as during exercise, the person is less able to increase and maintain ventilation at high levels due to these physiologic changes.

Airway Assessment

Objectives 5, 6

You must perform a primary survey on *every* patient (see Chapter 17). The purpose of the primary survey is to find and care for immediate life-threatening problems. The primary survey begins after the scene or situation has been found or made safe and you have gained access to the patient.

As you approach the patient, you will first form a general impression of her to determine if she appears "sick" or "not sick." You will also determine the urgency of further assessment and care. Using your senses of sight and hearing (look and listen), quickly determine if the patient is ill (a medical patient) or injured (a trauma patient). Look at the patient and determine if she has a life-threatening problem. If a life-threatening condition is found, you must treat it immediately. Examples of life-threatening conditions include:

- Unresponsiveness
- An obstructed airway
- Absent breathing (respiratory arrest)
- Severe bleeding

After forming a general impression of your patient, you must assess the patient's level of responsiveness. Begin by speaking to her. If the patient appears to be awake, tell the patient your first name and identify yourself as an EMT. Explain that you are there to help. You may ask, "Why did you call 9-1-1 today?" If the patient appears to be asleep, gently rub her shoulder and ask, "Are you okay?" or "Can you hear me?" Do not move the patient. If there is no response, determine whether the patient responds to a painful stimulus, such as pinching the skin on the back of the hand or earlobe. The patient is unresponsive if she does not respond to a verbal or painful stimulus.

Signs of adequate and inadequate airways are:

Signs of an *adequate* airway:
- The airway is open, and you can hear and feel air move in and out.
- The patient is talking clearly and speaking in full sentences or crying without difficulty.
- The sound of the voice is normal for the patient.

Not every sign listed below is present in every patient who has an inadequate airway.

Signs of an *inadequate* airway:
- Unusual sounds are heard with breathing, such as stridor or snoring (**stridor** is a harsh, high-pitched sound that is associated with upper-airway obstruction; **snoring** is a loud breathing sound that suggests the upper airway is partially blocked by the tongue).
- The awake patient is unable to speak, or the voice sounds hoarse.
- There is no air movement.
- The airway is obstructed due to the tongue, food, vomit, blood, teeth, or a foreign body.
- Swelling is present due to trauma or infection.

If your patient is awake but appears to have trouble breathing, ask, "Can you speak?" "Are you choking?" If she is able to speak or make noise, air is moving past her vocal cords. If she is unresponsive, open her airway. If a complete airway obstruction is present, you may initially see a rise and fall of the chest but you will not hear or feel air movement. If the patient's heart stops, you may see irregular, gasping breaths (**agonal breathing**) just after this occurs. Do not confuse gasping respirations with adequate breathing.

Opening the Airway

A patient without an open airway has no chance of survival. If the airway is not open, there is no breathing. Without breathing, the patient's heart will stop beating unless you open the airway and begin breathing for the patient. Therefore, one of the most important actions that you can perform is opening the airway of an unresponsive patient. An unresponsive patient loses the ability to keep his own airway open because he loses muscle tone. This loss of muscle tone causes the soft tissues of the throat and the base of the tongue to relax. If the patient is lying on his back, the tongue falls into the back of the throat, blocking the airway (Figure 12-2). Because the tongue is attached to the lower jaw, moving the jaw forward will lift the tongue away from the back of the throat.

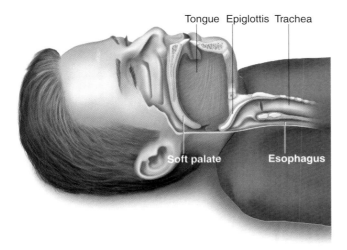

Tongue Epiglottis Trachea

Soft palate   Esophagus

FIGURE 12-2 ▲ An unresponsive patient loses the ability to keep his own airway open because he loses muscle tone. The tongue falls into the back of the throat, blocking the airway.

Stop and Think!

Because the risk of exposure to blood, vomitus, or potentially infectious material is high, you must remember to take appropriate standard precautions when managing a patient's airway.

Opening the Mouth

The crossed-finger technique may be used to open the mouth of an *unresponsive* patient (Figure 12-3).

To perform the crossed-finger technique:
- Kneel above and behind the patient.
- Cross the thumb and forefinger of one gloved hand.
- Place your thumb on the patient's lower front teeth and your forefinger on the upper front teeth.
- Use a scissors motion or finger-snapping motion to open the mouth.

Head Tilt–Chin Lift

Objectives 7, 8

The **head tilt–chin lift maneuver** is the most effective method for opening the airway in a patient with no known or suspected trauma to the head or neck. It requires no equipment and is simple to perform. When done correctly, the base of the tongue will be displaced

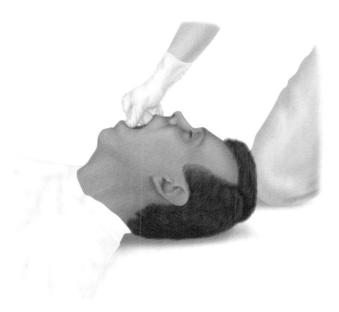

FIGURE 12-3 ▲ Opening the mouth by using the crossed-finger technique.

from blocking the back of the throat (Figure 12-4). Examples of patients who are likely to need the head tilt–chin lift maneuver include:

- An unresponsive patient with no known or suspected trauma to the head or neck
- A patient who is not breathing with no known or suspected trauma to the head or neck
- A patient who is not breathing and has no pulse (cardiac arrest) with no known or suspected trauma to the head or neck

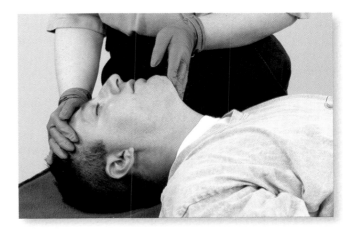

FIGURE 12-4 ▲ The head tilt–chin lift.

Steps in performing a head tilt–chin lift:

- Position the patient on his back.
- Place your hand that is closest to the patient's head on his forehead. Apply downward pressure with your palm, gently tilting the patient's head backward.
- Place the fingers of your hand that is closest to the patient's feet under the bony part of his chin. Do not compress the soft tissues under the chin; doing so can result in an airway obstruction.
- Lift the chin forward and support the jaw.
- Make sure the patient's mouth is open. If the patient is wearing dentures and they fit well, leave them in place. If the dentures are loose or do not fit well, remove them.
- Look, listen, and feel for breathing.

A variation of the conventional head tilt–chin lift is the **modified chin lift,** sometimes called the *trauma chin lift.* This procedure is best done by two rescuers. One rescuer stabilizes the patient's head and cervical spine in a neutral position to minimize movement. The second rescuer grasps the patient's chin and lower incisors with gloved fingers and then lifts to pull the lower jaw forward.

Jaw Thrust

Objectives 8, 9

An unresponsive patient's airway can be opened by placing your fingers behind the angle of the patient's jaw, displacing the jaw forward toward the patient's face, and performing a gentle head tilt while thrusting the jaw forward. This technique is called the *jaw thrust maneuver.*

Use a **modified jaw thrust maneuver** to open the airway of an unresponsive patient when trauma to the head or neck is suspected (Figure 12-5). The modified jaw thrust maneuver is also called the *jaw thrust without head tilt maneuver, trauma jaw thrust,* or the *jaw thrust without head extension maneuver.* The modified jaw thrust is a variation of the conventional jaw thrust. With this procedure, the patient's lower jaw is moved forward while the head and cervical spine are stabilized in a neutral position to minimize movement.

Although this method of opening the airway is effective, it is less effective than the head tilt–chin lift and is more tiring for rescuers. Because this technique requires the use of both hands, a second rescuer will be needed if the patient requires ventilation. Examples of patients who are likely to need the modified jaw thrust maneuver include:

- An unresponsive trauma patient
- An unresponsive patient with an unknown mechanism of injury

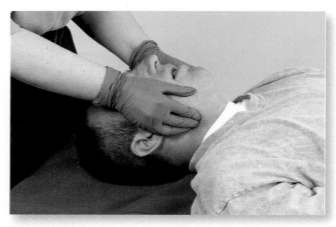

FIGURE 12-5 ▲ The modified jaw thrust maneuver.

Steps in performing a modified jaw thrust maneuver:

- Position the patient on his back, and kneel at the top of the patient's head.
- While keeping the patient's head and neck in line with the rest of his body, place your hands on each side of the patient's lower jaw. It may be helpful to rest your elbows on the surface on which the patient is lying.
- While stabilizing the patient's head in a neutral position, gently grasp the angles of the patient's lower jaw. Lift with both hands, gently moving the lower jaw forward. Make sure the patient's mouth is open. If the patient's lips close, gently pull back the lower lip with your gloved thumb.
- Look, listen, and feel for breathing.

You Should Know

The head tilt–chin lift and jaw thrust maneuvers may cause some movement of the cervical spine when they are performed. Healthcare professionals should use the modified jaw thrust maneuver to open the airway of a trauma victim if cervical spine injury is suspected. However, if the airway is not open and the modified jaw thrust does not open the airway, use the head tilt–chin lift maneuver.

Inspecting the Airway

After opening the airway, look in the mouth of every unresponsive patient and any responsive patient who cannot protect her airway. This can be done by opening the patient's mouth with your gloved hand. Look inside the patient's mouth for an actual or potential airway obstruction, such as a foreign body, blood, vomitus, teeth, or the patient's tongue. If you see a foreign body in the patient's mouth, attempt to remove it with your gloved fingers. If there is blood, vomitus, or other fluid in the patient's airway, clear it with suctioning.

Remember This

When resuscitating a patient, it is important to know the definitions of an infant, a child, and an adult:

- *Infant:* younger than 1 year of age
- *Child:* 1 year to 12 to 14 years of age (puberty)
- *Adult:* older than 12 to 14 years of age (puberty)

Airway Obstruction

Objective 10

A **foreign body airway obstruction (FBAO)** is a partial or complete blockage of the conducting airways due to a foreign body. For example, a piece of food, bleeding into the airway, or vomitus can block the airway. If the obstruction is not cleared, the heart, brain, and other organs of the body will be deprived of oxygen. When the heart stops, a patient is said to be in **cardiac arrest.** The longer the heart goes without oxygen, the greater the likelihood of cardiac arrest. The longer a patient is in cardiac arrest, the lower the patient's chance of survival. In addition to experiencing the cardiac arrest, the patient can suffer irreversible brain damage due to a lack of oxygen.

A foreign body airway obstruction can also result from a cardiac arrest. When a person becomes unresponsive, the jaw and tongue relax. The tongue falls into the back of the throat, obstructing the airway. Consequently, the tongue is the most common cause of upper airway obstruction in an unresponsive patient. In a breathing patient, snoring respirations can be heard when the upper airway is partially obstructed by the tongue. Loose dentures, vomitus, or trauma to the head, face, or neck can also block the airway. You may be able to correct an airway obstruction caused by the patient's tongue by properly positioning the patient's head and neck to open the airway.

The signs and symptoms of an airway obstruction caused by a foreign body depend on the following:

- The size of the foreign body
- The composition of the foreign body
- Where the foreign body is located (for example, in the patient's upper airway or lower airway)
- How long the foreign body has been present
- Whether the obstruction produced by the foreign body is partial or complete

In adults, an FBAO most often occurs during eating. Meat is the most common cause of obstruction. Older adult patients who have difficulty swallowing are at risk for an FBAO. Choking in adults is often associated with the following:

- Attempts to swallow large, poorly chewed pieces of food
- Alcohol use
- Loose or poorly fitting dentures

Most episodes of choking in infants and children occur during eating or play. FBAOs in children are often caused by the following:

- Small foods such as nuts, raisins, sunflower seeds, and popcorn
- Poorly chewed pieces of meat, grapes, hot dogs, raw carrots, or sausages
- Items commonly found in the home, including disk-shaped batteries, pins, rings, nails, buttons, coins, plastic or metal toy objects, and marbles

Other causes of airway obstruction in children include infection, such as croup and pneumonia. If you suspect an infection is the cause of an airway obstruction in an infant or child, transport the child as quickly as possible to the closest appropriate medical facility. Do not waste time on the scene in a useless and possibly dangerous attempt to relieve this type of obstruction.

Remember This

- A choking adult or child may hold her neck with the thumb and fingers. This sign is the universal distress signal for choking.
- Infants and children are at risk of FBAO because they are like little vacuum cleaners—everything goes into their mouth.
- Infants and children 6 months to 5 years of age are at the highest risk of an FBAO.
- Suspect an obstruction caused by infection when an infant or child presents with fever and congestion.

A patient who is alert and talking clearly or crying without difficulty has an open airway. If you suspect a foreign body airway obstruction but the patient is responsive, can speak or make sounds, and can cough forcefully, the patient has a mild airway obstruction. You may hear wheezing between coughs (**wheezing** is a high- or low-pitched whistling sound that is usually heard on exhalation; wheezing suggests that the lower airways are partially blocked with fluid or mucus). If unable to speak, cry, cough, or make any other sound, the patient has a severe airway obstruction. Death due to suffocation will follow rapidly if you do not take prompt action.

When caring for a conscious patient who is choking, it is important to remember that the patient's level of responsiveness will change as the amount of oxygen in the patient's blood decreases. The patient will usually be very anxious and restless and may even be combative. Reassure the patient and any family members who are present that you are going to help him. If the obstruction is not quickly relieved and the patient remains conscious, remember to remain calm and continue to provide reassurance while providing emergency care.

You Should Know

Signs of an Airway Obstruction

Mild Airway Obstruction
- Is responsive
- Is able to speak or make sounds
- Can cough forcefully
- May wheeze between coughs

Severe Airway Obstruction
- Has weak, ineffective cough, or may be unable to cough
- Emits high-pitched noise on inhalation or no sounds
- Has difficulty breathing or speaking or may be unable to speak
- May turn blue (cyanosis)

Clearing the Airway

Manual Maneuvers

Objective 11

The removal of foreign material from the airway is critical for patient survival. Manual techniques that may be used to clear a foreign body airway obstruction from the upper airway include backslaps, abdominal/chest thrusts, and finger sweeps. Finger sweeps are discussed below. Backslaps and abdominal/chest thrusts are shown in Appendix A.

You should use a finger sweep only when you can *see* solid material blocking the upper airway of an unresponsive patient. A finger sweep is *not* performed on responsive patients or on unresponsive patients who have a gag reflex.

Steps in performing a finger sweep:
- If the patient is uninjured, roll her to her side.
- Wipe out liquids from the airway, using your index and middle fingers covered with a cloth.

- Remove solid objects, using your gloved index finger positioned like a hook. Use your little finger when performing a finger sweep in an infant or child.

Remember This

A "blind" finger sweep is performed without first seeing foreign material in the airway. Blind finger sweeps should *never* be performed. Doing so may cause the object to become further lodged in the patient's throat.

You Should Know

If you are choking and no one is around to help you, perform abdominal thrusts on yourself to try and clear the obstruction. Make a fist with one hand. Place your fist, thumb side in, above your navel. (Make sure your hands are below the lowest part of your breastbone). Grab your fist tightly with your other hand. Pull your fist quickly inward and upward. You may need to do this several times to relieve the obstruction. If this action is unsuccessful, bend over the back of a chair or the side of a table, countertop, or railing. Press your upper abdomen against the edge with a quick thrust. Repeat this movement until the object is expelled.

Suctioning

Objectives 12, 13, 14

Suctioning is a procedure used to vacuum vomitus, saliva, blood, food particles, and other material from the patient's airway. You should always have suction equipment available when you are managing a patient's airway or assisting a patient's breathing. Having the equipment available means having it within arm's reach. If you hear a gurgling sound as a patient breathes, she needs to be suctioned immediately (**gurgling** is a wet sound that suggests that fluid is collecting in the patient's upper airway).

Suction Units

Suctioning requires the use of a device that creates negative pressure. Suction units consist of tubing, a collection chamber, and a manual or electrical power source. Some suction units also have a regulator. Most suction units are inadequate for removing solid objects, such as teeth, foreign bodies, and food.

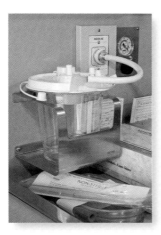

FIGURE 12-6 ▲ A stationary (or fixed) suction device is mounted (built in) on the wall of an ambulance and is usually powered by the vehicle's battery.

Mounted suction devices are built in on ambulance walls and are usually powered by the vehicle's battery (Figure 12-6). Mounted suction devices are also called *fixed suction units*. They provide a vacuum that is strong and adjustable. The parts of the suction unit that come in contact with body fluids are disposable. Disadvantages of mounted suction devices are that they are not portable and cannot be used with an alternative power source.

Battery-operated portable suction units are often used in Emergency Medical Services systems. They are lightweight and generally have good suction power (Figure 12-7). The suction unit must be checked daily to make sure it functions properly. Because most of these devices use rechargeable batteries, it is important that the suction unit be kept charged when not in use. Over time, rechargeable batteries will lose their ability to hold a charge and will need to be replaced. In most battery-operated suction units, the parts that come in contact with body fluids are disposable. However, in others the parts are not disposable and must be cleaned after each use.

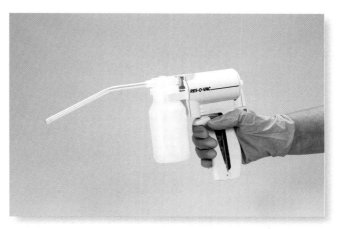

FIGURE 12-8 ▲ To create the vacuum necessary for suctioning, hand-powered units must be pumped or squeezed.

Hand-powered devices are lightweight, portable, and reliable (Figure 12-8). They are easy to use and relatively inexpensive. To create the vacuum necessary for suctioning, hand-powered units must be pumped or squeezed. This limits the length of time suctioning can be applied. The collection chamber of a hand-powered device is small. This limits the volume that can be suctioned. In most hand-powered suction units, the parts that come in contact with body fluids are disposable.

Suction Catheters

Suction catheters may be rigid or soft. Rigid suction catheters are able to quickly suction large amounts of fluid (Figure 12-9). A rigid suction catheter is also called a *hard suction catheter*, a *Yankauer catheter*, a *tonsil tip catheter*, or a *tonsil sucker*. Use a rigid suction catheter to remove secretions from a patient's mouth.

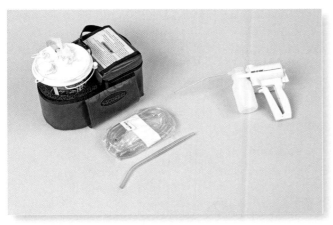

FIGURE 12-7 ▲ A battery-powered and a manual (hand-powered) suction unit.

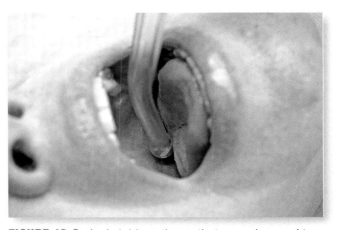

FIGURE 12-9 ▲ A rigid suction catheter can be used to remove secretions from a patient's mouth. This type of catheter should be inserted no deeper than the base of the tongue.

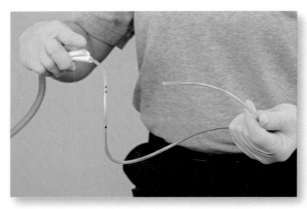

FIGURE 12-10 ▲ A soft suction catheter is used to clear the mouth and throat and remove secretions from a tracheal tube in an intubated patient.

Soft suction catheters are also called *flexible, whistle-tip,* or *French suction catheters* (Figure 12-10). These catheters are used to clear the mouth and throat. Advanced life support personnel may use a soft suction catheter to remove secretions from a tracheal tube in intubated patients. Soft suction catheters are available in many sizes. The inside diameter of soft suction catheters is smaller than that of rigid catheters.

Suctioning Technique

Objective 15

Steps in suctioning a patient's upper airway:
- If possible, give the patient 100% oxygen for 2 to 3 minutes before suctioning.
- Turn on the suction unit, and make sure it is working. If the unit is equipped with a pressure gauge, be sure it can generate a vacuum of 300 millimeters of mercury (mm Hg).
- Attach the suction catheter.
- *Without* applying suction, place the tip of the catheter in the patient's mouth. Gently advance the catheter tip along one side of the mouth. Insert the catheter tip only as far as you can see. Do not touch the back of the airway. Doing so can cause vomiting and/or changes in the patient's heart rate.
- Apply suction while moving the tip of the catheter from side to side as you withdraw it from the patient's mouth. Because you are removing air (oxygen) from the patient when suctioning, do not suction an adult for more than 15 seconds at a time. When suctioning an infant or child, do not apply suction for more than 10 seconds at a time.
- If the patient has secretions or vomit that cannot be removed quickly and easily by suctioning, log roll

her and clear the mouth manually. If the patient produces blood or secretions as rapidly as suctioning can remove, suction for 15 seconds, artificially ventilate for 2 minutes, then suction for 15 seconds, and continue in that manner. Consult medical direction when this situation occurs.
- If necessary, rinse the catheter and tubing with water to prevent blockage of the tubing from dried or large (chunky) material.

Because suctioning can cause serious changes in your patient's heart rate, you must watch your patient closely when you perform this procedure. The patient's heart rate may become slow or irregular because of a lack of oxygen or stimulation by the catheter of the back of the tongue or throat. These changes in the heart rate can occur in any patient. However, they are particularly common in infants and children. If the patient's heart rate slows, stop suctioning and provide ventilation with oxygenation.

The Recovery Position

Objective 16

The **recovery position** involves positioning an uninjured patient on his side (Figure 12-11). There are several variations of the recovery position. The 2005 Resuscitation Guidelines from the American Heart Association note that no single position is perfect for all victims. In the recovery position, gravity allows fluid to flow from the mouth and helps keep the airway clear.

Steps in placing a patient in the recovery position:
- Raise the patient's left arm above his head and then cross the patient's right leg over his left leg. (Use the opposite side if the patient has a contraindication to lying on one side.)
- While supporting the patient's face, grasp his right shoulder and roll him toward you onto his left side. The patient's head should be in as close to a midline position as possible. The patient's head, torso, and shoulders should move at the same time without twisting.

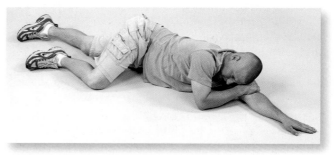

FIGURE 12-11 ▲ The recovery position.

- Place the patient's right hand under the side of his face.
- Continue to monitor the patient while he is in your care.

Remember This

- Do *not* place a patient with a known or suspected spinal injury in the recovery position, but assess the need for suctioning frequently.
- There is a potential risk for nerve and vessel injury if the patient lies on one arm for a prolonged period in the recovery position. To avoid these types of injuries, it may be necessary to roll the patient to the other side.

Keeping the Airway Open: Airway Adjuncts

Airway adjuncts are devices used to help keep a patient's airway open. When using an airway adjunct, you must first open the patient's airway by using one of the techniques already described. You should then insert the airway adjunct and maintain the proper head position while the device is in place.

Remember This

The use of an airway adjunct does not eliminate the need for maintaining proper head positioning.

Oral Airway

Objective 17

An **oral airway** is a curved device made of rigid plastic. An oral airway is also called an **oropharyngeal airway (OPA).** An OPA is inserted into the patient's mouth and used to keep the tongue away from the back of the throat. It may be used only in unresponsive patients without a gag reflex.

OPAs are available in a variety of sizes (Figure 12-12). Before inserting an OPA, you must determine the correct size for your patient. To select the correct size, hold the OPA against the side of the patient's face. Select an OPA that extends from the corner of the patient's mouth to the tip of the earlobe, or from the center of the patient's mouth to the angle of the jaw. If you select an airway of the wrong size, you can cause an airway obstruction. An airway that is too long can press the epiglottis against the entrance of the larynx, resulting in a complete airway obstruction (Figure 12-13a). An OPA that is too short may come out of the mouth or it may push the tongue into the back of the throat, causing an airway obstruction

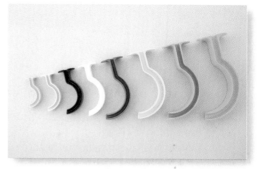

FIGURE 12-12 ▲ Oral airways are available in a variety of sizes.

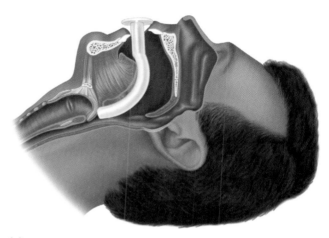

(a)

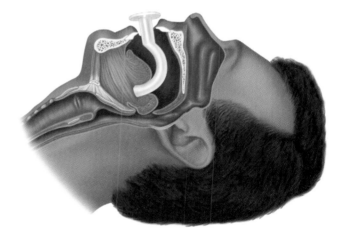

(b)

FIGURE 12-13 ▲ **(a)** An oral airway that is too long can press the epiglottis against the entrance of the larynx, resulting in a complete airway obstruction. **(b)** An oral airway that is too short may come out of the mouth or it may push the tongue into the back of the throat, causing an airway obstruction.

(Figure 12-13b). A properly sized OPA is one of the best tools for maintaining an open airway (Figure 12-14).

Skill Drill 12-1 shows the steps for sizing and inserting an oral airway.

Sizing and Inserting an Oral Airway

Use Steps 1–4 to insert an oral airway in an unresponsive adult.

STEP 1 ▶
- Place the patient on his back. Position yourself at the patient's head.
- Open the patient's airway with a head tilt–chin lift maneuver. If trauma is suspected, use the modified jaw thrust maneuver to open the airway.
- Select the correct-size oral airway. An oral airway is the correct size if it extends from the corner of the patient's mouth to the tip of the earlobe, or from the center of the mouth to the angle of the jaw.

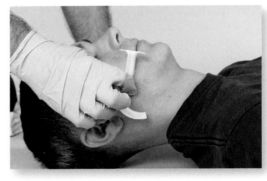

STEP 2 ▶
- Open the patient's mouth. Suction any secretions from the mouth, if present.
- Insert the airway upside down, with the tip pointing toward the roof of the patient's mouth. Advance the oral airway gently along the roof of the mouth.

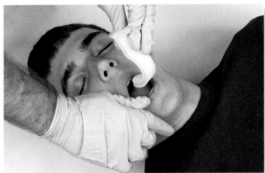

STEP 3 ▶ When the tip of the airway approaches the back of the throat, rotate the airway 180 degrees so that it is positioned over the tongue. Be careful not to push the tongue into the back of the throat.

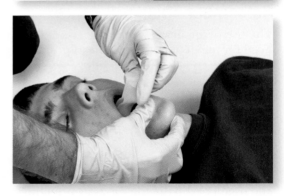

STEP 4 ▶
- When the oral airway is correctly positioned, the flange end should rest on the patient's lips or teeth. Remove the device immediately if the patient begins gagging as you slide it between the tongue and the back of the throat.
- Ventilate the patient.

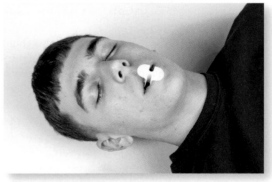

Use the following steps to insert an oral airway in an unresponsive infant or child:

STEP 5 ▶
- Place the patient on her back. Position yourself at the patient's head.
- Open the patient's airway.
- Select the correct-size oral airway.
- Open the patient's mouth. Suction any secretions from the patient's mouth, if present.
- Use a tongue blade to press the tongue down.
- Insert the oral airway with the tip following the base of the tongue.
- Advance the device until the flange rests on the patient's lips or teeth.
- Remove the oral airway immediately if the patient begins gagging as you slide it between the tongue and the back of the throat.
- Ventilate the patient.

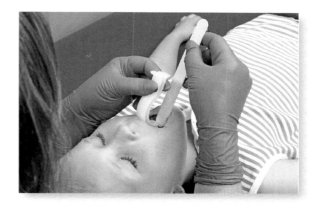

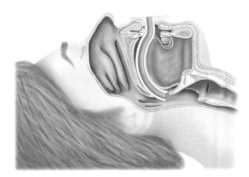

FIGURE 12-14 ▲ A properly placed oral airway is one of the best tools to maintain an open airway.

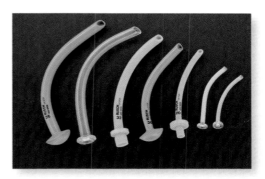

FIGURE 12-15 ▲ Nasal airways are available in different sizes.

Special Considerations

An oral airway should not be used in a patient who has a gag reflex. If you try to use an OPA in a patient with a gag reflex, she may vomit and aspirate the vomitus into her lungs. Use of an oral airway does not eliminate the need for maintaining proper head position.

Nasal Airway

Objective 18

A **nasal airway** is a soft, rubbery tube with a hole in it that is placed in the patient's nose (Figure 12-15). A nasal airway is also called a **nasopharyngeal airway (NPA)** or *trumpet airway*. The NPA allows air to flow from the hole in the NPA down into the lower airway. To select

Sizing and Inserting a Nasal Airway

STEP 1 ▶
- Place the patient on his back. Position yourself at the patient's head.
- Open the patient's airway.
- Choose the proper-size nasal airway.
- To select an airway adjunct of proper size, hold the nasal airway against the side of the patient's face. Select an airway that extends from the tip of the patient's nose to his earlobe.

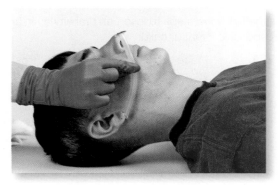

STEP 2 ▶ Lubricate the outside of the nasal airway with a water-soluble lubricant, if available.

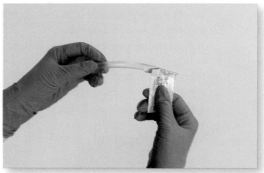

an NPA of proper size, hold the NPA against the side of the patient's face. Select an airway that extends from the tip of the patient's nose to his earlobe. When an NPA of the proper size is correctly positioned, the tip rests in the back of the throat. This positioning helps keep the tongue from blocking the upper airway (Figure 12-16). It can be placed in either nostril to help maintain an open airway. Remember that the bevel of the NPA needs to be kept against the nasal septum.

This airway can be used in an unresponsive patient. A nasal airway may be useful in semiresponsive patients who have a gag reflex. Situations in which a semiresponsive patient may need this type of airway include the following:

- Intoxication
- Drug overdose
- Stroke
- After a seizure
- Low blood sugar

Skill Drill 12-2 shows the steps for sizing and inserting a nasal airway.

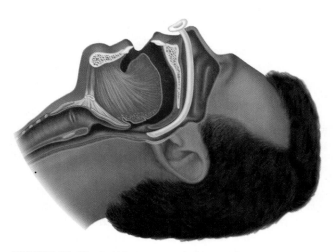

FIGURE 12-16 ▲ When a nasal airway of the proper size is correctly positioned, the tip rests in the back of the throat. This positioning helps to keep the tongue from blocking the upper airway.

STEP 3 ▶
- Gently push the tip of the patient's nose back slightly.
- Gently insert the nasal airway with the bevel pointing toward the nasal septum. During insertion, do not direct the airway upward. Do not force the device into position. Serious bleeding that is hard to control can result.

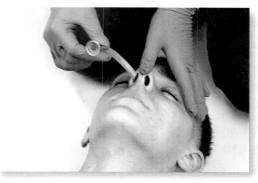

STEP 4 ▶
- Stop advancing the NPA when the bevel of the device is flush against the opening of the nostril.
- Assess placement by feeling for air coming from the device.

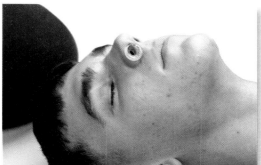

Special Considerations

Use of a nasal airway does not eliminate the need for maintaining proper head position. If the airway cannot be inserted into one nostril, try the other nostril. A nasal airway should be inserted gently into the nose along the "floor" of the nasal cavity. Do not try to insert the nasal airway up the nose along the "roof" of the nasal cavity.

Forceful insertion of a nasal airway may cause cuts or tears of the delicate mucous membranes of the nose. In some cases this can result in significant bleeding that may not be controlled by direct pressure.

If the nasal airway is too long, it may enter the esophagus. This can cause gastric distention and inadequate ventilation. A nasal airway does not prevent aspiration. This means that although a nasal airway may be properly positioned, it is still possible for blood, vomitus, or other secretions to enter the patient's lungs if they are not quickly removed with suctioning.

A nasal airway should not be used in situations involving trauma to the middle of the face or those in which a skull fracture is suspected (blood or clear fluid coming from the nose or ears). Check your local protocols in these situations.

On the Scene Wrap-Up

You and your partner work quickly to remove the patient from the toilet and into the next room where you can assess and treat him. Recognizing that the sound of stridor is a sign of an inadequate airway, you lay the patient on his back, noting that he is unresponsive. You perform a head tilt–chin lift and listen carefully for air movement from his nose or mouth. After you open the patient's airway, the high-pitched sound you heard earlier is gone. As you look at his chest, you can see that his rate of breathing is now within normal limits and his color is improving. Within minutes his eyes are open, and he is trying to sit up. As you assess the patient's vital signs, you realize that if his sister had waited a few more minutes to call, it is likely that he would have been in cardiac arrest. ■

▶ As an EMT, you must maintain an open airway in order to allow a free flow of air into and out of the patient's lungs. You must be familiar with the structures of the upper and lower airways. You must also understand the mechanisms of breathing.

▶ One of the most important actions that you can perform is to open the airway of an unresponsive patient. You must become familiar with the two main methods of opening an airway: the head tilt–chin lift and the modified jaw thrust maneuver. The head tilt–chin lift maneuver is used to open the airway if trauma to the head or neck is not suspected. When trauma to the head or neck of an unresponsive patient is suspected, you should use the modified jaw thrust maneuver to open the patient's airway. However, use a head tilt–chin lift maneuver if the jaw thrust does not open the airway.

▶ You should always have suction equipment within arm's reach when you are managing a patient's airway or assisting a patient's breathing. *Suctioning* is a procedure used to vacuum vomitus, saliva, blood, food particles, and other material from the patient's airway.

▶ If you see foreign material in the patient's mouth, you must remove it immediately. If foreign material is seen in an unresponsive patient's upper airway, a finger sweep may be used to remove it. A "blind" finger sweep is never performed. Performing a blind finger sweep may cause the object to become further lodged in the patient's throat.

▶ In some situations, the recovery position can be used to help maintain an open airway in an unresponsive patient. This position involves positioning a patient on her side. As an EMT, you must become familiar with placing a patient in this position. You must also remember not to place a patient with a known or suspected spinal injury in the recovery position.

▶ After you have opened a patient's airway, you may need to use an airway adjunct to keep it open. After the airway adjunct is inserted, maintain the proper head position while the device is in place.

- An oral airway (also called an oropharyngeal airway) is a device that is used only in unresponsive patients without a gag reflex. An OPA is inserted into the patient's mouth and used to keep the tongue away from the back of the throat.

- A nasal airway (also called a nasopharyngeal airway) is a device that is placed in the patient's nose. An NPA keeps the patient's tongue from blocking the upper airway. It also allows air to flow from the hole in the NPA down into the patient's lower airway.

Respiration

By the end of this chapter, you should be able to:

Knowledge Objectives ▶

1. Explain residual volume and vital capacity.
2. Define hypoventilation and hyperventilation.
3. Define oxygenation and oxygen saturation.
4. Define and differentiate between hypoxia and hypoxemia.
5. List and describe the factors necessary for optimal respiration.
6. Discuss conditions that can cause a disruption in airway patency.
7. Discuss conditions that can disrupt nervous control of the respiratory system.
8. Discuss conditions that can cause dysfunction of the thorax, nerves, or respiratory muscles.
9. Give examples of situations in which the percentage of oxygen in the air is likely to be inadequate.
10. Discuss conditions that affect alveolar function.
11. Describe the assessment of breath sounds.
12. Differentiate normal and abnormal breath sounds.
13. List the signs of adequate and inadequate ventilation.
14. Differentiate among respiratory distress, respiratory failure, and respiratory arrest.
15. List the signs of adequate and inadequate oxygenation.
16. Explain how pulse oximetry works.
17. Describe the indications for pulse oximetry.
18. Describe the pulse oximetry readings that reflect normal oxygen saturation, mild hypoxemia, moderate hypoxemia, and severe hypoxemia.
19. Discuss the limitations of pulse oximetry.
20. Define the components of an oxygen delivery system.
21. Identify types of oxygen cylinders and pressure regulators.
22. Explain safety considerations of oxygen storage and delivery.
23. List the steps for delivering oxygen from a cylinder and regulator.
24. Describe the use of an oxygen humidifier.
25. Identify a nonrebreather mask, and state the oxygen flow requirements needed for its use.
26. Identify a partial rebreather mask, and state the oxygen flow requirements needed for its use.
27. Identify a Venturi mask, and state the oxygen flow requirements needed for its use.

28. Identify a nasal cannula, and state the flow requirements needed for its use.
29. Describe the technique of giving blow-by oxygen.

Attitude Objectives ▶ 30. Defend the need to oxygenate a patient.
31. Defend the necessity of establishing and/or maintaining patency of a patient's airway.
32. Comply with standard precautions to protect against infectious and communicable diseases.
33. Communicate with empathy to patients with a problem related to respiration, oxygenation, or ventilation, as well as with family members and friends of the patient.

Skill Objectives ▶ 34. Perform pulse oximetry.

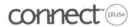

35. Perform oxygen delivery from a cylinder and regulator with an oxygen delivery device.
36. Perform oxygen delivery with an oxygen humidifier.
37. Deliver supplemental oxygen to a breathing patient using the following devices: nonrebreather mask, partial rebreather mask, Venturi mask, and nasal cannula.
38. Demonstrate the correct operation of oxygen tanks and regulators.
39. Demonstrate how to administer oxygen to the infant and child patient.
40. Demonstrate the technique of giving blow-by oxygen.

On the Scene

You and you partner are dispatched to a local motocross track for an injured person. On arrival at the scene, a security guard escorts you to the track where you find a 16-year-old male lying on the ground near a small mound of dirt. The patient states he missed the jump, landed on his right side, and now "it hurts to breathe." He reluctantly allows you to assess his chest and abdomen, which reveals an intact thoracic cage with abrasions over the right lower ribs. Both sides of the chest rise and fall equally. You note that he is able to speak in full sentences but is taking shallow, panting breaths about 30 times per minute. His skin is pink and dry. ■

THINK ABOUT IT

As you read this chapter, think about the following questions:

- How might the patient's injury affect respiration?
- What findings suggest that he is not breathing adequately?
- What do you expect to find when you assess his breath sounds?

Introduction

Respiration is the exchange of gases between a living organism and its environment. Because cells use oxygen to produce energy, a properly functioning respiratory system is necessary for cell metabolism. Without oxygen, cell metabolism becomes less efficient and eventually stops. This leads to cell, tissue, organ, and organ system damage and eventual death. If carbon dioxide is not adequately removed, acid builds up and changes in cell function result. In this chapter we discuss the conditions that must be present for optimal gas exchange, illnesses or injuries that can affect respiration, assessment of adequate and inadequate respiration and ventilation, and methods of delivering supplemental oxygen.

Physiology of Respiration

Pulmonary Ventilation

Objectives 1, 2

You will recall from Chapter 6 that breathing (pulmonary ventilation) is the movement of air in and out of the lungs. Inspiration (inhalation) is the process of breathing in and moving air into the lungs. Expiration (exhalation) is the process of breathing out and moving air out of the lungs. **Residual volume** is the amount of air left in the lungs after maximal expiration. **Vital capacity** is the amount of air that can be forcefully expelled from the lungs after breathing in as deeply as possible.

Tidal volume is the amount of air moved into or out of the lungs during a normal breath. At rest, a healthy adult moves about 500 mL of air with each breath. Of the 500 mL, about 150 mL remains in the anatomic dead space, where gas exchange does not take place. Patients with adequate ventilation are moving normal or near-normal volumes of air into and out of the lungs.

Minute volume, the amount of air moved in and out of the lungs in 1 minute, is determined by multiplying the tidal volume by the respiratory rate. For example, if the tidal volume is 500 mL and the patient's respiratory rate is 16 breaths/min, the minute volume is 8,000 mL/min, or 8 L/min. In a healthy adult, a minute volume between 5 and 8 L/min is needed to maintain adequate oxygenation and effectively eliminate carbon dioxide.

The amount of oxygen that reaches the cells can be changed by altering respiratory rate and depth. An inadequate tidal volume or respiratory rate can result in inadequate ventilation. Illnesses and injuries can affect the rate of ventilation, depth of ventilation, or both.

Hypoventilation is a minute volume that is below normal. Breathing that is too shallow or too slow can result in hypoventilation. The lower the minute volume, the lower the amount of carbon dioxide the person is exhaling. Many conditions can cause hypoventilation. For example, chest trauma, such as rib fractures, can impair the ability to adequately expand the chest wall, affecting the depth of ventilation.

Hyperventilation is a minute volume that is higher than normal. Breathing that is too deep or too fast can result in hyperventilation. A high minute volume indicates the individual is exhaling too much carbon dioxide. Causes of hyperventilation include stress, anxiety, stroke, head trauma, and aspirin overdose, among other conditions.

Remember This

Adequate ventilation is necessary for adequate respiration. However, adequate ventilation does not ensure adequate respiration.

Oxygenation

Objectives 3, 4

The oxygen content of the blood includes the oxygen in the body that is carried by hemoglobin molecules and dissolved in the plasma. **Oxygenation** is the process of loading oxygen molecules onto hemoglobin molecules in the bloodstream. A hemoglobin molecule can carry up to four oxygen molecules. When four oxygen molecules are bound to the hemoglobin molecule, the hemoglobin molecule is said to be saturated. Thus, **oxygen saturation** is a relative measure of the percentage of hemoglobin bound to oxygen.

Oxygen saturation can be measured by a machine called a **pulse oximeter.** A small sensor is clipped like a clothespin to an area of the patient's body (such as a fingertip). The sensor is connected to the oximeter, which calculates the amount of hemoglobin saturated with oxygen and displays this value as a percentage on its screen. Pulse oximetry is discussed in more detail later in this chapter.

Hypoxemia is a lack of oxygen in the arterial blood. Causes of hypoxemia include chronic obstructive pulmonary disease (COPD), a blood clot in the lungs (pulmonary embolism), fluid in the lungs (pulmonary edema), severe pneumonia, congenital heart disease, and inadequate oxygen in the surrounding air (such as in confined spaces). Hypoxemia leads to **hypoxia,** which is a lack of oxygen available to the tissues. Hypoxia may result from decreased amounts of oxygen in the air, loss of hemoglobin or hemoglobin function, decreased production of red blood cells, poisoning of substances within the cells, or diseases of the respiratory or cardiovascular systems.

External Respiration

External respiration is the exchange of gases between the alveoli and the red blood cells in the pulmonary capillaries. For optimal gas exchange, there must be good ventilation of the alveolus and good perfusion of its capillaries. When an individual is at rest, each red blood cell spends about 0.75 second in the alveolar-capillary network where oxygen and carbon dioxide are exchanged. During vigorous exercise, a red blood cell spends about 0.3 second in the alveolar-capillary network because of rapid blood flow through the area. Under normal conditions, it only takes about 0.25 second for loading of oxygen and off-loading of carbon dioxide to occur.

Internal Respiration

Internal respiration is the movement of oxygen from the red blood cells and into the tissue cells. During internal respiration, energy is released from molecules such as glucose and made available for use by the cells and tissues of the body. This process is called *cellular respiration*. During cellular respiration, oxygen and carbohydrates produce energy and create carbon dioxide and water as a by-product of metabolism.

An intact circulatory system and normal cardiac output are necessary to deliver oxygenated blood to the tissues. Pulmonary veins deliver the oxygenated blood to the left side of the heart for distribution to the body tissues via the arterial circulation. The carbon dioxide produced in the cell during internal respiration is absorbed by the blood, transported via the venous circulation to the right side of the heart, and eliminated through the lungs.

Remember This

The right heart receives systemic circulation and drives the pulmonary circulation. The left heart receives pulmonary circulation and drives the systemic circulation.

Pathophysiology of Respiration

Objective 5

Optimal respiration requires the following:

- Open (patent) airway
- Intact central nervous system
- Intact chest wall, pleura, respiratory organs, respiratory muscles, and nerves that supply these muscles
- Sufficient number of functioning alveoli
- Open pulmonary vessels
- Intact circulatory system and adequate cardiac output

Illness or injury affecting any one of these components can result in respiratory distress, respiratory failure, or respiratory arrest, which are discussed later in this chapter.

Pulmonary Ventilation
Disruption of Airway Patency

Objective 6

The conducting airways must be open and intact for normal ventilation to occur. An obstruction in the upper or lower airway can affect oxygenation and elimination of carbon dioxide. For example, unconsciousness generally results in a loss of muscle tone, which allows the tongue to fall back against the posterior wall of the pharynx. A head tilt–chin lift or jaw thrust maneuver is used to relieve this type of upper airway obstruction by lifting the base of the tongue away from the back of the throat. Material such as vomitus or blood must be suctioned from the upper airway. A foreign body can obstruct the upper airway requiring the use of back slaps and abdominal or chest thrusts to relieve the obstruction.

Swelling of the upper airway secondary to infection can cause an airway obstruction. **Croup**, a respiratory infection that primarily affects children ages 6 months to 3 years, is usually caused by a virus that causes swelling around the larynx and trachea. Rarely, croup may be caused by a bacterial infection. **Epiglottitis** is a bacterial infection of the upper airway that involves inflammation and swelling between the base of the tongue and the epiglottis. Epiglottitis can occur at any age, but typically affects children 3 to 7 years of age. Continued inflammation and swelling may progress to complete airway obstruction.

Swelling of structures within the upper airway can occur from burns and allergic reactions. An allergic reaction may occur in sensitive individuals when exposed to substances such as pollens, foods (i.e., shellfish, eggs, nuts, chocolate, tomatoes, milk, and berries), medications, molds, bee stings, or dyes.

Trauma to the airway can also result in an airway obstruction. For example, trauma to the face can cause an obstruction because of hemorrhage; aspiration of teeth, tissue, vomitus, or other secretions; injury to the tongue; or fracture of the mandible. Trauma to the neck can cause bruising, swelling, or fracture of the larynx or trachea, resulting in obstruction. Examples of conditions that can affect the patency and/or integrity of the airway are shown in the following *You Should Know* box.

You Should Know

Conditions That Can Affect the Patency and/or Integrity of the Airway

- Loss of muscle tone
- Foreign body
- Infection (croup, epiglottitis)
- Swelling (trauma, burns)
- Hemorrhage
- Allergic reactions
- Trauma to the face or neck

Interruption of Nervous Control

Objective 7

Respiratory centers in the brain control the rate and depth of breathing. An inadequate rate and/or depth of breathing can result in inadequate gas exchange. Stroke, brain injury, and drugs are examples of conditions that can affect nervous control of the respiratory system by slowing the rate and/or decreasing the depth of ventilation. When a stroke occurs, an artery in the brain is blocked or bursts, causing a change in the blood supply to a part of the brain. Respiration may be altered, depending on the blood vessel affected.

After an injury to the brain, bleeding or brain swelling can increase pressure within the cranium and compress the brainstem. This can result in changes in the rate, depth, and rhythm of respiration.

Some substances affect the respiratory centers of the brain. For example, alcohol and narcotics depress respiratory system function, lowering the respiratory rate and tidal volume, thereby decreasing minute volume.

You Should Know

Conditions That Can Affect Nervous Control of the Respiratory System

- Stroke
- Brain injury
- Drugs

Dysfunction of the Thorax, Nerves, or Respiratory Muscles

Objective 8

Adequate ventilation is dependent on an adequate rate and depth of movement of the thoracic cage by the respiratory muscles. The spinal cord and nerves transmit messages from the respiratory centers in the brain to the respiratory muscles. Trauma to the thorax and trauma or disease of the nerves that supply the respiratory muscles can result in insufficient respiratory muscle power for adequate breathing. For example, hypoventilation secondary to respiratory muscle weakness can occur in patients who have muscular dystrophy. Infections such as poliomyelitis can damage the nerves that supply the respiratory muscles, producing limited movement of the diaphragm and muscle weakness.

Trauma to the spinal cord in the area of the cervical spine can result in serious injury. The phrenic nerve that stimulates the diaphragm exits the spinal cord between the third and fifth vertebrae in the neck. If this nerve is severed or compressed, the patient will be unable to breathe on her own because her diaphragm is paralyzed. A spinal cord injury involving the lower neck or upper chest may result in paralysis of the muscles between the ribs.

Trauma to the thorax may result in inadequate respiration due to:

- Bruising of the underlying lung and associated hemorrhage of the alveoli, reducing the amount of lung tissue available for gas exchange
- Instability of the chest wall and pain associated with breathing, leading to decreased ventilation and hypoxia
- Interference with the normal "bellows" action of the chest, resulting in inadequate gas exchange

Examples of conditions that can cause dysfunction of the thorax, nerves, or respiratory muscles are shown in the following *You Should Know* box.

You Should Know

Conditions That Can Cause Dysfunction of the Thorax, Nerves, or Respiratory Muscles

- Muscular dystrophy
- Poliomyelitis
- Spinal cord injury
- Thoracic trauma

External and Internal Respiration

Objectives 9, 10

An adequate percentage of oxygen in the inspired air must be present for adequate respiration. Examples of situations in which the percentage of oxygen in the air is likely to be inadequate include high altitudes, confined spaces (such as underground vaults, tanks, storage bins, manholes, pits, silos, process vessels, and pipelines), and toxic or poisonous environments.

Adequate respiration requires a sufficient number of functioning alveoli, where gas exchange occurs. **Emphysema** is a respiratory disease that causes destruction of the alveolar walls; damage to the adjacent capillary walls; abnormal, permanent enlargement of the alveoli; and a loss of lung elasticity. Although the alveoli are enlarged, there are fewer of them, decreasing the number available for gas exchange. Because emphysema destroys the walls of the alveoli, air becomes trapped in the lungs during exhalation. The volume of air in the chest increases, giving the patient a barrel-chest appearance. Unable to exhale carbon dioxide normally, the patient uses accessory muscles to force air out of the lungs.

Off-loading of oxygen from the red blood cells to tissue cells is impaired when the presence of excess fluid increases the distance between the red blood cells and the capillaries. Pulmonary edema is an example of a condition in which this occurs. Left heart failure, inhalation of toxic fumes, and drowning are among the causes of pulmonary edema.

Pneumonia is another condition that affects gas exchange. It is an infection that may involve the lower airways and alveoli, part of a lobe, or an entire lobe of the lung. Once the organisms enter the lungs, they usually inhabit the alveoli and rapidly grow in number. White blood cells attack the invading organisms, resulting in inflamed alveoli that are filled with fluid and pus, hindering gas exchange.

Asthma is a condition associated with bronchospasm, swelling of the mucous membranes in the bronchial walls, and excessive mucus secretion. During an asthma attack, muscles around the bronchioles constrict, narrowing the airways and increasing airway resistance. Resistance refers to the opposition to gas flow in the airways. Swollen mucous membranes and the presence of excess mucus cause further narrowing of the airways, impeding ventilation and gas exchange. Examples of conditions affecting alveolar function are listed in the following *You Should Know* box:

> **You Should Know**
>
> **Examples of Conditions Affecting Alveolar Function**
>
> - Emphysema
> - Pulmonary edema
> - Pneumonia
> - Asthma

Circulation Compromise

Adequate respiration requires open pulmonary vessels, which transport blood to the alveoli to pick up oxygen and eliminate carbon dioxide. A balance between ventilation and perfusion must exist to ensure adequate gas exchange, and an adequate cardiac output is necessary to deliver oxygenated blood to the tissues.

Blockage of a pulmonary artery by an embolus results in alveoli that are ventilated but not perfused, severely impairing gas exchange. Obstruction of blood flow also occurs in such conditions as tension pneumothorax, cardiac tamponade, and heart failure. Hypovolemic shock and cardiogenic shock are examples of conditions that reduce cardiac output. Decreased blood flow to the tissue cells results in hypoxia.

Assessment of Ventilation

Is the Patient Breathing?

After making sure that the patient's airway is open, check for breathing. Breathing is the mechanical process of moving air into and out of the lungs. Normal breathing is quiet, painless, and occurs at a regular rate. Both sides of the chest rise and fall equally. Normal breathing does not require excessive use of the muscles between the ribs, above the collarbones, or in the abdomen during inhalation or exhalation. These muscles are called **accessory muscles for breathing.**

Remember This

Quiet breathing is not always a good sign. Breathing becomes quiet when a partial airway obstruction becomes a complete obstruction. Quiet breathing in a patient with asthma may indicate a decrease in air movement.

Breath Sounds

Objectives 11, 12

Breathing assessment requires evaluation of the patient's breath sounds (Figure 13-1). To do this, you

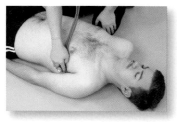

FIGURE 13-1 ▲ Assessment of ventilation requires listening for breath sounds.

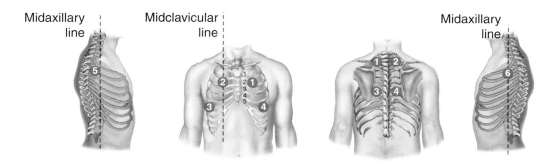

FIGURE 13-2 ▲ Listen at the top (apices) of the lungs in the midclavicular line on both sides of the chest. Listen at the bottom (bases) of the lungs and in the midaxillary line on both sides of the chest. Compare from side to side.

will use a stethoscope to listen to the movement of air into and out of the patient's lungs. Starting at the top (apices) of the lungs (about the second intercostal space), listen for breath sounds in six places (Figure 13-2):

1, 2. At the apices, midclavicular line on each side of the chest

3, 4. At the bases on each side of the chest

5, 6. In the midaxillary line on each side of the chest

Listen to one full respiratory cycle (inhalation and exhalation) in each location, comparing from side to side. Breath sounds should be assessed on the front and back of the patient's chest. While assessing breath sounds, watch and listen to see if the patient has any signs of difficulty breathing or pain with breathing.

Determine if breath sounds are present, diminished, or absent; equal or unequal; and/or clear, muffled, or noisy. Normal breath sounds are clear and equal on both sides of the chest. Diminished or absent lung sounds may be caused by spasm of the bronchioles, a foreign body, pneumonia, a completely or partially collapsed lung (pneumothorax), or blood in the pleural space (hemothorax). A hemothorax can produce muffled breath sounds, which appear distant. Trauma, infection, pneumothorax, and hemothorax are examples of conditions that can produce unequal breath sounds.

Normal breathing is quiet. Noisy breathing is usually abnormal breathing and a sign that the patient is in distress. **Stridor** is a harsh, high-pitched sound that suggests the upper airway is partially blocked. It is usually heard during inhalation. The sound of **snoring** suggests the upper airway is partially blocked by the tongue or soft tissue of the palate. **Gurgling** is a wet sound that suggests that fluid is collecting in the patient's upper airway.

Abnormal breath sounds may include crackles, rhonchi, and wheezes. **Crackles** (also called *rales*)

indicate the presence of fluid in the alveoli or larger airways. Crackles can be heard in patients with congestive heart failure, pulmonary edema, pneumonia, or trauma. They sound like hair rolled between the thumb and forefinger close to one's ear. **Rhonchi** are sounds produced when air flows through passages narrowed by mucus or fluid. They sound like "rattling" or "rumbling" in the lungs. Rhonchi can be heard in patients with pneumonia, upper respiratory infection, and chronic obstructive pulmonary disease. **Wheezing** is high- or low-pitched whistling sounds caused by the movement of air through narrowed airways that are partially blocked with fluid or mucus. An absence of wheezing in the asthmatic patient with breathing difficulty suggests that airflow is so diminished (the patient is moving too little air) that wheezing is not produced. Possible causes of wheezing are listed in the following *You Should Know* box.

You Should Know

Possible Causes of Wheezing

- Anaphylaxis
- Asthma
- Bronchiolitis
- Bronchospasm
- Chronic bronchitis
- Croup
- Emphysema
- Foreign body obstruction
- Heart failure
- Inhalation injury
- Pulmonary edema
- Pneumonia
- Tumor

Is Ventilation Adequate or Inadequate?

Objectives 13, 14

If your patient is awake and is able to speak or make noise, air is moving past the vocal cords. If the patient is unresponsive, open the airway, then place your ear close to the patient's mouth and nose. Look, listen, and feel for breathing:

- Look for a rise and fall of the chest.
- Listen for air escaping during exhalation.
- Feel for air coming from the mouth or nose.

If the patient is breathing, quickly determine whether ventilation is adequate or inadequate. To do this, you need to be able to see the rise and fall of the patient's chest and abdomen. If the patient has on many layers of clothing or bulky clothing, such as a jacket or coat, you will need to uncover him enough to watch him as he breathes.

Signs of adequate ventilation include the following:

Signs of *adequate* ventilation:
- Ability to breathe at a regular rate and within normal limits for the patient's age
- An equal rise and fall of the chest with each breath
- An adequate depth of breathing (tidal volume)
- Ability to speak in full sentences without pausing to catch his breath
- Clear breath sounds on both sides of the chest

Signs of inadequate ventilation include the following:

Signs of *inadequate* ventilation:
- Anxious appearance, concentration on breathing
- Confusion, restlessness
- Inability to speak in complete sentences
- Abnormal work (effort) of breathing (retractions, nasal flaring, accessory muscle use, sweating, tripod position, flared nostrils, or pursed lips)
- Abnormal breath sounds (stridor, wheezing, crackles, silent chest, unequal)
- Depth of breathing that is unusually deep or shallow
- A breathing rate that is too fast or slow for the patient's age
- An irregular breathing pattern
- Inadequate chest wall movement or damage due to trauma
- Pain with breathing

Respiratory distress is increased work of breathing (respiratory effort). A patient who has signs and symptoms of inadequate respiration must be considered to be experiencing respiratory distress. A patient who is having difficulty breathing is working hard (laboring) to breathe. She may be gasping for air. You may see her use the muscles in her neck to assist with inhalation. She may use her abdominal muscles and the muscles between the ribs to assist with exhalation. You may see **retractions** (a "sinking in") of the soft tissues between and around the ribs or above the collarbones.

Remember This

The best way to learn how to assess a patient's normal work of breathing is to watch a person without medical problems breathing while he or she is asleep. This is a good baseline to see comfortable breathing without signs of respiratory distress. It is also a good picture to recall when you have to artificially ventilate a patient.

A patient who is having difficulty breathing often naturally assumes a position to improve his breathing. For example, the patient may instinctively avoid lying down if he feels as if he is suffocating or if it is harder to breathe when he does so. If the increase in difficulty breathing occurs slowly over a period of days or weeks, the patient may increase the number of pillows used at night in order to breathe more easily. As breathing becomes more difficult, a patient may prefer to sit and sleep in a chair, such as a recliner. When breathing is particularly difficult, the patient may prefer to sit up and lean forward, with the weight of his upper body supported by his hands on his thighs or knees. This is called the **tripod position.** The patient's chin may be thrust forward with his mouth open. The tripod position allows the patient to draw in more air and better expand his lungs than if he is lying on his back or leaning back in a sitting position.

When assessing your patient, look to see if he is breathing through pursed (sometimes called puckered) lips. Pursed lip breathing may be seen in patients who have a history of long-term respiratory illnesses, such as emphysema.

Many factors affect a person's rate of breathing. For example, breathing slows during sleep. The rate of breathing increases with fever, pain, and emotions. Drugs may increase or decrease a person's breathing rate depending on the actions of the drug. A patient who has experienced trauma to the head or brain may have an abnormal breathing pattern. This occurs as the brain swells and pushes on lower structures in the brain. Other conditions in which an abnormal breathing pattern may be seen include stroke, diabetic emergencies, and toxic exposures.

Observe the rise and fall of the patient's chest. Unequal chest expansion may occur when part of the lung is obstructed or collapsed because of injury (such as a flail chest or pneumothorax) or illness (such as pneumonia). **Flail chest** occurs when two or more adjacent ribs are broken in two or more places or when the sternum is detached. The section of the chest wall between the broken ribs becomes free-floating because it is no longer in continuity with the thorax. This free-floating section of the chest wall is called the *flail segment.* **Paradoxical chest movement** is a sign of a flail segment. When paradoxical chest movement is present, a part of the chest wall moves in an opposite direction during breathing. When the patient breathes in, the flail segment is drawn inward instead of moving outward. When the patient breathes out, the flail segment moves outward instead of moving inward with the rest of the chest.

Inadequate respiration must be treated aggressively before it becomes absent respiration (respiratory arrest). A patient who is showing signs of respiratory distress will often progress to respiratory failure if you do not work quickly to relieve the symptoms. In **respiratory failure,** there is inadequate blood oxygenation and/or ventilation to meet the demands of body tissues. A patient in respiratory failure looks very sick and often very tired. Signs of greatly increased work of breathing are usually present. The patient's skin may appear pale, mottled, or blue. If respiratory failure is not corrected, it will usually progress to **respiratory arrest**, which is an absence of breathing. If not corrected, respiratory arrest will, in turn, rapidly lead to cardiac arrest. **Agonal breathing** is slow and shallow breathing that is sometimes seen just before the onset of respiratory arrest.

Other signs and symptoms of respiratory arrest:
- Unresponsiveness
- No air movement from the mouth or nose
- No chest rise and fall
- Changes in skin color caused by a lack of oxygen

Remember This

Think of respiratory distress, failure, and arrest as increasing levels of severity of a respiratory problem. If you do not move quickly to resolve it, the respiratory problem will also become a cardiac problem.

Assessment of Oxygenation

Objective 15

Internal respiration is necessary for life. It is sometimes difficult to assess internal respiration. When assessing a patient, it may be difficult to determine if you have a respiration, ventilation, or oxygenation

problem as they may coexist and one can cause the other.

Signs of adequate and inadequate oxygenation include the following:

Signs of *adequate* oxygenation:
- Does not appear to be in distress
- Has a mental status that is normal for that patient
- Has normal skin color

Signs of *inadequate* oxygenation:
- Oxygen concentration in surrounding air is abnormal (enclosed space, poisonous gas, high altitude)
- Color of the patient's skin and mucous membranes is abnormal (skin looks flushed, pale, gray, or blue)

Pulse Oximetry

Objectives 16, 17, 18, 19

Pulse oximetry is a method of measuring the amount of oxygen saturated in the blood. Pulse oximetry is commonly referred to as *pulse ox.* An oximeter is a small machine used to obtain this measurement (Figure 13-3). A small sensor is placed on an area of the patient's body in which pulsation can be detected, such as a fingertip or ear lobe. The sensor is connected to the oximeter, which is a computer. The sensor passes red and infrared light waves through the tissue to which it is attached.

Most of the body's oxygen is attached to hemoglobin molecules in the arterial blood. Hemoglobin absorbs red and infrared light waves differently when it is bound with oxygen than when it is not. The oximeter calculates the amount of hemoglobin saturated with

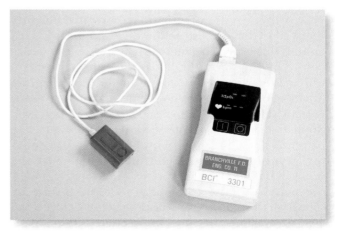

FIGURE 13-3 ▲ A pulse oximeter is used to check the amount of oxygen in the patient's blood.

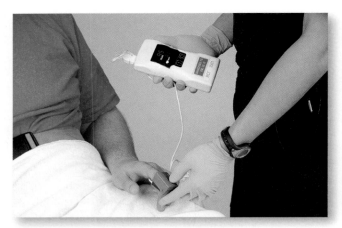

FIGURE 13-4 ▲ Clean the tissue to which the oximeter will be attached, such as the fingertip. Remove any dark or metallic nail polish, if present. Attach the pulse oximeter to the patient by inserting the patient's finger into the oximeter. Make sure the patient's tissue is centered over the light and detector. Turn the pulse oximeter on.

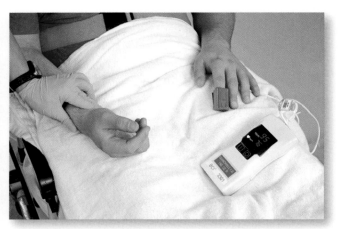

FIGURE 13-5 ▲ To make sure the pulse oximeter's measurements are accurate, check the patient's pulse to be sure that the pulse rate shown on the oximeter is consistent with what you feel when assessing the patient.

oxygen. This calculation is called the **saturation of peripheral oxygen (SpO_2).** The oximeter displays this value as a percentage on its screen, as well as the patient's pulse rate.

Pulse oximetry is a routine vital sign that should be obtained on *all* patients. It is used to detect and provide warnings about low levels of oxygen in the blood:

- A reading between 95% and 100% generally indicates adequate oxygenation.
- A reading between 91% and 94% suggests a mild lack of oxygen (hypoxemia).
- A reading between 86% and 90% suggests moderate hypoxemia.
- A reading below 85% generally indicates severe hypoxemia.

To use a pulse oximeter, start by making sure there is no dirt or obstruction on the oximeter's red light. If dirt is present, remove it and clean the device before putting it on the patient. Clean the tissue to which the oximeter will be attached, such as the fingertip or earlobe. Attach the pulse oximeter to the patient (Figure 13-4). If the fingertip is used, insert the patient's finger into the oximeter. Make sure the patient's tissue is centered over the light and detector. Turn the pulse oximeter on. To make sure the pulse oximeter's measurements are accurate, check the patient's pulse to be sure that the pulse rate shown on the oximeter is consistent with what you feel (palpate) when assessing the patient (Figure 13-5). Methods for assessing a patient's pulse are discussed in Chapter 17.

You Should Know

Indications for Pulse Oximetry

- Routine vital sign
- Altered mental status
- Respiratory rate outside the normal range for age
- Increased work of breathing
- Chief complaints are respiratory or cardiac
- History of respiratory difficulty or respiratory disease
- During delivery of supplemental oxygen
- During and after endotracheal intubation
- During transport of a sick or injured child

Pulse oximeter readings may be inaccurate in the following circumstances:

- Poor capillary blood flow
- Abnormal hemoglobin concentration
- Abnormal shape of the hemoglobin molecule

Examples of conditions that may cause these situations, resulting in misleading pulse oximetry readings, include the following:

- Cardiac arrest
- Shock
- Hypothermia
- Carbon monoxide poisoning
- Sickle cell disease
- Patient movement, shivering
- Patient use of nail polish

Supplemental Oxygen

Objective 20

The primary gases contained in ambient air are oxygen, nitrogen, and carbon dioxide. Supplemental oxygen therapy replaces some of the inert gas with oxygen and can improve internal respiration.

When administered to a patient, oxygen is considered a medication. An oxygen delivery system is used to deliver oxygen from an oxygen cylinder to the patient. An oxygen delivery system consists of an oxygen cylinder, cylinder valve, pressure regulator, flow meter, oxygen delivery tubing (connecting tubing) to carry oxygen to the patient's face, and an oxygen mask or cannula to deliver the oxygen to the patient's airway (Figure 13-6).

Oxygen Cylinders

Objective 21

Oxygen is stored in steel or aluminum cylinders. Oxygen cylinders (also called O_2 *tanks* or *bottles*) may be green, or they may be silver or chrome with green around the valve stem. Despite their characteristic color, it is best to identify the contents of a cylinder by checking its label or tag.

Letters are used to identify the size of an oxygen cylinder. D and E O_2 cylinders are small and portable and are and often used by EMTs. They weigh between 10 and 17 pounds when full. **Onboard oxygen** refers to the large oxygen cylinders (H, G, and M O_2 cylinders) carried on an ambulance. The amount of oxygen in various size cylinders is noted in Table 13-1.

A medical oxygen cylinder sold in the United States will accept a regulator designed only for use with oxygen. In this way, gases such as acetylene, ni-

TABLE 13-1	Oxygen Cylinders
Cylinder Type	**Amount of Oxygen, in Liters**
Portable	
D	350
E	625
Onboard	
M	3,450
G	5,300
H	6,900

trogen, or helium cannot be used with a medical oxygen regulator. There are two types of cylinder valves available in the United States. Small, portable cylinders (D and E cylinders, for example) use a pin-index valve (CGA-870). Large, nonportable cylinders (such as H and M O_2 cylinders) use a thread-index valve (CGA-540).

Oxygen cylinders must be handled carefully because their contents are under pressure. It is important to take the steps necessary to make sure an oxygen tank is secure, including when moving a patient. The federal Department of Transportation requires that oxygen cylinders be hydrostatically tested every 5 years to make sure they are safe to use.

Objective 22

Remember This

Using Oxygen Safely

- Never use combustible materials around oxygen equipment.
- Never place an oxygen cylinder where it may become part of an electrical circuit.
- Never use oil, grease, or other petroleum-based products on oxygen equipment.
- Never use adhesive tape or similar materials to seal connections or repair leaks.
- Never allow smoking around oxygen equipment.
- Never use oxygen around an open flame or spark.
- Never store oxygen cylinders in areas of extreme temperature.
- Never position any part of your body in front of or behind the cylinder's valve.
- Never leave an oxygen cylinder unattended.

Continued

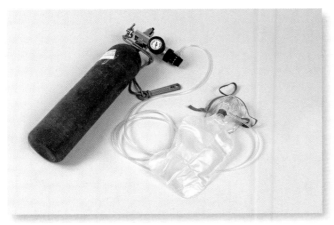

FIGURE 13-6 ▲ An oxygen delivery system.

- Never drag, roll, slide, or drop an oxygen cylinder.
- Never lift an oxygen cylinder by its cap; the sole purpose of the cap is to protect the valve.
- Never carry an oxygen cylinder by its attached regulator.
- Always store oxygen cylinders in well-ventilated areas.
- Always secure an oxygen cylinder when moving a patient.
- Always secure cylinders upright to keep them from falling or being knocked over.
- Always store full and empty cylinders separately. Avoid storing full cylinders for long periods.
- Always "crack" cylinder valves (open the valve just enough to let gas escape for a very short time) to expel foreign matter from the outlet port of the valve.
- Always follow the regulator manufacturer's instructions for attaching the regulator to an oxygen cylinder.
- Always use the sealing gasket specified by the regulator manufacturer.

Pressure Regulators

Objective 23

The tank pressure of a fully pressurized cylinder is approximately 2,000 pounds per square inch (psi), but tank pressure varies with the temperature. Tank pressure increases with increased temperature and decreases with decreased temperature. Because 2,000 psi is too high a pressure to be delivered to a patient, a **pressure regulator** is used to release oxygen from the oxygen cylinder in a controlled manner (Figure 13-7). It reduces pressure in the oxygen cylinder to a safe range, about 40–70 psi. Regulators may decrease the cylinder pressure in one or two stages. A one-stage (also called a *single-stage*) regulator decreases the cylinder

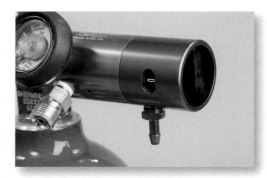

FIGURE 13-8 ▲ An oxygen flow meter.

pressure to a preset working pressure of about 40–70 psi. A two-stage (also called a *double-stage*) regulator creates two steps in the pressure drop. The pressure is first decreased as the gas leaves the cylinder and enters the regulator. It is reduced again when it meets the liter flow gauge.

A pressure regulator contains a gauge that tells you how much oxygen is left in the cylinder. An oxygen cylinder should be changed when the pressure gauge reading is below 500 psi. Some regulators also have a flow meter connected to them. A **flow meter** is a valve that controls the liters of oxygen delivered per minute (Figure 13-8). Oxygen flow is measured in liters per minute. The range of the flow meter is usually from 0 to 25 L/min. Skill Drill 13-1 shows the steps needed to set up an oxygen delivery system. Skill Drill 13-2 shows the steps in discontinuing oxygen administration.

Humidifiers

Objective 24

Medical oxygen is very drying to airway and lung tissue. A **humidifier** is a bottle filled with sterile water (Figure 13-9). When the bottle is connected to oxygen, oxygen

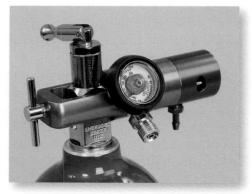

FIGURE 13-7 ▲ An oxygen pressure regulator.

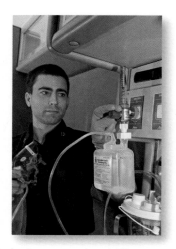

FIGURE 13-9 ▲ An oxygen humidifier.

Setting Up an Oxygen Delivery System

STEP 1 ▶
- Place the cylinder in an upright position and position yourself to the side of the cylinder. Verify the contents of the cylinder by checking the label or tag.
- After making sure that it is an oxygen cylinder, remove the protective seal covering the inlet.

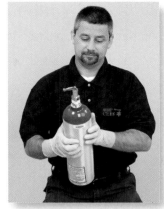

STEP 2 ▶
- Check the regulator and cylinder valve to make sure they are in good operating condition and free of dust and debris, such as oil and grease.
- Make sure that a washer or gasket is in place at the opening of the cylinder or regulator.

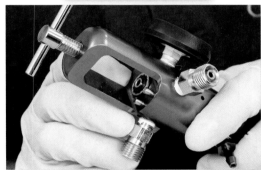

STEP 3 ▶ After making sure that the cylinder valve is aimed away from people or objects, quickly crack (open and close) the main valve on the top of the cylinder to blow out any dust and debris from its opening that might cause the valve to stick. You may need to use an oxygen wrench to open the valve. Then close the valve.

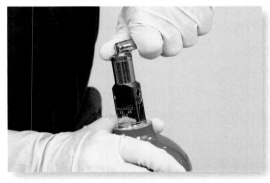

STEP 4 ▶
- Attach the pressure regulator to the cylinder. Carefully line up the pins on the regulator with the holes in the cylinder valve.
- Use an appropriate washer or gasket between the regulator and cylinder valve to ensure an airtight fit.

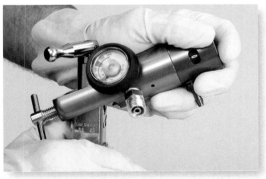

Continued

Setting Up an Oxygen Delivery System *Continued*

STEP 5 ▶ Hand-tighten the clamp on the regulator.

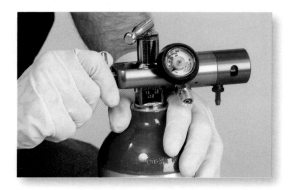

STEP 6 ▶ • Open the cylinder valve by turning it counterclockwise.
- Check the pressure in the cylinder and listen for leaks. If you hear a leak, close the valve.
- Verify that the regulator is properly attached and the washer or gasket is properly placed and in good condition. Then repeat Steps 5 and 6.

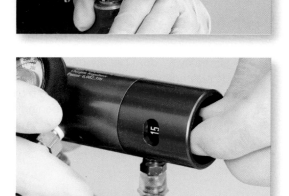

STEP 7 ▶ • Attach the oxygen delivery device to the regulator.
- Adjust the liter flow to the desired setting by turning the appropriate valve or knob on the regulator.

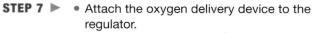

STEP 8 ▶ Apply the oxygen delivery device to the patient. Secure the oxygen cylinder.

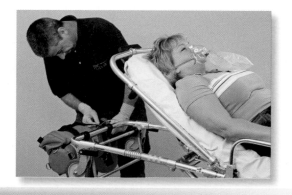

Discontinuing an Oxygen Delivery System

STEP 1 ▶ Remove the oxygen delivery device from the patient. Turn off the flow of oxygen.

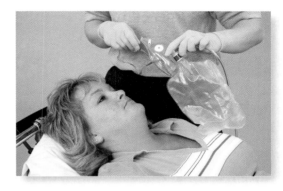

STEP 2 ▶ Turn off (clockwise) the main valve on the top of the cylinder.

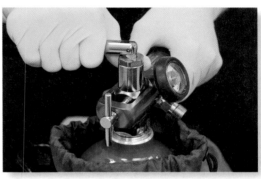

STEP 3 ▶ • Bleed oxygen out of the system by opening the flow meter valve until the flow stops.
• Close the flow meter valve.

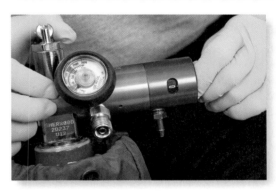

STEP 4 ▶ • If the cylinder is empty, loosen the clamp and remove the regulator from the cylinder.
• Store the oxygen cylinder appropriately.

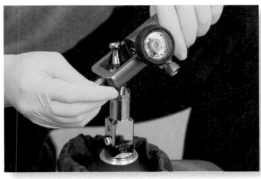

passes through the water to gather moisture. In some EMS systems, humidified oxygen is used when caring for patients with smoke inhalation, when caring for children with certain respiratory conditions (such as croup or epiglottitis), and during long transports. When a humidifier is used, it should be changed after each use to prevent the growth of bacteria in the container.

Making A Difference

Make it a habit to check the pressure remaining in an oxygen cylinder at the start of *every* shift and after *every* call in which oxygen was given. Replace an oxygen cylinder when the pressure within it is low. It is unacceptable to respond to an emergency and find out that your oxygen cylinder is empty.

You Should Know

To figure out how long the oxygen in an oxygen cylinder will last, divide the cylinder volume in liters by the flow rate used.

Oxygen Delivery Devices
Nonrebreather Mask

Objective 25

A **nonrebreather (NRB) mask** has one or more one-way disks covering the side ports of the mask that allow exhaled air to escape the mask but prevent room air from being breathed in (Figure 13-10). The mask is connected to a soft plastic bag that functions as a reservoir for oxygen. The reservoir bag has a one-way valve that prevents exhaled air from entering it. The bag is filled with oxygen *before* placing the mask on the patient and must never be less than two-thirds full while in use. This helps make sure that there is enough supplemental oxygen available for each breath. Adjust the oxygen flow rate so that the bag does not completely deflate when the patient inhales (usually 10-15 L/min). At 10-15 L/min, the oxygen concentration delivered is about 60% to 95%.

In most situations, an NRB mask is the preferred method of oxygen delivery in the field for a patient who is breathing adequately because it allows the delivery of high-concentration oxygen.

The NRB mask must fit snugly on the patient's face to prevent room air from mixing with the oxygen from the reservoir bag. Make sure the mask makes a good seal by forming the metal nosepiece to the patient's nose. Adjust the mask's elastic straps so that the mask is secure against the patient's face but not pressing so tightly that it leaves impressions in the skin.

Partial Rebreather Mask

Objective 26

Like the nonrebreather mask, a partial rebreather mask has an attached reservoir bag that is filled with oxygen *before* patient use. One-way disks are present on the side ports of the partial rebreather mask to prevent the entry of room air (Figure 13-11). An oxygen flow rate of 6 to 10 L/min is needed to deliver an oxygen concentration of about 35% to 60% and prevent excessive carbon dioxide buildup from the patient's exhaled air.

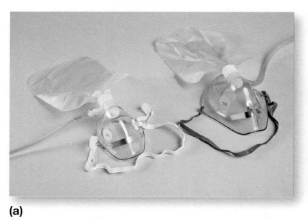
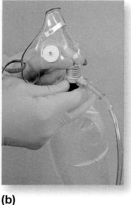
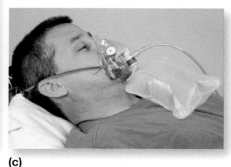

(a)   (b)   (c)

FIGURE 13-10 ▲ **(a)** Pediatric and adult nonrebreather masks. **(b)** Before placing it on the patient, attach the nonrebreather mask to an oxygen regulator. Set the flow rate so that when the patient inhales, the bag does not collapse (usually 10-15 L/min). Prefill the oxygen reservoir on the nonrebreather mask by placing two clean, gloved fingers inside the mask and closing off the valve. Hold the valve closed until the bag is full. **(c)** Apply the mask to the patient's face. Make sure the mask makes a good seal by forming the metal nosepiece to the patient's nose. Secure the mask to the patient's face.

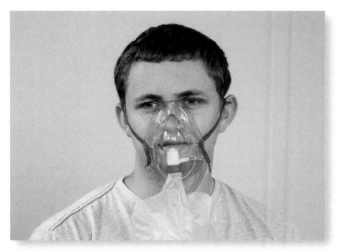

FIGURE 13-11 ▲ A partial rebreather mask is used for patients requiring moderate to high oxygen concentrations.

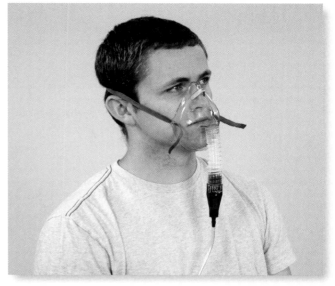

FIGURE 13-12 ▲ A Venturi mask.

Venturi Mask

Objective 27

A **Venturi mask**, also called an *air-entrainment mask* or *venti-mask*, is applied over the patient's nose and mouth and delivers a consistent mixture of oxygen and air, regardless of the patient's rate and depth of breathing. This type of mask is most often used for patients who have chronic obstructive pulmonary disease. A Venturi mask is supplied with removable color-coded adapters of different sizes that are positioned between the base of the mask and the oxygen source. The adapters are used to change the size of the opening in the mask, adjusting the mixture of room air and 100% oxygen entering the mask. Commonly available masks deliver 24%, 28%, 35%, 40%, or 50% oxygen (Figure 13-12). Recommended oxygen flow rates vary by manufacturer, ranging from 5 to 15 L/min.

Nasal Cannula

Objective 28

A **nasal cannula** is a piece of plastic tubing with two soft prongs that stick out from the tubing (Figure 13-13). The prongs are inserted into the patient's nostrils, and the tubing is secured to the patient's face. This oxygen delivery device is used for patients who require supplemental oxygen and are breathing adequately.

A nasal cannula can deliver an oxygen concentration of 25–45% at 1–6 L/min. Flow rates of more than 6 L/min are irritating to the nasal passages. This method of oxygen delivery will provide little benefit to the patient who is breathing through the mouth and not the nose. A nasal cannula is also ineffective if the patient's nose is plugged with mucus or blood. A summary of the oxygen delivery devices discussed in this chapter is shown in Table 13-2.

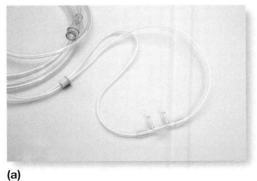

(a)

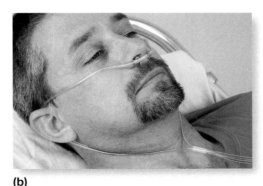

(b)

FIGURE 13-13 ▲ (a) A nasal cannula. (b) Place the prongs of the nasal cannula in the patient's nostrils. Place the tubing around the patient's ears and under the chin.

TABLE 13-2   Oxygen Delivery Systems

	Indications	Contraindications	Oxygen Flow	Approximate Inspired Oxygen Concentration
Nonrebreather mask	• Delivery of high-concentration oxygen • Moderate and severe hypoxemia	• Nonbreathing patient • Patient who has poor respiratory effort	10–15 L/min	60–95%
Partial rebreather mask	• Delivery of moderate- to high-concentration oxygen • Moderate and severe hypoxemia	• Nonbreathing patient • Patient who has poor respiratory effort	6–10 L/min	35–60%
Venturi mask	• Delivery of high-concentration oxygen • Moderate hypoxemia	• Nonbreathing patient • Patient who has poor respiratory effort	5–15 L/min; varies by mask manufacturer	24–50%
Nasal cannula	• Delivery of low- to medium-concentration oxygen • Mild hypoxemia	• Nonbreathing patient • Patient who is unable to breathe through the nose • Patient who has poor respiratory effort	1–6 L/min	25–45%

Blow-By Oxygen

Objective 29

Some patients will not tolerate oxygen delivered by means of a nasal cannula or face mask. If you are faced with a situation like this, consider **blow-by oxygen.** When oxygen is delivered using this method, the device used to deliver the oxygen does not make actual contact with the patient. For example, oxygen tubing can be attached to a toy or inside a paper cup. If a toy or paper cup is not available, the rescuer's cupped palm may be used (Figure 13-14). Oxygen is then "blown by" when the toy or cup is held near the patient's face. If the patient is sitting up, the blow-by device should be positioned above the level of the patient's nose and mouth. Oxygen will "pour out" (instead of "blow out") of the device because it is heavier than the surrounding gases. Although this method is not ideal for delivering oxygen, it is better than breathing room air.

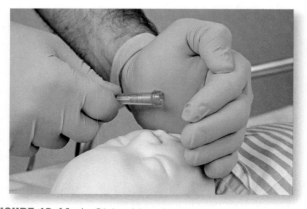

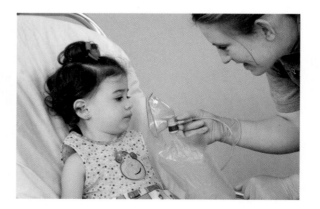

FIGURE 13-14 ▲ Giving blow-by oxygen.

On the Scene   Wrap-Up

The patient's shallow breathing is most likely the result of the blunt trauma sustained to his right chest and abdomen. There are many ways in which chest trauma can affect respiration. In this case, the pain associated with breathing leads to decreased ventilation and hypoxia. If the right lung is bruised from the injury and there is associated hemorrhage of the alveoli, less lung tissue will be available for gas exchange. Signs of inadequate ventilation in this patient include shallow breathing, a breathing rate that is too fast for the patient's age, and pain with breathing. Breath sounds should be carefully assessed. Based on the location of his injury and depth of breathing, expect breath sounds to be diminished in the base of the right lung. ■

Sum It Up

▶ Respiration is the exchange of gases between a living organism and its environment. Because cells use oxygen to produce energy, a properly functioning respiratory system is necessary for cell metabolism. Without oxygen, cell metabolism becomes less efficient and eventually stops. This leads to cell, tissue, organ, and organ system damage and eventual death.

▶ Breathing (pulmonary ventilation) is the movement of air in and out of the lungs. Inspiration (inhalation) is the process of breathing in and moving air into the lungs. Expiration (exhalation) is the process of breathing out and moving air out of the lungs.

▶ Residual volume is the amount of air left in the lungs after maximal expiration. Vital capacity is the amount of air that can be forcefully expelled from the lungs after breathing in as deeply as possible.

▶ Tidal volume is the amount of air moved into or out of the lungs during a normal breath. At rest, a healthy adult moves about 500 mL of air with each breath. Of the 500 mL, about 150 mL remains in the anatomic dead space, where gas exchange does not take place.

▶ Minute volume, the amount of air moved in and out of the lungs in 1 minute, is determined by multiplying the tidal volume by the respiratory rate.

▶ Hypoventilation is a minute volume that is below normal. Breathing that is too shallow or too slow can result in hypoventilation. Hyperventilation is a minute volume that is higher than normal. Breathing that is too deep or too fast can result in hyperventilation.

▶ The oxygen content of the blood includes the oxygen in the body that is carried by hemoglobin molecules and dissolved in the plasma. Oxygenation is the process of loading oxygen molecules onto hemoglobin molecules in the bloodstream. Oxygen saturation is a relative measure of the percentage of hemoglobin bound to oxygen. Oxygen saturation can be measured by a machine called a pulse oximeter.

▶ Hypoxemia is a lack of oxygen in the arterial blood. Hypoxemia leads to hypoxia, which is a lack of oxygen available to the tissues.

▶ Optimal respiration requires an open (patent) airway; intact central nervous system; intact chest wall, pleura, respiratory organs, respiratory muscles, and nerves that supply these muscles; sufficient number of functioning alveoli; open pulmonary vessels; and an intact circulatory system and adequate cardiac output. Illness or injury affecting any one of these components can result in respiratory distress, respiratory failure, or respiratory arrest.

▶ The conducting airways must be open and intact for normal ventilation to occur. An obstruction in the upper or lower airway can affect oxygenation and elimination of carbon dioxide. Examples of conditions that can affect the patency and/or integrity of the airway include a loss of muscle tone, foreign body, infection (croup, epiglottitis), swelling (trauma, burns), hemorrhage, allergic reactions, and trauma to the face or neck.

▶ Respiratory centers in the brain control the rate and depth of breathing. An inadequate rate and/or depth of breathing can result in inadequate gas exchange. Stroke, brain injury, and drugs are examples of conditions that can affect nervous control of the respiratory system by slowing the rate and/or decreasing the depth of ventilation.

▶ Adequate ventilation is dependent on an adequate rate and depth of movement of the thoracic cage by the respiratory muscles. The spinal cord and nerves transmit messages from the respiratory centers in the brain to the respiratory muscles. Trauma to the thorax and trauma or disease of the nerves that supply the respiratory muscles can result in insufficient respiratory muscle power for adequate breathing.

▶ An adequate percentage of oxygen in the inspired air must be present for adequate respiration. Examples of situations in which the percentage of oxygen in the air is likely to be inadequate include high altitudes, confined spaces (such as underground vaults, tanks, storage bins, manholes, pits, silos, process vessels, and pipelines), and toxic or poisonous environments.

▶ Adequate respiration requires a sufficient number of functioning alveoli, where gas exchange occurs. Examples of conditions that affect alveolar function include emphysema, pulmonary edema, pneumonia, and asthma.

- Adequate respiration requires open pulmonary vessels, which transport blood to the alveoli to pick up oxygen and eliminate carbon dioxide. A balance between ventilation and perfusion must exist to ensure adequate gas exchange, and an adequate cardiac output is necessary to deliver oxygenated blood to the tissues.

- Breathing assessment requires evaluation of the patient's breath sounds using a stethoscope. Listen to one full respiratory cycle (inhalation and exhalation) in each location, comparing from side to side. Breath sounds should be assessed on the front and back of the patient's chest. Determine if breath sounds are present, diminished, or absent; equal or unequal; and/or clear, muffled, or noisy.

- If the patient is breathing, quickly determine whether ventilation is adequate or inadequate. Signs of adequate ventilation include that the patient breathes at a regular rate and within normal limits for her age, has an equal rise and fall of the chest with each breath, has an adequate depth of breathing (tidal volume), speaks in full sentences without pausing to catch her breath, and has clear breath sounds on both sides of the chest. Signs of inadequate ventilation include an anxious appearance and/or concentration on breathing; confusion, restlessness; inability to speak in complete sentences; abnormal work (effort) of breathing; abnormal breath sounds; unusually deep or shallow depth of breathing; a breathing rate that is too fast or slow for the patient's age; an irregular breathing pattern; inadequate chest wall movement or damage due to trauma; and pain with breathing.

- Respiratory distress is increased work of breathing (respiratory effort). A patient who is showing signs of respiratory distress will often progress to respiratory failure if you do not work quickly to relieve the symptoms. In respiratory failure, there is inadequate blood oxygenation and/or ventilation to meet the demands of body tissues. If respiratory failure is not corrected, it will usually progress to respiratory arrest, which is an absence of breathing. If not corrected, respiratory arrest will, in turn, rapidly lead to cardiac arrest.

- Signs of adequate oxygenation include a patient who does not appear to be in distress, has a mental status that is normal for that patient, and has normal skin color.

- Inadequate oxygenation may occur because the oxygen concentration in surrounding air is abnormal (enclosed space, poisonous gas, high altitude). Signs of inadequate oxygenation include an abnormal color of the patient's skin and mucous membranes.

- A pulse oximeter calculates the amount of hemoglobin saturated with oxygen. This calculation is called the saturation of peripheral oxygen. Pulse oximetry should be obtained on all patients. It is used to detect and provide warnings about low levels of oxygen in the blood.
  - A reading between 95% and 100% generally indicates adequate oxygenation.
  - A reading between 91% and 94% suggests mild hypoxemia.
  - A reading between 86% and 90% suggests moderate hypoxemia.
  - A reading below 85% generally indicates severe hypoxemia.

- You may need to give patients supplemental oxygen. Become familiar with the features and functioning of oxygen cylinders. Remember to always keep combustible materials away from oxygen equipment.

- In most situations, a nonrebreather mask is the preferred method of oxygen delivery. It allows the delivery of high-concentration oxygen to a breathing patient. At 15 L/min, the oxygen concentration delivered is about 60% to 95%. A partial rebreather mask can deliver an oxygen concentration of about 35% to 60% with an oxygen flow rate of 6 to 10 L/min. A Venturi mask delivers a consistent mixture of oxygen and air, regardless of the patient's rate and depth of breathing. Commonly available masks deliver 24%, 28%, 35%, 40%, or 50% oxygen. Recommended oxygen flow rates vary by manufacturer, ranging from 5 to 15 L/min.

- The nasal cannula is often used for patients who have chest pain and are breathing adequately. It is also the preferred method of oxygen delivery in some EMS systems for patients showing signs and symptoms of a possible stroke (and who are breathing adequately). A nasal cannula can deliver an oxygen concentration of 25–45% at 1–6 L/min.

- Some patients will not tolerate oxygen delivered by means of a nasal cannula or face mask. In situations like this, consider blow-by oxygen. When oxygen is delivered using this method, the device used to deliver the oxygen does not make actual contact with the patient.

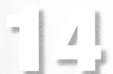

CHAPTER 14

Artificial Ventilation

By the end of this chapter, you should be able to:

Knowledge Objectives ▶

1. Describe differences between normal ventilation and positive-pressure ventilation.
2. Describe the purpose of cricoid pressure and how to perform this procedure.
3. Describe how to ventilate a patient with a resuscitation mask or barrier device.
4. List the parts of a bag-mask system.
5. Describe the steps in artificially ventilating a patient with a bag-mask for one and two rescuers.
6. Describe the signs of adequate artificial ventilation using the bag-mask.
7. Describe the signs of inadequate artificial ventilation using the bag-mask.
8. Describe the steps in artificially ventilating a patient with a flow-restricted, oxygen-powered ventilation device.
9. List the steps in performing mask-to-stoma artificial ventilation.
10. Describe how ventilating an infant or child is different from ventilating an adult.

Attitude Objective ▶

11. Explain the rationale for artificial ventilation and airway protective skills taking priority over most other basic life support skills.

Skill Objectives ▶

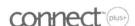

12. Demonstrate how to provide mouth-to-barrier device ventilation.
13. Demonstrate how to provide mouth-to-mask ventilation.
14. Demonstrate the assembly of a bag-mask unit.
15. Demonstrate the steps in artificially ventilating a patient with a bag-mask for one and two rescuers.
16. Demonstrate the steps in artificially ventilating a patient with a bag-mask while using the jaw thrust maneuver.
17. Demonstrate how to artificially ventilate a patient with a flow-restricted, oxygen-powered ventilation device.
18. Demonstrate how to artificially ventilate a patient with a stoma.
19. Demonstrate how to artificially ventilate the infant and child patient.

On the Scene

You and your partner are called to a farm where a 20-year-old man was thrown from his horse. You find him unresponsive on the ground surrounded by family and friends. You observe a 3-inch abrasion on the right parietal area and note that his breathing is shallow, irregular, and appears to stop for long periods. You can feel a strong pulse. ■

THINK ABOUT IT

As you read this chapter, think about the following questions:

- What findings suggest that he is not breathing adequately?
- Based on the information provided, what is the most appropriate method to oxygenate and ventilate this patient?

Introduction

In Chapter 12 you learned how to open a patient's airway and when to use airway adjuncts to keep the airway open. In Chapter 13 you learned the signs of adequate and inadequate oxygenation. You also learned about the delivery devices that may be used to administer supplemental oxygen. In this chapter we review the signs of adequate and inadequate ventilation and discuss the methods and devices used to manage inadequate ventilation.

Is Respiration Adequate or Inadequate?

In previous chapters you learned signs and symptoms of an adequate and inadequate airway, oxygenation, and ventilation, which are summarized in Table 14-1. Familiarity with this information is important in order to provide appropriate emergency care.

Positive-Pressure Ventilation

Objective 1

After you have opened a patient's airway, you may need to use an airway adjunct to keep it open. After the airway adjunct is inserted, maintain the proper head position while the device is in place. After ensuring that your patient has an open and adequate airway, you must assess breathing. If your patient's breathing is inadequate or absent, you will need to begin breathing for her immediately. When a patient is not breathing, she has only the oxygen-rich blood remaining in her lungs and bloodstream to survive on. You can assist breathing by forcing air into the patient's lungs. This

action is called **positive-pressure ventilation.** Mouth-to-mask ventilation, mouth-to-barrier ventilation, and bag-mask ventilation are some of the methods used to deliver positive-pressure ventilation.

There are differences between normal ventilation and positive-pressure ventilation. During normal ventilation, negative pressure is created inside the chest and air is sucked into the lungs. During positive-pressure ventilation, a healthcare professional is pushing air into the patient's lungs. During normal ventilation, blood returns to the heart from the body and blood is pulled back to the heart. During positive-pressure ventilation, blood return to the heart is decreased when the lungs are inflated. As a result, less blood is available for the heart to pump, and the amount of blood pumped out of the heart is reduced. During normal ventilation, the esophagus remains closed and no air enters the stomach. During positive-pressure ventilation, air is pushed into the stomach during ventilation. Excess air in the stomach (gastric distention) may lead to vomiting and subsequent aspiration. If enough air builds up in the patient's stomach to push on the lungs and diaphragm, effective breathing can be compromised. When delivering positive-pressure ventilation, avoid using too much volume. Use only enough volume to cause a gentle chest rise. An excessive rate or depth of positive-pressure ventilation can harm the patient. For example, ventilating too fast or too deep may cause low blood pressure, vomiting, and decreased blood flow when the chest is compressed during CPR.

Applying Cricoid Pressure

Objective 2

If positive-pressure ventilation is performed too rapidly or with too much volume, air can enter the stomach. The cricoid cartilage is the lowermost cartilage of the larynx (Figure 14-1), and it is the only complete ring of cartilage in the larynx. When pressure is applied to the

TABLE 14-1 Signs and Symptoms of Adequate and Inadequate Airway, Oxygenation, and Ventilation

	Adequate	Inadequate
Airway	• Airway open, air can be heard and felt moving in and out • Cries or talks clearly and speaks in full sentences without difficulty • Sound of the voice normal for the patient	• Unusual sounds heard with breathing, such as stridor or snoring • Awake patient unable to speak or voice sounds hoarse • No air movement • Airway obstruction due to the tongue, food, vomit, etc. • Swelling due to trauma or infection
Oxygenation	• Does not appear to be in distress • Has a mental status that is normal for that patient • Has normal skin color	• Oxygen concentration in surrounding air abnormal (enclosed space, poisonous gas, high altitude) • Color of the patient's skin and mucous membranes abnormal (skin looks flushed, pale, gray, or blue)
Ventilation	• Breathes at a regular rate and within normal limits for age • Has an equal rise and fall of the chest with each breath • Has an adequate depth of breathing (tidal volume) • Speaks in full sentences without pausing to catch breath	• Anxious appearance, concentration on breathing • Confusion, restlessness • Unable to speak in complete sentences • Abnormal work (effort) of breathing • Depth of breathing is unusually deep or shallow • A breathing rate that is too fast or slow for the patient's age • An irregular breathing pattern • Inadequate chest wall movement or damage due to trauma • Pain with breathing

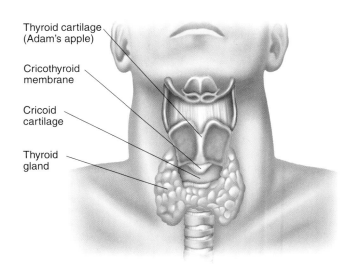

Thyroid cartilage (Adam's apple)

Cricothyroid membrane

Cricoid cartilage

Thyroid gland

FIGURE 14-1 ▲ The cricoid cartilage is the lowermost cartilage of the larynx.

cricoid cartilage, the trachea is pushed backward and the esophagus is compressed (closed) against the cervical vertebrae. This compression helps decrease the amount of air entering the stomach during positive-pressure ventilation, thus reducing the likelihood of vomiting and aspiration. **Cricoid pressure** (also called the *Sellick maneuver*) should be used only in unresponsive patients (Figure 14-2). It is usually applied by a third person during positive-pressure ventilation. The earlier cricoid pressure is applied, the less likely it is that air will enter the stomach during ventilations. Be sure to release cricoid pressure if the patient begins to vomit.

Steps in applying cricoid pressure:

• Using your index finger, locate the patient's thyroid cartilage on the front of the neck. Slowly move your finger downward until you feel a depression. Just below this depression is a firm ring of cartilage. This is the cricoid cartilage.

• Make sure the cricoid cartilage is between your thumb and index finger, and apply firm pressure.

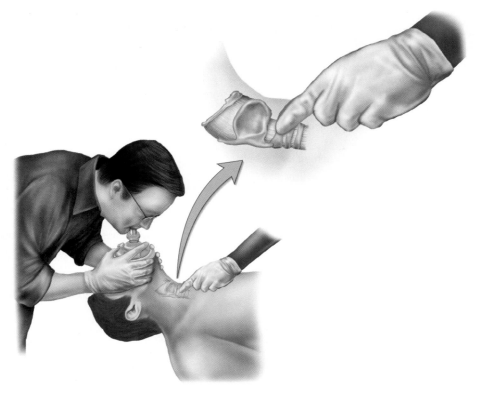

FIGURE 14-2 ▲ Applying cricoid pressure.

Pressure is applied in a downward direction (toward the patient's back). The cricoid cartilage should remain in the midline position; it should not move to either side.

- Maintain pressure until the patient begins breathing on her own, a tube has been inserted in the patient's trachea by appropriately trained personnel, or the patient becomes responsive as evidenced by moving, coughing, or gagging.

You Should Know

- The cricoid cartilage may be difficult to find in women, obese patients, and patients with thick necks.
- Applying too much pressure on the cricoid cartilage can cause an airway obstruction.
- An advanced level provider may ask you to apply cricoid pressure when inserting an endotracheal tube.
- Do not use cricoid pressure if the patient is vomiting or starts to vomit or is responsive or if an endotracheal tube has already been placed by advanced level providers.

Mouth-to-Mask Ventilation

Objective 3

The piece of equipment used for **mouth-to-mask ventilation** is the **pocket mask,** also called a *pocket face mask, ventilation face mask*, or *resuscitation mask.* The mask provides a physical barrier between you and the patient's nose, mouth, and secretions. The mask used should have a one-way valve that directs the patient's exhaled breath away from you (Figure 14-3). This helps prevent exposure

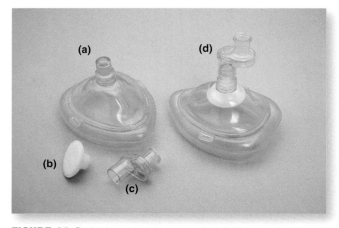

FIGURE 14-3 ▲ A pocket face mask. **(a)** The mask; **(b)** HEPA filter; **(c)** one-way valve; **(d)** pocket face mask assembled with mask, HEPA filter, and one-way valve.

TABLE 14-2 Rates for Positive-Pressure Ventilation

Patient	Breaths per Minute	Length of Each Breath
Adult	10 to 12 (1 breath every 5 to 6 seconds)	1 second
Infant/child	12 to 20 (1 breath every 3 to 5 seconds)	1 second
Newborn	40 to 60 (1 breath every 1 to 1.5 seconds)	1 second

to infectious disease. The mask should also have a disposable high-efficiency particulate air (HEPA) filter. A HEPA filter snaps inside the mask and is used to trap respiratory particles from patients with diseases such as tuberculosis. All masks should be transparent so that vomitus can be seen and suctioned from the airway. Some pocket masks have an oxygen inlet on the mask that allows oxygen delivery. When the mask is connected to oxygen with a minimum flow of 10 L/min, about 50% oxygen can be delivered to the patient.

Mouth-to-mask ventilation is very effective because you can use two hands to hold the mask in place on the patient's face and maintain proper head positioning at the same time. It also allows you to get a better face-to-mask seal, reducing the likelihood that air will leak from the mask. With a pocket mask you can adjust the volume of air to meet the patient's needs. You can do this by increasing or decreasing your own breath. When ventilating the patient through the mask, watch the rise and fall of her chest to determine if you need to adjust the volume of your breath. Rates for positive-pressure ventilation are shown in Table 14-2. Skill Drill 14-1 shows the steps for mouth-to-mask ventilation.

Making a Difference

Use the following guidelines when providing mouth-to-mask ventilation:

- Position the narrow portion of the mask over the bridge of the patient's nose. The wide portion of the mask should rest in the groove between the patient's lower lip and chin. The position of the mask is critical. If the mask is too large, turn it upside down and place the patient's nose in the chin piece of the mask.
- You are providing adequate ventilation if you see the patient's chest gently rise and fall with each breath.

Mouth-to-Barrier Device Ventilation

Objective 3

A **barrier device** is a thin film of plastic or silicone that is placed on the patient's face. It is used to pre-

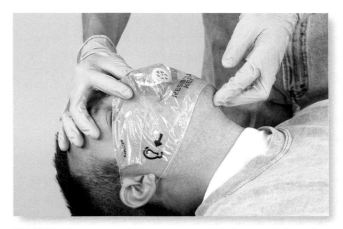

FIGURE 14-4 ▲ Mouth-to-barrier device ventilation.

vent direct contact with the patient's mouth during **mouth-to-barrier device ventilation** (Figure 14-4). Face shields, a type of barrier device, are compact and portable. Some face shields are equipped with a short tube (1 to 2 inches) that is inserted into the patient's mouth. Use a barrier device if a pocket mask is not available.

You Should Know

Air leaks are common when a barrier device is used.

Although their features vary, most barrier devices have a one-way valve or filter in the center of the face shield. This allows the patient's exhaled air to escape between the shield and the patient's face when you lift your mouth off the shield between breaths.

Steps in mouth-to-barrier device ventilation:
- Place the patient on her back. Open her airway with a head tilt–chin lift maneuver. If trauma is suspected, use the jaw thrust maneuver to open the airway.
- Position yourself at the patient's head. Place the barrier device over the patient's mouth and nose. The opening at the center of the device should be placed over the patient's mouth. If a tube is present on the device, insert the tube into the patient's mouth over the tongue.
- Gently close the patient's nostrils with your thumb and index finger. Take a normal breath and place

Skill Drill 14-1

Mouth-to-Mask Ventilation

STEP 1 ▶
- Connect a one-way valve to the mask. Place the patient on his back. Open his airway with a head tilt–chin lift maneuver. If trauma is suspected, use the jaw thrust maneuver to open the airway.
- Position yourself at the top of the patient's head. Lower the mask over the patient's nose and mouth. Create a face-to-mask seal by forming a C around the ventilation port with your thumb and index finger. Place the third, fourth, and fifth fingers of the same hand along the bony portion of the lower jaw. (These fingers form an E.) Lift up slightly on the jaw with these fingers.

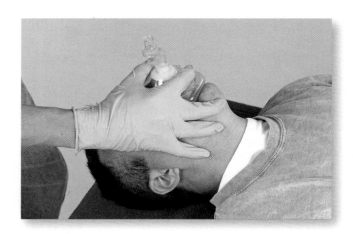

STEP 2 ▶
- Take a deep breath, and place your mouth around the one-way valve. Exhale slowly with just enough volume to make the chest rise. Deliver each breath over 1 second. (See Table 14-2.)
- Watch for the rise and fall of the patient's chest with each ventilation. Stop ventilation when adequate chest rise is observed. Remove your mouth from the one-way valve, and allow the patient to exhale between breaths.
- If air does not go in or the chest does not rise, reposition the patient's head. Reapply the mask to the patient's face, and try again to ventilate. If the air still does not go in, suspect an airway obstruction.
- Ventilate once every 3 to 5 seconds for an infant or child and once every 5 to 6 seconds for an adult.

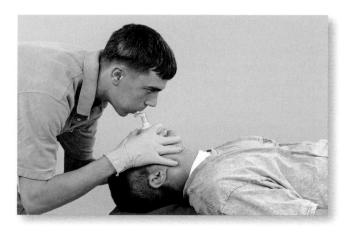

your mouth over the mouthpiece on the barrier device. Give a breath over 1 second, with just enough volume to make the chest gently rise.

- Watch for the rise and fall of the patient's chest with each ventilation. Stop ventilation when an adequate chest rise is observed. Too large a volume of air or a breath given too fast will cause the air to enter the stomach. Remove your mouth from the one-way valve, and allow the patient to exhale between breaths. Continue ventilation at the proper rate.
- If the patient's chest does not rise, ventilation is not effective. In this case the airway is obstructed or more volume or pressure is needed to provide effective ventilation. Readjust the position of the patient's head, make sure the mouth is open, and try again to ventilate. If the chest still does not rise, suspect an airway obstruction.

Bag-Mask Ventilation

Bag-Mask Features

Objective 4

A **bag-mask** (**BM**) **device** is a self-inflating bag with a one-way valve and mask used for **bag-mask ventilation** (using a self-inflating bag to force air into a patient's lungs). Most are equipped with an oxygen reservoir. The one-way valve on the BM prevents the patient's exhaled air from reentering the bag. The reservoir is an oxygen collector, allowing the delivery of a higher concentration of oxygen to the patient. A see-through mask with an air-filled cuff is attached to the bag (Figure 14-5). The see-through mask allows you to notice blood, vomit, or other secretions in the patient's mouth. The mask on most BMs has an inflatable cushion. A syringe is used to increase or decrease the amount of air in the cushion. Adjusting the amount of air in the cushion is important. Too much air in the cushion will not allow a tight seal

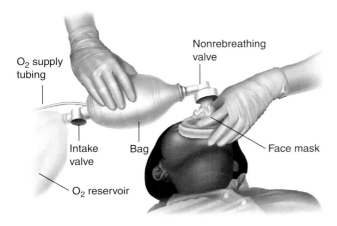

FIGURE 14-5 ▲ The components of a bag-mask (BM) device.

between the patient's face and the mask. Inflate the cushion with air so that it is flexible enough to make a tight seal over the patient's mouth and nose. This will limit the amount of room air that enters or oxygen that escapes from the mask.

You Should Know

A BM device is also called a *bag-valve-mask (BVM) device.*

It is important to select a mask of the proper size. A properly sized mask extends from the bridge of the patient's nose to the groove between his lower lip and chin. If a mask of the proper size is not used, air will leak from between the mask and the patient's face. This will result in less oxygen being delivered to the patient.

BM devices are available in adult, child, and infant sizes. Most adult BM devices can hold a volume of about 1,600 mL. BM devices used in the field today are disposable, and many come equipped with a built-in oxygen reservoir. When connected to oxygen, the reservoir collects a volume of 100% oxygen equal to the capacity of the bag. When the bag is squeezed, oxygen is delivered to the patient. When pressure on the bag is released, the bag expands and refills with oxygen.

A BM that is used during a cardiac arrest should not have a pop-off (pressure-release) valve, or if a pop-off valve is present, it should be one that can be manually disabled during resuscitation. To disable a pop-off valve, depress the valve with a finger during ventilation or twist the pop-off valve into the closed position. Failure to disable a pop-off valve may result in inadequate artificial ventilation.

Ventilating with a Bag-Mask Device

Objective 5

Ventilation performed with a BM device is often referred to as *bagging.* Although BM ventilation can be done using one person, it is best performed with two rescuers. It is not easy for one person to maintain the proper position of the patient's head, make sure the mask is sealed tightly on the patient's face, and compress the bag at the same time. When two people are available, one takes responsibility for compressing the bag. The other is responsible for maintaining the patient's head in the proper position and making sure the mask is sealed tightly on the patient's face.

One of the advantages of ventilating a patient with a BM device is the ability to feel the compliance of the patient's lungs. **Compliance** refers to the ability of the patient's lung tissue to distend (inflate) with ventilation. A patient who has healthy lungs requires relatively little pressure with the BM device (or other device used to deliver positive-pressure ventilation) to inflate the lungs. However, some diseases and injuries can cause changes in the patient's lung compliance. Compliance is considered good if the patient's lung inflate easily with positive-pressure ventilation. Poor compliance refers to increased resistance met when attempting to ventilate the lungs. When delivering positive-pressure ventilation, it is important to notice if there is a change in the ease with which you can ventilate the patient. For example, if it was initially easy to ventilate a patient with a BM but you now notice that it is becoming increasingly difficult to ventilate her, the patient's condition is changing. You will need to reassess the patient and search for the cause of this change.

Although a BM device can be used to assist ventilations in a patient with inadequate breathing, it is more commonly used to ventilate a nonbreathing patient. When a BM device is not connected to supplemental oxygen, 21% oxygen (room air) is delivered to the patient (Figure 14-6a). If a BM device is connected to supplemental oxygen set at a flow rate of 15 L/min but no reservoir is used, about 40% to 60% oxygen can be delivered to the patient, provided there is a good face-to-mask seal (Figure 14-6b). If the BM device is connected to supplemental oxygen at a flow rate of 15 L/min and a reservoir is present on the bag, about 90% to 100% oxygen can be delivered to the patient, provided there is a good face-to-mask seal (Figure 14-6c).

Steps in using a BM device by yourself to ventilate a nonbreathing patient:

- Connect the bag to the mask.
- Place the patient on his back. Open his airway with a head tilt–chin lift maneuver. If trauma is suspected, use the jaw thrust maneuver to open the airway. Size and insert an oral or nasal airway.
- Position the narrow portion of the mask over the bridge of the patient's nose. Position the wide portion of the mask between the patient's lower lip and chin. Lower the mask over the patient's nose and mouth.
- Create a face-to-mask seal by forming a C around the ventilation port with your thumb and index finger. Place the third, fourth, and fifth fingers of the same hand along the bony portion of the lower jaw, avoiding the soft tissue area. (These fingers form an E.) If no injury to the head or spine is suspected, lift up slightly on the jaw with these fingers, bringing the patient's jaw up to the mask as you tilt his head backward. If injury to the head or spine *is* suspected, do *not* tilt the patient's head backward. Instead, bring the patient's jaw up to the mask without moving the head or neck.

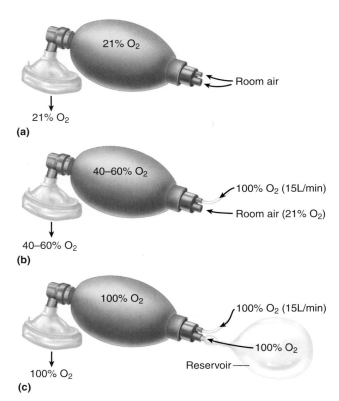

FIGURE 14-6 ▲ **(a)** A bag-mask device without supplemental oxygen will deliver 21% oxygen (room air) to the patient. **(b)** A bag-mask device used with supplemental oxygen at a flow rate of 15 L/min will deliver about 40% to 60% oxygen to the patient, provided there is a good face-to-mask seal. **(c)** A reservoir (an oxygen-collecting device) is attached to this bag-mask device. The reservoir collects a volume of 100% oxygen equal to the capacity of the bag. When the bag refills, 100% oxygen is drawn into the bag from the reservoir. With the oxygen flow rate set at 15 L/min, a bag-mask can deliver about 90% to 100% oxygen to the patient, provided there is a good face-to-mask seal.

- With your other hand, squeeze the bag until you see a gentle chest rise (Figure 14-7a). Deliver each ventilation over 1 second. Watch for a gentle rise and fall of the patient's chest with each ventilation. Stop ventilation when you see a gentle chest rise. Allow the patient to exhale between breaths.
- Ventilate at an age-appropriate rate: once every 3 to 5 seconds for an infant or child and once every 5 to 6 seconds for an adult.
- When possible, connect the bag to oxygen at a flow rate of 15 L/min and attach the reservoir.

You Should Know

Creating a face-to-mask seal by using your fingers to form a C and an E is only one of many acceptable methods of performing this skill.

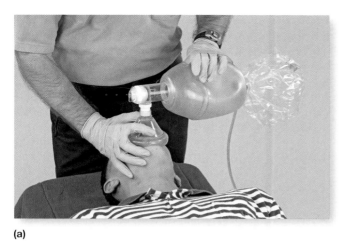

(a)

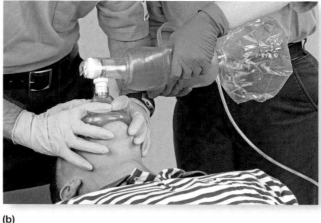

(b)

FIGURE 14-7 ▲ Bag-mask device ventilation. **(a)** One-person technique; **(b)** two-person technique.

Spontaneously Breathing Patients

There are times that you will need to assist the breathing of a patient who is breathing on her own but whose breathing is too slow or shallow to be effective. For example, a patient in respiratory distress or respiratory failure is likely to need assisted ventilation to improve her oxygenation and ventilation. The patient will usually show assessment findings and symptoms of inadequate breathing that may include any of the following:

- Altered mental status
- Decreased rate of breathing
- Greatly increased rate of breathing
- Inadequate depth of breathing
- Fatigue from work of breathing
- Abnormal skin color

Assisting a patient's breathing requires patience and practice. If the patient is awake, be sure to explain what you are going to do. For instance, "Mrs. __, I'm going to use this special bag and mask to help you breathe." Connect supplemental oxygen to the BM device. Because a patient who is having difficulty breathing may feel smothered when a mask is applied, begin by holding the mask near the patient's face. While explaining what you are doing, squeeze the bag a couple of times so the patient can feel the air escape from the bag. Then apply the mask to the patient's face. Match squeezing the bag with the patient's inspiration. As the patient starts to breathe in, gently squeeze the bag. Stop squeezing as the chest starts to rise. If the patient's breathing rate is too slow, insert artificial breaths between the patient's own breaths. The effectiveness of this technique is limited if the patient is combative (due to hypoxia) or if there is an inadequate face to mask seal.

Remember This

You can deliver a greater tidal volume with a pocket mask than with a BM device. There are two reasons for this. First, you can use both hands to hold a pocket mask securely in place and keep the patient's head in proper position at the same time. Second, you can adjust the depth of your breaths to make up for any leaks between the mask and the patient's face. This allows greater lung ventilation.

Steps in using a BM device with a second rescuer:
- Connect the bag to the mask.
- Place the patient on his back. Open his airway with a head tilt–chin lift maneuver. If trauma is suspected, use the jaw thrust maneuver to open the airway. Size and insert an oral or nasal airway.
- Position the narrow portion of the mask over the bridge of the patient's nose. Position the wide portion of the mask between his lower lip and chin. Lower the mask over the patient's nose and mouth.
- Create a face-to-mask seal by forming a **C** around the ventilation port with your thumb and index finger. Place the third, fourth, and fifth fingers of the same hand along the bony portion of the lower jaw, avoiding the soft tissue area. (These fingers form an **E**.) Lift up slightly on the jaw with these fingers, bringing the patient's jaw up to the mask. If injury to the head or spine is suspected, do *not* tilt the patient's head backward. Instead, bring the patient's jaw up to the mask without moving the head or neck.
- Have an assistant squeeze the bag with two hands until you see gentle chest rise (Figure 14-7b). Deliver each ventilation over 1 second. Watch for the rise and fall of the patient's chest with each

ventilation. Stop ventilation when you see a gentle chest rise. Allow the patient to exhale between breaths.

- Ventilate once every 3 to 5 seconds for an infant or child and once every 5 to 6 seconds for an adult.
- When possible, connect the bag to oxygen at a flow rate of 15 L/min, and attach the reservoir.

Making a Difference

The ability to provide positive-pressure ventilation is a very important EMT skill. You must practice this skill in order to do it effectively. During your initial training program and in later continuing education classes, take advantage of all opportunities to practice this important skill.

Adequate and Inadequate Artificial Ventilation

Objectives 6, 7

Adequate artificial ventilation (also called *rescue breathing*):
- The chest rises and falls with each artificial ventilation.
- The rate of ventilations is sufficient. Sufficient rates are:
  —About 10 to 12 times per minute for adults (once every 5 to 6 seconds)
  —About 12 to 20 times per minute for infants and children (once every 3 to 5 seconds)
- The patient's heart rate improves.
- The patient's color improves.

Inadequate artificial ventilation:
- The chest does not rise and fall with each ventilation.
- The ventilation rate is too slow or too fast.
- The heart rate does not improve with ventilation.
- The patient's color does not improve.

Troubleshooting Bag-Mask Ventilation

If the chest does not rise and fall with BM ventilation, reassess the patient. Start by reassessing the patient's head position. Reposition the airway and try again to ventilate.

The tidal volume delivered to the patient depends on a tight mask seal and adequate compression of the bag. If an air leak is present because of an improper mask seal, an inadequate tidal volume will be delivered to the patient. If air is escaping from under the mask, reposition your fingers and the mask.

Incomplete bag compression will also result in the delivery of an inadequate tidal volume to the patient. This can occur if the bag is large or the EMT's hands are small and only one hand is used to squeeze the bag. If the patient's chest does not rise and fall during BM ventilation, recheck the technique you are using to squeeze the bag. If the patient's chest does not rise, check for an obstruction. Lift the patient's jaw and suction the airway as needed. If the chest still does not rise, use a different method of artificial ventilation, such as a pocket mask or flow-restricted, oxygen-powered ventilation device.

Remember This

Situations in which ventilation with a BM device is most likely to be difficult include the following:

- Patients older than 55 years of age
- Patients with facial trauma
- Large patients
- Presence of a beard
- Lack of teeth or ill-fitting dentures

If the patient has dentures and they do not fit well, remove them so that they do not block the airway.

Flow-Restricted, Oxygen-Powered Ventilation Device

Objective 8

A **flow-restricted, oxygen-powered ventilation device (FROPVD)** is also called a *manually triggered ventilation (MTV) device* (Figure 14-8). A FROPVD is used to give positive-pressure ventilation with 100% oxygen. It can be attached to a face mask, tracheal tube, or tracheostomy tube.

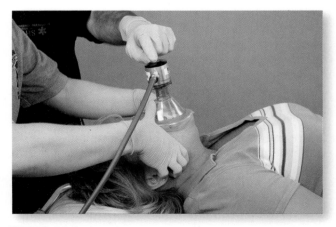

FIGURE 14-8 ▲ A flow-restricted, oxygen-powered ventilation device (FROPVD).

A FROPVD consists of high-pressure tubing that connects the oxygen supply and a valve that is activated by a lever or push button. When the valve is open, oxygen flows into the patient. The major advantages of this device are that it provides high concentrations of oxygen and allows the EMT to use two hands to maintain a tight face-to-mask seal. Although the FROPVD is easy to use, it is not carried on every EMS vehicle. In addition, a special unit and additional training are required for use in infants and children. The FROPVD can cause gastric distention in patients who are not intubated. When using this device, you will be unable to feel the compliance of the patient's lungs. Because a FROPVD delivers oxygen under high pressure, pressure injury (barotrauma) to the lungs is a possible complication of this device. Skill Drill 14-2 shows the steps to use a flow-restricted, oxygen-powered ventilator for a nonbreathing patient.

Making a Difference

A common phrase in EMS is "BLS before ALS": basic life support before advanced life support. This is particularly true when managing a patient's airway. Common problems in airway management involve the use of poor technique. Examples include improperly positioning the patient's head, failing to obtain (and maintain) a good seal with a bag-mask device, and delivering ventilations at an improper rate (usually too fast). Another common problem is failing to reassess the patient after each intervention. Rise above these common mistakes. Aspire to provide excellent care. Practice your skills often, perform them to the best of your ability, and reassess the patient who is in your care.

Special Considerations

Tracheal Stomas

Objective 9

A **laryngectomy** is the surgical removal of the larynx. A person who has had a laryngectomy breathes through a stoma. A **stoma** is an artificial opening. A **tracheal stoma** is a permanent opening at the front of the neck that extends from the skin surface into the trachea. It opens the trachea to the atmosphere. A **tracheostomy** is the surgical formation of an opening into the trachea. There are many reasons why a person may have a tracheal stoma:

- A throat tumor or infection
- A severe injury to the neck or mouth
- A disease or infection that affects swallowing
- The need for long-term breathing assistance with a mechanical ventilator

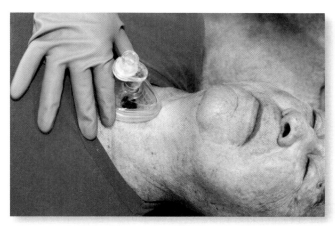

FIGURE 14-9 ▲ Mask-to-stoma breathing.

Patients who have a tracheal stoma breathe through this opening in the neck because it is their airway. If artificial ventilation is required, it should be delivered through the stoma.

Steps in performing mask-to-stoma breathing:
- Remove any garment (scarf, neck tie) covering the stoma.
- Place a barrier device or pediatric resuscitation mask on the patient's neck over the stoma. Make an airtight seal around the stoma (Figure 14-9).
- Slowly blow into the one-way valve on the mask until the chest rises.
- Remove your mouth from the mask to allow the patient to exhale.

Steps in performing BM-to-stoma breathing:
- Remove any garment (scarf, necktie) covering the stoma.
- Connect oxygen to the BM device. If the patient has a tracheostomy tube in place, remove the mask from the device. Connect the bag-mask device to the patient's tracheostomy tube (Figure 14-10). Squeeze the bag while watching for chest rise. Allow the patient to exhale passively.

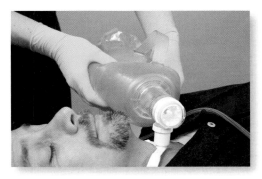

FIGURE 14-10 ▲ Ventilating through a tracheostomy tube.

Skill Drill 14-2

Flow-Restricted, Oxygen-Powered Ventilation for a Nonbreathing Patient

STEP 1 ▶ Prepare the flow-restricted, oxygen-powered ventilator. Select a mask of the correct size while another EMT ventilates the patient using another method. Connect the ventilator to the mask.

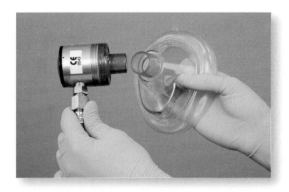

STEP 2 ▶ Position yourself at the patient's head. Position the mask on the patient's face. Seal the mask in place with one hand.

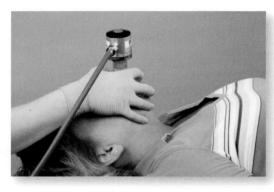

STEP 3 ▶ While holding the mask in place, open the patient's airway. If no trauma is suspected, use a head tilt–chin lift (as shown here). If trauma is suspected, open the airway using a jaw thrust maneuver.

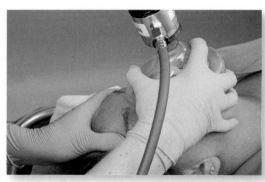

STEP 4 ▶ Trigger the valve (depress the button) on the ventilator to inflate the patient's lungs. Inflate only until you see adequate chest rise. Repeat once every 5 seconds. Watch for gastric distention. If seen, reposition the patient's head and recheck ventilation.

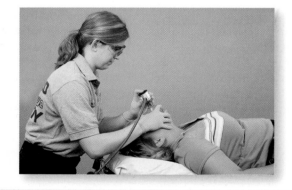

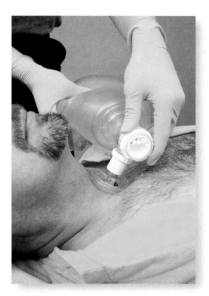

FIGURE 14-11 ◀ Bag-mask-to-stoma breathing.

- If a stoma is present (but no tracheostomy tube), attach a pediatric mask to the BM device. Center the mask over the stoma, and make an airtight seal around the stoma (Figure 14-11). If the chest does not rise and fall, seal the patient's mouth and nose, and try again to ventilate. Release the seal to allow the patient to exhale.

Dental Appliances

Dentures that fit well in the patient's mouth should be left in place. If they become loose or dislodged, remove them from the mouth because they can become a foreign body obstruction. Note that when you ventilate a patient with his dentures removed, it is harder to obtain a seal.

Infants and Children

Objective 10

Ventilating an infant or a child with a BM device requires special consideration. The flat bridge of an infant's or a child's nose makes it more difficult to obtain a good mask seal. Place the head in neutral position for an infant and in a slightly extended position for a child. Extending the head too far back may kink the airway, resulting in an airway obstruction. An oral airway may be needed when other procedures fail to provide a clear airway.

Use a pediatric BM device for full-term newborns, infants, and children. Use an adult bag for larger children and adolescents. Gastric distention is common when ventilating infants and children. To help avoid this, do not use excessive bag pressure when ventilating an infant or a child. Use only enough pressure to make the chest gently rise. Watch for improvement in skin color

and/or heart rate. When using a BM device during a cardiac arrest, make sure it does not have a pop-off valve. If a pop-off valve is present, it must be disabled (placed in the closed position) for adequate ventilation.

Sum It Up

▶ As an EMT, you must maintain an open airway in order to allow a free flow of air into and out of the patient's lungs. After you have opened a patient's airway, you may need to use an airway adjunct to keep it open. After the airway adjunct is inserted, maintain the proper head position while the device is in place.

▶ After making sure that the patient's airway is open, you must check for breathing. If the patient is breathing, you must determine if the patient is breathing adequately or inadequately. You must also be able to recognize the sounds of noisy breathing, which include stridor, snoring, gurgling, and wheezing.

▶ If your patient's breathing is inadequate or absent, you will need to assist the patient by forcing air into the patient's lungs during inspiration. This action is called positive-pressure ventilation and includes the following: mouth-to-mask ventilation, mouth-to-barrier ventilation, and bag-mask ventilation. As an EMT, you must be familiar with performing all these ventilation methods.

▶ Cricoid pressure helps decrease the amount of air entering the stomach during positive-pressure ventilation, which reduces the likelihood of vomiting and aspiration. This technique should be used only in unresponsive patients. It is usually applied by a third person during positive-pressure ventilation.

- A pocket mask is an effective means of delivering positive-pressure ventilation. When the mask is connected to oxygen with a minimum flow of 10 L/min, about 50% oxygen can be delivered to the patient.

- A barrier device is a thin film of plastic or silicone that is placed on the patient's face and used to prevent direct contact with the patient's mouth during positive ventilation.

- A bag-mask device is a self-inflating bag with a one-way valve and mask that is used to deliver positive-pressure ventilation. BM devices are available in adult, child, and infant sizes. Although BM ventilation can be done using one person, it is best performed with two rescuers. One of the advantages of ventilating a patient with a BM device is the ability to feel the compliance of the patient's lungs. Compliance refers to the ability of the patient's lung tissue to distend (inflate) with ventilation.

- A flow-restricted, oxygen-powered ventilation device is used to give positive-pressure ventilation with 100% oxygen. It can be attached to a face mask, tracheal tube, or tracheostomy tube.

- A tracheal stoma is a permanent opening at the front of the neck that extends from the skin surface into the trachea. A tracheostomy is the surgical formation of an opening into the trachea. If artificial ventilation is required, it should be delivered through the stoma.

- Gastric distention (swelling) is common when ventilating infants and children. When providing positive-pressure ventilation, avoid using excessive volume. Use only enough volume to cause a gentle chest rise.

Module 5

Patient Assessment

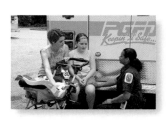

▶ CHAPTER 15

Therapeutic Communications and History Taking 294

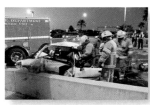

▶ CHAPTER 16

Scene Size-Up 310

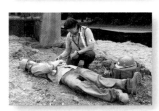

▶ CHAPTER 17

Patient Assessment 325

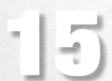

CHAPTER 15

Therapeutic Communications and History Taking

By the end of this chapter, you should be able to:

Knowledge Objectives ▶

1. Discuss the basic elements of the communication process.
2. Identify nonverbal behaviors that are used in patient interviewing.
3. Discuss common patient responses to illness or injury.
4. Discuss the communication skills that should be used to interact with the patient.
5. Discuss developmental considerations of various age groups that influence patient interviewing.
6. Discuss techniques that may be necessary when interviewing patients who have special needs.
7. Discuss the communication skills that should be used to interact with family members and bystanders.
8. Identify and explain each of the components of the patient history.
9. Provide examples of open-ended and closed or direct questions.
10. Discuss the need to search for additional medical identification.
11. Explain the standardized approach to history taking using the OPQRST and SAMPLE acronyms.
12. Give examples of pertinent positive and pertinent negative findings.
13. Differentiate between a sign and a symptom.

Attitude Objectives ▶

14. Exhibit professional nonverbal behaviors.
15. Advocate development of proper patient rapport.
16. Value strategies to obtain patient information.
17. Exhibit professional behaviors in communicating with patients in special situations.
18. Exhibit professional behaviors in communicating with patients from different cultures.

Skill Objective ▶

19. Demonstrate the skills that should be used to obtain information from the patient, family, or bystanders at the scene.

You are excited about having just completed your emergency medical technician training. You were issued a pager and radio for the local fire department earlier in the day. Later that evening your pager goes off, notifying you of your first call. A million thoughts run through your head as you inform dispatch of your response to the scene. At the scene, you and your partner are the first EMS personnel to arrive. Your gloves are already on as you knock on the door. An elderly man greets you at the door of the residence and leads you into the kitchen where his wife is seated. You immediately think of the questions needed to gather a thorough patient history. You begin asking the patient questions and move on to the next question with barely a pause for breath. ∎

THINK ABOUT IT

As you read this chapter, think about the following questions:

- How does your ability to be an active listener affect patient care?
- What is the most effective method of interviewing a patient?
- What questions are pertinent to a patient interview and how quickly should the questions be asked?
- Is there a benefit to establishing rapport with your patient?
- How do the answers to your questions affect your treatment plan?

Introduction

Your patients are individuals of varying ages with a wide range of life experiences, knowledge, reasoning abilities, skills, and medical needs. To communicate effectively with them, you must understand that communication requires more than knowing the proper words and their meaning. Communicating in a respectful manner may mean the difference between acquiring information and missing it. This chapter focuses on the basic requirements for successfully communicating with your patients.

The Communication Process

Objectives 1, 2

In Chapter 1 you learned that communication is the exchange of thoughts and messages that occurs by sending and receiving information. The communication process involves six basic elements (Figure 15-1):

1. A source (the sender)
2. Encoding
3. The message
4. The channel
5. A receiver (decoder)
6. Feedback

Problems with communication can occur at any step in this process.

The Sender

Communication starts with an information source. The source of verbal communication is spoken or written words. A **message** is the information to be communicated. The sender decides the message she wants to convey and then encodes it. **Encoding** is the act of placing a message into words or images so that it is understood similarly by the sender and receiver. Successful communication depends, in part, on the sender's ability to convey information clearly and simply. When you ask questions of a patient or relay information to her, you are the sender. To ensure that the message you are sending is clear, give careful thought to the words you choose and be confident that the information you relay to the patient is accurate.

The sender selects the path (channel) for transmitting the message to the receiver. Examples of channels include air, light, electricity, radio waves, paper, and postal systems. When communicating with a patient, you use your mouth (sound) and body (gesture) to create and alter your message. In face-to-face communication, the communication channels used consist of air (sound) and light (gesture), enabling the exchange of information between you and the patient.

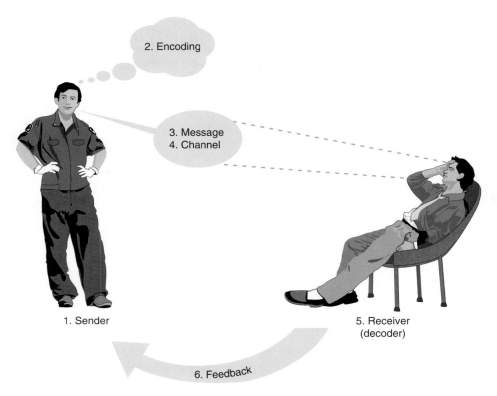

FIGURE 15-1 ◄ The six steps of the communication process: In this example, the EMT is the (1) sender and is (2) encoding his (3) message in words. He transmits his message through the (4) channels of air (sound) and light (gesture). The patient is the (5) receiver who decodes the message and provides (6) feedback to the EMT. In the feedback loop, the patient becomes the sender and the EMT becomes the receiver.

When interacting with patients and their families, awareness of nonverbal behavior is also important. Examples of nonverbal behaviors include actions, body language, and active listening. Actions and body language include physical appearance, posture, and gestures. Good grooming and a professional appearance are important characteristics of EMS professionals and help build the patient's trust. Your posture during a patient interview should be relaxed but reflect interest in the message the patient is relaying to you. Gestures should be natural, such as nodding in response to a patient's statement. Active listening requires your complete attention and the frequent use of verbal encouragement. This important skill requires practice.

The Receiver

The **receiver** is the person or group for whom the sender's message is intended. When a message is received, the receiver must interpret (decode) the sender's message. **Noise** is anything that obscures, confuses, or interferes with the communication. Communication is successful if the sender and the receiver understand the same information. However, just as errors can occur during encoding, they can also arise during **decoding.** For example, if the receiver was not actively listening to the message sent or if the words used in the message were not understood by the receiver, the message may be misinterpreted and result in confusion. For instance, if you ask a patient experiencing breathing difficulty when his dyspnea started, it is likely that he will not understand the word "dyspnea." If he attempts to answer your question without first asking for clarification of the misunderstood word, his answer will probably be inaccurate because he did not understand the question from the start. When communicating with your patients, do not use medical terms. Appropriate medical terminology should be used in your written reports and verbal communication with other healthcare professionals.

Feedback is the response from the receiver (verbal or nonverbal) that allows the sender to know how her message is being received. In the feedback loop, the receiver becomes the sender and the sender becomes the receiver. The switch from sender to receiver and back again occurs often during the communication process.

Communicating with the Patient

Strategies to Ascertain Information

When obtaining a patient history, patients generally relay information to healthcare professionals in three ways:

1. By "pouring out" the information in the form of complaints

2. By revealing some problems while concealing others that they believe are embarrassing

3. By hiding the most embarrassing parts of their problem from the interviewer (and themselves)

Obtaining information from the patient regarding a complaint is accomplished using open-ended and closed (direct) questions, which are discussed later in this chapter.

You may encounter resistance when attempting to interview a patient. There are two main reasons for resistance: (1) The patient wishes to maintain an image and fears losing that image, and (2) the patient is uncertain about your response and fears rejection or ridicule. Therefore, it is important to be nonjudgmental if you expect to obtain information from these patients. You must also be willing to talk with a patient about any condition the person may have.

In some situations, the patient may be hesitant to discuss a complaint. In order to explore the problem, it may be necessary to shift your questions away from the problem, and then return to it from a different angle. For example, a woman complaining of abdominal pain may be uncomfortable answering questions from a male EMT related to her menstrual cycle. A male patient with a possible urinary tract infection may be uncomfortable answering a female EMT's questions pertaining to his complaint. In these situations, shifting your line of questioning away from the problem and later returning to it with a slightly different approach will often result in obtaining the needed information.

Ill or injured patients often use defense mechanisms (also called *coping mechanisms*) to help them deal with the situation. For example, denial is a common defense mechanism used by patients experiencing chest pain. The patient may refuse to believe that the chest pain she is experiencing may be related to a heart attack. It is important to be aware of the patient's defense mechanisms, anticipate them in advance, and confront the patient if necessary to obtain necessary medical information.

If a patient is acting out and hostile, maintain a professional, nonthreatening demeanor. Calmly point out his behavior to him, ask him if his behavior is intentional, and let him know that this behavior is self-defeating. This distraction may allow the patient sufficient time to regroup and regain self-control.

The Patient's Response to Illness or Injury

Objective 3

What a patient considers an emergency may not appear to be an emergency to a person with medical training. Some medical personnel become irritated or annoyed when they feel they have been summoned to assist a person who does not appear particularly ill or who has a minor complaint. Keep in mind that pain is what the *patient* says it is and an emergency is what the

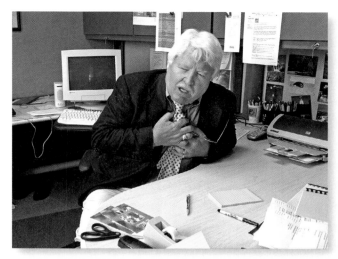

FIGURE 15-2 ▲ As an EMT, you must be prepared for a variety of emotions and behaviors from your patients.

patient perceives it to be. It is important that, as an Emergency Medical Services professional, you accept every call for assistance without prejudice. Provide the best emergency care you can for every patient—without questioning the validity of the complaint.

Because patients react differently to an illness or injury, you must be prepared for a variety of emotions and behaviors (Figure 15-2). Depending on the nature of the illness or the severity of the injury, your patient may experience a number of emotions. Your patient's response to these emotions may be seen as distrust, resentment, despair, anger, or regression. **Regression** is a return to an earlier or former developmental state. For example, an adult patient's behavior may appear child-like. This reaction is common and natural because an ill or injured patient, like a child, depends on others for survival.

You Should Know

Common Patient Responses to Illness or Injury

- Fear
- Embarrassment
- Frustration
- Pain
- Regression
- Feeling of being powerless or helpless
- Anxiety
- Anger
- Sorrow
- Depression
- Guilt, shame, or blame

It is important to understand these emotions in order to be tolerant of them. For example, a busy executive experiences a heart attack. She may feel helpless because she finds herself dependent on medical professionals whose experience and skills she cannot easily

TABLE 15-1   Interpersonal Distance in the United States

Zone	Distance	Notes
Public space	12 feet or more	Interaction with others is impersonal in this space; speaker's voice must be projected; subtle facial expressions imperceptible.
Social space	4–12 feet	Used for impersonal business transactions, hearing and vision are the primary senses used in this space; much of a patient interview occurs at this distance.
Personal space	1½–4 feet	This is the distance used when interacting with friends, perceived as extension of self; hearing and vision are important at this distance, voice is moderate, body odors are not apparent, no visual distortion; much of a physical assessment occurs in this space.
Intimate space	Touching to 1½ feet	Senses of smell and touch are the primary senses involved at this distance; visual distortion occurs; this distance is best for assessing breath and other body odors.

evaluate. She may be angry because her life has been disrupted. She may experience fear and anxiety because her independence is threatened. She may also wonder what the next few minutes, hours, days, and months will bring. Her concerns might include the following:

- "Why is this happening to me?"
- "Am I going to be disabled?"
- "How will I provide for my family if I can't work?"
- "Am I going to die?"

Approaching the Ill or Injured Patient

Objective 4

Introduce Yourself

When communicating with a patient, begin by identifying yourself and establishing your role by saying, "My name is ___. I am an emergency medical technician trained to provide emergency care. I am here to help you." Address the patient by proper name, Mr. __ or Mrs. __. Ask the patient what he or she wishes to be called, and then ask for permission to use this name. Do not use words such as "hon," "dear," or "sweetheart" when speaking to a patient. Phrases such as these are disrespectful and unprofessional.

Be considerate of your patient's personal space, physical condition, and feelings. **Personal space** is the invisible area immediately around each of us that we declare as our own. The size of your personal space can change depending on your cultural norms and the people you are with, but you may feel threatened when others invade your personal space without your consent.

When talking with a patient, it is important to consider the distance between you and the patient and recognize that a "comfortable distance" differs among cultures. For example, the Japanese typically have a larger personal space than North Americans do, whereas Italians have a much smaller one. Examples of the interpersonal distance common in the United States are listed in Table 15-1.

Many of the tasks you will perform as an EMT will often occur within the boundaries of another's personal space. It is helpful to take the time to explain procedures that intrude on that personal space before beginning the procedure. If you do not, the patient may become agitated, nervous, or even aggressive because of your actions.

While talking with the patient, family members, or bystanders, look at the person with whom you are talking instead of looking at your chart (Figure 15-3). Although this takes practice, nothing else conveys a greater sense of your understanding and control of the situation.

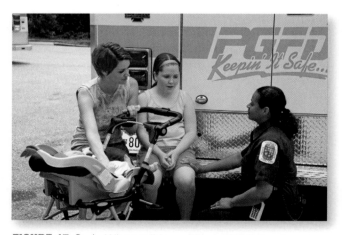

FIGURE 15-3 ▲ When talking with a patient, family members, or bystanders, be confident, calm, and respectful and look at the person with whom you are talking instead of looking at your chart.

TABLE 15-2 Responses to Facilitate a Good Patient Interview

Response	Description	Example
Facilitation	Encourages patient to provide more information	"Can you tell me more about your chest pain?"
Silence	Gives the patient more time to gather thoughts	The use of silence is a useful communication technique but can become uncomfortable for some patients.
Reflection	Echoing the patient's words back and using slightly different words	"You look anxious. Is it related to the chest pain you are experiencing?"
Empathy	Patient feels accepted and more open to talking	"That must have been difficult for you."
Clarification	Used when the patient uses a word which is confusing to the interviewer	"I am not sure what you mean. Could you explain it to me again?"
Confrontation	Focuses the patient's attention on one specific factor of the interview	"You said that you have a history of high blood pressure. When was the last time you took your medication?"
Interpretation	Based on observation or conclusion; linking events, making associations, or implying a cause	"The emergency department physician will let you know if your high blood pressure today is the result of not taking your medication for the past 3 days."
Explanation	Informing the patient and sharing factual or objective information	"It is important to take your blood pressure medication daily as prescribed—even when you are feeling fine and your blood pressure is within normal limits."
Summary	Reviewing the interview by asking openended questions that allow the patient to clarify details	"During the past few minutes you said . . . Is this correct? Did I leave anything out?"

Be confident and remain calm. Know what you are going to say before you say it. Have all the information you need before you start talking. Speak clearly and at an appropriate speed or pace, not too rapidly and not too slowly. Avoid the tendency to get excited. Speaking in a calm and professional manner gives the impression that you are in control of the situation.

Listen carefully to what your patient is telling you. Responses that the EMT can use to facilitate a good patient interview are shown in Table 15-2.

Help ease your patient's fears by explaining what you are about to do, how you will do it, and why it must be done. Use common terms (not medical terminology) when asking questions and explaining the care you will provide.

Be aware of your body position. Most patients find it intimidating if you are standing over them. Sit or kneel down so that you are at eye level with your patient. Be truthful. Patients have a legal right to know about their condition. This does not mean you have to be brutal, but do not lie to patients about their medical condition.

The following script is an example of possible communication between you and a patient as you enter the patient's home.

Medic 51: [As you enter the home.] "Hello, ambulance [or fire department] here. Did someone call 9-1-1?"

Patient: "Yes! In here."

Medic 51: [As you approach and kneel next to the patient.] "Hi! My name is Joe. I am an emergency medical technician with the ambulance [or fire department]. I am here to help you. Can you tell me about the emergency today?"

Patient: "Hard to breathe."

Medic 51: "My partner and I will be glad to take care of you. Could you please tell me your name and what you prefer to be called?"

Patient: "Mrs. Jones. Call me Linda."

Medic 51: "Linda, when did your trouble breathing start?"

Patient: "Yesterday."

Medic 51:	"I would like to give you some oxygen to help your breathing."
Patient:	"OK."
Medic 51:	"I am going to put this oxygen mask on your face. I want you to breathe normally. The oxygen will help your breathing."

Making a Difference

Do not assume that an unresponsive patient cannot hear what is being said. If your patient is unresponsive, speak in a normal tone of voice. Talk to the patient as if he or she were awake. Provide reassurance, offer words of comfort, and explain what you are doing. Many healthcare professionals have been embarrassed when a patient is successfully resuscitated and is able to accurately relay what was said by those caring for him or her.

Treat the Patient with Respect

Recognize the patient's need for privacy, preserve the patient's dignity, and treat the patient with respect. Most patients are uncomfortable about being examined. In our culture, clothing is ordinarily removed in front of another only in situations of trust or intimacy. Be aware that your patient will be anxious about having his clothing removed and having an examination performed by a stranger. Some patients will view these actions as an invasion of their privacy. Help ease your patient's fears by explaining what you are about to do and why it must be done (Figure 15-4). When performing a

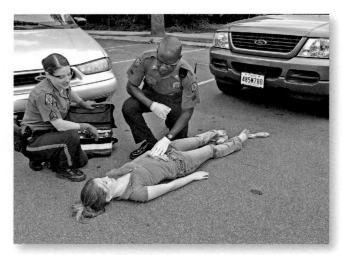

FIGURE 15-4 ▲ Explaining what you are about to do and why it must be done will help ease your patient's fears.

physical examination, be sure to properly drape or shield an unclothed patient from the stares of others. Conduct the examination professionally and efficiently. Talk with the patient throughout the procedure. These actions will build trust and help reduce the patient's anxiety. If your patient is a child, ask for help from a parent or family member to lessen the child's anxiety. Working with children will be covered in more detail in Chapter 44, "Pediatrics."

You Should Know

Traps of Interviewing

- Providing false assurance or reassurance
- Giving advice
- Showing approval or disapproval
- Using professional jargon
- Talking too much
- Changing the subject
- Using "why" questions (viewed as accusatory)
- Asking leading or biased questions
- Distancing
- Interrupting

Recognize the Patient's Need for Control

Although many patients will feel a sense of relief when you arrive, the lights, sirens, and flurry of activity involved in providing emergency care can be frightening. Even though your patient may be ill or injured, he will usually feel the need to show independence. When possible, allow the patient to make choices, such as the hospital to which he prefers to be transported.

Listen with Empathy

Remain calm, be sympathetic, and listen with empathy. Having **empathy** means understanding, being aware of, and being sensitive to the feelings, thoughts, and experiences of another. Effective listening requires concentration (Figure 15-5). Do not interrupt before your patient has finished telling you what the problem is. Do not anticipate what the patient is going to say and finish her sentences. Allow the patient time to explain what is wrong in her own words.

Do Not Give False Hope

Do not give false hope or false reassurance. You should not say, "Everything is going to be okay" when that is obviously not true. Similarly, you should not say you understand when you have not had the same experience as your patient. Instead, reassure the patient by saying, "We will do everything we can to help."

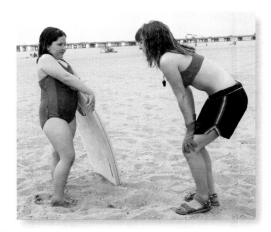

FIGURE 15-5 ▲ Effective listening requires concentration.

Use a Reassuring Touch

If appropriate, use a reassuring touch. Touch is a sensitive means of communication. It can be used to express feelings that cannot be expressed well with words. It is important to assess your level of comfort and that of your patient regarding the use of touch. Some healthcare professionals are uncomfortable touching patients to display concern, caring, and reassurance. Most patients will accept a reassuring touch and will respond positively to it. Others are uncomfortable when touched in this way and may misunderstand your intentions. Be sensitive to the patient's acceptance of touch. Learn to recognize when the use of compassionate touch is appropriate.

Children

Objective 5

Young infants (birth to 6 months of age) are unafraid of strangers and have no modesty. Older infants (6 months to 1 year of age) do not like to be separated from their caregiver (separation anxiety). They may be threatened by direct eye contact with strangers. If possible, assess the baby on the caregiver's lap. Avoid loud noises; bright lights; and quick, jerky movements. Smile and use a calm, soothing voice. Allow the baby to suck on a pacifier for comfort, if appropriate and if the child is willing to take it. Do not force the pacifier if the child does not want it.

Toddlers (1 to 3 years of age) respond appropriately to an angry or a friendly voice. When separated from their primary caregiver, most toddlers experience strong separation anxiety. Toddlers can answer simple questions and follow simple directions. However, you cannot reason with toddlers. Toddlers are likely to be more cooperative if they are given a comfort object like a blanket, stuffed animal, or toy.

Making a Difference

Cultural Considerations

Effective communication with persons of different cultures requires sensitivity and awareness. It is important to refrain from using offensive language and to avoid speaking in ways that are disrespectful to your patient's cultural beliefs. For example, you should be aware of the amount of personal space that is considered acceptable, the degree of eye contact considered acceptable, and acceptable touching.

- When speaking with most patients, 18 inches between people is usually considered a comfortable distance. Hispanics, Asians, and Middle Easterners generally stand closer together when talking.
- Many American Indians and patients of Mexican descent avoid direct eye contact to show respect. Sustained direct eye contact is considered rude or disrespectful. Mexican-Americans have a high respect for authority and the elderly. They should be addressed formally (by title). The Vietnamese avoid eye contact when speaking with someone they consider an authority figure or someone who is older. European-Americans use firm eye contact and look for the impact of what is being said.
- Hispanics typically find a touch on the arm, shoulder, or back comforting. Asian and Arab patients generally find touch acceptable only between members of the same gender, except within the family. Because Asians consider the area of the body below the waist private, it is almost never exposed. In addition, Asian-Americans prefer to be addressed by position and role, such as "mother" or "teacher." An individual's name is considered private and is used only by family and close friends.
- Mexican-American women may be reluctant to undress, even in the presence of a healthcare professional of the same gender.
- Pacific Islanders (native Hawaiians and Samoans) and Asian-Americans are often reluctant to ask questions or express emotion to others. They may be overly agreeable in their communications. Arab-Americans may be reluctant to reveal information about themselves to strangers. Hispanic-Americans are often vocal about illness or pain.

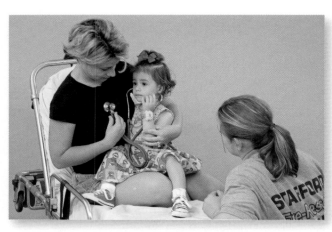

FIGURE 15-6 ▲ Encourage the trust of a young child by gaining the cooperation of her caregiver. By talking with the caregiver first, you may put the child more at ease if she sees that the adult is not threatened.

Toddlers are distrustful of strangers. They are likely to resist examination and treatment. When touched, they may scream, cry, or kick. Toddlers do not like having their clothing removed and do not like anything on their face. Encourage a child's trust by gaining the cooperation of the caregiver. Talk with the caregiver first: The child may be more at ease after seeing that the adult is not threatened (Figure 15-6). When possible, allow an infant or young child to remain on the caregiver's lap. If this is not possible, try to keep the caregiver within the child's line of vision. Approach the child slowly and address her by name. Talk to the child at eye level, using simple words and short phrases. Speak in a calm, reassuring tone of voice. Although young children may not understand your words, they will respond to your tone.

Remember This

Do not threaten a child who is uncooperative.

Preschoolers (3 to 5 years of age) are afraid of the unknown, the dark, being left alone, and adults who look or act mean. They may think their illness or injury is punishment for bad behavior or thoughts. Approach preschoolers slowly and talk to them at eye level. Use simple words and phrases and a reassuring tone of voice. Assure preschoolers that they were not bad and are not being punished.

Preschoolers may feel vulnerable and out of control when lying down. Assess and treat them in an upright position when possible. Preschoolers are modest. They do not like being touched or having their clothing removed. When assessing a child, keep in mind that she has probably been told not to let a stranger

touch her. Remove clothing, assess the child, and then quickly replace clothing. Allow the caregiver to remain with the child whenever possible.

Preschoolers are curious and like to "help." Encourage them to participate. Tell them how things will feel and what you are doing just before doing it. For example, a preschooler may fear being suffocated by an oxygen mask. It may be helpful to use a doll or a stuffed animal to explain the procedure. The child may want to hold or look at the equipment first.

Preschoolers are highly imaginative. When talking with a preschooler, choose your words carefully. Avoid baby talk and frightening or misleading terms. For example, avoid words such as "take," "cut," "shot," "deaden," or "germs." Instead of saying, "I'm going to take your pulse," you might say, "I'm going to see how fast your heart is beating."

When caring for school-age children (6 to 12 years of age), approach them in a friendly manner and introduce yourself. Talk directly to the child about what happened, even if you also obtain a history from the caregiver. Explain procedures before carrying them out. Allow school-age children to see and touch equipment that may be used in their care.

Honesty is very important when interacting with school-age children. If you are going to do something to a child that may cause pain, warn the child just before you do it. Give a simple explanation of what will take place, and do this just before the procedure so that the child does not have long to think about it. For example, if a child has a possible broken leg and you must move the leg to apply a splint, warn the child just before you move the leg.

Adolescents (13 to 18 years of age) expect to be treated as adults. Talk to adolescents in a respectful, friendly manner, as if speaking to an adult. If possible, obtain a history from the patient instead of from a caregiver. Expect an adolescent to have many questions and want detailed explanations about what you are planning to do or what is happening to her. Explain things clearly and honestly. Allow time for questions. Do not bargain with an adolescent in order to do what you need to do. Recognize the tendency for adolescents to overreact. Do not become angry with an emotional or hysterical adolescent.

Older Adults

Objective 5

An older adult may have difficulty hearing and poor vision. Assume a position directly in the patient's line of vision and speak directly toward him. Begin speaking to the patient in a normal tone of voice. If the patient has difficulty hearing, speak a little more loudly until he can hear you. Speak slowly and say each word clearly. Be careful not to "talk down" to the patient. Ask the patient one question at a time, and allow the patient time to respond. If it is necessary to repeat the question, phrase it exactly as it was asked the first time. Provide reassurance with a soothing voice and calm manner.

Non-English-Speaking Patients

Objective 6

Communication with non-English-speaking patients may require the use of an interpreter. Explain to the interpreter the type of questions that will be asked. Avoid interrupting a family member (or bystander) and interpreter when they are communicating. If an interpreter is not present at the scene, contact dispatch or medical direction. Telephone companies often have interpreters who are available 24 hours a day.

Hearing-Impaired Patients

Objective 6

You Should Know

Not all hearing-impaired people hear the same sounds in the same way.

Having a hearing impairment does not mean that the person lacks mental intelligence. Many deaf patients do not consider a lack of hearing a disability. In fact, they often resent being treated as if they have a disability. A common mistaken belief of some healthcare professionals is that they must speak more slowly and loudly for the patient to understand them. Not only does this not work, but it may actually confuse the patient. When you speak more slowly than normal, you have a tendency to overemphasize the way you move your mouth when you speak. This can lead to a greater misunderstanding if the patient is trying to read your lips. Try not to drastically change the way you speak. Use your normal tone of voice and speak at your normal speed—as if you were carrying on a conversation with any other patient (Figure 15-7). If the patient has a sound amplification device or hearing aid, you may need to help her put it in place.

You may have to get your patient's attention with a gentle touch on the shoulder. Face your patient directly so that she can see your face and mouth. Make sure that there is adequate lighting so that the patient can see your face and mouth clearly. When speaking, do not move your head around. Doing so makes it difficult for the patient to follow what you are saying. If the patient has some limited ability to hear, try to reduce any unnecessary background noise. For example, shut off televisions, radios, dish-

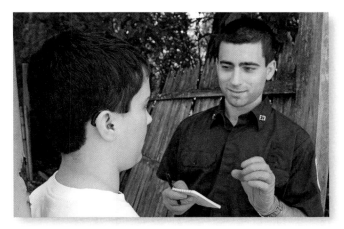

FIGURE 15-7 ▲ When speaking to a hearing-impaired patient, use your normal tone of voice and speak at your normal speed—as if you were carrying on a conversation with any other patient.

washers, or other noisy appliances while talking with the patient. You may even resort to the use of paper and pen to communicate.

When questioning your patient about his condition, think about the questions you want to ask. Then ask him short, direct questions that require a very specific answer. Make sure to actually speak or say every word in your question. Ask one question at a time, and follow up on the answer before starting another line of questioning. Doing so will allow you and the patient to focus on one problem at a time. It can even lead to a better interview. Avoid the use of sign language unless you are very skilled.

Remember to explain any procedure before providing care. Be sure to inform the EMS crew arriving on the scene of the patient's hearing impairment.

Visually Impaired Patients

Objective 6

The term *visual impairment* applies to a variety of vision disturbances. Visual impairments range from blindness and lack of usable sight to low vision. **Low vision** is a visual impairment that interferes with a person's ability to perform everyday activities.

If the patient is visually impaired, approach the patient from the front and introduce yourself. Identify any persons with you. Speak in a normal voice. Most blind persons are not hearing impaired so there is no need to raise your voice or shout when talking to them. If family members or others are present, address the patient by name so that it is clear to whom you are talking. Clearly explain any care you are going to provide before doing so. In this way, you do not surprise or startle the patient. Be sure to talk directly to the patient, not through a family member. Do not avoid the use of words such as "see" and "blind." These words are parts of normal speech.

A very strong bond can form between a visually impaired patient and her service dog. Make every attempt to keep them together if at all possible. Do not pet or otherwise distract a service dog. A blind person's safety depends on the animal's full attention.

You Should Know

When walking with a visually impaired patient, make sure that the pathway is free of clutter. Offer the patient your arm and let her hold on just above your elbow. Guide the patient by leading her. It can be very helpful to "verbalize" the location of your equipment. When giving directions, indicate left and right according to the way the patient is facing.

Speech-Impaired Patients

Objective 6

A brain injury or a lack of oxygen to the brain can cause many patients to experience speech difficulties but not affect other cognitive abilities. For example, a stroke patient may be unable to speak but may be able to understand your questions. You may be able to establish some other means of communication, such as a hand squeeze or even eye blinks. If your patient appears to understand your questions but is unable to answer, stop asking the questions but continue to talk to the patient. Let him know that you understand he is unable to talk. It may be comforting to the patient to know that you are aware of his situation.

Making a Difference

Never assume that a person who cannot speak clearly lacks mental intelligence. A severe speech deficit can be completely unrelated to intelligence.

Children and adults may have language problems that stem from a hearing impairment, a congenital learning disorder, a speech delay, autism, or cerebral palsy. Other speech problems may occur when a patient has difficulty with a speech pattern, such as stuttering. A patient who has cancer of the larynx may have a hoarseness or harshness in her voice. Such patients may have only a limited ability to respond to your questions. Try to keep your questions short and

to the point. In some situations, it may be helpful to ask questions that can be answered with a yes or no. Allow the patient time to respond and to do so in her own way. Rushing the patient to answer may only increase the person's anxiety and frustration. Pay attention and listen carefully to what the patient has to say. She may even use hand gestures or a notepad to communicate her needs.

Responses of Family, Friends, or Bystanders to Injury or Illness

Objective 7

Family members, friends, or bystanders at the scene of an ill or injured patient may have many of the same responses as the patient. Depending on the nature of the illness or the severity of the patient's injury, family members, friends, and bystanders may be anxious, angry, sad, demanding, or impatient. A bystander's anger often results from feelings of guilt. At the scene, the family, friends, or bystanders may pressure you to move the patient to the hospital before you have completed your assessment and provided initial emergency care.

Dealing with the patient's family or friends or with bystanders requires many of the same approaches you use in dealing with patients:

- Identify yourself and take control of the situation. Use a gentle but firm tone of voice, and briefly explain what you are doing to help the patient.
- Speak clearly and use common words (avoid using medical terms). Speak at an appropriate speed or pace, not too rapidly and not too slowly.
- Assume a helpful posture, and face the person speaking. Maintain eye contact while listening carefully. Clarify information that is unclear.
- Avoid interrupting when they are talking.
- Allow them to have and express their emotions, but do not let them distract you from treating the patient's illness or injury.
- Comfort them by being sympathetic, listening empathetically, and reassuring them that everything that can be done to help will be done.
- Do not give false hope or reassurance.
- Keep emotionally distraught individuals away from the patient. If possible, assign another EMT to care for them and their grief. You can reduce interference by well-meaning family, friends, and bystanders by assigning them a simple task to keep them occupied. Feeling useful frequently helps lessen a person's anxiety.

Remember This

When dealing with patients from different cultures, remember the following key points:

- An individual is the "foreground"—the culture is the "background."
- Different generations and individuals within the same family may have different sets of beliefs.
- Not all people identify with their ethnic cultural background.
- All people share common problems or situations.
- Respect the integrity of cultural beliefs.
- Recognize your personal cultural assumptions, prejudices, and belief systems, and do not let them interfere with patient care.
- Realize that people may not share your explanations of the causes of their ill health, but may accept conventional treatments.
- You do not have to agree with every aspect of another's culture, nor does the person have to accept everything about yours for effective and culturally sensitive healthcare to occur.

Patient History

Objective 8

The **patient history** is the part of the patient assessment that provides pertinent facts about the patient's current medical problem and medical history. Components of a patient history include the patient's chief complaint, history of the present illness, past medical history (pertinent to the medical event), and current health status (pertinent to the medical event).

Techniques of History Taking

Objectives 9, 10

With ill (medical) patients, take the patient's history before performing the physical exam. With injured (trauma) patients, perform the physical exam first. When possible, ask the questions of the patient directly, instead of communicating through a family member.

When asking questions to find out the patient's medical history, use open-ended questions when possible. **Open-ended questions** require that the patient answer with more than a yes or no. For example, you might ask, "What is troubling you today?" or "How can I help you?" or "Can you tell me why you called us today?" Open-ended questions give the patient an opportunity to express his thoughts, feelings, and ideas and they encourage the patient to describe and explain what is wrong. After asking a question, allow the patient time to answer. Do not anticipate what the patient is going to say and finish sentences for him. *Listen* closely to what the patient tells you, instead of thinking ahead to the next question you want to ask.

Making a Difference

Taking a medical history is not simply a matter of asking a series of rapid-fire questions in order to complete a report. Obtaining a useful medical history is an art. It requires thoughtful questions, good listening skills, and practice.

Questions that can be answered with yes or no or with one- or two-word responses are called **closed** or **direct questions.** There are times when asking questions that require a simple yes or no answer is appropriate. For instance, when asking the patient if he has a history of high blood pressure, diabetes, and other illnesses, a yes or no answer is appropriate, as it is when the patient is having difficulty communicating (because of severe pain or difficulty breathing or a language barrier). This type of questioning is also useful for focusing on specific points. For example, "Do you have any allergies?" and "Is this the first time you have ever had chest pain?" However, closed questions do not allow an opportunity for the patient to explain what is wrong.

In some situations, the patient will not be able to answer your questions. For example, the patient may be unresponsive or too short of breath to provide detailed answers. If a patient loses consciousness, knowing what his symptoms were before he lost consciousness can help identify possible causes of his condition. If the patient is unresponsive, gather as much information as possible by looking at the scene. Also look for medical identification tags (on a necklace or bracelet or in a wallet), and question family members, neighbors, coworkers, or others present at the scene.

In some situations, the patient's condition will be so critical that there is no time to collect detailed information. Ask the important questions while on the scene and as you are providing care. For example, you should ask the patient about any allergies while providing care at the scene. It is important that this information be documented and relayed to the healthcare professionals who assume patient care. Leave the less important questions to ask while providing patient care during transport.

To obtain a good history, it is best to use an organized approach so that key information is not overlooked.

Chief Complaint

Objective 8

A **chief complaint** is a very brief description, usually in the patient's own words, of the reason EMS was called. In some cases, the patient's chief complaint may turn out to be different from the reason EMS was called. For example, a family member may call 9-1-1 and tell the dispatcher that the patient is complaining of difficulty breathing. When you arrive and speak directly to the patient, you may find that she is complaining of chest pain and has no complaint of difficulty breathing. It is best to document the chief complaint by using the patient's own words in quotes. For example, "I can't catch my breath."

Some patients who call for medical help will have a history of a medical condition that is related to their current complaint. For instance, a patient whose chief complaint is difficulty breathing may have a history of asthma or heart failure. However, some patients will have a chief complaint that they have never experienced before. Some patients will have more than one chief complaint. In each case, listen carefully to what the patient's concerns are, and then ask questions that will help you form an accurate **field impression,** which is the conclusion you reach about what is wrong with your patient.

History of the Present Illness

Objectives 8, 11, 12

The **history of the present illness (HPI)** is a chronological record of the reason a patient is seeking medical assistance. It includes a detailed evaluation of the patient's chief complaint and the patient's answers to questions about the circumstances (including signs and symptoms) that led up to the request for medical help.

Ask the patient to tell you what happened. This information can provide important clues about the patient's current situation. For example, you arrive on the scene of a motor vehicle crash. After making sure there are no immediate life threats, you ask the patient what happened. She tells you she is a diabetic. She remembers taking her insulin this morning. She was running late for her doctor's appointment and did not have time to eat breakfast. She thinks she may have "blacked out." The information provided by the patient tells you that although you must look for possible injuries caused by the motor vehicle crash, some of the signs you will find during your physical exam may be caused by her medical condition.

If your patient is complaining of pain or discomfort, OPQRST is a memory aid that may help identify the type and location of the patient's complaint:

Onset: "How long ago did the problem or discomfort begin?" "What were you doing when the problem started?" "Did the problem begin suddenly (acutely) or slowly (gradually)?"

Provocation/palliation/position: "What makes the problem better or worse?" In what position was the patient found? Should the patient remain in that position?

Quality: "What does the pain feel like (dull, burning, sharp, stabbing, shooting, throbbing, pressure, or tearing)?"

Region/radiation: "Where is the pain?" "Is the pain in one area or does it move?" "Is the pain located in any other area?"

Severity: "On a scale of 0 to 10, with 0 being no pain and 10 being the worst, what number would you give your pain or discomfort?"

Time: "How long has your discomfort been present?" "Have you ever had this discomfort before?" "When?" "How long did it last?"

You Should Know

Ask your patient about the frequency with which the symptoms occur. Use this guide to help pinpoint symptom frequency:

- *Constant* means about 90% to 100% of the time.
- *Frequent* means about 75% of the time.
- *Intermittent* means about 50% of the time.
- *Occasional* means about 25% of the time.

To assess pain in a child 3 years or older, use the Wong-Baker FACES Pain Rating Scale (Figure 15-8). This scale shows six cartoon faces ranging from a smiling face representing "no hurt" to a tearful, sad face representing "worst hurt." To use the scale, explain to the child that each picture is a person's face. "Face 0 is very happy because he doesn't hurt at all. Face 1 hurts just a little bit. Face 2 hurts a little more. Face 3 hurts even more. Face 4 hurts a whole lot. Face 5 hurts as much as you can imagine, although you don't have to be crying to feel this bad." Ask the child to point to the face that best describes how he is feeling. Document the number indicated by the child. For example, "Patient rates pain 4 out of 10 on FACES Pain Scale." In real life, this is usually simplified when documenting on a prehospital care report to, "Pain 4/10 on FACES Pain Scale."

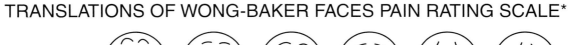

0–5 coding	0	1	2	3	4	5
0-10 coding	0	2	4	6	8	10

FIGURE 15-8 ▲ Wong-Baker FACES Pain Rating Scale.

Making a Difference

Cultural Considerations

Some healthcare professionals end an interview with a child by patting her on the head. Although this gesture is meant to show friendliness, it may be viewed differently by people of other cultures. For example, this gesture is considered an insult by Southeast Asians. They believe the head is the seat of the soul and the most sacred part of the body. Intentionally touching a child's head without the consent of the parents may make the parents or relatives angry.

When you are caring for patients, a "yes" answer pertaining to an illness or injury indicates a **pertinent positive** or positive finding. A "no" indicates a **pertinent negative** or negative finding. For example, when you are caring for a patient who has asthma, pertinent positive findings would include shortness of breath and/or a feeling of tightness in the throat or chest. Pertinent negative findings would include no history of a recent cold, bronchitis, pneumonia, or other infection. When you are caring for a female patient who is complaining of abdominal pain, pertinent positive findings include a sexually active woman whose last menstrual period was 6 weeks ago. Pertinent negative findings include no recent abdominal trauma or illness and no recent history of abdominal surgery or a vaginal infection.

Another important part of the HPI is the relevant family history. As you learned in Chapter 7, heredity is an important risk factor for some diseases. Ask the patient about related problems of family members. For example, if the patient is complaining of difficulty breathing and has a history of asthma, ask if there is a family history of asthma. If the patient is complaining of chest pain, ask if there is a family history of heart disease. Document the family member's relationship to the patient so that this information can be relayed to the receiving facility. For instance, a 46-year-old man is complaining of chest pain. When asked if there is a history of heart disease in his family, he informs you that his brother died at the age of 54 of a heart attack and that his father died at the age of 63 of the same condition. This information is relevant to the patient's current complaint and important to document and relay to the receiving facility.

Past Medical History

Ask the patient about conditions he may have that may help you determine what the problem is today. If time permits, ask about childhood illnesses and immunizations, adult illnesses, accidents and injuries, physical disability due to previous illness or injury, and recent hospitalizations or surgical procedures. If the patient is unresponsive or has an altered mental status (which will be discussed in the Chapter 17), look for a medical identification tag. Examples of questions to ask include the following:

- Are you seeing a doctor for any medical or psychological condition?
- Do you have a history of heart problems, respiratory problems, high blood pressure, diabetes, epilepsy, or any ongoing medical condition?
- Have you been in the hospital recently? Have you had any recent surgery?

Current Health Status

Objective 8

The current health status part of a patient history focuses on the patient's present state of health. If time permits, questions pertaining to the following topics should be asked.

Allergies

Allergies are common and may be the reason you were called to the scene. Find out if the patient has an allergy to any medications, foods, environmental factors (such as pollen or bees), or products (such as latex).

Ask the patient (or bystanders if the patient is unresponsive):

- Do you have any allergies to medications?
- Are you allergic to latex?
- Do you have any food allergies or allergies to insect stings, pollen, dust, or grass?

Check for a medical identification tag. The patient may be wearing a bracelet or necklace, or carrying a wallet card that identifies a serious medical condition, allergies, or medications she is taking.

Medications

Find out if the patient is currently taking any medications. You will need to ask specific questions because some patients do not consider some substances medications, such as vitamins or aspirin. Examples of questions to ask include:

- Do you take any prescription medications? Is the medication prescribed for you? What is the medication for? When did you last take it? (If applicable, ask one of the next two questions.) Are you taking medication for birth control (pills or injections)? Do you take medication for erectile dysfunction?
- Do you take any over-the-counter medications, such as aspirin, allergy medications, cough syrup, or vitamins? Do you take any herbs?
- Have you recently started taking any new medications? Have you recently stopped taking any medications?
- Do you use any recreational substances (cocaine, marijuana, or alcohol)?

If the patient is taking medication, send the medication containers to the hospital with the patient. This action helps the hospital staff determine what the patient's medical condition is, if he sees a doctor regularly and if he has been taking his medication correctly.

Personal Habits

Ask the patient about tobacco use, type (cigarette, cigar, pipe, and/or chewing), and years of use. If not already done, ask about the use of alcohol, including type (beer, wine, hard liquor) and the number of bottles or glasses per day. Ask about the frequency of use of coffee, cola, and tea and the number of cups or ounces per day. If not already done, ask about the use of recreational drugs, including type, frequency, and duration of use.

Diet and Last Oral Intake

In some situations, asking about the patient's diet is important. For example, if the patient has diabetes or appears malnourished, it will be essential for you to ask about the number of meals or snacks the patient consumes per day.

It is also important to determine when the patient last ate or had anything to drink. This is especially important if the patient is a diabetic or may need immediate surgery. Determine what she last ate or drank, how much she ate or drank, and when.

SAMPLE History

Objectives 11, 13

In EMS, SAMPLE is a memory aid used to standardize the approach to history taking. It is important to obtain a SAMPLE history from all responsive patients. SAMPLE stands for:

> **S**igns and symptoms
> **A**llergies
> **M**edications
> **P**ast medical history
> **L**ast oral intake
> **E**vents leading to the injury or illness

With the exception of signs and symptoms, the components of the SAMPLE memory aid have been previously discussed. You will recall from Chapter 7 that a sign is any medical or trauma condition displayed by the patient that can be seen, heard, smelled, measured, or felt. A symptom is any condition described by the patient. Signs and symptoms will be discussed in more detail in Chapter 17.

On the Scene | Wrap-Up

As you prepare to interview the patient, you force yourself to take a deep breath and slow down. You begin the patient assessment by kneeling next to the patient's knee, remembering not to kneel directly in front of the patient. You proceed to introduce yourself and ask the patient for her name. She responds by asking you to call her "Linda" and then tells you that she has felt dizzy most of the morning. You assure her that you are there to help her and all the crews will take good care of her. She smiles and thanks you for understanding how she feels. You are able to ask her all the proper questions, pausing politely after each question to allow her time to answer. You also know that your questions should not "lead" the patient to an answer and that you should not answer the question for her. You are able to comfort your patient and begin the proper treatment based on your interaction. The patient expresses her thanks, stating she is thankful that you were there to help her. ■

- The communication process involves six basic elements: a source, encoding, the message, channel, receiver (decoder), and feedback. The source of verbal communication is spoken or written words. A message is the information to be communicated. The sender decides the message to send and then encodes it. Encoding is the act of placing a message into words or images so that it is understood by the sender and receiver. The sender selects the path (channel) for transmitting the message to the receiver. The receiver is the person or group for whom the sender's message is intended. When a message is received, the receiver must interpret (decode) the sender's message. Noise is anything that obscures, confuses, or interferes with the communication. Feedback is the response from the receiver (verbal or nonverbal) that allows the sender to know how the message is being received.

- When communicating with a patient, identify yourself and explain that you are there to provide assistance. Recognize the patient's need for privacy, preserve the patient's dignity, and treat the patient with respect.

- When talking with family members and bystanders, avoid interrupting when they are talking. Speak clearly and use common words (avoid using medical terms). Speak at an appropriate speed or pace, not too rapidly and not too slowly.

- The patient history is part of the patient assessment during which you find out pertinent facts about the patient's medical history. Components of the patient history include the chief complaint, history of the present illness, past medical history (pertinent to the medical event), and current health status (pertinent to the medical event).

- When asking questions to find out the patient's medical history, use open-ended questions when possible. Open-ended questions require the patient to answer with more than a yes or no. Questions that require a yes or no answer are called direct questions.

- The chief complaint is the reason the patient called for assistance. The history of the present illness is a chronological record of the reason a patient is seeking medical assistance. It includes the patient's chief complaint and the patient's answers to questions about the circumstances that led up to the request for medical help. The conclusion you reach about what is wrong with your patient is called a field impression.

- OPQRST is a memory aid that may help identify the type and location of a patient's pain or discomfort. OPQRST stands for **O**nset, **P**rovocation/palliation/position, **Q**uality, **R**egion/radiation, **S**everity, and **T**ime.

- The Wong-Baker FACES Pain Rating Scale is a tool used to assess pain in children 3 years or older.

- SAMPLE is a memory aid used to standardize the approach to history taking. SAMPLE stands for **S**igns and symptoms, **A**llergies, **M**edications, **P**ast medical history, **L**ast oral intake, and **E**vents leading to the injury or illness. It is important to obtain a SAMPLE history from all responsive patients. A sign is any medical or trauma condition displayed by the patient that can be seen, heard, smelled, measured, or felt. A symptom is any condition described by the patient.

Scene Size-Up

By the end of this chapter, you should be able to:

Knowledge Objectives ▶
1. Determine if the scene is safe to enter.
2. Recognize hazards and potential hazards.
3. Describe common hazards found at the scene of a trauma patient and a medical patient.
4. Discuss common mechanisms of injury and nature of illness.
5. Discuss the reason for identifying the total number of patients at the scene.
6. Explain the reason for identifying the need for additional help or assistance.

Attitude Objectives ▶
7. Explain the rationale for crew members to evaluate scene safety before entering.
8. Serve as a model for others by explaining how patient situations affect your evaluation of mechanism of injury or illness.

Skill Objective ▶
9. Observe various scenarios and identify potential hazards.

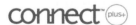

On the Scene

You are dispatched to a private residence for a "welfare check." Law enforcement personnel are already on the scene, and they are requesting your assistance for a 56-year-old man. Although there is no additional information available at the time of dispatch, you recognize the address as a house that you and your partner have been to several times in the past. As you arrive at the scene, you note three police cruisers. Officers are standing in the entryway of the house. You and your partner note two newspapers on the driveway. As you walk up the sidewalk, an officer tells you that a friend of the patient called the police department because he was concerned about the health of the man inside but gave no other information. The officers do not have any other information except that there are no immediate safety concerns that they can find. Officers are inside the house. You take the information, relay it to your partner, and enter the house to speak with the patient. ■

As you read this chapter, think about the following questions:

- What is scene size-up, and why is it important to the emergency medical technician?
- What are the components of an effective scene size-up?
- Who is responsible for the scene size-up?
- Why is it important to note subtle details in every emergency scene?

Introduction

Scene size-up is the first and most important aspect of patient assessment. Scene size-up begins as an EMT approaches the scene. During this phase, you will survey the scene to determine if any threats may cause injury to you, other rescuers, the patient, or bystanders. This evaluation also allows you to determine the nature of the call and the need for additional resources as necessary. Scene size-up is an ongoing process. Because conditions may change, you must remain aware of the situation for the duration of the call.

An Overview of Scene Size-Up

As an EMT, you will be called to provide emergency care to patients in many different settings. Your patients will include infants, children, young adults, middle-aged adults, the elderly, and patients with special healthcare needs. These patients may experience an emergency resulting from trauma or a medical condition. These emergencies may occur in a person's home, on a busy highway, in a shopping mall, or in an office. In every situation, you must quickly look at the entire scene before approaching the patient (Figure 16-1). You must size up the scene to find out if there are any threats that may cause injury to you, other rescuers, or bystanders, or that may cause additional injury to the patient.

The five parts of the first phase of patient assessment include:

1. Taking standard precautions
2. Evaluating scene safety
3. Determining the mechanism of injury or the nature of the patient's illness
4. Determining the total number of patients
5. Determining the need for additional resources

The scene size-up begins with the information received about the emergency. The information given to

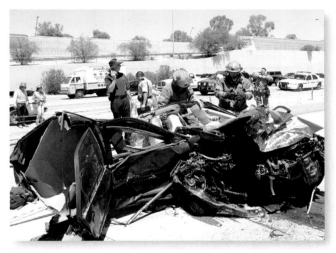

FIGURE 16-1 ▲ You must quickly survey the entire scene for safety on every emergency call.

the EMS dispatcher by the caller may help you determine the following:

- The location of the emergency
- If the call is a trauma emergency (such as a motor vehicle crash) or a medical emergency (such as a seizure)
- The number of vehicles involved
- The number of patients involved
- The ages and genders of all patients (if known)
- When the emergency occurred
- If the call involves fire or other potential hazards such as leaking materials, downed power lines, broken gas lines, hazardous materials, a violent patient, or dangerous pets
- If law enforcement or fire department personnel are on the scene
- If advanced life support (ALS) personnel have been sent to the scene
- If special resources will be required, such as a hazardous materials team, a confined space rescue team, a water rescue team, extrication equipment, or air medical transport

En route to the scene, try to create a mental picture of the call by using the information given to you by the dispatcher. Be prepared for the unexpected. What additional help might be needed on the scene? Law enforcement personnel? The fire department? A utility company? ALS personnel? How will you gain access to the patient? What questions will you ask the patient or family?

Remember This

The information given to you by a dispatcher is often limited to that provided by the caller. You may arrive at the scene of an emergency to find the patient with injuries or a complaint that differs from that reported by the caller to the dispatcher.

Standard Precautions Review

You must take appropriate standard precautions on *every* call. Consider the need for standard precautions before you approach the patient. Put on appropriate personal protective equipment on the basis of the information the dispatcher gives you and your initial survey of the scene (Figure 16-2). This equipment includes gloves, eye protection, mask, and gown, if necessary. Consider the following examples of real emergency situations:

- You are called to a fitness club for a woman with a rapid heart rate. The dispatcher tells you that the woman was using the treadmill when she felt weak, became dizzy, and felt her heart race. Because gloves should be worn before physical

contact with *every* patient, put on gloves while en route to the scene.

- You are called to respond to a single-vehicle rollover. The bystander who called 9-1-1 said the vehicle rolled twice and is resting on its side. There is heavy damage to the vehicle. He believes there are three patients. En route to the scene, put on gloves because it is likely that blood will be present on the scene. Once on the scene, put on a chin-length face shield (or protective eyewear and mask) if you see serious bleeding that could spray or splash into your eyes, nose, or mouth. Put on a gown if there is a chance of splashing blood or other body fluids and your clothing is likely to be soiled. If you are trained in fire or rescue techniques and will be responsible for that role during the rescue, wear appropriate clothing to protect yourself from fire, glass, sharp edges and fragments, and other debris at the scene. Protective clothing includes turnout gear, puncture-proof gloves, a helmet, eye protection (safety glasses or goggles), and boots with steel toes.

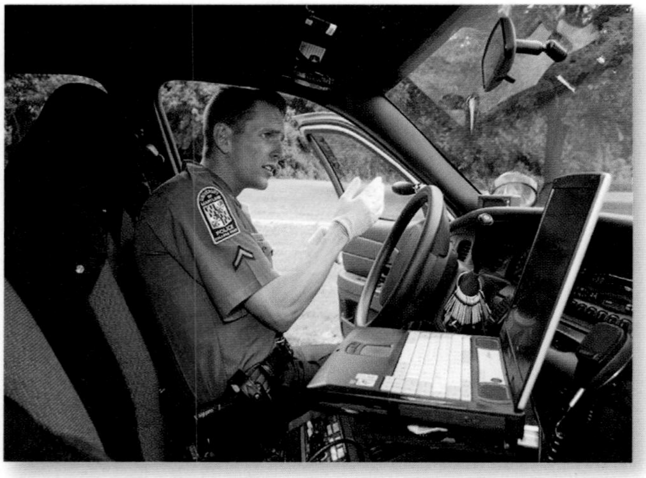

You Should Know

Components of Scene Size-Up
- Taking standard precautions
- Evaluating scene safety
- Determining the mechanism of injury (including considerations for stabilization of the spine) or the nature of the patient's illness
- Determining the total number of patients
- Determining the need for additional resources

Remember This

The scene size-up will help determine what PPE is needed. Be prepared. Every EMS call will pose a different set of challenges.

FIGURE 16-2 ▲ Put on appropriate personal protective equipment on the basis of the dispatch information received and your initial survey of the scene.

Scene Safety

Objective 1

Scene safety is an assessment of the entire scene and surroundings to ensure your well-being and that of other rescuers, the patient(s), and bystanders. Remember, you are of no help to the patient if you become a patient yourself!

Personal and Other Rescuer Safety

Objectives 2, 3

Study the scene before approaching the patient (Figure 16-3).

Questions to consider at a crash or rescue scene:
- Is the area marked by safety lights or flares?
- Is traffic controlled by law enforcement personnel?
- Does the vehicle, aircraft, or machinery appear stable?
- Do you see any leaking fluids?
- Are downed power lines present?
- Do you see fire, smoke, or potential fire hazards?
- Do you see entrapped victims?

At a scene involving toxic substances, obvious hazards may be present. At other scenes, the hazards may not be as obvious.

Clues suggesting the presence of hazardous materials:
- Placards on railroad cars, storage facilities, or vehicles
- Vapor clouds or heavy smoke
- Unusual odors
- Spilled solids or liquids
- Leaking containers, bottles, or gas cylinders
- Chemical transport tanks or containers

When you arrive at a scene, park at a safe distance that is upwind or uphill from the incident. Contact your local hazardous materials response team immediately. Do not enter the area unless you are trained to handle hazardous materials and are fully protected with proper equipment. Do not walk or drive an emergency vehicle through spilled liquids. Keep unnecessary people away from the area. Provide emergency care only after the scene is safe and the patient is decontaminated.

Emergencies that occur in a confined space such as a mine, well, silo, or an unreinforced trench may be low in oxygen (Figure 16-4). Rescues in these situations require specially trained personnel and equipment. Do not enter the area unless you have all the necessary equipment and have been trained in this type of rescue.

At a crime scene or hostile situation, assess the potential for violence.

Clues indicating the potential for violence:
- A knowledge of prior violence at a particular location
- Evidence of alcohol or other substance use
- Weapons visible or in use
- Loud voices, pushing, or fighting
- Hostile bystanders

Never enter a potential crime scene or a scene involving a family dispute, fight, attempted suicide, drugs, alcohol, or weapons until law enforcement personnel have secured the scene and declared it safe for you to enter and provide patient care.

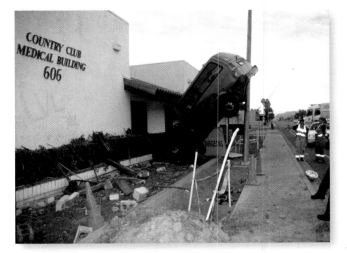

FIGURE 16-3 ▲ Study the scene before approaching the patient. Look for possible hazards.

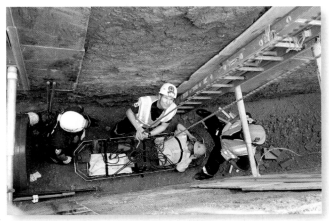

FIGURE 16-4 ▲ Confined space rescue requires specially trained personnel and equipment.

Notify appropriate law enforcement personnel immediately in the event that a crime scene is suspected. It is important to realize that, as a healthcare professional, your primary responsibility is to the patient. At the same time, law enforcement personnel need to protect any evidence that may be associated with the crime scene. In such situations, it is important that EMS and law enforcement personnel work cooperatively together.

Considering the environment before approaching the patient:

- If a surface or slope is unstable or if water, ice, fire, or downed power lines are present, call for specially trained personnel as needed.
- Do not enter a body of water unless you have been trained in water rescue and the necessary safety measures are in place.
- Do not enter fast-moving water or venture out on ice unless you have been trained in this type of rescue.
- If the scene is safe but extremes of heat or cold are a concern, move the patient to an ambulance as quickly as possible.

Patient Safety

You are responsible for ensuring the patient's safety. This responsibility includes:

- Protecting the patient from curious onlookers
- Assessing traffic and other hazards
- Protecting the patient from glass and other debris during extrication procedures (Figure 16-5)
- Protecting the patient from environmental temperature extremes

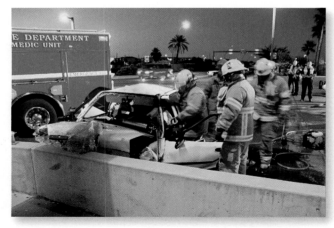

FIGURE 16-5 ▲ You are responsible for ensuring the patient's safety, including protecting the patient from glass and other debris during extrication procedures.

Bystander Safety

At the scene of an emergency, bystanders may become so engrossed in the situation that they fail to watch out for themselves. Look for bystanders who may be in danger or who may endanger your safety or that of the patient. Help bystanders avoid becoming patients by preventing them from getting too close to the scene. If the scene is safe and you need assistance, ask bystanders to help you. Reassure your patient and bystanders by working confidently and efficiently.

The Mechanism of Injury or the Nature of the Illness

During the scene size-up, try to determine the nature of the patient's problem. A **trauma patient** is one who has experienced an injury from an external force. In trauma situations, look for the mechanism of injury. A **medical patient** is one whose condition is caused by an illness.

In medical situations, try to determine the nature of the patient's illness.

Making a Difference

Trauma and medical emergencies can occur at the same time. For example, a patient with low blood sugar may be involved in a motor vehicle crash, or a patient may have had a seizure before falling. A patient with a history of asthma may develop difficulty breathing after an airbag deploys in a motor vehicle crash. Don't get tunnel vision!

The Mechanism of Injury

Mechanism of injury (MOI) refers to the way in which an injury occurs, as well as the forces involved in producing the injury. **Kinetic energy** is the energy of motion. The amount of kinetic energy an object has depends on the mass (weight) and speed (velocity) of the object. **Kinematics** is the science of analyzing the mechanism of injury and predicting injury patterns. The amount of injury is determined by the following three elements:

1. The type of energy applied
2. How quickly the energy is applied
3. The part of the body to which the energy is applied

Physical injury is the result of different sources of energy (Table 16-1). Injuries may be intentional or

TABLE 16-1 Sources of Energy and Mechanisms of Injury

Energy Source	Mechanism of Injury
Kinetic (mechanical) energy	Motor vehicle crashes
	Motorcycle crashes
	Firearms
	Falls
	Assaults
Thermal energy	Heat
	Steam
	Fire
Radiant energy	Rays of light (sun rays)
	Sound waves (explosions)
	Electromagnetic waves (x-ray exposure)
	Radioactive emissions (nuclear leak)
Chemical energy	Plant and animal toxins
	Chemical substances
Electrical energy	Lightning
	Exposure to wires, sockets, plugs

Source: Adapted from *Trauma Nursing Core Course Provider Manual,* 5th ed. (Des Plaines, IL: Emergency Nurses Association, 2000), p. 27.

TABLE 16-2 Examples of Unintentional and Intentional Injuries

Unintentional Injuries	Intentional Injuries
• Motor vehicle crash	• Assault
• Motorcycle crash	• Suicide
• Bicycle crash	• Homicide
• Pedestrian injuries	
• Fire, burn	
• Fall	
• Farm machinery (pin, crush, fall, runover, rollover)	
• Ejection from motor vehicle (including motorcycles, mopeds, all-terrain vehicles, or open bed of pickup trucks)	
• Snowmobile injuries	
• Snow or skiing injuries	
• Poisoning	
• Water-related incident (near drowning, diving)	
• Choking	
• Explosion	
• Electrocution	
• Entrapment	
• Ejection from a horse	

unintentional (Table 16-2). If you understand the types of forces that were involved in producing an injury, you will be able to look for specific injuries and injury patterns. On a trauma scene, you must quickly decide if the MOI is significant or not. If the patient is unresponsive, considering the mechanism of injury may be the only way you can determine what the injuries (or medical situation) might be. Survey the scene, and talk to the patient, family, and bystanders to determine the mechanism of injury.

Making a Difference

When providing care for a seriously injured trauma patient, make every effort to limit your time on the scene to 10 minutes or less. These patients require definitive care at the hospital. The longer it takes to deliver seriously injured patients to the hospital, the less likely they are to survive.

Blunt and Penetrating Trauma

Objective 4

Trauma is generally divided into two categories: blunt and penetrating. **Blunt trauma** is any mechanism of injury that occurs without actual penetration of the body. Examples of mechanisms of injury causing blunt trauma include motor vehicle crashes, falls, sports injuries, or assaults with a blunt object (Figure 16-6). Blunt trauma produces injury first to the body surface and then to the body's contents. This results in compression and/or stretching of the tissue beneath the skin. The amount of injury depends on how long the compression occurred, the force of the compression, and the area compressed.

Penetrating trauma is any mechanism of injury that causes a cut or piercing of the skin. Examples of mechanisms of injury causing penetrating trauma include gunshot wounds, stab wounds, and blast injuries (Figure 16-7). Penetrating trauma usually affects organs and tissues in the direct path of the wounding object.

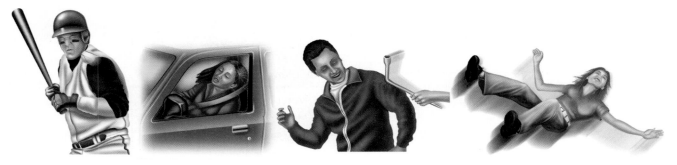

FIGURE 16-6 ▲ Blunt trauma is any mechanism of injury that occurs without actual penetration of the body. Examples of mechanisms of injury causing blunt trauma include motor vehicle crashes, falls, sports injuries, or assaults with a blunt object.

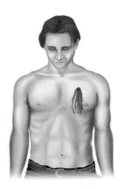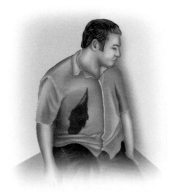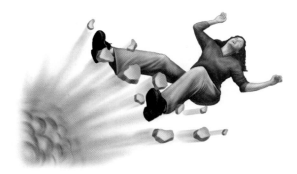

FIGURE 16-7 ▲ Penetrating trauma is any mechanism of injury that causes a cut or piercing of the skin. Examples of mechanisms of injury causing penetrating trauma include gunshot wounds, stab wounds, and blast injuries.

Making a Difference

The extent and seriousness of a patient's injuries may not be obvious. When evaluating the mechanism of injury, try to picture the organs that may have been damaged. This technique will help you predict the patient's injuries.

Motor Vehicle Crashes

A motor vehicle crash (MVC) can involve automobiles, motorcycles, all-terrain vehicles (ATVs), and tractors. Most motor vehicle crashes (75%) occur within 25 miles of home. Most crashes also occur in areas where the speed limit is 40 mph or less. In an MVC, three separate impacts occur as kinetic energy is transferred (Figure 16-8):

1. The vehicle strikes an object.
2. The occupant collides with the interior of the vehicle. Interior elements include seat belts, airbags, and the dashboard.

3. Internal organs collide with other organs, muscle, bone, or other structures inside the body. The lungs, brain, liver, and spleen are particularly vulnerable to trauma.

Note that a fourth impact may occur if loose objects in the vehicle become projectiles.

A motor vehicle crash is classified by the type of impact. The five types of impact include head-on (frontal), lateral, rear end, rotational, and rollover (Figure 16-9 on p. 318). The injuries that result depend on the type of collision, the position of the occupant inside the vehicle, and the use or nonuse of active (such as seat belts) or passive (such as airbags) restraint systems. Restraint systems are used to absorb the energy of the impact before the occupant hits something hard. They also limit the distance the body has to travel.

In a frontal impact, such as a head-on collision, the vehicle stops and the occupants continue to move forward by one of two pathways: down and under or up and over. In the down and under pathway, the victim's knees hit the vehicle's dashboard. The

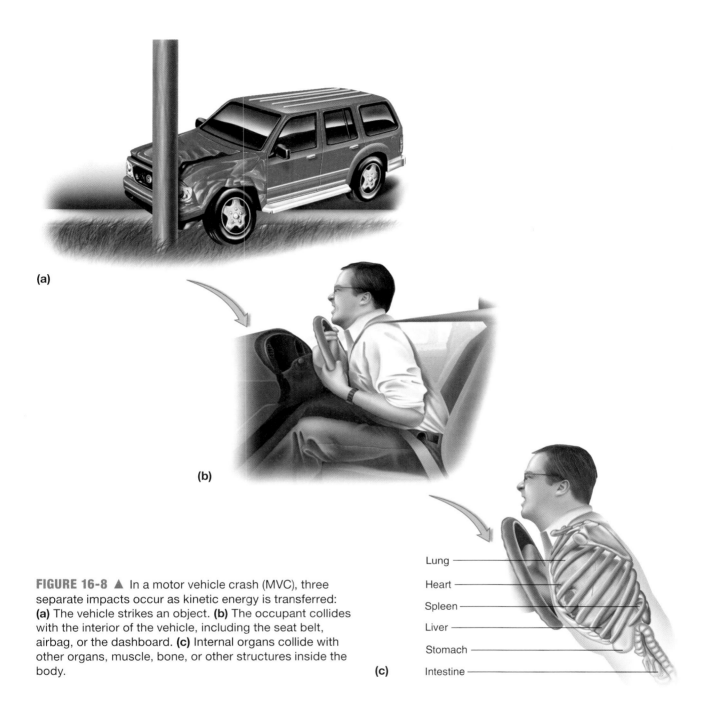

FIGURE 16-8 ▲ In a motor vehicle crash (MVC), three separate impacts occur as kinetic energy is transferred: **(a)** The vehicle strikes an object. **(b)** The occupant collides with the interior of the vehicle, including the seat belt, airbag, or the dashboard. **(c)** Internal organs collide with other organs, muscle, bone, or other structures inside the body.

(a)

(b)

(c)

Lung ————
Heart ————
Spleen ————
Liver ————
Stomach ————
Intestine ————

down and under pathway may be seen when the occupant is not wearing a lap and shoulder restraint system, or when the occupant is wearing only the shoulder harness and not a lap belt. Predictable injuries include a knee dislocation and/or patella fracture. The impact may also result in fractures of the femur or hip or a posterior dislocation of the hip socket (acetabulum).

In the up and over pathway, the victim's upper body strikes the steering wheel, resulting in injuries to the head, chest, abdomen, pelvis, and/or spine.

The up and over pathway may be seen when the occupant is not wearing a lap and shoulder restraint system or when the occupant is wearing only a lap restraint (not the shoulder harness). Predictable injuries based on common mechanisms of injury are listed in Table 16-3.

Other Considerations

Although mechanism of injury is important, it is not the only factor to consider when assessing a trauma patient and determining whether or not he is a priority

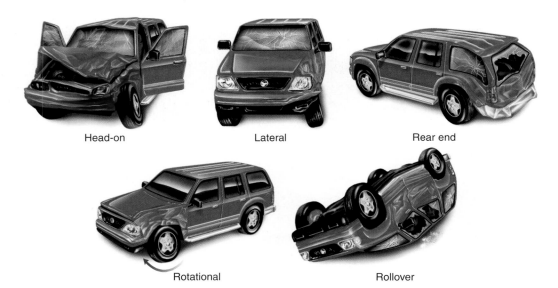

Head-on   Lateral   Rear end

Rotational   Rollover

FIGURE 16-9 ▲ A motor vehicle crash is classified by the type of impact. The five types of impact include head-on (frontal), lateral, rear end, rotational, and rollover.

TABLE 16-3 Predictable Injuries Based on Common Mechanisms of Injury		
Mechanism of Injury		**Predictable Injuries**
Motor vehicle crashes	Head-on collision	Below the steering wheel: • Lower-extremity fractures • Dislocated knees and hips At the level of and above the steering wheel: • Trauma to the head, brain, and face • Serious chest injuries
	Lateral (side) collision	• Head and cervical spine injuries • Injuries to the chest and pelvis • Internal injuries that may be present without outward signs of injury
	Rear-end collision	• Head, brain, and cervical spine injuries • Possible chest, abdomen, long bone, and soft tissue injuries
	Rotational collision	• Head and cervical spine injuries • Internal injuries that may be present without outward signs of injury
	Rollover	• Head and cervical spine injuries • Crushing injuries • Soft tissue injuries, multiple broken bones
Motor vehicle–pedestrian crashes	Adult	• Injuries to both lower legs • Secondary injuries that may occur when the body strikes the hood of the car and then the ground

Continued

TABLE 16-3 Predictable Injuries Based on Common Mechanisms of Injury *Continued*

Mechanism of Injury		Predictable Injuries
Motor vehicle–pedestrian crashes	Child	• Trauma to the lower extremities from the bumper • Chest and abdominal trauma from striking the hood • Injuries to the head and face from hitting the hood or windshield
Falls	Adult	• Compression injuries of the spine • Upper- or lower-extremity trauma
	Child	• Head, face, and neck trauma (young children tend to fall head first) • Upper- or lower-extremity trauma
Bicycle crashes	Without helmet	• Injuries to head, face, and spine; broken clavicles, and ribs • Extremity fractures • Abdominal injuries (from striking the handlebars)
	With helmet	• Upper- or lower-extremity trauma • Abdominal injuries (from striking the handlebars)
Motorcycle crashes	Head-on collision	• At the level of and above the handlebars: lower-extremity fractures with serious soft tissue injuries and blood loss • Head, face, and neck trauma likely on landing
	Lateral collision	• Pelvic or lower-extremity injuries; crushing injuries
	Ejection	• Type and severity of injuries dependent on how the victim lands and the nature of the object struck
	Laying down the bike	• Scrapes, burns, possible fractures of lower extremities
Penetrating traumas	Low-velocity weapons (knife, ice pick)	• Injury that is usually limited to the area penetrated • Blood loss
	Medium- and high-velocity weapons (shotgun, high-powered rifle, assault weapon)	• An injured area that is larger than the area penetrated • Fluid-filled organs (bladder, heart, great vessels, and bowel), which can burst because of the pressure waves generated • Liver, spleen, and brain, which are easily injured

patient. For some patients, the risk of significant injury is increased because of their age or a preexisting medical condition, despite what may appear to be a minor mechanism of injury.

In some EMS systems, other factors for designating "priority" status are considered in addition to the mechanism of injury (Table 16-4). These include anatomy, physiology, and patient factors. For instance, consider a patient who was involved in a motor vehicle crash (mechanism). The appearance of a bent steering wheel and starred windshield would lead you to suspect he experienced blunt trauma to his chest and head (anatomy). Your initial assessment reveals the patient has an altered mental status (physiology). Until a SAMPLE history has been obtained, you do not know if there are other patient factors to consider. Some trauma experts have also noted that significant injury may also be suspected from key phrases said by patients (Table 16-5). The more of these factors that are present, the more likely the patient has experienced a serious injury.

TABLE 16-4 Factors to Consider When Identifying Priority Trauma Patients

Mechanism of Injury	Anatomy	Physiology	Patient Factors
• Motor vehicle crash • Motorcycle crash • Bicycle crash • All-terrain vehicle (ATV) crash • Pedestrian injuries • Fire, burn • Fall • Farm machinery (pin, crush, fall, runover, rollover) • Ejection from motor vehicle (including motorcycles, mopeds, ATVs, or open bed of pickup trucks) • Poisoning • Water-related incident (near drowning, diving) • Choking • Explosion • Electrocution • Entrapment	• Penetrating trauma • Blunt trauma • Fracture • Burn • Significant soft tissue injury • Significant deformity • Injury to eyes, hands, feet, genitalia	• Altered mental status • Slow heart rate • Fast heart rate • Nausea/vomiting • Sweating • Shortness of breath • Chest pain • Headache • Severe pain • Hypotension • Respirations <10 or >40 • Fever >101° • Abdominal pain • Inability to walk	• Age <5 or >55 • Cardiac disease • Respiratory disease • Seizure disorder • Liver disease • Insulin-dependent diabetes • Obesity • Pregnancy • Immunosuppressed patients • Patients with a bleeding disorder or patients on blood thinners • Use of alcohol or drugs • Recent surgery/illness

TABLE 16-5 Patient Complaints and Possible Significant Injury

Possible Significant Injury	Patient Complaint
Compromised airway	"I can't breathe." "I can't swallow." "I'm choking."
Breathing problem, lack of oxygen, cardiac tamponade	"Let me sit up."
Blood loss, lack of oxygen	"Please help me." "I'm going to die."
Blood loss	"I'm thirsty."
Spinal cord injury	"I can't move my legs."
Irritation of the abdominal lining	"My belly hurts."
Significant injury	"Please do something for my pain."

Source: Adapted from M. Rhodes, "Trauma Resuscitation," in *The Trauma Manual*, A. Peitzman, M. Rhodes, C. W. Schwab, and D. M. Yealy, eds. (Philadelphia: Lippincott-Raven, 1998), p. 82.

You Should Know

Motor Vehicle Crash Statistics

- One out of four of all occupant deaths among children ages 0 to 14 years involve a drinking driver.
- Of children ages 0 to 14 years who were killed in motor vehicle crashes in the United States during 2002, 50% were unrestrained.
- Restraint use among young children often depends upon the driver's restraint use. Almost 40% of children riding with unbelted drivers were themselves unrestrained.
- Physical frailty increases the injury risk of older adults in a crash. A crash that results in nonfatal injuries to a younger person may result in the death of an older adult driver or passenger.

Motor Vehicle–Pedestrian Crashes

Adult pedestrians will typically turn away if they are about to be struck by an oncoming vehicle. This action results in injuries to the side or back of the body. A child will usually face an oncoming vehicle; this results in injuries to the front of the body.

Among children 5 to 9 years of age, pedestrian injuries are the most common cause of death from trauma.

Children are susceptible to pedestrian injuries because of the following factors:
- They have less accurate depth perception.
- They tend to "dart" into traffic.
- They cannot accurately judge the speed of a vehicle.

Children under the age of 5 years are at risk of being run over in the driveway. Most pedestrian injuries occur during the day, peaking in the period after school. About 30% of pedestrian injuries occur while the child is in a marked crosswalk.

Falls

Falls are a common mechanism of injury.

Factors to consider in a fall include:
- The height from which the patient fell
- The patient's weight
- The surface the patient landed on
- The part of the patient's body that struck first

Infants are more likely to fall from changing tables, countertops, and beds. Preschool children usually fall from windows. Older children fall more often from playground equipment. Adults who have jumped rather than fallen from a height tend to land on their feet and then fall onto their buttocks or outstretched hands. Of older adults who fall, 20–30% suffer moderate to severe injuries, such as hip fractures or head trauma.

You Should Know

Fall Statistics
- Falls are a leading cause of traumatic brain injuries.
- More than one-third of adults aged 65 years and older fall each year.
- Among children, preschoolers are at greatest risk for falls.

Bicycle Crashes

Most severe and fatal bicycle injuries involve head trauma. Other injuries associated with bicycle crashes include trauma to the face, limbs, and abdomen (from striking the handlebars).

The most common bicycle crashes include:
- Riding into a street without stopping
- Turning left or swerving into traffic that is coming from behind
- Running a stop sign
- Riding against the flow of traffic

Bicycle helmets can reduce the risk of head injury. A helmet absorbs some of the energy and disperses the blow over a larger area for a slightly longer time. It is estimated that helmets reduce the risk of head injury by 85% and brain injury by 88%.

The Nature of the Illness

The **nature of the illness (NOI)** describes the medical condition that resulted in the patient's call to 9-1-1. Examples include fever, difficulty breathing, chest pain, headache, and vomiting. Try to find out the nature of the illness by talking to the patient, family, coworkers, and bystanders. If the patient is uncooperative or unresponsive, look to family members or others at the scene as a source of information. Look for clues that may help explain the patient's condition, such as pills, spilled medicine containers, medical identification jewelry, or household or gardening chemicals.

While in a patient's home, look around you. Note the orderliness, cleanliness, and safety of the home (Figure 16-10). Sometimes homes are hazardous because of large collections of paper, trash, or animal waste. Look at the general appearance of the patient and other members of the family.

Check if there are any medical devices that may be used by the patient, such as home oxygen equipment or a breathing machine. Look for DNRs, advance directives, or Physician Orders for Life-Sustaining Treatment (POLST) documents.

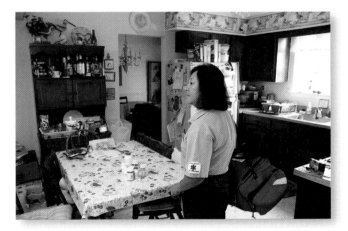

FIGURE 16-10 ▲ While in a patient's home, look around and note the orderliness, cleanliness, and safety of the home.

The Number of Patients

Objective 5

At the scene, you should take appropriate standard precautions, evaluate scene safety, and determine the mechanism of injury or the nature of the patient's illness. After taking these steps, determine the number of patients. The need for additional resources is based on the correct count of patients at any emergency scene. The number of patients for a medical call in which the patient complains of chest pain may be easy to answer. However, a rollover accident with multiple persons involved may be more difficult to assess. Be alert for patients in addition to the first patient you observe at the scene. Look for clues that other patients may be present. Clues might include toys, diapers, bottles, schoolbooks, a purse, or a child safety seat.

It is important to quickly find out the number of patients on the scene in order to request additional resources if necessary. In most situations, one EMS professional is needed for each patient, with one additional professional designated to drive each transporting vehicle. If a patient is severely ill or injured, two or more EMS professionals may be needed to provide emergency care. If there are more patients than you can effectively handle, call for additional help.

Remember This

Call for additional help *before* you make contact with the patient. Once you begin patient care, you will have fewer chances to make the call.

While waiting for the arrival of more resources, determine which patients should be treated first. The process of sorting patients by the severity of their illness or injury is called **triage.** This information is covered in more detail in Chapter 49.

Additional Resources

Objective 6

Determine if more help is needed at the scene. Types of additional help that may be needed are shown in Table 16-6. Contact the dispatcher as soon you recognize the need for more resources.

Remember This

Scene size-up is an ongoing process. Alter your plan of action as necessary based on the information obtained at the scene, your patient assessment findings, and available resources.

TABLE 16-6 Scene Hazards and Possible Resources

Scene Hazard	Possible Resources
Traffic control, crime, or violent scene	Law enforcement personnel
Complex extrication	Fire department, special rescue team
Hazardous materials	Fire department, hazardous materials team
Confined space	Fire department, special rescue team
Swift-water rescue	Fire department, special rescue team
High-angle rescue	Fire department, special rescue team
Trench rescue	Fire department, special rescue team
Downed power lines	Fire department, electric utility company
Natural gas leak	Fire department, gas utility company
Dangerous pets	Animal control
Mass-casualty incident	Law enforcement, fire department, advanced life support personnel, ground ambulances, air ambulances, municipal and public school bus services (if needed), Federal Emergency Management Agency (if needed), National Guard (if needed)

On the Scene   Wrap-Up

In each of the emergencies that an EMT responds to, the safety of the crew, the patient, and bystanders rests solely with the concept that scene size-up will dictate the course of action leading to the safest outcome for all personnel on the scene. This is a call where you must pay particular attention to details about the scene. There are newspapers in the driveway. There is no technical rescue or access problem.

As you enter the house, you notice a man lying on the living room sofa. You approach him and shake him gently as you say, "I'm an EMT. Sir, are you all right?" There is no response. You place a hand on his forehead, lift his chin, and look, listen, and feel for breathing. He is breathing quietly, about 16 times per minute. When you reach to feel his radial pulse, you notice his skin is cool, dry, and pale. His heart rate is about 100 beats per minute. Your partner tells you the patient's blood pressure is 114/66. You do not find any other abnormal findings in your examination. A police officer performs a quick search of the patient's home and finds a number of prescribed medicines for a heart condition but nothing that is unusual.

You apply oxygen by nonrebreather mask at 15 L/min. You quickly check the patient's blood sugar, which is normal. You contact medical direction and are instructed to load the patient immediately and transport to the closest appropriate hospital. You leave the scene with lights and sirens on to hasten your arrival to the hospital. When transporting another patient to the same hospital later in your shift, you learn that the patient had a stroke. He was transferred to the critical care unit. ■

Sum It Up

▶ As an EMT, you must quickly look at the entire scene before approaching the patient. You must size up the scene to find out if there are any threats that may cause injury to you, other rescuers, or bystanders or that may cause additional injury to the patient.

▶ Scene size-up is the first phase of patient assessment and is made up of five parts:
1. Taking standard precautions
2. Evaluating scene safety
3. Determining the mechanism of injury (including considerations for stabilization of the spine) or the nature of the patient's illness
4. Determining the total number of patients
5. Determining the need for additional resources

▶ You must take appropriate standard precautions on every call. Consider the need for standard precautions before you approach the patient. Put on appropriate PPE on the basis of the information the dispatcher gives you and your initial survey of the scene. This equipment includes gloves, eye protection, mask, and gown, if necessary.

▶ Scene safety is an assessment of the entire scene and surroundings to ensure your well-being and that of other rescuers, the patient(s), and bystanders.

▶ During the scene size-up, try to determine the nature of the illness or mechanism of injury.

▶ A medical patient is one whose condition is caused by an illness. The nature of the illness describes the medical condition that resulted in the patient's call to 9-1-1. Examples include fever, difficulty breathing, chest pain, headache, and vomiting. You should try to find out the nature of the illness by talking to the patient, family, coworkers, and bystanders.

▶ Mechanism of injury refers to the way in which an injury occurs as well as the forces involved in producing the injury. Kinetic energy is the energy of motion. The amount of kinetic energy an object has depends on the mass (weight) and speed (velocity) of the object. Kinematics is the science of analyzing the mechanism of injury and predicting injury patterns. The amount of injury is determined by the following three elements: (1) the type of energy applied, (2) how quickly the energy is applied, and (3) to what part of the body the energy is applied.

▶ A trauma patient is one who has experienced an injury from an external force. Traumatic situations include motor vehicle crashes, motor vehicle–pedestrian crashes, falls, bicycle crashes, motorcycle crashes, and penetrating traumas.

▶ Blunt trauma is any mechanism of injury that occurs without actual penetration of the body. Examples of mechanisms of injury causing blunt trauma include motor vehicle crashes, falls, sports injuries, or assaults with a blunt object. Blunt trauma produces injury first to the body surface and then to the body's contents.

▶ Penetrating trauma is any mechanism of injury that causes a cut or piercing of the skin. Examples of mechanisms of injury causing penetrating trauma include gunshot wounds, stab wounds, and blast injuries. Penetrating trauma usually affects organs and tissues in the direct path of the wounding object.

▶ A motor vehicle crash is classified by the type of impact. The five types of impact include head-on (frontal), lateral, rear end, rotational, and rollover.

▶ In a frontal impact, such as a head-on collision, the vehicle stops and the occupants continue to move forward by one of two pathways: down and under or up and over.
- In the down and under pathway, the victim's knees hit the vehicle's dashboard. The down and under pathway may be seen when the occupant is not wearing a lap and shoulder restraint system, or when the occupant is wearing only the shoulder harness and not a lap belt.
- In the up and over pathway, the victim's upper body strikes the steering wheel, resulting in injuries to the head, chest, abdomen, pelvis, and/or spine. The up and over pathway may be seen when the occupant is not wearing a lap and shoulder restraint system, or when the occupant is wearing only a lap restraint (not the shoulder harness).

▶ Although mechanism of injury is important, it is not the only factor to consider when assessing a trauma patient and determining whether or not she is a priority patient. For some patients, the risk of significant injury is increased because of their age or a preexisting medical condition, despite what may appear to be a minor mechanism of injury. In some EMS systems, other factors for designating priority status are considered in addition to the mechanism of injury. These include anatomy, physiology, and patient factors.

▶ Adult pedestrians will typically turn away if they are about to be struck by an oncoming vehicle. This action results in injuries to the side or back of the body. A child will usually face an oncoming vehicle, which results in injuries to the front of the body.

▶ Falls are a common mechanism of injury. Factors to consider in a fall include the height from which the patient fell, the patient's weight, the surface the patient landed on, and the part of the patient's body that struck first.

17

Patient Assessment

By the end of this chapter, you should be able to:

Knowledge Objectives ▶

1. Differentiate between a sign and a symptom.
2. Identify the components of vital signs.
3. State the importance of accurately reporting and recording the baseline vital signs.
4. Differentiate between central and peripheral pulses.
5. Differentiate among obtaining a pulse in an adult, child, and infant patient.
6. Describe the methods to obtain a pulse rate.
7. Identify the information obtained when assessing a patient's pulse.
8. Differentiate between a strong, weak, regular, and irregular pulse.
9. Describe the methods to obtain a breathing rate.
10. Identify the attributes that should be obtained when assessing breathing.
11. Differentiate between shallow, labored, and noisy breathing.
12. Describe the methods to assess the skin color, temperature, moisture, and capillary refill (in infants and children).
13. Describe normal and abnormal findings when assessing skin color.
14. Differentiate between pale, blue, red, and yellow skin color.
15. Describe normal and abnormal findings when assessing skin temperature.
16. Differentiate between hot, cool, and cold skin temperature.
17. Describe normal and abnormal findings when assessing skin moisture.
18. Describe normal and abnormal findings when assessing capillary refill in the infant or child patient.
19. Describe the methods to assess the pupils.
20. Identify normal and abnormal pupil size.
21. Differentiate between dilated (big) and constricted (small) pupil size.
22. Differentiate between reactive and nonreactive pupils and equal and unequal pupils.
23. Describe the methods to assess blood pressure.
24. Define systolic pressure.
25. Define diastolic pressure.
26. Explain the difference between auscultation and palpation for obtaining a blood pressure.
27. Discuss the examination techniques used during patient assessment.
28. List and describe the components of patient assessment and the purpose of each component.
29. Summarize the reasons for forming a general impression of the patient.

30. Define chief complaint and give examples.
31. Discuss methods of assessing the airway in the adult, child, and infant patient.
32. Discuss methods of assessing altered mental status in the adult, child, and infant patient.
33. State reasons for management of the cervical spine once the patient has been determined to be a trauma patient.
34. Describe methods used for assessing if a patient is breathing.
35. State what care should be provided to the adult, child, and infant patient with adequate breathing.
36. State what care should be provided to the adult, child, and infant patient with inadequate breathing.
37. Discuss the need for assessing the patient for external bleeding.
38. Explain the reason for prioritizing a patient for care and transport.
39. Discuss the purpose and components of the secondary survey.
40. State the areas of the body that are evaluated during the secondary survey.
41. Recite examples and explain why patients should receive a rapid trauma assessment.
42. Discuss the reason for performing a focused history and physical exam.
43. Distinguish between the secondary survey that is performed on a trauma patient and the one performed on a medical patient.
44. Discuss the purpose of patient reassessment.
45. Describe the components of the reassessment.
46. Discuss the reasons for repeating the primary survey as part of reassessment.
47. Describe trending of assessment components.

Attitude Objectives ▶

48. Explain the value of measuring the baseline vital signs.
49. Recognize and respond to the feelings patients experience during assessment.
50. Defend the need for obtaining and recording an accurate set of vital signs.
51. Explain the rationale of recording additional sets of vital signs.
52. Explain the importance of forming a general impression of the patient.
53. Explain the value of performing a primary survey.
54. Recognize and respect the feelings that patients might experience during assessment.
55. Explain the value of patient reassessment.
56. Explain the value of trending assessment components to other healthcare professionals who assume care of the patient.

Skill Objectives ▶

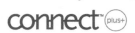

57. Demonstrate the techniques for assessing mental status.
58. Demonstrate the techniques for assessing the airway.
59. Demonstrate the techniques for assessing if the patient is breathing.
60. Demonstrate the techniques for assessing if the patient has a pulse.
61. Demonstrate the techniques for assessing the patient for external bleeding.
62. Demonstrate the techniques for assessing the patient's skin color, temperature, moisture, and capillary refill (infants and children only).
63. Demonstrate the ability to prioritize patients.
64. Demonstrate the patient assessment skills that should be used to assist with a patient who is unresponsive or has an altered metal status.
65. Demonstrate the skills involved in performing the secondary survey.
66. Demonstrate the techniques for assessing the pupils.
67. Demonstrate the techniques for obtaining a blood pressure.

68. Demonstrate the skills that should be used to obtain information from the patient, family, or bystanders at the scene.

69. Demonstrate the skills involved in reassessing a patient.

On the Scene

You are dispatched to a local park for a person who has an unknown problem. Upon arrival, you find a 20-year-old man lying next to his bicycle. He has a severely angulated left forearm and is bleeding from a cut on his left forehead. You notice that his lips are slightly blue and his respiratory rate is 30 breaths per minute. He is responsive and responds to your questions but cannot remember what happened. He keeps asking the same questions repeatedly. ■

THINK ABOUT IT

As you read this chapter, think about the following questions:

- What do you suspect happened?
- How does the size-up of the scene give you information about the patient's condition or possible injuries? Is that information pertinent to your initial assessment?
- What does your patient's mental status indicate?
- Should you be concerned about the patient's respiratory rate and the bluish color of his lips?

Introduction

As an EMT, you must be able to accurately assess and record a patient's vital signs. This chapter explains the difference between assessment findings and symptoms and discusses vital signs, including pulse, respirations, skin findings, pupils, and blood pressure.

You will be taught many skills during your EMT course. Of all the skills you will learn, the most important skill is patient assessment. Every decision you make about the care of your patient is based on what you find during your patient assessment. In this chapter you will learn about the primary and secondary surveys and differences in the assessment of trauma and medical patients.

Vital Signs

Signs, Symptoms, and Vital Signs

Objectives 1, 2, 3

A **sign** is a medical or trauma condition of the patient that can be seen, heard, smelled, measured, or felt by the examiner. Examples of signs include unusual chest movement, bleeding, swelling, pale skin, and a fast pulse. A **symptom** is a condition described by the patient. Shortness of breath,

nausea, abdominal pain, chills, chest pain, and dizziness are examples of symptoms.

You Should Know

Because signs can be seen, heard, smelled, measured, or felt, they are considered **objective findings.** Some of the ways signs (also called *clinical findings*) can be determined include physical or psychological examination, laboratory tests, and imaging studies (such as x-rays). Symptoms are **subjective findings** because they are dependent on (subject to) the patient's interpretation and description of his complaint.

Vital signs are measurements of breathing, pulse, skin temperature, pupils, and blood pressure. Measuring vital signs is an important part of patient assessment. Vital signs are measured to:

- Detect changes in normal body function
- Recognize life-threatening situations
- Determine a patient's response to treatment

Baseline vital signs are an initial set of vital sign measurements. Later measurements are compared against baseline vital signs. When possible, take two or more sets of vital signs. Doing so will allow you to note changes (trends) in the patient's condition and response to treatment. For example, after obtaining the first set of vital signs (the baseline), you will be able to spot if the patient's heart rate is increasing, staying about the same, or decreasing when you take them a second or third time. Watching these trends in your patient's condition is very important. With this information and your patient assessment findings, you will be able to recognize life-threatening emergencies, such as shock.

Items for taking a patient's vital signs include:

- A watch with a second hand or a digital watch that shows seconds. The watch will be used to count your patient's respirations and pulse as well as to note the time of events for your documentation.
- A penlight or flashlight. This will be used to look at your patient's pupils.
- A **stethoscope.** A stethoscope is an instrument used to hear sounds within the body, such as respirations. It is also used to measure blood pressure.
- A **sphygmomanometer** (blood pressure cuff) to take your patient's blood pressure.
- A pen and paper to record your findings.

Pulse

Objectives 4, 5, 6, 7, 8

Arteries are large blood vessels that carry blood away from the heart to the rest of the body. Blood is forced into the arteries when the heart contracts. A pulse is the rhythmic contraction and expansion of the arteries with each beat of the heart. A pulse can be felt anywhere an artery passes near the skin surface and can be pressed against firm tissue, such as a bone (Table 17-1).

TABLE 17-1	Central and Peripheral Pulses
Central Pulses	
Carotid	• Major artery of the neck • Supplies the head with blood • Pulsations can be found on either side of the trachea in the neck • Check this pulse first when assessing an *unresponsive* adult or child 1 year of age or older • Avoid applying excess pressure • Never assess the carotid pulse on both sides of the neck at the same time, this can decrease blood flow to the brain and slow the patient's heart rate
Femoral	• Located in the fold between the thigh and pelvis • In the field, not often used because of the presence of patient clothing • To adequately feel, may require more pressure than at other sites
Peripheral Pulses	
Radial	• Located in the wrist at base of the thumb • Used to assess circulation in the upper extremities • Check this pulse first when assessing a *responsive* adult or a child 1 year of age or older
Brachial	• Located on the inside of the upper arm, midway between the shoulder and the elbow • Used to assess circulation in the upper extremities • Always check this pulse in an infant
Posterior tibial	• Located on the inside of the ankle, just behind the ankle bone • Used to assess circulation in the lower extremities
Dorsalis pedis	• Located on the top surface of the foot • Used to assess circulation in the lower extremities

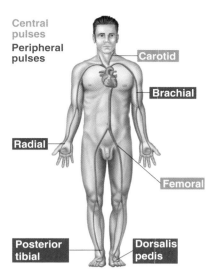

FIGURE 17-1 ▲ Location of central (carotid and femoral) and peripheral pulses (radial, brachial, posterior tibial, and dorsalis pedis).

A **central pulse** is a pulse found close to the trunk of the body (Figure 17-1). Examples of central pulses are the carotid pulse and femoral pulse.

- The carotid artery is the major artery of the neck. It supplies the head with blood. Pulsations can be found on either side of the trachea. To find the carotid pulse, place your index and middle fingers in the soft hollow area just to the side of the patient's trachea.
- The femoral artery is located in the fold between the thigh and pelvis. In the field, a femoral pulse is not often used because the patient's clothing prevents easy access to the femoral artery. To adequately feel a femoral pulse, you may have to apply more pressure than is required at other sites.

A peripheral pulse is located further from the trunk of the body than a central pulse. A peripheral pulse can be felt at several locations:

- The radial pulse is located in the wrist at the base of the thumb. Check for a radial pulse first when assessing a responsive adult or a child 1 year of age or older.
- The brachial pulse is located on the inside of the upper arm, midway between the shoulder and the elbow. Always check for a brachial pulse in an infant.
- The posterior tibial pulse is located on the inside of the ankle, just behind the ankle bone.
- The dorsalis pedis pulse is located on the top surface of the foot.

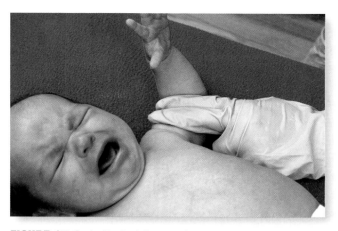

FIGURE 17-2 ▲ To feel for a pulse, use the pads of your index and middle fingers and apply gentle pressure to the artery.

To feel for a pulse:

- Use the pads of your index and middle fingers and apply gentle pressure to the artery (Figure 17-2). The pads on the tips of the finger are used because they are the most sensitive areas. Do not use your thumb to assess a pulse—it has a pulse of its own and could be mistaken for the patient's pulse. If you use too much pressure, you will cut off blood flow through the artery and will not be able to feel a pulse.
- Count the number of beats for 30 seconds. Then multiply the number by 2 to determine the number of beats per minute. If the pulse is irregular, count it for 1 full minute. Normal pulse rates for patients at rest are shown in Table 17-2.

A patient's pulse rate varies with age and physical condition. When checking the pulse, note if the pulse rate feels very slow, very fast, or within the normal

TABLE 17-2	Normal Pulse Rates at Rest	
Life Stage	**Age**	**Beats per Minute**
Newborn	Birth to 1 month	120 to 160
Infant	1 to 12 months	80 to 140
Toddler	1 to 3 years	80 to 130
Preschooler	4 to 5 years	80 to 120
School-age child	6 to 12 years	70 to 110
Adolescent	13 to 18 years	60 to 100
Adult	19 years and older	60 to 100

range for the patient's age. Also note if the rhythm of the pulse is regular or irregular. A slow heart rate may be normal in well-conditioned athletes. However, a slow heart rate may occur because of a medical- or trauma-related problem. A fast heart rate occurs as a normal response to the body's demand for more oxygen.

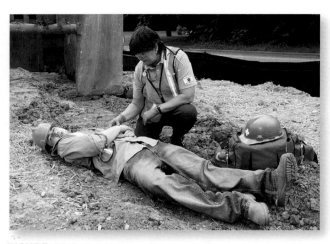

FIGURE 17-3 ▲ To count the respiratory rate, place the patient's arm across his chest or abdomen. Hold the patient's wrist as if you were assessing the radial pulse. Watch the rise and fall of the chest or abdomen. Begin counting when the chest or abdomen rises. Count each rise and fall of the chest or abdomen as one respiration.

> ### You Should Know
>
> **Possible Causes of a Slow Heart Rate**
> - Coughing
> - Vomiting
> - Straining to have a bowel movement
> - Heart attack
> - Head injury
> - Very low body temperature (hypothermia)
> - Sleep apnea
> - Some medications
>
> **Possible Causes of a Rapid Heart Rate**
> - Fever
> - Fear
> - Pain
> - Anxiety
> - Infection
> - Shock
> - Exercise
> - Heart failure
> - Substances such as caffeine and nicotine
> - Cocaine, methamphetamines, "ecstasy"
> - Some medications

Pulse "quality" refers to the strength of the heartbeat felt when taking a pulse. A normal pulse is easily felt, and the pressure is equal for each beat. This kind of pulse is said to be a "strong" pulse. A pulse is said to be "weak" if it is hard to feel. A pulse that is weak and fast is called a "thready" pulse. Pulses are normally of equal strength on both sides of the body.

Respirations

Objectives 9, 10, 11

Recall that a single respiration consists of one inhalation and one exhalation. Inspiration (inhalation) is the process of breathing in and moving air into the lungs. Expiration (exhalation) is the process of breathing out and moving air out of the lungs.

To count the patient's respirations:

- Place the patient's arm across his chest or abdomen. Hold the patient's wrist as if you were assessing the radial pulse. Watch the rise and fall of the chest or abdomen. Begin counting when the chest or abdomen rises. Count each rise and fall of the chest or abdomen as one respiration (Figure 17-3). Watch to see if respirations are regular and if the chest rises equally. Ask the patient not to speak during this time.

- Count respirations for 30 seconds. Multiply the number by 2 to determine the rate for 1 minute. If the patient's respirations are irregular or slow, count the rate for 1 full minute.

- In infants and young children, it is often easier to observe the rise and fall of the abdomen to determine the respiratory rate. Count an infant's respirations for 1 full minute.

Remember This

- Do not tell the patient you are counting her respiratory rate. If she knows that it is being assessed, she may vary her breathing without realizing it.

- Make it a habit to count the patient's pulse first. When you have finished, keep your hands in place but shift your attention to the patient's chest and abdomen and count her respiratory rate.

TABLE 17-3	Normal Respiratory Rates at Rest	
Life Stage	Age	Breaths per Minute
Newborn	Birth to 1 month	30 to 50
Infant	1 to 12 months	20 to 40
Toddler	1 to 3 years	20 to 30
Preschooler	4 to 5 years	20 to 30
School-age child	6 to 12 years	16 to 30
Adolescent	13 to 18 years	12 to 20
Adult	19 years and older	12 to 20

The normal respiratory rates for an adult, child, and infant at rest are shown in Table 17-3. The number of respirations per minute can be influenced by many factors. For example, exercise, stress, anxiety, pain, fever, and the use of stimulants can increase the respiratory rate. The use of narcotics or sedatives decreases the respiratory rate.

Normal respirations are evenly spaced and of adequate depth. Infants and young children tend to breathe less regularly than adults do. Irregular respirations may be associated with conditions such as a diabetic emergency or head injury. A patient is said to breathe "shallowly" if it is difficult to see movement of the chest or abdomen during breathing. Only a small volume of air is exchanged during shallow breathing.

Normal breathing is relaxed and effortless. "Labored" breathing is an increase in the work (effort) of breathing. If a patient is having difficulty breathing, he is usually irritable, anxious, or restless (Figure 17-4).

Possible signs of labored breathing include:
- Gasping for air
- Excessive widening of the nostrils with respiration (nasal flaring)
- The use of neck muscles to assist with inhalation
- The use of the abdominal muscles and the muscles between the ribs (intercostal muscles) to assist with exhalation
- A "sinking in" of the soft tissues between and around the ribs or above the collarbones (retractions)
- Skin color changes (blue or cyanotic skin)

Normal breathing is quiet. While counting the patient's respirations, listen for any abnormal respiratory sounds. Abnormal respiratory sounds include stridor, snoring, wheezing, gurgling, and crowing. **Crowing** is a long, high-pitched sound heard on inhalation.

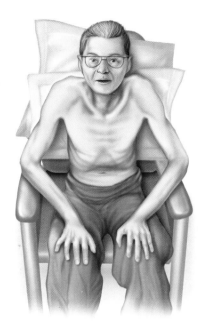

Gasping for air

Excessive widening of the nostrils with respiration (nasal flaring)

Use of muscles in the neck to assist with inhalation

Skin color changes (cyanosis around the mouth)

"Sinking in" of the soft tissues between and around the ribs or above the collarbones (retractions)

Use of the abdominal muscles and muscles between the ribs to assist with exhalation

FIGURE 17-4 ▲ Signs of respiratory distress.

Skin Color, Temperature, and Moisture

While assessing the patient's pulse, quickly check the patient's skin. Assessing the patient's skin condition can provide important information about the flow of blood through the body's tissues **(perfusion).**

Assess perfusion be evaluating:
- Skin color
- Skin temperature
- Skin moisture (moist, dry)
- Capillary refill (in infants and children younger than 6 years of age)

Skin Color

Objectives 12, 13, 14

Assess the patient's skin color by looking at areas of the body that are not usually exposed to the sun. For example, look at the palms of the hands, soles of the feet, oral mucosa (mucous membranes of the mouth), and conjunctiva (mucous membrane that lines the inner surface of the eyelid).

Abnormal skin colors include the following:
- Pale (whitish color) skin occurs when the blood vessels in the skin have severely narrowed (constricted) (Figure 17-5a). This condition may be seen in shock, fright, and anxiety, and with other causes.
- **Cyanosis,** a blue-gray color of the skin or mucous membranes, suggests inadequate breathing or poor perfusion (Figure 17-5b). It often appears first in the fingertips or around the mouth. Nail

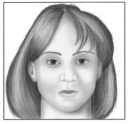
(a) Pale skin

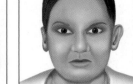
(b) Cyanosis

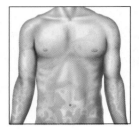
(c) Mottled skin

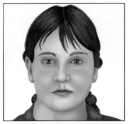
(d) Flushed skin

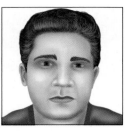
(e) Jaundice

FIGURE 17-5 ▲ Assess an adult patient's skin color in the palms of the hands and soles of the feet, inside the mouth, and inside the eyelids.

beds are an unreliable site to assess skin color. They are easily affected by air temperature and many medical conditions. Cyanosis may be seen in respiratory distress, airway obstruction, exposure to cold, blood vessel disease, shock, or cardiac arrest.

- **Mottling** refers to an irregular or patchy skin discoloration that is usually a mixture of blue and white (Figure 17-5c). Mottled skin is usually seen in patients in shock, with hypothermia, or in cardiac arrest.

- Flushed (red) skin may be caused by heat exposure, late stages of carbon monoxide poisoning, allergic reaction, alcohol abuse, or high blood pressure (Figure 17-5d).

- Jaundiced (yellow) skin may be seen in patients with liver or gallbladder problems (Figure 17-5e).

Skin Temperature

Objectives 15, 16

Assess skin temperature by placing the back of your hand against the patient's face, neck, or abdomen (Figure 17-6). The back surfaces of the hands and fin-

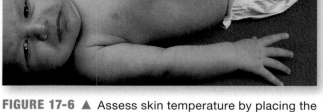

FIGURE 17-6 ▲ Assess skin temperature by placing the back of your hand against the patient's face, neck, or abdomen.

gers are used because the skin in these areas is thin and sensitive to temperature changes. Normal skin temperature is warm. Hot skin may be caused by fever or heat exposure. Cool skin may be caused by inadequate circulation or exposure to cold. Cold skin may be caused by extreme exposure to cold or shock. Clammy (cool and moist) skin may be caused by shock, among many other conditions. An infection, inflammation, or burn can cause localized warmth. Localized coolness may occur because of poor arterial blood flow to a limb.

Skin Moisture

Objective 17

Assess the moisture of the patient's skin:

- Normal skin is dry.

- Wet or moist skin may indicate shock, a heat-related illness, or a diabetic emergency.

- Warm and moist skin may be seen with anxiety, a warm environment, or exercise.

- Excessively dry skin may indicate dehydration.

Abnormal skin findings and possible causes are shown in Table 17-4.

Capillary Refill

Objective 18

Assess **capillary refill** in infants and children younger than 6 years of age. To assess capillary refill, firmly press on the child's nail bed until it blanches (turns white) and then release (Figure 17-7). Observe the time it takes for the tissue to return to its original color. If the temperature of the environment is normal to warm, color should return within 2 seconds. Other sites may be used to assess capillary refill, including the forehead, chest, abdomen, or fleshy part of the palm. A capillary refill time of 3 to 5 seconds is said to be *delayed*. This may indicate poor perfusion or exposure to cool temperatures. A capillary refill time of more than 5 seconds is said to be *markedly delayed* and suggests shock.

TABLE 17-4 Abnormal Skin Findings and Possible Causes

Skin Finding	Possible Cause
Color	
Pale (white) skin	Shock, fright, anxiety
Cyanotic (blue) skin	Respiratory distress, airway obstruction, exposure to cold, blood vessel disease, shock
Mottled (patchy blue and white) skin	Shock, hypothermia, cardiac arrest
Jaundice (yellow)	Liver or gallbladder problems
Flushed (red) skin	Heat exposure, late stages of carbon monoxide poisoning, allergic reaction, alcohol abuse, high blood pressure
Temperature and Moisture	
Hot and dry or moist	Heat exposure
Warm and moist	Anxiety, warm environment, exercise
Cool and dry	Inadequate peripheral circulation, exposure to cold
Cool or cold and moist	Shock
Localized warmth	Infection, inflammation, or burn
Localized coolness	Poor arterial blood flow to a limb

Remember This

Capillary Refill

- Normal: Less than 2 seconds
- Delayed: Refill time of 3 to 5 seconds
- Markedly delayed: Refill time of more than 5 seconds

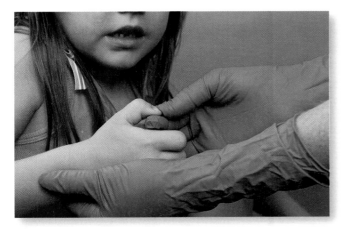

FIGURE 17-7 ▲ Assess capillary refill in infants and children less than 6 years of age.

Pupils

Objectives 19, 20, 21, 22

Examine the patient's pupils. The pupils are normally equal in size, round, and equally reactive to light (Figure 17-8).

Briefly shine light into the patient's eyes to assess the size, equality, and reactivity of the patient's pupils:

- *Size.* Dilated (very big) pupils in the presence of bright light may be caused by trauma, fright, poisoning, eye medications, or glaucoma. Constricted (small) pupils in a darkened area may be caused by narcotics, treatment with eye drops, or a nervous system problem.
- *Equality.* Unequal pupils, a condition called **anisocoria,** are a normal finding in 2% to 4% of the population. In most patients, unequal pupils suggest a head injury, a stroke, the presence of an artificial eye, or cataract surgery on one eye.
- *Reactivity.* Reactivity refers to whether or not the pupils change in response to light. Normally, a light that is shined into the pupil of one eye will cause the pupils of both eyes to constrict. Nonreactive

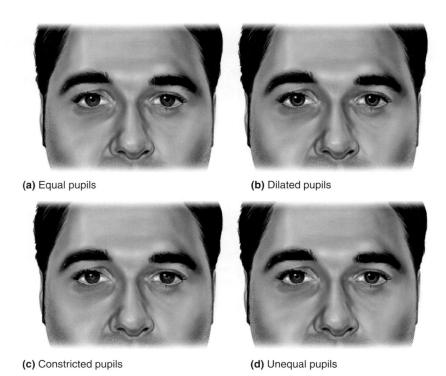

(a) Equal pupils   **(b)** Dilated pupils

(c) Constricted pupils   **(d)** Unequal pupils

FIGURE 17-8 ▲ Assess the size, equality, and reactivity of your patient's pupils.

pupils do not change when exposed to light. This condition may occur because of medications or cardiac arrest. Unequally reactive pupils (one pupil reacts but the other does not) may occur because of a head injury or stroke.

Abnormal pupil findings and possible causes are shown in Table 17-5.

Blood Pressure

Objectives 23, 24, 25, 26

Blood pressure (BP) is the force exerted by the blood on the walls of the arteries. Blood pressure is usually assessed using a blood pressure cuff and stethoscope.

This method of taking a blood pressure is called *blood pressure by auscultation* because it involves the use of a stethoscope. Electronic sphygmomanometers, which do not require the use of a stethoscope, are also available.

When a blood pressure cuff is applied to a patient's arm and inflated, blood flow in the artery under the cuff is momentarily cut off. If a stethoscope is applied over the artery, sounds can be heard that reflect the patient's blood pressure. As the cuff is slowly deflated, blood flow resumes through the partially compressed artery. The first sound heard is the systolic pressure. Systolic pressure is the pressure in an artery when the heart is pumping blood. As the pressure in the cuff continues to drop, a point is reached

TABLE 17-5 Abnormal Pupil Findings and Possible Causes	
Pupil Finding	**Possible Cause**
Constricted (small)	Narcotics, treatment with eye drops, head injury, exposure to organophosphate insecticides (such as malathion), some mushrooms, nerve agents
Dilated (very wide)	Trauma, fright, poisoning, eye medications, glaucoma, use of amphetamines, caffeine, cocaine, methamphetamine
Unequally reactive (one pupil that reacts but the other does not)	Normal finding in some individuals; head injury, stroke, presence of an artificial eye, cataract surgery on one eye
Nonreactive (pupils that do not change when exposed to light)	Medications, cardiac arrest

where sounds are no longer heard because the artery is no longer compressed. The point at which the sound disappears is the diastolic pressure. Diastolic pressure is the pressure in an artery when the heart is at rest.

A blood pressure measurement is made up of both the systolic and the diastolic pressure. It is written as a fraction (116/78), with the systolic number first. The blood pressure is recorded as an even number since most gauges have a scale marked in increments of 2 millimeters of mercury (mm Hg). If you are using a digital blood pressure device, the readings obtained may include both odd and even numbers.

A noninvasive blood pressure (NIBP) monitor does not require the use of a stethoscope to measure blood pressure. The machine's blood pressure cuff is applied to the patient's arm. As the cuff is deflated, the machine monitors the changes in pressure caused by the flow of blood through the artery.

Using a Stethoscope

A **stethoscope** is an instrument that is used to listen to body sounds. It consists of four major parts: the chest piece, tubing, binaurals, and earpieces (Figure 17-9). The earpieces should fit snugly but comfortably in the ears. For the best sound reception, the earpieces should normally point toward the EMT's face as the stethoscope is put on. The earpieces should be cleaned before and after use. The **binaurals** are the metal pieces of the stethoscope that connect the earpieces to the plastic or rubber tubing. When you are using a stethoscope, the binaurals should be angled so the earpieces remain in the ears without causing discomfort. The stethoscope's plastic or rubber tubing should be flexible and about 12 to 18 inches in length. Longer tubing decreases sound wave transmission.

The chest piece of the stethoscope may consist of a diaphragm and/or bell. The diaphragm is the circular, flat part at the end of the tubing. It has a thin plastic disk on the end. Although the diaphragm is used to detect high-pitched sounds, such as breath sounds, it is also commonly used when obtaining a blood pressure by auscultation. The diaphragm should be firmly held against the patient's skin with the fingertips of the index and middle fingers.

Some stethoscopes are also equipped with a bell. The bell has a deep, hollow, cuplike shape. It is used to detect low-pitched sounds such as those heard during blood pressure measurement. The bell should be lightly held against the patient's skin, with just enough pressure to form a seal. When possible, the stethoscope should be placed directly on the patient's skin because clothing makes sounds harder to hear. Skill Drill 17-1 explains how to assess a patient's blood pressure by auscultation.

Remember This

Obtain a blood pressure by auscultation before applying an NIBP monitor.

Sometimes the presence of noise on the scene makes it impossible to hear sounds through a stethoscope. In situations like this, assess the patient's blood pressure by palpation. Skill Drill 17-2 explains how to assess a patient's blood pressure by using this method. When a blood pressure is obtained by palpation, the diastolic pressure cannot be measured. Document the patient's blood pressure as the systolic pressure over a capital "P," such as 110/P.

Many factors can influence a patient's blood pressure. For example, anxiety, fear, fever, pain, emotional stress, and obesity increase blood pressure. Blood loss may decrease blood pressure. Table 17-6 on p. 338 shows normal blood pressures for patients of different ages.

When taking a blood pressure, it is important to use a blood pressure cuff of the correct size. The width of the cuff should not be more than two-thirds the length of the patient's upper arm. Blood pressure readings will be wrong if the cuff is the wrong size.

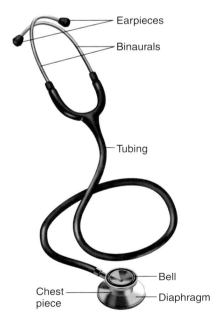

FIGURE 17-9 ▲ A stethoscope consists of four major parts: the chest piece, tubing, binaurals, and earpieces.

Measuring Blood Pressure by Auscultation

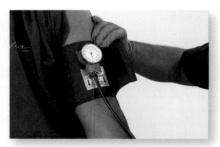

STEP 1 ▲
- Expose the patient's upper arm. Select the correct-size blood pressure cuff for the patient.
- Wrap the pressure cuff evenly around the patient's upper arm at least 1 inch above the elbow. Place the arrow on the cuff over the patient's brachial artery.

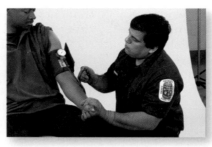

STEP 2 ▲
- Locate the patient's radial artery.
- Rapidly inflate the cuff until you can no longer feel the radial pulse. Inflate the cuff 30 mm Hg beyond the point at which you last felt the pulse.

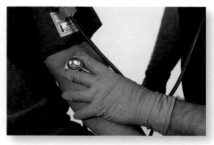

STEP 3 ▲
- Place the stethoscope in your ears.
- Place the bell or diaphragm of the stethoscope over the brachial artery, and hold it in place.

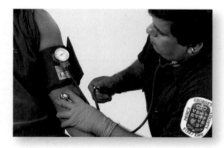

STEP 4 ▲
- While watching the gauge, deflate the cuff slowly and evenly at a rate of 2 to 3 mm Hg per second.
- Listen for sounds. The first sound is the systolic pressure and should be near the point where the radial pulse disappeared.

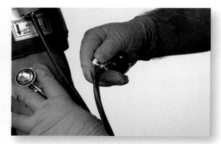

STEP 5 ▲ Continue to deflate the cuff, noting the point where the sound disappears. This is the diastolic pressure.

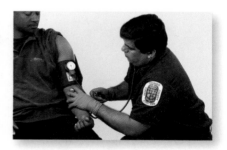

STEP 6 ▲
- Deflate the cuff completely.
- Record the blood pressure as systolic/diastolic pressure.

Measuring Blood Pressure by Palpation

STEP 1 ▶ • Expose the patient's upper arm. Select the correct-size blood pressure cuff for the patient.
     • Wrap the pressure cuff evenly around the patient's upper arm at least 1 inch above the elbow. Place the arrow on the cuff over the patient's brachial artery.

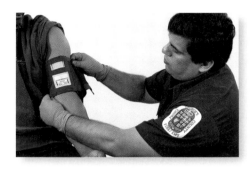

STEP 2 ▶ • Locate the patient's radial artery.
     • Rapidly inflate the cuff until you can no longer feel the radial pulse. Inflate the cuff 30 mm Hg beyond the point at which you last felt the pulse.

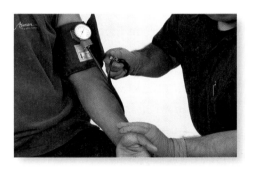

STEP 3 ▶ • While watching the gauge, deflate the cuff slowly and evenly at a rate of 2 to 3 mm Hg per second.
     • Note the point on the gauge when you feel the return of the radial pulse. This is the systolic pressure and should be near the point where the radial pulse disappeared. The diastolic pressure cannot be accurately measured by palpation.

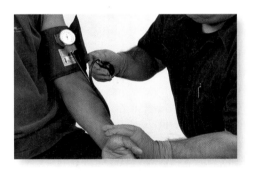

STEP 4 ▶ • Deflate the cuff completely.
     • Record the blood pressure as systolic/P (for example, 148/P).

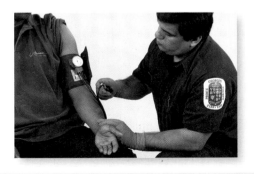

TABLE 17-6 Normal Blood Pressure at Rest

Life Stage	Age	Systolic Pressure	Diastolic Pressure
Newborn	Birth to 1 month	74 to 100	50 to 68
Infant	1 to 12 months	84 to 106	56 to 70
Toddler	1 to 3 years	98 to 106	50 to 70
Preschooler	4 to 5 years	98 to 112	64 to 70
School-age child	6 to 12 years	104 to 124	64 to 80
Adolescent	13 to 18 years	100 to 119	60 to 79
Adult	19 years and older	118 to 132	70 to 82

Remember This

Common Errors in Blood Pressure Measurement

Errors That Produce a False Low

- The patient's arm is above the level of the heart.
- The cuff is too wide.

Errors That Produce a False High

- The cuff is deflated too slowly.
- The patient's arm is unsupported.
- The cuff is too narrow.
- The cuff is wrapped too loosely or unevenly.

Errors That Produce Either a False High or Low

- Retaking a blood pressure too quickly may produce a falsely high systolic or low diastolic reading. Wait 2–3 minutes before reinflating the cuff.
- Deflating the cuff too quickly may produce a falsely low systolic and high diastolic reading. Deflate the cuff at a rate of 2–3 mm Hg per second.

For an unstable patient, vital signs should be assessed and recorded at least every 5 minutes. At a minimum, for a stable patient, vital signs should be assessed and recorded every 15 minutes. Remember, a stable patient can become unstable very quickly. Reassess frequently!

Remember This

Learning to take accurate vital signs is very important. Because vital signs allow you to detect changes in your patient's condition, take them often.

Additional Vital Signs

Pulse Oximetry

You will recall from Chapter 13 that pulse oximetry is a method of measuring the amount of oxygen saturated in the blood. Pulse oximetry is considered a routine vital sign and should be performed on all patients (Figure 17-10).

Exhaled Carbon Dioxide

Some EMS agencies consider exhaled carbon dioxide an additional vital sign. An **exhaled carbon dioxide detector**, also called an *end-tidal carbon dioxide (ETCO$_2$) detector,* measures a person's exhaled carbon dioxide (Figure 17-11). Although an exhaled CO$_2$ detector is most often used to confirm the position of a tube that has been placed in a patient's trachea, some detectors

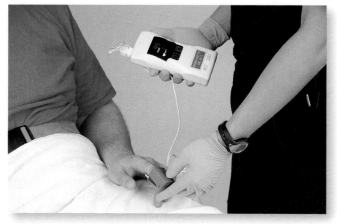

FIGURE 17-10 ▲ Consider pulse oximetry a routine vital sign and obtain oxygen saturation readings on all patients.

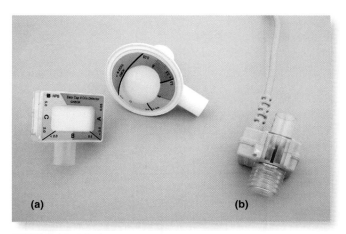

FIGURE 17-11 ▲ Exhaled carbon dioxide detectors. **(a)** Colorimetric CO$_2$ detector; **(b)** electronic CO$_2$ detector.

can be used with oxygen delivery devices, such as a nasal cannula or bag-mask device.

Pain Assessment

Some regulatory agencies consider an assessment of a patient's pain an additional vital sign. EMS and other healthcare professionals often underestimate a patient's pain. Some of the reasons for this may include the following:

- Some healthcare professionals believe it is a "waste of time" to ask a patient about pain.
- Because pain is unique to the person experiencing it, it is difficult for another person to accurately tell how severe the pain is.
- The patient may be unable to relay any needs about the pain. For example, it may be difficult to adequately assess pain in an infant or young child. It may also be difficult to assess pain if the patient speaks a language different from your own or has an illness that prevents her from verbalizing her needs.

If the patient is able to express pain, the way in which it is expressed varies. A patient may have tremendous pain, yet show no outward signs of any discomfort. On the other hand, a patient may cry, be very loud and expressive, or revert to childlike behavior when in pain. To assess pain in children 3 years or older, use the Wong-Baker FACES Pain Rating Scale (see Chapter 15). To assess pain in adults, ask patients to rate their pain using a scale from 0 to 10: "On a scale of 0 to 10, with 0 being no pain and 10 being the worst, what number would you give your pain or discomfort?" Remember to document your findings.

An Overview of Patient Assessment

Objectives 27, 28

The ability to properly assess a patient is one of the most important skills you can master. The components of patient assessment are shown in Table 17-7. You must learn to work quickly and efficiently in all types of situations. Some situations may include poor lighting conditions, temperature extremes, and large numbers of people. To work efficiently, you must approach patient assessment systematically. The emergency care you provide to your patient will be based on your assessment findings.

While assessing your patient, you will discover signs and symptoms. You must provide emergency medical care based on those signs and symptoms. Discovering the patient's signs and symptoms requires you to use your senses of sight (look), sound (listen), touch (feel), and smell.

- ***Look (inspect).*** You will use your sense of sight to assess parts of the patient's body and behavior. Does he look sick or poorly nourished? Do you see obvious problems such as a rash, external bleeding, vomiting, seizures, an arm or leg deformity, pale or flushed skin, or sweating?
- ***Listen (auscultate).*** You will use your sense of hearing to find out why your patient called for assistance. You will also listen to find out if the patient is breathing normally, if she is having difficulty breathing, or if breathing is absent. You will use a stethoscope to listen to the patient's lung sounds. You will use a stethoscope and blood pressure cuff to take a blood pressure.
- ***Feel (palpate).*** You will use your sense of touch to find out important information about your patient. Using your hands or forearms, you can find out if the patient's skin is hot, warm, cool, or cold. You can also determine if a body part is

TABLE 17-7 Components of Patient Assessment

Initial Assessment

Scene size-up	• Take standard precautions. • Evaluate scene safety. • Determine the mechanism of injury or the nature of the patient's illness. • Determine the total number of patients. • Determine the need for additional resources.

Primary survey	• Form general impression.
	  —Appearance
	  —(Work of) breathing
	  —Circulation
	• Check:
	  —**A**irway, level of responsiveness, cervical spine protection
	  —**B**reathing (Ventilation)
	  —**C**irculation (Perfusion)
	  —**D**isability (minineurological exam)
	  —**E**xpose
	• Identify priority patients.

Secondary survey	• Obtain vital signs. • Gain focused SAMPLE history, OPQRST. • Perform head-to-toe or focused physical examination.

Reassessment

	• Repeat the primary survey. • Reassess vital signs. • Repeat the focused assessment regarding patient complaint or injuries. • Reevaluate emergency care.

hard, soft, or swollen. You will also determine if touching a part of the patient's body causes pain.

- *Smell.* Your will use your sense of smell to identify odors associated with specific problems. For example, a sweetish (fruity) breath odor can indicate a diabetic problem. The smell of alcohol may explain why a patient is slow to answer your questions.

The **primary survey** is a rapid assessment to find and treat all immediate life-threatening conditions. During this phase of patient assessment, you will look for and treat life-threatening conditions as you discover them ("find and fix"; "treat as you go") and decide if the patient needs immediate transport or additional on-scene assessment and treatment.

The **secondary survey** is a physical examination performed to discover medical conditions and/or injuries that were not identified in the primary survey. During this phase of the patient assessment, you will also obtain vital signs, reassess changes in the patient's condition,

and determine the patient's chief complaint, history of present illness, and significant past medical history. The secondary survey does not begin until the primary survey has been completed and treatment of life-threatening conditions has begun.

You Should Know

An organized approach to patient assessment helps make certain that no significant findings or problems were missed.

Performing the Primary Survey

As mentioned above, the primary survey is a rapid assessment of the patient to find and care for immediate life-threatening conditions. You must perform a primary survey on *every* patient. The primary survey begins after the scene or situation has been found safe or

PATIENT ASSESSMENT

Initial Assessment

Scene Size-up

Primary Survey	Secondary Survey
General impression: Appearance (Work of) Breathing Circulation	Vital signs
Airway + Level of responsiveness Cervical spine protection	Focused history (SAMPLE, OPQRST)
	Head-to-toe (or focused) physical exam

Breathing (Ventilation)

Circulation (Perfusion)

Disability (Minineurological exam)

Expose

Reassessment

FIGURE 17-12 ▲ Patient assessment.

made safe and you have gained access to the patient (Figure 17-12). It usually requires less than 60 seconds to complete. However, it may take longer if you must provide emergency care to correct an identified problem. Remember to wear appropriate personal protective equipment before approaching the patient.

The primary survey has several parts:
- General impression
- Airway, level of responsiveness, cervical spine protection
- Breathing (ventilation)
- Circulation with bleeding control (perfusion)
- Disability (minineurological exam)
- Expose (for examination)
- Identification of priority patients

General Impression

Objective 29

Whenever you meet someone for the first time, you form a first impression—sometimes without realizing it. You will do the same thing with every patient. A **general**

impression (also called a *first impression*) is an "across-the-room" assessment. As you approach a patient, you will form a general impression of her complaint without her telling you what it is. You can complete it in 60 seconds or less. The purpose of forming a general impression is to decide whether the patient looks "sick" or "not sick." A variation of the sick or not sick approach consists of three questions:

- Does the patient appear stable?
- Does the patient appear stable but is potentially unstable?
- Does the patient appear unstable?

If the patient looks sick (unstable), you must act quickly. As you gain experience, you will develop an instinct for quickly recognizing when a patient is sick.

Remember This

Your patient's condition can change at any time. A patient that initially appears not sick may rapidly worsen and become sick. Reassess your patient often.

Before you speak to your patient and find out what is wrong, stop a short distance from her (Figure 17-13).

Look and listen:
- What things stand out in your mind when you first see her?
- Does the patient look ill (medical patient) or injured (trauma patient)? If the patient looks ill, are there clues around you that suggest the nature of the illness? For example, the presence of an oxygen tank suggests that someone in the home has a chronic medical condition. If the patient is injured, what is the mechanism of injury?

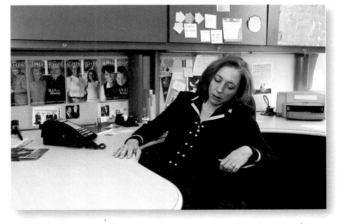

FIGURE 17-13 ▲ Form a general impression by pausing a short distance from the patient.

- How old do you think the patient is? Is the patient male or female?
- Does the patient look sick? If she looks sick, she may have a life-threatening problem. Life-threatening problems must be treated immediately. Examples of life-threatening problems include unresponsiveness, a blocked airway, absent breathing (respiratory arrest), and severe bleeding. If you find a life-threatening condition, you must treat it before going on to the next step.

Making a Difference

Some say that your "intuition" helps you form a general impression of a patient. Actually, a combination of knowledge, careful observation, effective communication, and experience is what forms that intuition.

You will base your general impression of a patient on three main areas: (1) appearance, (2) breathing, and (3) circulation. Remember: Approach a patient only after making sure that the scene is safe.

1. *Appearance.* Unless the patient is sleeping, his eyes should be open. His eyes should follow you as you move. If he looks agitated, limp, or appears to be asleep, approach him immediately and begin the primary survey.

2. *(Work of) breathing.* With normal breathing, both sides of the chest rise and fall equally. Normal breathing is quiet, painless, and occurs at a regular rate. Approach the patient immediately and begin the primary survey if the patient:
   - Looks as if he is struggling (laboring) to breathe
   - Has noisy breathing
   - Is breathing faster or more slowly than normal
   - Looks as if his chest is not moving normally

3. *Circulation.* The patient's skin color should be normal for his ethnic group. Approach the patient immediately and begin the primary survey if the patient's skin looks flushed (red), pale (whitish color), gray (ashen), or blue (cyanotic).

Some refer to the general impression as the "big picture." If your general impression reveals an urgent problem, move quickly. Begin emergency care, and arrange for immediate patient transport. If your general impression does not reveal an urgent problem, work at a reasonable pace and continue your patient assessment. Remember to explain what you are doing to the patient and family.

Remember This

During the Primary Survey, Find the Answers to Five Questions

1. Is the patient awake and alert?
2. Is the patient's airway open?
3. Is the patient breathing?
4. Does the patient have a pulse?
5. Does the patient have severe bleeding?

Airway, Level of Responsiveness, and Cervical Spine Protection

Objective 30

After forming a general impression, begin the primary survey by assessing the patient's airway and level of responsiveness. Assessment of a patient's airway and level of responsiveness *occurs at the same time.* If the patient appears to be awake, start by telling her your first name. Let her know you are an EMT. Explain that you are there to help. Next, ask your patient a question like, "Why did you call 9-1-1 today?" Her answer will give you some important information. First, it will tell you whether her airway is open. Second, it will tell you her level of responsiveness. Third, the patient's answer should be her chief complaint. A **chief complaint** is the reason EMS was called.

You Should Know

In a textbook, the steps of patient assessment are listed separately for purposes of discussion, although some steps are performed at the same time. For example, it is important to reemphasize that assessment of a patient's airway and level of consciousness (LOC) occurs *simultaneously.* In this book, the information presented pertaining to assessment of the airway could have been positioned after the information pertaining to level of responsiveness. The information about assessment of the patient's airway is presented first to help you recall the ABCDE memory aid. A slight modification to this well-known memory aid may more accurately reflect these simultaneous steps: LOC/ABCDE.

Airway

Objective 31

The human body must have a continuous supply of oxygen to survive. Air containing oxygen enters the body through the nose and mouth. It travels down the pharynx (throat), through the trachea (windpipe),

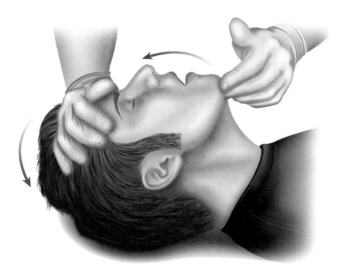

FIGURE 17-14 ▲ If you do not suspect trauma, use the head tilt–chin lift maneuver to open the airway of a patient who is unresponsive.

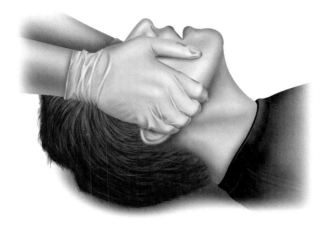

FIGURE 17-15 ▲ If you suspect trauma, use the jaw thrust maneuver to open the airway of a patient who is unresponsive.

and into the lungs. In the lungs, oxygen is transferred to the blood. The oxygen-rich blood is circulated to every cell in the body. The cells of the body cannot live long without oxygen. Therefore, a life-threatening emergency can result if the flow of air is blocked (obstructed) or if oxygen-rich blood is not circulated throughout the body.

A patient who is alert and talking clearly or crying without difficulty has a **patent** (open) airway. The airway is the pathway from the nose and mouth to the lungs. If the patient is unable to speak, cry, cough, or make any other sound, his airway is completely obstructed. If the patient has noisy breathing, such as snoring or gurgling, he has a partial airway obstruction.

If the patient is unresponsive and you do not suspect trauma, open his airway by using the head tilt–chin lift maneuver (Figure 17-14). If the patient is unresponsive and you suspect trauma, open his airway by using the modified jaw thrust maneuver (Figure 17-15). Both these maneuvers lift the tongue away from the back of the throat, allowing air to enter the lungs. If you are unable to open the airway (or maintain an open airway) by using the jaw thrust, use the head tilt–chin lift maneuver. If the patient is an unresponsive infant or child, do not hyperextend the neck when opening the airway.

Look for an actual or potential airway obstruction, such as a foreign body, blood, vomitus, teeth, or the patient's tongue. The tongue is the most common cause of a blocked airway in an unresponsive patient. If there is a solid object visible in the airway, remove it with a finger sweep. If there is blood, vomitus, or other fluid in the patient's airway, clear it with suctioning.

Level of Responsiveness (Mental Status)

Objective 32

Level of responsiveness is also called *level of consciousness (LOC)* or *mental status.* These terms refer to a patient's level of awareness. A patient's mental status is "graded" using a scale called the **AVPU scale** as follows.

> **A**lert
> Responds to **V**erbal stimuli
> Responds to **P**ainful stimuli
> **U**nresponsive

If the patient looks as if she is sleeping, gently rub her shoulder and ask, "Are you okay?" or "Can you hear me?" Unresponsiveness may indicate a life-threatening condition. If the patient does not answer, family or bystanders may be able to supply information. You may ask, "Can you tell me what happened?"

Determine whether the patient is awake and responds appropriately to questions. Evaluate her orientation to the following:

- Person (The patient can tell you her name.)
- Place (The patient can tell you where she is.)
- Time (The patient can tell you the day, date, or time.)
- Event (The patient can tell you what happened.)

A patient who is speaking or crying is responsive (conscious), breathing, and has a pulse. A patient who is oriented to person, place, time, and event is said to be *alert and oriented × (times) 4,* or *A&O×4.* If your patient is awake but cannot answer these questions correctly, the patient is said to be confused or disoriented. For example, if your patient is awake and knows his name (alert and oriented to person) and where he is

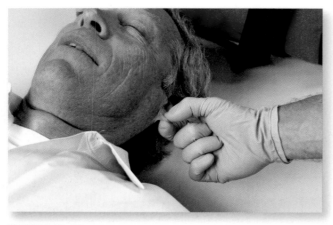
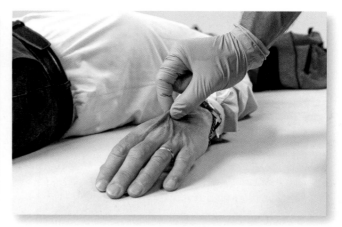

FIGURE 17-16 ▲ Determining the response to a painful stimulus.

(alert and oriented to place) but does not know what day it is and cannot tell you what happened, he is said to be *alert and oriented* × 2.

If the patient is not awake but responds appropriately when spoken to, he is said to "respond to verbal stimuli." For example, the patient will respond correctly to a request such as "squeeze my fingers." If the patient is not awake but responds to a painful stimulus, such as pinching the skin on the back of the hand or ear lobe, he is said to "respond to painful stimuli" (Figure 17-16). The patient is unresponsive if he does not respond to a verbal or painful stimulus. Again, it is important to note what kind of stimulus is applied and what the patient's response to it is.

As you continue your assessment, note any changes in the patient's mental status. The brain requires a constant supply of oxygen and sugar. Changes in the patient's level of responsiveness may result from a decreased supply of oxygen or sugar. These changes may also come from the use of alcohol or drugs, brain swelling caused by injury, or other causes. In a trauma patient, agitation and combativeness may be caused by a decreased supply of oxygen.

It is important to document (and report) which realms of orientation the patient is disoriented to. If advanced life support personnel arrive on the scene, be sure to tell them about any changes in the patient's mental status. Otherwise, relay this information to the staff person who takes the report from you at the hospital. In your prehospital care report, document the patient's response to a specific stimulus and any changes in mental status, for example, "The patient opened her eyes on command," "The patient moaned in response to a pinch on the wrist," or "The patient knows her name but does not know the date, where she is, or what happened."

An alert infant or young child (younger than 3 years of age) smiles, orients to sound, follows objects

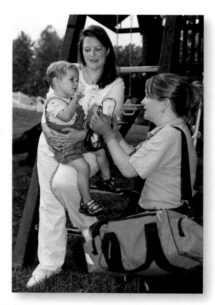

FIGURE 17-17 ▲ An alert infant or young child smiles, orients to sound, follows objects with her eyes, and interacts with those around her.

with his eyes, and interacts with those around him (Figure 17-17). As the infant or young child's mental status decreases, the following changes may be seen (in order of decreasing mental status):

- The child may cry but can be comforted.
- The child may show inappropriate, persistent crying.
- The child may become irritable, agitated, and restless.
- The child may have no response (unresponsive).

Assessing the mental status of a child older than 3 years of age is the same as assessing the mental status of an adult.

Making a Difference

Assessing a young child can be difficult. Toddlers distrust strangers and are likely to resist your attempts to examine them. They do not like having their clothing removed. They fear pain, separation from their caregiver, and separation from their favorite blanket or toy. When possible, assess the child in the arms or lap of her caregiver. Approach the child slowly and talk to her at eye level. Use simple words and phrases and a reassuring tone of voice. The child will understand your tone even if she does not understand your words.

Cervical Spine Protection

Objective 33

For trauma patients or unresponsive patients with an unknown nature of illness, take **spinal precautions.** Spinal precautions are used to stabilize the head, neck, and back in a neutral position. This stabilization is done to minimize movement that could cause injury to the spinal cord. The technique used to minimize movement of the head and neck is called **in-line stabilization.** The term *in-line* refers to keeping the head and neck anatomically in line with the body. In-line stabilization is first performed by using your hands. This is called *manual stabilization.* Manual stabilization is a temporary maneuver. The patient's head is not considered stabilized until it is secured to a long backboard.

If the patient is awake and you suspect trauma to the head, neck, or back, face the patient so that he does not have to turn his head to see you. Instruct him not to move his head or neck. Position your hands on both sides of the patient's head and spread your fingers apart (Figure 17-18). Place the patient's head in a

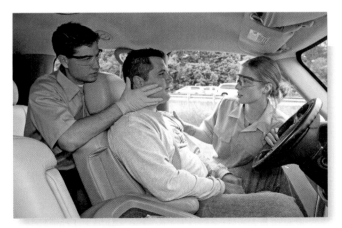

FIGURE 17-18 ▲ In-line stabilization requires keeping the head and neck anatomically in line with the body.

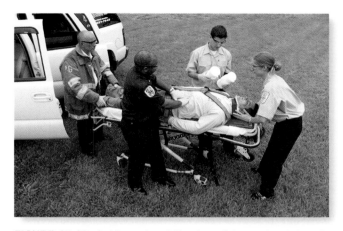

FIGURE 17-19 ▲ Manual stabilization of the patient's head and neck must be continued until the patient is properly secured to a long backboard with the head stabilized.

neutral position (eyes facing forward and level) and in line with the body. If the patient complains of pain or you meet resistance when moving his head and neck to a neutral position, stop and stabilize the head and neck at the point just before resistance was met. Once begun, manual stabilization of the patient's head and neck must be continued without interruption until the patient is properly secured to a backboard with the head and neck stabilized (Figure 17-19).

You Should Know

Examples of emergency care that may be needed to manage the patient's airway during the primary survey include the following:

- Spinal stabilization (also called spinal motion restriction) as needed for trauma
- Head tilt–chin lift or jaw thrust maneuver
- Suctioning
- Repositioning
- Removal of a foreign body
- Insertion of an oral or nasal airway

Breathing

Objectives 34, 35, 36

The priorities for assessing breathing and providing necessary treatment for infants and children are the same as for adults. After you have made sure that the patient's airway is open, assess her breathing. If the patient is responsive, watch and listen to her as she breathes. Quickly determine whether her breathing is adequate or inadequate. Keep in mind that normal respiratory rates for infants and children are faster than for adults.

Assessment findings and symptoms of inadequate breathing may include any of the following:

- Altered mental status
- Decreased rate of breathing
- Greatly increased rate of breathing
- Inadequate depth of breathing
- Fatigue from work of breathing
- Nasal flaring
- Tripod position
- Pursed lip breathing
- Abnormal skin color

If the patient is unresponsive, look, listen, and feel for breathing (Figure 17-20). Look for a rise and fall of the chest. Because the diaphragm is the main muscle used for breathing in infants and young children, watch the abdomen when assessing breathing. Look at the chest to assess breathing in older children and adults. Listen for air movement. Determine whether breathing is absent, quiet, or noisy. Feel for air movement from the patient's nose or mouth against your chin, face, or palm. If breathing is present, quickly determine whether it is adequate or inadequate. Breathing that is too fast or too slow for the patient's age is a red flag that requires a search for the cause.

If breathing is adequate and the patient is responsive, allow him to assume a comfortable position. Remember that emergency care for life-threatening conditions is given during the primary survey. For example, if your primary survey reveals that the patient needs oxygen, give oxygen by means of a nonrebreather mask or other oxygen delivery device before continuing the rest of the steps in the assessment.

If the patient is unresponsive and her breathing is adequate, maintain an open airway. Use airway adjuncts, such as an oral airway, if needed. Place the patient in the recovery position if there are no contraindications.

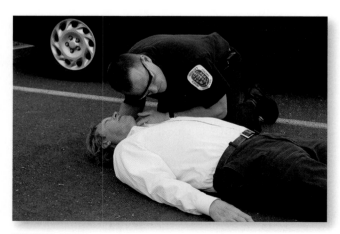

FIGURE 17-20 ▲ If the patient is unresponsive, look, listen, and feel for breathing.

Provide oxygen, and watch the patient closely to make sure that adequate breathing continues.

If the patient is unresponsive and breathing is inadequate or if the patient is not breathing, begin positive-pressure ventilation using a pocket mask, mouth-to-barrier device, or bag-mask (BM) device. Give breaths with just enough force to see the patient's chest rise gently with each breath. If the patient has dentures and they fit well, leave them in place to help provide a good mask seal. If the dentures are loose, remove them so that they do not fall back into the throat and obstruct the airway. Watch the patient's chest while you ventilate the patient. If your ventilations are going in, you should see the patient's chest rise gently with each breath. Continue breathing for the patient until he begins to breathe adequately on his own or another trained rescuer takes over.

If your initial breath does not go in, gently reposition the patient's head and breathe for her again. If there is still no chest rise, begin cardiopulmonary resuscitation (CPR). Check the patient's mouth for a foreign body each time you open the airway to give rescue breaths. (See Appendix A.)

You Should Know

Examples of emergency care that may be needed to manage the patient's breathing during the primary survey include the following:

- Giving of oxygen
- Suctioning
- Repositioning
- Removal of a foreign body
- Insertion of an oral or nasal airway
- Positive-pressure ventilation

Circulation

The assessment of circulation involves looking for signs of obvious bleeding and feeling for central and peripheral pulses. Evaluation of perfusion involves assessment of the patient's skin color, temperature, and moisture and assessment of capillary refill (in children less than 6 years of age).

Obvious Bleeding

Objective 37

Look from head to toes for signs of significant external bleeding. Control major bleeding, if present, by applying direct pressure over the bleeding site. Apply a pressure bandage if needed. If bleeding cannot be controlled from an extremity with direct pressure and the patient is showing signs and symptoms of shock, apply a tourniquet.

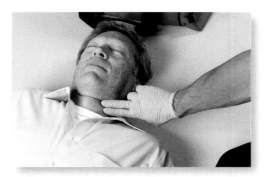

FIGURE 17-21 ▲ Use the carotid artery to check the pulse of an unresponsive adult or child older than 1 year of age.

Pulses

When assessing a *responsive* adult or a child 1 year of age or older, first check the radial pulse in the wrist. Use the carotid artery in the neck to check the pulse of an *unresponsive* adult or child older than 1 year of age (Figure 17-21). Feel for a brachial pulse in the upper arm in an infant (Figure 17-22). Feel for a pulse for at least 5 but no more than 10 seconds. A heart rate that is too fast or too slow for the patient's age is a red flag that requires a search for the cause. If there is no pulse, you must begin chest compressions.

Making a Difference

Practice finding pulses on adults and children of various ages. Knowing how to find a normal pulse in a healthy patient will help you recognize what is abnormal.

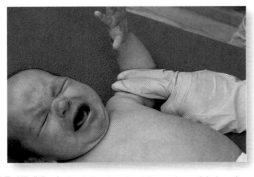

FIGURE 17-22 ▲ In infants, feel for a brachial pulse.

Skin Color, Temperature, and Moisture

While assessing the patient's pulse, quickly check the patient's skin. Assessing the patient's skin condition can provide important information about the flow of blood through the body's tissues (perfusion). Remember that adequate perfusion requires a functioning pump (the heart), adequate blood volume (fluid), and an intact vascular system (container). In the primary survey, perfusion is assessed by evaluating skin color, temperature, and condition (moist, dry).

Capillary Refill

In infants and children younger than 6 years of age, capillary refill is also used to assess perfusion. Capillary refill in adults is an unreliable indicator of perfusion because it is easily affected by medications, chronic medical conditions, cold weather, and smoking.

Disability

Altered mental status means a change in a patient's level of awareness. Altered mental status is also called an *altered level of consciousness (ALOC)*. Common causes of an altered mental status are shown in the following *You Should Know* box. A patient who has an altered mental status is at risk of an airway obstruction. As awareness decreases, muscle tone decreases. When this occurs, the tongue can fall back into the throat and cause an airway obstruction. The breathing muscles may not expand and contract as strongly as normal. This can result in inadequate breathing, low blood oxygen, and respiratory failure.

The AVPU scale is used early in the primary survey to assess responsiveness. Most EMS systems use the **Glasgow Coma Scale (GCS)** during the disability phase of the primary survey to obtain a more detailed assessment of the patient's neurological status. This minineurological examination is used to establish a baseline level of responsiveness and note any obvious problem with central nervous system (brain and spinal cord) function. Three categories are assessed with the GCS: (1) eye opening, (2) verbal response, and (3) motor response (see Table 17-8). The Glasgow Coma Scale score is the sum of the scores in three cat-

egories. The lowest possible score is 3. The highest possible score is 15. A patient who has a score in the range of 3 to 8 is usually said to be in a coma. When relaying GCS information to the healthcare professional assuming care of your patient, do not provide only the sum of the three categories. Instead, provide the sum in each category and the total score. For example, "Eye opening = 3, verbal response = 4, and motor response = 4. Total GCS score = 11." In this way, improvement or worsening of the patient's condition can be more closely assessed.

If the patient has an altered mental status and cannot maintain her own airway, open (or position) the airway by using a manual maneuver and insert an oral or nasal airway as needed. Suction as necessary. Give oxygen. If the patient's breathing is adequate, apply oxygen by mask at 10 to 15 L/min. If the patient's breathing is inadequate, assist her breathing with a BM

TABLE 17-8 Adult, Child, and Infant Glasgow Coma Scale

Glasgow Coma Scale	Adult or Child	Score	Infant
*E*ye opening	Spontaneous, opens with blinking	4	Spontaneous
	Responds to verbal command, speech, or shout	3	Responds to verbal
	Responds to pain	2	Responds to pain
	No response	1	No response
Best *V*erbal response	Oriented	5	Coos, babbles
	Confused, but able to answer questions	4	Irritable cry, but can be comforted
	Confused; answers with inappropriate words	3	Inappropriate crying or screaming
	Incomprehensible sounds	2	Grunting or agitated, restless
	No response	1	No response
Best *M*otor response	Obeys commands	6	Spontaneous
	Purposeful response to pain	5	Purposeful response to touch
	Withdraws from pain	4	Withdraws from pain
	Abnormal flexion (decorticate)	3	Abnormal flexion (decorticate)
	Abnormal extension (decerebrate)	2	Abnormal extension (decerebrate)
	No response	1	No response
	Total = E + V + M	(3 to 15)	

or mouth-to-mask device. Position the patient. If the patient is sitting or standing, help her to a position of comfort on a firm surface. If there is no possibility of trauma to the head or spine, place her in the recovery position. Assess the patient's blood glucose level per local protocol (see Chapter 20).

Remember This

When assessing a patient who has an altered mental status, keep in mind that the patient's usual mental status may be different from the average person. It is important to ask the family if the patient's mental status appears different from what is normal for him.

You Should Know

Emergency care that may be needed to manage the patient's neurological status during the primary survey includes the following:
- Maintaining the airway
- Giving oxygen
- Ensuring adequate breathing
- Suctioning
- Positioning patient
- Stabilizing spine

Expose

When assessing a patient, you can't treat what you don't find. Expose pertinent areas of the patient's body for examination. Factors that you must consider when exposing the patient include protection of the patient's modesty, the presence of bystanders, and environment and weather conditions.

Removing the clothing of a medical patient may reveal a medical identification bracelet or necklace, implanted pacemaker or defibrillator, surgical scars, swollen tissue, or other important findings. Removing the clothing of a trauma patient may reveal injured areas that would otherwise go unnoticed. Clothing that might impair patient movement, respirations, or distal circulation should be removed. Remember to keep the patient warm.

Identifying Priority Patients

Objective 38

Upon completion of the primary survey, determine whether the patient is stable, potentially unstable, or unstable. Patients who require immediate transport ("load and go") include the following:

- Patients who give a poor general impression
- Unresponsive patients
- Responsive patients who cannot follow commands
- Patients who have difficulty breathing
- Patients who are in shock
- Women who are undergoing a complicated childbirth
- Patients with chest pain and a systolic blood pressure less than 100 mm Hg
- Patients with uncontrolled bleeding
- Patients with severe pain anywhere

Performing the Secondary Survey

Objectives 39, 40, 41, 42, 43

A secondary survey should be completed on *all* patients following the primary survey. The reason the secondary survey is performed is to locate and begin the initial management of the signs and symptoms of illness or injury. This examination is performed only after you have found and treated all life-threatening injuries or illnesses.

The phrase **physical examination** implies a head-to-toe assessment of the patient's entire body. A secondary survey is typically a head-to-toe examination. However, the secondary survey is patient-, situation-, and time-dependent. A quick secondary survey (head-to-toe assessment) of a trauma patient with a significant mechanism of injury (MOI) is called a **rapid trauma assessment.** A significant MOI is one that is likely to produce serious injury. A quick secondary survey of a medical patient who is unresponsive or has an altered mental status is called a **rapid medical assessment.** The phrase **focused physical examination** is used to describe an assessment of specific body areas that relate to the patient's illness or injury. For instance, a patient with an isolated injury, such as a painful ankle, would typically not require a head-to-toe physical examination. This patient would require a physical examination focused on the injured area of the body.

General Approach

Examine the patient systematically, placing special emphasis on areas suggested by the chief complaint and present illness. When examining your patient, keep in mind that most patients view a physical exam with apprehension and anxiety—they feel vulnerable and exposed. Ease your patient's fears by explaining what you are about to do and why it must be done. Remember to properly shield an unclothed patient from the view of others. Conduct the exam professionally and efficiently while displaying compassion and talking with the patient throughout the procedure. If your patient is a child, ask a parent or family member to help you. Doing so should lessen the child's anxiety.

The procedure for performing a secondary survey is the same for trauma and medical patients. However, the physical findings that you are looking for and discover may have a different meaning depending on whether the patient is a trauma or medical patient. For instance, a swollen ankle in a trauma patient may be a sign of a sprain or broken bone. Swollen ankles in a patient with difficulty breathing and a history of a heart condition are more likely to be a sign of heart failure.

When examining your patient, first look (inspect), listen (auscultate), and then feel (palpate) body areas to identify potential injuries. Use your sense of smell to identify unusual odors during the exam, such as alcohol on the patient's breath, body, or clothing. Because it can cause pain, palpation should be performed last. **DCAP-BTLS** is a helpful memory aid to remember what to look and feel for during the physical exam:

> **DCAP-BTLS**
>
> **D**eformities
>
> **C**ontusions (bruises)
>
> **A**brasions (scrapes)
>
> **P**unctures/penetrations
>
> **B**urns
>
> **T**enderness
>
> **L**acerations (cuts)
>
> **S**welling

Another memory aid that may be helpful is **DOTS**:

> **D**eformities
>
> **O**pen injuries
>
> **T**enderness
>
> **S**welling

Depending upon the severity of the patient's injury or illness, a secondary survey may not be completed. This is because treatment of life-threatening conditions takes priority over performing this examination. A secondary survey is usually performed en route to the receiving facility. However, the exam should be performed on the scene if transport is delayed.

Making a Difference

You must be able to tell the difference between a seriously ill or injured patient who needs a rapid secondary survey and a less seriously ill or injured patient who needs a focused exam. If a life threat is discovered during the secondary survey, stop and treat it and repeat the primary survey.

Assessment of Vital Signs

Obtain vital signs after managing life-threatening problems found in primary survey. Remember to take two or more sets of vital signs. Doing so will allow you to note changes (trends) in the patient's condition and response to treatment. Reassess and record vital signs at least every 5 minutes in an unstable patient and at least every 15 minutes in a stable patient.

Assess respirations by evaluating rate, depth/equality, and rhythm. Assess any changes in respiration, including abnormal respiratory sounds. Assess the patient's pulse. Initially, a radial pulse should be assessed in all patients 1 year of age or older. In patients younger than 1 year of age, a brachial pulse should be assessed. If a pulse is present, assess its rate and quality. The quality of a pulse includes assessment of pulse strength (absent, weak, strong/full [normal], or bounding), rhythm, and equality. Assess skin color, temperature, and moisture. Assess capillary refill in infants and children younger than 6 years of age. Assess the pupils for size, equality, and reactivity. Assess the patient's blood pressure. Blood pressure should be assessed in any patient older than 3 years of age. Whenever possible, blood pressure should be assessed by auscultation. If available, attach a pulse oximeter and monitor the patient's oxygen saturation.

The Head-to-Toe Examination

Remember that patient assessment requires a consistent, organized approach. Begin the head-to-toe exam by reassessing the patient's mental status and then checking the patient's head. Then examine the neck, chest, abdomen, pelvis, lower extremities, upper extremities, and the back. Compare one side of the body with the other. For example, if an illness or injury involves one side of the body, use the unaffected side as the normal finding for comparison.

Although the steps for performing a head-to-toe exam are presented in this chapter in a specific order, keep in mind that some tasks are usually performed at the same time. For example, your partner may be taking the patient's vital signs while you perform the physical exam. If you find a life-threatening condition or injury, treat it when you find it. Remember that a focused physical examination may be more appropriate than a head-to-toe exam, based on the patient's chief complaint, your primary survey findings, and the mechanism of injury or nature of illness. Additional information about assessment of medical and trauma patients will be covered in Modules 6 and 8, respectively.

Keep the following points in mind during the head-to-toe exam:

- If the patient's condition worsens during the physical exam, go back and repeat the primary survey.

In situations like this, you may never complete the physical exam.

- If the patient appeared stable at the end of the primary survey, but becomes unstable during the secondary survey, expedite patient transport to the closest appropriate medical facility.

- If you found life-threatening injuries in the primary survey, it is possible that you may never get to perform the head-to-toe exam. In situations like this, ask another EMT to perform the head-to-toe exam while you manage the life-threatening injuries already identified.

- In a responsive infant or child, use a toes-to-head or trunk-to-head approach. This approach should help reduce the infant's or the child's anxiety.

- Remember that when caring for patients, a yes pertaining to an illness or injury is considered a pertinent positive or positive finding. A no is considered a pertinent negative or negative finding. Keep this in mind when examining your patient and obtaining the patient's history. Document your findings accordingly. For example, the absence of swelling in the legs and feet of a patient complaining of shortness of breath is a pertinent negative that should be documented.

Reassessment of Mental Status

As you begin the head-to-toe exam, it is very important to note any changes in a patient's mental status. Decreased blood flow to the brain can cause the patient's mental status to worsen. For example, if the patient was alert during the primary survey and now responds only to voice or pain, his mental status has worsened. On the other hand, if the patient was unresponsive during the primary survey and now responds to pain, his mental status has improved.

If the patient is alert, she can direct the physical exam with her complaints and response. A patient who is not awake may still react during the physical examination. For example, the patient may respond to your voice or may withdraw from pain. A patient displays *purposeful movement* when she attempts to remove the stimulus. *Nonpurposeful movement* is displayed when the patient moves in response but does not attempt to remove the stimulus. Be sure to document the patient's response to a specific stimulus. For example, "The patient responded to a pinch on the wrist by pulling both arms toward her chest."

Changes in a patient's level of responsiveness are important findings that must be relayed to the healthcare professionals to whom you transfer care. It is also important to document these findings in the prehospital care report.

Head and Face

The head contains many blood vessels. Wounds of the face or scalp may bleed heavily. Before examining the head of a trauma patient, have someone manually stabilize the patient's head and neck to keep him from moving—if this has not already been done. Using your gloved hands, gently feel the patient's scalp for deformities, depressions, tenderness, and swelling (Skill Drill 17-3, Step 1). Look for any open wounds or discolored areas. Run your fingers through the patient's hair and examine your gloves for the presence of blood. Gently slide your gloved hands behind the patient's head and feel for tenderness, swelling, or depressions that may indicate a skull fracture. If you feel a depression or an indentation in the skull, you may hear and feel crackling. This is called **crepitation** or *crepitus*. It is caused by the grating of broken bone ends against each other. Control bleeding from a scalp wound by applying gentle, direct pressure with a dry, sterile dressing. If you suspect a skull fracture, do not apply direct pressure to the center of the wound. Doing so could force bone fragments down into the brain. Instead, apply gentle pressure around the edges of the wound and over a broad area.

Remember This

Assume that any patient who has significant facial trauma also has a cervical spine and head injury until proved otherwise.

Assess the face for DCAP-BTLS (Skill Drill 17-3, Step 2). Swelling of the face is often first seen around the eyes and cheeks because the subcutaneous tissue is relatively loose in these areas. Look at the patient's face for **symmetry** (evenness). Assess for symmetry by comparing one side of the face with the other. Examples of **asymmetry** (unevenness) of facial movements that may be seen include an eye on one side of the face that does not close completely or drooping of the lower eyelid and mouth (Figure 17-23 on p. 358). These are signs of a possible stroke.

Gently palpate the facial bones—eye sockets (orbits), nasal bones, cheek bones, maxilla (upper jaw bone), and mandible (lower jaw bone)—for instability or tenderness (Skill Drill 17-3, Steps 3–6). The orbits are often fractured in patients who have experienced facial trauma. Assess for crepitation. If the patient is responsive and has experienced facial trauma, ask him if he has any facial numbness. If facial numbness or weakness is present, the patient may have possible nerve damage associated with the facial injury.

Performing the Secondary Survey

STEP 1 ▶ Using your gloved hands, gently feel the patient's scalp for deformities, depressions, tenderness, and swelling. Look for any open wounds or discoloration.

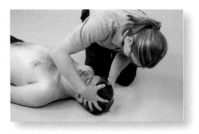

STEP 2 ▶ Assess the face for DCAP-BTLS. Look at the patient's face for symmetry (evenness).

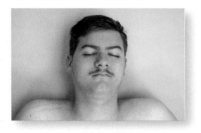

STEP 3 ▶ Gently palpate the eye sockets (orbits) for instability or tenderness.

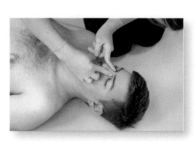

STEP 4 ▶ Gently palpate the nasal bones for instability or tenderness.

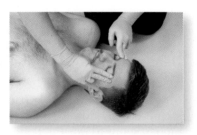

STEP 5 ▶ Gently palpate the cheek bones for instability or tenderness.

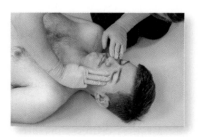

STEP 6 ▶ Gently palpate the upper jaw bone (maxilla) and lower jaw bone (mandible) for instability or tenderness.

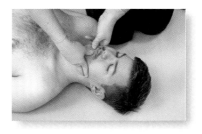

STEP 7 ▶ Look for blood or fluid from the nose and singed nasal hairs. Also look for nasal flaring (widening of the nostrils).

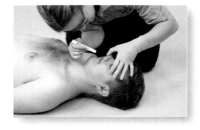

STEP 8 ▶ Look in the mouth for blood; vomitus; absent, broken, or loose teeth; an injured or swollen tongue; or foreign material. Note the color of the patient's lips and the mucous membrane of the mouth.

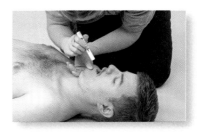

STEP 9 ▶ Note the presence of any unusual odors on the patient's breath, body, or clothing.

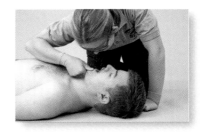

STEP 10 ▶ Assess the size and shape of the pupils and their response to light. Look at the eyelids for discoloration, cuts, or swelling. Look at the whites of the eyes for discoloration. Look at the conjunctivae for redness, pus, and foreign bodies.

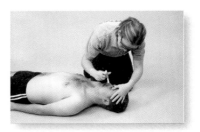

Continued

Performing the Secondary Survey   *Continued*

STEP 11 ▶ Look for blood or fluid leaking from the ears.

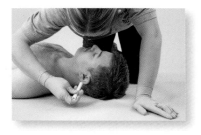

STEP 12 ▶ Look for bruising behind the ears.

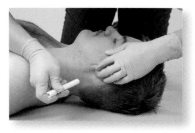

STEP 13 ▶ Assess the neck for DCAP-BTLS, open wounds, a laryngeal stoma, use of accessory muscles, and jugular venous distention.

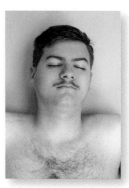

STEP 14 ▶ Medical alert tags may be worn on a necklace or bracelet. These ID tags contain important medical information, including the patient's medical condition, important prescription medications, and allergies.

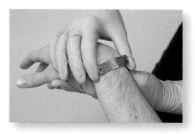

STEP 15 ▶ Gently feel the front and back of the neck to detect areas of tenderness or deformity.

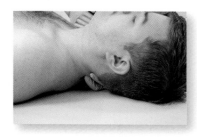

STEP 16 ▶ Feel the position of the trachea just above the manubrium in the suprasternal notch.

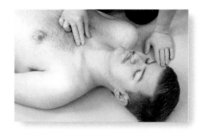

STEP 17 ▶ Assess the chest for DCAP-BTLS. Note the shape of the patient's chest. Assess the patient's work of breathing, including the use of accessory muscles during breathing. Look for surgical scars, an equal rise and fall of the chest, bruises, open wounds, obvious deformities, or signs of a rash.

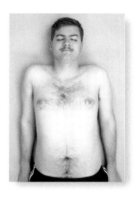

STEP 18 ▶ Listen for breath sounds. Listen at the top (apices) of the lungs in the midclavicular line on both sides of the chest. Listen at the bottom (bases) of the lungs and in the midaxillary line on both sides of the chest. Compare from side to side.

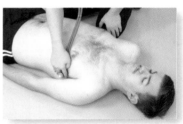

STEP 19 ▶ Feel the collarbones, shoulders, breastbone, and ribs for tenderness and deformity. Check for subcutaneous emphysema. Gently reach under the patient to assess the back of the chest.

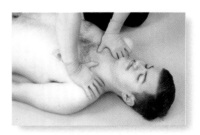

STEP 20 ▶ Using the pads of your fingers, gently feel the upper and lower areas of the abdomen for injuries or tenderness.

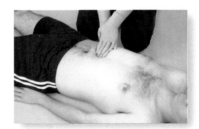

Continued

Performing the Secondary Survey *Continued*

STEP 21 ▶ Gently reach under the patient to assess the lower back.

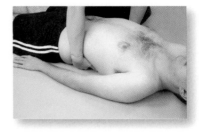

STEP 22 ▶ If the patient has not complained of pain and there are no obvious signs of pelvic injury, assess the pelvis by applying gentle downward pressure on the pubic bone. Press the iliac crests of the pelvis inward toward each other and posteriorly toward the back.

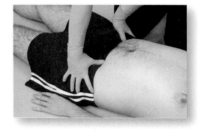

STEP 23 ▶ • Examine the upper leg.

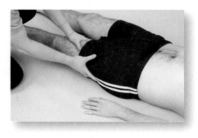

• Examine the lower leg.

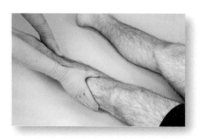

• Assess the dorsalis pedis pulse in each lower extremity at the same time. Note any difference in pulse strength, regularity, or rate between locations. Remember to assess movement and sensation in each extremity.

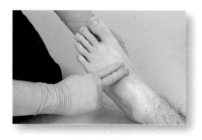

STEP 24 ▶ • Examine the upper arm.

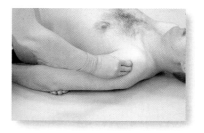

• Examine the lower arm.

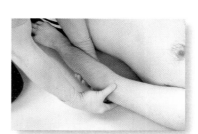

• Assess the radial pulse in each upper extremity at the same time. Note any difference in pulse strength, regularity, or rate between locations.

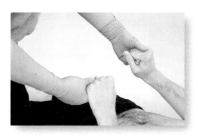

STEP 25 ▶ If the patient is awake, assess movement by asking the patient to squeeze your fingers.

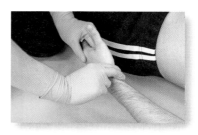

STEP 26 ▶ Logroll the patient to assess the patient's back.

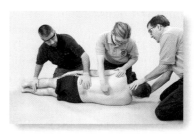

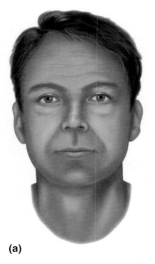 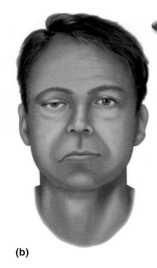

(a)   **(b)**

FIGURE 17-23 ▲ Examples of asymmetrical facial movements that may be seen include an eye on one side of the face that does not close completely or drooping of the lower eyelid and mouth. **(a)** Symmetrical; **(b)** asymmetrical.

Look for blood or fluid from the nose and singed nasal hairs (Skill Drill 17-3, Step 7). Singed facial hairs suggest a possible airway burn. Do not insert a nasal airway if the patient has known or suspected trauma to the midface. Look for signs of increased breathing effort, such as **nasal flaring** (widening of the nostrils). Complaints of nasal stuffiness and drainage from the nose can be caused by environmental allergies. Although swelling around the nose and eyes may be seen in a patient who has experienced trauma to the face, these findings may also be seen in a patient who has a medical condition (such as a sinus infection). A patient who has a sinus infection may complain of pain or tenderness when you feel the areas just above or below the eyes.

Look in the mouth for blood; vomitus; absent, broken, or loose teeth; an injured or swollen tongue; and foreign material (Skill Drill 17-3, Step 8). Suction as needed. Note the color of the patient's lips and the mucous membrane of the mouth. They should appear pink and moist. A bluish tinge of the lips and mucous membranes is common in dark-skinned patients. Swelling of the lips may be caused by trauma or an allergic reaction to medications, foods, or other allergens. Lips that are dry and cracked may be caused by exposure to the sun, wind, or a dry environment, or dehydration. Note the presence of any unusual odors on the patient's breath, body, or clothing (see the following *You Should Know* box and Skill Drill 17-3, Step 9). If the patient is coughing up sputum, note its color, amount, and consistency. If the patient is unresponsive, insert an oral airway to maintain an open airway. Suction the mouth to clear the airway if necessary.

Eyes and Ears

Look for injury to the eyes, but do not touch the eyes to find out if an injury is present. Assess for DCAP-BTLS. Look for **ecchymosis** (bluish discoloration) around the eyes, a condition known as **raccoon eyes.** This sign can occur because of direct trauma to the face. It can also be associated with a possible skull fracture. Look for the presence of blood in the anterior chamber of the eye **(hyphema).** Look for the presence of redness, contact lenses, or a foreign body. Use a penlight or flashlight to check the pupils for size, shape, equality, and reactivity (Skill Drill 17-3, Step 10). The pupils are normally equal, round, and react briskly to light. Unequal pupils in the presence of head trauma suggest **edema** (swelling) of the brain. Do a quick check of the patient's vision by asking, "How many fingers am I holding up?"

Look at the eyelids for discoloration, cuts, or swelling. Assess the sclerae (whites of the eyes) for discoloration. A yellow discoloration (jaundice) of the sclerae suggests liver disease. Red or bloodshot sclerae may be caused by allergies, trauma, or an infection. The sclera is lined with a paper-thin mucous membrane called the **conjunctiva.** If the conjunctiva becomes infected (conjunctivitis), it can produce a red eye with pus, mucus, or watery discharge.

Remember This

Use a penlight or flashlight to look in the ears, nose, and mouth and to examine the eyes.

Look for blood or fluid leaking from the ears (Skill Drill 17-3, Step 11). If fluid is seen in the ears, do not attempt to stop the flow. Cover the ear with a loose, sterile dressing. A bluish discoloration of the mastoid process (behind the ear) is called **Battle's sign** and is a sign of a possible skull fracture (Skill Drill 17-3, Step 12). Note the color of the earlobes. They may appear pale or blue in a cold environment. Excessive redness may indicate inflammation, fever, or high blood pressure in some patients.

Patients who have an infection of the external or middle ear often pull or tug at the affected ear. Middle ear infections are common, particularly in patients who have seasonal allergies. Inflammation of the outer ear can be caused by an allergic reaction to personal care products, such as hair dye and perfume.

You Should Know

Raccoon eyes and Battle's sign are signs of a possible skull fracture. These signs may not be present for several hours after the injury.

Neck

Examine the front and back of the neck. Assess for DCAP-BTLS. Look to see if the patient has a **laryngeal stoma** (surgical opening in the neck). Is the patient using the accessory muscles in the neck during breathing? Look at the jugular veins on the side of the neck (Skill Drill 17-3, Step 13). The jugular veins run from the angle of the jaw to the shoulders. The neck veins normally bulge slightly when a patient is supine. Flat neck veins in a supine patient suggest decreased blood volume. **Distention** (bulging) of the neck veins when the patient is placed in a sitting position at a 45-degree angle indicates a backup of blood from the heart because of fluid overload or an injury to the chest, lungs, or heart. Distention of the neck veins is commonly called **jugular venous distention (JVD).**

Look for open wounds and for medical identification (Skill Drill 17-3, Step 14). Medical alert tags may be worn on a necklace or bracelet. These ID tags contain important medical information, such as the patient's medical condition, important prescription medications, and allergies. Do not consider the information on a medical alert tag a complete listing of the patient's medication or medical history.

Gently feel the front and back of the neck to detect areas of tenderness or deformity (Skill Drill 17-3, Step 15). Feel for tenderness or crepitation of the cervical spine. Feel the position of the trachea just above the manubrium in the suprasternal notch (Skill Drill 17-3, Step 16). It should be in a midline position. Shifting of the trachea from a midline position is called **tracheal deviation.** When a **tension pneumothorax** is present, the trachea deviates away from the injured lung (see Chapter 35). Feel for **subcutaneous emphysema** (air trapped beneath the skin), which feels like a crackling sensation under the fingers while palpating the chest. It feels and sounds like crisped rice cereal or bubble wrap. The presence of subcutaneous emphysema suggests a collapsed lung or ruptured bronchial tube and the leakage of air into the pleural space.

If there is an open wound of the neck, cover the wound with an **occlusive** (airtight) dressing to prevent air from entering the wound. Apply a cervical immobilization device if a spinal injury is suspected or if the patient is unresponsive and the MOI is unknown. Ask another EMT to continue to maintain in-line spinal stabilization while you continue the assessment. *Remember:* Once begun, manual stabilization must continue until the patient has been completely immobilized on a long backboard. If the patient has difficulty swallowing, monitor the patient's airway closely. Be prepared to suction if needed.

Chest

To examine the chest, it is usually necessary to remove the patient's clothing. Protect the patient's privacy and shield him from curious onlookers. Assess for DCAP-BTLS (Skill Drill 17-3, Step 17). Assess the patient's work of breathing. Check for the use of accessory muscles during breathing. Look for surgical scars, an equal rise and fall of the chest, bruises, open wounds, or obvious deformities. The presence of a long scar over the patient's breastbone indicates a cardiac history. Unequal chest expansion may occur when part of the lung is obstructed or collapsed because of injury (such as a flail chest, pneumothorax) or illness (such as pneumonia). Observe if paradoxical chest movement is present, which is a sign of a flail segment.

You Should Know

Paradoxical chest wall movement may be most easily seen in an unresponsive patient. In patients with thick or muscular chest walls, it may be hard to see paradoxical movement. In some conscious patients, spasm and splinting of the chest muscles may cause paradoxical motion to go unnoticed.

If you see an open chest wound, immediately cover it with your gloved hand and then apply an occlusive dressing. Tape the dressing to the chest on three sides. Leave the fourth side open to allow air to escape but not enter the wound. If the patient appears to worsen after covering the wound with the dressing (or your hand), remove it to let air escape. Then reapply your hand or the dressing to the wound. If you see an object impaled in the chest, such as a knife, do not try to remove it. Removing it can result in bleeding and the entry of air into the chest. Leave the object where it is, and stabilize it in place with bulky dressings. If a flail segment is present, the patient will usually need positive-pressure ventilation with a bag-mask device.

Note the shape of the patient's chest. A barrel-shaped chest suggests a history of chronic lung disease.

Look at the skin for signs of a rash. The presence of a rash may indicate the patient's problem is the result of an allergic reaction.

Use a stethoscope to listen to the movement of air into and out of the patient's lungs. Starting at the apices of the lungs (about the second intercostal space), listen for breath sounds in six places (Skill Drill 17-3, Step 18):

- At the apices, midclavicular line on each side of the chest
- At the bases on each side of the chest
- In the midaxillary line on each side of the chest

Listen to one full respiratory cycle (inhalation and exhalation) in each location, comparing from side to side. Determine whether breath sounds are present, diminished, or absent; equal or unequal; and/or clear, muffled, or noisy. Breath sounds on the back of the chest are best assessed later in the physical exam when the rest of the back is examined. Watch and listen to see if the patient has any signs of difficulty breathing or pain with breathing.

A patient who has experienced trauma to the head or brain may have an abnormal breathing pattern. This occurs as the brain swells and pushes on lower structures in the brain. An abnormal breathing pattern is an important assessment finding. Be sure to document this finding and relay it to the healthcare professional to whom you transfer patient care.

Gently feel the collarbones, shoulders, breastbone, and ribs for tenderness and deformity (Skill Drill 17-3, Step 19). Check for subcutaneous emphysema. Gently reach under the patient to assess the back of the chest. Examine your gloves for the presence of blood.

Abdomen

Remember that the abdominal cavity is divided into four imaginary quadrants (Figure 17-24). These quadrants are created by drawing two imaginary lines that intersect with the midline through the navel (umbilicus). The abdomen contains solid and hollow organs. Solid organs, such as the liver and spleen, bleed. When hollow organs are cut or burst, their contents spill into the abdominal cavity. This results in pain and soreness. Hollow organs include the stomach, intestines, and gallbladder.

Assess the abdomen for DCAP-BTLS. When assessing the abdomen, look for the following:

- Surgical scars
- Bruising
- Open wounds
- Obvious bleeding
- Protruding abdominal organs
- An impaling object
- Distension

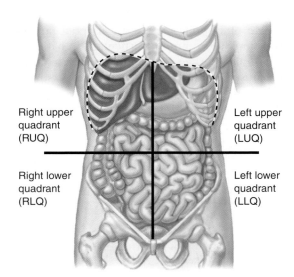

FIGURE 17-24 ▲ The abdominal cavity is divided into four imaginary quadrants created by drawing two imaginary lines that intersect with the midline through the navel (umbilicus).

- Generator for an implantable cardioverter-defibrillator
- Catheter for an insulin pump
- Signs of obvious pregnancy

Look to see if abdominal distention is present (the abdomen appears larger than normal). Abdominal distention can be caused by blood, fluid, or air. It is difficult to assess in obese patients. If exposed abdominal organs are present, do not attempt to reinsert them into the abdominal cavity. Cover them with a moist, sterile dressing. If you see an object impaled in the abdomen, leave the object in place and stabilize it in place with bulky dressings.

The abdomen is normally soft and is not painful or tender to touch. To examine the abdomen, place one hand on top of the other. Use the pads of the fingers of the lower hand and gently feel the upper and lower areas of the abdomen for injuries or tenderness (Skill Drill 17-3, Step 20). If the patient is responsive, ask her to point to the area that hurts (point tenderness). Assess the area that hurts last. Watch the patient's face while you palpate the abdomen. A grimace may indicate tenderness over a particular abdominal area. Determine if the abdomen feels soft or hard (rigid). Note the presence of any masses or pulsations. In a pregnant patient, note movement or the absence of movement in the fetus. Gently reach under the patient to assess the lower back (Skill Drill 17-3, Step 21). Examine your gloves for the presence of blood.

Patients with abdominal pain may present in different positions. Patients with **peritonitis** (inflammation of the abdominal lining) usually prefer to lie absolutely still. Patients with a bowel obstruction are often restless and often move in an attempt to find a position of comfort. Patients may also present with their knees in a flexed position (fetal position) to decrease tension on the abdominal muscles.

Abdominal pain is not always felt directly over the affected organ. For example, gallbladder pain may radiate to the right scapula and shoulder. Pancreatic pain may radiate to the back and improve when the patient sits forward. A ruptured aortic aneurysm may present with pain radiating to the back.

Pelvis

The pelvic area contains large blood vessels. Therefore, an injury to the pelvic ring can result in life-threatening internal and external bleeding. Assess the pelvis for DCAP-BTLS. If the patient complains of pain in the pelvic area or if obvious deformity is present, do *not* palpate or compress the pelvis. If the patient has not complained of pain and there are no obvious signs of pelvic injury, assess the pelvis by directing gentle downward pressure on the pubic bone, using the heel of one hand. Press the iliac crests of the pelvis inward toward each other and posteriorly toward the back (Skill Drill 17-3, Step 22). Do *not* rock the pelvis. If applying pressure results in tenderness, instability, or crepitation, suspect a pelvic fracture. When examining the pelvic area, check to see if the patient lost control of his bowels or bladder. Examples of situations in which this may occur include seizures, stroke, or cardiac arrest.

Severe blood loss may occur from a break in the continuity of the pelvis. If tenderness, instability, or crepitation of the pelvis is present, give oxygen and secure the patient to a long backboard. The patient will need rapid transport to the closest appropriate facility.

Remember This

If the patient complains of pain in the pelvic area or if obvious deformity is present, do *not* palpate or compress the pelvis.

Extremities

Assess the extremities for DCAP-BTLS. Look for open wounds, swelling, and abnormal positioning, such as an unequal length, etc. Look at the wrists and ankles for a medical ID tag. Look for swelling (edema) of the hands, feet, and ankles. Look for signs of a possible insect bite or sting, signs of possible intravenous drug abuse, or the presence of a dialysis shunt/fistula.

Assess pulses, motor function, and sensation in each extremity. Feel the dorsalis pedis pulse (on the top of the foot) in each lower extremity (See Skill Drill 17-3, Step 23). Assess the radial pulse in each upper extremity (Skill Drill 17-3, Step 24). Gently feel the upper and lower portion of each extremity for bone or joint deformities.

Assess movement and sensation in each extremity. If the patient is awake, assess movement of the lower extremities by asking if she can push both her feet into your hands at the same time. Assess movement of the upper extremities by asking the patient to squeeze your fingers using both of her hands at the same time (Skill Drill 17-3, Step 25). Compare the strength of her grips and note if they are equal or if one side appears weaker. If the patient is awake, assess sensation by touching the hands and toes of each extremity and asking her to tell you where you are touching. If the patient is unresponsive, assess movement and sensation by applying a pinch to each foot and hand. See if the patient responds to pain with facial movements or movement of the extremity.

A fractured femur (open or closed) may result in significant blood loss. Injury to both femurs may cause life-threatening bleeding. Even if there is no break in the skin, internal bleeding may be present. Comparing one extremity to the other may reveal differences in size as blood builds up in the soft tissues. If you suspect a femur fracture, give oxygen, control significant bleeding if present, and immobilize the patient on a long backboard. Transport to the closest appropriate medical facility. If the patient has experienced multiple injuries or his vital signs are unstable, a splint should be applied during transport if time permits. If the patient's injuries are not critical and his vital signs are stable, immobilize the injured body part with an appropriate splint before transport.

Remember This

Check **PMS** in each extremity:
  Pulse
  Movement
  Sensation

(Some EMS systems prefer use of the acronym *circulation, movement, and sensation,* or *CMS*). Compare each extremity to the opposite extremity. Assess PMS in each of your patient's extremities *before* and *after* immobilization. Be sure to document your findings.

Posterior Body

After making sure that there are enough personnel to assist you, logroll the patient to assess the patient's back (Skill Drill 17-3, Step 26). Make sure to maintain in-line spinal stabilization while rolling the patient. Assess the back for DCAP-BTLS. Look for swelling in the sacral area. In patients confined to bed, fluid collects in this area. If possible, listen to breath sounds on the posterior chest. Feel for swelling, tenderness, instability, and crepitation. If any open wounds are present, cover them with an airtight dressing. Control significant bleeding if present. Immobilize the patient to a long backboard.

Emergency Care During the Secondary Survey

Life-threatening conditions must be managed as soon as they are found. Less critical conditions can be managed as they are found during or after completing the secondary survey. Examples include:

- Abrasions, burns, and lacerations: Provide wound care.
- Swollen, discolored, deformed extremity: Provide immobilization.
- Minor bleeding: Control bleeding and provide wound care.

You Should Know

Patient assessment has been described as an input-output process. The assessment findings are the input. The treatment you provide to the patient is the output.

Reassessment

Purpose of Reassessment

Objective 44

You must frequently reevaluate your patients to make sure that you deliver appropriate emergency care. These reevaluations are called **reassessments.** A reassessment should be performed on *every* patient.

Reassessment allows you to:
- Reevaluate the patient's condition.
- Assess the effectiveness of the emergency care provided.
- Identify any missed injuries or conditions.
- Observe subtle changes or trends in the patient's condition.
- Alter emergency care as needed.

Components of Reassessment

Objective 45

Reassessment consists of the following components:

- Repeating the primary survey
- Reassessing and documenting vital signs
- Repeating the focused assessment
- Reevaluating the emergency care provided

Repeating the Primary Survey

Objective 46

Begin reassessment by repeating the primary survey (Skill Drill 17-4, Step 1). This is done in order to identify and treat life-threatening injuries that may have been missed. Reassess the patient's level of responsiveness, and note any changes in the patient's mental status. If the patient has an altered mental status, document the patient's response to a specific stimulus. Communicate any changes in mental status to the healthcare professionals to whom you transfer patient care. Document any changes in mental status in the prehospital care report.

Reassess the patient's airway. If the patient is able to talk clearly and without difficulty, assume her airway is open. If the patient is unresponsive, look in the patient's mouth for an actual or potential obstruction (such as a foreign body, blood, vomitus, or broken teeth). Check placement of any airway adjuncts that are inserted. If necessary, insert one to maintain an open airway. Document and communicate any changes or trends to those to whom you transfer patient care.

Reassess the patient's breathing rate and quality. Assess the rise and fall of the patient's chest, respiratory rate, depth and equality of breathing, and rhythm of respirations. Look for signs of increased work of breathing (respiratory effort) and signs of chest trauma. Note if the patient's respirations are absent, quiet, or noisy. Give appropriate treatment as necessary. For instance, give oxygen (if not already done), and suction the airway if needed. Document and communicate any changes or trends to those to whom you transfer patient care.

Reassess the patient's circulation by assessing the patient's pulse rate and quality. Reassess the patient's perfusion by assessing the patient's skin temperature, color, and moisture. Note any changes since you last assessed the patient's pulse. For example, if the patient's pulse was initially strong and regular and is now weak and irregular, this important finding suggests the patient's condition is worsening. In contrast, if the patient's pulse was initially hard to feel and is now strong, this finding suggests the patient's condition is improving. If you were initially able to feel a carotid pulse but were unable to feel a radial pulse, be sure to reassess the patient's radial pulse to see if there has been a change in this finding. Look for changes in skin color. Feel for changes in skin temperature and moisture. Remember to reassess capillary refill in infants and children younger than 6 years of age. Reassess the patient for signs of obvious external bleeding. Major bleeding should have been controlled during the primary survey. If there are any

Reassessment

STEP 1 ▶ Repeat the primary survey.

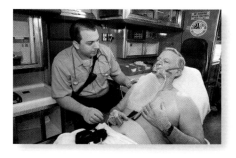

STEP 2 ▶ Reassess and document the patient's vital signs.

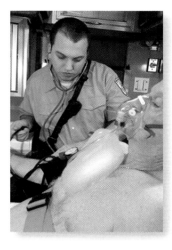

STEP 3 ▶ Repeat the focused assessment of the patient's specific complaint or injury.

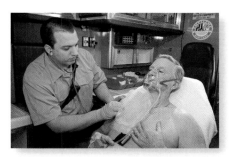

STEP 4 ▶ Reassess the treatments you have provided to be sure that they are effective.

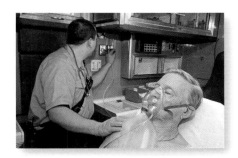

sites of minor bleeding, bleeding should be controlled and dressings applied as needed. Document and communicate any changes or trends to those to whom you transfer patient care. If applicable, reconsider your transport decision (patient destination and mode of transport) on the basis of your assessment findings.

Reassessing Vital Signs

Objective 47

Reassess and document the patient's vital signs (Skill Drill 17-4, Step 2). Reassess each of the following:

- Respiratory rate and quality
- Pulse rate and quality
- Blood pressure
- Pupils
- Skin color, temperature, and moisture
- Capillary refill in infants and children younger than 6 years of age

Compare the vital signs taken during reassessment with the baseline vital signs taken earlier. Having two or more sets of vitals allows you to note changes (trends) in the patient's condition and response to treatment. For example, by comparing the values obtained for the patient's heart rate, you will be able to see if it is increasing, staying about the same, or decreasing. Watching these trends will enable you to recognize life-threatening emergencies, such as shock.

Repeating the Focused Assessment

Repeat the focused assessment of the patient's specific complaint or injury (Skill Drill 17-4, Step 3). If the patient develops a new complaint or if a previously identified symptom changes, perform a focused assessment on the area of complaint.

Reevaluating Emergency Care Interventions

Reassess the treatments you have provided to be sure that they are effective (Skill Drill 17-4, Step 4).

Remember This

When providing patient care, always make sure that suction is within arm's reach.

Airway and Breathing

After making sure that the patient's airway is open, check to see if the method you chose to deliver oxygen during the initial assessment is still appropriate. For example, if the patient was initially breathing adequately and was placed on oxygen by nonrebreather mask but is now breathing shallowly at a rate of 6 breaths per minute, you will need to remove the nonrebreather mask and assist the patient's breathing with a bag-mask device that is connected to supplemental oxygen. In contrast, if you were assisting a patient's breathing with a bag-mask device but his respiratory effort and rate are now adequate, consider switching to a nonrebreather mask to deliver oxygen. In any case, close monitoring of the patient's airway and breathing is essential.

If the patient is unresponsive and an oral or nasal airway was inserted, check to make sure that the device is properly positioned. If the patient is being ventilated with a bag-mask device, make sure it is connected to oxygen at 10 to 15 L/min. If a reservoir bag is used, make sure that the reservoir is inflated. Reassess the effectiveness of bag-mask ventilation by ensuring there is adequate rise and fall of the chest. Check to make sure that there is an adequate face-to-mask seal. Reassess the patient's lung compliance (resistance to ventilation). Increasing resistance suggests an airway obstruction.

If oxygen is being delivered by mask, make sure the mask is connected to oxygen at the appropriate flow rate. Make sure the reservoir bag (if a nonrebreather or partial rebreather mask is used) is not pinched off and remains inflated. Make sure the inhalation valve is not obstructed.

If oxygen is being delivered by nasal cannula, make sure the oxygen flow rate is set at no more than 6 L/min. Make sure the prongs are properly placed in the patient's nose. Make sure open chest wounds have been properly sealed with an airtight dressing taped on three sides. Also, make sure that there is no trapped air under the fourth side of the dressing. Loosen it if needed.

Remember This

Regardless of the method used to deliver it, be sure to check the amount of oxygen left in the tank often.

Circulation

If the patient is injured, make sure that bleeding from previously identified wounds is controlled and there is no fresh bleeding. If time and the patient's condition permits, make sure that open wounds are properly dressed and bandaged and the patient is properly positioned.

Other Interventions

If the patient is injured and a head or spinal injury is suspected, make sure the patient's spine is adequately stabilized. Make sure the cervical collar used is of appropriate size and fits properly. Make sure that the patient remains properly secured to a long backboard.

Make sure injured extremities are effectively immobilized. Check to make sure that dressings, bandages, and splints applied to an extremity are not too tight.

Reassess the patient's response to any medications you may have given. For example, if you assisted the patient in taking prescribed nitroglycerin (NTG) for chest discomfort, assess the patient's response, vital signs, and degree of discomfort after taking the medication. If glucose was given to a patient experiencing a diabetic emergency, reassess the patient's mental status and vital signs. If you assisted a patient with asthma in taking a prescribed metered dose from an inhaler, reassess the patient's breath sounds, degree of breathing difficulty, and vital signs.

How often you need to reassess is guided by the length of time spent with the patient or the patient's condition. Reassess at least every 15 minutes for a stable patient and every 5 minutes for an unstable patient. Reassess the patient's mental status and maintain an open airway. Monitor the patient's breathing, pulse, skin color, temperature, and moisture. Repeat the physical exam as needed. Continue to calm and reassure the patient.

Remember This

It is important that your documentation and verbal report to other healthcare professionals accurately reflects your assessment findings and the emergency care provided. Be sure to accurately record all times associated with the care given.

On the Scene Wrap-Up

The scene size-up provides clues that point to a bicycle crash with traumatic injuries. On the basis of your scene size-up, you should suspect head, neck, and spine trauma in addition to the visible injuries. Your general impression and primary survey will confirm these suspicions and help you prioritize your treatment plan. You must also consider that this patient may have an altered mental status because of another problem, such as low blood sugar.

It cannot be stated too frequently that the purpose of the primary survey is to "find and fix" life-threatening injuries. This patient has signs and symptoms of potentially life-threatening problems to both the nervous system and the respiratory system. When you remove the patient's shirt, you see a wound on his chest that appears to be "bubbling." You immediately call an ALS unit for an intercept. The patient is transported rapidly to the closest trauma center. The patient survives because you recognized this deadly chest injury. ■

Sum It Up

► Vital signs are assessments of breathing, pulse, temperature, pupils, and blood pressure. Measuring vital signs is an important part of patient assessment. Vital signs are measured to detect changes in normal body function, recognize life-threatening situations, and determine a patient's response to treatment. Remember to take two or more sets of vital signs. Doing so will allow you to note changes (trends) in the patient's condition and response to treatment. Additional vital signs include pulse oximetry, exhaled carbon dioxide, and pain assessment.

► A sign is any medical or trauma condition displayed by the patient that can be seen, heard, smelled, measured, or felt. A symptom is any condition described by the patient.

► The ability to properly assess a patient is one of the most important skills you can master. As an EMT, you must learn to work quickly and efficiently in all types of situations. To work efficiently, you must approach patient assessment systematically. The emergency care you provide to your patient will be based on your assessment findings.

► While assessing your patient, you will discover signs and symptoms. You must provide emergency medical care based on those signs and symptoms. Discovering the patient's signs and symptoms requires you to use your senses of sight (look), sound (listen), touch (feel), and smell.

► Patient assessment consists of the following components:
- Initial assessment
  —Scene size-up
    - Take standard precautions.
    - Evaluate scene safety.
    - Determine the MOI or the nature of the patient's illness.
    - Determine the total number of patients.
    - Determine the need for additional resources.
  —Primary survey
    - General impression
      1. Appearance
      2. (Work of) breathing
      3. Circulation
    - *A*irway, level of responsiveness, cervical spine protection
    - *B*reathing (ventilation)
    - *C*irculation (perfusion)
    - *D*isability (minineurological exam)

- **E**xpose
  - Identify priority patients
- —Secondary survey
  - Vital signs
  - SAMPLE history, OPQRST
  - Head-to-toe or focused physical examination
- Reassessment
  - —Repeat the primary survey.
  - —Reassess vital signs.
  - —Repeat the focused assessment regarding patient complaint or injuries.
  - —Reevaluate emergency care.

▶ The primary survey is a rapid assessment to find and treat all immediate life-threatening conditions. It begins after the scene or situation has been found safe or made safe and you have gained access to the patient. During this phase of patient assessment, you will look for and treat life-threatening conditions as you discover them ("find and fix"; "treat as you go") and decide if the patient needs immediate transport or additional on-scene assessment and treatment. You must perform a primary survey on every patient.

▶ The secondary survey is a physical examination performed to discover medical conditions and/or injuries that were not identified in the primary survey. During this phase of the patient assessment, you will also obtain vital signs; reassess changes in the patient's condition; and determine the patient's chief complaint, history of present illness, and significant past medical history. The secondary survey does not begin until the primary survey has been completed and treatment of life-threatening conditions has begun.

▶ A general impression (also called a first impression) is an across-the-room assessment. As you approach the patient, you will form a general impression without the patient's telling you what the complaint is. You can complete it in 60 seconds or less. The purpose of forming a general impression is to decide if the patient looks "sick" or "not sick." If the patient looks sick, you must act quickly. As you gain experience, you will develop an instinct for quickly recognizing when a patient is sick. You will base your general impression of a patient on three main areas: (1) appearance, (2) breathing, and (3) circulation.

▶ After forming a general impression, begin the primary survey by assessing the patient's airway and level of responsiveness. Assessment of a patient's airway and level of responsiveness occurs at the same time. Level of responsiveness is also called level of consciousness or mental status. These terms refer to a patient's level of awareness. A patient's mental status is "graded" using a scale called the AVPU scale as follows: A = **A**lert; V = responds to **V**erbal stimuli; P = responds to **P**ainful stimuli; U = **U**nresponsive.

▶ A patient who is oriented to person, place, time, and event is said to be alert and oriented × (times) 4, or A&O×4. Assessing the mental status of a child older than 3 years of age is the same as that of an adult.

▶ For trauma patients or unresponsive patients with an unknown nature of illness, take *spinal precautions*. Spinal precautions are used to stabilize the head, neck, and back in a neutral position. This stabilization is done to minimize movement that could cause injury to the spinal cord.

▶ After making sure that the patient's airway is open, assess the patient's breathing to determine if breathing is adequate or inadequate. If the patient is unresponsive and breathing is inadequate or if the patient is not breathing, begin rescue breathing by using a pocket mask, mouth-to-barrier device, or BM device.

▶ Assessment of circulation involves evaluating for signs of obvious bleeding, central and peripheral pulses; skin color, temperature, and condition; and capillary refill (in children less than 6 years of age). Look from the patient's head to toes for signs of significant external bleeding. Control major bleeding, if present.

▶ Altered mental status means a change in a patient's level of awareness. Altered mental status is also called an altered level of consciousness (ALOC). A patient who has an altered mental status is at risk of an airway obstruction. Most EMS systems use the Glasgow Coma Scale during the disability phase of the primary survey to obtain a more detailed assessment of the patient's neurological status. This minineurological examination is used to establish a baseline level of responsiveness and note any obvious problem with central nervous system (brain and spinal cord) function. Three categories are assessed with the GCS: (1) eye opening, (2) verbal response, and (3) motor response.

▶ Expose pertinent areas of the patient's body for examination. Factors that you must consider when exposing the patient include protecting the patient's modesty, the presence of bystanders, and environment and weather conditions.

▶ Determine if the patient requires on-scene stabilization or immediate transport (load-and-go situations) with additional emergency care en route to a hospital.

▶ The secondary survey is patient-, situation-, and time-dependent. For instance, a patient with an isolated injury, such as a painful ankle, would typically not require a head-to-toe physical examination. However, a secondary survey should be performed in the following situations:

- Trauma patients with a significant MOI
- Trauma patients with an unknown or unclear MOI
- Trauma patients with an injury to more than one area of the body
- All unresponsive patients
- All patients with an altered mental status
- Some responsive medical patients, as indicated by history and focused physical examination findings

▶ A quick secondary survey (head-to-toe assessment) of a trauma patient with a significant MOI is called a rapid trauma assessment. A significant MOI is one that is likely to produce serious injury. A quick secondary survey of a medical patient who is unresponsive or has an altered mental status is called a rapid medical assessment. The phrase focused physical examination is used to describe an assessment of specific body areas that relate to the patient's illness or injury. The procedure for performing a secondary survey is the same for trauma and medical patients. However, the physical findings that you are looking for and discover may have a different meaning depending on whether the patient is a trauma or medical patient.

▶ When examining your patient, first look (inspect), listen (auscultate), and then feel (palpate) body areas to identify potential injuries.

▶ DCAP-BTLS is a helpful memory aid to remember what to look and feel for during the physical exam: **D**eformities, **C**ontusions (bruises), **A**brasions (scrapes), **P**unctures/penetrations, **B**urns, **T**enderness, **L**acerations (cuts), **S**welling.

▶ Reassessment consists of four main areas:
- Repeating the primary survey
- Reassessing vital signs
- Repeating the focused assessment
- Reevaluating emergency care

▶ Reassessment should be performed on every patient. It is performed after the secondary survey, if a secondary survey is performed. In some situations, the patient's condition may prevent performance of a secondary survey.

▶ Reassess at least every 15 minutes for a stable patient and every 5 minutes for an unstable patient. Continue to calm and reassure the patient.

Module 6

Medical Emergencies

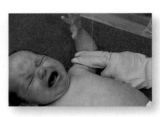

► CHAPTER **18**
Medical Overview   371

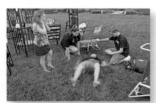

► CHAPTER **19**
Neurological Disorders   376

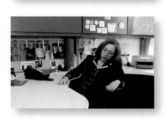

► CHAPTER **20**
Endocrine Disorders   393

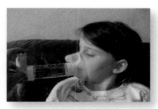

► CHAPTER **21**
Respiratory Disorders   406

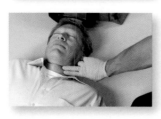

► CHAPTER **22**
Cardiovascular Disorders   426

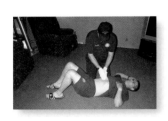

► CHAPTER **23**

Abdominal and Gastrointestinal Disorders 456

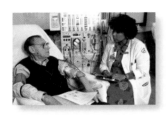

► CHAPTER **24**

Genitourinary and Renal Disorders 467

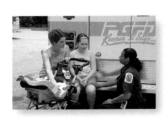

► CHAPTER **25**

Gynecologic Disorders 477

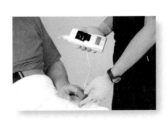

► CHAPTER **26**

Nontraumatic Musculoskeletal Disorders 486

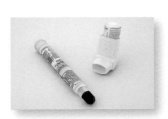

▶ CHAPTER **27**
Immunology 494

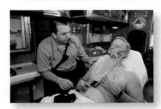

▶ CHAPTER **28**
Toxicology 504

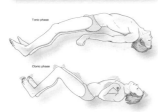

▶ CHAPTER **29**
Psychiatric Disorders 520

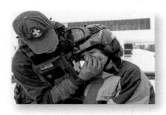

▶ CHAPTER **30**
Diseases of the Nose 530

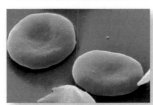

▶ CHAPTER **31**
Hematology 533

Medical Overview

By the end of this chapter, you should be able to:

Knowledge Objectives ▶

1. Describe the approach to the assessment of a responsive medical patient.
2. Describe the unique needs for assessing an individual who is unresponsive or has an altered mental status.
3. Recite examples and explain why patients should receive a rapid medical assessment.

Attitude Objective ▶

4. Attend to the feelings that the medical patient might be experiencing.

Skill Objective ▶

5. Demonstrate the techniques for performing a medical patient assessment.

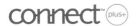

On the Scene

Your crew responds to a local high school for a report of abdominal pain. You arrive to find a 17-year-old female lying on her right side on a bed in the school nurse's office. The school nurse reports that the patient reported to her office complaining of severe abdominal pain. You approach the patient and find that she is awake, alert, and oriented to person, place, time, and event. ■

THINK ABOUT IT

As you read this chapter, think about the following questions:

- Is this patient ill or injured?
- What are possible causes of abdominal pain?
- Is this patient's condition life threatening or potentially life threatening?

Introduction

In this chapter we discuss assessment of the medical patient. A medical patient is a person whose complaint is related to an illness. For the medical patient, the patient's level of responsiveness is the first important factor in determining the type of physical examination you need to perform (Figure 18-1). A **focused physical exam** is usually performed for a responsive medical patient because he or she can usually tell you what is wrong that prompted a call for medical help. If the patient is unresponsive or has an altered mental status, a **rapid medical assessment** (head-to-toe examination) needs to be done to find out what is wrong.

Remember This

The patient's level of responsiveness is the first important factor when determining whether a medical patient needs a rapid medical assessment or a focused exam.

The Responsive Medical Patient

Objective 1

If your patient is responsive and ill (not injured), spend a few minutes learning about his or her medical history before beginning your physical examination. If your patient is complaining of pain or discomfort, remember to use the OPQRST memory aid to help identify the type and location of the patient's complaint. Finding out the patient's medical history will often help you pinpoint the patient's present problem. The information you collect will help guide where you look and what you are looking for in the focused physical exam. For example, if your patient is complaining of abdominal pain, your physical exam will be focused on that area. Performing the physical exam helps establish the accuracy of your initial assumption.

Remember This

OPQRST Assessment of Pain/Discomfort

Onset

Provocation/palliation/position

Quality

Region/radiation

Severity

Time

After the focused physical exam, obtain vital signs. Assess the patient's pulse, respirations, blood pressure, and oxygen saturation. Assess the skin for color, temperature, and moisture. Assess the pupils for size, equality, and reactivity. Check capillary refill in infants and children younger than 6 years of age.

Table 18-1 shows a few examples of the body areas that should be assessed on the basis of the patient's chief complaint. Although it may seem overwhelming right now, knowing the body areas to assess on the basis of a patient's chief complaint will become easier as you learn more about specific illnesses and injuries.

You Should Know

Importance of a Thorough History

- It is the primary component of the overall assessment of the medical patient.
- It requires a balance of knowledge and skill to obtain a thorough and accurate history.
- It helps to ensure that proper care will be provided for the patient.

Putting It All Together

You are called for a 75-year-old man complaining of difficulty breathing. Your first impression reveals an elderly man sitting in a chair. He is awake and appears anxious. You see beads of sweat on his forehead. His breathing looks faster than normal and is labored. His skin looks pink.

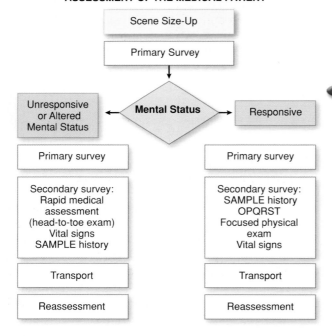

FIGURE 18-1 ▲ Assessment of the medical patient flowchart.

TABLE 18-1 Focused Medical Assessment by Chief Complaint

Chief Complaint	Body Area	Possible Medical Condition
Abdominal pain	Abdomen, pelvis	Ectopic pregnancy, heart attack, appendicitis, gallbladder disease, disease of the colon, bowel obstruction, spontaneous abortion
Altered mental status	Head, neck, chest, abdomen, back, extremities	Stroke, low blood sugar, overdose, seizure, heat-related illness, hypothermia, anaphylaxis, hypoxia, shock
Arm complaint	Head, neck, chest, upper extremities	Heart attack–related pain, insect stings, musculoskeletal problems
Back pain	Back	Kidney stone, back strain, aortic aneurysm
Chest discomfort	Neck, chest, abdomen, extremities	Heart attack, respiratory infection, gallbladder disease, anxiety disorder
Difficulty breathing/ shortness of breath	Head, neck, chest, lower extremities	Asthma, emphysema, heart failure, heart attack, anxiety disorder, toxic exposure, pulmonary embolism, anaphylaxis
Dizziness	Head, chest	Dehydration, abnormal heart rhythm, viral infection
Fainting	Head, chest (and any body part that may have been injured if the patient fell)	Dehydration, low blood sugar, abnormal heart rhythm
Headache	Head, neck	Stroke, seizure, meningitis
Leg complaint	Head, neck, chest, lower extremities	Heart failure, bite or sting, blood clot, stroke, peripheral vascular disease
Nausea/vomiting	Chest, abdomen	Heart attack, bowel obstruction, toxic exposure, anaphylaxis, viral illness, pregnancy, foodborne illness, dehydration
Neck pain or stiffness	Head, neck	Meningitis
Palpitations	Neck, chest	Abnormal heart rhythm, anxiety
Weakness	Head, chest	Shock, abnormal heart rhythm, nervous system disorder, anemia, electrolyte imbalance

In response to your questions, you learn that the patient's shortness of breath has been present for about 2 days but became noticeably worse this afternoon. He has a history of "heart problems" (pertinent positive). The patient has no allergies. He takes furosemide (a "water pill") and atenolol ("for my heart") daily (pertinent positive). He says that sitting up helps his breathing and activity worsens his shortness of breath (pertinent positives). Because of his severe shortness of breath, he can only speak to you using phrases instead of sentences (pertinent positive). He denies chest pain or discomfort (pertinent negative). He rates his difficulty breathing 9/10.

When you finish gathering the history of the present illness, you have a pretty good idea that the patient's current problem is related to his known heart problem. You recognize that the patient's symptoms, medical history, and medications are consistent with a patient who has congestive heart failure (CHF). CHF is your **general impression** (also called a *first impression*) at this point. Your field impression may change, depending on what you find during the focused physical exam. However, based on the information available so far, you begin the focused physical exam looking for signs that support your field impression of CHF.

When you listen to the patient's chest with a stethoscope, you hear crackling sounds in the lower lobes of his lungs on both sides of his chest (pertinent positive). Examination of the patient's legs reveals swelling of both ankles and calves (pertinent positive). The patient's blood pressure is 158/100. His pulse is 144 and his respirations are 28. The patient's history of the present illness (HPI) and physical findings are consistent with a field impression of CHF. Equipped with this information, you are able to provide appropriate emergency care and prepare the patient for transport.

The Unresponsive Medical Patient

Rapid Medical Assessment

Objectives 2, 3

After you perform a scene size-up and make sure the scene is safe to enter, an unresponsive medical patient or a patient who has an altered mental status needs a primary survey and then a rapid head-to-toe physical examination, similar to a rapid trauma assessment. Because the rapid assessment is performed on a medical patient, it is called a *rapid medical assessment.* Performing a quick head-to-toe physical exam will help you identify the patient's problem. Treat problems as you find them. The DCAP-BTLS memory aid used for the rapid trauma assessment is also used for the rapid medical assessment. Remember that DCAP-BTLS stands for deformities, contusions, abrasions, punctures or penetrations, burns, tenderness, lacerations, and swelling.

As you begin the rapid medical assessment, it is important not to have "tunnel vision." For instance, although you may have been called for a diabetic emergency, do not assume that this is the actual (or only) problem. If you approach the patient looking only for assessment findings and symptoms consistent with a diabetic emergency, you may miss important indicators of other illnesses or injuries. An unresponsive patient who is known to have a history of diabetes may have fallen when she lost consciousness. In situations like this, you must consider the possibility of an injury to the head, neck, or back. Assign another rescuer to manually stabilize the head and neck in a neutral position while you examine the patient.

A detailed discussion of a head-to-toe examination was provided in Chapter 17. Information pertaining to assessment of the medical patient is repeated below and expanded upon where appropriate.

Head and Neck

Begin the rapid medical assessment by reassessing the patient's mental status and then checking the patient's head. The skull normally feels smooth and symmetric.

There is normally no tenderness to palpation. Check for DCAP-BTLS. Look and feel for signs of trauma from a previous injury. Look at the patient's face for symmetry, focusing on the symmetry of the eyebrows, eyelids, and sides of the mouth. Asymmetry, such as drooping on one side of the face, is a sign of a possible stroke. Examine the sclerae, which are normally white in color. Note any color change, such as jaundice, which suggests liver disease.

Look in the ears and nose for leakage of blood or fluid. Note if the patient is wearing a hearing aid. Note any deformity of the nose and look for signs of nasal flaring. Check the pupils for size, reactivity, and equality. Assess the conjunctiva, which should be pink and moist.

Reassess the mouth for blood, vomitus, a foreign body, or secretions. Suction as needed. The oral mucosa should be pink and moist. Note the presence of any unusual odors on the patient's breath, body, or clothing.

Assess the neck and look at the neck veins. Flat neck veins may be a sign of dehydration or blood loss. The presence of jugular venous distention when the patient's torso is at a 45-degree angle suggests fluid overload, which may be seen in heart failure. Look to see if the patient has a laryngeal stoma (surgical opening in the neck). Is the patient using the accessory muscles in the neck during breathing? Check to see if the patient is wearing a medical identification necklace or other medical jewelry.

Chest

Expose the patient's chest. Check for DCAP-BTLS. Assess the ease of the patient's respiratory effort. Is the patient using accessory chest muscles during breathing? Note if the chest rises and falls symmetrically. Note the shape of the patient's chest. Look at the skin for signs of a rash and surgical scars. Listen to breath sounds and determine if they are present, diminished, or absent; equal or unequal; and clear or noisy. Note the presence of any medical devices, such as a pacemaker, or medication patches.

Abdomen and Pelvis

Assess the abdomen. Check for DCAP-BTLS. If applicable, look for signs of obvious pregnancy. Look to see if abdominal distention is present. Also, note the presence of any surgical scars. Using the pads of your fingers, palpate all four quadrants of the abdomen. Watch the patient's face while you palpate. A grimace may indicate tenderness over a particular abdominal area. Determine if the abdomen is soft or hard (rigid). Note the presence of any masses, pulsations, or medical devices. In a pregnant patient, note movement or the absence of movement in the fetus.

Assess the pelvis for DCAP-BTLS. Look for signs of obvious bleeding or incontinence of urine or stool.

Extremities

Check for DCAP-BTLS. Look for a medical identification bracelet. Assess pulses, motor function, and sensation in each extremity. Look for edema of the hands, feet, and ankles. Look for signs of a possible insect bite or sting, or signs of possible intravenous drug abuse.

Posterior Body

Assess the posterior body for DCAP-BTLS. Look for swelling in the sacral area. In patients confined to bed, fluid collects in this area. If possible, listen to breath sounds on the posterior chest.

After the rapid medical assessment, assess the patient's vital signs, and then proceed with getting the patient's medical history from family and friends and from clues such as medical jewelry, pill containers, and medical devices. Provide emergency care based on your physical exam findings.

Do not forget about family members at the scene. Explain to the family the emergency care provided and where the patient will be transported for further care.

Putting It All Together

You are called to a private residence for an "ill woman." You are met at the door by the patient's anxious husband. He quickly leads you to the bedroom where you can see his wife lying in bed. From the doorway, the patient appears to be sleeping. You can see her chest rise and fall easily with each breath. Her skin looks pale.

As you quickly perform a primary survey and rapid medical assessment, the husband tells you that his 59-year-old wife had a kidney transplant 6 months ago and her body may be rejecting the kidney. The doctors have been trying different medications over the past few months. His wife took her first dose of a new medication about 2 hours ago. The husband says he entered the bedroom about 10 minutes ago and his wife would not answer him when he called her name. He then called 9-1-1.

Your exam reveals that the patient is unresponsive. Her airway is open and she is breathing about 24 times/min. She has strong radial and carotid pulses at rates of about 110 beats/min. Her skin is pale, cool, and moist.

The physical exam is unremarkable except for swelling around both the patient's eyes and in both hands. You ask the patient's husband how long this has been present. He says it wasn't there this morning, but the same thing happened about 3 months ago. The doctors felt that it was a result of an allergic reaction. You ask about the patient's allergies and the medications that she is currently taking. You learn that she is allergic to codeine and Darvon, but she has not had either medication recently. She takes Prograf, cyclosporine, prednisone, Imuran, and Bactrim regularly for her kidney transplant. The husband does not know the name of the medication she took for the first time today.

The patient's blood pressure is 190/116. Her respiratory rate is 24, and her heart rate is 110 beats/min. Her oxygen saturation is 96% on room air. Recognizing that the history of the present illness and physical exam findings are consistent with an allergic reaction, your partner places the patient on 100% oxygen by nonrebreather mask. As you contact medical direction for instructions, your partner begins preparing the patient for transport.

On the Scene   Wrap-Up

There are many possible causes of abdominal pain including ectopic pregnancy, heart attack, appendicitis, gallbladder disease, disease of the colon, bowel obstruction, and spontaneous abortion. After assessing and interviewing your patient, you suspect the patient has an ectopic pregnancy. Recognizing that this is a potentially life-threatening problem, you immediately contact dispatch and request ALS personnel to the scene. Your prompt recognition of this medical emergency will make a difference in this patient's outcome. ■

Sum It Up

▶ A responsive medical patient can usually tell you what is wrong. After performing a scene size-up and primary survey, obtain the history of the present illness and SAMPLE history. Then perform a focused physical exam that is guided by the patient's chief complaint and signs and symptoms. After the focused exam, take the patient's vital signs and provide appropriate emergency care based on your findings.

▶ After you perform a scene size-up and primary survey, an unresponsive medical patient, or a patient who has an altered mental status, needs a rapid medical assessment. A rapid medical assessment is a quick head-to-toe exam that is performed using the same DCAP-BTLS approach used for trauma patients. Take the patient's vital signs, and try to find out what happened from family members or bystanders at the scene. Provide appropriate emergency care based on your findings.

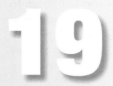
Neurological Disorders

By the end of this chapter, you should be able to:

Knowledge Objectives ▶
1. Define altered mental status.
2. List and explain possible causes of altered mental status.
3. Establish the relationship between airway management and the patient with altered mental status.
4. Define seizure and status epilepticus.
5. Discuss the pathophysiology of seizures.
6. Describe and differentiate the major types of seizures.
7. Describe the phases of a generalized seizure.
8. Discuss the assessment findings associated with seizures.
9. Describe the emergency medical care for the patient with seizures.
10. Define stroke and transient ischemic attack.
11. Describe and differentiate the types of strokes.
12. Discuss the pathophysiology of stroke.
13. Discuss the assessment findings associated with stroke.
14. Describe the emergency medical care for the patient experiencing a stroke.
15. Define syncope and near syncope.
16. Discuss the pathophysiology of syncope.
17. Discuss the assessment findings associated with syncope.
18. Discuss the emergency medical care for the patient with syncope or near syncope.
19. Discuss the pathophysiology of headache.
20. Discuss the assessment findings associated with headache.
21. Discuss the emergency medical care for the patient experiencing a headache.

Attitude Objectives ▶
22. Attend to the feelings that a patient with a neurological emergency might be experiencing.
23. Develop methods of conveying empathy to patients whose ability to communicate is limited by their condition.

Skill Objectives ▶
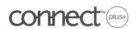
24. Demonstrate the steps in the assessment and emergency medical care for the patient with an altered mental status.
25. Demonstrate the steps in the assessment and emergency medical care for the patient with seizures.
26. Demonstrate the steps in the assessment and emergency medical care for the patient experiencing a stroke.

27. Demonstrate the steps in the assessment and emergency medical care for the patient with syncope or near syncope.

28. Demonstrate the steps in the assessment and emergency medical care for the patient with a headache.

On the Scene

You are responding to a call to "check welfare." A woman called 9-1-1. She says she is worried. Her elderly neighbor has not been seen in 2 days, and his newspapers are stacked up on the front walk. Law enforcement personnel are on the scene and tell you it is safe to enter the residence. You see the patient, an elderly man, lying on the floor. You shake him gently as you say, "I'm an emergency medical technician. Sir, are you all right?" There is no response. You place a hand on his forehead, lift his chin, and look, listen, and feel for breathing. He is breathing quietly, about 16 times per minute. When you reach to feel his radial pulse, you notice how cold and pale his skin is. His heart rate is 128 beats per minute. ■

THINK ABOUT IT

As you read this chapter, think about the following questions:

- What are some possible causes of this patient's altered mental status?
- What additional assessment should you perform?
- Is there more information that you should look for in the patient's home?
- What treatment measures would be appropriate for this patient?

Introduction

A patient with an altered mental status can be challenging to care for because she usually cannot tell you what is wrong. You must obtain a careful history from the patient, family, or others to find out the underlying cause of the patient's altered mental status. An altered mental status should be treated as a medical emergency. Regardless of cause, emergency care of the patient with an altered mental status focuses on the patient's airway, breathing, and circulation.

Altered Mental Status

Objectives 1, 2

Altered mental status means a change in a patient's level of awareness. Altered mental status is also called an *altered level of consciousness (ALOC)*. The change in the patient's mental status may occur gradually or suddenly. A patient with an altered mental status may appear confused, agitated, combative, sleepy, difficult to awaken, or unresponsive. The length of the patient's altered mental status may be brief or prolonged. Examples of conditions that can cause an altered mental status are shown in the following *You Should Know* box.

You Should Know

Common Causes of Altered Mental Status
AEIOU-TIPPS

- Alcohol, abuse
- Epilepsy (seizures)
- Insulin (diabetic emergency)
- Overdose, (lack of) oxygen (hypoxia)
- Uremia (kidney failure)
- Trauma (head injury), temperature (fever, heat- or cold-related emergency)
- Infection
- Psychiatric conditions
- Poisoning (including drugs and alcohol)
- Shock, stroke

Emergency Care

Objective 3

When assessing patients who have an altered mental status, keep in mind that the patients' usual mental status may be different from that of the average person. It is important to ask the families if the patients' mental status appears different from what is normal for them. Regardless of the cause, emergency care of patients with an altered mental status focuses on their airway, breathing, and circulation.

To treat a patient with altered mental status:

- A patient who has an altered mental status is at risk of an airway obstruction. As awareness decreases, muscle tone decreases. When this occurs, the tongue can fall back into the throat and cause an airway obstruction. The breathing muscles may not expand and contract as strongly as normal. This can result in inadequate breathing, hypoxia, and respiratory failure.
- Establish and maintain an open airway. Stabilize the cervical spine if there is any possibility of trauma. If the patient cannot maintain his own airway, insert an oral or nasal airway as needed. Suction as necessary.
- Give oxygen. If the patient's breathing is adequate, apply oxygen by mask at 10 to 15 L/min. If the patient's breathing is inadequate, assist breathing with a bag-mask (BM) or mouth-to-mask device.
- Position the patient. If the patient is sitting or standing, help her to a position of comfort on a firm surface. If there is no possibility of trauma to the head or spine, place the patient in the recovery position.
- Remove or loosen tight clothing.
- Assess the patient's vital signs, including oxygen saturation. Assess the patient's blood glucose level (see Chapter 20).
- Maintain body temperature.
- Comfort, calm, and reassure the patient and the family.
- Reassess for signs that the patient is responding to interventions as often as indicated during transport. Record all patient care information, including the patient's medical history and all emergency care given, on a prehospital care report (PCR).

You Should Know

In some Emergency Medical Services systems, off-line protocols (algorithms) are used to outline the care you can provide for specific patient situations. If the patient's condition does not stray from the criteria set in the algorithm, then you may treat the patient according to the algorithm without having to make phone or radio contact with medical direction. If the patient's condition differs from the algorithm in any way, then contact with medical direction must be made immediately. Check with your instructor and EMS coordinator to learn about your local protocols.

Seizures

Objectives 4, 5

Seizures are another possible cause of altered mental status. A **seizure** is a temporary change in behavior or consciousness caused by abnormal electrical activity within one or more groups of brain cells. A seizure is a symptom (not a disease) of an underlying problem within the central nervous system.

The most common cause of adult seizures in a patient with a known seizure disorder is the failure to take antiseizure medication. The most common cause of seizures in infants and young children is a high fever. **Epilepsy** is a condition of recurring seizures in which the cause is usually irreversible. Known causes of seizures are shown in the following *You Should Know* box. The cause of seizures is unknown in 30% of cases.

You Should Know

Known Causes of Seizures

- Failure to take antiseizure medication
- Rapid rise in body temperature (febrile seizure)
- Infection
- Hypoxia
- Head trauma
- Brain tumor
- Poisoning
- Low blood sugar level (hypoglycemia)
- Seizure disorder
- Previous brain damage
- Electrolyte disturbances
- Alcohol or drug withdrawal
- Eclampsia (seizures associated with pregnancy)
- Abnormal heart rhythm
- Genetic and hereditary factors
- Stroke

Types of Seizures

Objective 6

Although there are many different types of seizures, they can be categorized into two main areas—generalized seizures and partial seizures. Partial seizures can evolve into generalized seizures.

Generalized Seizures

A **generalized seizure** begins suddenly and involves a period of altered mental status. In this type of seizure, nerve cells in both hemispheres of the brain begin firing abnormally. There are two main types of generalized seizures: tonic-clonic seizures and absence seizures.

Tonic-Clonic Seizures

Objective 7

When most people hear the word "seizure," they think of the kind of seizure that involves stiffening and jerking of the patient's body. This type of generalized seizure is called a **tonic-clonic seizure** and is very common. Tonic-clonic seizures are also called *generalized motor seizures* or *grand mal seizures*. A tonic-clonic seizure usually has four phases:

1. Aura
2. Tonic phase
3. Clonic phase
4. Postictal phase

An **aura** is a peculiar sensation that comes before a seizure. Not all seizures are preceded by an aura. Common auras are listed in the next *You Should Know* box. The aura is followed by a loss of consciousness. During the tonic phase, the body's muscles stiffen (Figure 19-1). The patient's breathing may be noisy, and he may turn blue. This phase usually lasts 15 to 20 seconds. During the clonic phase, alternating jerking and relaxation of the body occur. The jerking movements during the clonic phase are often called **convulsions.** This is the longest phase of the seizure. It may last several minutes. The patient's heart rate and blood pressure are increased, and respirations are usually absent (apneic). His skin is usually warm, flushed, and moist. He may lose control of his bowels and bladder. Bleeding may occur if the patient bites his tongue or cheek.

The **postictal phase** is the period of recovery that follows a seizure. During this period, the patient often appears limp, has shallow breathing, and has an altered mental status. This altered mental status may appear as confusion, sleepiness, memory loss, unresponsiveness, or difficulty talking. During this phase the patient slowly awakens. She may complain of a headache and muscle soreness. This phase may last minutes to hours.

You Should Know

Common Auras

- Unusual taste
- Dreamy feeling
- Feeling of fear
- Visual disturbance such as a flashing or floating light
- Unpleasant odor
- Stomach pain
- Rising or sinking feeling in the stomach

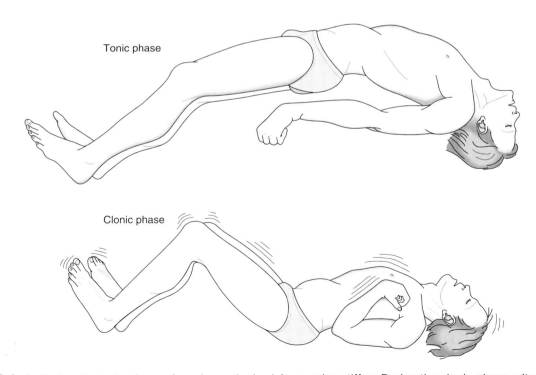

FIGURE 19-1 ▲ During the tonic phase of a seizure, the body's muscles stiffen. During the clonic phase, alternating jerking and relaxation of the body occur.

Absence Seizures

Absence seizures (also called *petit mal seizures*) are another type of generalized seizure. They usually occur in children more than 5 years of age and can occur in adults. An absence seizure is characterized by a brief loss of consciousness (for 5 to 10 seconds) without a loss of muscle tone. The patient may have a blank stare accompanied by slight head turning or eye blinking. This type of seizure does not cause muscle contractions and is not associated with an aura or postictal state.

Partial Seizures

In a **partial seizure**, nerve cells fire abnormally in one hemisphere of the brain. There are two main categories of partial seizures: simple partial seizures and complex partial seizures. A partial seizure may progress into a generalized seizure.

Simple Partial Seizures

A **simple partial seizure** (also called a *focal seizure* or *focal motor seizure*) involves motor or sensory symptoms with no change in mental status. This type of seizure usually lasts about 10 to 20 seconds. Examples of motor symptoms include stiffening or jerking of muscles in one part of the body. For instance, the patient's face or an extremity may begin to twitch or jerk. Sensory symptoms may include pain, numbness, or tingling localized to a specific area.

Complex Partial Seizures

A **complex partial seizure** (also called a *temporal lobe seizure* or *psychomotor seizure*) is a partial seizure in which the patient's consciousness, responsiveness, or memory is impaired. This type of seizure is often preceded by an aura and generally lasts for less than 30 minutes (averaging about 1 to 3 minutes). A complex partial seizure may be associated with repeat behaviors (**automatisms**) such as lip smacking, chewing or swallowing movements; fumbling of the hands; or shuffling of the feet. Postictal confusion or sleep may follow the seizure.

Status Epilepticus

Objective 4

Status epilepticus is recurring seizures without an intervening period of consciousness. Status epilepticus is a medical emergency. It can cause brain damage or death if it is not treated. Complications associated with status epilepticus include the following:

- Aspiration of vomitus and blood
- Long bone and spine fractures
- Dehydration
- Brain damage caused by a lack of oxygen or a depletion of glucose (sugar)

Remember This

Brain damage can occur in as little as 5 minutes of sustained seizure activity; therefore, emergency ALS intervention should occur as quickly as possible. Do not delay transport while waiting for the seizure activity to abate in cases of prolonged seizures.

Patient Assessment

Objective 8

When you arrive on the scene, perform a scene size-up before starting emergency medical care. If the scene is safe, approach the patient and try to find out if the seizure is the result of trauma or an illness. Remember to put on appropriate personal protective equipment. Check for medical jewelry. Look for evidence of burns or suspicious substances that might indicate poisoning or a toxic exposure. Are there signs of recent trauma? Perform a primary survey and a physical exam. Demonstrate a caring attitude when performing your assessment and providing care.

Depending on its severity, injuries can occur during a seizure. Because a patient may bite her tongue or cheek during a seizure, be sure to look in the patient's mouth for bleeding when the seizure is over. You may see scrapes on her head, face, or extremities because of the seizure. Fractures of the skull, arm, or leg can also occur.

When taking the patient's SAMPLE history, speak with kindness to the family members and friends of the patient. Show concern about the patient's condition and well-being. Find out if the patient has any allergies. Also find out if he is taking any medications (prescription and over the counter). Has there been any recent change in his medications (a new medication, a medication that he has stopped taking, or a change in dosage)? When finding out the patient's past medical history, ask the following questions:

- Is this the patient's first seizure?
- If the patient has a history of seizures, is she on an antiseizure medication? Did the patient take the prescribed medication today? How often do the seizures usually happen? Does this seizure look like those the patient has had before?
- Does the patient have a history of stroke or diabetes? (Low blood sugar can cause seizures.)
- Does she have a history of heart disease? (An irregular heart rhythm can cause a low oxygen level and lead to seizures.)
- Does the patient use or abuse alcohol or drugs? (Alcohol or drug withdrawal can result in seizures).

When finding out the events that led to the seizure, think about the questions in the following bulleted list. If the seizure has stopped by the time you arrive, be sure to ask what the seizure looked like. If the seizure is in progress when you arrive, keep these questions in mind while watching the patient. You will need to describe what you saw (or what the family or bystanders describe to you) to ALS personnel who arrive on the scene or to the staff at the receiving facility. Your description of the seizure may be important in finding the cause of the seizure.

- What was the patient doing at the time of the seizure? Did he hit his head or fall?
- Did the patient cry out or attract your attention in any way?
- What did the seizure look like? When did the seizure start? How long did it last?
- Did the seizure begin in one area of the body and progress to others?
- Did the patient lose bowel or bladder control?
- When the patient woke up, was there any change in his speech? Was he able to move his arms and legs normally?
- Did the patient exhibit any unusual behavior before, during, or after the seizure?

You Should Know

- Many cardiac arrests are called in to 9-1-1 as a seizure.
- More than 30% of new patients with epilepsy will never know what causes their seizures.

Emergency Care

Objective 9

Treating a patient experiencing a seizure can be difficult. If the patient is postictal, she is sometimes combative or confused. The patient may not let you perform the skills that are necessary. As a result, frustration can set in on both sides. Keep in mind that you are on the scene for a purpose. That purpose is to provide the best emergency care possible. It may take you several attempts to get answers to questions, put oxygen on the patient, or get the patient loaded into the ambulance. Remember that, as a patient becomes conscious in the postictal phase, confusion and combativeness are normal. No matter what caused the seizure, your emergency care must focus on the patient's airway, breathing, and circulation.

To treat a patient with seizures:
- Protect the patient's privacy. Ask bystanders (except the patient's family or caregiver) to leave the area.

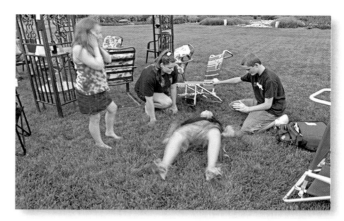

FIGURE 19-2 ▲ Protect a person who is having a seizure from harm by moving furniture and other objects away from him. If he is wearing eyeglasses, remove them. Undo any tight clothing.

- Position the patient. If the patient is sitting or standing, help him to the floor.
- If the patient is actively seizing, protect the patient from harm by moving furniture and other objects away from the patient (Figure 19-2). Roll the patient to his side (lateral recumbent position) to prevent aspiration of blood, vomitus, or other secretions. Protect the patient's head with a pillow or other soft material. Do not insert anything into the patient's mouth. This includes your fingers, an oral airway, a padded tongue blade, or a bite block. Undo any tight clothing. Remove eyeglasses. Do not try to restrain body movements during the seizure.
- As soon as the seizure is over, make sure the patient's airway is open. Be sure to have suction available because the patient may vomit during or after the seizure. Gently suction the patient's mouth if secretions are present. If the patient's breathing is adequate, apply oxygen by mask at 10 to 15 L/min. If the seizure is prolonged or if the patient's breathing is inadequate, assist him breathing with a BM or mouth-to-mask device. If the patient is confused or agitated, he may not tolerate an oxygen mask. In this case, blow-by oxygen is acceptable. When the patient is able to tolerate a mask, it should be applied. Place the patient in the recovery position if no trauma is suspected.
- Comfort, calm, and reassure the patient and his family. Watch the patient very closely for repeat seizures.
- When ALS personnel arrive at the scene (or when transferring patient care at the receiving facility), pass on any patient information that you have gathered. You should include what the patient looked like when you first arrived on the scene, the care you gave, and the patient's response to your care. You should also include in your report any background information obtained from

friends and family about the nature and appearance of the seizure.

- Some patients are light sensitive (photophobic) after a seizure. Take care to reduce the patient's exposure to bright lights and loud noises. Although rapid transport may be the best course of action, take care not to stimulate the patient more than necessary.

Stroke

Objective 10

A **stroke** is caused by the blockage or rupture of an artery supplying the brain (Figure 19-3). A stroke is also called a *cerebrovascular accident (CVA)* or *brain attack.* Strokes cause brain injury because the blood supply to the brain is reduced or cut off. The brain is deprived of necessary oxygen and nutrients, resulting in injury to the brain cells.

> **You Should Know**
>
> Although stroke is common in older adults, it can occur at *any* age—including infants, children, and young adults.

Types of Stroke

Objectives 10, 11, 12

There are two main forms of stroke: ischemic and hemorrhagic. An **ischemic stroke** is caused by a blood clot that decreases blood flow to the brain. Eighty percent of all strokes are ischemic strokes. Ischemic strokes can be further classified as either thrombotic or embolic (Figure 19-4). In a **thrombotic stroke,** a **thrombus** (blood clot) forms in a blood vessel of, or leading to, the brain. The blood vessel may be partially or completely blocked by the blood clot. Symptom onset is gradual. A thrombotic stroke is the most common cause of stroke in persons over 50 years of age.

In an **embolic stroke,** a blood clot breaks up and travels through the circulatory system where it lodges in a vessel within or leading to the brain. The blood clot is now called an **embolus.** A cerebral embolus results from blockage of a vessel within the brain by a fragment of a foreign substance originating from outside the central nervous system, usually the heart or a carotid artery. Other types of emboli include tumor fragments, an air embolus (from injury to the chest), or a fat embolus (from an injury to a long bone). An embolism can occur in persons of any age, but it is commonly seen in young or middle-aged adults and in persons with preexisting diseases. Onset of symptoms is usually sudden.

A **hemorrhagic stroke** (also called a *cerebral hemorrhage*) is caused by bleeding into the brain (Figure 19-5). They account for the remaining 20% of all strokes. There are two forms of hemorrhagic stroke. **Subarachnoid hemorrhage** is caused by a ruptured blood vessel in the subarachnoid space, usually caused by an **aneurysm** (an abnormal bulging of a blood vessel). **Intracerebral hemorrhage** is caused by a ruptured blood vessel within the brain itself (usually a result of chronic high blood pressure).

A **transient ischemic attack (TIA)** is sometimes called a *ministroke.* A TIA is a temporary interruption of the blood supply to the brain. The patient's signs and

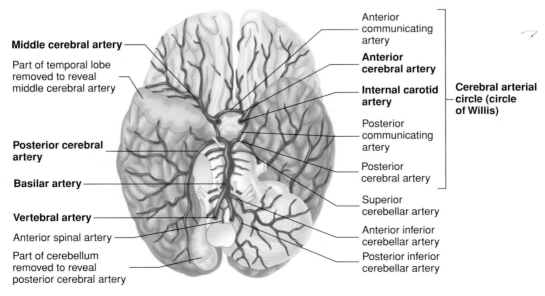

FIGURE 19-3 ▲ A stroke is caused by the blockage or rupture of an artery supplying the brain.

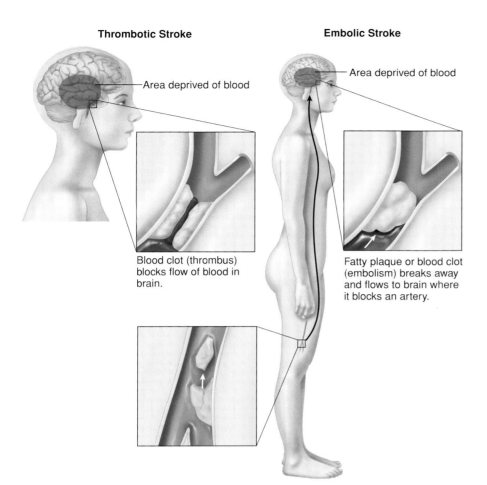

Thrombotic Stroke

Area deprived of blood

Blood clot (thrombus) blocks flow of blood in brain.

Embolic Stroke

Area deprived of blood

Fatty plaque or blood clot (embolism) breaks away and flows to brain where it blocks an artery.

FIGURE 19-4 ◄ Ischemic strokes are caused by a blood clot that decreases blood flow to the brain. The blood vessel may be partially or completely blocked by the blood clot.

Hemorrhagic Strokes

Subarachnoid hemorrhage

Intracerebral hemorrhage

Arachnoid

Area of bleeding

Ruptured aneurysm

Area of bleeding

Ruptured blood vessel

FIGURE 19-5 ▲ A hemorrhagic stroke is caused by bleeding into the brain.

symptoms resemble those of a stroke but are temporary. Signs and symptoms typically last less than 1 hour, completely resolving within 24 hours, with no permanent damage. While the patient is exhibiting symptoms, it is not possible to tell whether the patient is having a TIA or a stroke. Patients who experience a TIA may be at increased risk for eventual stroke.

Risk Factors

Risk factors for stroke include:

- Hypertension
- Cigarette smoking
- Cardiovascular diseases, such as atherosclerosis, myocardial infarction (heart attack), and heart rhythm disorders (such as atrial fibrillation)
- Diabetes mellitus
- TIA
- Cocaine or amphetamine abuse

Assessment Findings and Symptoms

Objective 13

The patient's signs and symptoms are related to the artery affected and the part of the brain deprived of oxygen, glucose, and other nutrients. A stroke occurring on the right side of the brain will produce symptoms on the left side of the body. A stroke occurring on the left side of the brain will affect the right side of the body. Warning signs of a stroke are listed in the following *You Should Know* box.

You Should Know

Warning Signs of a Stroke

- Sudden weakness or numbness of the face, arm, or leg on one side of the body
- Sudden facial drooping, inability to swallow, or tongue deviation
- Sudden dimness, blurriness, or loss of vision, particularly in one eye
- Loss of speech or trouble talking or understanding speech
- Sudden, severe headache with no known cause
- Unexplained dizziness, unsteadiness, or sudden falls, especially with any of the previous symptoms
- Confusion, agitation, combativeness, decreasing level of consciousness, coma
- Seizures
- Inappropriate behavior, such as excessive laughing or crying

The FAST assessment is a useful tool for finding out if a person who has an altered mental status might be having a stroke.

FAST assesses four main areas:

Face. Ask the patient to show his teeth. Both sides of the face should move equally. Does one side of the face droop?

Arms. Ask the patient to raise her arms out in front of her (with eyes closed). Both arms should move the same or both arms should not move at all. Does one arm drift downward?

Speech. Ask the patient to repeat a simple sentence. The patient should be able to say the right words without slurring or forgetting or substituting words. Are the words slurred? Can he repeat the sentence correctly?

Time. Ask the patient or family members what time the patient's symptoms began, and document this information.

"Give Me 5 for Stroke" is a joint campaign of the American Academy of Neurology, the American College of Emergency Physicians, and the American Heart Association–American Stroke Association to encourage Americans to recognize stroke symptoms, call 9-1-1, and get to the emergency department.

Give Me 5 for Stroke:
1. *Walk.* Is their balance off?
2. *Talk.* Is their speech slurred or face droopy?
3. *Reach.* Is one side weak or numb?
4. *See.* Is their vision all or partly lost?
5. *Feel.* Is their headache severe?

The Cincinnati Prehospital Stroke Scale is another assessment tool that can be used to find out if the patient might be having a stroke.

The Cincinnati Prehospital Stroke Scale tests three areas:
1. Ask the patient to smile.

   Normal finding: Both sides of face move equally.

   Abnormal finding: One side of face does not move at all.
2. Ask the patient to close her eyes, raise her arms out in front of her, and hold the position for 10 seconds.

   Normal finding: Both arms move equally or not at all.

   Abnormal finding: One arm drifts compared to the other.

3. Ask the patient to say a simple sentence, for example, "You can't teach an old dog new tricks" or "The sky is blue in Cincinnati."

Normal finding: The patient should be able to say the correct words with no slurring.

Abnormal finding: The patient's words are slurred, inappropriate words are used, or the patient is unable to speak.

If the patient's response is not normal in any area (with any assessment tool used) and the patient's symptoms began within the last 3 hours, contact medical direction and/or begin transport to the closest stroke center.

Emergency Care

Objective 14

To treat a patient with stroke symptoms:
- Maintain spinal stabilization (spinal motion restriction) if trauma is suspected.
- Establish and maintain an open airway. Remove ill-fitting dentures, if present. Insert an oral or nasal airway as needed. Have suction equipment readily available, and suction as necessary.
- Give oxygen as specified by your local protocol. If the patient's breathing is inadequate, provide positive-pressure ventilation with 100% oxygen and assess the adequacy of the ventilations delivered.
- Position the patient. If the patient is unresponsive and there is no possibility of cervical spine trauma, place the patient in the recovery (lateral recumbent) position to aid drainage of secretions. If the patient is immobilized because of suspected trauma and vomits, the patient and backboard should be turned as a unit and the patient's airway cleared with suctioning.
- Protect paralyzed extremities from injury.
- Explain procedures to the patient. Although unresponsive or responsive but unable to speak, the patient may still be able to hear and understand. This is called *expressive aphasia*. If unable to understand your words or speech, the patient may be experiencing *receptive aphasia*.
- Assess and monitor the patient's vital signs and oxygen saturation. Assess the patient's blood glucose level (per local protocol). Treat for low blood sugar if indicated (see Chapter 20).
- Do not give the patient anything to eat or drink.
- Attempt to find out from the patient, family members, friends, or bystanders:
  —If the patient sustained trauma to the head or neck

  —If the patient is taking any medications, including prescription, over-the-counter (such as aspirin), and illicit drugs
  —When the patient's symptoms began
  —Whether the onset of symptoms was gradual or sudden
  —Whether the patient had any seizure activity
  —Pertinent past medical history (such as a previous stroke, TIA, diabetes mellitus, angina, heart attack, heart rhythm disorder, smoking, and/or high blood pressure)

- Because medications ("clot-busting drugs") given at the hospital for treating thrombotic strokes must be given within 3 hours of onset of symptoms, it is very important to determine when the patient's symptoms began. If the patient's symptoms began within the last 3 hours, contact medical direction. At the beginning of your communication with medical direction, let them know that you have a "stroke alert" patient. A "stroke alert" patient is any patient with a sudden onset of neurological deficits such as facial asymmetry, arm drift, or slurred speech who is known to have had symptom onset within 3 hours. Medical direction will advise you of the facility to transport the patient to, which is usually the closest stroke center. Give medical direction an estimated time of arrival to the specified facility. The "stroke alert" terminology is also used in the hospital to notify a group of professionals who specialize in stroke care (stroke team) of the patient's impending arrival. Stroke centers specialize in diagnosing and treating diseases of the blood vessels of the brain. The stroke team at a stroke center works very quickly to determine the cause of the stroke, where it is located, and give appropriate care.
- If possible, have family accompany the patient to the hospital, or obtain a cell phone contact number for the family member to answer questions that the patient may not be able to answer.
- Reassess the patient as often as indicated during transport. Record all patient care information, including the patient's medical history and all emergency care given, on a PCR.

Syncope

Objectives 15, 16

Because the brain is unable to store important nutrients such as oxygen and glucose, disruption of the blood flow to the brain for more than 5 to 10 seconds will result in unresponsiveness. **Syncope (fainting)** is a brief loss of responsiveness caused by a temporary decrease in blood flow to the brain. Syncope is sometimes called a *blackout*. Common causes of syncope are listed in the following *You Should Know* box.

Common Causes of Syncope

- Low blood sugar
- Bearing down when urinating or having a bowel movement
- Strenuous coughing
- Breath holding or hyperventilation
- Blood drawing or the sight of blood
- Standing in one place too long
- Bleeding, dehydration
- Some drugs used for anxiety, high blood pressure, nasal congestion, and allergies
- Sudden drop in blood pressure
- Sudden standing up from a lying position
- Head trauma
- Hot and humid conditions
- Crowded places
- Eating of a heavy meal
- Fasting
- Heart rate that is too fast or too slow
- Stroke
- Witness to violence or other disturbing experiences
- Exposure to painful or noxious stimuli

Before a person faints, she often has warning signs or symptoms (see the following *You Should Know* box). These warning signs and symptoms are called **near syncope** or **presyncope**. Syncope usually results within a few seconds of the onset of symptoms. The patient usually recovers shortly after lying down.

Assessment Findings and Symptoms of Near Syncope

- Dizziness
- Anxiety
- Lightheadedness
- Pale skin
- Sweating
- Weakness
- Nausea
- Thready pulse
- Low blood pressure
- Partial or complete loss of vision or hearing

Patient Assessment

Objective 17

Perform a primary survey. If there is any possibility of trauma, stabilize the spine. Assess the patient's mental status, airway, breathing, and circulation. Just before fainting, the patient's skin is often cool, pale, and moist. This is the sympathetic nervous system's attempt to restore blood flow to the brain. The patient's skin usually returns to normal color and temperature when he is placed in a lying position and his blood pressure returns to normal. Suspect hypovolemic shock or a heart problem if the patient's skin remains cool and clammy after he is placed in a lying position. Look inside the patient's mouth, and assess the elasticity of the patient's skin (skin turgor). Dry mucous membranes and poor skin turgor suggest dehydration and hypovolemia.

Perform a secondary survey. If the patient is unresponsive, perform a rapid medical assessment. Follow with evaluation of baseline vital signs and gathering of the patient's medical history. If the patient is responsive, gather information about the patient's medical history and then perform a focused medical assessment. Examples of questions to ask the patient, family members, friends, and bystanders at the scene are shown in the following *Making a Difference* box. Provide all information obtained to the ALS personnel who arrive on the scene or to the staff at the receiving facility.

Making a Difference

Questions to ask a patient with near syncope or syncope include:

- When did the patient's symptoms begin?
- What was the patient doing when her symptoms began?
- Is this the first time the patient has fainted?
- Were there any symptoms before the event? For example, did the patient complain of weakness, lightheadedness, dizziness, visual disturbances, headache, chest pain, or pounding in her chest before she fainted?
- Did anyone see what happened? Did you see any jerking muscle movements? Did the patient lose control of her bowels or bladder?
- If the patient fainted, how long was the patient unresponsive? Did the patient appear confused after awakening?
- Did the patient fall? Are there any signs of trauma?
- What is the patient's past medical history? Does the patient have a history of diabetes, seizures,

high blood pressure, heart problems, or any other condition?

- When was the patient's last meal or snack?
- Is the patient taking any medications (prescription or over the counter)? When did the patient last take her medications?

Remember This

You can generally tell the difference between a seizure and syncope. With syncope, the patient regains consciousness within a couple of minutes and is completely alert after the event.

Emergency Care

Objective 18

To treat a patient with syncope:
- Establish and maintain an open airway. Stabilize the cervical spine if there is any possibility of trauma. If the patient cannot maintain his own airway, insert an oral or nasal airway as needed. Suction as necessary.
- Give oxygen. If the patient's breathing is adequate, apply oxygen by mask at 10 to 15 L/min. If the patient's breathing is inadequate, assist his breathing with a BM or mouth-to-mask device.
- Position the patient supine, and remove or loosen tight clothing.
- Assess and monitor the patient's vital signs and oxygen saturation. Assess the patient's blood glucose level (per local protocol). Treat for low blood sugar if indicated.
- Maintain body temperature.
- Comfort, calm, and reassure the patient and his family.
- Reassess for signs that the patient is responding to interventions as often as indicated during transport. Record all patient care information, including the patient's medical history and all emergency care given, on a PCR.

Headache

Types of Headaches

Objective 19

Headache is a common complaint in patients of all ages. There are many types of headaches including sinus headaches, tension-type headaches, migraine headaches, cluster headaches, medication-induced headaches, and organic headaches.

Sinus Headaches

You will recall that the sinuses (air-filled spaces lined with mucous membranes inside some cranial bones) drain into the nose. Sinuses are located in the frontal bone of your skull, on each side of the cheek bone, and behind the bridge of your nose. Sinuses produce mucus and trap bacteria and provide additional surface area to nasal passages for warming and humidifying air. If the sinus passages are blocked and mucus cannot drain, the sinuses can become swollen and inflamed (sinusitis). Infection can result when bacteria become entrapped in the sinus tissues. **Sinus headaches** can be triggered by the resulting pressure changes in the sinuses. An upper respiratory infection (such as a cold), allergies (such as hay fever), or smoking may precipitate or contribute to sinusitis. It can also result from structural problems in the nasal cavity.

Tension-Type Headaches

Tension-type headaches, also called *muscle contraction headaches, ordinary headaches,* or *stress headaches,* are the most common type of headache. They can occur at any age, but onset during adolescence or young adulthood is common. The discomfort of tension-type headaches is described as mild to moderate pain that feels like a tight band around the head. Although their exact cause is unknown, they are sometimes associated with muscle spasms of the neck and shoulder. Tension-type headaches are not associated with an aura and are not aggravated by physical activity, but may be accompanied by photophobia.

Tension-type headaches may be associated with anxiety and stress, but factors that can contribute to them include the following:

- Poor posture
- Eye strain, poor lighting conditions
- Lack of sleep or changes in sleep routine
- Skipping meals
- Cramps from assuming an unnatural head or neck position for long periods
- Excessive noise
- Bright lights
- Misalignment of the teeth or jaws

Migraine Headaches

Migraine headaches were once believed to be the result of changes in the diameter or size of blood vessels that supply the brain. Today, most medical experts believe they are caused by changes in a major pain pathway in the nervous system and imbalances in brain chemicals. These changes affect blood flow in the brain and surrounding tissues.

Migraines can occur with or without an aura. Most patients who have migraines report a family history of them, and women experience migraines more often than men. Children also experience migraines, with migraine without an aura being the most common. Most patients who experience migraines report a headache that occurs on one side of the head. The pain associated with a migraine generally lasts from 1 to 3 hours, but may last as long as 24 hours. Possible migraine triggers are shown in the following *You Should Know* box.

Cluster Headaches

Cluster headaches are attacks of severe pain that is primarily localized to the eye, temple, forehead, or cheek area. The attacks occur in cyclical patterns, or clusters, and their cause is uncertain. Cluster periods may occur several times a day and last from weeks to months, followed by periods of weeks, months, or years when the individual is free of headaches. Episodes often occur during sleep and awaken the patient. Cluster headaches occur more often in men than in women and can affect people at any age, but most commonly between the ages of 20 and 40 years.

A cluster headache typically begins quickly, usually without warning. Within minutes, excruciating pain develops and reaches a peak within 10 to 15 minutes. Each episode lasts 10 minutes to 3 hours. The pain is usually located on the same side of the head during a cluster period and has been described as an excruciating sharp, penetrating, burning, or boring pain behind one eye that feels like a hot poker being stuck in the eye or that the eye is being pushed out of its socket. Facial swelling and tearing of the eye on the affected side is typically present, and the cheek on the affected side may be flushed and warm. Although uncommon, it is possible for a person to experience both migraine and cluster headaches.

Medication-Induced Headaches

Medication-induced headaches, also called *rebound headaches,* can result from overuse of medications or substances. For example, overuse of caffeine-containing substances such as coffee, tea, or soft drinks can precipitate rebound headaches. Exceeding the recommended dose of over-the-counter medications such as aspirin, acetaminophen (Tylenol) and ibuprofen (Advil, Motrin), and prescription medications such as narcotics that are a combination of codeine and acetaminophen (Tylenol with Codeine No. 3 and No. 4) may also contribute to rebound headaches. Headaches can also be an adverse effect of medications used to treat conditions such as depression or high blood pressure.

Organic Headaches

Organic headaches, also called *structural headaches*, are the result of an abnormality in the brain or skull. Possible causes include infection (such as meningitis, which is an inflammation of the meninges, the membranes covering the brain and spinal cord), cerebral hemorrhage, benign or malignant brain tumor, or a cerebral aneurysm (an abnormal bulging of a blood vessel).

Remember This

Headaches can be a symptom of a more serious underlying condition. Examples of signs and symptoms accompanying a headache that are red flags indicating that a more thorough assessment is warranted include the following:

Red Flags

- Sudden onset of the "worst headache of my life"
- Headache that awakens the patient from sleep
- Fever
- Rash
- Severe hypertension
- Seizures
- Stiff neck
- Altered mental status
- Vomiting
- Headache upon exertion

Remember that the skull is a rigid container that houses the brain, its blood vessels, and cerebrospinal fluid (CSF). An increase in the volume of fluid or tissue within the cranial cavity will result in an increase in pressure within it (intracranial pressure, or ICP) unless something else gives. For example, the presence of a tumor, aneurysm, or bleeding within the brain will cause a headache due to increased pressure if the amount of CSF or the volume of the brain (or both) is not decreased to offset it.

Patient Assessment

Objective 20

When you arrive on the scene, perform a scene size-up before starting emergency medical care. If the scene is safe, put on appropriate personal protective equipment, approach the patient, and try to find out if the headache is the result of trauma or an illness. Perform a primary survey. If there is any possibility of trauma, stabilize the spine. Assess the patient's mental status, airway, breathing, and circulation.

Perform a secondary survey. If the patient is unresponsive, perform a rapid medical assessment. Follow with evaluation of baseline vital signs and gathering of the patient's medical history. If the patient is responsive, gather information about the patient's medical history and then perform a focused medical assessment. Possible signs and symptoms pertaining to the types of headaches discussed in this chapter are listed in Table 19-1. Examples of questions to ask the patient, family members,

TABLE 19-1 Possible Signs and Symptoms of Headaches	
Headache Type	**Possible Assessment Findings and Symptoms**
Sinus	Dull pressurelike pain in one specific area of the face or head, such as behind the eyes Facial tenderness to touch Pain that may worsen with sudden movement of the head or bending forward Yellow-green or blood-tinged nasal discharge Possible fever
Tension-type	Mild to moderate pain that feels like a tight band around the head Headache occurring primarily in the forehead, temples, back of the head and/or neck Tightness in the neck, as if the head and neck were in a cast
Migraine	Can occur with or without an aura Typical headache occurs on one side of the head Headache pain generally lasts 1 to 3 hours
Cluster	Sudden onset of excruciating pain described as sharp, penetrating, boring, or burning; pain is so intense that most patients cannot sit still Tearing of the eye, swelling around the eye, possible drooping eyelid, and a stuffy or runny nose on the affected side of the face Flushing on the affected side of the face Sweaty, pale skin
Medication-induced	Typically a daily occurrence Start of the headache generally the worst, as the medication wears off Nausea Anxiety, restlessness, irritability, difficulty concentrating Depression Trouble sleeping
Organic	Sudden sharp, intense, or severe headache Sudden lack of balance or falling Confusion Inappropriate behavior Seizures Difficulty speaking

friends, and bystanders at the scene are shown in the following *Making a Difference* box. Provide all information obtained to the ALS personnel who arrive on the scene or to the staff at the receiving facility.

Making a Difference

Following are possible questions to ask a patient with a headache:

- When did your symptoms begin?
- What were you doing when your symptoms began?
- Do you have a history of headaches? If so, is this headache similar to or different from those you have previously experienced? If it is different, how is it different?
- How often do you have headaches (daily, weekly, monthly)? Is your headache pain constant throughout the day, or does it come and go?
- Can you point to where the pain is?
- How long do your headaches usually last (minutes, hours)?
- Were there any symptoms before the event? For example, did you experience an aura?
- What associated symptoms are you experiencing (nausea, vomiting, sensitivity to light or sound, pain worsened by movement, visual or speech disturbances, tingling or numbness, temporary weakness of an extremity)?
- Are you taking any medications (prescription or over the counter)? When did you last take your medications? What types of medications do you take to manage your headaches (over-the-counter medications, sinus medications, prescription pain medications)? Have you ingested any alcohol or used any recreational drugs?
- Do you take medications to prevent headaches?
- What methods have you tried to control your headaches (massage, acupuncture, special diet, herbal preparations, hot or cold packs)?
- What is your past medical history? Do you have a history of diabetes, seizures, high blood pressure, heart problems, or any other condition?
- When was your last meal or snack?

Emergency Care

Objective 21

To treat a patient with headache:
- Maintain spinal stabilization (spinal motion restriction) if trauma is suspected.
- Establish and maintain an open airway.

- Give oxygen. If the patient's breathing is adequate, apply oxygen by mask at 10 to 15 L/min. If the patient's breathing is inadequate, assist her breathing with a BM or mouth-to-mask device.
- Assist the patient to a position of comfort.
- Assess and monitor the patient's vital signs and oxygen saturation. Assess the patient's blood glucose level (per local protocol). Treat for low blood sugar if indicated (see Chapter 20).
- Attempt to find out from the patient, family members, friends, or bystanders:
  —If the patient sustained trauma to the head or neck
  —If the patient is taking any medications, including prescription, over-the-counter, and illicit drugs.
  —When the patient's symptoms began
  —Whether the onset of symptoms was gradual or sudden
  —Whether the patient had any seizure activity
  —Pertinent past medical history (such as seizures, diabetes, high blood pressure)
- Comfort, calm, and reassure the patient and family.
- Reassess the patient as often as indicated during transport. Record all patient care information, including the patient's medical history and all emergency care given, on a PCR.

On the Scene ▸ Wrap-Up

By the time the paramedic crew arrives, you have obtained the patient's blood pressure and applied oxygen by nonrebreather mask. The patient's blood pressure is 96/54. You did not find any other abnormal findings in your examination. The paramedics start an IV, assess the patient's blood sugar, and recheck his vital signs. They notice that his breathing is now more labored, so they insert an oral airway and instruct you to assist the patient's breathing with a bag-mask device while they prepare to insert an endotracheal tube. While the tube is inserted in the patient's airway, a police officer performs a quick search of the patient's home and finds the prescribed medicines but nothing else that is unusual. The paramedics leave the scene with lights and sirens on to hasten their arrival to the hospital.

You wonder what caused this patient's condition. Later, the paramedics tell you that he had a stroke with bleeding in his brain. Apparently, the stroke happened a day or two ago. His body temperature was low from lying immobile on the floor for so long. Unfortunately, his condition rapidly worsened at the hospital, and he died an hour after arrival. ■

▶ A seizure is a temporary change in behavior or consciousness caused by abnormal electrical activity within one or more groups of brain cells. A seizure is a symptom of an underlying problem within the central nervous system. The most common cause of adult seizures in patients with a known seizure history is the failure to take antiseizure medication. The most common cause of seizures in infants and young children is a high fever. Epilepsy is a condition of recurring seizures; the cause is usually irreversible.

▶ The type of seizure that involves stiffening and jerking of the patient's body is called a tonic-clonic seizure (formerly called a grand mal seizure). This type of seizure typically has four phases:

 1. Aura: A peculiar sensation that comes before a seizure.
 2. Tonic phase: The body's muscles stiffen, the patient's breathing may be noisy, and the patient may turn blue.
 3. Clonic phase: Alternating jerking and relaxation of the body occur.
 4. Postictal phase: The period of recovery that follows a seizure; the patient often appears limp, has shallow breathing, and has an altered mental status.

▶ Status epilepticus is recurring seizures without an intervening period of consciousness. Status epilepticus is a medical emergency. It can cause brain damage or death if it is not treated.

▶ A stroke is caused by the blockage or rupture of an artery supplying the brain. There are two main forms of stroke: ischemic and hemorrhagic.

 • Ischemic strokes are caused by a blood clot that decreases blood flow to the brain. Ischemic strokes can be further classified as either thrombotic or embolic. In a thrombotic stroke, a blood clot (thrombus) forms in a blood vessel of, or leading to, the brain. In an embolic stroke, a blood clot breaks up and travels through the circulatory system where it lodges in a vessel within or leading to the brain.

 • Hemorrhagic strokes (also called cerebral hemorrhages) are caused by bleeding into the brain. Subarachnoid hemorrhage is caused by a ruptured blood vessel in the subarachnoid space, usually a result of an aneurysm (an abnormal bulging of a blood vessel). Intracerebral hemorrhage is caused by a ruptured blood vessel within the brain itself (usually a result of chronic high blood pressure).

▶ A transient ischemic attack is a temporary interruption of the blood supply to the brain. Signs and symptoms typically last less than 1 hour, completely resolving within 24 hours, with no permanent damage.

▶ The FAST assessment is a useful tool for finding out if a person who has an altered mental status might be having a stroke. The scale assesses four main areas:

 1. Face: Ask the patient to show his teeth. Both sides of the face should move equally. Does one side of the face droop?
 2. Arms: Ask the patient to raise her arms out in front of her (with eyes closed). Both arms should move the same or both arms should not move at all. Does one arm drift downward?
 3. Speech: Ask the patient to repeat a simple sentence. The patient should be able to say the right words without slurring or forgetting or substituting words. Are the words slurred? Can he repeat the sentence correctly?
 4. Time: What time did the patient's symptoms begin?

▶ "Give Me 5 for Stroke" is a joint campaign of the American Academy of Neurology, the American College of Emergency Physicians, and the American Heart Association–American Stroke Association to encourage Americans to recognize stroke symptoms, call 9-1-1, and get to the emergency department.

 1. Walk: Is their balance off?
 2. Talk: Is their speech slurred or face droopy?
 3. Reach: Is one side weak or numb?
 4. See: Is their vision all or partly lost?
 5. Feel: Is their headache severe?

▶ The Cincinnati Prehospital Stroke Scale is another assessment tool that can be used to find out if the patient might be having a stroke. It tests three areas:

 1. Ask the patient to smile. Normal finding: Both sides of the face move equally. Abnormal finding: One side of the face does not move as well as the other side.
 2. Ask the patient to close his eyes, raise his arms out in front of him, and hold the position for 10 seconds. Normal finding: Both arms move equally or not at all. Abnormal finding: One arm drifts compared to the other.
 3. Ask the patient to say a simple sentence, for example, "You can't teach an old dog new tricks" or "The sky is blue in Cincinnati." Normal finding: The patient should be able to say the correct words with no slurring. Abnormal finding: The patient's words are slurred, inappropriate words are used, or the patient is unable to speak.

- If the patient's response is not normal in any area (with any stroke assessment tool used) and the patient's symptoms began within the last 3 hours, contact medical direction and/or begin transport to the closest stroke center.
- Syncope (fainting) is a brief loss of responsiveness caused by a temporary decrease in blood flow to the brain. Syncope is sometimes called a blackout. Before fainting, a person often has warning signs or symptoms. These warning signs and symptoms are called near syncope or presyncope. Syncope usually results within a few seconds of the onset of symptoms. The patient usually recovers shortly after lying down.
- Headache is a common complaint in patients of all ages. Types of headaches include sinus headaches, tension-type headaches, migraine headaches, cluster headaches, medication-induced headaches, and organic headaches. The emergency care provided for a patient experiencing a headache is primarily supportive—such as administering oxygen, assisting the patient in assuming a position of comfort, and providing comfort and reassurance during transport.

Endocrine Disorders

By the end of this chapter, you should be able to:

Knowledge Objectives ▶

1. Discuss the role of glucose in the body.
2. Identify normal blood glucose levels, and describe how blood glucose levels are regulated in the body.
3. Describe the relationship of insulin to blood glucose levels.
4. Discuss the hormones released from pancreatic cells and their function.
5. Describe the pathophysiology of each type of diabetes mellitus.
6. Discuss the possible complications of diabetes mellitus.
7. Discuss the pathophysiology of hypoglycemia.
8. Recognize the assessment findings and symptoms of the patient with hypoglycemia.
9. Discuss the pathophysiology of hyperglycemia.
10. Recognize the assessment findings and symptoms of the patient with hyperglycemia.
11. Describe the emergency care of the patient experiencing a diabetic emergency.
12. Describe the indications and steps in performing a blood glucose test.
13. Evaluate the need for medical direction in the emergency medical care of a diabetic patient.
14. Discuss the pathophysiology of hypothyroidism.
15. Recognize the assessment findings and symptoms of the patient with hypothyroidism.
16. Discuss the pathophysiology of hyperthyroidism.
17. Recognize the assessment findings and symptoms of the patient with hyperthyroidism.
18. Describe the emergency care of the patient experiencing a thyroid-related emergency.

Attitude Objectives ▶

19. Explain the rationale for performing a blood glucose test.
20. Explain the rationale for administering oral glucose.

Skill Objectives ▶

21. Demonstrate the steps in the emergency medical care of the patient with altered mental status and a history of diabetes.
22. Demonstrate the steps in performing a blood glucose test.
23. Demonstrate the steps in the administration of oral glucose.
24. Demonstrate the assessment and documentation of the patient's response to oral glucose.
25. Demonstrate the steps in the emergency medical care of the patient with a thyroid disorder.

Your rescue crew is called to the home of a 54-year-old woman for a "diabetic emergency." The patient is found responsive but confused in her kitchen. She complains of intense hunger, a headache, and extreme weakness and informs you that she is a diabetic. Her skin is pale, cool, and moist. ■

THINK ABOUT IT

As you read this chapter, think about the following questions:

- What physical signs, if present when examining this patient, would lead you to believe that she has had a long bout with uncontrolled diabetes?
- Can you give examples of situations in which a diabetic patient's blood glucose level may become too low?
- What additional assessments should you perform?
- What treatment measures would be appropriate for this patient?

Introduction

Diabetic emergencies are one of the possible causes of **altered mental status.** Because a lack of glucose can cause permanent brain damage, you must be able to recognize the signs and symptoms of a diabetic emergency and quickly provide appropriate emergency care. In this chapter we review the functions of glucose and insulin, types of diabetes mellitus, common signs and symptoms of diabetic emergencies, and how to obtain a blood glucose reading and render appropriate care.

Glucose

Objectives 1, 2, 3, 4

Glucose, a sugar, is the basic fuel for body cells. The level of sugar in the blood (the "blood sugar") must remain fairly constant to ensure proper functioning of the brain and body cells. The brain must be constantly supplied with glucose because it cannot store it. The brain is very sensitive to changes in glucose levels. Changes in glucose levels can result in changes in the patient's behavior.

The body's blood glucose level is primarily regulated by the pancreas (Figure 20-1). Normal blood glucose levels generally range between 70 and 120 milligrams/deciliter (mg/dL). A rise in the blood glucose level (such as after a meal) stimulates beta cells in the pancreas to secrete the hormone insulin. Because glucose is a large molecule, it cannot easily enter the body's cells where it is needed. **Insulin** helps glucose

enter the body's cells to be used for energy. As the blood glucose level drops toward normal, the release of insulin slows. Excess glucose is stored in the liver

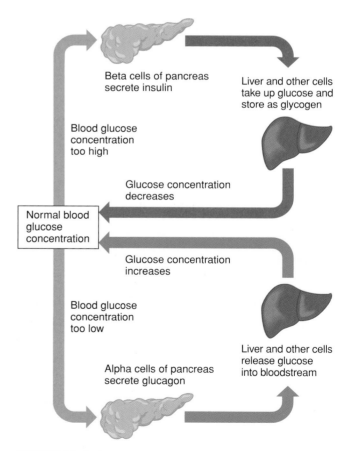

Beta cells of pancreas secrete insulin

Liver and other cells take up glucose and store as glycogen

Blood glucose concentration too high

Glucose concentration decreases

Normal blood glucose concentration

Glucose concentration increases

Blood glucose concentration too low

Liver and other cells release glucose into bloodstream

Alpha cells of pancreas secrete glucagon

FIGURE 20-1 ▲ The body's blood glucose level is primarily regulated by the pancreas.

TABLE 20-1 Pancreatic Cell Function

Pancreatic Cells	Hormone Released	Hormone Function
Alpha	Glucagon	Stimulates cells in the liver to break down stores of glycogen into glucose; increases blood sugar
Beta	Insulin	Helps glucose enter body cells to be used for energy; decreases blood sugar
Delta	Somatostatin	Inhibits release of insulin and glucagon

and muscles as glycogen. A drop in the blood glucose level stimulates the release of glucagon from alpha cells in the pancreas. **Glucagon** is a hormone that stimulates cells in the liver to break down stores of glycogen into glucose. This increases the blood glucose level. As the blood glucose level rises toward normal, the release of glucagon slows. **Somatostatin** is a hormone that is released by delta cells in the pancreas. This hormone inhibits the release of insulin and glucagon (Table 20-1).

For cells to use sugar properly, there must be an adequate supply of insulin. In a healthy person, insulin secretion increases after eating. Insulin helps transport glucose from the blood into cells, including muscle, liver, and fat cells where the glucose is stored or used as fuel.

You Should Know

The values used for a normal blood glucose level vary. Some references state the normal range is from 70 to 120 mg/dL. Others state that the normal range is from 80 to 120 mg/dL. Although both are acceptable, be aware that these norms may vary. In addition, it is important to note that when these tests are performed in a laboratory, the norms may vary by lab.

Types of Diabetes Mellitus

Objective 5

Diabetes mellitus is a disease involving the pancreas. There are three major types of diabetes mellitus (Table 20-2). The pancreas either produces too little insulin or stops producing it completely. Sugar builds up in the blood. The body's cells do not have enough sugar for energy and do not perform properly.

Type 1 Diabetes Mellitus

In **type 1 diabetes mellitus**, little or no insulin is produced by beta cells in the pancreas. This results in a buildup of glucose in the blood. Despite the buildup of glucose in the blood, the body's cells are starved for glucose because, without insulin, glucose is unable to enter most body cells.

Although it may occur at any age, type 1 diabetes usually begins during childhood or young adulthood. Signs and symptoms vary widely and may develop suddenly or gradually over days to weeks. Common assessment findings and symptoms are shown in the following *You Should Know* box. Because the patient's pancreas isn't producing insulin, the patient with type 1 diabetes

TABLE 20-2 Major Types of Diabetes Mellitus

Diabetes Type	Other Names	Possible Causes
Type 1	Insulin-dependent diabetes mellitus (IDDM) Juvenile diabetes	Usually unknown Viral infection Injury to pancreas Immune system disorder
Type 2	Non-insulin-dependent diabetes mellitus (NIDDM) Adult-onset diabetes	Insulin resistance and relative insulin shortage
Gestational	Diabetes during pregnancy	Changes in body metabolism caused by pregnancy

mellitus requires treatment with insulin. Some patients also require treatment with oral medication to manage their blood glucose level.

You Should Know

Common Assessment Findings and Symptoms of Type 1 Diabetes

- "Three polys"
  - **Polyuria** (increased urination)
  - **Polydipsia** (increased thirst)
  - **Polyphagia** (increased appetite)
- Abdominal pain with vomiting
- Fruity breath odor
- Blurred vision
- Tiredness

You Should Know

According to the American Diabetes Association, most Americans who are diagnosed with diabetes have type 2 diabetes.

Type 2 Diabetes Mellitus

Objective 5

Type 2 diabetes mellitus is the most common type of diabetes. It usually affects people older than 40 years of age, especially those who are overweight. Type 2 diabetes is caused by a combination of insulin resistance and relative insulin shortage. **Insulin resistance** refers to a condition in which the pancreas releases insulin, but the normal effect of insulin on the tissue cells of the body is diminished. In an attempt to counteract this resistance, the pancreas releases more insulin into the bloodstream. Insulin levels rise. In some cases, glucose builds up in the bloodstream despite the increased amount of insulin. This results in high blood glucose levels or type 2 diabetes. Major causes of insulin resistance include obesity, genetics, sedentary lifestyle, and stress. Type 2 diabetes mellitus can often be managed by diet, exercise, and oral medications that lower blood sugar levels (see Table 20-3). Some people require insulin.

Gestational Diabetes

Objective 5

When a woman develops diabetes during pregnancy, it is called **gestational diabetes.** Gestational diabetes does not include previously diabetic pregnant patients.

TABLE 20-3 Examples of Oral Diabetes Medications

Generic name	Trade name
tolbutamide	Orinase
chlorpropamide	Diabinese
tolazamide	Tolinase
glyburide	Micronase
glipizide	Glucotrol
glimepiride	Amaryl
repaglinide	Prandin
metformin	Glucophage
rosiglitazone maleate	Avandia
pioglitazone hydrochloride	Actos

According to the American Diabetes Association, gestational diabetes affects about 4% of all pregnant women. Hormones released during pregnancy can change the effectiveness of insulin. These changes usually begin in the fifth or sixth month of pregnancy. Diabetes develops if the pancreas cannot make enough insulin to control the level of glucose in the blood. Treatment for gestational diabetes includes a special diet; regular, moderate exercise (according to physician instructions); and daily blood glucose testing. Some patients require insulin injections.

Gestational diabetes usually goes away after the baby is born, but it may take several weeks. The mother is at increased risk for gestational diabetes in her next pregnancy and for type 2 diabetes later in life.

Complications of Diabetes Mellitus

Objective 6

If diabetes is not controlled, high glucose levels can cause complications, particularly to blood vessels and cells of the nervous system (see the next *You Should Know* box). One of the ways people can limit the progression of this disease is to regularly monitor their blood sugar and follow their doctor's instructions regarding diet, exercise, and prescribed medications to help regulate their blood sugar level.

Hypoglycemia

Objectives 7, 8

Hypoglycemia is a lower-than-normal blood sugar level. In adults, hypoglycemia is a blood glucose level less than 70 mg/dL.

Hypoglycemia is the most common diabetic emergency. The onset of hypoglycemia symptoms is sudden (minutes to hours). Early signs and symptoms of hypoglycemia include signs of stimulation of the sympathetic division of the autonomic nervous system. For example, the presence of sweating, palpitations, increased heart rate, tremors, pale color, hunger, and nervousness serves as an early warning system.

Remember that the brain cannot store glucose. If hypoglycemia is not corrected, signs and symptoms reflecting the brain's lack of an adequate glucose supply will quickly follow. These signs and symptoms may include tiredness, irritability, visual disturbances, difficulty concentrating, confusion, combativeness, fainting, seizures, and loss of consciousness. Prolonged hypoglycemia can lead to irreversible brain damage. Common signs and symptoms of hypoglycemia are shown in Table 20-4.

Remember This

Hypoglycemia is also called *insulin shock*. Keeping this in mind may help you remember the later signs and symptoms of hypoglycemia.

The blood sugar level may become too low if the diabetic patient:

- Has taken too much insulin
- Has not eaten enough food

TABLE 20-4 Hypoglycemia and Hyperglycemia

	Hypoglycemia	Hyperglycemia
Onset	Sudden (minutes to hours)	Gradual (hours to days)
Assessment findings and symptoms	Altered mental status (varies from nervousness to coma) *Early signs* • Sweating • Palpitations • Increased heart rate • Tremors • Pale color • Hunger • Headache • Nervousness *Later signs* • Confusion, combativeness, irritability, difficulty concentrating • Tiredness • Staggering walk • Visual disturbances • Cool, pale, clammy skin • Fainting • Seizures • Coma	Altered mental status (varies from drowsiness to coma) • Rapid, deep breathing (Kussmaul respirations) • Sweet or fruity (acetone) breath odor • Loss of appetite • Thirst • Dry skin • Abdominal pain • Nausea and/or vomiting • Increased heart rate • Normal or slightly decreased blood pressure • Weakness

- Has overexercised and burned off sugar faster than normal
- Experiences significant physical (such as an infection) or emotional stress

Remember This

Many patients with serious medical conditions such as diabetes, a drug allergy, or a heart condition carry information with them about their condition. If your patient is unable to answer questions, look for a medical identification card or a medical identification necklace or bracelet so that you can provide proper emergency care.

Hyperglycemia

Objectives 9, 10

Hyperglycemia is a higher-than-normal blood sugar level. The onset of hyperglycemia symptoms is gradual (hours to days).

Normally, the body metabolizes carbohydrates for energy. As hyperglycemia worsens, body cells become starved for sugar. Although sugar is present in the blood, it cannot be transported into the body's cells without insulin. The buildup of sugar causes the kidneys to increase urine output, which leads to dehydration. Signs of dehydration include warm, dry skin and a loss of skin elasticity (poor skin turgor). Increased urine output results in the loss of large amounts of sodium, potassium, and other electrolytes. This can result in abnormal heart rhythms, abdominal pain, vomiting, and muscle cramping. The body begins breaking down fats and proteins to provide energy. The breakdown of fats and proteins produces waste products, including acids. The patient begins breathing deeply and rapidly in an attempt to get rid of the excess acid by "blowing off" carbon dioxide. This breathing pattern is called **Kussmaul respirations.** The patient's breath may have a fruity (acetone) odor. It has been estimated that 25–30% of the population can't smell ketones on a patient's breath, so you cannot use the absence of this sign to rule out hyperglycemia. Signs and symptoms of hyperglycemia are shown in Table 20-4.

Diabetic ketoacidosis (DKA) is severe, uncontrolled hyperglycemia (usually over 300 mg/dL). DKA usually occurs in people who have type 1 diabetes but may also occur in those who have type 2 diabetes. DKA is also called *diabetic coma.*

The blood sugar level may become too high when the diabetic patient:

- Has not taken insulin or oral diabetic medication, or has taken an incorrect dose
- Has eaten too much food that contains or produces sugar
- Has lost a large amount of fluid, such as through vomiting
- Experiences physical (such as infection, pregnancy, or surgery) or emotional stress that affects the body's insulin production

You Should Know

Family or friends who may be on the scene of a diabetic emergency can usually direct you to the location of any medications being taken by the patient. If the patient is taking insulin, it is usually stored in the refrigerator with the patient's name and dosage clearly marked on the container.

Patient Assessment

Observe the patient's environment for clues to the cause of the patient's altered mental status. Look for medical identification indicating a history of diabetes and current use of insulin or oral diabetic medication. Assess the patient's abdomen and belt for the presence of an insulin pump. If the patient is in a private residence, look in the refrigerator for insulin.

Perform a primary survey. Stabilize the spine if needed. Assess the patient's mental status, airway, breathing, and circulation. Identify any life-threatening conditions, and provide care based on those findings. Establish patient priorities. Priority patients include:

- Patients who give a poor general impression
- Unresponsive patients with no gag reflex or cough
- Responsive patients who are unable to follow commands

Advanced life support (ALS) assistance should be requested as soon as possible. If ALS personnel are not available, the patient should be transported promptly to the closest appropriate facility.

Perform a physical examination. If the patient is unresponsive, perform a rapid medical assessment. Follow with evaluation of baseline vital signs and gathering of the patient's medical history. If the patient is responsive, gather information about the patient's medical history and then perform a focused medical assessment. Sources of information for a patient who has an altered mental status include the scene, family members, friends, and bystanders. Information obtained from the patient may be unreliable. Examples of questions to ask when caring for a patient who has an altered mental status are shown in the following *Making a Difference* box. Provide all information obtained to the receiving facility.

Making a Difference

Questions to ask about a patient experiencing a possible diabetic emergency:

- Does the patient have a history of diabetes?
- What time did the patient's symptoms begin? Did the patient's symptoms begin suddenly or gradually?
- What was the patient doing when the symptoms began?
- When was the patient's last meal or snack? How much did the patient eat (or drink)? Did the patient vomit after eating? Has the patient skipped any meals?
- Is the patient taking any medications (prescription and over the counter)?
- When did the patient last take any medications? For patients taking insulin, ask whether they have taken their insulin today and how much insulin was taken. Has the patient's insulin (or oral diabetic medication) dosage changed recently?
- Does the patient have any associated symptoms (such as nausea, vomiting, weakness)?
- Has the patient performed an unusual exercise or physical activity today?
- Has the patient had a recent infection or surgery?
- Has the patient experienced any psychological stress?
- Has the patient consumed any alcohol?
- What is the patient's normal blood glucose level? What was the patient's blood sugar level the last time it was measured?

Age-Related Considerations

Assessment and management of the pediatric and older adult patient experiencing a diabetic emergency may vary from that of other patients. A pediatric patient who has diabetes is usually insulin-dependent. It is important to keep in mind that children who have diabetes are prone to dehydration and seizures and may have cerebral edema (brain swelling) in the late stages of hyperglycemia. Some children may have diabetes but be undiagnosed.

An older adult who has diabetes is prone to dehydration, poor peripheral circulation, and infections. Signs and symptoms of a heart attack can be masked in the patient with diabetes, a circumstance commonly referred to as a *silent myocardial infarction (MI)*.

Emergency Care

Objective 11

To treat a patient with a possible diabetic emergency:
- Stabilize the spine if trauma is suspected.
- Any patient who has an altered mental status is at risk of not being able to manage her own airway. It is critical for you to aggressively assess the need for an oral or nasal airway and to continuously monitor and reassess the patient's airway. Suction as necessary.
- Give oxygen. If the patient's breathing is adequate, apply oxygen by nonrebreather mask at 15 L/min if not already done. If the patient's breathing is inadequate, provide positive-pressure ventilation with 100% oxygen and assess the adequacy of the ventilations delivered.
- Position the patient. If there is no possibility of cervical spine trauma, place the patient in a lateral recumbent (recovery) position to aid drainage of secretions. If the patient who is immobilized because of suspected trauma vomits, the patient and backboard should be turned as a unit and the patient's airway cleared with suctioning.
- Remove or loosen tight clothing. Maintain body temperature.
- Perform a blood glucose test (if permitted by state and local protocol).
- If the patient is responsive, determine if the patient is alert enough to swallow. Give oral glucose according to local or state medical direction or protocol.
- Transport. Reassess often until patient care is turned over to ALS personnel or medical personnel at the receiving facility.

Remember This

Because a lack of glucose can cause permanent brain damage, any diabetic patient with an altered mental status should be considered to have hypoglycemia until proved otherwise.

Remember This

Patients who have had diabetes for some time are often familiar with the EMS system. After receiving glucose for hypoglycemia, the patient's mental status usually quickly returns to normal. Some patients then refuse transport to the hospital. In these situations, you should contact medical direction for instructions about how to proceed. In specific cases, medical direction will allow the patient to refuse transport if you make sure that an adult is present and the patient eats a substantial meal. If these conditions are met and medical direction authorizes the patient's refusal, complete a refusal form. The patient's signature should be obtained on the form and a witness signature should be obtained at the same time. Ideally, this will be the person taking responsibility for the patient. Be sure to document the advice the patient was given, the patient's understanding of the risks of refusal, and the patient's understanding of the possible outcome if the advice given is not followed.

Performing a Blood Glucose Test

Objective 12

Blood glucose testing is used to assist in the management of patients with specific signs and symptoms. The results obtained from the test help determine if the patient's glucose level is too high, too low, or within normal limits. Patient care, treatment, and outcome may be improved with its use.

Indications:

1. Unresponsive patient, cause unknown (any age group, including trauma)
2. Known diabetic patient with any of the following assessment findings and symptoms:
   - Altered mental status (confusion, change in usual behavior)
   - Unresponsiveness
   - Slurred speech
   - Cold and clammy skin or hot, dry skin and/or mucous membranes
   - Pale or flushed color
   - Sweating
   - Headache, dizziness
   - Palpitations and/or abnormal heart rhythm seen on heart monitor
   - Visual disturbances
   - Shakiness or patient states he "feels funny"
   - Excessive urination and/or thirst
   - Acetone (fruity) breath
   - Rapid, deep breathing (Kussmaul respirations)
   - Seizures
3. Patients with altered mental status, cause unknown (including trauma), especially if showing signs and/or symptoms listed above
4. Special situations
   - Infant or child having seizures or an altered mental status
   - Pregnancy with signs and symptoms listed previously or signs and symptoms of pregnancy-induced hypertension (see Chapter 42)
   - Older adults
   - Patients with a history of alcoholism
   - Overweight patients
   - Malnourished patients
   - Patients on long-term drug therapies, such as steroids or hormonal therapy

Procedure

To check a patient's glucose level, you will take a blood sample from the patient. In adults, the most common site used is the side of a finger. Pricking the side of a finger (or toe) is less painful than pricking the pad of a finger or toe. The device used to prick the patient's finger is called a **lancet.** Some lancets are adjustable, allowing you to change how deeply the lancet pierces the patient's skin. This is important if alternate sites are used, such as the fleshy part of the hand, base of the thumb, upper arm, thigh, or back of the calf.

The device used to measure the amount of glucose in a blood sample is called a **blood glucose meter** or **glucometer.** A drop of blood is placed on a patch on a test strip. The test strip is inserted into the glucometer. The glucometer analyzes the specimen and gives a digital display of the patient's glucose level. Many patients who have diabetes have a glucometer to regularly check their glucose levels. Physicians and diabetes educators usually tell their patients to check their glucose level before meals, before bed, and 1 to 2 hours after meals. If the patient has type 1 diabetes, the patient is usually asked to check his glucose level at 2 a.m. or 3 a.m. at least once a week. In addition to these "routine" tests, the patient may need to check his glucose level before exercising, if showing signs or symptoms of low blood sugar, and when sick.

Skill Drill 20-1 shows how to perform a blood glucose test with a glucometer. Because the features of glucometers vary, be sure you are familiar with the devices approved for use in your EMS system.

Performing a Blood Glucose Test with a Glucometer

STEP 1 ▶
- Put on appropriate personal protective equipment.
- Identify the need for blood glucose testing on the basis of your assessment findings, the patient's chief complaint, and past medical history.

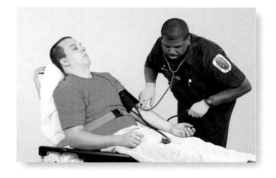

STEP 2 ▶
- Assemble and prepare the necessary equipment.
- Explain the procedure to the patient.

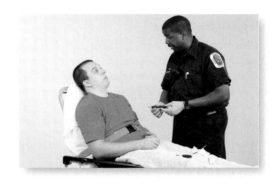

STEP 3 ▶
- Select and cleanse the puncture site. Be sure to allow the area to dry before pricking the skin. Any alcohol present on the skin will interfere with the test results.
- Prick the skin quickly with the lancet to get a small drop of blood. Apply a drop of blood on the test strip. Be sure to completely cover the patch on the test strip with blood.

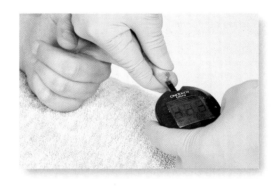

STEP 4 ▶
- Turn on the glucometer. Insert the test strip. (Some manufacturers have the test strip placed in the machine before the drop of blood is obtained. Follow the manufacturer's instructions).
- Wait for the glucometer to analyze the sample and display the patient's glucose reading.
- Apply a small adhesive bandage to the puncture site.

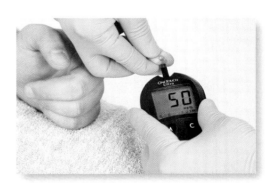

Blood Glucose Testing: Equipment

- Blood glucose test strips
- Glucometer
- Disposable lancets
- Disposable gloves
- Gauze pads
- Alcohol swabs
- Small adhesive bandage
- Watch or clock with second hand (if using color-changing strips)
- Sharps container

Oral Glucose

Objective 13

If approved by medical direction (and your state and local EMS system), you may give oral glucose to a patient who has an altered mental status and a history of diabetes controlled by medication and is able to swal-

low. Oral glucose given to a patient with an altered mental status and a known history of diabetes can make a difference between the development of coma (unconsciousness) and ability to maintain consciousness. If oral glucose is not available (and if approved by medical direction), other quick-sugar mixtures can be used. It has been estimated that quick-sugar foods (see the following *Remember This* box) can increase a person's blood sugar about 30 mg/dL in about 20 minutes.

Remember This

Quick-Sugar Foods

- Fruit juice, such as orange or apple juice (½ cup)
- Water mixed with 1 tablespoon of table sugar
- Jam or jelly (2 tablespoons)
- Honey or corn syrup (1 tablespoon)
- Regular (nondiet) soft drink (½ cup)

Before giving any medication, specific criteria must be met (Table 20-5). These criteria include making sure that the medication to be given is indicated for

TABLE 20-5 Oral Glucose

Generic name	oral glucose
Trade name	Glutose, Insta-Glucose
Mechanism of action	Increases the amount of sugar available for use as energy by the body
Indications	Patients with altered mental status who have a known history of diabetes controlled by medication and can swallow
Dosage	One tube
Adverse effects	• Nausea • May be aspirated by the patient without a gag reflex
Contraindications	• No permission from medical direction • Unresponsiveness • Inability to swallow • Known allergy to the glucose preparation
Special considerations	• Ensure that the patient has signs and symptoms of altered mental status with a known history of diabetes. • Make sure the patient is responsive, can swallow, and can protect her airway. • Obtain an order from medical direction to give the medication. • Use appropriate personal protective equipment. • Practice the six rights of drug administration. • Although the body readily absorbs glucose, keep in mind that it is also rapidly metabolized and your patient will need additional care.

the patient. You must also make sure that the patient does not have any allergies to the medication. Even though you are giving glucose, it is possible that the patient may have an allergy to the way the drug is packaged or manufactured. If a drug contains any preservatives, it is possible the patient may have an adverse reaction to the preservative in the medication. Next, you must make sure that the patient is responsive, has an open airway, and can swallow. Because any patient who has an altered mental status has the potential to become unresponsive without warning, it is essential to make sure the patient has (and maintains) an open airway. If all these criteria are met and medical direction has given the order to administer the drug, oral glucose can be given. The steps for giving oral glucose were shown in Skill Drill 11-2 in Chapter 11.

Thyroid Disorders

The thyroid gland secretes two thyroid hormones and the hormone calcitonin (Figure 20-2). Thyroid hormones are primarily responsible for controlling the rate at which cellular metabolism occurs. For example, increasing the rate at which cellular metabolism occurs increases the speed with which energy is available to perform body functions. Calcitonin lowers the concentration of calcium in the blood and promotes bone formation.

Hypothyroidism

Objectives 14, 15

Inadequate secretion of thyroid hormones is called **hypothyroidism** (also called *underactive thyroid*). There are many causes of hypothyroidism including inflammation of the thyroid gland, surgical removal of the thyroid gland, and a low dietary intake of iodine. Sometimes the thyroid gland enlarges, resulting in a painless mass in the neck called a goiter (Figure 20-3). Although once common, hypothyroidism resulting from a lack of iodine in the diet is uncommon in the United States today because iodized salt is readily available.

Assessment findings and symptoms associated with hypothyroidism are consistent with those of a slow metabolic rate and include the following:

- Fatigue, sluggishness
- Hair loss
- Increased sensitivity to cold
- Unexplained weight gain or difficulty losing weight
- Coarse, dry hair
- Heavier than normal menstrual periods
- Brittle fingernails
- Depression
- Muscle cramps and weakness

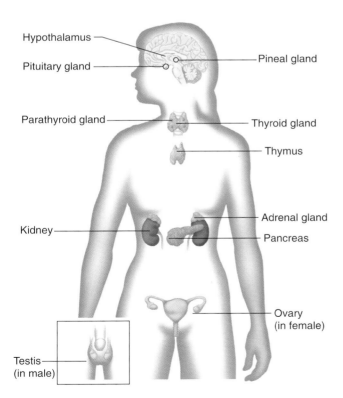

FIGURE 20-2 ▲ The thyroid gland is located in the neck.

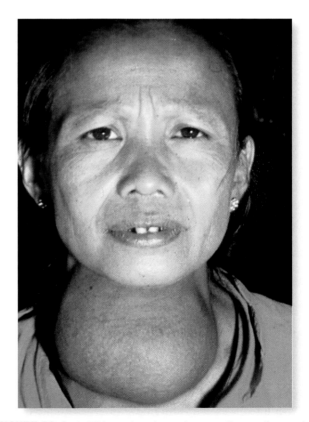

FIGURE 20-3 ▲ This patient has a large goiter on the neck.

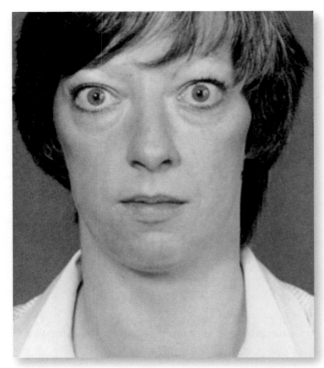

FIGURE 20-4 ▲ Hyperthyroidism can cause protruding eyes.

Hyperthyroidism

Objectives 16, 17

Hyperthyroidism (also called *overactive thyroid*) results from an oversecretion of thyroid hormones, which markedly increases the rate of cellular metabolism. Assessment findings and symptoms associated with hyperthyroidism are consistent with those of a rapid metabolic rate and include the following:

- Increased sensitivity to heat
- Nervousness, agitation
- Unexplained weight loss
- Decreased concentration
- Irregular menstrual periods
- Increased heart rate

Some patients who have hyperthyroidism have protruding eyeballs, which is partially due to swelling of tissue at the back of the eye socket (Figure 20-4).

Emergency Care

Objective 18

To treat a patient with a possible thyroid-related emergency:

- Stabilize the spine if trauma is suspected.
- Assess the patient's mental status and ability to maintain his own airway. Assess the need for an oral or nasal airway, and reassess often while the patient is in your care. Suction as necessary.
- Give oxygen. If the patient's breathing is adequate, apply oxygen by nonrebreather mask at 15 L/min if not already done. If the patient's breathing is inadequate, provide positive-pressure ventilation with 100% oxygen and assess the adequacy of the ventilations delivered.
- Place the patient in a position of comfort.
- Remove or loosen tight clothing. Maintain body temperature.
- Transport. Reassess often until patient care is turned over to ALS personnel or medical personnel at the receiving facility.

On the Scene　Wrap-Up

Severely uncontrolled diabetes can wreak havoc on the body, resulting in blindness, kidney failure, nerve damage, and circulatory disorders. A patient who has uncontrolled diabetes may be missing fingers, toes, hands, feet, and even portions of the leg. The blood sugar level may become too low if the diabetic patient has taken too much insulin, has not eaten enough food, has over-exercised and burned off sugar faster than normal, or experiences significant physical stress (such as an infection) or emotional stress. The brain does not have any stored glucose, and the longer it is deprived of sugar, the more damage results. All indications in this patient point to a low blood sugar. You administer oxygen, obtain the patient's vital signs and oxygen saturation, and perform a blood glucose test using a glucometer, which is 42 mg/dL. You quickly administer oral glucose, and her mental status improves within minutes. The patient agrees to be transported for physician evaluation. ∎

Sum It Up

▶ Glucose, a sugar, is the basic fuel for body cells. The level of sugar in the blood (the blood sugar) must remain fairly constant to ensure proper functioning of the brain and body cells. Changes in glucose levels can result in changes in the patient's behavior.

▶ The body's blood glucose level is primarily regulated by the pancreas. Normal blood glucose levels generally range between 70 and 120 mg/dL.

▶ Insulin helps glucose enter the body's cells to be used for energy. As the blood glucose level drops toward normal, the release of insulin slows. Glucagon is a hormone that stimulates cells in the liver to break down stores of glycogen into glucose. This increases the blood glucose level. Somatostatin is a hormone that is released by delta cells in the pancreas. This hormone inhibits the release of insulin and glucagon.

► Diabetes mellitus is a disease involving the pancreas. There are three major types of diabetes mellitus.

- In type 1 diabetes mellitus, little or no insulin is produced by beta cells in the pancreas. This results in a buildup of glucose in the blood. Despite the buildup of glucose in the blood, the body's cells are starved for glucose because, without insulin, glucose is unable to enter most body cells. Although it may occur at any age, type 1 diabetes usually begins during childhood or young adulthood.

- Type 2 diabetes mellitus is the most common type of diabetes. It usually affects people older than 40 years of age, especially those who are overweight. Type 2 diabetes is caused by a combination of insulin resistance and relative insulin shortage. Insulin resistance refers to a condition in which the pancreas releases insulin, but the normal effect of insulin on the tissue cells of the body is diminished. In an attempt to counteract this resistance, the pancreas releases more insulin into the bloodstream. Insulin levels rise. In some cases, glucose builds up in the bloodstream despite the increased amount of insulin. This results in high blood glucose levels or type 2 diabetes.

- When a woman develops diabetes during pregnancy, it is called gestational diabetes. Gestational diabetes does not include previously diabetic pregnant patients. Hormones released during pregnancy can change the effectiveness of insulin. These changes usually begin in the fifth or sixth month of pregnancy. Diabetes develops if the pancreas cannot make enough insulin to control the level of glucose in the blood.

► Hypoglycemia is a lower-than-normal blood sugar level. In adults, hypoglycemia is a blood glucose level less than 70 mg/dL. Hypoglycemia is the most common diabetic emergency. The onset of hypoglycemia symptoms is sudden (minutes to hours). Prolonged hypoglycemia can lead to irreversible brain damage.

► Hyperglycemia is a higher-than-normal blood sugar level. The onset of hyperglycemia symptoms is gradual (hours to days). As hyperglycemia worsens, body cells become starved for sugar. Although sugar is present in the blood, it cannot be transported into the body's cells without insulin. The buildup of sugar causes the kidneys to increase urine output, which leads to dehydration. The body begins breaking down fats and proteins to provide energy. The breakdown of fats and proteins produces waste products, including acids. The patient begins breathing deeply and rapidly in an attempt to get rid of the excess acid by "blowing off" carbon dioxide. This breathing pattern is called Kussmaul respirations.

► Diabetic ketoacidosis is severe, uncontrolled hyperglycemia (usually over 300 mg/dL). DKA usually occurs in people who have type 1 diabetes but may also occur in those who have type 2 diabetes. DKA is also called diabetic coma.

► Blood glucose testing is used to assist in the management of patients with specific signs and symptoms. The results obtained from the test help determine if the patient's glucose level is too high, too low, or within normal limits. The device used to measure the amount of glucose in a blood sample is called a blood glucose meter or glucometer.

► If approved by medical direction (and your state and local EMS system), you may give oral glucose to a patient who has an altered mental status and a history of diabetes controlled by medication and is able to swallow. Oral glucose given to a patient with an altered mental status and a known history of diabetes can make a difference between development of coma (unconsciousness) and ability to maintain consciousness.

► Inadequate secretion of thyroid hormones is called hypothyroidism (also called underactive thyroid). There are many causes of hypothyroidism including inflammation of the thyroid gland, surgical removal of the thyroid gland, and a low dietary intake of iodine. Hyperthyroidism (also called overactive thyroid) results from an oversecretion of thyroid hormones, which markedly increases the rate of cellular metabolism.

Respiratory Disorders

By the end of this chapter, you should be able to:

Knowledge Objectives ▶
1. Describe assessment of the patient with breathing difficulty.
2. Explain orthopnea and paroxysmal nocturnal dyspnea.
3. Describe abnormal breath sounds and what they mean.
4. Explain possible questions to ask a patient with breathing difficulty.
5. Describe a method of categorizing a patient's level of respiratory distress.
6. List examples of trauma and medical conditions that may cause breathing difficulty.
7. Identify the pathophysiology, assessment findings, and emergency care for croup.
8. Identify the pathophysiology, assessment findings, and emergency care for epiglottitis.
9. Identify the pathophysiology, assessment findings, and emergency care for pertussis.
10. Identify the pathophysiology, assessment findings, and emergency care for cystic fibrosis.
11. Identify the pathophysiology, assessment findings, and emergency care for asthma.
12. Identify the pathophysiology, assessment findings, and emergency care for chronic bronchitis.
13. Identify the pathophysiology, assessment findings, and emergency care for emphysema.
14. Identify the pathophysiology, assessment findings, and emergency care for pneumonia.
15. Identify the pathophysiology, assessment findings, and emergency care for acute pulmonary embolism.
16. Identify the pathophysiology, assessment findings, and emergency care for acute pulmonary edema.
17. Identify the pathophysiology, assessment findings, and emergency care for spontaneous pneumothorax.

Attitude Objectives ▶
18. Defend emergency medical technician treatment regimens for various respiratory disorders.
19. Explain the rationale for assisting a patient with a prescribed inhaler.

Skill Objective ▶
20. Demonstrate the emergency medical care for a patient with breathing difficulty.

You are working as an EMT on a basic life support (BLS) ambulance with a BLS partner. At 2:00 a.m. you are dispatched to a call for a child in respiratory distress. Although you use lights and siren en route to the call, your response time to the scene is 8 minutes. You make a mental note that you are 20 minutes from the nearest hospital.

Upon arrival, you find a 3-year-old girl in moderate respiratory distress. Her parents are very anxious. They tell you that their daughter has been diagnosed with reactive airway disease and has been prescribed an inhaler to be given every 4 hours with a spacer. They filled the prescription today, but are not sure they are using it correctly.

The child's color is pink, and she is coughing frequently. She is breathing 22 times per minute. Her heart rate is 120. When you listen to her lungs, you hear slight expiratory wheezing that is scattered throughout both lung fields. ■

THINK ABOUT IT

As you read this chapter, think about the following questions:

- What emergency care can you give to help this child?
- Could you set up a metered-dose inhaler with a spacer and instruct the parents and patient on the appropriate technique?

Introduction

As an EMT, you will often encounter patients with respiratory disorders. The anatomy and physiology of the respiratory system was discussed in Chapters 6, 7, 12, 13, and 14 and should be reviewed before reading this chapter, if necessary. In this chapter we discuss assessment of the patient with breathing difficulty and the assessment findings and symptoms and emergency care for specific respiratory disorders.

Assessing the Patient with Breathing Difficulty

Scene Size-Up

Objective 1

When you are called for a patient with breathing difficulty, determine if it is caused by trauma or a medical condition. If the scene suggests trauma might be a cause, determine the mechanism of injury from the patient, family members, or bystanders and your inspection of the scene. If trauma is suspected, be sure to maintain spinal stabilization while you assess the patient. If the scene suggests a medical cause, determine the nature of the illness from the patient, family members, or bystanders. Observe the patient's environment for clues to the cause of the patient's breathing difficulty.

Primary Survey

Objectives 1, 2, 3

After making sure that the scene is safe and putting on appropriate personal protective equipment, form a general impression before approaching your patient. You should use this method when evaluating all respiratory emergencies.

Assess the patient's appearance (mental status and body position), work of breathing, and skin color. If the patient looks agitated or limp or appears to be asleep, approach her immediately and begin the primary survey. Observe the patient's position. Patients with dyspnea (difficulty breathing) often sit or stand to inhale adequate air. In a **tripod position,** the patient prefers to sit up and lean forward, with the weight of her upper body supported by her hands on her thighs or knees. **Orthopnea** is breathlessness when lying flat that is relieved or lessened when the patient sits or stands. **Paroxysmal nocturnal dyspnea** is a sudden onset of difficulty breathing that occurs at night. It occurs because of a buildup of fluid in the alveoli or pooling of secretions during sleep.

Remember that normal breathing is quiet, painless, and occurs at a regular rate.

Approach the patient immediately and begin the primary survey if the patient:

- Looks as if he is struggling (laboring) to breathe
- Has noisy breathing
- Is breathing faster or more slowly than normal
- Looks as if his chest is not moving normally
- Has skin that looks flushed (red), pale (whitish color), gray (ashen), or blue (cyanotic)

As respiratory distress increases, the patient will typically have a decrease in oxygenated blood. This causes the patient's skin, nail beds, and mucous membranes to look bluish-gray (cyanotic) in color. This is a late sign of hypoxia. Earlier indications of hypoxia include confusion, anxiety, irritability, restlessness, an increased respiratory rate, increased heart rate, and mild respiratory distress. Oxygen should be given when a patient presents with respiratory distress.

After forming a general impression, assess the patient's mental status. As the amount of oxygen in the blood decreases, the patient may become anxious, restless, confused, and combative. As the amount of carbon dioxide in the blood increases, the patient may become increasingly difficult to arouse.

Assess the patient's airway and breathing. Observe how many words the patient can speak before she needs to take a breath. Can the patient answer questions in full sentences? Or can she speak only a few words before needing to take a breath? If your patient is awake but appears to have trouble breathing, ask, "Can you speak?" or "Are you choking?" If she is able to speak or make noise, air is moving past her vocal cords. If a complete airway obstruction is present, you may initially see rise and fall of the chest, but you will not hear or feel air movement. If the patient's heart stops, you may see irregular, gasping breaths (agonal respirations) just after this occurs. Do not confuse gasping respirations with adequate breathing.

When assessing the patient's breathing, note the rise and fall of the chest. Estimate the respiratory rate. The patient with breathing difficulty often has a respiratory rate outside the normal limits for his age. The normal respiratory rate for an adult at rest is 12 to 20 breaths/min. If the rate is below 12, it is called **bradypnea.** If the rate is above 20, it is called **tachypnea.** If the respiratory rate falls out of the normal range, look for possible causes for this abnormal vital sign. An increase in a patient's respiratory rate is an early sign of respiratory distress. **Agonal breathing** (slow, gasping respirations) may be observed just before death. The patient with agonal breathing requires immediate positive-pressure ventilation with 100% oxygen. Possible causes of changes in respiratory rate are shown in Table 21-1.

Note the depth and equality of the patient's breathing. In an adult, a normal breath is about 7 to 8 mL per kilogram of patient weight. This amount is called the

TABLE 21-1 Possible Causes of Changes in Respiratory Rate

Decreased Respiratory Rate	Increased Respiratory Rate
Drug overdose	Fever
Respiratory distress	Pain
Respiratory failure	Anxiety
Head injury	Respiratory distress
Hypothermia	Respiratory failure
	Certain drugs
	Increased metabolic rate
	Hypoxia
	Trauma
	Diabetic ketoacidosis

tidal volume. Remember that **minute volume** is the total amount of air breathed in and out in 1 minute. Minute volume = tidal volume × respiratory rate. Think of *tidal volume* as the depth of a patient's breathing. When a patient has a tube inserted into her trachea, tidal volume can be measured directly. When a patient is not intubated (does not have an airway tube in her trachea), we must learn to assess the patient's tidal volume using our eyes and ears. You can indirectly assess tidal volume by watching the rise and fall of the patient's chest. Assess whether the chest rise and fall appear normal, increased, or decreased. The patient with difficulty breathing often has inadequate or shallow respirations. Place your stethoscope on the patient's chest and listen closely. You should hear air movement during the whole time the chest expands, as well as while it contracts. This is important to note because it is possible to see rise and fall of a patient's chest with little or no air exchange. For example, shallow respirations, even in the presence of an increased respiratory rate, may be inadequate to ventilate the patient. Comparing from side to side, determine if breath sounds are present or absent, equal or unequal, and clear or noisy. The patient with inadequate breathing requires immediate positive-pressure ventilation with 100% oxygen. Table 21-2 lists common abnormal breath sounds and their significance.

Note the rhythm of the patient's respirations. Conditions that may cause irregular breathing include a head injury, drug overdose, and diabetic emergency. Note any signs of increased work of breathing (respiratory effort). A patient who is having difficulty breathing is working hard (laboring) to breathe. She may be gasping for air. You may see her use the muscles in her neck to assist with inhalation. She may use her abdominal muscles and muscles between the ribs to assist with exhalation. You may see **retractions** ("sinking in" of the soft tissues between and around the ribs or above the

TABLE 21-2 Abnormal Breath Sounds and What They Mean

Breath Sound	Description	What It Means
Crackles (rales)	• Short popping or crackling sounds • Heard more often on inhalation than on exhalation	Movement of air through moisture or fluid
Rhonchi	• "Rattling" or "rumbling" sounds	Movement of air through passages narrowed by mucus or fluid
Wheezes	• High- or low-pitched whistling sounds • Usually heard at the end of inhalation or on exhalation	Movement of air through narrowed lower airways

collarbones). Indentations of the skin above the collarbones (clavicles) are called **supraclavicular retractions.** Indentations of the skin between the ribs are called **intercostal retractions.** Indentations of the skin below the rib cage are called **subcostal retractions.**

Note if the patient's respirations are quiet, absent, or noisy. Normal breathing is quiet. However, quiet breathing is not always a good sign. Breathing becomes quiet when a partial airway obstruction becomes a complete obstruction. Quiet breathing in a patient with asthma may indicate a decrease in air movement. Noisy breathing is usually abnormal breathing and a sign that the patient is in distress. Noisy breathing is indicated by stridor, snoring, wheezing, gurgling, or grunting (see Chapter 13).

Assess the patient's circulation and perfusion. While feeling the patient's pulse, estimate the heart rate. Note its regularity and strength. Note the color, temperature, and moisture of the patient's skin. Observe the nail beds, earlobes or tops of the ears, lips, base of the tongue, and the area around the mouth for pallor or cyanosis. Cyanosis is a very late finding in infants and children. If cyanosis is present, the child may require positive-pressure ventilation. In infants and children younger than 6 years of age, assess capillary refill. If appropriate, evaluate for possible major bleeding.

Priority patients include the following:
- Those in whom an open airway cannot be established or maintained
- Those who are experiencing difficulty breathing or who exhibit signs of respiratory distress
- Those with absent or inadequate breathing and who require continuous positive-pressure ventilation

A summary of the assessment findings and symptoms of breathing difficulty is shown in the following *You Should Know* box.

You Should Know

Assessment Findings and Symptoms of Breathing Difficulty
- Shortness of breath
- Restlessness, anxious appearance, concentration on breathing
- Possible altered mental status (with fatigue or obstruction)
- Breathing rate too fast or slow for age
- Irregular breathing pattern
- Depth of breathing unusually deep or shallow
- Noisy breathing
- Sitting upright, leaning forward to breathe
- Unable to speak in complete sentences
- Pain with breathing
- Retractions, use of accessory muscles
- Abdominal breathing (diaphragm only)
- Coughing
- Increased pulse rate
- Unusual anatomy (barrel chest)
- Skin that looks flushed, pale, gray, or blue and feels cold or sweaty
- Drowsiness, decreased pulse rate as patient tires

Remember This

When a patient experiences a respiratory emergency, advanced life support (ALS) assistance should be requested as soon as possible. If ALS personnel are not available, the patient should be transported promptly to the closest appropriate facility.

Secondary Survey

Objective 4

If your patient is responsive, find out her medical history first before performing the physical examination. Consider initiating treatment (at least oxygen administration) before taking a long history. Remember to use OPQRST to recall important questions to ask when obtaining the history of the present illness. The patient should be your primary source of information. Additional sources of information include the scene, family members, friends, and bystanders. If the patient is unable to speak in complete sentences, limit your questions to those that require a yes or no answer. In situations like this, the family becomes an important source of information. The information you collect will help guide where you look and what you are looking for in the focused physical exam. Examples of questions to ask a patient who is having breathing difficulty are shown in the following *Making a Difference* box.

Making a Difference ~~~~~~

Possible Questions to Ask a Patient with Difficulty Breathing

SAMPLE

- Can you tell me why you called us today?
- Do you have any allergies to medications, dust, pollen, pets, perfume, or foods?
- Do you have a prescribed inhaler? What is the name of the medication? How many times per day do you use it? When did you last use it? Do you take any other medications? Has the dosage of any of your medications been changed recently? Have you ever been on steroids, such as prednisone, for your asthma?
- Do you have a history of asthma? How often do you have asthma attacks? Compared with other attacks, would you describe this one as mild, moderate, or severe?
- Do you have a history of congestive heart failure or chronic obstructive pulmonary disease (COPD)?
- Have you had a recent cold, flu, bronchitis, pneumonia, or other infection?
- Do you smoke? How many packs per day?
- Have you ever been hospitalized or had a tube inserted into your airway for your breathing difficulty?
- When did you last have anything to eat or drink?
- What were you doing when your symptoms began?

OPQRST

- **O**nset: How long ago did your symptoms begin?
- **P**rovocation/palliation/position: What makes the problem better or worse? Does anything you do relieve your symptoms?
- **Q**uality: Can you describe your discomfort? (If the patient is having pain, ask him what it feels like, e.g., dull, burning, sharp, stabbing, shooting, throbbing, pressure, or tearing.)
- **R**egion/radiation: Do you have any pain associated with your breathing? Where is the pain? Is the pain in one area, or does it move? Is the pain located in any other area?
- **S**everity: On a scale of 0 to 10, with 0 being the least and 10 being the worst, what number would you give your breathing difficulty? (If the patient is having pain, ask him to rate his pain using the 0 to 10 scale.)
- **T**ime: How long has your breathing difficulty been present? Did your symptoms begin suddenly or gradually? Have you ever had these symptoms before? When? How long did they last?

~~~~~~

After the primary survey, an unresponsive medical patient (or a patient with an altered mental status) needs a rapid medical assessment. This quick head-to-toe physical exam will help you identify the patient's problem. Treat problems as you find them.

Infant and Child Assessment Considerations

A child's nasal passages are very small, short, and narrow. It is easy for children to develop obstruction of these areas with mucus or foreign objects. If an infant or child is having difficulty breathing, you may see nasal flaring. **Nasal flaring** refers to widening of the nostrils when the patient breathes in. This sign is the body's attempt to increase the size of the airway and increase the amount of available oxygen.

Newborns are primarily nose breathers. A newborn will not automatically open her mouth to breathe when her nose becomes obstructed. As a result, any obstruction of the nose will lead to respiratory difficulty. You must make sure the newborn's nose is clear to avoid breathing problems. **Head bobbing** is an indicator of increased work of breathing in infants. When the baby breathes out, the head falls forward. The baby's head comes up when the baby breathes in and its chest expands.

Although the opening of the mouth is usually small, a child's tongue is large in proportion to the mouth. The tongue is the most common cause of upper airway obstruction in an unconscious child because the immature muscles of the lower jaw allow the tongue to fall to the back of the throat.

In children, the opening between the vocal cords (glottic opening) is higher in the neck and more toward the front than in an adult. As we grow up, our neck gets longer and the glottic opening drops down. The flap of cartilage that covers this opening, the epiglottis, is larger proportionally and floppier in children. Therefore, any injury to or swelling of this area can block the airway.

In children, the trachea is softer and more flexible and has a smaller diameter and shorter length than in adults. The trachea has rings of cartilage that keep the airway open. In children, this cartilage is soft and collapses easily, which can then obstruct the airway. Extending or flexing the neck too far can result in crimping of the trachea and a blocked airway. To avoid blocking the airway, place the head of an infant or young child in a neutral or "sniffing" position. This may require slight elevation of the shoulders.

A child's ribs are soft and flexible because they are made up mostly of cartilage. The muscles between the ribs (intercostal muscles) help lift the chest wall during breathing. Because these muscles are not fully developed until later in childhood, the diaphragm is the primary muscle of breathing. As a result, the abdominal muscles move during breathing. During normal breathing, the abdominal muscles should move in the same direction as the chest wall. If they are moving opposite each other, this is called **seesaw breathing** and is abnormal. A child's respiratory rate is normally faster than an adult's and decreases with age. Because the muscles between the ribs are not well developed, a child cannot keep up a rate of breathing that is more rapid than normal for very long.

The stomach of an infant or child often fills with air during crying. Air can also build up in the stomach if rescue breathing is performed. As the stomach swells with air, it pushes on the lungs and diaphragm. This action limits movement and prevents good ventilation. Because infants and young children depend on the diaphragm for breathing, breathing difficulty results if movement of the diaphragm is limited.

The skin of an infant or child will more reliably show changes related to the amount of oxygen in the blood. Pale (whitish) skin may be seen in shock, fright, or anxiety. A bluish (cyanotic) tint, often seen first around the mouth, suggests inadequate breathing or poor perfusion. This is a critical sign that requires immediate treatment.

Determining the Patient's Level of Respiratory Distress

Objective 5

When determining the patient's level of respiratory distress, find out as much patient information as possible and apply the most appropriate interventions and treatments. This needs to be done rapidly and accurately. The patient should be placed in one of four categories.

Categories of respiratory distress:
1. No breathing difficulty or shortness of breath
2. Mild breathing difficulty
3. Moderate breathing difficulty
4. Severe breathing difficulty

Remember This

Ask the patient with breathing difficulty to count to 10. This will give you an idea of the patient's level of respiratory distress. A person with no breathing difficulty can count to 10 easily. A person who is having severe breathing difficulty will usually be unable to count to 10 due to shortness of breath.

No Breathing Difficulty

A patient who has no breathing difficulty has no signs of respiratory distress. The patient appears relaxed and denies shortness of breath. Breathing is quiet and unlabored. The patient is able to speak in full sentences without pausing to catch her breath. Breathing is regular and at a rate within normal limits for her age. The patient's breathing pattern is smooth and regular. There is equal rise and fall of the chest with each breath. The patient may have occasional sighing respirations. The patient's depth of breathing (tidal volume) is adequate. The color of the patient's skin and the mucous membranes of her mouth are normal. They do not appear pale, flushed, or bluish-gray.

Mild Breathing Difficulty

A patient who has mild breathing difficulty may be hypoxic but can move an adequate amount of air. His heart rate and respiratory rate may be increased. He is alert and can answer your questions in complete sentences. This patient should be given high-concentration oxygen by nonrebreather mask. If indicated, start to treat the underlying cause of the patient's breathing difficulty with the patient's prescribed metered-dose inhaler (MDI).

Remember This

Always have resuscitation equipment within arm's reach when caring for a patient who presents with respiratory distress. Examples of equipment that should be available include oxygen, oral and nasal airways, bag-mask (BM) device, suction unit and suction catheters, and an automated external defibrillator (AED).

Do not insert a nasal airway into the nose of a patient with trauma to the nose or midface.

Moderate Breathing Difficulty

A patient who has moderate breathing difficulty may be hypoxic, but she can still move an adequate amount of air (although her tidal volume may be decreased). Hypoxia can make patients irritable, anxious, or frightened. Increased carbon dioxide levels can cause confusion, lethargy, and lack of concentration. Bradycardia is an ominous sign, indicating that respiratory arrest is likely to ensue.

The patient with moderate breathing difficulty will have an increased heart rate and respiratory rate. She will have difficulty answering questions and will be unable to speak in complete sentences. With this in mind, ask questions that require only a short answer. Try to keep the patient calm and relaxed. Give high-concentration oxygen by nonrebreather mask. Pulse oximetry should be used on all patients receiving oxygen— especially on *all* respiratory patients, not just those with moderate to severe difficulty breathing. Check vital signs, level of responsiveness, and the patient's response to your treatment.

Making a Difference

Respiratory distress is very frightening for patients. Your remaining calm and appearing to have a plan of action can be very comforting to patients in respiratory distress.

If the patient's condition does not improve, prepare to assist ventilations. Assisted ventilation requires skill. The patient with moderate breathing difficulty may resist your attempts to assist her breathing. Explain to the patient that you are going to help her breathing. As the patient starts to breathe in, gently squeeze the bag. Stop squeezing as the chest starts to rise. When squeezing the bag, match the patient's breathing—do not try to take over. Ask the patient to try to breathe with you. Interpose extra ventilations, if necessary. Some patients may require only an extra breath or a slightly larger volume. Allow the patient to exhale before giving the next breath. Feel for changes in the patient's lung compliance with the BM device. Signs of adequate and inadequate artificial ventilation are listed in Table 21-3.

Attempt to treat the underlying cause of the patient's breathing difficulty. If the patient has a prescribed inhaler, have the patient try to use it if possible. The patient's ability to use the inhaler will depend on the level of respiratory distress. Assisting a patient with a prescribed inhaler is discussed later in this chapter.

Severe Breathing Difficulty

A patient who has severe breathing difficulty may be sleepy or unresponsive. The patient may have been wild and combative but now appears quiet. This is a sign of respiratory failure. The patient is wearing out. If the patient is responsive, he may be unable to speak or may only be able to speak in short phrases of one to two words. The patient may assume a tripod position and may need support to maintain a sitting position as he tires. His breathing rate may initially be rapid with periods of slow breathing. As he tires and his condition worsens, his breathing rate will slow and then become agonal (gasping) respirations. As his breathing muscles tire, his breathing will become shallow. The patient's skin may appear blue or mottled despite being given oxygen.

Remember This

- An unresponsive patient is unable to protect her own airway.
- Do not try to insert an oral airway in a semiresponsive patient. This can cause gagging and vomiting.
- If necessary, assist an unresponsive patient's breathing by using a bag-mask device connected to 100% oxygen.

TABLE 21-3 Signs of Adequate and Inadequate Artificial Ventilation	
Signs of *Adequate* Artificial Ventilation	**Signs of *Inadequate* Artificial Ventilation**
• Chest rise and fall are seen with each artificial ventilation • Rate of ventilation is sufficient, about once every 3 to 5 seconds for an infant or child, once every 5 to 6 seconds for an adult • Heart rate improves with artificial ventilation	• Chest does not rise and fall with artificial ventilation • Rate of ventilation is too slow or too fast • Heart rate does not return to normal with artificial ventilation

Specific Respiratory Disorders

Objective 6

Dyspnea is a common chief complaint that you will encounter. **Dyspnea** is a sensation of shortness of breath or difficulty breathing. The patient may express his breathing difficulty in different ways. For example, the patient may say that he is "short of breath," "short-winded," or "can't get my breath." Causes include trauma (see Chapter 35) and medical conditions, such as those listed in Table 21-4.

Croup

Objective 7

Croup is an infection, usually caused by one of the same viruses responsible for common colds. The virus affects the larynx and the area just below it (Figure 21-1). It is spread from person to person by droplets from coughing and sneezing. Although there are many types of viruses responsible for croup, one cause is respiratory syncytial virus (RSV). Some viruses that cause croup are most widespread in late fall and early winter. Croup caused by RSV usually peaks in the middle of winter, although some cases occur in the spring.

Assessment Findings and Symptoms

Viral croup most commonly occurs in children between the ages of 6 months and 3 years, although it can occur in older children. The child's caregiver usually relays symptoms of a cold for 2 to 3 days, such as a fever and a stuffy or runny nose. The virus that causes croup causes the walls of the trachea and larynx to become inflamed and swell. Inflammation and swelling in this area narrow the upper airway passages. As the upper airway passages narrow, the child may develop stridor, hoarseness, and a loud cough that sounds like the barking of a seal. Signs and symptoms of croup often worsen at night. Episodes of mild croup often break when air the child breathes is cooler than body temperature and humid but less than 100% saturated with water vapor. This cools the mucous membranes and constricts blood vessels in the affected area, decreasing swelling. Assessment findings and symptoms are listed in the following *You Should Know* box.

You Should Know

Assessment Findings and Symptoms of Croup

- Gradual onset, usually over 2 to 3 days
- Stridor
- Barking cough
- Hoarse voice
- Low-grade fever (usually less than 102.2°F)

TABLE 21-4 Possible Causes of Difficulty Breathing	
Trauma Condition	**Medical Condition**
• Flail chest	• Croup
• Inhalation injury	• Epiglottitis
• Drowning incident	• Pertussis
• Pulmonary contusion	• Cystic fibrosis
• Diaphragm injury	• Reactive airway disease/asthma
• Tracheobronchial tree injury	• Allergic reaction
• Simple pneumothorax	• Heart attack
• Open pneumothorax	• Partial airway obstruction
• Tension pneumothorax	• Chronic obstructive pulmonary disease (chronic bronchitis, emphysema)
• Traumatic asphyxia	• Abnormal heart rhythm
• Scapula fracture	• Lung cancer
• Rib fractures	• Congestive heart failure or acute pulmonary edema
• Cervical spine injury	• Pneumonia
	• Foreign body airway obstruction
	• Acute pulmonary embolism

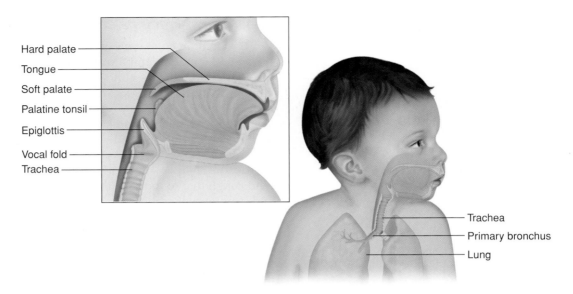

FIGURE 21-1 ▲ Croup affects the larynx and the area just below it.

Emergency Care

Allow the child to assume a position of comfort. Avoid agitating the child. Allow the child to have her favorite blanket, doll, stuffed animal, or toy to help her feel secure. If possible, allow the caregiver to hold the child while giving supplemental oxygen. If the child will not tolerate a mask, give blow-by oxygen. If the child shows signs of respiratory failure or respiratory arrest, assist her breathing by using a bag-mask with 100% oxygen. Transport to the hospital for further evaluation. Record all patient care information, including the patient's medical history, emergency care given, and the patient's response to your care, on a prehospital care report (PCR).

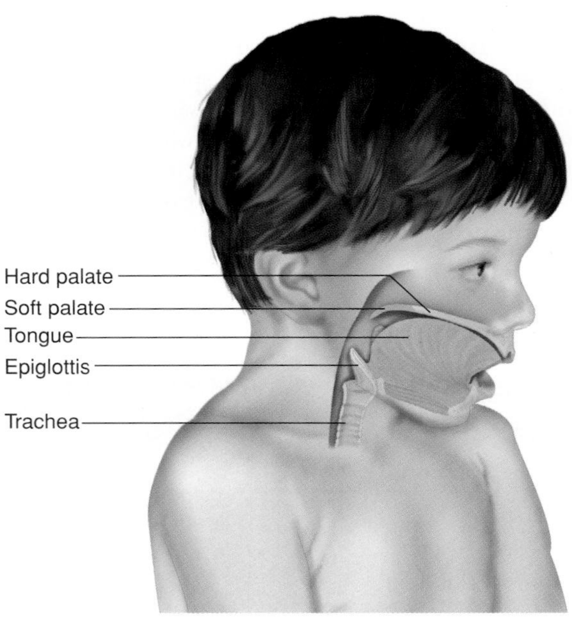

Remember This

In general, a patient who is having difficulty breathing instinctively assumes a position of comfort to improve breathing. Do not force the patient to lie down. This may compromise the airway and cause immediate obstruction.

FIGURE 21-2 ▲ Epiglottitis is a bacterial infection of the epiglottis.

Epiglottitis

Objective 8

Epiglottitis is a bacterial infection of the epiglottis (Figure 21-2). When epiglottitis occurs in children, it typically affects children between 3 and 7 years of age. Since there is now a vaccine for epiglottitis, it is uncommon in children and more commonly seen in adults. The onset of symptoms is usually sudden, developing over a few hours. Respiratory arrest may occur because of a complete airway obstruction or a combination of partial airway obstruction and fatigue.

Assessment Findings and Symptoms

A patient who has epiglottitis is and looks very sick. Assessment findings and symptoms are listed in the next *You Should Know* box. A comparison of croup and epiglottitis is shown in Table 21-5.

TABLE 21-5 Comparison of Croup and Epiglottitis

	Croup	Epiglottitis
Age	6 months to 3 years	3 to 7 years, and in adults
Cause	Viral	Bacterial
Onset	Gradual	Sudden
Signs/symptoms	• Stridor • Barking cough • Hoarse voice • Low-grade fever (usually less than 102.2°F)	• Stridor • Restlessness • Sore throat, drooling • Muffled voice • High fever (usually 102°F to 104°F) • Tripod position, unwilling to lie down • Difficulty swallowing • Dyspnea

You Should Know

Assessment Findings and Symptoms of Epiglottitis

- Restlessness
- Tripod position, unwilling to lie down
- Sudden onset of high fever, usually 102° to 104°F
- Sore throat
- Muffled voice
- Drooling
- Difficulty swallowing
- Dyspnea
- Stridor

Emergency Care

A patient with suspected epiglottitis must be observed closely at all times. Avoid upsetting the patient. If the patient is a child, the child to assume a position of comfort with his favorite toy or blanket, if available. Allow the caregiver to hold the child while you give supplemental oxygen. If the child will not tolerate a mask, give blow-by oxygen. Do not attempt to look into the patient's mouth or throat. This may agitate the patient and worsen his respiratory distress. If respiratory arrest occurs, give positive-pressure ventilations with 100% oxygen. Rapidly transport the child to the closest appropriate medical facility. Record all patient care information, including the patient's medical history, emergency care given, and the patient's response to your care, on a PCR.

Pertussis

Objective 9

Pertussis, also called whooping cough, is a highly contagious bacterial infection of the respiratory tract. The bacterium that causes pertussis is found in the mouth, nose, and throat of an infected person. The disease is spread from person to person by droplets from coughing and sneezing. Pertussis can affect persons of any age. Childhood vaccines in the United States include immunization against pertussis. However, the immunity to the disease does not last forever, which is why some older children and adults become infected.

Assessment Findings and Symptoms

The initial signs and symptoms of pertussis are similar to those of a cold—runny nose, sneezing, low-grade fever, and a mild, nonproductive, occasional cough. About 7 to 14 days later, the patient experiences severe coughing spasms in which the patient often cannot inhale between coughs. Gagging is common and thick mucus may be expelled. When the coughing spasm is over, the patient struggles to inhale with the trachea severely narrowed by mucus, resulting in a high-pitched whooping sound. Assessment findings and symptoms are listed in the next *You Should Know* box.

Complications of the disease include hypoxia, apnea, pneumonia, seizures, and malnutrition. In the United States, most pertussis-related deaths occur among unvaccinated children or children too young to be vaccinated.

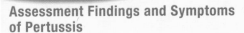
Assessment Findings and Symptoms of Pertussis

- Runny nose
- Sneezing
- Low-grade fever
- Severe coughing spasms
- Gagging
- High-pitched whooping sound or crowing
- Vomiting

Emergency Care

Emergency care for a patient with pertussis is primarily supportive. Avoid upsetting the patient and allow her to assume a position of comfort. If the patient is a child, allow the caregiver to hold the child while you give supplemental oxygen. If the patient will not tolerate a mask, give blow-by oxygen. If the patient shows signs of respiratory failure or respiratory arrest, assist her breathing by using a bag-mask with 100% oxygen. Transport to the hospital for further evaluation. Record all patient care information, including the patient's medical history, emergency care given, and the patient's response to your care, on a PCR.

You Should Know

The pertussis vaccine is combined with diphtheria and tetanus and given at specific intervals during childhood (2 months, 4 months, 6 months, 15–18 months, and 4–6 years). In addition to diphtheria, pertussis, and tetanus, one childhood vaccine (Pediarix) also protects against hepatitis B and polio. Another vaccine (TriHIBit) protects against diphtheria, tetanus, pertussis, and haemophilus influenzae type B.

Cystic Fibrosis

Objective 10

Cystic fibrosis (CF) is an inherited disease that appears in childhood. A defective gene inherited from each parent results in an abnormality in the glands that produce or secrete sweat and mucus.

The defective gene affects a protein that controls the movement of sodium and chloride in and out of cells that line various organs, such as the lungs and the pancreas. Because sodium and chloride are components of salt, the defective gene ultimately disturbs the salt balance in the body.

Mucus that is present in the body is normally watery, keeping the lining of certain organs moist and preventing them from drying out or becoming infected. In CF, there is too little salt and water on the outside of the cells. As a result, mucus in the lining of the bronchi becomes very thick and sticky, making it difficult to remove with coughing. The mucus builds up in the lungs, blocking the airways, and creating an environment where bacteria can grow. This leads to repeated respiratory infections and breathing difficulty. In addition, the thick, sticky mucus can also block tubes, or ducts, in the pancreas of a patient with CF. As a result, enzymes produced by the pancreas that are required for the breakdown of fats cannot reach the small intestine. Without them, the intestines cannot fully absorb fats and proteins, which can result in malnutrition.

Assessment Findings and Symptoms

The symptoms and severity of CF vary from person to person. Typical assessment findings and symptoms are listed in the following *You Should Know* box. Many patients with CF survive into adulthood, although poor health is common.

You Should Know

Assessment Findings and Symptoms of Cystic Fibrosis

- Nasal congestion
- Very salty-tasting skin
- Frequent respiratory infections
- Persistent cough
- Use of accessory muscles for respiration
- Wheezing
- Shortness of breath
- Increased respiratory rate
- Cyanosis
- Poor growth/weight gain in spite of a good appetite ("failure to thrive")
- Abdominal distention
- Abdominal pain/discomfort
- Thin extremities
- Widening and rounding (clubbing) of the tips of the fingers and toes due to hypoxia
- Diarrhea or frequent greasy, foul-smelling, bulky stools

Emergency Care

Older patients and parents of children with CF are generally aware of their disease. Some patients may be oxygen-dependent and will require respiratory support and suctioning to clear the airway of mucus and secretions. Respiratory failure is the most common cause of death in people with CF.

Emergency care is primarily supportive. Allow the patient to assume a position of comfort, which is usually sitting up. Be sure to have suction within arm's reach and suction as necessary. Give supplemental oxygen and monitor the patient's vital signs and oxygen saturation. If the patient will not tolerate a mask, give blow-by oxygen. If the patient shows signs of respiratory failure or respiratory arrest, assist his breathing by using a bag-mask with 100% oxygen. Transport to the hospital for additional care. Record all patient care information, including the patient's medical history, emergency care given, and the patient's response to your care, on a PCR.

Asthma

Objective 11

Asthma (also known as *reactive airway disease*, or *RAD*) is widespread, temporary narrowing of the air passages that transport air from the nose and mouth to the lungs. Asthma may be triggered by many allergens or irritants. Asthma that is triggered by an allergic reaction is called **allergic asthma.** Asthma that is triggered by factors not related to allergies is called **nonallergic asthma.** Possible asthma triggers are shown in the next *You Should Know* box and Figure 21-3. After exposure to the trigger, the smooth muscles surrounding the

bronchioles spasmodically contract (bronchospasm) and swell, and mucus secretion increases. The mucus secreted is abnormally thick. Airway passages are narrowed because of smooth muscle contraction, excessive mucus secretion, or a combination of both. This results in the trapping of air in the bronchioles. Exhalation becomes prolonged as the patient tries to exhale the trapped air. This has been described as trying to blow air through a straw filled with cotton.

At present, there is no cure for asthma. However, symptoms can be managed with proper prevention and treatment.

You Should Know

Possible Triggers of Asthma

- Allergens such as dust mites, cockroaches, pollens, molds, pet dander, dust, shellfish, some medications
- Environmental irritants such as smoke, dust, paint fumes, smog, aerosol sprays, perfumes
- Weather factors such as extremes of heat, cold, humidity
- Exercise
- Colds, flu, sore throat, sinus infection
- Emotional stress

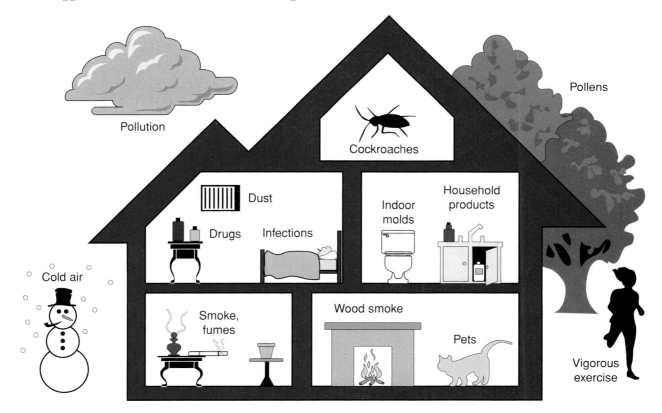

FIGURE 21-3 ▲ Possible asthma triggers.

Assessment Findings and Symptoms

Wheezing is the most common asthma symptom. However, in the asthmatic patient, an absence of wheezing is a serious sign that suggests that airflow is so diminished (the patient is moving too little air) that wheezing is not produced. Children with asthma will often have spells of frequent coughing, rather than wheezing. Other assessment findings and symptoms associated with asthma are shown in the following *You Should Know* box.

You Should Know

Assessment Findings and Symptoms of Asthma

- Wheezing
- Restlessness
- Dry cough
- Dyspnea
- Chest tightness
- Rapid breathing
- Increased heart rate
- Retractions
- Use of accessory muscles

Emergency Care

Allow the patient to assume a position of comfort. Give 100% oxygen, preferably by nonrebreather mask. Provide calm reassurance to help reduce the patient's anxiety. Encourage the patient to cough and breathe deeply to assist in the removal of secretions. If instructed to do so by medical direction, assist the patient in using her prescribed inhaler. Transport to the closest appropriate medical facility for further evaluation. Record all patient care information, including the patient's medical history, emergency care given, and the patient's response to your care, on a PCR.

You Should Know

Patients with reactive airway disease have problems with air trapping. In these patients, positive-pressure ventilation can trigger further bronchoconstriction. It can also cause complications such as barotrauma and breath stacking. **Barotrauma** is injury to tissue caused by excess pressure. **Breath stacking,** a series of breaths without adequate exhalation, can lead to excessive inflation, tension pneumothorax, and low blood pressure. As a result, a slower respiratory rate (6 to 10 breaths/min) and smaller tidal volume (6 to 8 mL/kg) should be used for positive-pressure ventilation than that used for nonasthmatic patients. Be sure to allow the patient time to exhale before giving the next breath. The patient should have at least twice as long to exhale as he does to inhale. A slow, assisted ventilation may be all he can tolerate.

Chronic Bronchitis

Objective 12

Chronic bronchitis is defined as sputum production for 3 months of a year for at least 2 consecutive years. The major cause of chronic bronchitis is cigarette smoking. Respiratory irritants, such as smoke, irritate the airways and cause an increase in mucus production (Figure 21-4). Prolonged exposure to respiratory irritants eventually causes distortion and scarring of the bronchial wall, decreasing the size of the airway opening. Excessive mucus production in the bronchi causes a chronic or recurrent productive cough (sometimes of colored sputum). Because the size of the airway opening is decreased, some secretions are trapped in the alveoli and smaller air passages.

Some individuals with chronic bronchitis retain carbon dioxide. In healthy persons, the main stimulus to increase ventilation is an increase in carbon dioxide. Over time, patients with chronic bronchitis adapt to the retention of carbon dioxide, and their main stimulus to breathe becomes a decrease in oxygen (hypoxic drive). The term *blue bloater* has been used to describe these individuals because the patient is often obese with a cyanotic complexion.

Remember This

Never withhold oxygen from a patient who needs it. Be prepared to assist ventilations if necessary.

Assessment Findings and Symptoms

Signs and symptoms depend on severity of the disease and whether or not there are other problems in addition to the chronic bronchitis. Common assessment findings and symptoms are shown in the following *You Should Know* box.

You Should Know

Assessment Findings and Symptoms of Chronic Bronchitis

- Productive cough
- Cyanosis
- Labored breathing
- Use of accessory muscles
- Increased respiratory rate
- Peripheral edema
- Inability to speak in complete sentences without pausing for a breath

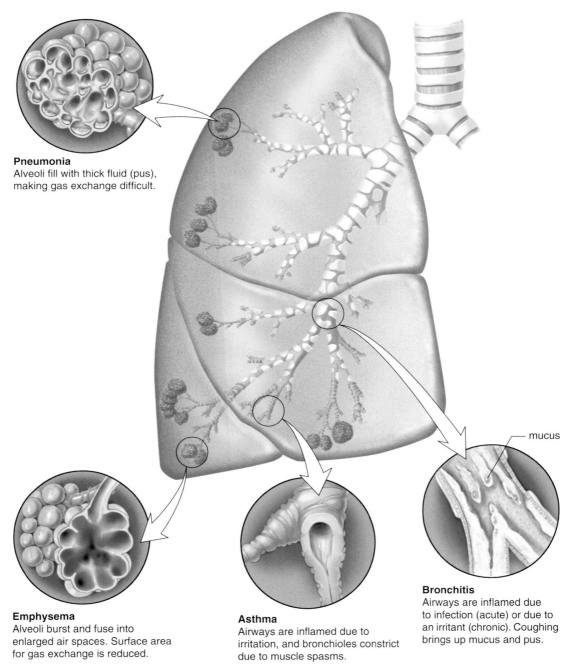

Pneumonia
Alveoli fill with thick fluid (pus), making gas exchange difficult.

mucus

Emphysema
Alveoli burst and fuse into enlarged air spaces. Surface area for gas exchange is reduced.

Asthma
Airways are inflamed due to irritation, and bronchioles constrict due to muscle spasms.

Bronchitis
Airways are inflamed due to infection (acute) or due to an irritant (chronic). Coughing brings up mucus and pus.

FIGURE 21-4 ▲ Disorders of the lower respiratory tract.

Emergency Care

Allow the patient to assume a position of comfort. If signs of breathing difficulty are present, give oxygen by nonrebreather mask at 10 to 15 L/min or as ordered by medical direction. If no signs of respiratory distress are evident, give oxygen by nasal cannula at 2 L/min or as ordered by medical direction. Monitor the patient closely, reassessing every 5 minutes, and be prepared to assist ventilations as necessary. Provide calm reassur-ance to help reduce the patient's anxiety. Encourage the patient to cough and breathe deeply to help in the removal of secretions. If instructed to do so by medical direction, help the patient use her prescribed inhaler. Transport to the closest appropriate medical facility for further evaluation. Record all patient care informa-tion, including the patient's medical history, emer-gency care given, and the patient's response to your care, on a PCR.

In the United States, chronic obstructive pulmonary disease includes emphysema and chronic bronchitis. Other names for COPD include *chronic obstructive airway disease* and *chronic obstructive lung disease*. According to the National Heart, Lung, and Blood Institute, most people with COPD have both chronic bronchitis and emphysema.

Emphysema

Objective 13

Emphysema is an irreversible enlargement of the air spaces distal to the terminal bronchioles. This disease leads to destruction of the walls of the alveoli, distention of the alveolar sacs, and loss of lung elasticity. The patient with emphysema may be called a *pink puffer* because she can often increase her respiratory rate to maintain a relatively normal amount of oxygen (pink color), although her work of breathing is increased during exhalation (puffer). Carbon dioxide levels are often normal in patients with emphysema because they hyperventilate to maintain normal oxygen levels.

Assessment Findings and Symptoms

In emphysema, the lungs inflate easily, but air becomes trapped in the lungs because of the lack of elastic recoil. The volume of air in the chest increases, giving the patient a barrel-chest appearance. The loss of elasticity causes exhalation to become an active (rather than passive) process, increasing the work of breathing. Assessment findings and symptoms of emphysema are shown in the following *You Should Know* box.

Assessment Findings and Symptoms of Emphysema

- Barrel chest
- Use of accessory muscles
- Pursed-lip breathing
- Chronic cough
- Prolonged exhalation
- Increased respiratory rate
- Dyspnea with exertion

Emergency Care

If signs of breathing difficulty are present, give oxygen by nonrebreather mask at 10 to 15 L/min or as ordered by medical direction. If no signs of respiratory distress are evident, give oxygen by nasal cannula at 2 L/min or as ordered by medical direction. Monitor the patient closely, reassessing every 5 minutes. Be prepared to assist ventilations as necessary. Provide calm reassurance to help reduce the patient's anxiety. Encourage the patient to cough and breathe deeply to assist in the removal of secretions. If instructed to do so by medical direction, assist the patient in using her prescribed inhaler. Transport to the closest appropriate medical facility for further evaluation. Record all patient care information, including the patient's medical history, emergency care given, and the patient's response to your care, on a PCR.

Pneumonia

Objective 14

Pneumonia is an infection that often affects gas exchange in the lung. It may involve the lower airways and alveoli, part of a lobe, or an entire lobe of the lung. Pneumonia is most often caused by bacteria and viruses, although it may also be caused by fungi and parasites. Bacterial pneumonia can occur in any part of the lung. It usually causes inflammation and swelling of the alveoli. Viral pneumonia often begins in the bronchioles and then spreads to the alveoli.

Assessment Findings and Symptoms

Assessment findings and symptoms are listed in the following *You Should Know* box.

Assessment Findings and Symptoms of Pneumonia

- Fever
- Chills
- Increased respiratory rate
- Increased heart rate
- Possible cough
- Shortness of breath
- Malaise
- Possible pleuritic (sharp, stabbing) chest pain

Emergency Care

Allow the patient to assume a position of comfort. Give oxygen by nonrebreather mask at 10 to 15 L/min. Transport to the hospital for further evaluation and treatment. Record all patient care information, including the patient's medical history, emergency care given, and the patient's response to your care, on a PCR.

Pulmonary Embolism

Objective 15

A **pulmonary embolus** is usually the result of a clot that forms in the deep veins in the leg and then travels through the veins to the heart and then to the pulmonary circulation. The clot becomes trapped in the smaller branches of the pulmonary arteries, causing partial or complete blood flow obstruction. As a result, a portion of the lung is ventilated but not perfused. To compensate, the patient's respiratory rate increases. If the area involved is large, respiratory failure will occur.

Factors that increase the risk for pulmonary embolism include the following:

- Obesity
- Prolonged bed rest or immobilization
- Recent surgery, particularly of the legs, pelvis, abdomen, or chest
- Leg or pelvic fractures or injuries
- Use of high-estrogen oral contraceptives
- Pregnancy
- Chronic atrial fibrillation (a heart rhythm disorder)

Assessment Findings and Symptoms

Signs and symptoms depend on the:

- Size and location of the embolus
- Number of emboli
- Presence or absence of underlying cardiac and pulmonary disease

You Should Know

Assessment Findings and Symptoms of Pulmonary Embolism

Common findings and symptoms:
- Sudden onset of dyspnea
- Apprehension, restlessness
- Increased respiratory rate
- Increased heart rate

Possible findings and symptoms:
- Pleuritic chest pain
- Cough
- Blood-tinged sputum
- Hypotension

Emergency Care

Allow the patient to assume a position of comfort unless hypotension is present. If the patient is alert but showing signs of breathing difficulty, give oxygen by nonrebreather mask at 10 to 15 L/min. Provide positive-pressure ventilation with 100% oxygen as necessary. Reassess the patient frequently. Transport promptly to the closest appropriate medical facility. Record all patient care information, including the patient's medical history, emergency care given, and the patient's response to your care, on a PCR.

Acute Pulmonary Edema

Objective 16

Pulmonary edema is most commonly caused by failure of the left ventricle of the heart. When the left ventricle fails, fluid is forced into the lung tissue as the right ventricle continues to pump blood into the pulmonary circulation. The alveoli fill with fluid, limiting their ability to effectively exchange oxygen and carbon dioxide. Other (noncardiac) conditions can result in pulmonary edema, including:

- Drowning
- Narcotic overdose
- Trauma
- High altitude
- Poisonous gases

Assessment Findings and Symptoms

Assessment findings and symptoms are listed in the following *You Should Know* box.

You Should Know

Assessment Findings and Symptoms of Acute Pulmonary Edema

- Restlessness, anxiety
- Dyspnea on exertion
- Orthopnea
- Paroxysmal nocturnal dyspnea
- Frothy, blood-tinged sputum
- Cool, moist skin
- Use of accessory muscles
- Jugular venous distention
- Wheezing
- Crackles (rales)
- Rapid, labored breathing
- Increased heart rate
- Increased or decreased blood pressure (depending on severity of edema)

Emergency Care

Help the patient sit up (unless hypotension is present) to promote lung expansion. If breathing is adequate, administer oxygen by nonrebreather mask at 10 to 15 L/min. If breathing is inadequate, provide positive-pressure ventilation with 100% oxygen. Reassess frequently, monitoring vital signs at least every 5 minutes. Be prepared to assist ventilations as necessary. Provide calm reassurance to help reduce the patient's anxiety. Transport promptly to the closest appropriate medical facility. Record all patient care information, including the patient's medical history, emergency care given, and the patient's response to your care, on a PCR.

Spontaneous Pneumothorax

Objective 17

A **pneumothorax** is a collection of air or gas between the lung and the chest wall. A **spontaneous pneumothorax** is a type of pneumothorax that does not involve trauma to the lung. There are two types of spontaneous pneumothorax. A **primary spontaneous pneumothorax** occurs in people with no history of lung disease. This condition most commonly occurs in tall, thin men between the ages of 20 and 40. It rarely occurs in persons older than 40 years. A **secondary spontaneous pneumothorax** most often occurs as a complication of lung disease. Chronic obstructive pulmonary disease is the most common underlying disorder. Other lung diseases associated with this condition include asthma, pneumonia, tuberculosis, and lung cancer. A secondary spontaneous pneumothorax usually occurs in older persons. A spontaneous pneumothorax typically occurs while the patient is at rest or during sleep. It is usually caused by the rupture of a **bleb** (a small air- or fluid-filled sac) in the lung.

Assessment Findings and Symptoms

The patient's signs and symptoms depend on the size of the pneumothorax and the patient's general health.

Emergency Care

If spinal injury is suspected, maintain manual in-line stabilization until the patient is secured to a long backboard. If spinal injury is not suspected, place the patient in a position of comfort. Most patients will be more comfortable sitting up. Establish and maintain an open airway. Give oxygen. If the patient's breathing is adequate, apply oxygen by nonrebreather mask at 10 to 15 L/min if not already done. If the patient's breathing is inadequate, provide positive-pressure ventilation with 100% oxygen. Assess the adequacy of the ventilations delivered. Transport promptly to the closest appropriate facility. Reassess frequently. Record all patient care information, including the patient's medical history, emergency care given, and the patient's response to your care, on a PCR.

Metered-Dose Inhalers

A patient who has a prescribed metered-dose inhaler (MDI) typically has reversible constriction of his airways. An MDI is used to deliver inhaled respiratory medications. Inhaled steroids are another type of medication that may be given by means of an MDI. Inhaled steroids help decrease inflammation in the airways. Advair (fluticasone and salmeterol) is an example of a drug that is both a bronchodilator and inhaled steroid. Fluticasone is a steroid that helps reduce inflammation. Salmeterol is a bronchodilator that relaxes bronchial smooth muscle to improve breathing.

You will recall from Chapter 11 that an MDI is small and consists of two parts, the medication canister and a plastic dispenser with a mouth piece (Figure 21-5). Because some patients find it hard to coordinate breathing in and pressing the inhaler at the same time, a physician will often prescribe a "spacer" to be used with the MDI. The spacer increases the amount of medication delivered into the respiratory tract. The spacer can also be attached to a resuscitation mask to aid medication delivery for a young child (Figure 21-6). Table 21-6 lists important information about prescribed MDIs that you should know. The procedure for assisting a patient with his prescribed MDI was shown in Skill Drill 11-4.

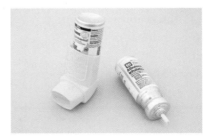

FIGURE 21-5 ▲ A metered-dose inhaler is small and consists of two parts, the medication canister and a plastic dispenser with a mouthpiece.

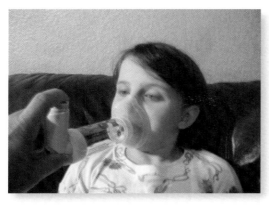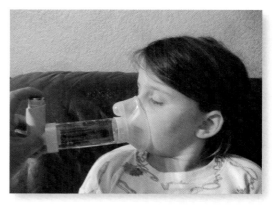

FIGURE 21-6 ▲ MDI use by children is very common. Children will often have a spacer with the device. A spacer used for a young child may be equipped with a mask, such as the one shown here. In these photos, the child's father is assisting her with a dose from her inhaler.

TABLE 21-6	Prescribed Metered-Dose Inhaler
Generic (trade) name	• albuterol (Proventil, Ventolin) • isoetharine (Bronkosol) • metaproterenol (Alupent, Metaprel) • fluticasone and salmeterol (Advair)
Mechanism of action	Inhaled bronchodilators relax bronchial smooth muscle, reducing airway resistance. • terbutaline (Brethine, Bricanyl) • ipratropium bromide (Atrovent)
Indications	An EMT can assist a patient in using a prescribed inhaler if *all* the following criteria are met: • The patient has signs and symptoms of a respiratory emergency. • The patient has a physician-prescribed handheld inhaler. • There are no contraindications to giving the medication. • The EMT has specific authorization by medical direction.
Dosage	Number of inhalations based on medical direction's order or physician's order based on consultation with the patient
Adverse effects	• Increased heart rate • Shaking or tremors • Restlessness • Nervousness • Nausea • Headache • Dizziness
Contraindications	• Medical direction does not give permission • Patient is unable to use device • Inhaler is not prescribed for the patient • Patient has already met maximum prescribed dose before EMT arrival
Special considerations	• Assist the patient in finding his MDI if it is not readily available • Assess the patient's lung sounds and oxygen saturation before administration of an MDI to establish a baseline. Assess lung sounds and oxygen saturation again after administration of the MDI, and compare your findings. • Wait at least 3 minutes before assisting with another dose from the MDI. • Reassess lung sounds, vital signs, oxygen saturation, and patient's degree of breathing difficulty.

Whenever you are dealing with patients in respiratory distress, remain calm and professional. This will help calm the patient and family members and decrease the patient's level of distress. Remember that any patient in respiratory distress will benefit from oxygen. Give oxygen by any means tolerated by the patient.

This child will benefit from oxygen and an MDI given appropriately. Teach the patient and parents that the spacer increases the amount of medication delivered into the respiratory tract. Have the patient depress the inhaler to inject the medication dose into the chamber of the spacer. Have the patient do this before placing the mouthpiece of the spacer in her mouth. Ask the patient to depress the inhaler, breathe in and hold her breath, breathe out, and then take another deep breath through the mouthpiece of the spacer and hold her breath. Explain to the patient (and parents) that a patient who is using a spacer should try to take two deep breaths from the spacer and hold them for each puff from the inhaler.

Reapply oxygen, recheck the patient's vital signs and oxygen saturation, and reassess the patient's degree of breathing difficulty. If ordered by medical direction, repeat the dose after 1 to 3 minutes. When finished with the inhaler, wipe off the mouthpiece with an alcohol swab and replace the cap. To decrease the possibility of adverse effects from the medication, have the patient rinse her mouth out with water. ■

Sum It Up

▶ After making sure that the scene is safe, form a general impression before approaching the patient with a respiratory emergency. If the patient looks agitated or limp or appears to be asleep, approach him immediately and begin the primary survey. Approach the patient immediately and begin the primary survey if the patient looks as if he is struggling (laboring) to breathe, has noisy breathing, is breathing faster or more slowly than normal, or looks as if his chest is not moving normally. Approach the patient immediately and begin your primary survey if the patient's skin looks flushed, pale, gray, or cyanotic.

▶ Patients with dyspnea often sit or stand to inhale adequate air. In a tripod position, the patient prefers to sit up and lean forward, with the weight of her upper body supported by her hands on her thighs or knees. Orthopnea is breathlessness when lying flat that is relieved or lessened when the patient sits or stands. Paroxysmal nocturnal dyspnea is a sudden onset of difficulty breathing that occurs at night. It occurs because of a buildup of fluid in the alveoli or pooling of secretions during sleep.

▶ The normal respiratory rate for an adult at rest is 12 to 20 breaths/min. If the rate is below 12, it is called bradypnea. If the rate is above 20, it is called tachypnea.

▶ Retractions are "sinking in" of the soft tissues between and around the ribs or above the collarbones. Indentations of the skin above the collarbones (clavicles) are called supraclavicular retractions. Indentations of the skin between the ribs are called intercostal retractions. Indentations of the skin below the rib cage are called subcostal retractions.

▶ Head bobbing is an indicator of increased work of breathing in infants. When the baby breathes out, the head falls forward. The baby's head comes up when the baby breathes in and its chest expands.

▶ When determining the patient's level of respiratory distress, find out as much patient information as possible and apply the most appropriate interventions and treatments. This needs to be done rapidly and accurately. The patient should be placed in one of four categories: (1) no breathing difficulty or shortness of breath, (2) mild breathing difficulty, (3) moderate breathing difficulty, or (4) severe breathing difficulty.

▶ Croup is an infection, usually caused by one of the same viruses responsible for common colds. The virus affects the larynx and the area just below it. It is spread from person to person by droplets from coughing and sneezing. Viral croup most commonly occurs in children between the ages of 6 months and 3 years, although it can occur in older children.

▶ Epiglottitis is a bacterial infection of the epiglottis. When epiglottitis occurs in children, it typically affects children between 3 and 7 years of age. Since there is now a vaccine for epiglottitis, it is uncommon in children and more commonly seen in adults. The onset of symptoms is usually sudden, developing over a few hours. Respiratory arrest may occur because of a complete airway obstruction or a combination of partial airway obstruction and fatigue. Do not attempt to look into the child's mouth or throat. This may agitate the child and worsen respiratory distress.

▶ Pertussis, also called whooping cough, is a highly contagious bacterial infection of the respiratory tract. The bacterium that causes pertussis is found in the mouth, nose, and throat of an infected person. The disease is spread from person to person by droplets from coughing and sneezing. Pertussis can affect persons of any age.

▶ Cystic fibrosis is an inherited disease that appears in childhood. A defective gene inherited from each parent results in an abnormality in the glands that produce or secrete sweat and mucus. In CF, mucus in the lining of the bronchi becomes very thick and sticky, making it difficult to remove with coughing. The mucus builds up in the lungs, blocking the airways and leading to repeated respiratory infections and breathing difficulty.

▶ Asthma (also known as reactive airway disease) is widespread, temporary narrowing of the air passages that transport air from the nose and mouth to the lungs. After exposure to a trigger, the smooth muscles surrounding the bronchioles spasmodically contract and swell, and mucus secretion increases. Airway passages are narrowed because of smooth muscle contraction, excessive mucus secretion, or a combination of both. This results in the trapping of air in the bronchioles. Exhalation becomes prolonged as the patient tries to exhale the trapped air.

▶ Chronic bronchitis is defined as sputum production for 3 months of a year for at least 2 consecutive years. The major cause of chronic bronchitis is cigarette smoking. Excessive mucus production in the bronchi causes a chronic or recurrent productive cough. Because the size of the airway opening is decreased, some secretions are trapped in the alveoli and smaller air passages.

▶ Emphysema is an irreversible enlargement of the air spaces distal to the terminal bronchioles. This disease leads to destruction of the walls of the alveoli, distention of the alveolar sacs, and loss of lung elasticity.

▶ Pneumonia is an infection that often affects gas exchange in the lung. It may involve the lower airways and alveoli, part of a lobe, or an entire lobe of the lung. Pneumonia is most often caused by bacteria and viruses, although it may also be caused by fungi and parasites.

▶ A pulmonary embolus is usually the result of a clot that forms in the deep veins in the leg and then travels through the veins to the heart and then to the pulmonary circulation. The clot becomes trapped in the smaller branches of the pulmonary arteries, causing partial or complete blood flow obstruction. As a result, a portion of the lung is ventilated but not perfused.

▶ Pulmonary edema is most commonly caused by failure of the left ventricle of the heart. When the left ventricle fails, fluid is forced into the lung tissue as the right ventricle continues to pump blood into the pulmonary circulation. The alveoli fill with fluid, limiting their ability to effectively exchange oxygen and carbon dioxide.

▶ A spontaneous pneumothorax is a type of pneumothorax that does not involve trauma to the lung. A primary spontaneous pneumothorax occurs in people with no history of lung disease. This condition most commonly occurs in tall, thin men between the ages of 20 and 40. It rarely occurs in persons older than 40 years. A secondary spontaneous pneumothorax most often occurs as a complication of lung disease.

▶ A patient who has a prescribed MDI typically has reversible constriction of her airways. An MDI is used to deliver inhaled respiratory medications, such as bronchodilators and/or inhaled steroids.

Cardiovascular Disorders

By the end of this chapter, you should be able to:

Knowledge Objectives ▶

1. Describe the structure and function of the cardiovascular system.
2. Define cardiovascular disease, coronary heart disease (CHD), and coronary artery disease (CAD).
3. Define acute coronary syndromes (ACSs).
4. Describe the pathophysiology of coronary artery disease and the processes of atherosclerosis and arteriosclerosis.
5. Define peripheral artery disease (PAD).
6. Define and give examples of modifiable, nonmodifiable, and contributing risk factors for heart disease.
7. Define and differentiate stable and unstable angina pectoris.
8. Define acute myocardial infarction (MI), and describe possible assessment findings and symptoms associated with this condition.
9. Describe atypical assessment findings and symptoms associated with acute coronary syndromes.
10. Define congestive heart failure (CHF), and describe possible assessment findings and symptoms associated with this condition.
11. Define pulmonary edema, and describe its relationship to left ventricular failure.
12. Define hypertension, prehypertension, essential hypertension, secondary hypertension, and hypertensive emergencies.
13. Define cardiogenic shock, and describe possible assessment findings and symptoms associated with this condition.
14. Explain the importance of advanced life support intervention, if it is available, when caring for a patient with a cardiovascular emergency.
15. Describe the emergency medical care of the patient experiencing a cardio-vascular emergency.
16. Discuss the position of comfort for patients with various cardiac emergencies.
17. Discuss the use of oxygen, aspirin, and nitroglycerin in patients experiencing an acute coronary syndrome.
18. Define cardiac arrest and its possible causes.
19. Define sudden cardiac death.
20. Describe the links in the chain of survival.
21. Discuss the EMT's role in the chain of survival.
22. Define defibrillation.
23. Differentiate between a manual defibrillator, an implantable cardioverter-defibrillator, and an automated external defibrillator.
24. Differentiate between the fully automated and the semiautomated defibrillator.

25. Describe AED use in adults and children.
26. List the indications for automated external defibrillation.
27. Explain that not all patients with chest pain will experience cardiac arrest, nor do all patients with chest pain need to be attached to an AED.
28. Discuss the advantages of AEDs.
29. Discuss the use of remote defibrillation through adhesive pads.
30. Discuss the goal of quality management in automated external defibrillation.
31. Discuss the procedures that must be taken into consideration for standard operation of the various types of AEDs.
32. Explain the role medical direction plays in the use of automated external defibrillation.
33. List the steps in the operation of the AED.
34. Discuss the circumstances that may result in inappropriate shocks.
35. Explain the considerations for interruption of cardiopulmonary resuscitation when you are using an AED.
36. Discuss the importance of postresuscitation care.
37. List the components of postresuscitation care.

Attitude Objectives ▶ 38. Value the sense of urgency for assessment and intervention for the patient with cardiac compromise.

39. Explain the rationale for administering oxygen, aspirin, and nitroglycerin to a patient with chest pain or discomfort that is suspected to be of cardiac origin.

Skill Objectives ▶ 40. Demonstrate the assessment and emergency medical care of a patient experiencing chest pain or discomfort.

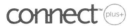

41. Demonstrate the application and operation of the AED.
42. Demonstrate the assessment and documentation of patient response to the AED.
43. Practice completing a prehospital care report for patients with cardiac emergencies.

On the Scene

Your quiet shift as on-duty EMT for a casino ends abruptly when you see an elderly woman slump forward onto a nickel slot machine. "Code 99, slot machines," you radio to the other EMTs. Donning your gloves, you move quickly to the patient. She doesn't respond to your voice or a shoulder shake, so you lower her limp body gently onto her back on the floor. "Call 9-1-1 and then bring the AED," you tell the next arriving officer. Carefully tilting her head back, you lower your ear above her nose and mouth and look to see if her chest rises. She is not breathing, so you pull a pocket mask from your uniform pants and deliver two breaths, just enough to make her chest rise. Then sliding your fingers into the groove beside her trachea, you feel for a carotid pulse. There is none, so you place your hands over her breastbone and begin chest compressions. You scan the room, hoping another EMT will arrive quickly with the AED. ■

THINK ABOUT IT

As you read this chapter, think about the following questions:

• What could have caused the patient's heart to stop beating?
• What ratio of compressions to breaths will you provide?
• Why is it important for the AED to arrive quickly?
• How will you know if her circulation resumes?

Cardiac emergencies are the most common type of medical emergency in the United States. As an EMT, you must know the signs and symptoms of cardiac compromise and give appropriate patient care based on your assessment findings. When authorized by medical direction, an EMT may assist a patient in taking aspirin and prescribed nitroglycerin. EMTs and automated external defibrillators (AEDs) are important links in the successful resuscitation of a patient in cardiac arrest away from the hospital.

Review of Circulatory System Anatomy and Physiology

Circulatory System

Components

Objective 1

The circulatory system is made up of the cardiovascular and lymphatic systems. The cardiovascular system is made up of three main parts: a pump (the heart), fluid (blood), and a container (the blood vessels). If there is a problem within this system, the problem will stem from one of these three parts.

The lymphatic system consists of lymph, lymph nodes, lymph vessels, tonsils, the spleen, and the thymus gland. The spleen, liver, and bone marrow are also associated with the circulatory system because they form and store blood.

Function

- *Transport.* Blood carries oxygen, food, hormones, minerals, and other essential substances to all parts of the body. Blood carries carbon dioxide and other waste material from the body's cells to the lungs, kidneys, or skin for elimination.
- *Maintenance of body temperature.* Blood vessels narrow (constrict) and widen (dilate) as needed to retain or dissipate heat at the skin's surface.
- *Protection.* The blood and lymphatic system protect the body against invasion by foreign microorganisms through the immune (defense) system.

The Cardiovascular System

The Heart

The heart lies in the chest cavity (mediastinum) behind the sternum and between the lungs. The heart has four chambers (Figure 22-1). The two upper chambers are the right and left atria. The atria are thin-walled chambers that receive blood from the systemic circulation and lungs. The two lower chambers are the right and left ventricles. The ventricles pump blood to the lungs and systemic circulation (body). The right ventricle pumps blood to the lungs. The left ventricle pumps blood to the body. The ventricles are larger and have thicker walls than the atria.

Four heart valves prevent the backflow of blood and keep blood moving in one direction (Figure 22-2). The tricuspid and mitral (bicuspid) valves are called **atrioventricular (AV) valves** because they lie between an atrium and ventricle. The **tricuspid valve** is located between the right atrium and right ventricle. The **mitral (bicuspid) valve** is located between the left atrium and left ventricle.

The pulmonic and aortic valves are called **semilunar valves** because they are shaped like half-moons. The **pulmonic valve** is located at the junction of the right ventricle and pulmonary artery. The **aortic valve** is located at the junction of the left ventricle and aorta (see the following *You Should Know* box).

You Should Know

Heart Valves

Atrioventricular valves
- Tricuspid
- Mitral (bicuspid)

Semilunar valves
- Aortic
- Pulmonic

The heart is more than a muscle. It contains specialized contractile and conductive tissue that allows the generation of electrical impulses. Unlike other cells of the body, specialized electrical (pacemaker) cells in the heart can produce an electrical impulse without being stimulated by another source, such as a nerve. This property is called **automaticity.** The electrical (pacemaker) cells in the heart are arranged in a system of pathways called the *conduction system* (Figure 22-3). Normally, an impulse begins in the sinoatrial (SA) node. The SA node is the heart's primary pacemaker. The impulse leaves the SA node and travels through the atrial muscle and down to the atrioventricular (AV) node. The impulse spreads from the AV node to the bundle of His, to the right and left bundle branches, and then to the Purkinje fibers. The Purkinje fibers penetrate the ventricular muscle and cause the ventricles to contract. Blood is then pumped to the lungs and through the aorta to the body.

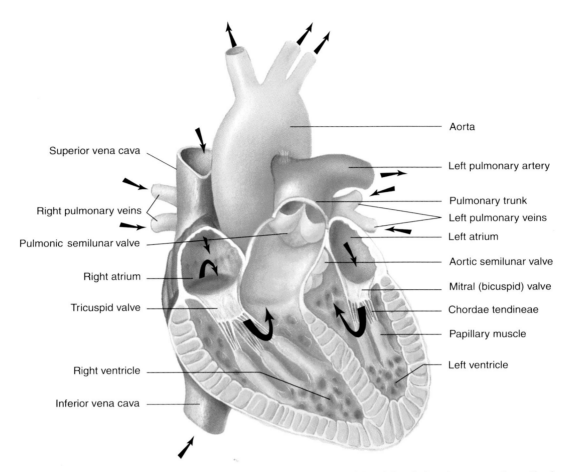

Superior vena cava

Right pulmonary veins

Pulmonic semilunar valve

Right atrium

Tricuspid valve

Right ventricle

Inferior vena cava

Aorta

Left pulmonary artery

Pulmonary trunk

Left pulmonary veins

Left atrium

Aortic semilunar valve

Mitral (bicuspid) valve

Chordae tendineae

Papillary muscle

Left ventricle

FIGURE 22-1 ▲ Blood flow through the heart. The right atrium receives blood that is low in oxygen from the body. Blood passes through the tricuspid valve into the right ventricle. The right ventricle pumps blood through the pulmonary valve to the lungs. The left atrium receives blood rich in oxygen from the lungs. Blood passes through the mitral valve into the left ventricle. The left ventricle pumps blood through the aortic valve to the aorta and out to the body.

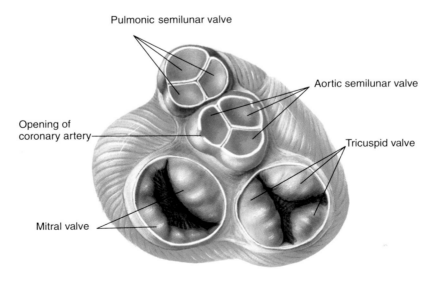

Pulmonic semilunar valve

Opening of coronary artery

Mitral valve

Aortic semilunar valve

Tricuspid valve

FIGURE 22-2 ▲ The valves of the heart.

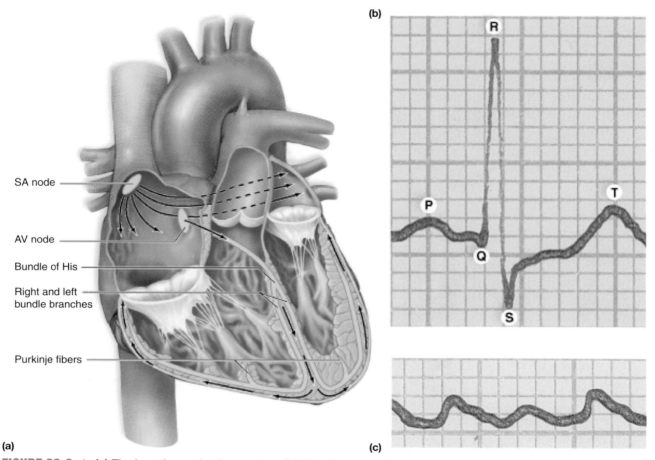

(a)   (b)   (c)

FIGURE 22-3 ▲ **(a)** The heart's conduction system. **(b)** Waveforms produced by normal electrical conduction through the heart. **(c)** This is an example of ventricular fibrillation (VF). A patient in VF is unresponsive, not breathing, and has no pulse.

SA node
AV node
Bundle of His
Right and left bundle branches
Purkinje fibers

Major Blood Vessels

Blood flow from the heart through the body moves through the following vessels: arteries → arterioles → capillaries → venules → veins. Major veins and arteries are shown in Figure 22-4.

Arteries have thick walls because they transport blood under high pressure (Figure 22-5). They carry blood away from the heart to the rest of the body. All arteries, except the pulmonary arteries, carry oxygen-rich blood. Arteries help maintain blood pressure through vasoconstriction and vasodilation.

All arteries are direct or indirect branches of the aorta. The aorta is the largest artery of the body and is the major artery originating from the heart. It lies in front of the spine in the chest and abdominal cavities. It divides at the level of the navel into the iliac arteries.

Like the other organs of the body, the heart must have its own source of oxygen-rich blood. The heart depends on two coronary arteries and their branches for its supply of oxygenated blood (Figure 22-6). Most arteries receive blood when the left ventricle contracts. However, the valve leaflets cover the openings to the coronary arteries when the left ventricle contracts. As a result, blood flows into the coronary arteries when the left ventricle is relaxed. During times of stress, the heart needs more oxygen and depends on widening (dilation) of the arteries to increase blood flow through the coronary arteries.

The carotid arteries arise from the top of the aorta (aortic arch) and are the major arteries of the neck (Figure 22-7a). They supply the head and neck with oxygen-rich blood. The pulsations of these arteries can be felt on either side of the larynx in the grooves created by the large neck muscles.

The only arteries in the body that do not carry oxygen-rich blood are the pulmonary arteries. They arise out of the right ventricle where they deliver oxygen-poor blood to the lungs for gas exchange.

The brachial artery supplies the upper arm with blood. A brachial pulse can be felt on the inside of the arm between the elbow and the shoulder. This artery is used when determining a blood pressure (BP) with a blood pressure cuff and stethoscope (Figure 22-7b). The radial artery is the major artery of the lower arm. A radial pulse can be felt on the thumb side of the wrist (Figure 22-7c).

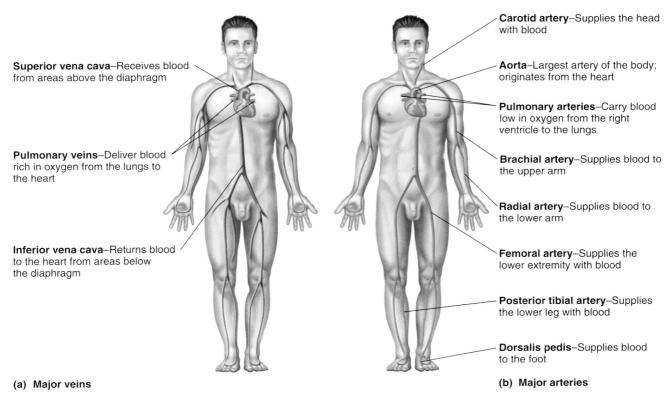

Superior vena cava–Receives blood from areas above the diaphragm

Pulmonary veins–Deliver blood rich in oxygen from the lungs to the heart

Inferior vena cava–Returns blood to the heart from areas below the diaphragm

Carotid artery–Supplies the head with blood

Aorta–Largest artery of the body; originates from the heart

Pulmonary arteries–Carry blood low in oxygen from the right ventricle to the lungs

Brachial artery–Supplies blood to the upper arm

Radial artery–Supplies blood to the lower arm

Femoral artery–Supplies the lower extremity with blood

Posterior tibial artery–Supplies the lower leg with blood

Dorsalis pedis–Supplies blood to the foot

(a) Major veins

(b) Major arteries

FIGURE 22-4 ▲ **(a)** Major veins and **(b)** major arteries.

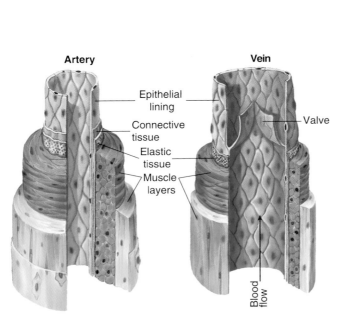

Artery

Vein

Epithelial lining

Connective tissue

Elastic tissue

Muscle layers

Valve

Blood flow

FIGURE 22-5 ▲ The walls of arteries are much thicker than the walls of veins.

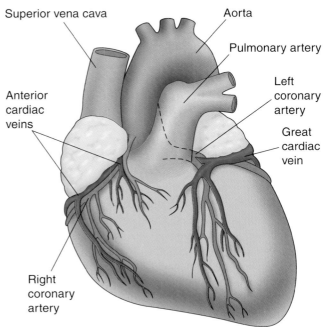

Superior vena cava

Aorta

Pulmonary artery

Anterior cardiac veins

Left coronary artery

Great cardiac vein

Right coronary artery

FIGURE 22-6 ▲ The heart depends on two coronary arteries and their branches for its supply of oxygenated blood.

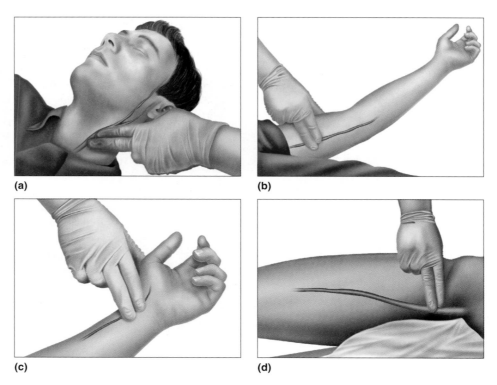

FIGURE 22-7 ▲ Major arteries and pulses: **(a)** Neck, or carotid, pulse; **(b)** arm, or brachial, pulse; **(c)** wrist, or radial, pulse; **(d)** groin, or femoral, pulse.

Remember This

The right and left carotid arteries should never be felt at the same time. Doing so can cause severe lowering of the heart rate and decrease blood flow to the brain.

The femoral arteries are the major arteries of the thigh. They supply the upper leg with blood. A femoral pulse can be felt in the groin area (the crease between the abdomen and thigh; Figure 22-7d.) The posterior tibial artery supplies the lower leg with blood. The posterior tibial pulse is located just behind the ankle bone (medial malleolus). The dorsalis pedis artery is an artery in the foot. A pedal pulse can be felt on the top surface of the foot.

Arterioles are the smallest branches of arteries leading to the capillaries. Capillaries are microscopic vessels whose walls are one cell thick. They serve as vessels for exchange of wastes, fluids, and nutrients between the blood and tissues. They connect arterioles and venules. All tissues except cartilage, hair, nails, and the cornea of the eye contain capillaries.

Venules are the smallest branches of veins leading from the capillaries. Veins are low-pressure vessels that collect blood for transport back to the heart. The major veins of the body include the pulmonary veins and the superior and inferior vena cavae (see Figure 22-4 a).

Veins contain valves to prevent backflow of blood. All veins, except the pulmonary veins, carry deoxygenated (oxygen-poor) blood. The pulmonary veins deliver blood rich in oxygen from the lungs to the left atrium of the heart. The superior vena cava receives blood from areas above the diaphragm, such as the head and upper extremities. The inferior vena cava returns blood to the heart from areas below the diaphragm, such as the torso and lower extremities. Both the superior and inferior vena cavae drain into the right atrium of the heart.

Blood

Formed elements of the blood include red blood cells (erythrocytes), white blood cells (leukocytes), and platelets (thrombocytes). Plasma is the liquid part of blood.

Red blood cells transport oxygen to body cells. Each red blood cell contains hemoglobin, an iron-containing protein. Hemoglobin carries oxygen from the lungs to the tissues and gives blood its red color. Red blood cells also transport carbon dioxide away from body cells. White blood cells defend the body from microorganisms, such as bacteria and viruses that have invaded the bloodstream or tissues of the body. Platelets are essential for the formation of blood clots. They function to stop bleeding and repair ruptured blood vessels.

Plasma is the clear, straw-colored liquid component of blood (blood minus its formed elements). Plasma carries nutrients to the cells and waste products from the cells.

Physiology of Circulation

The heart has two very important jobs. It must pump blood low in oxygen to the lungs, where the blood gives up carbon dioxide and takes on oxygen. It must also pump oxygen-rich blood to all the body's cells. To understand how the heart achieves these tasks, think of the heart as a double pump. The pumps are the right heart (lung or pulmonary circuit) and the left heart (body or systemic circuit) (Figure 22-8).

For the purposes of understanding blood flow through the body, let's use the right atrium as our reference point. Blood low in oxygen enters the right atrium and flows through the tricuspid valve and into the right ventricle. From the right ventricle, blood is pumped through the pulmonic valve into the pulmonary arteries (pulmonary circuit) and then to the lungs where red blood cells are oxygenated. From the lungs, oxygen-rich blood flows through the pulmonary veins and into the left atrium. From the left atrium, blood flows through the mitral (also called the *bicuspid*) valve and into the left ventricle. From the left ventricle, blood is pumped through the aortic valve and into the aorta (systemic circuit). From

the aorta, blood flows to the rest of the body through arteries, arterioles, capillaries, venules, and veins. Cells use the oxygen, along with nutrients from food, to make energy. Then veins carry the blood (now low in oxygen) from the body cells back to the right heart. The superior and inferior vena cavae deliver oxygen-poor blood from the body to the right atrium. Understanding the concept of blood flow and how the cardiovascular system operates will help your assessment of a patient experiencing a cardiovascular emergency.

When the left ventricle contracts, a wave of blood is sent through the arteries, causing them to expand and recoil. A pulse is the regular expansion and recoil of an artery caused by the movement of blood from the heart as it contracts. A pulse can be felt anywhere the blood in an artery simultaneously passes near the skin surface and over a bone. Central pulses are located close to the heart and include the carotid and femoral pulses. Peripheral pulses are located farther from the heart and include the radial, brachial, posterior tibial, and dorsalis pedis pulses.

Blood pressure is the force exerted by the blood on the inner walls of the heart and blood vessels. Systolic blood pressure is the pressure exerted against the walls of the arteries when the left ventricle contracts. Diastolic blood pressure is the pressure exerted against the walls of the arteries when the left ventricle is at rest.

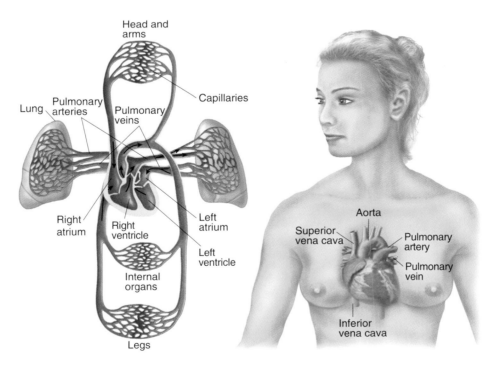

FIGURE 22-8 ▲ The heart works as a double pump. The right heart (pulmonary circuit) pumps blood to the lungs. The left heart (systemic circuit) pumps blood to the cells of the body. Red represents oxygen-rich blood and blue oxygen-poor blood.

Perfusion is the circulation of blood through an organ or a part of the body. **Shock (hypoperfusion)** is inadequate circulation of blood through an organ or a part of the body. It is a state of profound depression of the vital processes of the body. Signs and symptoms of shock are listed in the following *You Should Know* box.

You Should Know

Signs and Symptoms of Shock

- Restlessness, anxiety, or altered mental status
- Pale, cyanotic, cool, clammy skin
- Rapid, weak pulse
- Rapid, shallow breathing
- Nausea and vomiting
- Reduction in total blood volume
- Low or decreasing blood pressure

Cardiovascular Disease

Objective 2

The American Heart Association estimates that more than 70 million Americans suffer from some sort of cardiovascular disease. **Cardiovascular disease** is disease of the heart and blood vessels. **Coronary heart disease (CHD)** is disease of the coronary arteries and the complications that result, such as angina pectoris or a heart attack. **Coronary artery disease (CAD)** is a term used for diseases that slow or stop blood flow through the arteries that supply the heart muscle with blood.

Acute Coronary Syndromes

Objectives 3, 4, 5, 6

The heart depends on two coronary arteries and their branches for its supply of oxygen-rich blood. During relaxation (diastole) of the left ventricle, blood flows into the coronary arteries, supplying oxygen and nutrients to the heart. During times of stress, the heart requires more oxygen and depends on widening (dilation) of the arteries to increase blood flow through the coronary arteries.

Acute coronary syndromes (ACSs) are conditions caused by temporary or permanent blockage of a coronary artery as a result of coronary artery disease. ACSs include unstable angina pectoris and myocardial infarction. These conditions will be described in more detail later. Common causes of CAD include arteriosclerosis and atherosclerosis. **Arteriosclerosis** means hardening (*-sclerosis*) of the walls of the arteries (*arterio-*). As the walls of the arteries become hardened, they lose their elasticity. Arteriosclerosis usually begins early in life and progresses slowly with age. In **atherosclerosis,** the inner

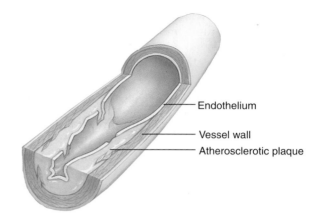

FIGURE 22-9 ▲ In atherosclerosis, the inner lining (endothelium) of the walls of large- and medium-size arteries become narrowed and thicken. Narrowing of the vessel occurs because of a buildup of plaque.

lining (endothelium) of the walls of large and medium-size arteries becomes narrowed and thickens. Narrowing of the vessel occurs because of a buildup of plaque (Figure 22-9). Plaque is usually made up of calcium, fats (lipids), cholesterol, and other substances. Although it is not known for certain how atherosclerosis starts, researchers think that inflammation causes damage to the inner lining of an artery. For example, tobacco smoke causes inflammation, damaging the inner lining of blood vessels. This speeds up the process of atherosclerosis.

When atherosclerosis affects a coronary artery, angina or a heart attack may result. When it affects the carotid arteries that supply the brain, a transient ischemic attack (TIA) or stroke may result. When atherosclerosis affects arteries that supply the arms, legs, and feet, the condition is called **peripheral artery disease (PAD).** When it affects arteries that supply the kidneys, kidney failure may result.

Conditions that may increase a person's chance of developing a disease are called **risk factors.** While some risk factors can be changed, others cannot. Risk factors that can be changed are called **modifiable risk factors.** Risk factors that cannot be changed are called **nonmodifiable risk factors.** Factors that can be part of the cause of a person's risk of heart disease are called **contributing risk factors.** Heart disease risk factors are shown in Table 22-1.

When a coronary artery becomes narrowed or blocked, the part of the heart muscle it supplies is starved for oxygen and nutrients (becomes ischemic). **Ischemia** is a reduced blood supply to an organ or tissue. Ischemia can result from narrowing or blockage of an artery or spasm of an artery. Atherosclerosis is a common reason for narrowing of a coronary artery. Body cells that lack oxygen (are ischemic) produce lactic acid. Lactic acid irritates nerve endings in the affected area, causing pain or discomfort.

TABLE 22-1 Heart Disease Risk Factors

Modifiable Factors	Nonmodifiable Factors	Contributing Factors
Diabetes mellitus	Family history	Stress
High blood pressure	Gender	Depression
Elevated blood cholesterol	Race	Heavy alcohol intake (three or more drinks per day)
Tobacco smoke	Increasing age	
Lack of exercise		
Obesity		

You Should Know

Ischemia can be reversed if treated promptly.

Angina Pectoris

Objective 7

Angina pectoris (literally, "choking in the chest") is a symptom of CAD that occurs when the heart's need for oxygen exceeds its supply. Examples of conditions that may increase the heart's demand for oxygen include physical exertion and emotional upset. In these situations, the coronary arteries normally widen to allow more blood to reach the heart muscle. When a person has CAD, the affected artery (or arteries) is unable to widen adequately because of narrowing, thickening, or blockage.

You Should Know

Angina most often occurs in patients who have disease involving one or more coronary arteries. However, it can also occur in persons who have other cardiac problems.

A person is said to have **stable angina pectoris** when the symptoms are relatively constant and predictable in terms of severity, precipitating events, and response to therapy. A person who has **unstable angina pectoris** has angina that is progressively worsening, occurs at rest, or is brought on by minimal physical exertion. A person with unstable angina has episodes of chest discomfort that occur with increased frequency or are different from her typical pattern of angina. The person's discomfort usually lasts longer than stable angina (up to 30 minutes) and may radiate more widely. Examples of situations that may lead to ischemia of the heart muscle and anginal discomfort are shown in the following *You Should Know* box.

You Should Know

Angina Pectoris: Possible Triggers
- Physical exertion
- Emotional upset
- Eating of a heavy meal
- Exposure to extreme hot or cold temperatures
- Cigarette smoking
- Sexual activity
- Stimulants, such as caffeine or cocaine

Acute Myocardial Infarction

Objectives 8, 9

An **acute myocardial infarction** (**acute MI** or "heart attack") occurs when a coronary artery becomes severely narrowed or is completely blocked, usually by a blood clot (thrombus). When the affected portion of the heart muscle (myocardium) is deprived of oxygen long enough, the area dies (infarcts) (Figure 22-10). Death of portions of the heart muscle may occur as early as 20 minutes after the onset of symptoms. The blockage within the affected coronary artery must be removed as soon as possible to prevent ischemic tissue from becoming dead tissue. If too much of the heart muscle dies, shock and cardiac arrest will result.

When the heart muscle lacks oxygen (becomes ischemic), lactic acid and carbon dioxide build up. This usually results in chest pain or discomfort that starts in the center of the chest, behind the breastbone. Anginal discomfort may be accompanied by difficulty breathing, sweating, nausea, vomiting, weakness, and palpitations. The discomfort associated with stable angina typically lasts 2 to 5 minutes. It is usually quickly relieved (less than 5 minutes) by rest and/or drugs, such as nitroglycerin (NTG). Episodes of unstable angina are usually more severe and prolonged.

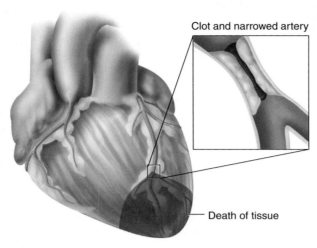

Clot and narrowed artery

Death of tissue

FIGURE 22-10 ▲ A heart attack (myocardial infarction) occurs when a coronary artery becomes severely narrowed or is completely blocked, usually by a blood clot (thrombus). When the affected portion of the heart muscle (myocardium) is deprived of oxygen long enough, the area dies (infarcts).

Typical Signs and Symptoms of Heart Attack

- Uncomfortable squeezing, ache, dull pressure, or pain in the center of the chest lasting more than a few minutes
- Discomfort in one or both arms, the back, neck, jaw, or stomach
- Anxiety, dizziness, irritability
- Abnormal pulse rate (may be irregular)
- Abnormal blood pressure
- Nausea, vomiting
- Lightheadedness
- Fainting or near fainting
- Breaking out in a cold sweat (diaphoresis)
- Weakness
- Difficulty breathing (dyspnea)
- Palpitations
- Feeling of impending doom

Remember This

Because their assessment findings and symptoms are similar, you will not be able to tell the difference between unstable angina and a heart attack in the field. Treat a patient with unstable angina with the same urgency as a patient with a possible heart attack.

Assessment findings and symptoms of a heart attack vary. Typical signs and symptoms are shown in the next *You Should Know* box. Although chest discomfort is the most common symptom of a heart attack, studies have shown than about 20% of patients who are diagnosed as having a heart attack never have chest pain. When chest discomfort is present, the patient usually describes it as located under the breastbone (substernal), but it may be present across the chest or in the upper abdomen (epigastric pain). It may radiate to the neck, jaw, teeth, back, shoulders, arms, elbows, wrists, and, occasionally, to the back between the shoulder blades. Pain usually radiates down the left arm. The patient may describe symptoms of discomfort (rather than pain) such as "pressing," "tight," "squeezing," "viselike," "aching," "heaviness," "dull," "burning," "crushing," "smothering," or indigestion-type symptoms.

As with angina, a patient who is having a heart attack may have associated symptoms such as palpitations, fainting, sweating, shortness of breath, or nausea. **Palpitations** are an abnormal awareness of one's heartbeat. Patients may describe palpitations as, "My heart is racing," "My heart is pounding," or "My heart skipped a beat." The patient may experience **fainting (syncope)** or near

fainting (near syncope). Fainting is a sudden, temporary loss of consciousness that occurs when one or both sides of the heart do not pump out a sufficient amount of blood, resulting in inadequate blood flow to the brain.

Older adults, diabetic individuals, and women often have assessment findings and symptoms of acute coronary syndromes that differ from those of a "typical" patient. This is called an *atypical presentation* or *atypical signs and symptoms*. See Table 22-2 for examples of signs and symptoms that may be seen in these patients.

Patients who experience an ACS may receive treatment to open the blocked or partially blocked coronary artery. Clot-busting drugs (fibrinolytics) are sometimes used for this purpose. In some EMS systems, paramedics can give clot-busting drugs. In others, these drugs are given in the hospital. Some patients may undergo angioplasty to open the affected coronary artery. During **angioplasty,** a balloon-tipped catheter is inserted into a partially blocked coronary artery. When the balloon is inflated, plaque is pressed against the walls of the artery, improving blood flow to the heart muscle. About 20–30% of the time, the artery closes up again within 6 months and another angioplasty needs to be done. Drug-coated stents are now used to help decrease the rate in which a vessel renarrows. A **stent** is a small plastic or metal tube that is inserted into a vessel or duct to help keep it open and maintain fluid flow through it. In some cases, the patient's cardiologist may recommend bypass surgery. A **coronary artery bypass graft (CABG)** (pronounced "cabbage") is a surgical procedure.

TABLE 22-2 Atypical Signs and Symptoms of Acute Coronary Syndromes

Older Adults	Diabetic Individuals	Women
Unexplained new onset of or worsened difficulty breathing with exertion	Change in mental status	Pain or discomfort in the chest, arms, back, shoulders, neck, jaw, or stomach
Unexplained nausea, vomiting	Weakness	Anxiety, dizziness
Sweating	Fainting	Shortness of breath
Unexplained tiredness	Lightheadedness	Weakness
Change in mental status	Shoulder and/or back pain	Unusual tiredness
Weakness		Cold sweats
Fainting		Nausea, vomiting
Abdominal discomfort		Numbness or tingling in one or both upper extremities

When a CABG is performed, a graft is created from a healthy blood vessel from another part of the patient's body. One end of the graft may be attached to the aorta and the other end to the coronary artery beyond the blockage. In this way, the graft reroutes blood flow around the diseased coronary artery.

When caring for a patient who is experiencing an acute coronary syndrome, keep in mind that "time is muscle." Studies have shown that the risk of death from a heart attack is related to the time elapsed between the onset of symptoms and start of treatment. The earlier the patient receives emergency care, the greater the chances of preventing ischemic heart tissue from becoming dead heart tissue. The American College of Cardiology and the American Heart Association recommend that eligible heart attack patients should receive treatment with clot-busting drugs within 30 minutes or angioplasty within 90 minutes from the time they present to EMS personnel or the emergency department.

Making a Difference

Because the benefits of treatment for a heart attack lessen quickly over time, it is important that patients seek medical attention as soon as possible after the onset of symptoms. Most patients experiencing an ACS do not seek medical care for 2 hours or more. When patients recognize that they are having an acute coronary syndrome, fewer than 60% use EMS for treatment and transportation to the hospital. Most patients are driven by someone else or drive themselves to the hospital.

Take the time to teach your patients, family, friends, and community how to recognize signs and symptoms associated with acute coronary syndromes. Teach them the importance of calling 9-1-1 as soon as they recognize these signs.

Congestive Heart Failure

Objectives 10, 11

When a person has **congestive heart failure (CHF),** one or both sides of the heart fail to pump efficiently. When the left ventricle fails as a pump, blood backs up into the lungs (pulmonary edema). When the right ventricle fails, blood returning to the heart backs up and causes congestion in the organs and tissues of the body. Swelling of the feet and ankles is often one of the first visible signs of CHF in patients who can walk. In patients confined to bed, swelling is seen around the lower back. Distention of the veins of the neck (jugular venous distention, or JVD) may also be seen. Possible assessment findings and symptoms are listed in the following *You Should Know* box.

You Should Know

Possible Assessment Findings and Symptoms of Heart Failure

- Fatigue
- Nausea
- Palpitations
- Swelling of the feet, ankles
- Swelling of the sacral area in bedridden patients
- Unexplained weight gain
- Shortness of breath
- Dyspnea with exertion
- Paroxysmal nocturnal dyspnea
- Orthopnea
- Jugular venous distention
- Pulmonary edema

Hypertensive Emergencies

Objective 12

Hypertension is a sustained elevation of the systolic or diastolic blood pressure. For adults 18 and older, a sustained systolic blood pressure of 140 mm Hg or higher or a diastolic pressure of 90 mm Hg or higher indicates hypertension. A person who has diabetes or chronic kidney disease has high blood pressure if his or her blood pressure is 130/80 mm Hg or higher. **Prehypertension** exists when the systolic blood pressure is between 120 and 139 or the diastolic blood pressure is between 80 and 89 on multiple readings.

In hypertension, excessive pressure is exerted on the arteries. Over time, this can result in damage to the heart, brain, eyes, blood vessels, and kidneys. Many factors can contribute to hypertension, including salt intake, hormone levels, and the condition of the individual's kidneys, nervous system, and blood vessels. When hypertension has no identifiable cause, it is called **essential hypertension** or **primary hypertension.** Hypertension that has an identifiable cause is called **secondary hypertension.** Possible causes of secondary hypertension are listed in the following *You Should Know* box. Because hypertension increases the risk of stroke, heart attack, heart failure, and kidney failure, the patient's physician will prescribe lifestyle changes and medications to reduce blood pressure and lower the patient's risk of complications.

You Should Know

Possible Causes of Secondary Hypertension

- Anxiety
- Appetite suppressants
- Atherosclerosis or arteriosclerosis
- Birth control pills
- Cocaine use
- Diabetes
- Kidney disease
- Migraine medications
- Obesity
- Pregnancy (gestational hypertension)

Hypertensive emergencies are situations that require rapid lowering of blood pressure to prevent or limit damage to organs such as the heart, brain, and kidneys. A hypertensive emergency is determined by assessment findings and symptoms of organ dysfunction, and not just by blood pressure numbers. Possible assessment findings and symptoms are listed in the following *You Should Know* box. Hypertensive emergencies usually occur in patients with a history of hypertension and may be caused by failure to take blood pressure medications or other treatments as prescribed or toxemia of pregnancy.

You Should Know

Possible Assessment Findings and Symptoms of Hypertensive Emergencies

- Responsive, altered mental status, or unresponsiveness
- Strong, bounding pulse
- Skin color may be normal, pale, or flushed
- Skin hydration may be dry or moist
- Skin temperature may be warm or cool
- Headache
- Ringing in the ears (tinnitus)
- Nausea or vomiting
- Dizziness
- Shortness of breath
- Paroxysmal nocturnal dyspnea
- Orthopnea
- Nosebleed (epistaxis)
- Seizures

Cardiogenic Shock

Objective 13

You will recall that shock is the inadequate circulation of blood through an organ or a part of the body. Because the presence of shock affects the body's ability to oxygenate and perfuse cells, shock can lead to death if it is not corrected.

The amount of blood the heart pumps throughout the body depends on how many times the heart beats and the force of the contractions. **Cardiogenic shock** is a condition in which the heart fails to function effectively as a pump. As a result, the heart does not pump enough blood to maintain adequate perfusion. Possible assessment findings and symptoms are listed in the next *You Should Know* box. Cardiogenic shock may be due to disease of or injury to the conduction system, abnormal heart rhythms (such as when the heart beats too quickly or too slowly), or an injury to the heart.

Patient Assessment

Objective 14

Patient assessment begins with doing a scene size-up and putting on appropriate personal protective equipment. Form a first impression and perform a primary survey. Assess the patient's mental status, airway, breathing, and circulation. Note the rate and rhythm of respirations and any signs of increased work of breathing (respiratory effort). Listen for air movement and note if respirations are quiet, absent, or noisy. If the patient is responsive, allow the patient to assume a position of comfort. Give 100% oxygen, preferably by nonrebreather mask. Provide calm reassurance to help reduce the patient's anxiety.

Assess the patient's pulse. If the patient has no pulse, begin cardiopulmonary resuscitation (CPR) unless there are signs of obvious death or the patient has an advance directive. If a pulse is present, estimate the heart rate. Assess pulse regularity and strength. A weak pulse may indicate a decrease in the amount of blood pumped out by the left ventricle as a result of a heart attack or CHF. An absent pulse in an extremity may indicate blockage of an artery in the extremity or severely low blood pressure.

Assess perfusion. Note the color, temperature, and moisture of the patient's skin. Cool extremities may occur from blood vessel narrowing (constriction). Sweating may indicate pain, anxiety, or shock. Pale or cyanotic (blue) skin may indicate a decrease in the amount of blood pumped out by the left ventricle as a result of a heart attack.

If appropriate, evaluate for possible major bleeding. If you have not already done so, establish patient priorities, determine the need for additional resources, and make a transport decision. Is there time to provide on-scene care, or should the patient be loaded into the ambulance and rapidly transported? Priority cardiac patients include those with severe chest pain with a systolic blood pressure of less than 100 mm Hg, those with severe respiratory distress, and pulseless patients. Additional resources for any patient experiencing a cardiovascular emergency include activation of advanced life support (ALS) assistance. ALS personnel will apply a cardiac monitor to the patient and look for signs of ischemia or injury to the patient's heart muscle. They will also start an intravenous line and give drugs for pain and abnormal heart rhythms, if present. Care should be taken to evaluate the time it will take for an ALS unit to arrive and the time that it would take to load the patient into the ambulance and transport rapidly to the closest appropriate hospital. Another consideration is meeting the ALS unit to transfer care to ALS before arrival at the hospital. In rural areas, this is often the safest way to initiate ALS care. Remember: Time is muscle.

Once you have made a transport decision, obtain a SAMPLE history from the patient if he is responsive. Remember to use the OPQRST tool if he is complaining of pain or discomfort. Examples of questions to ask a patient who is experiencing an acute coronary syndrome are shown in the following *Making a Difference* box. If the patient is unresponsive or has an altered mental status, quickly size up the scene, form a general impression, perform a primary survey, and then proceed to the rapid medical assessment.

Making a Difference

OPQRST

- **O**nset: How long ago did your symptoms begin? Did your symptoms begin suddenly or gradually? What were you doing when your symptoms began? Were you resting, sleeping, or doing some type of physical activity?
- **P**rovocation/palliation/position: What have you done to relieve the pain or discomfort? Does the discomfort disappear with rest? Have you taken any medications (such as nitroglycerin) to relieve the problem before we arrived? Is your discomfort worsened when you take a deep breath in, or does it stay the same? Does it get better or worse when you change positions, or does it stay the same?
- **Q**uality: What does the pain or discomfort feel like? (Ask the patient to describe the pain or discomfort in his own words, which may include *dull, burning, sharp, stabbing, shooting, throbbing, pressure,* or *tearing*).
- **R**egion/radiation: Where is your discomfort? Is it in one area or does it move? Is it located in any other area?
- **S**everity: On a scale of 0 to 10, with 0 being the least and 10 being the worst, what number would you give your discomfort?

Continued

- **T**ime: How long has the discomfort been present? Have you ever had these symptoms before? When? How long did they last? Compared with other episodes, would you describe this one as mild, moderate, or severe?

Additional Questions
- Do you have any allergies?
- Do you have high blood pressure, diabetes, or high cholesterol? Do you have a history of any heart problems? For example, have you ever had a heart attack, angina, congestive heart failure, or an abnormal heart rhythm? Have you ever had angioplasty, bypass surgery, stent insertion, or a heart transplant? Do you have a pacemaker or implanted defibrillator?
- Do you have a history of lung, liver, or kidney disease or any other medical condition?
- What medicines do you take? Do you take any medicines for your blood pressure or cholesterol? Do you take any water pills or medicines for your heart? When did you last take them? Do you take aspirin? When did you last take it? Do you take nitroglycerin? When did you last use it? Has the dose of any of your medications been changed recently? Do you take any medications for sexual enhancement?
- When did you last have anything to eat or drink?
- Do you smoke? How many packs per day?
- Are you having any other symptoms? For example, do you feel nauseated, more tired than usual, lightheaded, or weak? Do you feel short of breath? Have you vomited?

Patients who have heart problems are often prescribed medications. Diuretics ("water pills") may be prescribed for high blood pressure or CHF. Drugs that widen (dilate) blood vessels, such as NTG, may be prescribed to relieve chest pain and reduce the heart's workload. Antiarrhythmics ("heart pills") may be prescribed to control abnormal heart rates or rhythms. Find out if the patient takes her medications regularly and her usual response to them. Ask if there have been any recent changes in medications (additions, deletions, or change in dosages).

Find out the patient's pertinent past medical history. Patients who smoke are at an increased risk for diseases of the heart and blood vessels. Patients with a family history of heart or blood vessel disease are at increased risk for developing these conditions. Provide all information obtained to the paramedics who arrive on the scene or to the staff at the receiving facility.

If the patient is responsive, perform a focused physical examination. Remember, the focused exam is guided by the patient's chief complaint and presenting signs and symptoms. When a patient is complaining of chest discomfort, important body areas to assess include the neck, chest, abdomen, and extremities. If the patient is complaining of shortness of breath or difficulty breathing, assess the head, neck, chest, and lower extremities.

Look at the patient's face for signs of distress. Look at his neck for JVD. Look at his chest for use of accessory muscles, retractions, and equal rise and fall. Note the presence of secretions from the mouth and nose. If present, note if the secretions are blood tinged and/or foamy. These signs suggest pulmonary edema.

Observe the patient's position. The patient may place a clenched fist against her chest to indicate the location of her discomfort. The patient with CHF often sits upright with the legs in a dependent position, laboring to breathe. Assess the patient's extremities for swelling.

Listen to breath sounds. Crackles, with or without wheezes, may indicate failure of the left ventricle. If the patient can speak, note if he can speak in full sentences.

Obtain baseline vital signs. Assess the patient's pulse, respirations, blood pressure, and oxygen saturation. An increased heart rate may suggest anxiety, pain, CHF, or an abnormal heart rhythm. A decreased heart rate may suggest an abnormal heart rhythm or the effect of some heart medications. The patient's respiratory rate may be increased as a result of anxiety, pain, or CHF. An elevated blood pressure may be the result of anxiety, emotional stress, or pain or may indicate preexisting high blood pressure. A fall in blood pressure may indicate shock or the effect of some heart medications.

Emergency Care

Objectives 15, 16, 17

Provide calm reassurance to help reduce the patient's anxiety. Allow the patient to assume a position of comfort. Most patients will prefer a semi-Fowler's position. Do not allow any patient who has a heart- or breathing-related complaint to perform activities that require exertion, such as walking to the stretcher. Asking the patient to walk to a stretcher or ambulance *increases* the heart's need for oxygen. When providing emergency care to such patients, your goal is to *decrease* oxygen demand. Bring the stretcher to the patient—not the patient to the stretcher.

MONA is a memory aid used to recall the initial treatments often used by healthcare professionals when caring for patients experiencing an acute coronary syndrome.

MONA stands for:

Morphine

Oxygen

Nitroglycerin

Aspirin

Although morphine is given only by ALS personnel in the field, EMTs can begin treating the patient with the remaining three drugs. Start by giving 100% oxygen, preferably by nonrebreather mask. If the patient's breathing is inadequate, give positive-pressure ventilation with 100% oxygen. Assess the adequacy of the ventilations delivered.

Aspirin is indicated for chest pain or other signs and symptoms suspected to be of cardiac origin (see Table 22-3). Emergency medical dispatchers will generally ask the patient experiencing an acute coronary syndrome to chew aspirin while emergency personnel are en route to the scene. If ordered by medical direction (and there are no contraindications), aspirin should be given as soon as possible after the patient's onset of chest discomfort. Be sure to first verify that the patient is not allergic to aspirin. It should be used with caution in a patient who has a history of asthma, nasal

polyps, or nasal allergies. Severe allergic reactions in sensitive patients have occurred.

NTG is used to treat chest discomfort that is believed to be cardiac in origin. Find out if the patient has been prescribed NTG. If the patient does have prescribed NTG, find out if the medication is with the patient and when the last dose was taken.

Until 2004, patients were told to take up to three NTG tablets, 5 minutes apart, when they had a sudden onset of chest pain or discomfort before calling 9-1-1. This was changed to encourage earlier contacting of EMS by patients with symptoms suggestive of ACSs. Patients are now taught that if their pain or discomfort does not improve (or worsens) within 5 minutes of taking one NTG dose, the patient or a family member should call 9-1-1 right away. Patients are also taught to take a dose of the drug immediately before chest discomfort is expected to occur (such as before physical exertion) to prevent anginal symptoms.

Contact medical direction. If instructed to do so, assist the patient with the use of NTG and then continue with the focused exam. Remember to reassess the patient's vital signs after *each dose* of this drug. Table 22-4 summarizes important information about

TABLE 22-3 Aspirin

Generic name	acetylsalicylic acid
Trade name	Bayer, Ecotrin, Empirin, and others
Mechanism of action	Inhibits platelet clumping, thus interfering with blood clotting
Indications	Chest pain or other signs and symptoms suspected to be of cardiac origin
Dosage (adult)	Two to four 81-mg tablets (baby aspirin), chewed and swallowed
Adverse effects	• Rapid pulse • Dizziness • Flushing • Nausea, vomiting • Gastrointestinal bleeding
Contraindications	• Known allergy or sensitivity to aspirin • Bleeding ulcer or bleeding disorders • Children and adolescents
Special considerations	• Obtain an order from medical direction either on-line or off-line to give the medication. • If ordered by medical direction, aspirin should be given as soon as possible after the patient's onset of chest discomfort. • Use appropriate personal protective equipment. • Practice the six rights of drug administration. • Use with caution in the patient with a history of asthma, nasal polyps, or nasal allergies. Severe allergic reactions in sensitive patients have occurred.

TABLE 22-4 Nitroglycerin

Generic name	nitroglycerin
Trade names	Nitrostat, Nitro-Bid, Nitrolingual, Nitroglycerin Spray
Mechanism of action	• Relaxes blood vessels • Decreases the workload of the heart
Indications	An EMT can assist a patient in taking nitroglycerin if *all* the following criteria are met: • The patient has signs and symptoms of chest discomfort suspected to be of cardiac origin. • The patient has physician-prescribed sublingual tablets or spray. • There are no contraindications to giving nitroglycerin. • The EMT has specific authorization by medical direction.
Dosage	Dosage is one tablet or one spray under the tongue. This dose may be repeated in 3 to 5 minutes (maximum of three doses) if: • The patient experiences no relief. • The patient's systolic blood pressure remains above 100 mm Hg systolic. • The patient's heart rate remains between 50 and 100 beats per minute. • There are no other contraindications. • The EMT is authorized by medical direction to give another dose of the medication.
Adverse effects	Hypotension is a common and significant side effect. Other side effects include tachycardia, bradycardia, headache, palpitations, and fainting.
Contraindications	• Medical direction does not give permission • Medication not prescribed for the patient • Patient has already taken maximum prescribed dose before EMT arrival • Hypotension or blood pressure below 100 mm Hg systolic • Heart rate less than 50 beats/min or more than 100 beats/min • Head injury (recent) or stroke (recent) • Infants and children • Patient has taken a medication for sexual enhancement within the last 24 to 48 hours
Special considerations	• NTG is heat and light sensitive. If the patient has been carrying this medication in a pocket, it may no longer be effective. • Be watchful for a change in the patient's level of responsiveness after giving this medication. • Because NTG relaxes blood vessels, it has the potential to significantly decrease the patient's blood pressure. Reassess the patient's vital signs after *each dose* of this drug. • Recheck the patient's vital signs within 2 minutes. • Reassess the patient's degree of discomfort.

sublingual NTG that you should know. Skill Drills 11-5 and 11-6 in Chapter 11 show the procedure for assisting a patient with prescribed NTG.

If the patient does not have prescribed NTG, continue the focused exam. Transport promptly if:

• The patient has signs of cardiac compromise and no prior history of cardiac problems.

• The patient has a history of cardiac problems but does not have NTG.

• The patient has a systolic blood pressure of less than 100 mm Hg.

Reassess as often as indicated until patient care is turned over to ALS personnel or medical personnel at the receiving facility.

Cardiac Arrest

Objectives 18, 19

If the heart stops beating, no blood will flow. If no blood flows, oxygen cannot be delivered to the body's cells. When the heart stops, the patient is said to be in **cardiac arrest.** The signs of cardiac arrest include sudden unresponsiveness, absent breathing, and no signs of circulation. Possible causes of a cardiac arrest are shown in the following *You Should Know* box.

Because the organs of the body must have oxygen, chest compressions are used to circulate blood any time that the heart is not beating. Chest compressions are combined with rescue breathing to oxygenate the blood. The combination of rescue breathing and external chest compressions is called **cardiopulmonary resuscitation (CPR).** Rescue breathing should always be performed using a barrier device or pocket mask. Mouth-to-mouth breathing is not recommended.

Sudden cardiac death (SCD) is the unexpected death from cardiac causes early after symptom onset (immediately or within 1 hour) or without the onset of symptoms. About two-thirds of sudden cardiac deaths take place away from the hospital, usually in a private or residential setting.

The Chain of Survival

Objectives 20, 21

Survival of cardiac arrest depends on a series of critical actions called the *chain of survival*. The **chain of survival** is the ideal series of events that should take place immediately after recognition of an injury or the onset of sudden illness (Figure 22-11).

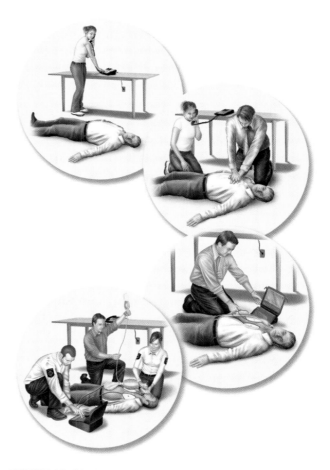

FIGURE 22-11 ▲ The chain of survival.

The chain of survival consists of four crucial steps:

1. **Early access (recognition of an emergency and calling 9-1-1).** The public must be educated to recognize the early warning signs of a heart attack. Many patients do nothing and hope their symptoms will go away. The average time between the onset of symptoms and admission to a medical facility is about 3 hours. Some patients may delay seeking help for more than 24 hours. A patient's collapse must be identified by a person who can activate the EMS system. CPR training teaches citizens how to contact the EMS system, decreasing the time to defibrillation. EMS personnel must arrive rapidly to the scene with all necessary equipment.

2. **Early CPR.** Bystander CPR is the best treatment the patient can receive until arrival of a defibrillator and advanced cardiac life support (ACLS) personnel.

3. **Early defibrillation. Defibrillation** is the delivery of an electrical shock to a patient's heart to end an abnormal heart rhythm, such as **ventricular fibrillation (VF or VFib).** When the heart is in VF, the electrical impulses are completely disorganized. As a result, the heart cannot pump blood effectively. If you were able to look at the heart while it is in VF, you would see it quivering like a bowl of gelatin. For every minute that the patient's heart is in VF, the chance of surviving the cardiac arrest decreases by about 10% without bystander CPR. When bystander CPR is provided, the decline in chance of survival is more gradual, averaging 3–4% per minute. The only effective treatments for VF are CPR and the delivery of electrical shocks to the heart with a machine called a *defibrillator.* The shock attempts to stop VF and allow the patient's normal heart rhythm to start again. CPR can keep oxygen-rich blood flowing to the heart and brain until the arrival of an *automated external defibrillator (AED)* and advanced care.

4. **Early advanced care.** Early advanced care provided by paramedics at the scene is a critical link in the treatment of cardiac arrest. Paramedics combine defibrillation by first-responding units with airway management and intravenous medications by the ALS units. If ALS units are not available, the patient should be transported rapidly to a facility for definitive cardiac care.

Time is critical when dealing with a victim of cardiac arrest. A break in any of the links in the chain can reduce the patient's chance of survival, despite excellence in the rest of the chain.

You are an important part of the chain of survival. As an EMT, you will rarely perform one-rescuer CPR while on duty. However, you may need to perform CPR alone while your EMT partner is preparing equipment or your partner is driving to a receiving facility.

When providing care for a patient in cardiac arrest, you must know:

- Appropriate use of standard precautions
- How to use an AED
- When to request available ALS backup
- How to suction the patient's airway
- How to use airway adjuncts
- How to use a bag-mask (BM) device with oxygen attached
- How to use a flow-restricted, oxygen-powered ventilation device
- Techniques for safe lifting and moving patients in cardiac arrest
- Techniques for interviewing bystanders and family members to obtain facts related to a cardiac arrest
- Techniques of effective CPR
- How to assist ALS personnel when requested (and allowed by state and regional authorities)

When you arrive at the scene of a cardiac arrest, you should start CPR immediately if the patient is unresponsive, breathless (apneic), and pulseless. The steps for CPR are shown in Appendix A. However, you should not perform CPR if there is a valid do not resuscitate (DNR) order or in cases of obvious death. If you arrive on the scene of a cardiac arrest and the DNR paperwork is unclear, the validity of the DNR order is questionable, or a written DNR order (or DNR bracelet) is not present, begin resuscitation efforts and call additional medical help to the scene.

Patient Assessment and Emergency Care

After determining that the scene is safe, form a general impression of the patient. A patient in cardiac arrest appears unresponsive and does not appear to be breathing. Skin color is usually pale, gray, or blue.

Assess Responsiveness

Begin the primary survey. Use the AVPU scale to quickly check the patient's level of responsiveness (mental status). Gently squeeze the patient's shoulders and shout, "Are you all right?" If the patient does not respond, shout for help. If you are alone and there is no response to your shout for help, contact your dispatcher and request additional resources, including an AED (if you do not have an AED with you).

A = Airway

If the patient is unresponsive and you do not suspect trauma, open her airway by using the head tilt–chin lift maneuver. If you suspect trauma, open the airway by using the modified jaw thrust maneuver. If trauma is suspected but you are unable to maintain an open airway by using the jaw thrust, open the airway by using the head tilt–chin lift maneuver. If the patient is an unresponsive infant or child, do not hyperextend the neck when opening the airway. Suction any blood, vomit, or other fluid that may be present from the patient's airway.

B = Breathing

After you have made sure that the patient's airway is open, assess his breathing. Place your face near the patient and look for the rise and fall of the chest. Listen and feel for air movement from the patient's nose or mouth. The assessment of breathing should take at least 5 seconds but no more than 10 seconds. If the patient's breathing is not adequate, begin rescue breathing by using a pocket mask, mouth-to-barrier device, or bag-mask device. If the patient has dentures and they fit well, leave them in place to help provide a good mask seal. If the dentures are loose, remove them so that they do not fall back into the throat and block the airway. Give two breaths (each breath over 1 second) with just enough force to make the chest rise with each breath.

Making a Difference

If the patient is breathing very slowly or has occasional, gasping breaths (agonal breathing), the breathing is inadequate. Provide emergency care as if the patient were not breathing at all.

Watch the patient's chest while you breathe into the patient. If your breaths are going in, you should see the chest rise with each breath. Be sure to pause between breaths. This pause allows you to take another breath. It also allows the patient's lungs to relax and air to escape. If the patient is unresponsive, insert an oral airway to help keep the patient's airway open. Continue breathing for the patient until she begins to breathe adequately on her own or another trained rescuer takes over.

If your first breath does not go in, gently reposition the patient's head and breathe for him again. If the breaths still do not go in, you must assume the airway is blocked. If the patient is unresponsive, check for a pulse.

Remember This

Ventilate the patient with just enough pressure to make the chest rise with each breath. If you give breaths too quickly or too forcefully, you will push air into the stomach. This causes the stomach to distend (swell) with air and the patient may vomit. If the patient vomits, roll the patient onto his side until the vomiting stops. Suction the vomitus from the patient's mouth. Then roll the patient onto his back and resume rescue breathing if needed.

C = Circulation

Once you have made sure that the patient's airway is open and have started rescue breathing, assess circulation. Use the carotid artery to check the pulse of an unresponsive adult or child older than 1 year of age. Feel for a brachial pulse in an unresponsive infant. Feel for a pulse for at least 5 seconds but no more than 10 seconds. If you definitely feel a pulse, give one breath every 5 to 6 seconds for an adult. Give one breath every 3 to 5 seconds for an infant or child. Reassess the patient's pulse about every 2 minutes. If you do not definitely feel a pulse within 10 seconds, or if you are uncertain, begin chest compressions.

Remember This

For chest compressions to be effective, the patient must be positioned on a firm, level surface. If you find the patient in bed, move her to the floor. Place her arms at her sides. If the patient is found facedown, ask your partner to help you carefully roll the patient, so that her head, shoulders, and chest move together as a unit without twisting. Once the patient is lying face-up, position yourself at the patient's side so that you can provide rescue breathing and chest compressions if necessary.

Chest Compressions—Adult

Kneel beside the patient's chest. Place the heel of one hand in the center of the patient's chest, between the nipples. Place your other hand on top of the first. Interlock the fingers of both hands to keep your fingers off the patient's ribs. If you have arthritis in your hands or wrists, give compressions by grasping the wrist of the hand that is on the patient's chest with your other hand and pushing down with both.

Position yourself directly above the patient's chest so that your shoulders are directly over your hands. With your arms straight and your elbows locked, press down about 1½ to 2 inches on the adult patient's breastbone with the heels of your hands. Release pressure (let up) after each compression to allow the patient's chest to recoil. Releasing pressure on the patient's chest allows blood to flow into the chest and heart. When performing adult CPR, deliver 30 compressions at a rate of about 100 compressions per minute. One cycle consists of 30 chest compressions and 2 rescue breaths. After 5 cycles (which is about 2 minutes), check for a pulse. If the patient has a pulse, check breathing. If the patient has a pulse but is not breathing, give rescue breaths at a rate of 1 breath every 5 to 6 seconds. If there is still no pulse, continue CPR. Check for a pulse again every few minutes.

Because performing chest compressions is tiring, rescuers should switch roles about every 2 minutes or five cycles of CPR. The "switch" should ideally take place in 5 seconds or less. Two-rescuer CPR is discussed in more detail in Appendix A.

Chest Compressions—Child

For the general public, CPR guidelines for a child pertain to a child from 1 to about 8 years of age. For healthcare professionals, a child is considered any youngster between 1 year old and the start of puberty (about 12 to 14 years of age). For children between the ages of 1 and 12 to 14, perform chest compressions if there is no pulse. You should also perform compressions if a pulse is present but the heart rate is less than 60 beats per minute with signs of poor perfusion (pale, cool, mottled skin). A child's chest may be compressed using the heel of one hand or the same technique as for an adult. Press down on the breastbone about one-third to one-half the depth of the chest. Give chest compressions at a rate of about 100 compressions per minute. After every 30 compressions, give 2 rescue breaths.

Chest Compressions—Infant

For an infant, perform chest compressions if there is no pulse. You should also perform compressions if a pulse is present but the heart rate is less than 60 beats per minute with signs of poor perfusion (pale, cool, mottled skin). Compress the infant's chest with two fingers. Press down on the breastbone about one-third to one-half the depth of the chest. Give chest compressions at a rate of about 100 compressions per minute. After every 30 compressions, give 2 rescue breaths.

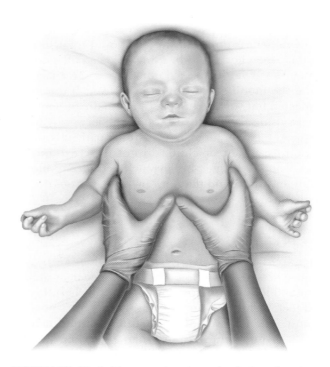

FIGURE 22-12 ▲ The two-thumb method of performing CPR on an infant. This method is used when two rescuers are available.

When two healthcare professionals are available to perform CPR on an infant, the two-thumb technique is preferred for performing chest compressions. Place your thumbs side by side or one on top of the other over the lower half of the infant's breastbone. Your thumbs should be placed about one finger's width below the nipple line (Figure 22-12). Encircle the infant's chest with the fingers of both hands. Use your thumbs to compress the chest about one-third to one-half the depth of the chest. The second EMT gives the rescue breaths.

CPR guidelines for adults, children, and infants are presented in Table 22-5.

D = Defibrillation

Types of Defibrillators

Objectives 22, 23, 24

A **defibrillator** is a device that delivers an electrical shock to a patient's heart to stop an abnormal heart rhythm. Defibrillation is the technique of administering the electrical shock. A **manual defibrillator** requires that the rescuer to analyze and interpret the patient's cardiac rhythm (Figure 22-13). If the rhythm requires defibrillation, the rescuer applies paddles or adhesive pads to the patient's chest to deliver the shock. This type of defibrillator is used by ALS and hospital personnel.

An **implantable cardioverter-defibrillator (ICD)** is a device that is surgically placed below the skin surface

TABLE 22-5 Cardiopulmonary Resuscitation Guidelines

	Adult	Child	Infant
Patient age	More than 12 to 14 years	1 through 12 to 14 years	Under 1 year
Rescue breaths	About 10–12 breaths/min 1 breath every 5–6 sec	About 12–20 breaths/min 1 breath every 3–5 sec	About 12–20 breaths/min 1 breath every 3–5 sec
Location of pulse check	Carotid	Carotid	Brachial
Method of chest compressions	Heel of 1 hand, other hand on top	Heel of 1 hand or same as for adult	2 fingers (1 rescuer) *or* 2 thumbs with the fingers of both hands encircling the chest (2 rescuers)
Depth of chest compressions	1½ to 2 inches	⅓ to ½ the chest depth	⅓ to ½ the chest depth
Rate of chest compressions	About 100/min	About 100/min	About 100/min
Ratio of chest compressions to rescue breaths (one cycle)	1 or 2 rescuers: 30 compressions to 2 breaths (30:2)	1 rescuer: 30 compressions to 2 breaths (30:2) 2 rescuers: 15 compressions to 2 breaths (15:2)	1 rescuer: 30 compressions to 2 breaths (30:2) 2 rescuers: 15 compressions to 2 breaths (15:2)

in the patient's chest wall (usually under the skin beneath the shoulder) or upper abdomen (Figure 22-14). A person who has an ICD has had, or is at high risk of having, heart rhythm problems. An ICD is programmed to recognize heart rhythms that are too fast or life-threatening (such as VF). When an ICD recognizes a too fast rhythm or VF, it delivers a shock to the heart to "reset" it. Because an ICD is in direct contact with the heart muscle by using wires, much less energy is needed to deliver a shock than is required when an external defibrillator is used.

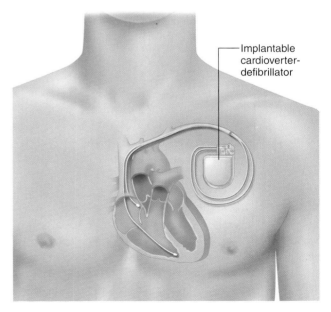

Implantable cardioverter-defibrillator

FIGURE 22-14 ▲ An implantable cardioverter-defibrillator (ICD) is surgically placed below the skin surface in the patient's chest wall (usually under the skin beneath the shoulder) or upper abdomen.

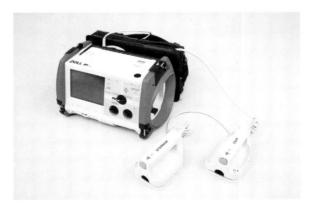

FIGURE 22-13 ▲ A manual defibrillator requires a healthcare professional to interpret the patient's heart rhythm.

An **automated external defibrillator (AED)** contains a computer programmed to recognize heart rhythms that should be shocked, such as VF (Figure 22-15). The accuracy of AEDs in rhythm analysis is high in detecting rhythms needing shocks and rhythms that do not need shocks. Accurate rhythm analysis is dependent on properly charged defibrillator batteries and proper defibrillator maintenance.

An AED is attached to the patient by means of connecting cables and two disposable adhesive pads. The adhesive pads have a thin metal pad covered by a thick layer of adhesive gel. The pads record the patient's heart rhythm and, if appropriate, deliver a shock. When the pads are placed on the patient's bare chest, the AED examines the patient's heart rhythm for any abnormalities.

There are many AED manufacturers. As a result, there are slight differences in AED screen layouts and controls and in the location to plug in the adhesive pads. There are also differences in color, weight, and voice instructions. It is essential that you understand and be familiar with the operation of the AED used by your EMS agency.

You must also know the difference between a fully automated external defibrillator and a **semiautomated external defibrillator (SAED).** When a fully automated external defibrillator is used, the power is turned on and the pads are attached to the patient. The AED then performs all the necessary steps to defibrillate the patient. A fully automated machine analyzes the patient's heart rhythm, warns everyone to stand clear of the patient if it recognizes a shockable rhythm, and then delivers a shock through the pads that were applied to the patient's chest.

An SAED is also called a *shock-advisory defibrillator*. When an SAED is used, the power is turned on and the adhesive pads are attached to the patient.

Some AEDs require that the rescuer press an "analyze" control to begin analyzing the patient's cardiac rhythm, while others automatically begin analyzing the patient's cardiac rhythm when the adhesive pads are attached to the patient's chest. The SAED, by means of a voice or visual message, "advises" the rescuer of the steps to take on the basis of its analysis of the patient's heart rhythm. For example, if an SAED detects a shockable rhythm, it will advise the rescuer to press the shock control to deliver a shock. Use of the letters AED in the remainder of this text implies use of an SAED because most AEDs in use today are SAEDs.

Older AEDs were monophasic defibrillators, which means that the current delivered by the defibrillator passed through the heart in one direction. Newer AEDs are biphasic defibrillators, in which the defibrillator delivers current in two phases. The current passes through the heart in one direction and then passes through the heart again in the opposite direction.

Adult and Pediatric Defibrillation

Objectives 25, 26, 27

A standard AED is used for a patient who is unresponsive, not breathing, pulseless, and greater than or equal to 8 years of age (about 55 pounds, or more than 25 kg). A special key or pad-cable system is available for some AEDs so that the machine can be used on children between 1 and 8 years of age. The key or pad-cable system decreases the amount of energy delivered to a dose appropriate for a child (Figure 22-16). If a child is in cardiac arrest and a key or pad-cable system is not available, use a standard AED.

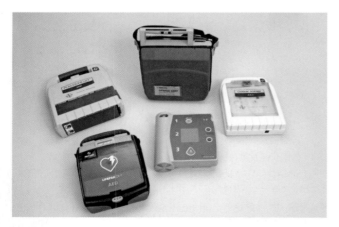

FIGURE 22-15 ▲ Examples of automated external defibrillators.

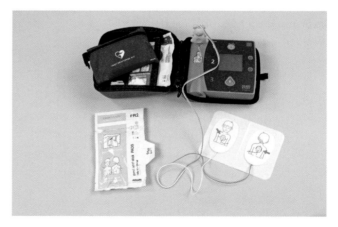

FIGURE 22-16 ▲ Special pads and cables are available for some AEDs for use on children between 1 and 8 years of age.

Not all patients who have chest pain experience a cardiac arrest. A patient who has chest pain or discomfort does not need to be attached to an AED. However, a patient who has signs of cardiac compromise is at increased risk of sudden cardiac death. With this in mind, make sure that you have oxygen, an oral airway, a bag-mask device, suction equipment, and an AED within arm's reach in case of cardiac arrest.

Under current resuscitation guidelines, an AED should be applied only to an adult or child who is unresponsive, breathless (apneic), and pulseless. Although AEDs exist for use in infants, current resuscitation guidelines make no recommendation for or against AED use in infants.

When an adult experiences a cardiac arrest caused by VF, prompt defibrillation is the most important treatment you can provide from the time of the arrest to about 5 minutes following the arrest. For example, if you arrive on the scene and see an adult collapse (witness a cardiac arrest), assess the patient's airway, breathing, and circulation, and then quickly apply an AED. Perform CPR until the AED is ready. Survival rates from witnessed cardiac arrest are highest when immediate CPR is provided and defibrillation occurs within 3 to 5 minutes.

When EMS personnel arrive more than 4 to 5 minutes after an adult cardiac arrest, studies have shown increased survival rates when CPR is performed for about 2 minutes before attempting defibrillation. Check with your medical director about your EMS agency's standard operating procedure in such situations. Your medical director may recommend that if you arrive at the scene of an adult cardiac arrest, you did not witness the patient's collapse, and your response time is more than 4 to 5 minutes, your operating procedure should be to provide five cycles of CPR (about 2 minutes) and then analyze the patient's rhythm with an AED.

Advantages of Automated External Defibrillators

Objectives 28, 29

- Learning to use and operate an AED is easy. The AED provides voice and visual prompts to the user. During training, rescuers learn to recognize a cardiac arrest (unresponsive, apneic, pulseless patient), learn how to properly attach the AED to the patient, and memorize the treatment sequence.
- Less training is required to operate an AED and maintain skills in its use than is the case with a manual defibrillator.
- AEDs use adhesive pads attached to the patient by connecting cables to deliver shocks to the patient.

This helps ensure rescuer safety because the rescuer is not in direct contact with the patient during the AED's analysis of the patient's rhythm or during the shock phase of AED operation. This feature permits what is called *remote, hands-free,* or *hands-off* defibrillation. The adhesive pads used cover a larger surface area than the paddles of manual defibrillators, delivering more effective shocks.

- Some AEDs are equipped with a screen that allows rescuers to view the patient's heart rhythm. This is often useful to ALS personnel because they can select specific drugs to give the patient on the basis of the rhythm seen. They can also continue monitoring the patient's heart rhythm with the AED after resuscitation.
- In some areas, studies have shown high survival rates (49% to 74%) for witnessed cardiac arrests away from a hospital when CPR and AEDs are used. Examples of areas showing improved survival rates include casinos, airports, and commercial passenger planes.

Special Considerations

Objective 30

- Before using the AED, make certain all personnel are clear of the patient, stretcher, and defibrillator.
- Before applying the AED pads, quickly look at the patient's chest and upper abdomen for a small lump under the skin that suggests the presence of a permanent pacemaker or ICD. Do not hesitate to apply an AED if the patient is in cardiac arrest and has a pacemaker or ICD in place. In such situations, place the AED pads at least 1 inch from the pacemaker or ICD.
- When applying AED pads to the patient's chest, make sure there are no air pockets between the pads and the patient's skin. Press from one edge of the pad across the entire surface to remove all air.
- If the patient has a hairy chest, the AED pads may not stick to the patient's chest. The AED will be unable to analyze the patient's heart rhythm and will give a "check electrodes" message. Try pressing down firmly on each AED pad, and see if that corrects the problem. If the "check electrodes" message from the AED persists (and you have a second set of AED pads available), quickly remove the AED pads. This will remove some of the patient's chest hair. Quickly look at the patient's chest. If a lot of chest hair remains, quickly shave the areas of the chest where the AED pads will be

placed. Put on a second set of AED pads. Follow the prompts by the AED.

- Before using an AED, familiarize yourself with the manufacturer's recommendations regarding the use of the device around water. If the patient is lying on a metal surface, remove the patient from contact with the surface before attaching the AED.

- If a medication patch is present on the patient's chest, make sure you are wearing gloves and then remove the patch. Do not place an AED pad over the medication patch and try to defibrillate through it. Examples of medications that may be worn in patch form by patients include NTG; nicotine; hormone replacement therapy; and medications for nausea, vomiting, dizziness, blood pressure, and pain control. After removing the patch, wipe the area clean with a dry cloth before applying the AED pads. Do not use alcohol or alcohol-based cleansers.

- Before delivering a shock with an AED, make sure that oxygen is not flowing over the patient's chest. Fire can be ignited by sparks from poorly applied AED pads in an oxygen-enriched atmosphere.

Medical Direction and Quality Management

Objectives 31, 32

Just as for the other skills you perform as an EMT, you will operate an AED under the authorization of a medical director. To ensure delivery of the best-quality patient care possible, the medical director (or designated representative) carefully reviews every call in which an AED is used. Quality management involves the performance of individuals using AEDs, the effectiveness of the EMS system in which AEDs are used, and data collection and review.

AEDs are equipped with memory modules that record important information for later review by medical direction. The data from the AED can be downloaded to a computer or pocket PC. Examples of information recorded by an AED include the patient's heart rhythm, number of shocks delivered, time of each shock delivered, and the energy level used for each shock. Some AEDs also document CPR compression data. Some AEDs have an audio recording feature that is voice-activated so that conversation during the call is recorded.

In addition to reviewing the data from the AED, the medical director will also review the prehospital care report pertaining to the call, voice recordings (if the AED is so equipped), and magnetic tape recordings stored in the AED (if so equipped). Each call is reviewed to determine if the patient was treated ac-

cording to professional standards and local standing orders. Other areas that may be evaluated include:

- Scene command
- Safety
- Efficiency
- Speed
- Professionalism
- Ability to troubleshoot
- Completeness of patient care
- Interactions with other professionals and bystanders

By reviewing each call in which an AED is used, problems within the EMS system can be identified, each link in the chain of survival can be evaluated, and EMS personnel can learn from their successes and mistakes.

Operation of the Automated External Defibrillator

Objective 33

Follow these steps to operate an AED:

1. **Power.** Be sure the patient is lying face-up, on a firm, flat surface. Start CPR if the AED is not immediately available. Place the AED next to the rescuer who will be operating it. Turn on the power. Depending on the brand of AED, this is done by either pressing the ON button or lifting up the AED screen or lid.

2. **Pads.** Open the package containing the AED pads. Connect the pads to the AED cables (if not pre-connected). Then apply the pads to the patient's bare chest. The correct position for the pads is usually shown on the package containing the pads. Alternately, it may be shown in a diagram on the AED itself. If the patient's chest is wet, quickly dry it before applying the pads. Briefly stop CPR to allow pad placement on the patient's chest. Connect the cable to the AED.

3. **Analyze.** Analyze the patient's heart rhythm. Some AEDs require that you press an "analyze" button. Other defibrillators automatically start to analyze when the pads are attached to the patient's chest. Do not touch the patient while the AED is analyzing the rhythm.

4. **Shock.** If the AED advises that a shock is indicated, check the patient from head to toe to make sure no one (including you) is touching the patient before pressing the shock control. Make sure oxygen is not flowing over the patient's chest. Remove oxygen-delivery devices, such as a bag-mask device, from around the patient and stretcher. Shout, "Stand clear!" Press the shock control once it is illuminated and the machine indicates it is ready to deliver the

shock. Resume CPR, beginning with chest compressions, immediately after delivery of the shock unless the patient regains consciousness or begins spontaneous movement. After five cycles of CPR, reanalyze the rhythm. Continue this sequence until the patient regains a pulse, the patient regains consciousness or begins spontaneous movement, or ALS personnel take over patient care. The decision to remain on scene for ALS personnel, transport to a rendezvous with ALS, or transport directly to a medical facility depends on local protocol, transport time, and medical direction.

The adult AED sequence is shown in Skill Drill 22-1.

Inappropriate Delivery of Shocks

Objective 34

In some cases, an AED may deliver inappropriate shocks. In all cases, this can be attributed to one of two things: mechanical or human error. Mechanical error, such as low batteries, can cause an inappropriate delivery of shocks. This is because accurate rhythm analysis is dependent on properly charged defibrillator batteries.

Human error, such as failure to follow the manufacturer's instructions in the use of an AED, can result in the delivery of inappropriate shocks. To avoid delivering inappropriate shocks:

- Attach an AED only to unresponsive, apneic, pulseless patients.
- Place an AED in the "analyze" mode *only* when cardiac arrest has been confirmed and all movement, including the movement of patient transport, has stopped. When transporting a patient, the AED may remain attached to the patient. However, do not press the "analyze" button while the patient is being moved. For example, if you are en route to the hospital with the patient in an ambulance, the vehicle must be brought to a stop before you press the "analyze" button.
- Avoid using cell phones, radios, or other devices that emit electrical signals during rhythm analysis. Signal noise may interfere with the AED's analysis of the patient's cardiac rhythm.

Interruption of Cardiopulmonary Resuscitation

Objective 35

Movement caused by CPR can cause the AED to stop its analysis of the patient's rhythm. No one should be touching the patient when the patient's cardiac rhythm is being analyzed and when shocks are delivered. Chest compressions and positive-pressure ventilations must be stopped when the rhythm is being analyzed and

when shocks are delivered. This prevents accidental shocks to rescuers and allows accurate rhythm analysis. Resume CPR immediately after delivering a shock or when the AED advises that no shock is indicated.

When chest compressions are stopped for even a few seconds (such as to give rescue breaths or perform other procedures), blood flow to the heart and brain drops quickly and drastically. To help improve your patient's chances of surviving a cardiac arrest, make sure that interruptions in chest compressions are kept to a minimum when performing CPR.

Postresuscitation Care

Objectives 36, 37

If the patient begins moving, check the patient's pulse and breathing. If the patient is breathing adequately, apply oxygen by nonrebreather mask at 15 L/min and transport. If the patient is not breathing adequately, provide positive-pressure ventilation with 100% oxygen. Secure the patient to a stretcher. Depending on local protocol, you may be expected to remain on scene for ALS personnel, begin transport and rendezvous with ALS personnel, or transport directly to a medical facility. Remember to use proper lifting and moving techniques when transferring the patient to the ambulance. Keep the AED attached to the patient during transport. En route, perform a focused physical exam, and then reassess every 5 minutes.

Recent studies have shown that inducing hypothermia for cardiac arrest victims may improve neurological outcome and survival to hospital discharge. By lowering body temperature to 89.6°F (32°C), the metabolic demands of the brain and the risk of cerebral swelling are reduced. Because studies have shown that some of the most important benefits of induced hypothermia are achieved if therapy is started within 15 minutes of resuscitation, many EMS systems have developed protocols that specify when and how hypothermia is to be induced in the field. For example, the protocol may specify that hypothermia be induced in the field if the patient has a return of spontaneous circulation but remains unresponsive after resuscitation from cardiac arrest that is not due to trauma or hemorrhage. Check with your instructor and EMS agency about the use of prehospital hypothermia in your area.

Cardiac Arrest During Transport

If you are transporting a patient who stops breathing and becomes pulseless, stop the vehicle. Start CPR and apply the AED. Analyze the rhythm as soon as the AED is ready. Deliver a shock, if indicated. Immediately resume CPR. Continue resuscitation (and transport) according to your local protocol.

Adult Automated External Defibrillator Sequence

STEP 1 ▶

- Be sure the patient is lying face-up, on a firm, flat surface.
- Place the AED next to the rescuer who will be operating it. Turn on the power of the AED.
- If more than one rescuer is present, one rescuer should continue CPR while the other readies the AED for use.
- One rescuer should apply the AED pads to the patient's bare chest.

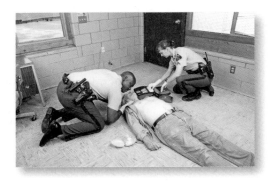

STEP 2 ▶

- Analyze the patient's heart rhythm. Do not touch the patient while the AED is analyzing the rhythm.
- If the AED advises that a shock is indicated, check the patient from head to toe to make sure no one (including you) is touching the patient before pressing the shock control. Make sure oxygen is not flowing over the patient's chest.
- Shout, "Stand clear!

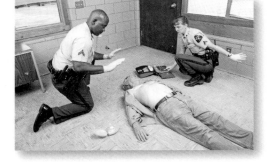

STEP 3 ▶ Press the shock control once it is illuminated and the machine indicates it is ready to deliver the shock.

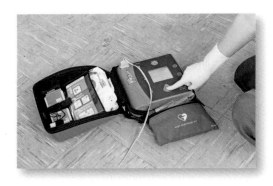

STEP 4 ▶

- After delivery of the shock, quickly resume CPR, beginning with chest compressions unless the patient regains consciousness or begins spontaneous movement.
- After five cycles of CPR, reanalyze the rhythm.

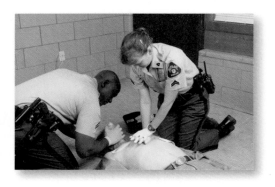

Support of the Family

Any emergency involving a cardiac arrest is a stressful situation, regardless of the cause of the arrest. Family members, friends, or bystanders at the scene may be anxious, angry, sad, hysterical, demanding, or impatient. Allow them to have and express their emotions. However, do not let others distract you from treating the patient. Accept their concerns, and recognize that their behavior stems from grief.

Identify yourself, and, using a gentle but firm tone of voice, let them know that everything that can be done to help will be done. Allow family members to be present, unless they are emotionally distraught and interfere with your efforts to resuscitate the patient. Comfort them by being sympathetic and listening with empathy, but do not give false hope or reassurance.

When to Stop Cardiopulmonary Resuscitation

You should stop CPR only if:

- The patient shows obvious signs of life, such as consciousness and spontaneous movement.
- Effective breathing and circulation have returned.
- The scene becomes unsafe.
- You are too exhausted to continue.
- You transfer patient care to a healthcare professional with equal or higher certification.
- A physician assumes responsibility for the patient.

Automated External Defibrillator Maintenance

Maintenance procedures for an AED should be performed according to the manufacturer's recommendations. Little maintenance is needed with newer AEDs because they perform automated self-tests. Some AEDs perform daily self-tests whereas others occur weekly. An AED self-tests when it is powered on. It may also self-test when batteries are installed. When an AED self-tests, it examines its internal circuitry, battery status, electronics used in heart rhythm analysis, defibrillator electronics, and microprocessor electronics. A manual AED self-test can be performed at any time. Check the policies of your EMS agency regarding requirements for regular maintenance schedules.

Failure of an AED is most often related to improper device maintenance, commonly battery failure. No defibrillator can work properly without properly functioning batteries. Always have extra batteries on hand.

Training and Sources of Information

Many organizations publish materials about CPR and automated external defibrillation, including the American Heart Association, American Safety and Health Institute, American Red Cross, and National Safety Council.

To maintain skill proficiency, most EMS systems permit a maximum of 90 days between practice drills to reassess proficiency in AED usage; many systems practice skills as often as once a month.

On the Scene   Wrap-Up

Another EMT arrives with the AED and turns it on. After the large electrode patches are applied, he tells you to stop CPR so that the machine can analyze the patient's heart rhythm. The machine's monotone voice states, "Shock advised, stand clear." The other EMT commands "Stand clear!" and scans the patient to be sure no one is touching her as he depresses the flashing shock button. You see her body twitch as the electric shock travels through your patient's heart. After the shock, you resume CPR for about 2 minutes and then wait as the machine again analyzes her heart rhythm. As the machine says, "No shock advised," you see her chest heave with a sudden intake of breath. You can feel a carotid pulse, weak at first, but stronger with each beat.

You carefully roll the patient onto her side. Your partner then takes a moment to explain the situation to the patient's husband. When the paramedics arrive, you give a brief report. The patient is trying to sit up, dazed and confused about what has happened. You cannot believe how exhilarated you feel as you help the paramedics wheel her out to the ambulance. ■

Sum It Up

▶ The circulatory system consists of the cardiovascular and lymphatic systems. The cardiovascular system is made up of the heart, blood, and blood vessels. The lymphatic system consists of lymph, lymph nodes, lymph vessels, the tonsils, the spleen, and the thymus gland. The circulatory system is responsible for transporting oxygen, water, and nutrients (such as sugar, electrolytes, and vitamins) throughout the body. It also carries away wastes produced by body cells (such as carbon dioxide) to the lungs, kidneys, or skin for removal from the body.

▶ The heart is divided into four chambers. The two upper chambers are the right and left atria. The atria receive blood from the body and lungs. The right atrium receives blood that is low in oxygen from the body. The left atrium receives blood rich in oxygen from the lungs. The two lower chambers of the heart are the right and left ventricles. The ventricles are larger and have thicker walls than the atria because their function is to pump blood to the lungs and body. The right ventricle pumps blood to the lungs. The left ventricle pumps blood to the body.

► Four heart valves prevent the backflow of blood and keep blood moving in one direction. The tricuspid and mitral (bicuspid) valves are called atrioventricular valves because they lie between the atria and ventricles. The aortic and pulmonic valves are called semilunar valves because they are shaped like half-moons.

► The liquid portion of the blood is called plasma. Plasma carries blood cells throughout the body. The formed elements of the blood include red blood cells, white blood cells, and platelets.

► Blood vessels that carry blood away from the heart to the rest of the body are called arteries. Arteries have thick walls because they transport blood under high pressure. Vessels that return blood to the heart are called veins. The walls of veins are thinner than arteries. Capillaries are the smallest and most numerous of the blood vessels.

► Acute coronary syndromes are conditions caused by temporary or permanent blockage of a coronary artery as a result of coronary artery disease. ACSs include unstable angina pectoris and myocardial infarction.

► Arteriosclerosis means hardening of the walls of the arteries. As the walls of the arteries become hardened, they lose their elasticity. In atherosclerosis, the inner lining (endothelium) of the walls of large- and medium-size arteries become narrowed and thicken.

► Conditions that may increase a person's chance of developing a disease are called risk factors. While some risk factors can be changed, others cannot. Risk factors that can be changed are called modifiable risk factors. Risk factors that cannot be changed are called nonmodifiable risk factors. Factors that can be part of the cause of a person's risk of heart disease are called contributing risk factors.

► Ischemia is decreased blood flow to an organ or tissue. Ischemia can result from narrowing or blockage of an artery or spasm of an artery. Atherosclerosis is a common reason for narrowing of a coronary artery.

► Angina pectoris (literally, "choking in the chest") is a symptom of CAD that occurs when the heart's need for oxygen exceeds its supply. A person is said to have stable angina pectoris when the symptoms are relatively constant and predictable in terms of severity, precipitating events, and response to therapy. A person who has unstable angina pectoris has angina that is progressively worsening, occurs at rest, or is brought on by minimal physical exertion.

► An acute myocardial infarction (or heart attack) occurs when a coronary artery becomes severely narrowed or is completely blocked, usually by a blood clot (thrombus). When the affected portion of the heart muscle (myocardium) is deprived of oxygen long enough, the area dies (infarcts). If too much of the heart muscle dies, shock (hypoperfusion) and cardiac arrest will result.

► The risk of death from a heart attack is related to the time elapsed between the onset of symptoms and start of treatment. The earlier the patient can receive emergency care, the greater the chances of preventing ischemic heart tissue from becoming dead heart tissue.

► When a person has congestive heart failure, one or both sides of the heart fail to pump efficiently. When the left ventricle fails as a pump, blood backs up into the lungs. When the right ventricle fails, blood returning to the heart backs up and causes congestion in the organs and tissues of the body.

► Signs and symptoms of a heart attack vary. Although chest discomfort is the most common symptom of a heart attack, some patients never have chest pain. Older adults, diabetic individuals, and women who have a heart attack are more likely to present with signs and symptoms that differ from those of a "typical" patient. This is called an atypical presentation or atypical signs and symptoms.

► Many states have passed legislation to include aspirin as a medication that can be carried on an EMS unit and given by EMTs. Check your state and local protocols for the appropriate use of this drug.

► As an EMT, you can assist a patient in taking prescribed NTG if the patient has signs and symptoms of chest pain or discomfort, the patient has physician-prescribed NTG, there are no contraindications to giving the medication, and you have specific authorization by medical direction (off-line or on-line).

► If the heart stops beating, no blood will flow. If no blood flows, oxygen cannot be delivered to the body's cells. When the heart stops, the patient is said to be in cardiac arrest. The signs of cardiac arrest include sudden unresponsiveness, absent breathing, and no signs of circulation. Chest compressions are used to circulate blood any time that the heart is not beating. Chest compressions are combined with rescue breathing to oxygenate the blood. The combination of rescue breathing and external chest compressions is called cardiopulmonary resuscitation.

► Sudden cardiac death is the unexpected death from cardiac causes early after symptom onset (immediately or within 1 hour) or without the onset of symptoms. Survival of cardiac arrest depends on a series of critical actions called the chain of survival. The chain of survival is the ideal series of events that should take place immediately after recognizing an injury or the onset of sudden illness. The chain consists of four steps:

1. Early access
2. Early CPR
3. Early defibrillation
4. Early advanced care

▶ An automated external defibrillator contains a computer programmed to recognize heart rhythms that should be shocked (defibrillated), such as ventricular fibrillation. A standard AED is used for a patient who is unresponsive, not breathing, pulseless, and greater than or equal to 8 years of age (about 55 pounds, or more than 25 kg). A special key or pad-cable system is available for some AEDs so that the machine can be used on children between 1 and 8 years of age. The key or pad-cable system decreases the amount of energy delivered to a dose appropriate for a child. If a child is in cardiac arrest and a key or pad-cable system is not available, use a standard AED.

▶ When an adult experiences a cardiac arrest as a result of VF, prompt defibrillation is the most important treatment you can provide from the time of the arrest to about 5 minutes following the arrest. If you witness a cardiac arrest, assess the patient's airway, breathing, and circulation, and then quickly apply an AED. Perform CPR until the AED is ready.

▶ To ensure delivery of the best-quality patient care possible, the medical director (or designated representative) carefully reviews every call in which an AED is used. Each call is reviewed to determine if the patient was treated according to professional standards and local standing orders.

▶ If the patient has a pacemaker or implantable cardioverter-defibrillator in place, place the AED pads at least 1 inch from the device.

▶ Before using an AED, familiarize yourself with the manufacturer's recommendations regarding the use of the device around water. If a medication patch is present on the patient's chest, make sure you are wearing gloves and then remove the patch.

▶ To operate an AED, place the AED next to the rescuer who will be operating it. Turn on the power. Connect the AED pads to the AED cables (if not preconnected). Then apply the pads to the patient's bare chest in the locations indicated on the pads. Connect the cable to the AED. Analyze the patient's heart rhythm. If the AED advises that a shock is indicated, check the patient from head to toe to make sure no one is touching the patient (including you) before pressing the shock control. Make sure oxygen is not flowing over the patient's chest. Shout, "Stand clear!" Press the shock control once it is illuminated and the machine indicates it is ready to deliver the shock. Resume CPR, beginning with chest compressions, immediately after delivery of the shock unless the patient regains consciousness or begins spontaneous movement.

▶ If you are transporting a patient who stops breathing and becomes pulseless, stop the vehicle. Start CPR and apply the AED. Analyze the rhythm as soon as the AED is ready. Deliver a shock, if indicated. Immediately resume CPR unless the patient regains consciousness or begins spontaneous movement. Continue resuscitation (and transport) according to your local protocol.

▶ Maintenance procedures for an AED should be performed according to the manufacturer's recommendations. Failure of an AED is most often related to improper device maintenance, commonly battery failure.

Abdominal and Gastrointestinal Disorders

By the end of this chapter, you should be able to:

Knowledge Objectives ▶

1. Describe the borders of the abdominal cavity.
2. Name the two major blood vessels in the abdomen.
3. Define peritoneum and retroperitoneal space.
4. Name the organs located in the right upper quadrant, left upper quadrant, right lower quadrant, and left lower quadrant.
5. List solid organs in the abdominal cavity and retroperitoneal space.
6. List hollow organs in the abdominal cavity and retroperitoneal space.
7. Describe and discuss the function of the primary gastrointestinal (GI) organs.
8. Describe and discuss the function of the gastrointestinal accessory organs.
9. Define acute abdomen and referred pain.
10. Discuss hemorrhagic causes of acute abdominal pain.
11. Describe assessment findings and symptoms of upper GI bleeding and lower GI bleeding.
12. Define hematemesis and melena.
13. Discuss nonhemorrhagic causes of acute abdominal pain.
14. Discuss assessment of the patient with abdominal pain.
15. Discuss the specific questions to ask to obtain a history of a patient with abdominal pain.
16. Discuss emergency care for the patient with abdominal pain.

Attitude Objective ▶

17. Defend emergency medical technician treatment regimens for various abdominal or gastrointestinal disorders.

Skill Objectives ▶

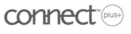

18. Demonstrate the ability to take a relevant history from the patient with an abdominal or GI disorder.
19. Demonstrate the ability to perform a physical assessment on the patient with an abdominal or GI disorder.
20. Practice completing a prehospital care report for patients with abdominal emergencies.

On the Scene

You and your EMT partner have just finished lunch when your station tones are activated, and you are dispatched to a private residence for a report of abdominal pain. Your knock at the door is answered by a woman who appears to be about 60 years of age. She greets you and asks you to step inside her home. You observe as she uses a walker to walk slowly in front of you to the couch. You note several clean towels have been placed over the seat cushions. The patient gently sits down, pausing a moment to make sure that she is seated on a towel. As you begin questioning her about her symptoms, it is obvious that she is uncomfortable talking to you about them. She reluctantly reports abdominal pain, frequent "gas pains," and dark stools. The patient also says, "Lately I just haven't had the energy I normally do." ■

THINK ABOUT IT

As you read this chapter, think about the following questions:

- What additional assessment should you perform?
- What emergency care would be appropriate for this patient?

Introduction

Abdominal pain is a common patient complaint. Although it is unnecessary for prehospital personnel to determine the specific cause of abdominal pain, it is important to understand the possible causes of the complaint. In this chapter we discuss common gastrointestinal disorders, assessment of the patient with abdominal discomfort, and the initial emergency care for a patient with an abdominal or gastrointestinal complaint.

Review of Digestive System Anatomy and Physiology

Basic Anatomy

Objectives 1, 2, 3, 4

The abdominal cavity is bordered superiorly by the diaphragm, inferiorly by the pelvis, posteriorly by the spine, and anteriorly by the abdominal wall. The major blood vessels of the abdomen are the **aorta** and **inferior vena cava.** Because the abdominal cavity is lined by a smooth membrane called the **peritoneum,** the abdominal cavity is sometimes called the **peritoneal cavity.** If the peritoneum becomes inflamed, the condition is called **peritonitis.** The area behind the peritoneal cavity is called the **retroperitoneum** or **retroperitoneal space.** The kidneys, ureters, and rectum are examples of structures located in the retroperitoneal space.

Remember that the abdominal cavity is divided into four quadrants to make things easier when identifying the abdominal organs and the location of pain or injury (Figure 23-1).

- *RUQ.* The right upper quadrant contains the liver, the gallbladder, portions of the stomach, the large and small intestines, part of the pancreas, and the major blood vessels.

- *LUQ.* The left upper quadrant contains the stomach, spleen, pancreas, and large and small intestines.
- *RLQ.* The right lower quadrant contains the cecum, appendix, and large and small intestines.
- *LLQ.* The left lower quadrant contains the large and small intestines.

In females, the right and left lower quadrants contain the ovaries and fallopian tubes. The uterus is in the midline superior to (above) the pelvis and just posterior to (behind) the bladder.

Solid and Hollow Organs

Objectives 5, 6

The abdomen contains solid and hollow organs. **Solid organs** of the abdomen and retroperitoneal space include the liver, spleen, pancreas, and kidneys. Solid organs bleed when injured. When hollow organs are cut

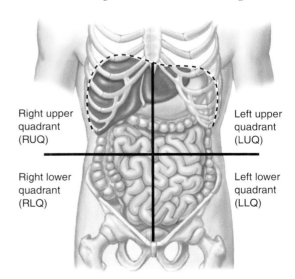

Right upper quadrant (RUQ)

Left upper quadrant (LUQ)

Right lower quadrant (RLQ)

Left lower quadrant (LLQ)

FIGURE 23-1 ▲ The abdominal cavity is divided into four quadrants.

or burst, their contents spill into the abdominal cavity causing pain and soreness. **Hollow organs** of the abdomen and retroperitoneal space include the stomach, intestines, appendix, gallbladder, and urinary bladder.

Digestive System Organs

Objectives 7, 8

The primary organs of the digestive system are the mouth, pharynx, esophagus, stomach, small intestine, large intestine, rectum, and anal canal. The accessory organs of digestion are the teeth and tongue, salivary glands, liver, gallbladder, and pancreas (Figure 23-2).

The mouth, teeth, and salivary glands begin the process of digestion. The tongue manipulates food for chewing and swallowing. The salivary glands moisten and lubricate food so it can be swallowed and secrete enzymes that begin the breakdown of food. The teeth mince food into small pieces so it can be swallowed when mixed with saliva. Swallowing moves food from the pharynx into the esophagus. The esophagus is a hollow, muscular tube through which food is moved from the pharynx to the stomach by **peristalsis,** which is the involuntary wavelike contraction of smooth muscle that moves material through the digestive tract. The stomach is a hollow organ found in the left upper quadrant of the abdomen that receives and stores food. It mixes food with gastric juices, breaking it down into partially digested food called **chyme.**

The intestines occupy a large portion of the abdominal cavity. The small intestine is composed of the duodenum, jejunum, and ileum and receives chyme from the stomach and secretions from the pancreas and liver. It selectively absorbs nutrients that can be used by the body. The large intestine (colon) consists of the cecum, ascending colon, transverse colon, descending colon, sigmoid colon, rectum, and anal canal. It absorbs water and electrolytes from the remaining chyme and changes it from a fluid to a semisolid mass. The appendix is a hollow, fingerlike appendage that is attached to the cecum. Inflammation of the appendix (appendicitis) can result in right lower quadrant abdominal pain.

The liver is the largest internal organ of the body and lies just below the diaphragm. It stores glycogen, detoxifies many substances, produces bile (which

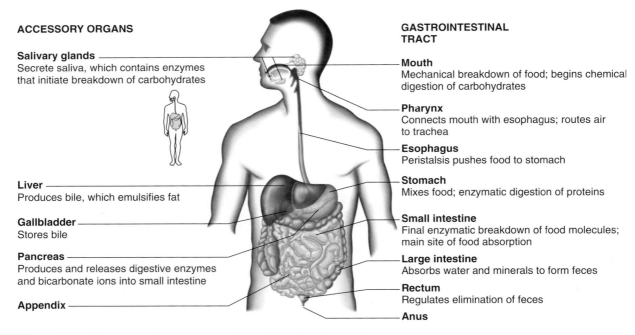

ACCESSORY ORGANS

Salivary glands
Secrete saliva, which contains enzymes that initiate breakdown of carbohydrates

Liver
Produces bile, which emulsifies fat

Gallbladder
Stores bile

Pancreas
Produces and releases digestive enzymes and bicarbonate ions into small intestine

Appendix

GASTROINTESTINAL TRACT

Mouth
Mechanical breakdown of food; begins chemical digestion of carbohydrates

Pharynx
Connects mouth with esophagus; routes air to trachea

Esophagus
Peristalsis pushes food to stomach

Stomach
Mixes food; enzymatic digestion of proteins

Small intestine
Final enzymatic breakdown of food molecules; main site of food absorption

Large intestine
Absorbs water and minerals to form feces

Rectum
Regulates elimination of feces

Anus

FIGURE 23-2 ▲ Primary and accessory organs of the digestive system.

emulsifies fats), and stimulates the gallbladder to secrete stored bile into the small intestine. Because the liver also stores blood, significant blood loss can result if it is lacerated as a result of an injury to the abdomen or lower chest. The gallbladder stores the bile produced by the liver until it is needed by the small intestine. Inflammation of the gallbladder (cholecystitis) or blockage of the bile ducts within it may produce severe right upper quadrant pain. The pancreas secretes glucagon, insulin, and somatostatin and powerful enzymes that aid in protein, carbohydrate, and fat digestion. Peritonitis can result if these enzymes spill into the abdominal cavity because of injury or disease, causing severe pain.

The Acute Abdomen

Objective 9

The phrase **acute abdomen** means a sudden onset of abdominal pain. Although there are many causes of abdominal pain including inflammation, loss of the blood supply to an organ, nerve sensitivity, spasm of the intestinal muscles, and stretching or distention of an organ,

sometimes the cause is unknown. The patient who has an acute abdomen often has associated findings and symptoms such as nausea and vomiting and abdominal tenderness and/or rigidity. Signs and symptoms of shock may also be present.

Although the abdomen is often the source of the problem when a patient has abdominal pain, sometimes the pain originates from another source, such as an organ that is near (but not within) the abdominal cavity. For example, abdominal pain due to a stomach problem is usually localized in the area of the stomach. However, disease affecting the kidneys can also cause abdominal pain. Therefore abdominal pain may or may not be the result of a problem involving an organ within the abdominal cavity.

It is also possible for the pain from an injured or diseased abdominal organ to be felt in areas distant from the original source. For example, pancreatic pain may be felt in the back and pain due to gallbladder disease may be felt in the area below or between the shoulders. Pain that is felt in a part of the body that is away from the tissues or organ that causes the pain is called **referred pain.** Examples of referred pain appear in Figure 23-3 and in the next *You Should Know* box.

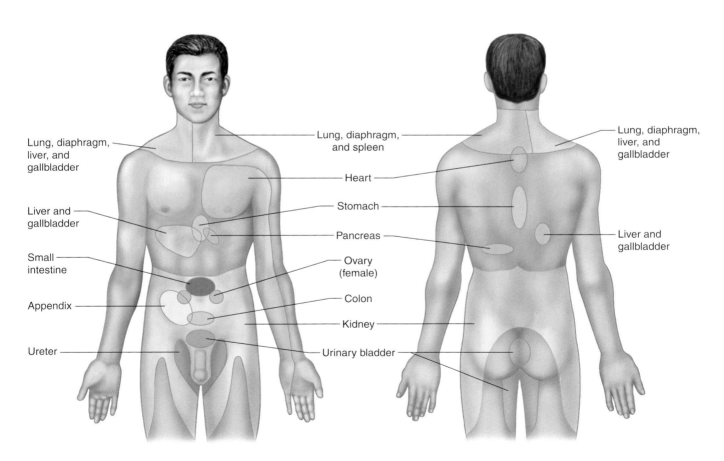

FIGURE 23-3 ▲ Sites of referred pain.

Hemorrhagic Causes of Acute Abdominal Pain

Gastritis

Objective 10

Gastritis is an inflammation of the stomach lining. Possible causes include increased gastric secretion associated with excessive consumption of alcohol, infection caused by a virus or bacteria (such as *Helicobacter pylori*, or *H. pylori*), and prolonged use of medications such as nonsteroidal anti-inflammatory drugs (NSAIDs), which include ibuprofen and aspirin. Gastritis can develop after severe physical stress, such as burns, severe infection, surgery, or trauma. Assessment findings and symptoms include belching, nausea and vomiting, and indigestion. The patient may complain of a burning sensation in the upper abdomen.

Peptic Ulcer Disease

Objective 10

A **peptic ulcer** is an open sore in the lining of the stomach (gastric ulcer), duodenum (duodenal ulcer), or esophagus (esophageal ulcer). The primary cause of peptic ulcer disease is a stomach infection caused by *H. pylori*. A contributing cause is excess secretion of digestive juices. Over time, the protective mucous lining of the stomach, duodenum, or esophagus is worn away by excess secretion of digestive juices, such as hydrochloric acid, by stomach cells. The lining of the stomach, duodenum, or esophagus can also be disrupted by prolonged use of medications (such as NSAIDs) or alcohol. Esophageal ulcers are typically associated with the reflux of stomach acid (gastroesophageal reflux disease, or GERD).

The patient who has a gastric ulcer usually complains of nausea, vomiting, and a burning pressure in the left upper quadrant of the abdomen and back that occurs 1 to 2 hours after meals. If the ulcer has penetrated the wall of the stomach, the discomfort may be aggravated with food.

The patient who has a duodenal ulcer typically complains of a burning, cramping, pressurelike pain across the upper abdomen that occurs 2 to 4 hours after meals, midmorning, midafternoon, and in the middle of the night. The discomfort of a duodenal ulcer is usually relieved with antacids and food. The patient may occasionally experience nausea and vomiting.

The patient who has an esophageal ulcer usually complains of indigestion, nausea, and abdominal cramping. These symptoms usually appear 2 to 3 hours after eating and may worsen if the patient does not ingest food. The discomfort of an esophageal ulcer is usually relieved with antacids and food.

Abdominal Aortic Aneurysm

Objective 10

An aneurysm is an abnormal bulging of a blood vessel. An abdominal aortic aneurysm (AAA) is a weakened area of the abdominal aorta that bulges. If the aneurysm ruptures, massive bleeding and death can result. Experts are not sure what causes an AAA to form, but contributing factors include smoking, high blood pressure, atherosclerosis, advanced age, and family history (immediate relative) of abdominal aortic aneurysm. Initially, the patient will most likely not have any symptoms. In fact, the presence of an aneurysm is often identified when the patient is undergoing tests for another medical problem. However, as the size of the aneurysm increases, the patient may develop symptoms including midabdominal and back pain and a pulsating sensation in the abdomen. Once an aneurysm reaches 2 inches (5 cm) in diameter, medical intervention is usually necessary to prevent rupture. When the aneurysm ruptures or is near rupturing, the patient will typically complain of sudden, severe ripping or tearing pain in the abdomen or lower back and may show signs of shock. Depending on the location of the aneurysm, femoral and pedal pulses may be unequal. Rapid transport or an ALS intercept is indicated if you suspect your patient has a ruptured abdominal aortic aneurysm.

Upper Gastrointestinal Bleeding

Objectives 10, 11, 12

Bleeding may occur from any part of the gastrointestinal (GI) tract. GI bleeding is a medical emergency. **Upper GI bleeding is** bleeding from the esophagus, stomach, or duodenum. Common causes include gastritis, peptic ulcer disease, tumors, esophagitis (inflammation of the esophagus), and esophageal varices (enlarged and twisted veins in the esophagus).

Assessment findings and symptoms include **hematemesis** (vomiting blood). Vomited blood may be bright red if it is recent or if bleeding is forceful. Forceful and repeated vomiting may cause hematemesis by tearing small blood vessels lining the stomach and esophagus. If blood accumulates in the stomach and is partially digested and then vomited, the vomited material may resemble coffee grounds. The patient may also present with syncope, fatigue, and shortness of breath.

Lower Gastrointestinal Bleeding

Objectives 10, 11, 12

Lower GI bleeding can originate in the small intestine, colon, or rectum. Common causes include tumors, hemorrhoids, and colitis (inflammation of the colon). Assessment findings and symptoms include rectal bleeding, increased frequency of stools, and cramping pain. The color of blood in the stool depends on the source of the bleeding and the amount of time the blood has spent in the GI tract. For example, black, tarry stool is called **melena** and reflects partially digested blood from the upper GI tract, whereas blood from the lower colon or rectum usually appears bright red. Stools streaked with blood and blood drops on toilet paper or in the toilet bowl may be caused by colon cancer, rectal trauma, or bleeding from internal or external hemorrhoids.

Nonhemorrhagic Causes of Acute Abdominal Pain

Appendicitis

Objective 13

Appendicitis is a condition in which the appendix becomes inflamed and generally requires surgical removal. It is most common in adolescents and young adults, but can occur at any age. Assessment findings and symptoms include the sudden onset of abdominal pain that typically starts around the umbilicus and then shifts to the right lower quadrant of the abdomen. Most patients also experience nausea, vomiting, fever, and a loss of appetite. The pain associated with appendicitis is described as unrelenting, usually increasing in intensity over 6 to 12 hours. The pain typically worsens with movement, coughing, and deep breathing. Most patients will prefer to lie still with one leg flexed to reduce tension on the abdominal muscles. Peritonitis can result if the appendix ruptures, causing severe pain and a tender, rigid abdomen.

Intestinal Obstruction

Objective 13

Intestinal obstruction is a blockage of the large or small intestine that prevents food and fluid from passing through. An intestinal obstruction may be partial (allowing some intestinal contents to pass) or complete (nothing can pass through the intestine). A complete obstruction is a medical emergency that requires immediate surgery to relieve the blockage.

Intestinal obstruction has many causes, including foreign objects (such as pins, bones, and small toys), narrowing of the intestinal opening caused by swelling and inflammation from abdominal trauma, radiation therapy, or an infection, but it is most often the result of adhesions (bands of scar tissue in the intestine that develop in some people after surgery), hernias (protrusion of tissue through a weak area or abnormal opening in the wall of the cavity in which it is normally contained, such as the abdomen), or tumors.

Assessment findings and symptoms of intestinal obstruction include intermittent, cramping abdominal pain; nausea, vomiting or diarrhea; gradual loss of appetite; abdominal distention and tenderness; decreased or no passage of stool; inability to pass gas; fever; and chills.

Pancreatitis

Objective 13

Pancreatitis (inflammation of the pancreas) is usually caused by gallstones or excessive alcohol use. Trauma, viral infections, and some drugs are among other possible causes of pancreatitis. In some cases the cause is never found. Pancreatitis can be acute or chronic. Acute pancreatitis begins suddenly and lasts for a few days. Chronic pancreatitis develops gradually and continues for many years.

Assessment findings and symptoms of pancreatitis include abdominal pain that typically radiates to the back and is described as severe, deep, piercing, and steady. The pain often begins when lying down, and the patient may assume many different positions in an attempt to relieve the pain. Pancreatic pain is aggravated by eating and is not relieved by vomiting. Nausea, vomiting, abdominal tenderness, fever, hypotension, and tachycardia may be present.

Cholecystitis

Objective 13

Inflammation of the gallbladder is called **cholecystitis.** It is usually caused by gallstones that lodge in the duct that drains the gallbladder or in the nearby bile duct.

Gallstones may or may not produce symptoms. The presence and severity of symptoms depends on whether the stones are stationary or mobile and whether they cause an obstruction.

Assessment findings and symptoms of cholecystitis include pain in the upper middle or right upper quadrant of the abdomen that occurs 3 to 6 hours after a heavy meal (such as a meal that is high in fat) and is unrelieved by antacids. The pain is described as severe and steady and worsens with movement. The pain generally lasts from 1 to 4 hours and may radiate to the area below or between the shoulders. The patient may also experience nausea, vomiting, constipation or diarrhea, and excessive belching.

Gastroenteritis

Objective 13

Gastroenteritis, also called the "stomach flu," is an inflammation of the lining of the intestinal tract, most often caused by a virus. Assessment findings and symptoms include diarrhea, abdominal pain and tenderness, vomiting, headache, fever, and chills.

Hepatitis

Objective 13

Hepatitis is an inflammation of the liver, most commonly caused by a viral infection. There are five main hepatitis viruses, referred to as types A, B, C, D, and E. Hepatitis A and hepatitis E are spread primarily through food or water contaminated by feces from an infected person. Hepatitis B is spread through contact with infected blood, through sex with an infected person, and from mother to child during childbirth. Hepatitis C is spread primarily through contact with infected blood and, less commonly, through sexual contact and childbirth. Hepatitis D is spread through contact with infected blood. Vaccines offer protection from hepatitis A and hepatitis B. Alcohol or substance abuse can also lead to hepatitis.

Although some people who have hepatitis have no symptoms, others may have dull right upper quadrant pain and tenderness (unrelated to food consumption), nausea and vomiting, loss of appetite, extreme fatigue, dark urine, clay-colored stools, and jaundice.

Kidney Stones

Objective 13

A kidney stone is a hard mass that forms from crystallization of excreted substances in the urine. A stone that lodges in a ureter can cause urine to back up behind it and into the kidney. The backup of urine causes the kidney to stretch, which increases pressure and causes pain. Assessment findings and symptoms can include excruciating pain that is usually located in the flank, radiating to the groin. Kidney stones are covered in more detail in Chapter 24.

Pelvic Inflammatory Disease

Objective 13

Pelvic inflammatory disease (PID) is an infection of the uterus, fallopian tubes, and other female reproductive organs. PID occurs when sexually transmitted bacteria enter a woman's vagina and spread upward into her cervix, uterus, fallopian tubes, and other reproductive organs. Common assessment findings and symptoms include fever and lower abdominal pain that may radiate to the lower back or right shoulder. PID is covered in more detail in Chapter 25.

Patient Assessment

Objectives 14, 15

Patient assessment begins with a scene size-up and putting on appropriate personal protective equipment. Form a general impression, and perform a primary survey. Assess the patient's mental status, airway, breathing, and circulation. If the patient is responsive, allow the patient to assume a position of comfort. Note the rate and rhythm of respirations and any signs of increased work of breathing (respiratory effort). Listen for air movement, and note if respirations are quiet, absent, or noisy. Assess the patient's heart rate, pulse regularity, and strength. Assess perfusion. Note the color, temperature, and moisture of the patient's skin. If appropriate, evaluate for possible major bleeding. Provide calm reassurance to help reduce the patient's anxiety. If you have not already done so, establish patient priorities, determine the need for additional resources, and make a transport decision.

Once you have made a transport decision, obtain a SAMPLE history from the patient, or from family members if the patient is unresponsive. Remember to use the OPQRST tool if the patient is complaining of pain or discomfort. Examples of questions to ask a patient who is experiencing abdominal discomfort are shown in the next *Making a Difference* box. If the patient is unresponsive or has an altered mental status, quickly size up the scene, form a general impression, perform a primary survey, and then proceed to the rapid medical assessment. Provide all information obtained to the paramedics who arrive on the scene or to the staff at the receiving facility.

Making a Difference

OPQRST

- **O**nset: How long ago did your symptoms begin? Did your symptoms begin suddenly or gradually? What were you doing when your symptoms began? What is new or different today about your discomfort that prompted your call for assistance?

- **P**rovocation/palliation/position: What is the relationship of your pain to meals (worse with eating, unaffected by food, begins about 2 hours after meals, begins after a high-fat meal)? What have you done to relieve the pain or discomfort? Have you taken any medications (such as antacids) to relieve the problem before we arrived? Does your pain get better or worse when you change positions, or does it stay the same?

- **Q**uality: What does the pain or discomfort feel like? (Is it constant, intermittent, sharp, dull, tearing, cramping, or burning?)

- **R**egion/radiation: Where is your discomfort? Is it in one area, or does it move (to the back, flank, neck, arm, or shoulder)?

- **S**everity: On a scale of 0 to 10, with 0 being the least and 10 being the worst, what number would you give your discomfort?

- **T**ime: How long has the discomfort been present? Have you ever had these symptoms before? When? How long did they last? Compared with other episodes, would you describe this one as mild, moderate, or severe?

Additional Questions

- Are you having any other symptoms (such as fever, nausea, weakness, fatigue)? Have you vomited? If yes, have you vomited blood?

- Do you have heartburn?

- Do you have rectal pain?

- How frequently do you have a bowel movement? What color is the stool? Since your symptoms began, have you noticed any blood in your stool?

- Do you have any allergies?

- What medicines do you take?

- Do you have a history of heart, lung, liver, or kidney disease or other medical condition?

- When did you last have anything to eat or drink?

If the patient is responsive, perform a focused physical examination. When a patient is complaining of abdominal discomfort, important body areas to assess include the abdomen and pelvis.

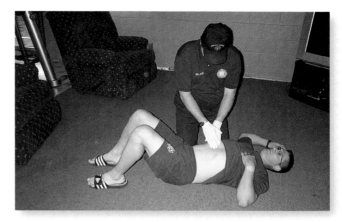

FIGURE 23-4 ▲ The best position for an abdominal examination is with the patient supine, head down, with knees slightly bent.

Begin the physical exam by observing the patient's position. Patients with peritonitis or appendicitis usually prefer to lie absolutely still because any motion causes further peritoneal irritation and pain. Patients with an intestinal obstruction are often restless and move in an attempt to find a position of comfort. Patients may also present with their knees in a flexed position (fetal position) to decrease tension on the abdominal muscles. Patients with a kidney stone may also move around trying to find a comfortable position.

Listen to breath sounds, and assess the patient's pulse, respirations, blood pressure, and oxygen saturation. Assess the abdomen for DCAP-BTLS. When assessing the abdomen, look to see if abdominal distention is present (the abdomen appears larger than normal). Abdominal distention can be caused by blood, fluid, or air.

Palpate the abdomen, placing one hand on top of the other (Figure 23-4). If the patient is responsive, ask him to point to the area that hurts (point tenderness). Use the pads of the fingers of the lower hand and gently feel the upper and lower areas of the abdomen for tenderness. Assess the area that hurts last. Watch the patient's face while you palpate the abdomen. A grimace may indicate tenderness over a particular abdominal area. Determine if the abdomen feels soft or hard (rigid). Note the presence of any scars, masses, or pulsations.

Emergency Care

Objective 16

Prehospital care for a patient experiencing abdominal discomfort is supportive. Allow the patient to assume a position of comfort and provide calm reassurance. Administer oxygen. If the patient's breathing is inadequate, give positive-pressure ventilation with 100%

oxygen. Assess the adequacy of the ventilations delivered. Be alert for signs and symptoms of shock and treat for shock as indicated. The patient who has abdominal pain needs to be transported for physician evaluation. Initiate an ALS intercept if needed, and transport as soon as possible. Reassess as often as indicated until patient care is turned over to ALS personnel or medical personnel at the receiving facility. The causes of abdominal pain discussed in this chapter are summarized in Table 23-1.

TABLE 23-1 Causes of Abdominal Pain

Condition	Possible Causes	Pain Location	Assessment Findings/Symptoms
Abdominal aortic aneurysm	Exact cause unknown; contributing factors include smoking, high blood pressure, atherosclerosis, advanced age, and family history (immediate relative) of abdominal aortic aneurysm	Midabdominal and back pain that is described as a sudden, severe ripping or tearing pain when the aneurysm ruptures or is near rupture	Femoral and pedal pulses that may be unequal and can be absent; signs of shock due to blood loss
Appendicitis	Inflammation of the appendix	Sudden onset of abdominal pain that typically starts around the umbilicus and then shifts to the right lower quadrant of the abdomen	Nausea, vomiting, fever, loss of appetite
Cholecystitis	Inflammation of the gallbladder	Pain in the upper middle or right upper quadrant of the abdomen that is often aggravated by ingestion of a fatty meal	Nausea, vomiting, constipation or diarrhea, belching
Gastritis	Excessive consumption of alcohol; infection caused by a virus or bacteria (such as *H. pylori*); prolonged use of nonsteroidal anti-inflammatory drugs; severe physical stress such as burns, severe infection, surgery, or trauma	Burning sensation in the upper abdomen	Belching, nausea and vomiting, and indigestion
Gastroenteritis ("stomach flu")	Inflammation of the lining of the intestinal tract usually caused by a virus	Generalized abdominal pain and tenderness	Diarrhea, vomiting, headache, fever, and chills
Hepatitis	Inflammation of the liver, most commonly caused by a viral infection	Dull right upper quadrant pain	Nausea and vomiting, loss of appetite, extreme fatigue, dark urine, clay-colored stools, jaundice
Intestinal obstruction	Tumor, intestinal inflammation, foreign body	Generalized intermittent, cramping abdominal pain	Nausea, vomiting or diarrhea, gradual loss of appetite, abdominal distention and tenderness, decreased or no passage of stool, inability to pass gas, fever, chills

continued

TABLE 23-1 Causes of Abdominal Pain *Continued*

Condition	Possible Causes	Pain Location	Assessment Findings/Symptoms
Kidney stones	Exact cause unknown; contributing causes include urinary tract infections, inadequate fluid intake, dehydration, excess calcium levels in the urine, family history of kidney stones	Excruciating pain that is usually located in the flank, radiating to the groin; common descriptions of pain: "coming in waves" (colicky pain) or "feeling like crushed glass going through my side"	Nausea, vomiting, sweating, blood in the urine, painful or burning urination, restlessness, inability to find a comfortable position
Pancreatitis	Inflammation of the pancreas; usually caused by gallstones or excessive alcohol use	Abdominal pain that typically radiates to the back	Pain aggravated by eating and not relieved by vomiting; nausea, vomiting, abdominal tenderness, fever, hypotension, tachycardia may be present
Pelvic inflammatory disease	Infection of the uterus, fallopian tubes, and other female reproductive organs; usually caused by sexually transmitted bacteria	Lower abdominal pain that may radiate to the lower back or right shoulder	Fever, vaginal discharge that may have a foul odor, painful intercourse, painful urination, increased heart rate secondary to pain and fever, normal or slightly elevated blood pressure (due to pain)

On the Scene Wrap-Up

You and your partner complete your assessment and find no immediate life-threatening conditions. Continuing patient care, you perform a focused history and physical exam. Your patient reports that her symptoms began about 1 hour ago and have not decreased in frequency. Your partner informs you that the patient's blood pressure is 158/80, pulse 102, and respirations 16. Her oxygen saturation on room air is 96%. You place the patient on supplemental oxygen and prepare her for transport. You later learn that the patient was admitted to the hospital with a diagnosis of lower GI bleeding. ■

Sum It Up

▶ The abdominal cavity is bordered superiorly by the diaphragm, inferiorly by the pelvis, posteriorly by the spine, and anteriorly by the abdominal wall. The major blood vessels of the abdomen are the aorta and inferior vena cava.

▶ The abdominal cavity is lined by a smooth membrane called the peritoneum. The area behind the peritoneal cavity is called the retroperitoneum or retroperitoneal space. The kidneys, ureters, and rectum are examples of structures located in the retroperitoneal space.

▶ The abdominal cavity is divided into four quadrants. The right upper quadrant contains the liver, the gallbladder, portions of the stomach, and the major blood vessels. The left upper quadrant contains the stomach, spleen, pancreas, and large and small intestines. The right lower quadrant contains the appendix. The left lower quadrant, along with the other three quadrants, contains the intestines.

▶ Solid organs of the abdomen and retroperitoneal space include the liver, spleen, pancreas, and kidneys. Hollow organs of the abdomen and retroperitoneal space include the stomach, intestines, gallbladder, and urinary bladder.

▶ The primary organs of the digestive system are the mouth, pharynx, esophagus, stomach, small intestine, large intestine, rectum, and anal canal. The accessory organs of digestion are the teeth and tongue, salivary glands, liver, gallbladder, and pancreas.

▶ The phrase acute abdomen means a sudden onset of abdominal pain.

▶ Abdominal pain may or may not be the result of a problem involving an organ within the abdominal cavity. Pain that is felt in a part of the body that is away from the tissues or organ that causes the pain is called referred pain.

► Gastritis is an inflammation of the stomach lining. Assessment findings and symptoms include belching, nausea and vomiting, and indigestion. The patient may complain of a burning sensation in the upper abdomen.

► A peptic ulcer is an open sore in the lining of the stomach (gastric ulcer), duodenum (duodenal ulcer), or esophagus (esophageal ulcer).

► Bleeding may occur from any part of the GI tract. GI bleeding is a medical emergency.

► Upper GI bleeding is bleeding from the esophagus, stomach, or duodenum. Assessment findings and symptoms include hematemesis (vomiting blood). Vomited blood may be bright red if it is recent or if bleeding is forceful. The patient may also present with syncope, fatigue, and shortness of breath.

► Lower gastrointestinal bleeding can originate in the small intestine, colon, or rectum. Assessment findings and symptoms include rectal bleeding, increased frequency of stools, and cramping pain.

► Appendicitis is a condition in which the appendix becomes inflamed and generally requires surgical removal. Assessment findings and symptoms include the sudden onset of abdominal pain that typically starts around the umbilicus and then shifts to the right lower quadrant of the abdomen. Most patients also experience nausea, vomiting, fever, and a loss of appetite.

► Intestinal obstruction is a blockage of the large or small intestine that prevents food and fluid from passing through. Assessment findings and symptoms include intermittent, cramping abdominal pain; nausea, vomiting, or diarrhea; gradual loss of appetite; abdominal distention and tenderness; decreased or no passage of stool; inability to pass gas; fever; and chills.

► Inflammation of the pancreas is usually caused by gallstones or excessive alcohol use. Assessment findings and symptoms of pancreatitis include abdominal pain that typically radiates to the back. Pancreatic pain is aggravated by eating and is not relieved by vomiting. Nausea, vomiting, abdominal tenderness, fever, hypotension, and tachycardia may be present.

► Inflammation of the gallbladder is called cholecystitis. Assessment findings and symptoms of cholecystitis include pain in the upper middle or right upper quadrant of the abdomen. The patient may also experience nausea, vomiting, constipation or diarrhea, and excessive belching.

► Gastroenteritis, also called the stomach flu, is an inflammation of the lining of the intestinal tract, most often caused by a virus. Assessment findings and symptoms include diarrhea, abdominal pain and tenderness, vomiting, headache, fever, and chills.

► Hepatitis is an inflammation of the liver, most commonly caused by a viral infection. Although some people who have hepatitis have no symptoms, others may have dull right upper quadrant pain and tenderness (unrelated to food consumption), nausea and vomiting, loss of appetite, extreme fatigue, dark urine, clay-colored stools, and jaundice.

► Assess the patient. Form a general impression, and perform a primary survey. If you have not already done so, establish patient priorities, determine the need for additional resources, and make a transport decision. Once you have made a transport decision, obtain a SAMPLE history from a responsive patient. Remember to use the OPQRST tool if she is complaining of pain or discomfort.

► If the patient is responsive, perform a focused physical examination. Observe the patient's position. Listen to breath sounds, and assess the patient's pulse, respirations, blood pressure, and oxygen saturation. Assess the abdomen for DCAP-BTLS. Look to see if abdominal distention is present. Palpate the abdomen, and determine if the abdomen feels soft or hard (rigid).

► If the patient is unresponsive or has an altered mental status, quickly size up the scene, form a general impression, perform a primary survey, and then proceed to the rapid medical assessment. Provide all information obtained to the paramedics who arrive on the scene or to the staff at the receiving facility.

► Prehospital care for a patient experiencing abdominal discomfort is supportive. Allow the patient to assume a position of comfort and provide calm reassurance. Administer oxygen. Be alert for signs and symptoms of shock. Initiate an ALS intercept if needed, and transport as soon as possible. Reassess as often as indicated.

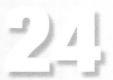

Genitourinary and Renal Disorders

By the end of this chapter, you should be able to:

Knowledge Objectives ▶
1. Discuss the anatomy and physiology of the genitourinary system.
2. Discuss the functions of the urinary system.
3. Identify the pathophysiology, assessment findings, and symptoms associated with kidney stones.
4. Identify the pathophysiology, assessment findings, and symptoms associated with a urinary tract infection.
5. Discuss types of urinary catheters and care of the patient with a urinary catheter during transport.
6. Identify the pathophysiology, assessment findings, and symptoms associated with pyelonephritis.
7. Identify the pathophysiology, assessment findings, and symptoms associated with renal failure.
8. Discuss types of dialysis.
9. Discuss complications related to dialysis.
10. Discuss assessment of the patient with a genitourinary disorder.
11. Discuss the specific questions to ask to obtain a history of a patient with a genitourinary disorder.
12. Describe the emergency care for a patient experiencing a kidney stone, urinary tract infection, pyelonephritis, or renal failure.

Attitude Objective ▶
13. Defend emergency medical technician treatment regimens for various genitourinary disorders.

Skill Objectives ▶
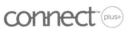
14. Demonstrate the ability to take a relevant history from the patient with a genitourinary disorder.
15. Demonstrate the ability to perform a physical assessment on the patient with a genitourinary disorder.
16. Practice completing a prehospital care report for patients with genitourinary disorders.

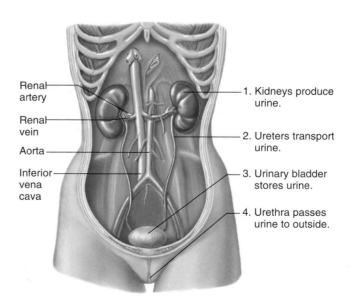

On the Scene

You and your partner are en route to a local restaurant for an "unknown medical problem." You arrive to find a 48-year-old woman supine on the floor and being cared for by several restaurant employees and some fellow diners. They tell you that the patient was about to sit down at a table and suddenly slumped to the floor. The patient is alert and oriented to person, place, time, and event. As you quickly perform a primary survey and simultaneously ask questions, she tells you that she is feeling very weak and dizzy. You observe an arteriovenous (AV) fistula in the patient's left forearm and ask the patient about it. She reports that she has a history of renal failure and completed a dialysis treatment about 2 hours ago. ■

THINK ABOUT IT

As you read this chapter, think about the following questions:

- What is an AV fistula?
- What important modifications must you make when obtaining vital signs from a patient with an AV fistula?
- What are some of the possible complications of hemodialysis?
- What level of transport is most appropriate for this patient?

Introduction

As an EMT, you will be called to provide emergency care for a patient experiencing a genitourinary disorder. Some conditions, such as a kidney stone, are relatively easy to recognize because the patient's description of the complaint combined with your assessment findings is usually straightforward. In contrast, other disorders can be difficult to recognize because the genitourinary system affects many body systems. As it was with gastrointestinal disorders, it is not necessary for you to determine the specific cause of the patient's complaint, but it is important to understand the possible causes of the complaint. In this chapter we discuss common genitourinary disorders and the assessment of initial emergency care for a patient with a genitourinary complaint.

Review of the Urinary System

General Anatomy

Objective 1

The urinary system consists of the kidneys, ureters, urinary bladder, and urethra (Figure 24-1). Humans typically have two bean-shaped kidneys that are about the size of a human fist. They are located in the retroperitoneal space (behind the abdominal cavity) on each side of the lumbar spine, at about the level of the twelfth rib. An adrenal gland is situated on top of each kidney. The surface of each kidney is surrounded by two layers of fat to help protect it from trauma. Each kidney has a renal artery, renal vein, and a ureter. The kidneys receive their blood supply from the renal arteries, which are branches of the abdominal aorta. Blood is returned to the inferior vena cava via the renal veins.

The kidneys' main roles are to filter water-soluble waste products from the blood; reabsorb water, electrolytes (such as sodium, potassium, and calcium), and

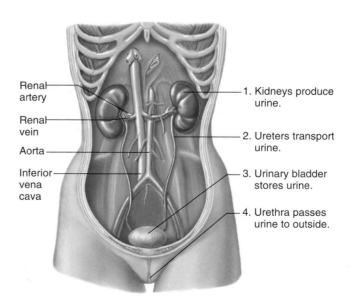

Renal artery

Renal vein

Aorta

Inferior vena cava

1. Kidneys produce urine.

2. Ureters transport urine.

3. Urinary bladder stores urine.

4. Urethra passes urine to outside.

FIGURE 24-1 ▲ The urinary system.

nutrients; and excrete what is not needed into the urine. Each kidney contains about 1 million filters called *nephrons*, which are the functional units of the kidney. Each nephron is made up of a network of capillaries and tubules through which the blood is filtered and nutrients reabsorbed. Urea, a waste product, is removed from the blood by the kidneys. Urea is produced when the liver breaks down foods containing protein, such as meat, poultry, and certain vegetables.

The ureters are tubes about 10 inches long that drain urine from the kidneys to the urinary bladder. The walls of the ureters contain smooth muscle that contracts and relaxes every 10 to 15 seconds, forcing urine away from the kidneys and sending it in small spurts into the urinary bladder, which serves as a temporary storage site for urine. The bladder is held in place by ligaments attached to other organs and the pelvic bones. The outlet of the bladder is controlled by a circular muscle called a sphincter. The wall of the bladder contains stretch receptors. The bladder swells and stretches as the amount of stored urine within it increases, stimulating the stretch receptors. When the bladder is full, the stretch receptors send a signal to the brain, which is felt as an urge to urinate. When urination begins, the bladder muscles tighten, squeezing urine from the bladder, and the sphincter muscle relaxes, allowing urine to flow.

Urine released from the bladder travels through a muscular tube called the *urethra* to the outside of the body. In males, the urethra also transports semen from the body. The male urethra measures up to 8 inches (20 cm) and is longer than that of females, which measures about 1.5 inches (3.8 cm).

Functions

Objective 2

The urinary system is responsible for the following functions:

- Maintaining a balance of salts and other substances in the blood
- Excreting waste products and foreign chemicals
- Assisting in regulating arterial blood pressure
- Producing a hormone that aids the formation of red blood cells

Renal Disorders

Kidney Stones

Objective 3

Kidney stones, also called **renal calculi,** are one of the most common genitourinary disorders. A kidney stone is a hard mass that forms from crystallization of excreted substances in the urine. The shape and size of a kidney stone varies. The stone may be smooth or jagged, as small as a grain of sand or, reportedly, as large as a golf ball. Stones that are very small often produce no symptoms and are passed easily out of the body in the urine. A stone may remain in the kidney or travel, lodging in a ureter, the bladder, or the urethra. Most stones do not cause a problem while they are in the kidney. However, a stone that lodges in a ureter can cause urine to back up behind it and into the kidney, which continues to produce urine. The backup of urine causes the kidney to stretch, which increases pressure and causes severe pain.

Experts do not agree as to why kidney stones form, but several factors increase the risk for developing kidney stones, including urinary tract infections (discussed later in this chapter), inadequate fluid intake, dehydration, and excess calcium levels in the urine. A person with a family history of kidney stones may be more likely to develop stones.

Assessment findings and symptoms can include excruciating pain that is usually located in the flank, radiating to the groin. The patient usually moves about writhing in pain, trying to find a comfortable position. Nausea, vomiting, and sweating are common. As the stone travels from the kidney into the ureter, the walls of the ureter contract in an attempt to move the stone into the bladder and relieve the obstruction. As the walls of the ureter contract the patient experiences pain that occurs in waves called *colic*. Irritation of the ureter by the stone can cause **hematuria** (blood in the urine). Blood in the urine may also be caused by trauma and kidney and bladder infections. The patient may feel the need to urinate more often and experience **dysuria** (painful or burning urination) as the stone nears the bladder.

You Should Know

Assessment Findings and Symptoms of Kidney Stones

- Excruciating pain in the flank, radiating to the groin
- Nausea, vomiting, and sweating
- Hematuria
- Dysuria
- Restlessness

Urinary Tract Infection

Objective 4

A **urinary tract infection (UTI)** is an infection that affects any part of the urinary tract. Inflammation or infection limited to the urethra is called **urethritis** and of the bladder is called **cystitis.** Inflammation or infection of the kidneys is called pyelonephritis and is discussed in the next section of this chapter. Although viruses, yeasts, and fungi can cause a UTI, bacteria are the usual cause.

Urinary tract infections are common in women (particularly sexually active women), probably because the opening to a woman's urethra lies close to both the vagina and the anus, and the short length of the urethra decreases the distance bacteria must travel to reach the bladder. In men, an enlarged prostate can interfere with urine flow, increasing the risk of a UTI. UTIs also occur in patients who have a urinary catheter in place. Urinary catheters are discussed later in this chapter.

Assessment findings and symptoms of a urinary tract infection are listed in the following *You Should Know* box.

Urinary Catheters

Objective 5

A **urinary catheter** is a tube that is inserted into the bladder to empty it of urine. It may be inserted before some surgical procedures, for some diagnostic tests, or as a means of urinary drainage for patients who have a chronic illness or are confined to bed.

Urinary catheters are available in many types and sizes. A **condom catheter** (also called a *Texas catheter*) is sometimes used for urine collection in male patients. This type of catheter consists of a condom or condom-like device with a tube attached to the distal end that is connected to a drainage bag. Condom catheters are made of several different materials, including latex. Some catheters have a Velcro attachment, and others have special double-sided tape that provides a surface on which the catheter is attached without impeding circulation. A condom catheter is easily removed for bathing or skin care. Because a condom catheter is an external urinary catheter, the patient is less likely to predispose to urinary tract infection.

A **straight catheter** is used to drain urine when a patient is temporarily unable to urinate or to obtain a urine specimen. This type of catheter has no balloon to inflate and no drainage bag.

A urinary catheter that remains in place for a longer period is called an **indwelling catheter** or **retention catheter**. The most commonly used indwelling urinary catheter is the Foley catheter. The **Foley catheter** is a flexible tube that is inserted through the urethra and into the bladder to drain urine. The tube is kept in place by a small balloon that is inflated with about 5 to 10 mL of sterile water once the tube is securely in the bladder. Urine is collected in an external drainage bag that is typically taped to the patient's thigh and hung on the side of the patient's bed by means of a plastic or metal hook. This helps prevent accidental dislodgment of the catheter.

Before transporting a patient with a urinary catheter, ensure that the catheter is securely taped to the patient's thigh. There should be some slack in the catheter tubing so the catheter will not be pulled when the patient's leg is moved, but there should be no kinks in the tubing. Assess the urine collection bag to ensure that there is no leakage from the bag. If the bag is full or leaking, inform the sending facility nurse. Note the color of the patient's urine, recognizing that some medicines and vitamins may change the color of urine. If the patient's urine does not appear to be a normal color, ask the sending facility nurse if this is normal for the patient at the time of transport. Note if the patient's urine is thick, cloudy, has mucus in it, or has red specks in it. Note if the patient's urine has a strong smell or if he complains of pain or burning in the urethra, bladder, or abdomen. After moving the patient to the gurney, make sure that the urine collection bag is positioned below the level of the patient's bladder so that urine will flow downward from the catheter, through the tubing, and into the bag.

A urine collection bag should be emptied when it is two-thirds full. After taking standard precautions, use a urinal to collect the urine. Remove the drain spout from its sleeve at the bottom of the urine bag without touching its tip. Open the slide valve on the spout. Let the urine flow out of the urine bag into the urinal, making sure that the drain tube does not touch anything. Close the slide valve, and put the drain spout into its sleeve at the bottom of the urine bag. Note the color and amount of urine collected. Ensure the clamp is secure and is not leaking. If you are transporting the patient a long distance, make sure you have sufficient collection urinals to remove the collection bag contents.

Your documentation should include the following:

- Patient assessment findings before and during transport
- At least two full sets of vital signs
- The amount (in milliliters) of any urine removed from the urine collection bag before or during transport
- The color of the patient's urine
- The location and patient's rating of any pain or discomfort using the 0 to 10 pain scale

Following is an example of documentation: "250 mL of dark yellow, clear urine emptied from the urine drainage bag. Catheter securely taped to patient's inner left thigh. Patient denies any discomfort."

Pyelonephritis

Objective 6

Pyelonephritis is an infection of the kidney. It is often the result of a bacterial bladder infection and a backflow of urine from the bladder into the ureters or kidney. Pyelonephritis is much more common in females than in males. Severe or recurring infections can cause permanent kidney damage. Assessment findings and symptoms of pyelonephritis are show in the following *You Should Know* box.

You Should Know

Assessment Findings and Symptoms of Pyelonephritis

- Fever, chills
- Fatigue
- Nausea, vomiting
- Dysuria
- Hematuria
- Cloudy or abnormal urine color
- Foul or strong urine odor
- Flank pain or lower back pain
- Warm, moist skin
- Increased urinary frequency
- Stationary preference (because movement causes pain)

Renal Failure

Objective 7

Renal failure, also called **kidney failure,** is a condition in which the kidneys fail to remove wastes adequately, concentrate urine, and conserve electrolytes to meet the demands of the body. There are acute and chronic forms of the disease. **Acute renal failure (ARF),** also called *acute kidney injury (AKI),* is a sudden deterioration of kidney function that is potentially reversible. There are many causes of ARF, including an obstruction or blockage along the urinary tract, kidney damage from severe dehydration or infection, and decreased blood flow to the kidneys from blood loss or shock. **Chronic renal failure (CRF)** develops over months and years and is usually irreversible. The most common causes of chronic renal failure are related to poorly controlled diabetes and poorly controlled hypertension. **End-stage renal disease (ESRD)** exists when kidney failure is permanent. Assessment findings and symptoms associated with acute and chronic renal failure and ESRD are shown in Table 24-1.

Dialysis

Objectives 8, 9

Patients who have acute or chronic renal failure or who have ESRD may undergo dialysis. **Dialysis** is a procedure, normally performed by the kidneys, that removes waste products from the blood. There are two types of dialysis: hemodialysis and peritoneal dialysis.

TABLE 24-1 Assessment Findings of Acute and Chronic Renal Failure and End-Stage Renal Disease

Acute Renal Failure	Chronic Renal Failure	End-Stage Renal Disease
• Reduced or no urinary output	• Headache	• Altered mental status
• Excessive urination at night	• Weakness	• Shortness of breath
• Lower extremity swelling	• Loss of appetite	• Peripheral edema
• Loss of appetite	• Vomiting	• Chest pain
• Altered mental status	• Increased urination	• Bone pain
• Metallic taste in mouth	• Rusty or brown-colored urine	• Itching
• Tremors or seizures	• Increased thirst	• Nausea, vomiting, diarrhea
• Easy bruising or prolonged bleeding	• Hypertension	• Bruising
• Flank pain	• Itching	• Muscle twitching, tremors, seizures
• Tinnitus		• Hallucinations
• Hypertension		
• Abdominal pain or discomfort		
• Dyspnea because of fluid retention		

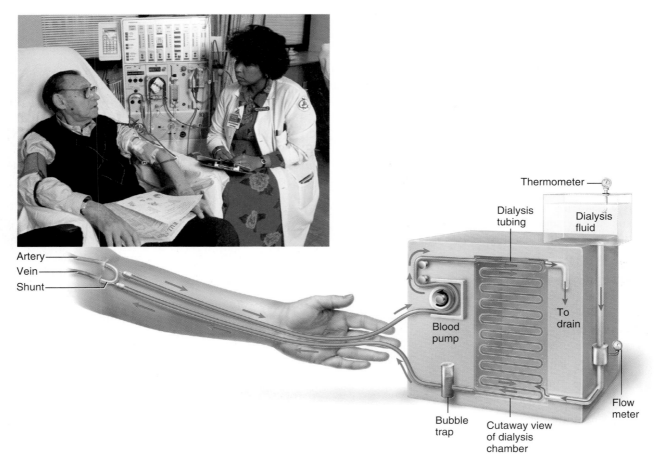

Artery
Vein
Shunt

Thermometer
Dialysis tubing
Dialysis fluid
Blood pump
To drain
Bubble trap
Cutaway view of dialysis chamber
Flow meter

FIGURE 24-2 ▲ Hemodialysis using an AV shunt.

Hemodialysis

During **hemodialysis,** the patient is connected to a machine called a *dialyzer* or *artificial kidney* (Figure 24-2). In order to connect the patient to the dialysis machine, a means of accessing her vascular system is required. For patients requiring short-term dialysis treatment, a surgeon creates an external **arteriovenous (AV) shunt.** The shunt consists of two pieces of flexible tubing, each with a tip on the end. One piece of the shunt tubing is placed in an artery in the patient's wrist or ankle, and the tip of the other is placed in a nearby vein. The tubing sticks out of two small incisions in the skin, enabling easy connection to the dialysis machine. When it is time for dialysis, each piece of tubing is clamped, separated, and connected to the dialyzer. When the patient is not receiving dialysis, the two pieces of tubing are connected to each other, allowing blood to flow through the tubes. In general, an AV shunt can be used for 6 months or less because it is prone to problems with clotting and infection. When it is no longer needed, it is surgically removed.

If the need for dialysis is long term, a surgeon creates an **arteriovenous fistula** in which a large artery and vein are joined, usually at the patient's wrist or near the elbow (Figure 24-3). Unlike an AV shunt, an AV fistula is under the patient's skin. Once the fistula is formed, arterial blood flows directly into the vein. Over a period of about 3 to 7 weeks, the vein enlarges and its walls thicken due to increased arterial pressure. This is beneficial because the patient's vein must be able to withstand repeated needle sticks associated with dialysis treatments. An AV fistula can often be used for years.

Sometimes a patient's blood vessels are too small for the surgeon to use to create an AV fistula. Examples of such patients include older adults and patients who have diabetes. In this situation, a surgeon may create an **arteriovenous graft.** Grafts are most commonly placed in the upper or lower arm. To form the graft, a blood vessel is created using artificial material, or a blood vessel from the patient's body is used, such as a vein from the thigh. The graft is created using the newly formed vessel to join an existing artery and vein.

Hemodialysis involves the transfer of a large volume of blood between the patient and the machine. The patient's AV shunt, fistula, or graft is connected by

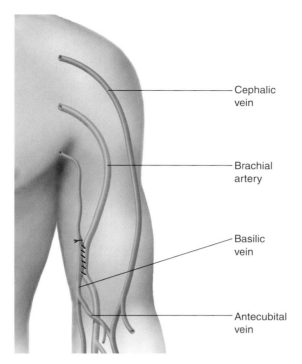

FIGURE 24-3 ▲ Arteriovenous fistula.

Cephalic vein

Brachial artery

Basilic vein

Antecubital vein

needles and tubing to the machine. A specialized chemical solution (dialysate) is used in the dialyzer to draw excess water, minerals, and waste products from the blood through a semipermeable membrane. The dialysate also balances the other electrolytes in the body. Although the dialysate and the patient's blood flow through the dialyzer at the same time, they are kept separate by the semipermeable membrane and never touch. The machine exchanges a few ounces of the patient's blood at a time and then returns the blood to his bloodstream.

Hemodialysis is usually performed two to three times per week and lasts for 4 to 5 hours. Although hemodialysis is often performed in a dialysis center or hospital, many patients have home dialysis units and can perform the procedure with the help of a family member or friend after receiving special training.

Possible complications of hemodialysis include shortness of breath, muscle cramps, nausea and vomiting, hypotension from too rapid fluid removal, dehydration, blood loss, sepsis, and cardiac arrest resulting from electrolyte disturbances. Infection and hemorrhage can occur at the vascular access site. Assessment and emergency care for the dialysis patient are discussed later in this chapter.

Peritoneal Dialysis

In **peritoneal dialysis,** a catheter is inserted into the patient's peritoneal cavity through a small abdominal incision below the umbilicus. The catheter remains per-

manently in the abdomen and is taped onto the outside of the body so that it does not interfere with everyday activities. During the dialysis process, known as an exchange or pass, dialysate is instilled into the patient's peritoneal cavity through the catheter and left in the abdomen for a designated period determined by the patient's physician. The patient's peritoneum serves as a semipermeable membrane across which wastes and excess fluids are exchanged. The fluid is then drained from the abdomen, measured, and discarded.

There are three different types of peritoneal dialysis: **continuous ambulatory peritoneal dialysis (CAPD), continuous cyclic peritoneal dialysis (CCPD),** and **intermittent peritoneal dialysis (IPD).** CAPD does not require a machine and is performed by the patient. The patient typically performs the exchange process three to five times per day while carrying out her normal daily activities. CCPD requires the use of a machine called a *cycler* that automates the exchange procedure. The machine fills the patient's abdomen with dialysate and then drains it at the end of the exchange. The cycler can be used in the home, allowing most exchanges to occur at night while the patient sleeps. IPD uses the same type of machine as CCPD, but treatments take longer, sometimes lasting up to 24 hours. IPD usually is done in the hospital but can be done at home. Because of the advantages of the other techniques, IPD is rarely used anymore.

Possible complications of peritoneal dialysis include peritonitis from bacteria entering the peritoneal cavity through or around the catheter, blockage of the catheter from clots, kinking of the catheter, hypotension, and hypovolemia.

Patient Assessment

Objectives 10, 11

Patient assessment begins with a scene size-up and putting on appropriate personal protective equipment. Form a general impression, and perform a primary survey. Assess the patient's mental status, airway, breathing, and circulation. The patient with renal disease may have an altered level of consciousness ranging from slight confusion to coma caused by an electrolyte imbalance and/or a buildup of waste products in the body. The patient may also show signs of irritability and an inability to concentrate. Note the rate and rhythm of respirations and any signs of increased work of breathing. Listen for air movement, and note if respirations are quiet, absent, or noisy. If the patient is responsive, allow the patient to assume a position of comfort. Give 100% oxygen, preferably by nonrebreather mask. Provide calm reassurance to help reduce the patient's anxiety.

Assess the patient's pulse, estimating the heart rate and assessing pulse regularity and strength. Assess perfusion by noting the color, temperature, and moisture of the patient's skin. Very warm skin suggests the presence of an infection. In the patient with kidney disease, yellowish or gray skin can indicate retention of waste products in the blood. The patient with chronic renal failure often has dry, itchy skin. If the patient complains of itching, ask when it began and what he has done to remedy the problem before your arrival. If appropriate, evaluate for possible major bleeding. Because the patient with acute or chronic renal failure can develop problems with blood clotting, assess the patient's skin for signs of bruising.

If you have not already done so, establish patient priorities, determine the need for additional resources, and make a transport decision. Is there time to provide on-scene care, or should the patient be loaded into the ambulance and rapidly transported?

Obtain a SAMPLE history from the patient if she is responsive and use the OPQRST memory aid if she is complaining of pain or discomfort. Examples of questions to ask a patient who is experiencing a genitourinary disorder are shown in the next *Making a Difference* box. If the patient is unresponsive or has an altered mental status, quickly size up the scene, form a general impression, perform a primary survey, and then proceed to the rapid medical assessment.

If the patient is responsive, perform a focused physical examination. Remember, the focused exam is guided by the patient's chief complaint and presenting signs and symptoms.

Observe the patient's position. Remember that the patient with a kidney stone is likely to move about, seeking a comfortable position. The patient who has renal failure or end-stage renal disease and has missed a dialysis appointment may develop pulmonary edema. This patient is likely to be sitting up and laboring to breathe. Look at his chest for use of accessory muscles, retractions, and equal rise and fall. Note the presence of secretions from the mouth and nose. If present, note if the secretions are blood tinged and/or foamy. Assess the patient's extremities for swelling, which is common in renal patients and usually caused by the retention of sodium and water.

Listen to breath sounds. When listening to breath sounds, remember to ask the patient to breathe in and out through his mouth, and listen for one full inspiration and expiration before moving your stethoscope to another position. Compare from side to side.

Assess the patient's pulse, respirations, blood pressure, and oxygen saturation. The patient with renal disease may have an abnormal heart rate or rhythm caused by an electrolyte imbalance. Her pulse may be weak if she has an inadequate fluid volume and bounding

Making a Difference
OPQRST

- **O**nset: How long ago did your symptoms begin? Did your symptoms begin suddenly or gradually? What were you doing when your symptoms began?
- **P**rovocation/palliation/position: What have you done to relieve the pain or discomfort? Does the discomfort disappear with rest? Is there anything that makes your symptoms better or worse?
- **Q**uality: What does the pain or discomfort feel like?
- **R**egion/radiation: Where is your discomfort? Is it in one area, or does it move?
- **S**everity: On a scale of 0 to 10, with 0 being the least and 10 being the worst, what number would you give your discomfort?
- **T**ime: How long has the discomfort been present? Have you ever had these symptoms before? When? How long did it last?

Additional Questions

- Do you have a history of kidney stones or urinary tract infections?
- Do you have burning with urination?
- Are you urinating more frequently than usual?
- Have you noticed blood in your urine?
- Do you have any allergies?
- Do you have a history of lung, liver, or kidney disease or other medical condition?
- What medicines do you take? Has the dose of any of your medications been changed recently?
- When did you last have anything to eat or drink?
- When was your last dialysis appointment? (if applicable)
- Have you been following your renal diet? (if the patient is in renal failure)

if she has excess fluid volume. If the patient is on hemodialysis, avoid taking a blood pressure in the arm with an AV shunt or fistula.

With the patient supine, assess the patient's abdomen noting if it is soft, rigid, tender or nontender, or distended. Assess the abdomen for DCAP-BTLS. The patient may have abdominal cramps, nausea, vomiting, and/or diarrhea caused by an electrolyte imbalance. If the patient receives peritoneal dialysis, look at the area around the dialysis catheter for redness, swelling, or discharge.

Provide all information obtained during your assessment to the paramedics who arrive on the scene or to the staff at the receiving facility. Carefully document all patient care information on a prehospital care report.

Emergency Care

Objective 12

Prehospital care for a patient experiencing a genitourinary emergency is supportive. Allow the patient to assume a position of comfort, and provide calm reassurance. Administer oxygen. If the patient's breathing is inadequate, give positive-pressure ventilation with 100% oxygen. Assess the adequacy of the ventilations delivered. If signs and symptoms of pulmonary edema are present, place the patient in a sitting position with the legs dependent, if possible. If the patient has an AV shunt or fistula and is bleeding from the vascular access site, control bleeding with direct pressure. Be alert for signs and symptoms of shock, and if present, keep the patient in a supine position. The patient experiencing a genitourinary emergency needs to be transported for physician evaluation. Initiate an ALS intercept if needed, and transport as soon as possible. Reassess as often as indicated until patient care is turned over to ALS personnel or medical personnel at the receiving facility.

On the Scene — Wrap-Up

You recall that an AV fistula is a large artery and vein that have been surgically joined and used for vascular access during long-term dialysis. As your partner obtains an initial set of vital signs, he is careful to avoid the arm with the AV fistula when taking the patient's blood pressure. Your initial assessment reveals the patient has a heart rate of 138 and a blood pressure of 80/50. You remember that muscle cramps, nausea and vomiting, and hypotension from too rapid fluid removal, dehydration, blood loss, or sepsis are possible complications of hemodialysis as well as infection or bleeding from the AV fistula. You examine the patient's fistula and confirm that there is no sign of bleeding. Recognizing that the patient's hypotension is most likely a complication of her dialysis, you immediately request an ALS unit for additional care and transport. While your partner administers oxygen and obtains another set of vital signs, you return to the patient and complete your physical examination, and then begin preparing her for transport. ■

Sum It Up

▶ The urinary system consists of the kidneys, ureters, urinary bladder, and urethra. The kidneys' main roles are to filter water-soluble waste products from the blood reabsorb water, electrolytes (such as sodium, potassium, and calcium), and nutrients and excrete what is not needed in the urine. The ureters are tubes about 10 inches long that drain urine from the kidneys to the urinary bladder. The urinary bladder serves as a temporary storage site for urine. Urine released from the bladder travels through a muscular tube called the urethra to the outside of the body. In males, the urethra also transports semen from the body.

▶ The urinary system is responsible for the following functions:
  • Maintaining a balance of salts and other substances in the blood
  • Excreting waste products and foreign chemicals
  • Assisting in regulating arterial blood pressure
  • Producing a hormone that aids the formation of red blood cells

▶ Kidney stones, also called renal calculi, are one of the most common genitourinary disorders. A kidney stone is a hard mass that forms from crystallization of excreted substances in the urine. A stone that lodges in a ureter can cause urine to back up behind it and into the kidney, which continues to produce urine. The backup of urine causes the kidney to stretch, which increases pressure and causes severe pain. Assessment findings and symptoms can include excruciating pain that is usually located in the flank, radiating to the groin. Nausea, vomiting, and sweating are common. Irritation of the ureter by the stone can cause hematuria (blood in the urine). The patient may experience dysuria (painful or burning urination) as the stone nears the bladder.

▶ A urinary tract infection is an infection that affects any part of the urinary tract. Inflammation or infection limited to the urethra is called urethritis and of the bladder is called cystitis. Inflammation or infection of the kidneys is called pyelonephritis.

▶ A urinary catheter is a tube that is inserted into the bladder to empty it of urine. It may be inserted before some surgical procedures, for some diagnostic tests, or as a means of urinary drainage for patients who have a chronic illness or are confined to bed.

▶ Pyelonephritis is often the result of a bacterial bladder infection and a backflow of urine from the bladder into the ureters or kidney. Severe or recurring infections can cause permanent kidney damage.

- Renal failure, also called kidney failure, is a condition in which the kidneys fail to remove wastes adequately, concentrate urine, and conserve electrolytes to meet the demands of the body. Acute renal failure, also called acute kidney injury, is a sudden deterioration of kidney function that is potentially reversible. Chronic renal failure develops over months and years and is usually irreversible. End-stage renal disease exists when kidney failure is permanent.

- Patients who have acute or chronic renal failure or who have ESRD may undergo dialysis. Dialysis is a procedure, normally performed by the kidneys, that removes waste products from the blood.

- Hemodialysis involves the transfer of a large volume of blood between the patient and the machine. The patient's AV shunt, fistula, or graft is connected by needles and tubing to the dialysis machine. A specialized chemical solution (dialysate) is used in the dialyzer to draw excess water, minerals, and waste products from the blood through a semipermeable membrane. The dialysate also balances the other electrolytes in the body. Possible complications of hemodialysis include muscle cramps, nausea and vomiting, hypotension from too rapid fluid removal, dehydration, blood loss, and sepsis. Infection and hemorrhage can occur at the vascular access site.

- In peritoneal dialysis, a catheter is inserted into the patient's peritoneal cavity through a small abdominal incision below the umbilicus. During the dialysis process, dialysate is instilled into the patient's peritoneal cavity through the catheter and left in the abdomen for a designated period determined by the patient's physician. The patient's peritoneum serves as a semipermeable membrane across which wastes and excess fluids are exchanged. The fluid is then drained from the abdomen, measured, and discarded. Possible complications of peritoneal dialysis include peritonitis from bacteria entering the peritoneal cavity through or around the catheter, blockage of the catheter from clots, kinking of the catheter, hypotension, and hypovolemia.

- Prehospital care for a patient experiencing a genitourinary emergency is supportive. Administer oxygen. If signs and symptoms of pulmonary edema are present, place the patient in a sitting position. If the patient has an AV shunt or fistula and is bleeding from the vascular access site, control bleeding with direct pressure. Be alert for signs and symptoms of shock, and if present, keep the patient in a supine position. The patient experiencing a genitourinary emergency needs to be transported for physician evaluation. Initiate an ALS intercept if needed, and transport as soon as possible. Reassess as often as indicated until patient care is turned over to ALS personnel or medical personnel at the receiving facility.

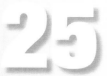
Gynecologic Disorders

By the end of this chapter, you should be able to:

Knowledge Objectives ▶
1. Identify the following structures: ovaries, uterus, cervix, labia, fallopian tubes, vagina, perineum, and endometrium.
2. Identify specific details of the medical history that should be obtained in the gynecologic patient.
3. Identify specific physical findings that should be assessed in the gynecologic patient.
4. Describe the typical assessment findings, symptoms, and emergency care for pelvic inflammatory disease.
5. Describe the typical assessment findings, symptoms, and emergency care for a suspected ectopic pregnancy.
6. Identify potential sources of trauma to the external genitalia and management of injuries.
7. Discuss the assessment of a sexual assault victim, and identify the ways in which it differs from usual assessment.
8. Identify principles of management for the sexual assault victim.

Attitude Objectives ▶
9. Value the importance of maintaining a patient's modesty and privacy while still being able to obtain necessary information.
10. Defend the need to provide care for a patient of sexual assault, while still preventing destruction of crime scene information.

Skill Objectives ▶

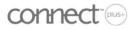

11. Demonstrate the ability to take a relevant history from the patient with a gynecologic emergency.
12. Demonstrate the ability to perform a physical assessment on the patient with a gynecologic emergency.
13. Demonstrate completing a prehospital care report for patients with a gynecologic emergency.

On the Scene

You and your partner are called to one of the local high schools for a student complaining of abdominal pain. You locate the nurse's office and find a 17-year-old female seated in a chair. She complains of "feeling hot, having chills, and stomach pain." Her skin is hot to the touch, and she is shivering. ■

As you read this chapter, think about the following questions:

- What questions should you ask this patient to help determine the cause of her complaint?
- What are the most common assessment findings and symptoms of a gynecologic emergency?
- What emergency care should you provide?

Introduction

Gynecology is the study of the female reproductive system. Gynecologic emergencies are conditions that affect the female reproductive organs. Patients experiencing a gynecologic emergency most often present with either abdominal pain or vaginal bleeding. In this chapter we discuss nontraumatic and traumatic causes of gynecologic emergencies and assessment and emergency care for the patient experiencing a gynecologic emergency.

Review of the Female Reproductive System

Objective 1

The female reproductive organs are found in the pelvic cavity (Figure 25-1). The **ovaries** are paired, almond-shaped organs located on either side of the uterus. The

ovaries perform two main functions: producing eggs and secreting hormones, such as estrogen and progesterone. Each ovary contains thousands of follicles. About once a month during a woman's reproductive years, a follicle matures to release an egg (**ovulation**). The fallopian tubes (also called *uterine tubes*) are hollow tubes that extend from each ovary to the uterus. They receive and transport the egg to the uterus after ovulation. Fertilization normally takes place in the upper third of the fallopian tube.

The uterus (womb) is a pear-shaped, hollow, muscular organ located in the pelvic cavity. It prepares for pregnancy each month of a woman's reproductive life. If pregnancy does not occur, the endometrium (the inner lining of the uterus) sloughs off and is discarded. This discharge of blood and tissue from the uterus is called **menstruation.** It is often referred to as a woman's *period*. If pregnancy does occur, the developing embryo implants in the uterine wall and develops there. The uterus stretches throughout pregnancy to adjust to the increasing size of the fetus. During labor, the uterus contracts powerfully and rhythmically to expel the infant from the mother's body. After delivery of

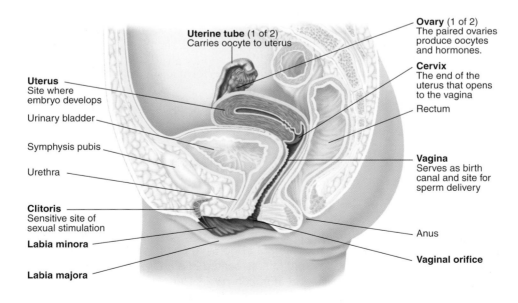

Uterine tube (1 of 2)
Carries oocyte to uterus

Ovary (1 of 2)
The paired ovaries produce oocytes and hormones.

Cervix
The end of the uterus that opens to the vagina

Rectum

Uterus
Site where embryo develops

Urinary bladder

Symphysis pubis

Urethra

Vagina
Serves as birth canal and site for sperm delivery

Clitoris
Sensitive site of sexual stimulation

Labia minora

Labia majora

Anus

Vaginal orifice

FIGURE 25-1 ▲ The structures of the female reproductive system.

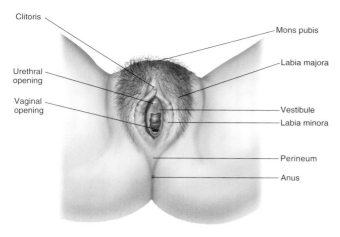

FIGURE 25-2 ▲ External female reproductive structures.

the infant, the uterus quickly clamps down to stop bleeding. (Labor and delivery will be covered in Chapter 42, "Obstetrics.")

The **cervix** is the narrow opening at the distal end of the uterus. It connects the uterus to the vagina. During pregnancy, it contains a plug of mucus. The mucus plug seals the opening to the uterus, keeping bacteria from entering. When the cervix begins to widen during early labor, the mucus plug, sometimes mixed with blood (bloody show), is expelled from the vagina. The vagina is also called the *birth canal*. It is a muscular tube that serves as a passageway between the uterus and the outside of the body (Figure 25-2). It receives the penis during intercourse. It also serves as the passageway for menstrual flow and the delivery of an infant. The **perineum** is the area between the vaginal opening and anus. The perineum may be torn during delivery. This most commonly occurs during first deliveries, explosive deliveries, and diabetic deliveries. The **labia** are structures that protect the vagina and urethra but are prone to soft tissue injury. The **labia major** is located laterally and the **labia minora** is located more medially.

Assessment of the Gynecologic Patient

Objectives 2, 3

Assessment of the patient experiencing a gynecologic emergency includes careful history taking skills.

Obtain a SAMPLE history to gather relevant medical information:

- **S**igns and symptoms: Ask the patient if she has had these same symptoms before. Common assessment findings and symptoms associated with gynecologic emergencies are shown in the next *You Should Know* box.

- **A**llergies: Ask if the patient has any allergies to medications or other materials, such as latex.

- **M**edications: Ask if the patient takes any prescription or over-the-counter medications. Also ask her about the use of alcohol or any recreational drugs.

- **P**ast medical history: Ask if the patient has a history of heart problems, respiratory problems, high blood pressure, diabetes, epilepsy, or any other ongoing medical conditions. Does she have a history of:
  —Urinary tract infections?
  —Gallbladder problems?
  —**Endometriosis** (a condition in which uterine tissue is located outside the uterus, causing pain and bleeding)?
  —Kidney stones?

- **L**ast oral intake: Find out when the patient last had something to eat or drink.

- **E**vents leading to the injury or illness: Ask about the events leading to the present situation by asking specific questions.

If the patient is complaining of abdominal pain, use OPQRST to identify the type and location of the patient's pain.

Examples of additional questions to ask include the following:

- Are you sexually active? Is it possible that you are pregnant (missed or late period, breast tenderness, urinary frequency, morning sickness)? Do you have any bleeding after intercourse?

- Do you use birth control?

- When was your last menstrual period? Was it a normal period? Are your periods usually regular? Did you have any bleeding after that period?

- Where is your pain exactly? (Ask the patient to point to the location.) What is it like (constant, comes and goes, dull, sharp, cramping)?

- Does your discomfort worsen when walking, with intercourse, or when having a bowel movement? Does a change of position or stopping activity relieve the discomfort?

If the patient is having vaginal bleeding, ask the following questions (in addition to those listed above):

- How long have you been bleeding?

- Is the blood dark red (like menstrual blood) or bright red?

- Is the bleeding heavier or lighter than a normal menstrual period? How many sanitary napkins or tampons have you used (in pads or tampons per hour)?

- Have you passed any clots?

- Do you feel dizzy when standing?

Common Assessment Findings and Symptoms of Gynecologic Emergencies

- Abdominal pain of sudden or gradual onset
- Abdominal tenderness
- Vaginal discharge
- Abnormal vaginal bleeding
- Fever, chills
- Fainting
- Sweating
- Increased heart rate
- Nausea, vomiting
- Pain during intercourse
- Pain that worsens with coughing or urination
- Pain in the tip of the shoulder (may be seen in ectopic pregnancy)

Perform a physical exam. Keep in mind that your patient may be anxious about having her clothing removed and having an examination performed by a stranger. Be certain to explain what you are about to do and why it must be done. Remember to properly drape or shield an unclothed patient from the stares of others. Conduct the examination professionally and efficiently, and talk with your patient throughout the procedure.

As an EMT, you must not visually inspect the vaginal area unless major bleeding is present or you anticipate that childbirth is about to occur. In these situations, it is best to have another healthcare professional or law enforcement officer present. If possible, include a female attendant or rescuer in your examination. The vaginal area is touched only during delivery and (ideally) when another healthcare professional or law enforcement officer is present.

Emergency Care of the Gynecologic Patient

Objectives 4, 5

To treat the patient with a gynecologic emergency, follow these steps:

- Take appropriate standard precautions. Assess baseline vital signs, and provide emergency care.
- Provide specific treatment based on the patient's assessment findings and symptoms.
- Establish and maintain an open airway. Give oxygen. If the patient's breathing is adequate, apply oxygen by nonrebreather mask at 15 L/min if not

already done. If the patient's breathing is inadequate, provide positive-pressure ventilation with 100% oxygen, and assess the adequacy of the ventilations delivered.

- Treat the patient for shock if signs are present by placing the patient in a supine position and keeping her warm.
- Document any vaginal discharge including the color, odor, amount, and the presence or absence of clots.
- If vaginal bleeding is present, apply external sanitary napkins as necessary. As the pad becomes blood-soaked, replace it with a new one. All blood-soaked garments and pads should accompany the patient to the hospital.
- Transport and reassess as often as indicated en route.
- Record all patient care information, including the patient's medical history and all emergency care given, on a prehospital care report.

Nontraumatic Gynecologic Conditions

Pelvic Inflammatory Disease

Objective 4

Pelvic inflammatory disease (PID) is an infection of the uterus, fallopian tubes, and other female reproductive organs. It is usually caused by sexually transmitted bacteria, such as chlamydia and gonorrhea. PID occurs when bacteria enter a woman's vagina and spread upward into her cervix, uterus, fallopian tubes, and other reproductive organs. An untreated infection can lead to septic shock and infertility. Common assessment findings and symptoms appear in the following *You Should Know* box.

Assessment Findings and Symptoms of Pelvic Inflammatory Disease

- Lower abdominal pain (may radiate to the lower back or right shoulder)
- Fever
- Vaginal discharge that may have a foul odor
- Painful intercourse
- Painful urination
- Increased heart rate secondary to pain and fever
- Normal or slightly elevated blood pressure (due to pain)

Using appropriate personal protective equipment, provide supportive care.

Allow the patient to assume a position of comfort. Document any vaginal discharge including the color, odor, and amount. Because appendicitis and cystitis can also present with lower abdominal pain, these conditions can be difficult to distinguish from PID. The patient should be transported for physician evaluation. Reassess as often as indicated en route. Record all patient care information, including the patient's medical history and all emergency care given, on a prehospital care report.

Sexually Transmitted Diseases

Chlamydia is a sexually transmitted disease (STD) caused by the bacterium *Chlamydia trachomatis*. STDs are also called sexually transmitted infections (STIs). Although signs and symptoms of chlamydia are usually mild or absent, complications (including infertility) can occur. According to the Centers for Disease Control and Prevention, chlamydia can be transmitted during vaginal, anal, or oral sex. It can also be passed from an infected mother to her baby during vaginal childbirth. It is estimated that about 75% of infected women and about 50% of infected men have no symptoms. When symptoms do occur in women, they typically include an abnormal vaginal discharge or a burning sensation when urinating. As the infection spreads from the cervix to the fallopian tubes, signs and symptoms can include lower abdominal pain, lower back pain, nausea, fever, pain during intercourse, or bleeding between menstrual periods. Signs and symptoms in infected men can include a discharge from the penis or a burning sensation when urinating. Chlamydia can be easily treated and cured with antibiotics.

Gonorrhea is an STD caused by the bacterium *Neisseria gonorrhoeae*. Gonorrhea multiplies in warm, moist areas of the reproductive tract such as the cervix, uterus, and fallopian tube in women and in the urethra in men and women. According to the Centers for Disease Control and Prevention, gonorrhea is spread through contact with the penis, vagina, mouth, or anus. Ejaculation does not have to occur for gonorrhea to be transmitted or acquired. Gonorrhea can also be spread from mother to baby during delivery. Like chlamydia, individuals infected with gonorrhea may have no symptoms. When signs and symptoms are present in men, they typically include a burning sensation when urinating; a white, yellow, or green discharge from the penis; or painful or swollen testicles. Signs and symptoms in women typically include a painful or burning sensation when urinating, increased vaginal discharge, or vaginal bleeding between periods. Several antibiotics are available that can successfully cure gonorrhea; however, the number of strains of gonorrhea that are resistant to drug therapy is increasing, making treatment more difficult.

Syphilis is an STD caused by the bacterium *Treponema pallidum*. The disease is transmitted through direct contact with a syphilis sore (called a *chancre*) during vaginal, anal, or oral sex. Syphilis can also be spread from mother to baby during pregnancy. If untreated, syphilis progresses in stages. During the primary stage of syphilis, a chancre appears at the site where syphilis entered the body, lasts 3 to 6 weeks, and heals on its own. If the disease is not recognized and treatment is not sought during this period, the infection progresses to the secondary stage, which is characterized by lesions on mucous membranes and a skin rash. Additional signs and symptoms during this stage can include fever, swollen lymph glands, sore throat, patchy hair loss, headaches, weight loss, muscle aches, and fatigue. If unrecognized and untreated, syphilis progresses to the latent (hidden) stage, which can last for years. During this phase, the patient has no signs or symptoms. The final (late) stages of the disease can develop 10 to 20 years after the initial infection and involve damage to the brain, nerves, eyes, heart, blood vessels, liver, bones, and joints. Syphilis is diagnosed by means of a blood test and, if caught in its early stages, can be successfully treated with antibiotics.

The most common sexually transmitted infection (STI) is genital human papillomavirus (HPV). There are more than 40 HPV types; some can cause genital warts, others can cause cervical cancer, and still others can cause cancers of the vulva, vagina, anus, and penis. Genital HPV is transmitted through genital contact, usually during vaginal or anal sex. According to the Centers for Disease Control and Prevention, there is no treatment for HPV itself, but there are treatments for the diseases that HPV can cause.

Ectopic Pregnancy

Objective 5

An **ectopic pregnancy** occurs when a fertilized egg implants outside the uterus. An ectopic pregnancy is a medical emergency. The most common site where this occurs is inside a fallopian tube (Figure 25-3). An ectopic pregnancy that occurs in a fallopian tube is called a *tubal pregnancy*. Less commonly, the egg implants in the abdomen, cervix, or an ovary. In an ectopic pregnancy, the growing fetus bursts through the tissue in which it has implanted. Severe bleeding can occur as a result of ruptured blood vessels.

The initial signs and symptoms of an ectopic pregnancy include a missed menstrual period or small amounts of vaginal bleeding that occur irregularly over 6 to 8 weeks. The patient may complain of mild cramping on one side of the pelvis, nausea, lower back pain, and lower abdominal or pelvic pain.

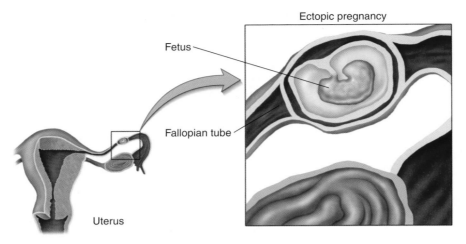

Ectopic pregnancy

Fetus

Fallopian tube

Uterus

FIGURE 25-3 ▲ An ectopic pregnancy occurs when a fertilized egg implants outside the uterus, usually inside a fallopian tube.

If rupture occurs, the patient often complains of a sudden onset of severe pain on one side of the lower abdomen. The pain can radiate to the back, rectum, vagina, and left shoulder (referred pain). Vaginal bleeding may or may not be present. The patient may feel faint or may actually faint. Severe internal bleeding may be present. The patient may have signs of shock, such as decreasing blood pressure, an increased heart rate, and cool, clammy skin.

The diagnosis of an ectopic pregnancy is made at the hospital, not in the field. Prepare for immediate transport to the closest appropriate facility. Keep on-scene time to a minimum. Request an early response of advanced life support (ALS) personnel to the scene or consider an ALS intercept while en route to the receiving facility. Do not delay transport for ALS arrival. Give oxygen by nonrebreather mask. Treat the patient for shock if signs are present by placing the patient in a supine position and keeping her warm. Remember to provide emotional support for the patient and family. Reassess as often as indicated during transport. Record all patient care information, including the patient's medical history and all emergency care given, on a PCR.

Remember This

Although there are many causes of abdominal pain, you must consider lower abdominal pain in any woman of childbearing age to be caused by an ectopic pregnancy until proved otherwise. An ectopic pregnancy is a medical emergency.

Ovarian Cyst

An **ovarian cyst** is a fluid-filled sac that develops on or within an ovary. The most common type of ovarian cyst

forms during the menstrual cycle and goes away on its own in 1 to 3 months. Although most ovarian cysts do not cause symptoms, others can cause symptoms if the cyst pushes on nearby structures, ruptures, or bleeds. Possible assessment findings and symptoms are listed in the following *You Should Know* box.

You Should Know

Assessment Findings and Symptoms of Ovarian Cyst

- Lower abdominal or pelvic pain that may be severe, sudden, and sharp
- Irregular menstrual periods
- Dull ache in the lower back and thighs
- Faintness, dizziness, or weakness
- Feeling of lower abdominal or pelvic pressure or fullness
- Pelvic pain after strenuous exercise or sexual intercourse
- Weight gain
- Pain or pressure with urination or bowel movements
- Difficulty passing urine completely
- Nausea and vomiting

Vaginitis

Vaginitis, an inflammation of the vagina, may be caused by an infection due to bacteria or yeast or from reduced estrogen levels after menopause. Signs and symptoms typically include vaginal discharge that varies in color, odor, and amount, depending on the cause of the vaginitis. Additional signs and symptoms can include light vaginal bleeding, vaginal itching or irritation, painful intercourse, and painful urination. Vaginitis usually responds well to appropriate medication therapy.

Cervicitis

Cervicitis, an inflammation of the cervix, is often caused by infection with sexually transmitted diseases, including gonorrhea and chlamydia. Because cervicitis may be present but produce no signs or symptoms, some women are unaware that they have it until they undergo testing for another medical condition and the infection is found. When signs and symptoms are present, they can include frequent, painful urination; pain during intercourse; gray or yellow vaginal discharge; or vaginal bleeding after intercourse, between menstrual periods, or after menopause. Treatment for cervicitis usually includes antibiotics to treat the underlying infection.

Cervical Cancer

Cervical cancer is one of the most common cancers that affect a woman's reproductive organs. Various strains of the human papillomavirus (HPV), a sexually transmitted infection, play a role in causing most cases of cervical cancer. Signs and symptoms can include pain during intercourse, bloody vaginal discharge that may have a foul odor, or vaginal bleeding after intercourse, between menstrual periods, or after menopause. Treatment for cervical cancer varies, depending on the number of layers of the cervix that are affected.

Uterine Fibroids

Many women develop uterine fibroids during their childbearing years. Uterine fibroids are growths that often cause no symptoms and seldom require treatment. When uterine fibroids do cause symptoms, they can include back or leg pain, heavy menstrual bleeding, pelvic pressure or pain, prolonged menstrual periods, or bleeding between periods. Treatment for uterine fibroids varies, ranging from medical observation to hysterectomy.

Regardless of the possible cause of the patient's gynecologic emergency, provide supportive care to the patient experiencing an emergency and allow the patient to assume a position of comfort. The patient should be transported for physician evaluation. Reassess as often as indicated en route. Record all patient care information, including the patient's medical history and all emergency care given, on a prehospital care report.

Traumatic Gynecologic Emergencies

Objective 6

Trauma to the external genitalia may occur from bicycle injuries, blows, foreign body insertion, childbirth lacerations, or sexual assault. Take appropriate standard precautions. Ensure and maintain an open airway. Give oxygen. Control bleeding with local pressure to the area, using trauma dressings or sanitary napkins. Do not pack or place dressings inside the vagina. Monitor the patient's vital signs closely and treat for shock if indicated. Provide additional care based on the patient's signs and symptoms. Provide reassurance and privacy. Transport to an appropriate medical facility for further care, reassessing as often as indicated during transport. Record all patient care information, including the patient's medical history and all emergency care given, on a PCR.

Apparent Sexual Assault

Objectives 7, 8

Criminal assault situations require initial and ongoing assessment and management, as well as psychological care. Take appropriate standard precautions. When possible, have an EMT of the same gender assess the sexual assault victim. Ensure and maintain an open airway. Maintain a nonjudgmental attitude during the SAMPLE history and focused assessment. Protect the crime scene, and document any pertinent findings. Discourage the patient from bathing, douching, urinating, or cleaning wounds until after transport and evaluation at the receiving facility. It is very important to explain that these actions remove evidence that can be helpful in the criminal or civil investigation. Do *not* allow the patient to do these things. Also, advise the patient to bring additional clothing to the hospital (if it is appropriate to wait on scene long enough for this to happen), or advise a family member or friend to bring additional clothing since the patient's clothing will be removed as evidence. Do not allow the patient to comb her hair or clean her fingernails. The patient should not be allowed to eat or drink because doing so washes away evidence.

You Should Know

Become familiar with your state's procedures and protocols regarding evidence handling.

Handle the patient's clothing as little as possible. Bag all items separately in paper bags, and seal with evidence tape (if available). Do not use plastic bags for bloodstained articles. Plastic holds in moisture, which can promote the growth of bacteria. Bacterial growth can contaminate evidence. Examine the genitalia only if profuse bleeding is present. Transport to an appropriate medical facility for further care. Reassess as often as indicated during transport. Record all patient care information, including the patient's medical history and all emergency care given, on a PCR.

On the Scene   Wrap-Up

You quickly obtain a SAMPLE history and then ask additional questions based on the patient's responses. She reports that she ate breakfast this morning (about 3 hours ago), has no allergies, and takes no medications. She started "feeling bad" about 1 hour ago and points to her lower abdomen as the site of her abdominal pain. In response to additional questions she admits to being sexually active and says she has had an unusual vaginal discharge "that smells" for about a week. Recalling that patients experiencing a gynecologic emergency most often present with either abdominal pain or vaginal bleeding, you explain to the patient that she will need to be transported for evaluation by a physician. As you assist the patient onto the gurney, you allow her to assume a position of comfort and provide supportive care en route to the hospital. ■

Sum It Up

▶ Gynecology is the study of the female reproductive system. Gynecologic emergencies are conditions that affect the female reproductive organs. Patients experiencing a gynecologic emergency most often present with either abdominal pain or vaginal bleeding.

▶ Assessment of the patient experiencing a gynecologic emergency includes careful history taking skills.

▶ When performing a physical exam, keep in mind that your patient may be anxious about having her clothing removed and having an examination performed by a stranger. Be certain to explain what you are about to do and why it must be done. Remember to properly drape or shield an unclothed patient from the stares of others. Conduct the examination professionally and efficiently, and talk with your patient throughout the procedure.

▶ As an EMT, you must not visually inspect the vaginal area unless major bleeding is present or you anticipate that childbirth is about to occur. In these situations, it is best to have another healthcare professional or law enforcement officer present. If possible, include a female attendant or rescuer in your examination. The vaginal area is touched only during

delivery and (ideally) when another healthcare professional or law enforcement officer is present.

▶ Pelvic inflammatory disease is an infection of the uterus, fallopian tubes, and other female reproductive organs. It is usually caused by sexually transmitted bacteria, such as chlamydia and gonorrhea. PID occurs when bacteria enter a woman's vagina and spread upward into her cervix, uterus, fallopian tubes, and other reproductive organs. An untreated infection can lead to septic shock and infertility.

▶ Chlamydia is a sexually transmitted disease that can be transmitted during vaginal, anal, or oral sex. It can also be passed from an infected mother to her baby during vaginal childbirth. Chlamydia can be easily treated and cured with antibiotics.

▶ Gonorrhea is an STD that multiplies in warm, moist areas of the reproductive tract such as the cervix, uterus, and fallopian tube in women and in the urethra in men and women. Several antibiotics are available that can successfully cure gonorrhea; however, the number of strains of gonorrhea that are resistant to drug therapy is increasing, making treatment more difficult.

▶ Syphilis is an STD transmitted through direct contact with a syphilis sore (called a chancre) during vaginal, anal, or oral sex. Syphilis can also be spread from mother to baby during pregnancy. Syphilis is diagnosed by means of a blood test and, if caught in its early stages, can be successfully treated with antibiotics.

▶ Genital human papillomavirus is a sexually transmitted infection that is transmitted through genital contact, usually during vaginal or anal sex. According to the Centers for Disease Control and Prevention, there is no treatment for HPV itself, but there are treatments for the diseases that HPV can cause.

▶ An ectopic pregnancy occurs when a fertilized egg implants outside the uterus. An ectopic pregnancy is a medical emergency. The most common site where this occurs is inside a fallopian tube. An ectopic pregnancy that occurs in a fallopian tube is called a *tubal pregnancy*. Severe bleeding can occur as a result of ruptured blood vessels. The patient may complain of mild cramping on one side of the pelvis, nausea, lower back pain, and lower abdominal or pelvic pain. If rupture occurs, the patient often complains of a sudden onset of severe pain on one side of the lower abdomen. Vaginal bleeding may or may not be present. Severe internal bleeding may be present. The patient may have signs of shock, such as decreasing blood pressure, an increased heart rate, and cool, clammy skin.

▶ Although there are many causes of abdominal pain, you must consider lower abdominal pain in any woman of childbearing age to be caused by an ectopic pregnancy until proved otherwise.

- An ovarian cyst is a fluid-filled sac that develops on or within an ovary. The most common type of ovarian cyst forms during the menstrual cycle and goes away on its own in 1 to 3 months. Although most ovarian cysts do not cause symptoms, others can cause symptoms if the cyst pushes on nearby structures, ruptures, or bleeds.

- Vaginitis, an inflammation of the vagina, may be caused by an infection due to bacteria or yeast or from reduced estrogen levels after menopause. Vaginitis usually responds well to appropriate medication therapy.

- Cervicitis, an inflammation of the cervix, is often caused by infection with sexually transmitted diseases, including gonorrhea and chlamydia. Treatment for cervicitis usually includes antibiotics to treat the underlying infection.

- Cervical cancer is one of the most common cancers that affect a woman's reproductive organs. Treatment for cervical cancer varies depending on the number of layers of the cervix that are affected.

- Uterine fibroids are growths that often cause no symptoms and seldom require treatment. When uterine fibroids do cause symptoms, they can include back or leg pain, heavy menstrual bleeding, pelvic pressure or pain, prolonged menstrual periods, or bleeding between periods.

- Trauma to the external genitalia may occur from bicycle injuries, blows, foreign body insertion, childbirth lacerations, or sexual assault. Trauma to the external genitalia should be treated as other bleeding soft tissue injuries. Control bleeding with local pressure to the area, using trauma dressings or sanitary napkins. Do not pack or place dressings inside the vagina. Monitor the patient's vital signs closely and treat for shock if indicated.

- Criminal assault situations require initial and ongoing assessment and management, as well as psychological care. When possible, have an EMT of the same gender assess the sexual assault victim. Maintain a nonjudgmental attitude during the SAMPLE history and focused assessment. Protect the crime scene, and document any pertinent findings. Discourage the patient from bathing, douching, urinating, or cleaning wounds until after transport and evaluation at the receiving facility. The patient should not be allowed to eat or drink because doing so washes away evidence. Handle the patient's clothing as little as possible. Bag all items separately in paper bags, and seal with evidence tape (if available). Examine the genitalia only if profuse bleeding is present. Transport to an appropriate medical facility for further care.

CHAPTER 26

Nontraumatic Musculoskeletal Disorders

By the end of this chapter, you should be able to:

Knowledge Objectives ▶

1. Briefly discuss the anatomy and physiology of the musculoskeletal system.
2. Discuss common nontraumatic musculoskeletal disorders including osteoporosis, arthritis, fibromyalgia, and overuse syndromes.
3. Define fracture.
4. Identify specific details of the medical history that should be obtained in the patient with a nontraumatic musculoskeletal disorder.
5. Identify specific physical findings that should be assessed in the patient with a nontraumatic musculoskeletal disorder.
6. Identify general principles of emergency care for the patient with a nontraumatic musculoskeletal disorder.

Attitude Objectives ▶

No attitude objectives are identified for this lesson.

Skill Objectives ▶

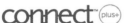

7. Demonstrate the ability to take a relevant history from the patient with a nontraumatic musculoskeletal disorder.
8. Demonstrate the ability to perform a physical assessment on the patient with a nontraumatic musculoskeletal disorder.
9. Demonstrate completing a prehospital care report for patients with a nontraumatic musculoskeletal disorder.

On the Scene

You and your partner are called to an assisted living facility for a report of hip pain. On arrival at the door of the appropriate room, you knock on the door and hear a woman tell you to "come on in." You find an 87-year-old woman sitting in a recliner complaining of pain in her right hip that she describes as "very painful." Your partner moves forward to manually stabilize her cervical spine while you ask the patient if she fell. She states that she did not fall; she simply went to sit down on her chair when she heard a "pop" and felt intense pain in her right hip. You decide to withhold cervical spinal stabilization and begin care for this patient. ■

THINK ABOUT IT

As you read this chapter, think about the following questions:

- Based on the information provided, what is the most likely cause of this patient's signs and symptoms?
- What emergency care should you provide?

Introduction

Nontraumatic musculoskeletal disorders are common. Although they are not life-threatening, they may be very painful. In this chapter we discuss some of the more common nontraumatic musculoskeletal disorders, typical assessment findings and symptoms associated with these conditions, and general emergency care.

Review of the Musculoskeletal System

Objective 1

The human skeleton provides the support for the body and provides a frame for other parts of the musculoskeletal system to attach to, including ligaments, tendons, and muscles (Figure 26-1).

Bones are living, growing tissues that are made up mostly of collagen and calcium. **Collagen** is a protein that provides a soft framework. **Calcium** is a mineral that strengthens and hardens the framework. New bone is constantly added to the skeleton, and old bone is removed. Bones become large, heavy, and thick during childhood and teenage years because new bone is added faster than old bone is removed. Maximum bone strength and thickness are reached at about age 30. After age 30, bone cells begin to die more rapidly than new cells are produced, resulting in a gradual decline in bone mass.

You will recall from Chapter 6 that skeletal muscles move the skeleton, produce the heat that helps maintain a constant body temperature, and maintain posture (Figure 26-2). Most skeletal muscles are attached to bones by means of **tendons,** which are cords of connective tissue that firmly attach the end of a muscle to a bone. **Ligaments** are tough groups of connective tissue that attach bones to bones and bones to cartilages. **Cartilage** provides cushioning between bones and allows easy movement of joints. Ligaments provide support and strength to joints and restrain excessive joint movement.

A **joint** is a place where two bones come together. Some joints do not move, while others allow limited movement, and others allow for movement that is more complicated. An **immovable joint,** or *fibrous joint*, is joined by fibrous connective tissue and does not move. The edges of the bones of the skull are held together by fibrous joints. **Cartilaginous joints** are joints in which the bones are attached by cartilage. These joints, found in the spine and ribs, allow

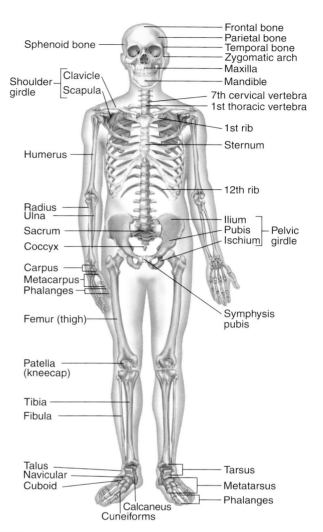

FIGURE 26-1 ▲ The human skeleton is made up of the axial skeleton (shown in gold), which consists of the skull, vertebral column, sternum, and ribs. The appendicular skeleton (shown in blue) is attached and includes the shoulder and pelvic girdle and the limb bones.

for only a little movement. Most of the joints of the body are **synovial joints,** which allow movement in many directions. This type of joint is found at the hip, shoulders, elbows, knees, wrists, and ankles. Synovial joints are broken down into groups according to their shape and movement. Examples include ball-and-socket joints (Figure 26-3), gliding joints, and hinge joints (Figure 26-4). The ends of the bones of a synovial joint are covered with a layer of smooth cartilage and connected by ligaments lined with synovial membrane to reduce friction. The synovial membrane secretes synovial fluid, which acts as a lubricant to help the joints move easily.

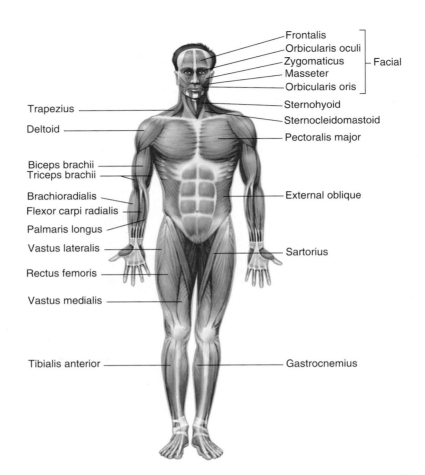

FIGURE 26-2 ▲ The human body has more than 600 skeletal muscles. A few of them are identified here.

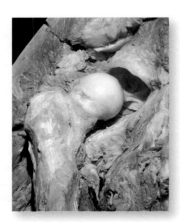

FIGURE 26-3 ▲ The hip joint is an example of a ball-and-socket joint.

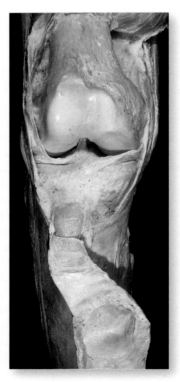

FIGURE 26-4 ▲ The knee joint is an example of a hinge joint.

Nontraumatic Musculoskeletal Conditions

Arthritis

Objective 2

Osteoarthritis (OA), also called *degenerative arthritis* or *degenerative joint disease,* is a chronic condition characterized by the breakdown of the joint's cartilage. When cartilage breaks down, bones rub against each other, causing pain, stiffness, and limitations in movement of the joint. Osteoarthritis commonly affects the hands, wrists, elbows, shoulders, spine, hips, knees, and ankles.

There are two different types of osteoarthritis: primary and secondary. Primary osteoarthritis is associated with aging and its cause is unknown. Secondary osteoarthritis is caused by another disease or condition. For example, diabetes, obesity, hormone disorders, and injury to joints can lead to secondary osteoarthritis.

Rheumatoid arthritis is a type of arthritis in which the lining of the joints is inflamed. In the initial stages of the disease, inflammation of the joint lining results in pain, warmth, stiffness, redness, and swelling around the joint. In later stages of the disease, the affected joint becomes misaligned and loses its shape, further limiting joint movement.

Osteoporosis

Objectives 2, 3

Osteoporosis is a disease of progressive bone loss in which bones become weak and brittle due to low levels of calcium, phosphorus, and other minerals in the bones. It is a common cause of fractures in women after menopause and older adults. A **fracture** is a break in a bone. If a bone is broken, chipped, cracked, or splintered, it is said to be fractured. Although osteoporosis can affect any bone, fractures are common in the spine, hip, or wrist. For some patients who have osteoporosis, everyday activities such as straining when lifting a child or vacuum cleaner, bending down to pick up a newspaper, walking, stepping off a curb, or even coughing or sneezing can result in a fracture.

Osteoporosis often goes unnoticed because bone loss occurs gradually and without symptoms. Once bones have been weakened by osteoporosis, collapse and fractures of the vertebrae produce back pain, a gradual loss of height, and **kyphosis** (severely stooped posture). Hip fractures usually occur because of a fall. Healing after surgery to repair the fracture may be slow and difficult because of poor bone quality.

Fibromyalgia

Objective 2

Fibromyalgia (FM) is a disorder characterized by general fatigue and widespread musculoskeletal pain and stiffness that often persists for months at a time. Although any body part can be affected, the most common sites of pain include the neck, back, shoulders, pelvis, and hands. Fibromyalgia can occur in children and older adults, but most often develops during early and middle adulthood. Women are affected more often than men. The cause of fibromyalgia is not known, although many theories exist. Common assessment findings and symptoms are listed in the following *You Should Know* box.

You Should Know

Common Assessment Findings and Symptoms of Fibromyalgia

- Musculoskeletal aches, pain, and stiffness
- Soft tissue tenderness
- Depression and anxiety
- Impaired concentration
- Problems with short- and long-term memory
- Headaches
- Bladder irritability and spasms
- Painful menstruation
- General fatigue
- Sleep disturbances
- Sensitivity to odors, noises, bright lights, and touch

Overuse Syndromes

Objective 2

Overuse syndromes are a group of conditions in which a part of the body is injured from repeated motions performed in the course of normal work or daily activities. Over time, overuse disorders can cause temporary or permanent damage to tendons, muscle, and ligaments. Other terms used to describe overuse syndromes include the following:

- Cumulative trauma disorder
- Occupational overuse syndrome
- Overuse disorder
- Overuse strain
- Repetitive motion disorders
- Repetitive strain injury
- Repetitive stress injury

The most commonly affected areas of the body are the hands, wrists, elbows, and shoulders, but the neck, back, hips, knees, feet, legs, and ankles can also be affected. Examples of common overuse disorders include the following:

- Hand and wrist: carpal tunnel syndrome, wrist tendonitis
- Elbow: tennis elbow, golfer's elbow
- Hip: snapping hip syndrome, hip bursitis
- Knee and leg: shin splints, kneecap bursitis
- Foot and ankle: Achilles tendonitis

Bursitis or tendonitis is common in overuse disorders. A bursa is a small, jellylike sac that is filled with a small amount of fluid and acts as a cushion, minimizing friction between bones and the soft tissues that overlie them. Bursa are found around various joints in the body, such as the shoulder, elbow, hip, knee, and heel. In **bursitis,** a bursa becomes swollen and inflamed, resulting in pain when the joint is moved. Bursitis usually results from repetitive movement or prolonged and excessive pressure. **Tendonitis,** which is an inflammation of a tendon or the covering of the tendon, is often associated with pain, tenderness, and (possibly) limited movement of the muscle attached to the affected tendon.

Common assessment findings and symptoms of overuse syndromes are listed in the following *You Should Know* box.

You Should Know

Common Assessment Findings and Symptoms of Overuse Syndromes

- Numbness
- Decreased joint motion
- Swelling
- Burning
- Pain
- Aching
- Redness
- Weakness
- Tingling
- Clumsiness
- Cracking or popping of joints

The carpal tunnel is a narrow passageway found at the inside center of the wrist. The passageway is surrounded by bone on three sides and a ligament on the other. Tendons and the median nerve, which runs from the forearm into the hand and conducts sensation to the palm side of the thumb and fingers (although not the little finger), pass through the carpal tunnel. The median nerve also conducts impulses to some small muscles in the hand that allow the fingers and thumb to move. When the wrist and fingers are used, tendons slide back and forth within the tunnel. If irritation of the tendons or their coverings results in swelling, the area within the tunnel narrows and the median nerve is compressed. Carpal tunnel syndrome is caused when pressure in the carpal tunnel compresses the median nerve. This can result in pain, burning, tingling, weakness, or numbness in the palm of the hand, fingers, and wrist that can extend up the arm. Symptoms of carpal tunnel syndrome can be aggravated by activities such as driving, typing, racquet sports, and weight lifting.

Wrist tendonitis is inflammation of one or more of the tendons around the wrist joint. Overuse of the joint when performing activities such as throwing, catching, bowling, hitting a tennis ball, typing, or sewing can result in pain, tenderness, and swelling over the area of inflammation.

Tennis elbow is a condition that affects the tendons that attach to the bone on the lateral part of the elbow. Although the exact cause is unknown, overuse of the muscles and tendons of the forearm occurs with activities such as lifting, gripping, and/or grasping, resulting in pain on the outside of the arm at the elbow joint. Sports such as tennis and fencing and professions such as meat cutting, plumbing, carpentry, painting, and weaving are commonly associated with tennis elbow.

Golfer's elbow is a form of tendonitis similar to tennis elbow but involves pain on the inside of the arm at the elbow joint. The pain of golfer's elbow is usually triggered when gripping an object.

Snapping hip syndrome, also called *dancer's hip,* is a condition characterized by an audible snapping or popping noise (or deep "clunk") over the tendon and a snapping sensation when the hip is moved from flexion to extension. Snapping hip syndrome typically occurs in individuals between the ages of 15 and 40 years during activities such as ballet, gymnastics, horseback riding, soccer, and running.

Pain and inflammation over the outside of the upper thigh may be caused by hip bursitis. Examples of conditions associated with hip bursitis include running-oriented sports such as soccer and football, bicycling, climbing stairs, or trauma such as falling onto the hip or bumping the hip on the edge of a table. Hip bursitis usually occurs in middle-aged or older adults and is more common in women than in men.

Medial tibial stress syndrome, also called *shin splints,* is a term used to describe pain over the front of the tibia. It is most commonly seen in runners and basketball and tennis players. An increase in the duration and intensity of training can cause an overload on the tibia and surrounding tissues, resulting in tenderness, soreness or pain, and swelling along the inner part of the lower leg.

Bursitis of the kneecap, also known as *housemaid's knee*, can cause swelling and pain on top of the kneecap and limited motion of the knee. This condition is common in professions that require prolonged kneeling, such as plumbing, roofing, carpet laying, and gardening.

The Achilles tendon, the largest and strongest tendon in the body, attaches the muscles of the calf to the heel bone. Because the Achilles tendon is used when walking, running, or jumping, Achilles tendonitis most commonly occurs in individuals who do a lot of walking, runners, dancers, and tennis and basketball players. Changes in or wearing inappropriate footwear, training on poor surfaces, and changes in the intensity of training schedules can contribute to Achilles tendonitis. The patient typically complains of pain over the back of the heel, usually after periods of inactivity, and may have swelling or a "bump" or "knot" on the tendon. In some patients, a crackling sound may be heard when the tendon is touched or moved.

Patient Assessment

Objectives 4, 5

Conduct a scene size-up and ensure your safety. Put on appropriate personal protective equipment. Perform a primary survey to identify and treat any life-threatening conditions. Take the patient's vital signs, and gather the patient's medical history. If the patient is complaining of pain, use OPQRST to identify the type and location of the patient's pain. Examples of questions to ask a patient who is experiencing a nontraumatic musculoskeletal disorder are shown in the next *Making a Difference* box.

Perform a physical examination. The assessment findings and symptoms of nontraumatic musculoskeletal conditions vary but typically include pain or tenderness, deformity, swelling, loss of or abnormal movement, sensation changes, and/or circulatory changes. Use the DCAP-BTLS memory aid to recall what to look and feel for during the physical exam:

> **D**eformities
> **C**ontusions (bruises)
> **A**brasions (scrapes)
> **P**unctures/penetrations
> **B**urns
> **T**enderness
> **L**acerations (cuts)
> **S**welling

Making a Difference

OPQRST

- **O**nset: How long ago did your symptoms begin? Did your symptoms begin suddenly or gradually? What were you doing when your symptoms began? Were you resting, sleeping, or doing some type of physical activity? Did you hear or feel a pop or snap when your symptoms began?
- **P**rovocation/palliation/position: What have you done to relieve the pain or discomfort? Does the discomfort disappear with rest? Does it get better or worse when you change positions, or does it stay the same?
- **Q**uality: What does the pain or discomfort feel like? (Ask the patient to describe the pain or discomfort in his own words, such as *dull, burning, sharp, stabbing, shooting, throbbing, pressure, or tearing.*)
- **R**egion/radiation: Where is your discomfort? Is it in one area or does it move? Is it located in any other area?
- **S**everity: On a scale of 0 to 10, with 0 being the least and 10 being the worst, what number would you give your discomfort?
- **T**ime: How long has the discomfort been present? Have you ever had these symptoms before? When? How long did they last?

Additional Questions

- Do you have any allergies?
- Do you have a history of heart problems, respiratory problems, high blood pressure, diabetes, epilepsy, or any other ongoing medical conditions?
- Do you have a history of lung, liver, kidney disease, or other medical condition?
- What medicines do you take?
- When did you last have anything to eat or drink?

Feel along the length of the extremity for deformities, tenderness, and swelling. Feel and listen for crepitus, which is the grating of broken bone ends against each other. Check the **p**ulse, **m**ovement, and **s**ensation (PMS) in each extremity. Compare each extremity to the opposite extremity. Perform a bilateral (right and left at the same time) assessment of the most distal extremities for pulses, movement, and sensation. While assessing the extremities bilaterally, note any differences in your findings. Assess the dorsalis pedis pulse (on top of the foot) in each lower extremity. Assess the radial pulse in each upper extremity.

Assess movement of the lower extremities by asking the patient if she can push her feet into your hands (plantar flexion). Ask the patient to flex her feet dorsally by instructing her to pull her toes toward her nose (dorsiflexion). Assess movement of the upper extremities by asking the patient to squeeze your fingers. Compare the strength of her grips, and note if they are equal or if one side appears weaker. Assess sensation by touching the fingers and toes of each extremity and asking her to tell you where you are touching. Assess the patient's thumb or pinky (or great toe or baby toe) to avoid the confusion of having to describe which "middle" digit is being touched.

Emergency Care

Objective 6

In general, emergency care for a patient with a nontraumatic musculoskeletal disorder is supportive. Take appropriate standard precautions, and provide specific treatment based on the patient's signs and symptoms. Allow the patient to assume a position of comfort. Maintain an open airway. Give oxygen if indicated.

In some cases, applying a splint can help relieve joint pain. Splinting is explained in detail in Chapter 37, "Orthopedic Trauma." Before applying a splint, you should manually stabilize the affected extremity. This will require another person, who will use his hands to gently support the extremity. To stabilize an injured joint, support the bones above and below it. Additional support may be needed underneath the injured area so that it does not sag. Do not release manual stabilization until the affected area has been properly immobilized. Pad a rigid or semirigid splint before applying it. Padding helps lessen patient discomfort caused by pressure, especially around bony areas. After the extremity is splinted, apply an ice bag or cold pack. Place a cloth or bandage between the patient's skin and the cold source.

Comfort, calm, and reassure the patient, family members, and friends of the patient. Transport and reassess as often as indicated en route. Record all patient care information, including the patient's medical history and all emergency care given, on a prehospital care report.

On the Scene   Wrap-Up

The patient tells you that she has been diagnosed with and is being treated for osteoporosis. Your physical exam reveals pain and swelling of the right hip and slight rotation of her right foot. You suspect that the patient has a hip or femur fracture and will require transport to the closest appropriate facility for additional care. You and your partner carefully place the patient on a long backboard and apply padding and splinting for the patient's comfort during the transport to the hospital. ∎

Sum It Up

▶ The human skeleton provides the support for the body and provides a frame for other parts of the musculoskeletal system to attach to, including ligaments, tendons, and muscles.

▶ Bones become large, heavy, and thick during childhood and teenage years because new bone is added faster than old bone is removed. Maximum bone strength and thickness is reached at about age 30. After age 30, bone cells begin to die more rapidly than new cells are produced resulting in a gradual decline in bone mass.

▶ Skeletal muscles move the skeleton, produce the heat that helps maintain a constant body temperature, and maintain posture. Most skeletal muscles are attached to bones by means of tendons.

▶ Ligaments are tough groups of connective tissue that attach bones to bones and bones to cartilage. Cartilage provides cushioning between bones and allows easy movement of joints. Ligaments provide support and strength to joints and restrain excessive joint movement.

▶ A joint is a place where two bones come together. Some joints do not move, while others allow limited movement, and others allow for movement that is more complicated.

▶ Osteoarthritis is a chronic condition characterized by the breakdown of the joint's cartilage. When cartilage breaks down, bones rub against each other, causing pain, stiffness, and limitations in movement of the joint. Osteoarthritis commonly affects the hands, wrists, elbows, shoulders, spine, hips, knees, and ankles.

▶ Rheumatoid arthritis is a type of arthritis in which the lining of the joints is inflamed. In the initial stages of the disease, inflammation of the joint lining results in pain, warmth, stiffness, redness, and swelling around the joint. In later stages of the disease, the affected joint becomes misaligned and loses its shape, further limiting joint movement.

▶ Osteoporosis is a disease of progressive bone loss in which bones become weak and brittle due to low levels of calcium, phosphorus, and other minerals in the bones. It is a common cause of fractures in women after menopause and in older adults. A fracture is a break in a bone. Although osteoporosis can affect any bone, fractures are common in the spine, hip, or wrist.

▶ Fibromyalgia is a disorder characterized by general fatigue and widespread musculoskeletal pain and stiffness that often persists for months at a time. Although any body part can be affected, the most common sites of pain include the neck, back, shoulders, pelvis, and hands.

▶ Overuse syndromes are a group of conditions in which a part of the body is injured from repeated motions performed in the course of normal work or daily activities. The most commonly affected areas of the body are the hands, wrists, elbows, and shoulders, but the neck, back, hips, knees, feet, legs, and ankles can also be affected. Over time, overuse disorders can cause temporary or permanent damage to tendons, muscle, and ligaments.

▶ Bursitis or tendonitis is common in overuse disorders. In bursitis, a bursa becomes swollen and inflamed, resulting in pain when the joint is moved. Bursitis usually results from repetitive movement or prolonged and excessive pressure. Tendonitis, which is an inflammation of a tendon or the covering of the tendon, is often associated with pain, tenderness, and (possibly) limited movement of the muscle attached to the affected tendon.

Immunology

By the end of this chapter, you should be able to:

Knowledge Objectives ▶

1. Define allergic reaction.
2. Discuss the routes by which a substance that causes an allergic reaction can enter the body.
3. List common causes of allergic reactions.
4. Discuss latex allergy among patients and healthcare professionals.
5. Define antigen, antibody, sensitization, and allergen.
6. Discuss the inflammatory process.
7. Define anaphylaxis.
8. Differentiate signs and symptoms of a mild allergic reaction from those of a moderate or severe allergic reaction.
9. Discuss assessment of the patient with an allergic reaction.
10. Identify specific details of the medical history that should be obtained from patient with an allergic reaction.
11. Describe the emergency medical care for the patient with an allergic reaction.

Attitude Objective ▶

12. Explain the rationale for administering epinephrine with an autoinjector.

Skill Objectives ▶

connect (plus+)

13. Demonstrate the ability to take a relevant history from the patient with an allergic reaction.
14. Demonstrate the ability to perform a physical assessment of the patient with an allergic reaction.
15. Demonstrate completing a prehospital care report for patients with an allergic reaction.

On the Scene

You and your partner are called to a local elementary school for a "possible allergic reaction." Upon your arrival, you find an anxious 6-year-old girl. You can see that her face is swollen. She says she "can't breathe right" and had this same problem last week at lunchtime. As you quickly assess the patient, your partner obtains the patient's vital signs. Her blood pressure is 100/64, pulse 110 (strong and regular). Her respirations are 20 breaths/min, shallow and labored. Her skin is flushed, warm, and dry. You can hear the patient wheezing with each breath. ■

As you read this chapter, think about the following questions:

- What are some of the common causes of an allergic reaction?
- Are the patient's signs and symptoms consistent with an allergic reaction?
- Can you provide emergency care for this child if her parents are not present?

Introduction

Allergic reactions can range from a mild rash to life-threatening anaphylaxis. You must be able to recognize the signs and symptoms of these conditions and provide appropriate patient care. Your ability to recognize and manage anaphylaxis may be lifesaving.

Causes of Allergic Reactions

Objectives 1, 2, 3, 4

An **allergic reaction** is an exaggerated response by the body's immune system to a substance. The substance that causes an allergic reaction can enter the body in four ways: ingestion, injection, inhalation, or absorption through the skin or mucous membranes (Figure 27-1). Common causes of allergic reactions are shown in Table 27-1.

One cause of allergic reactions deserves special mention. Latex allergy has become increasingly common among patients and healthcare professionals. Products that are commonly made of latex are shown in Table 27-2. The main source used to make natural rubber latex is the rubber tree. Several chemicals are added to the tree's milky fluid during the manufacture of commercial latex. Latex contains proteins that may be absorbed through the skin or inhaled. This can cause an allergic reaction in susceptible persons. Skin

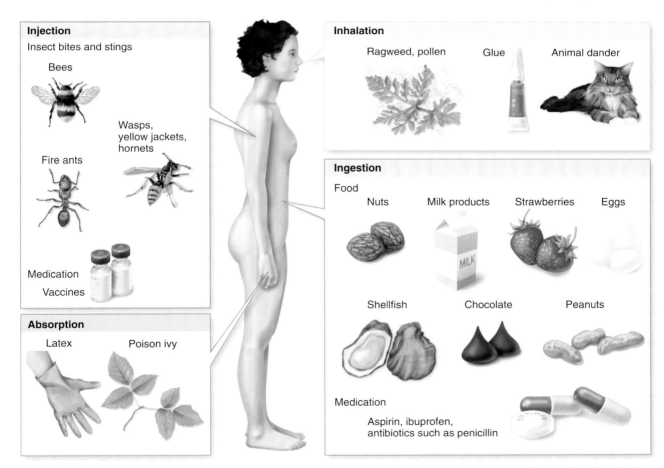

FIGURE 27-1 ▲ An allergen can enter the body in four ways: ingestion, injection, inhalation, or absorption through the skin or mucous membranes.

TABLE 27-1 Routes of Entry of Allergens and Possible Causes of Allergic Reactions

Ingestion	Injection	Inhalation	Surface Absorption
• Aspirin • Nonsteroidal anti-inflammatory drugs (ibuprofen [Advil, Motrin]) • Insulin • Antibiotics • Peanuts • Tree nuts • Milk products • Berries • Eggs • Seafood • Chocolate • Grains • Beans • Food preservatives (sulfites)	• Bees • Wasps • Hornets • Fire ants • Jellyfish • Antivenin • Dyes used in diagnostic x-rays and scans • Animal serums (or "sera") (vaccines) • Transfusion of blood or blood products	• Pollen • Mold • Dust • Grasses • Mildew • Paint • Perfume • Animal dander • Bug spray • Latex	• Pollen • Latex • Soap • Cleansers • Fertilizer • Poison ivy, oak, sumac

TABLE 27-2 Products That Commonly Include Latex

Household Products	Healthcare Products
• Erasers • Rubber bands • Dishwashing gloves • Balloons • Condoms • Diaphragms • Baby bottle nipples • Pacifiers • Diapers • Sanitary pads • Incontinence pads • Rubber toys and balls • Handles on tools, racquets • Tires • Hot water bottles • Shoe soles • Computer mouse pads • Expandable fabric (waistbands) • Motorcycle and bicycle handgrips • Swimming goggles • Some scuba diving suits	• Adhesive tape and bandages • Latex rubber gloves • Blood pressure cuff tubing • Stethoscope tubing • Tourniquets • Electrode pads • Oral and nasal airways • Airway masks • Thermometer probes • Suction tubing • Medication vial tops • Endotracheal tubes • Syringe plungers • Bulb syringes • Urinary catheters • Wound drains • Ostomy pouches • Material used to fill root canals • Wheelchair cushions • Crutch pads • Mattresses on stretchers

TABLE 27-3	Foods That May Cause an Allergic Reaction in People Who Have a Latex Allergy
Association with Latex Allergy	**Food**
High	Banana, avocado, chestnut
Moderate	Apple, celery, kiwi, papaya, potato, tomato
Low or uncertain	Cherry, fig, hazelnut, mango, nectarine, peach, peanut, pear, pineapple, walnut

absorption may increase when perspiration collects under latex gloves or other clothing that contains latex. Some latex gloves contain powder to make the gloves easier to put on and take off. The glove powder acts as a carrier of latex protein, which can become airborne when the gloves are put on or removed. Latex proteins can cause an allergic reaction when inhaled by individuals allergic to latex.

Among those who have the greatest chance of developing a latex allergy are people who have had many dental or medical procedures or surgeries, people with spina bifida, people with urinary system abnormalities, and healthcare workers. Some foods contain proteins that are similar to rubber (see Table 27-3). These foods may cause an allergic reaction in highly sensitive people who have a latex allergy.

What Happens in an Allergic Reaction

Objectives 5, 6, 7, 8

An **antigen** is any substance that is foreign to an individual and causes antibody production. When the body's immune system detects an antigen, white blood cells respond by producing antibodies specific to that antigen. An **antibody** is a substance produced by white blood cells to defend the body against bacteria, viruses, or other antigens. Antibodies are stored attached to mast cells, which are found in connective tissue. The mucous membranes of the respiratory and digestive tracts contain large numbers of mast cells. **Sensitization** is the formation of antigen-specific antibodies and occurs with the body's first exposure to an antigen. When the body is reexposed to the same antigen, the antigen attaches to the antibody on the sensitized mast cell. When an antigen causes signs and symptoms of an allergic reaction, the antigen is called an **allergen.**

The **inflammatory response** is a series of local cellular and vascular responses that are triggered when the body is injured or invaded by an antigen. During this protective response, the body attempts to wall off or contain the injury or invasion at the point of entry, preventing the spread of microorganisms or antigens to other areas of the body. Another function of the inflammatory response is to dispose of dead cells and bacteria. This job is performed by white blood cells that move in to the area and attempt to ingest and disable the invader.

Cells that have been damaged by injury or invasion release a number of chemicals, including histamine. Histamine moves into the capillaries, increasing blood flow to the area by causing local arterioles and capillaries to dilate. This increased blood flow is responsible for the redness and increased heat that is characteristic of inflammation. Increased heat makes the injured area unfavorable for microorganisms while increased blood flow to the area enables white blood cells to move in and attempt to ingest and disable the invader. Widespread dilation of arterioles and capillaries can cause a fall in blood pressure. Once the inflammatory response has begun, responding cells activate other cells of the immune system. This leads to a cascade of additional immune system reactions. Histamine and other chemicals cause the capillaries to leak plasma and fluid into the surrounding tissue, resulting in swelling. Swelling may be limited to one area of the body (localized) or affect multiple body systems (systemic). Histamine also causes constriction of bronchial smooth muscle producing dyspnea. Pressure on nerve cells caused by tissue swelling can cause pain in the affected area.

Remember This

The primary signs of inflammation are redness, heat, swelling, and pain.

Most allergic reactions happen soon after reexposure to an allergen. Some reactions are mild, causing symptoms that are annoying but not life-threatening. For example, inhaling an antigen such as plant pollen can result in irritation of the eyes, nose, and respiratory

TABLE 27-4 Assessment Findings and Symptoms of an Allergic Reaction*

Mild Allergic Reaction	Moderate or Severe Allergic Reaction
• Anxiety	• Anxiety, fright, altered mental status, unresponsiveness
• Runny nose	• Feeling of impending doom
• Stuffy nose	• Swelling of the face, eyes, lips, tongue, or throat
• Sneezing	• Hoarseness
• Red, watery eyes	• Difficulty swallowing or talking
• Red skin (flushing)	• Stridor
• Rash	• Difficulty breathing
• Hives	• Weakness
• Itching	• Continuous or strong cough
• Feeling of fullness in mouth or throat	• Wheezing
• Swelling of hands, feet	• Abdominal cramps, pain
• Tingling of hands, feet	• Nausea, vomiting
• Occasional or slight cough	• Dizziness, lightheadedness, unexplained fainting
• Urgency to urinate	• Low blood pressure
	• Chest discomfort or tightness

*Not all signs and symptoms are present in every case.

tract. Assessment findings and symptoms often include red, watery eyes; sneezing and a runny nose; and coughing. When an allergic reaction is severe and affects multiple body systems, it is called **anaphylaxis**. Anaphylaxis is a life-threatening emergency. Signs and symptoms of an allergic reaction may progress in minutes from mild to severe. In some cases, a severe reaction occurs without warning.

Remember This

The more rapid the onset of symptoms after exposure to an allergen, the more severe the allergic reaction is likely to be.

After reexposure to an allergen, the release of histamine and other chemicals cause serious signs and symptoms that affect many body systems. The initial symptoms of an allergic reaction usually include **pruritus** (itching) and swelling at the site of exposure to the allergen. Many patients also develop **urticaria** (hives) and a rash. Effects of histamine and other chemicals on the respiratory system can include swelling in the throat, narrowing of the lower airways, and increased mucus production. Swelling of the upper airway can result in hoarseness; stridor; and noisy, labored breathing. Narrowing of the lower airways results in wheezing that can sometimes be heard without the need of a stethoscope. Effects on the skin can include itching, hives, and a

rash. Effects on the gastrointestinal system can include nausea, vomiting, diarrhea, and abdominal pain or cramps. The patient's heart rate may be irregular. Because one of the effects of histamine is widening (dilation) of the blood vessels, effects on the cardiovascular system can cause lightheadedness, weakness, and an increased heart rate. The patient's blood pressure can drop quickly and drastically. Assessment findings and symptoms of an allergic reaction are shown in Tables 27-4 and 27-5.

Patient Assessment

Objectives 9, 10

When you are dispatched to a call for a possible allergic reaction, keep in mind that the patient's condition can worsen in minutes. When you arrive at the scene, perform a scene size-up and put on appropriate personal protective equipment. Be aware of possible hazards to yourself and your crew, such as bees or other insects or environmental hazards such as pool chemicals or cleaning fluids. Once the scene is determined to be safe to enter, quickly find out as much information as you can about the nature of the illness from the patient, family, or bystanders. Look at the patient's environment for clues about the cause of the patient's chief complaint.

Form a general impression of the patient. If your general impression indicates the patient has a de-

TABLE 27-5 Signs and Symptoms of an Allergic Reaction by Body System

Body System	Assessment Findings and Symptoms
Respiratory	Tightness in the throat ("lump in the throat") or chest Coughing Rapid breathing Labored breathing Noisy breathing Hoarseness Stridor Difficulty talking Wheezing Increased mucus production
Cardiovascular	Lightheadedness, fainting Weakness Increased heart rate Irregular heart rhythm Decreased blood pressure Circulatory collapse
Nervous	Restlessness Fear, panic, or a feeling of impending doom Headache Altered mental status, unresponsiveness Seizures
Skin (integumentary)	Warm, tingling feeling in the face, mouth, chest, feet, and hands Itching (pruritus) Rash Hives (urticaria) Red skin (flushing) Swelling of the face, neck, hands, feet and/or tongue
Gastrointestinal	Nausea Vomiting Abdominal cramps, pain Diarrhea
Generalized findings	Itchy, watery eyes Runny nose

creased level of responsiveness or shows signs of respiratory distress or failure, move quickly. Perform a primary survey, identify any life-threatening conditions, and provide care based on those findings.

Remember This

Before touching the patient, ask about the possibility of latex allergy so that you do not inadvertently worsen the patient's current condition.

Assess the patient's mental status. A patient experiencing an allergic reaction is often anxious. Provide calm reassurance to help reduce the patient's anxiety. If the patient has an altered or a decreasing mental status, move quickly. If the patient is unresponsive and there is any possibility of trauma, stabilize the patient's cervical spine.

Assess the patient's airway. The presence of stridor, hoarseness, difficulty swallowing, or swelling of the tongue suggests an impending airway obstruction. If any of these signs are present, request advanced life support (ALS) assistance as soon as possible. If ALS personnel are not available, complete your primary survey and then prepare the patient for prompt transport to the closest appropriate facility.

Assess the patient's breathing. Carefully assess for signs of respiratory distress or respiratory failure. A patient who is experiencing an allergic reaction may be coughing or wheezing or have an increased respiratory rate, difficulty breathing, and/or a feeling of chest tightness. Assess the patient's circulation. The patient may complain of lightheadedness or weakness. He may have an increased heart rate, irregular heart rhythm, and/or low blood pressure. Respiratory and skin symptoms often appear earlier in children than in adults. Cardiovascular and gastrointestinal symptoms often occur earlier in adults than in children. Although most anaphylaxis patients present with typical symptoms, some may present with unexplained fainting, a cardiac-related event, or low blood pressure.

You Should Know

Although anaphylaxis can occur with antigens that are ingested, inhaled, or absorbed, it is more common when an antigen is injected (such as an insect sting or intravenous antibiotics).

If you have not already done so, establish patient priorities and make a transport decision. Is there time to provide on-scene care, or should the patient be loaded into the ambulance and rapidly transported?

Priority patients include:
- Patients who give a poor general impression
- Patients experiencing difficulty breathing
- Patients with signs and symptoms of shock

- Unresponsive patients with no gag reflex or cough
- Responsive patients who are unable to follow commands

Request ALS personnel as soon as possible for a patient with signs and symptoms of anaphylaxis. Consider the time it will take for an ALS unit to arrive and the time that it will take to load the patient into the ambulance and transport rapidly to the closest appropriate hospital. If needed, contact medical direction for advice.

Once you have made a transport decision, obtain a SAMPLE history from a responsive patient. Examples of questions to ask a patient who is experiencing an allergic reaction are shown in the next *Making a Difference* box. If the patient is unresponsive or has an altered mental status, quickly size up the scene, perform a primary survey, and then proceed to the rapid medical assessment. Follow with evaluation of baseline vital signs and gathering of the patient's medical history. A family member, friend, coworker, or others at the scene may be able to provide important information about the cause of the patient's symptoms.

Quickly look to see if the patient is wearing medical identification that indicates the patient has an allergy. Patients who have known allergies usually know how to avoid whatever it is that triggers an allergic reaction. These patients are advised by their physician to wear medical identification that clearly identifies their allergies.

Patients who have severe allergic reactions may be prescribed an anaphylaxis kit. An anaphylaxis kit contains an epinephrine autoinjector (EpiPen) (Figure 27-2). Some kits also contain a metered-dose inhaler. When the patient is exposed to something to which she has a severe allergic reaction, the patient self-administers the epinephrine by means of an automatic injectable needle and syringe. People who have an allergy to latex are advised to carry an epinephrine autoinjector, wear medical identification, and carry extra pairs of nonlatex gloves

Making a Difference

Questions to Ask a Patient Who Is Experiencing an Allergic Reaction

- When did your symptoms begin?
- How were you exposed?
- What were you doing when the symptoms began?
- How soon after exposure did your symptoms begin?
- Do you have any allergies to medications, foods, or other substances or materials?
- Are you taking any medications (prescription and over the counter)? Do you take your medications regularly? Has there has been any recent change in medications (additions, deletions, or change in dosages)?
- Have you ever experienced an allergic reaction? If so, what were you exposed to that caused the reaction? How serious was the reaction? Were you hospitalized? Have you ever been intubated or "needed a breathing tube" because of an allergic reaction?
- Do you have a physician-prescribed epinephrine autoinjector or anaphylaxis kit? If so, have you given yourself a dose before we arrived?
- Have you taken any medications to relieve your symptoms before we arrived?
- Do you have a history of asthma, heart disease, high blood pressure, or other illness?

for emergency medical or dental care. In addition to looking for medical jewelry (such as a bracelet) indicating the patient has an allergy, also look for peel-and-stick plastic decals that may indicate a latex allergy. You may find decals such as the one shown in Figure 27-3 at the

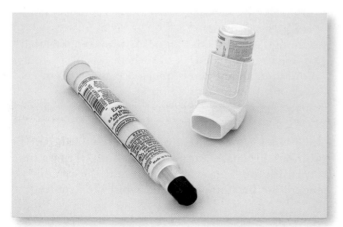

FIGURE 27-2 ▲ An anaphylaxis kit contains an epinephrine autoinjector. Some kits also contain a metered-dose inhaler.

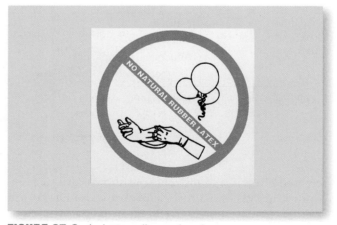

FIGURE 27-3 ▲ Latex allergy decal.

entrance to a patient's home and on a car window or windshield, alerting EMS personnel that someone inside is allergic to latex.

If the patient has a latex allergy, make a note of this on your prehospital care report. Write the words "LATEX ALLERGY" clearly on the report and include latex in the allergy section of the form. If your EMS agency has a latex-free kit, use latex-free supplies from the kit for patient care. Place a latex allergy wristband from the kit on the patient. If your EMS agency does not have a latex-free kit, wrap cotton gauze over blood pressure cuff tubing and stethoscope tubing to avoid contact with the patient. Wrap cotton gauze over the patient's upper arm before placing a blood pressure cuff on the patient. Remember to communicate the presence of the patient's latex allergy to ALS personnel arriving on the scene and/or to the staff at the receiving facility when transferring patient care.

Perform a focused physical exam, and obtain baseline vital signs. Assess the patient's pulse, respirations, and blood pressure. Assess oxygen saturation by using a pulse oximeter. Provide all information obtained to the ALS crew arriving on the scene or to the receiving facility staff.

Emergency Care

Objective 11

If the patient has come in contact with a substance that is causing an allergic reaction without signs of respiratory distress or shock:

- Maintain an open airway.
- Give oxygen.
- Transport and perform ongoing assessments often while en route.

A patient without wheezing or signs of respiratory compromise or hypotension should not receive epinephrine. However, keep in mind that the condition of a patient experiencing an allergic reaction can change rapidly. A patient who was initially stable can develop massive airway swelling and a possible airway obstruction in minutes. Remember that the presence of stridor, hoarseness, difficulty swallowing, or swelling of the tongue suggests an impending airway obstruction. Constant reassessment is essential.

If the patient has come in contact with a substance that caused a past allergic reaction and complains of respiratory distress or shows signs and symptoms of shock:

- Establish and maintain an open airway. The patient with an allergic reaction may initially present with airway or respiratory compromise, or airway or respiratory compromise may develop as the reaction progresses. Make sure suction equipment is within arm's reach.

- Give oxygen. If the patient's breathing is adequate, apply oxygen by nonrebreather mask at 10 to 15 L/min if not already done. If the patient's breathing is inadequate, provide positive-pressure ventilation with 100% oxygen and assess the adequacy of the ventilations delivered. Ventilation with a bag-mask device may be difficult because of narrowing of the patient's bronchioles.

- Find out if the patient has a prescribed epinephrine autoinjector available. An EMT may assist a patient with using an epinephrine autoinjector at the discretion of his or her program medical director (see Table 27-6). In some states, EMTs now carry epinephrine autoinjectors (EpiPens) on their EMS units and are not limited to administering the medication to patients who have been prescribed one. Obtain an order from medical direction either on-line or off-line to give (or assist the patient in giving) epinephrine by means of an autoinjector. After administration, reassess the patient in 2 minutes. Record reassessment findings and prepare for transport. If the patient does not have a prescribed epinephrine autoinjector or you do not carry this medication, transport immediately. The procedure for using an epinephrine autoinjector is shown in Skill Drill 11-3 in Chapter 11.

- Reassess every 5 minutes. Transport promptly to the closest appropriate medical facility.

- If the patient's condition improves, provide supportive care. Continue to give oxygen and treat for shock.

- If the patient's condition worsens, contact medical direction for orders to give an additional dose of epinephrine, if available. Signs that indicate the patient's condition is worsening include decreasing mental status, increasing breathing difficulty, and decreasing blood pressure. Treat for shock. Be prepared to begin cardiopulmonary resuscitation (CPR) and use the automated external defibrillator (AED), if necessary.

Age-Related Considerations

When providing care for a child experiencing an anaphylactic reaction, keep in mind that a pediatric weight-based autoinjector is available. An epinephrine autoinjector may be contraindicated in an older adult who has coronary artery disease. When providing care to an older adult who has coronary artery disease and is experiencing anaphylaxis, it is a good idea to consult medical direction before administration of epinephrine (if your protocols do not clearly address this situation).

TABLE 27-6 Epinephrine

Generic name	Epinephrine
Trade name	Adrenalin, EpiPen
Mechanism of action	Epinephrine works by relaxing the passages of the airway and constricting the blood vessels. The opening of the airway allows the patient to move more air into and out of the body, which will increase the amount of oxygen in the bloodstream. Constriction of the blood vessels slows the leakage of fluid from the blood vessels into the space around the cells of the body.
Indications	An EMT can assist a patient in using an epinephrine autoinjector if *all* of the following criteria are met: • The patient exhibits signs and symptoms of a severe allergic reaction, including respiratory distress and/or signs and symptoms of shock. • The medication is prescribed for the patient, or your EMS system authorizes EMTs to carry the medication. • Medical direction has authorized use for the patient.
Dosage	Adult: One adult autoinjector (0.3 mg) Infant and child: One infant or child autoinjector (0.15 mg)
Adverse effects	• Rapid heart rate • Anxiety • Excitability • Nausea, vomiting • Chest pain or discomfort • Headache • Dizziness
Contraindications	There are no contraindications when used in a life-threatening situation.
Special considerations	• Give the patient oxygen by nonrebreather mask before giving epinephrine. • Assess the patient's lung sounds before administration of epinephrine to establish a baseline. Assess lung sounds again after administration of epinephrine, and compare your findings. • Note any changes in patient condition and vital signs. • The patient will need to be transported for additional care.

Remember This

When caring for a patient experiencing an allergic reaction, quickly determine if ALS personnel are needed. ALS personnel will apply a cardiac monitor to the patient, start an intravenous line, and give drugs that can quickly help decrease the severity of the patient's symptoms. They will also perform advanced airway techniques if the patient's condition warrants it. Evaluate the time it will take for an ALS unit to arrive and the time that it would take to load the patient into the ambulance and transport rapidly to the closest appropriate facility. Another consideration is meeting the ALS unit to transfer patient care to ALS personnel before arrival at the hospital.

On the Scene Wrap-Up

You immediately recognize the child's signs and symptoms are consistent with an allergic reaction. The child tells you she is allergic to peanuts. The child's teacher tells you that the school has a signed consent form on file from the child's parents allowing the school to authorize care in an emergency.

While giving the child oxygen by nonrebreather mask, you learn that the patient traded her cookies for another child's cookies. It appears that the cookies she ate contained peanut butter. You ask the child if she has a prescribed epinephrine autoinjector. She nods that she does, but she forgot her kit and left it at home today. As you and your partner quickly load the patient into the ambulance, you notice that the patient's respiratory distress is worsening. Your partner asks the child's teacher to notify the child's parents of your destination and then begins rapid transport to the closest appropriate hospital. ■

Sum It Up

▶ An allergic reaction is an exaggerated immune response to any substance. The substance that causes an allergic reaction can enter the body in four ways: ingestion, injection, inhalation, or absorption through the skin or mucous membranes. Possible causes include insect bites or stings, food, plants, and medications, among others.

▶ An antigen is any substance that is foreign to an individual and causes antibody production. An antibody is a substance produced by white blood cells to defend the body against bacteria, viruses, or other antigens. The antibodies attach to mast cells, which are found in connective tissue. This process, called sensitization, occurs with the body's first exposure to the antigen. When an antigen causes signs and symptoms of an allergic reaction, the antigen is called an allergen. When an allergic reaction is severe and affects multiple body systems, it is called anaphylaxis. Anaphylaxis is a life-threatening emergency.

▶ Assessment findings pertaining to the respiratory system may include tightness in the throat ("lump in the throat") or chest, coughing, rapid breathing, labored breathing, noisy breathing, hoarseness, stridor, difficulty talking, and wheezing. Assessment findings pertaining to the cardiovascular system may include an increased heart rate, lightheadedness, fainting, weakness, irregular heart rhythm, decreased blood pressure, and circulatory collapse. Assessment findings pertaining to the nervous system may include restlessness, fear, panic or a feeling of impending doom, headache, an altered mental status, unresponsiveness, and seizures. Assessment findings pertaining to the skin may include itching (pruritus),

hives (urticaria), red skin (flushing), and swelling to the face, neck, hands, feet, and/or tongue. The patient may state he has a warm tingling feeling in the face, mouth, chest, feet, and hands. Assessment findings pertaining to the gastrointestinal system may include nausea, vomiting, abdominal cramps or pain, an urgency to urinate, and diarrhea. Generalized findings may include itchy, watery eyes and a runny nose.

▶ Assessment findings that reveal shock (hypoperfusion) or respiratory distress indicate the presence of a severe allergic reaction.

▶ If the patient has come in contact with a substance that caused a past allergic reaction and complains of respiratory distress or shows signs and symptoms of shock, form a general impression, perform an initial assessment, and perform a focused history and physical exam. Assess the patient's baseline vital signs and SAMPLE history. Give oxygen if not already done in the initial assessment. Find out if the patient has a prescribed epinephrine autoinjector available. With approval from medical direction, help the patient with administration of the epinephrine autoinjector. Reassess in 2 minutes. Record reassessment findings. If the patient does not have an epinephrine autoinjector available, transport immediately.

▶ If the patient has contact with a substance that causes an allergic reaction without signs of respiratory distress or shock, continue with a focused assessment. A patient without wheezing or signs of respiratory compromise or hypotension should not receive epinephrine.

▶ A patient experiencing an allergic reaction may initially present with airway or respiratory compromise, or airway or respiratory compromise may develop as the allergic reaction progresses.

▶ If the patient's condition improves, provide supportive care. Continue to give oxygen and treat for shock. If the patient's condition worsens, contact medical direction for orders to give an additional dose of epinephrine, if available. Signs that indicate the patient's condition is worsening include decreasing mental status, increasing breathing difficulty, and decreasing blood pressure. Treat for shock. Be prepared to begin CPR and use the AED, if necessary.

Toxicology

By the end of this chapter, you should be able to:

Knowledge Objectives ▶

1. Define poison, poisoning, toxin, antidote, and poison control center.
2. Discuss the role of the poison control center in the United States.
3. Describe the routes of entry of toxic substances into the body.
4. Define toxidrome, and discuss the signs and symptoms associated with various toxidromes.
5. Define substance abuse, substance misuse, tolerance, addiction, withdrawal, and overdose.
6. Give examples of stimulants and signs and symptoms of stimulant misuse or abuse.
7. Give examples of depressants and signs and symptoms of depressant misuse or abuse.
8. Give examples of signs and symptoms of alcohol misuse or abuse.
9. Define alcohol withdrawal syndrome and delirium tremens.
10. Give examples of hallucinogens and signs and symptoms of hallucinogen misuse or abuse.
11. Give examples of designer drugs and signs and symptoms of designer drug misuse or abuse.
12. Discuss assessment of the patient with a toxicological emergency.
13. Identify specific details of the medical history that should be obtained in the patient with a toxicological emergency.
14. Describe the emergency medical care for the patient with a toxicological emergency.
15. List common poisonings by ingestion and the signs and symptoms related to common poisonings by this route.
16. Discuss the emergency medical care for poisoning by ingestion.
17. List common poisonings by inhalation and the signs and symptoms related to common poisonings by this route.
18. Discuss the emergency medical care for poisoning by inhalation.
19. List common poisonings by injection and the signs and symptoms related to common poisonings by this route.
20. Discuss the emergency medical care for poisoning by injection.
21. List common poisonings by surface absorption and the signs and symptoms related to common poisonings by this route.
22. Discuss the emergency medical care for poisoning by surface absorption.

23. Explain the rationale for administering activated charcoal.

24. Demonstrate the ability to take a relevant history from the patient experiencing a toxicological emergency.

connect™ (plus+)

25. Demonstrate the ability to perform a physical assessment of the patient experiencing a toxicological emergency.

26. Demonstrate completing a prehospital care report for patients experiencing a toxicological emergency.

On the Scene

You and your emergency medical technician partner are dispatched to a private residence for a "possible overdose." On arrival at the scene, an anxious family member ushers you into a bedroom where you find a 35-year-old woman lying in bed. Your first impression reveals that the patient's eyes are closed and she is unaware of your approach. She is breathing about 8 to 10 breaths/min. Her breathing does not appear labored. Her skin looks pink and dry. Her face looks swollen, as if she has been crying. An empty bottle of Percocet tablets is on the nightstand. After you repeatedly call her name, the patient slowly opens her eyes and then goes back to sleep. The family member at your side says that the patient and her husband "have been having problems." ∎

THINK ABOUT IT

As you read this chapter, think about the following questions:

- What is the route of toxic exposure in this situation?
- If the patient took the Percocet tablets that were on the nightstand, what other signs and symptoms can you anticipate finding during your patient assessment?
- In what types of poisonings is activated charcoal used?
- Should activated charcoal be given to this patient? Why or why not?

Introduction

Poisoning and substance abuse calls are common emergencies. Many children are poisoned every year as they explore their environments. Many adults overdose on medication, either accidentally or deliberately. In this chapter we will discuss the routes by which poisons may enter the body, assessment findings and symptoms associated with poisoning and overdoses, and the emergency medical care for patients with toxicological conditions.

What Is a Poison?

Objectives 1, 2, 3, 4

A **poison** is any substance taken into the body that interferes with normal body function. **Poisoning** is exposure to a substance that is harmful in any dosage. A **toxin** is a poisonous substance. An **antidote** is a substance that neutralizes a poison.

You Should Know

- More than 80% of toxic exposures are accidental.
- More than 90% of toxic exposures occur in the home.
- More than 50% of poisonings occur in children younger than 6 years of age.
- More than 90% of poisonings involve only one substance.
- More than 75% of poisonings occur by ingestion.
- Most poisonings involve everyday household items, such as cleaning supplies, medicines, cosmetics, and personal care items.

A **poison control center (PCC)** is a medical facility that provides free telephone advice to the public and medical professionals in case of exposure to poisonous substances. In the United States, the national (toll-free) telephone number is 1-800-222-1222. This number is staffed 24 hours a day, 7 days a week, 365 days a year by pharmacists, physicians, nurses, and poison information providers. A PCC is an excellent resource that is often used by EMS personnel. When the substance involved is known, the medical professionals at a PCC can help determine the toxicity of the substance and give advice about the emergency care the patient should receive.

You Should Know

The ability to accept treatment orders or instructions from a PCC is based on local medical direction and local protocols. Be sure to check and find out if you are able to accept treatment orders from your local PCC.

A poison may be a solid, liquid, spray, or gas (Table 28-1). Toxins enter the body in four ways: ingestion, inhalation, injection, or absorption (Figure 28-1). Exposure to a toxin may be accidental or intentional. Most poisonings are accidental. Examples of accidental poisonings are listed in the following *You Should Know* box.

You Should Know

Examples of Accidental Poisonings

- Bites and stings
- Food poisoning
- Medication taken or given more than once by mistake
- Wrong medication taken or given
- Someone else's medication taken or given
- Medication doses given or taken too close together
- Exposure through breast milk
- Wrong dose or medication given by healthcare professional

Signs and symptoms of a toxic exposure can vary depending on the substance involved; the route of entry; the amount ingested, inhaled, injected, or absorbed; and the length of the exposure. Signs, symptoms, and characteristics that often occur together in toxic exposures are called **toxidromes** (Table 28-2 on p. 508). When the cause of a toxic exposure is unknown, knowing the "typical" signs and symptoms of certain toxic exposures can help you identify the poison and allow you to give appropriate care.

TABLE 28-1 Examples of Common Poisons

Form of Poison	Examples
Solid	Medicines, plants, granulated detergents, granular pesticides, fertilizers, pool chemicals, disc batteries, chalk, clay, fabric softeners, diaper pail deodorizers, toilet bowl deodorizers
Liquid	Syrup medicines, laundry soap, fabric softener, laundry bluing/brightening products, baby oil, bath oil, bubble bath, cream or lotion makeup, mouthwash, permanent wave solutions, hair removal products, rubbing alcohol, nail glue remover, furniture polish, lighter fluid, typewriter correction fluid, gasoline, kerosene, drain opener, disinfectants, toilet bowl cleaner, rust remover, pool chemicals, lamp oil, paint, antifreeze, windshield solution, brake fluid
Spray	Oven cleaner, glass cleaner, air freshener, insecticides, weed killer, spray paint, fabric softener, disinfectant
Gas	Carbon monoxide, automobile exhaust fumes, fumes from gas or oil burning stoves, tear gas, chlorine gas, pool chemicals, and chemicals that workers are exposed to at industrial plants

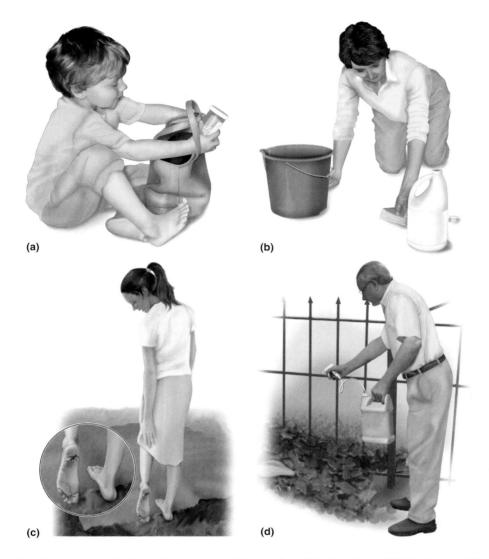

FIGURE 28-1 ▲ A toxin can enter the body in four ways: **(a)** ingestion, **(b)** inhalation, **(c)** injection, or **(d)** absorption through the skin or mucous membranes.

Commonly Misused and Abused Substances

Objective 5

Intentional poisonings may occur because of suicide or homicide (murder), substance abuse or misuse, or acts of terrorism. **Substance abuse** is the deliberate, persistent, and excessive self-administration of a substance in a way that is not medically or socially approved. Recreational use of substances is considered intentional abuse. **Substance misuse** is the self-administration of a substance for unintended purposes, for appropriate purposes but in improper amounts or doses, or without a prescription for the person receiving the medication. **Tolerance** occurs when an individual requires progressively larger doses of a drug to achieve the desired effect. **Addiction** is a psychological and physical dependence on a substance that has gone beyond voluntary control. **Withdrawal** is the condition produced when an individual stops using or abusing a drug to which he is physically or psychologically addicted. An **overdose** is an intentional or unintentional overmedication or ingestion of a toxic substance. Commonly misused and abused substances include stimulants, depressants, hallucinogens, and designer drugs.

TABLE 28-2 Common Toxidromes

Toxidrome	Signs and Symptoms	Examples
Sympathomimetic (produces signs and symptoms like those of the sympathetic division of the autonomic nervous system)	Agitation, rapid breathing, increased heart rate, increased blood pressure, fever, seizures, sweating	Amphetamines, methamphetamines Cocaine Phencyclidine (PCP) Ecstasy Caffeine, pseudoephedrine (found in OTC cold remedies)
Cholinergic	Altered mental status, decreased or increased heart rate, fever, seizures SLUDGEM • Salivation • Lacrimation (tearing) • Urination • Defecation • Gastrointestinal distress • Emesis (vomiting) • Miosis (pupil constriction)	Organophosphate and carbamate insecticides (ant sprays, flea sprays, and insect sprays, powders, and liquids) Some mushrooms Nerve agents (sarin gas)
Anticholinergic	Confusion; hallucinations; agitation; coma; blurred vision; warm, flushed, dry skin; dilated pupils, tachycardia, hypertension	Antihistamines such as diphenhydramine (Benadryl) Jimson weed Tricyclic antidepressants such as amitriptyline (Elavil), desipramine (Norpramin), nortriptyline (Aventyl, Pamelor)
Opioid (narcotics)	Altered mental status, coma, slow or absent breathing, slow heart rate, low blood pressure, constricted pupils (*Note:* Meperidine, propoxyphene, and diphenoxylate may cause *dilated* pupils.)	Morphine Codeine Heroin Oxycodone (Oxycontin) Fentanyl (Duragesic) Diphenoxylate (Lomotil) Meperidine (Demerol) Methadone (Dolophine) Propoxyphene (Darvon)
Sedative/hypnotic (substances used to aid sleep, reduce anxiety, and treat depression, epilepsy, and high blood pressure)	Slurred speech, hallucinations, confusion, coma, respiratory depression, low blood pressure, pupil dilation or constriction, blurred vision, dry mouth, decreased temperature, staggering walk	Lorazepam (Ativan) Alprazolam (Xanax) Barbiturates (phenobarbital) Benzodiazepines (diazepam [Valium]) Alcohol GHB (a date rape drug or "liquid x")

Stimulants

Objective 6

Stimulants increase mental and physical activity. Examples include cocaine, amphetamines, methamphetamines, and phencyclidine (PCP). Common legal stimulants include caffeine and nicotine. Stimulants produce feelings of alertness and well-being. They may produce violent behavior. Other signs and symptoms of stimulant misuse or abuse are listed in the following *You Should Know* box. When the effects of the drug wear off, the user is often exhausted and sleeps. On awakening, the user may be confused, depressed, or suicidal.

**Assessment Findings and Symptoms
of Stimulant Misuse or Abuse**

- Restlessness
- Irritability
- Combativeness
- Increased heart rate
- Increased respiratory rate
- Increased blood pressure
- Sweating
- Tremors
- Hallucinations
- Fever
- Headache
- Dizziness
- Moist or flushed skin
- Chest pain or discomfort
- Palpitations
- Nausea or vomiting
- Loss of appetite

Depressants

Objective 7

Depressants include alcohol, barbiturates, narcotics (opiates), and benzodiazepines. Signs and symptoms of depressant misuse or abuse are listed in the following *You Should Know* box.

**Assessment Findings and Symptoms
of Depressant Misuse or Abuse**

- Drowsiness
- Slurred speech
- Decreased heart rate
- Decreased blood pressure
- Decreased respiratory rate
- Poor coordination
- Confusion

Alcohol

Objectives 8, 9

Alcohol slows mental and physical activity. It affects judgment, vision, reaction time, and coordination. When approaching the patient who has ingested alcohol, observe the scene for evidence of trauma. In large quantities, alcohol can cause death.

Making a Difference

Signs and symptoms of alcohol misuse or abuse can mimic those of other medical conditions (such as a diabetic emergency, head injury, epilepsy, drug reaction, or central nervous system, or CNS, infection). In addition, alcohol abuse can often mask potentially lethal conditions such as a head injury. Do not *assume* the patient is intoxicated. Carefully assess the patient for the presence of other injuries or illnesses. Perform a blood glucose test (if permitted by state and local protocol).

Disulfiram (Antabuse) is a medication prescribed for alcoholics to discourage them from drinking. When combined with alcohol or alcohol-containing foods, medications, or products (such as over-the-counter cough medications, mouthwash, and facial cleaning products), Antabuse produces unpleasant, and sometimes serious, reactions. Reactions last 30 minutes to 8 hours (usually 3 to 4 hours) and include nausea, vomiting, abdominal discomfort, chest discomfort, palpitations, headache, dizziness, and blurred vision. Although rare, seizures, heart failure, heart attack, and cardiac arrest have occurred.

Alcohol withdrawal syndrome occurs 6 to 48 hours after a chronic alcoholic reduces or stops her alcohol consumption. Signs and symptoms of alcohol withdrawal include tremors ("the shakes"), anxiety, irritability, inability to sleep, sweating, nausea, and vomiting. The patient must be monitored closely by healthcare professionals, or **delirium tremens (DTs)** can occur. DTs usually begin 24 to 72 hours after a chronic alcoholic reduces or stops alcohol consumption. The diagnosis of DTs is made when symptoms of alcohol withdrawal progress beyond the usual symptoms of withdrawal. DTs are potentially fatal.

Signs and symptoms of DTs include those of alcohol withdrawal plus:

- Altered mental status (confusion, visual and/or auditory hallucinations, severe agitation)
- Seizures
- Increased heart rate
- Increased blood pressure
- Elevated body temperature

Symptoms may be present for several days. In general, seizures associated with alcohol withdrawal occur 6 to 48 hours after the last drink.

Barbiturates

Barbiturates are prescribed to relieve anxiety, promote sleep, control seizures, and relax muscles. Examples of barbiturates include pentobarbital (Nembutal), secobarbital (Seconal), amobarbital (Amytal), and phenobarbital (Luminal). Street names for these drugs include *yellow jackets, reds, blues, Amy's, rainbows, Barbs, downers, goof balls,* and *stumblers.* Barbiturates are particularly dangerous when combined with alcohol. Overdose can produce respiratory depression, coma, and death. Withdrawal can cause anxiety, tremors, nausea, fever, convulsions, and death.

Narcotics

Narcotics are prescribed drugs used to relieve moderate to severe pain, control diarrhea, and suppress cough. Narcotics include opium, opium derivatives, and artificial compounds that produce opiumlike effects (see the following *You Should Know* box). Overdose can result in respiratory depression, constricted (pinpoint) pupils, shock, and death. Withdrawal can cause tearing, nasal congestion, headache, joint pain, dilated pupils, abdominal cramps, increased heart rate, chills, fever, gooseflesh, tremors, loss of appetite, vomiting, diarrhea, sweating, confusion, and intense agitation.

You Should Know

Examples of Narcotics

- morphine
- oxycodone (Oxycontin)
- fentanyl (Duragesic)
- codeine
- paregoric
- diphenoxylate (Lomotil)
- hydrocodone
- acetaminophen and hydrocodone (Vicodin)
- hydromorphone (Dilaudid)
- meperidine (Demerol)
- methadone (Dolophine)
- acetaminophen and oxycodone (Percocet)
- aspirin and oxycodone (Percodan)
- propoxyphene (Darvon)
- butorphanol (Stadol)
- nalbuphine (Nubain)
- pentazocine (Talwin)

Benzodiazepines

Benzodiazepines are prescribed medications used to control anxiety and stress, aid sleep, and relax muscles. They are also used for sedation and to control seizures.

TABLE 28-3 Benzodiazepines

Generic Name	Trade Name
alprazolam	Xanax
chlordiazepoxide	Librium
clonazepam	Klonopin
clorazepate	Tranxene
diazepam	Valium
lorazepam	Ativan
midazolam	Versed
oxazepam	Serax

These drugs vary widely in their onset, indications, potency, and duration of effect. Table 28-3 lists common benzodiazepines. Overdose can result in respiratory depression and death. Respiratory depression may be especially significant if benzodiazepines are taken in combination with alcohol or other drugs. Withdrawal can cause anxiety, tremors, nausea, fever, seizures, and death.

You Should Know

Respiratory depression from benzodiazepines alone is somewhat rare. Most benzodiazepine-related deaths and serious consequences usually result from overdoses of benzodiazepines combined with another substance, often alcohol.

Hallucinogens

Objective 10

Hallucinogens include lysergic acid diethylamine (LSD), PCP (angel dust), and mescaline (street names include *buttons, mess,* and *peyote*). These drugs produce changes in mood, thought, emotion, and self-awareness. Recreational use of mushrooms (also called *magic mushrooms* or *shrooms*) is another example of a hallucinogen whose effects typically last from 3 to 7 hours, depending on a number of factors including dosage and method of preparation. Ingestion can produce such physical signs and symptoms as dizziness, nausea, vomiting, increased heart rate and blood pressure, and numbness of the mouth. Examples of sensory changes that have been described include seeing "halos" around lights, flashing lights, enhanced colors and textures, and feeling "bonded" with other people. Signs and symptoms of hallucinogen misuse and abuse include flushed face, sudden mood changes, fear, and anxiety.

They can also cause hallucinations, profound depression, and irrational and disruptive behavior that can make the user dangerous to himself and others.

Designer Drugs

Objective 11

Designer drugs are variations of federally controlled substances that have high abuse potential (such as narcotics and amphetamines). These drugs are produced by persons ranging from amateurs to highly skilled chemists (called *cookers*) and sold on the street. Designer drugs can be injected, smoked, snorted, or ingested. Signs and symptoms of designer drug misuse and abuse are unpredictable and depend on the drug that is being chemically altered. Because designer drugs are often much stronger than the original form of the drug, overdose occurs frequently.

Fentanyl (Duragesic), a narcotic analgesic, is one drug used to make designer narcotics. Street names include *china white, synthetic heroin,* and *Persian white.* Signs and symptoms of misuse or abuse include respiratory depression and mental status depression.

Designer amphetamines include Ecstasy. The chemical name for Ecstasy is MDMA—methylene-dioxymethamphetamine. It is also called *Adam, XTC,* and *Love Drug.* Signs and symptoms of misuse or abuse include increased heart rate, sweating, agitation, erratic mood swings, and increased blood pressure.

You Should Know

Toxic exposures that involve more than one substance (such as alcohol and recreational drugs) are often difficult to recognize and treat. In these situations, the patient will most likely not have signs and symptoms specific to only one toxidrome. In any case, do not delay providing emergency care in order to find the cause of the toxic exposure.

Patient Assessment
Scene Size-Up

Objective 12

When responding to a call involving a possible toxic exposure, you may or may not know the substance(s) involved. For example, a 9-1-1 caller may tell the dispatcher that her toddler ate rat poison or that a teenager took an overdose of sleeping pills. On the other hand, the 9-1-1 dispatcher may not have any information available from the caller other than an "unresponsive person" or a person who "is not acting right." Remember scene safety in *all* circumstances. Protecting yourself and your crew must be your primary concern so that you are not injured or poisoned.

Use appropriate protection or have trained rescuers remove the patient from the poisonous environment. Call for additional resources if needed. On arrival at the scene, observe the patient's environment for clues as to the source of the poisoning.

Clues for the source of poisoning:
- Unusual odors
- Smoke or flames
- Open medicine cabinet
- Open or overturned containers
- Syringes or other drug paraphernalia

Primary Survey

As with all patients, form a general impression, and then quickly assess the patient's mental status, airway, breathing, and circulation. Stabilize the patient's spine if needed.

Many toxic exposures result in mental status changes. For example, sedatives and alcohol cause CNS depression. Agitation or violent behavior may be caused by CNS stimulants, such as cocaine, amphetamines, and PCP. Some substances can cause CNS stimulation *or* depression, depending on the dose ingested. Some toxins can cause visual or auditory hallucinations and personality changes. Seizures are a complication of toxic exposures and should be anticipated. Any toxic exposure that results in mental status changes increases the patient's risk of problems with his ABCs.

When assessing the patient's airway, look for burns around the mouth and blisters of the lips or mucous membranes. Note if the patient has trouble swallowing or is drooling. Excessive salivation is one of the signs associated with organophosphate insecticide exposure (see Table 28-2). Listen for stridor and hoarseness. If any of these signs are present, the patient is at risk of an airway obstruction. You may need to use airway adjuncts, such as an oral or nasal airway to keep the patient's airway open. Because some substances increase airway secretions and others cause nausea and vomiting, have suction equipment within arm's reach while the patient is in your care.

You Should Know

Odors can provide clues about the possible cause of the patient's signs and symptoms. For example, cyanide exposure is associated with an odor of bitter almonds. However, it has been estimated that only about 50% of the population can smell the odor of bitter almonds. Exposure to arsenic or organophosphate insecticides is associated with the smell of garlic.

Many toxic exposures affect breathing. For instance, substances that can cause a decreased respiratory rate include sedatives, narcotics, and depressants, such as alcohol (see Table 28-2). Substances that can cause an increased respiratory rate include aspirin, amphetamines, methamphetamines, caffeine, cocaine, PCP, and carbon monoxide. Be prepared to provide positive-pressure ventilation. Narrowing of the lower airway because of swelling, mucus, or spasms of the bronchi may cause wheezing.

Toxic exposures can also affect the victim's heart rate and blood pressure. Drugs that stimulate the sympathetic division of the autonomic nervous system will result in an increased heart rate. For instance, expect to see an increased heart rate if the patient has been exposed to amphetamines, cocaine, and Ecstasy. When taken in excess, alcohol and some prescribed heart medications are examples of substances that can cause a decreased heart rate. Some plants such as lily of the valley, foxglove, and oleander contain substances that can slow the heart rate. An irregular heart rhythm and shock are complications of toxic exposures and should be anticipated.

Establish patient priorities.

Priority patients include the following:
- Patients who give a poor general impression
- Patients experiencing difficulty breathing
- Patients with signs and symptoms of shock
- Unresponsive patients with no gag reflex or cough
- Responsive patients who are unable to follow commands

If a patient with a suspected toxic exposure has any of the previous findings, provide initial emergency care and transport immediately to the closest appropriate medical facility, with advanced life support (ALS) backup if available.

Secondary Survey

Objective 13

Finding out as much information as you can about the circumstances surrounding a toxic exposure is important. In cases involving an intentional exposure, keep in mind that the history obtained from the patient may not be reliable. Relay all information you find out when transferring care to ALS personnel or the staff at the receiving facility.

Examples of questions to ask:
- What poison was involved? Find out (and document) the exact name of the substance.
- How much was taken?
- When was it taken (or when did the exposure occur)? The answer to this question influences patient symptoms and the emergency care that will be provided by ALS personnel and at the hospital. If

the patient is unresponsive, finding out the time of ingestion or exposure may be impossible unless someone witnessed the event. In such situations, an estimate of the time of ingestion or exposure can often be made by determining when the patient was last seen.
- Where was the patient found? Any witnesses?
- Over what period was the substance ingested (or did the exposure occur)?
- Why was it taken? Attempt to find out whether the ingestion was accidental, intentional, or recreational, or a suicide attempt.
- What else was taken? For instance, did the patient ingest any alcohol or take any acetaminophen (Tylenol)? Although many intentional ingestions involve more than one substance, your patient may not volunteer this information.
- Was any seizure activity observed?
- Has a PCC been contacted? If so, what instructions were received? What has already been done to treat the poisoning?
- How much does the patient weigh? In cases of ingested poisons, this information is necessary to determine the dose of activated charcoal.
- Does the patient have any allergies to medications or other substances or materials?
- What medications (prescription and over the counter) is the patient currently taking? Has there been any recent change in medications (additions, deletions, or change in dosages)?
- Does the patient have any underlying illnesses (such as heart disease, high blood pressure, diabetes, kidney disease, liver disease, or seizures)? Many ingested substances are broken down in the liver and prepared for removal from the body by the kidneys. Patients who have illnesses that affect these organs may receive a toxic dose without intentionally taking too much of a substance.
- Does the patient have a history of depression or mental health problems? Has the patient ever been treated at a mental health or rehabilitation facility? These questions are important in determining the possibility of a suicide attempt.

Remember This

Ask questions using "who, what, where, when, why, and how" as a memory aid.

The patient's vital signs and physical exam findings (toxidrome) can provide clues to help you identify the substance involved. For instance, if you find a patient unresponsive with pinpoint pupils and slow breathing, consider the possibility of a narcotic overdose. On the other hand, don't assume that all is well if the patient's vital signs are within normal limits. A poisoned patient's condition can change quickly.

A quick check of the patient's pupils can reveal important clues. Cocaine and amphetamines are examples of substances that can cause dilated pupils. Most narcotics, some sedatives, organophosphates, and PCP cause constricted pupils. Exposure to anticonvulsants, PCP, and sedatives can result in rapid, jerky eye movements (nystagmus).

Assess the patient's skin color, temperature, and moisture. Note any redness, blisters, or patient complaints of burning or itching. Look for liquids or powder on the patient's skin or clothing.

Common signs and symptoms of poisoning are shown in the following *You Should Know* box.

You Should Know

Common Assessment Findings and Symptoms of Poisoning

- Altered mental status
- Difficulty breathing
- Headache
- Nausea
- Vomiting
- Diarrhea
- Chest or abdominal pain
- Sweating
- Seizures
- Burns around the mouth
- Burns on the skin

Emergency Care

Objective 14

To care for a patient exposed to toxins:

- Have trained rescuers remove the patient from the source of the poison.
- Follow proper decontamination procedures, if necessary, and prepare the ambulance to receive the patient. Methods used for decontamination will depend on the toxin and type of exposure.
- Establish and maintain an open airway. Wearing gloves, remove pills, tablets, or fragments from the patient's mouth, as needed, without injuring yourself. Do not stick your fingers in the mouth of a conscious patient with a possible altered mental status. The patient may follow your instructions and spit the pill fragments out. If not, you may attempt to remove the fragments with a suction catheter or other appropriate device.
- Be alert for vomiting and have suction ready. Pills or fragments need to be transported to the hospi-

tal with the patient so that emergency department personnel can identify any unknown substances. Pills should be placed in a zip-closure bag and properly labeled.

- Apply a pulse oximeter and give oxygen. If the patient's breathing is adequate, apply oxygen by nonrebreather mask at 10 to 15 L/min if not already done. If the patient's breathing is inadequate, provide positive-pressure ventilation with 100% oxygen and assess the adequacy of the ventilations delivered. Pulse oximetry readings can be unreliable in some toxic exposures, such as those involving carbon monoxide.
- Call a poison center for advice about decontamination procedures and patient care as needed. Do not delay transport to contact poison control.
- If the patient has ingested a poison (and is awake), consult medical direction about giving activated charcoal.
- If the patient is unresponsive or seizing, consult medical direction about checking the patient's blood sugar.
- If possible, bring all containers, bottles, labels, and other evidence of suspected poisons to the receiving facility.
- If the patient vomits, save the vomitus in a container (such as a portable suction unit) and transport it to the receiving facility for analysis.
- Anticipate complications, including:
  —Seizures
  —Vomiting
  —Shock
  —Agitation
  —Irregular heart rhythm
- When ALS personnel arrive at the scene (or when transferring patient care at the receiving facility), pass on any patient information that you have gathered. You should include what the patient looked like when you first arrived on the scene, the care you gave, and the patient's response to your care.
- If the patient is stable, reassess every 15 minutes while the patient is in your care. If the patient is unstable, reassess every 5 minutes.

Remember This

When caring for a patient who intentionally exposed herself to a toxic substance, ensure the safety of yourself and your crew while on the scene *and* during patient transport. Watch for behavioral changes and unpredictability.

Ingested Poisons

Objective 15

Most toxic exposures that you will respond to are because of ingested poisons. In some cases, they will be the result of intentional overdoses. Examples of ingested poisons are shown in the following *You Should Know* box.

You Should Know

Examples of Ingested Poisons

- Heart, blood pressure medications
- Tranquilizers, nerve pills
- Antihistamines, cough and cold medicines
- Vitamins, iron pills
- Pain relievers, fever reducers
- Diabetes medicines
- Miniature batteries
- Arts, crafts, and office supplies
- Food, alcoholic beverages
- Mothballs
- Cigarettes, tobacco products
- Pesticides
- Antifreeze, windshield solution
- Indoor and outdoor plants (wild mushrooms, philodendron, foxglove, castor bean, dieffenbachia, pokeweed, holly berries)
- Cleaning products (drain cleaner, toilet bowl cleaner, oven cleaner, rust remover, laundry detergent, automatic dishwasher detergent)
- Cosmetics and personal care products (artificial nail remover, perfume, aftershave, mouthwash, facial cleansers, hair tonics)
- Hydrocarbons (gasoline, kerosene, lamp oil, motor oil, lighter fluid, furniture polish, paint thinner)

Patient Assessment

Objective 15

Signs and symptoms of ingested poisons are listed in the next *You Should Know* box. Because the patient's signs and symptoms are related to the drug ingested, the amount ingested, and the length of time since the ingestion, try to find out this information as quickly as possible. For example, how many pills were in the bottle before they were ingested? How many are left in the bottle? If the patient took a prescription medication,

when was the prescription last filled? Ingestions sometimes involve liquids. Attempt to obtain information about the product from the container's label. When possible, take the label with you to the hospital.

You Should Know

Assessment Findings and Symptoms of Ingested Poisons

- History of ingestion
- Nausea
- Vomiting
- Diarrhea
- Altered mental status
- Abdominal pain
- Chemical burns around the mouth
- Unusual breath odors

Emergency Care

Objective 16

To care for a patient who has ingested poison:

- Using gloves, remove pills, tablets, or fragments from the patient's mouth, as needed, without injuring yourself. Do not stick your fingers in the mouth of a conscious patient with a possible altered mental status. The patient may follow your instructions and spit the pill fragments out. If not, you may attempt to remove the fragments with a suction catheter or other appropriate device.
- Establish and maintain an open airway. Be alert for vomiting; have suction ready. When indicated (and if trauma is not suspected), position the patient in the recovery position to reduce the risk of aspiration.
- Give oxygen. If the patient's breathing is adequate, apply oxygen by nonrebreather mask at 10 to 15 L/min if not already done. If the patient's breathing is inadequate, provide positive-pressure ventilation with 100% oxygen. Assess the adequacy of the ventilations delivered.
- Consult medical direction about giving activated charcoal.
- Bring all containers, bottles, labels, and other evidence of suspected poisons to the receiving facility.
- Transport the patient to the closest appropriate facility, keeping the patient warm.
- En route to the receiving facility, reassess (including vital signs) as often as indicated.
- Carefully document all patient care information on a prehospital care report (PCR).

When ingestions cause death, the most common substances involved are pain relievers, antidepressants, stimulants and street drugs, sedatives, and cardiovascular medications.

Giving Activated Charcoal

Objective 16

If the patient is alert and cooperative, medical direction may instruct you to give the patient activated charcoal. Activated charcoal binds (adsorbs) with many (but not all) chemicals, slowing down or blocking absorption of the chemical in the gastrointestinal (GI) tract. Skill Drill 11-1 shows the procedure for giving a patient activated charcoal. Table 28-4 summarizes important information about activated charcoal that you must know.

Inhaled Poisons

Objective 17

A poison may be inhaled in the form of sprays, dust, droplets, vapors, gases, and fumes. Because the lungs have a large surface area and good blood supply, inhaled poisons can be quickly absorbed and distributed throughout the body. Some inhaled toxins cause significant and permanent damage to the lungs, brain, kidneys, liver, heart, blood, and bone marrow.

Some chemicals (such as ammonia and chlorine) produce fumes with a characteristic odor that can alert you to their presence. However, some gases have no odor. This makes them particularly dangerous because exposure to the poison can occur without the person even being aware of the exposure. Such is the case with many carbon monoxide poisonings. Carbon monoxide (CO) is a colorless, odorless gas that is the result of incomplete

TABLE 28-4   Activated Charcoal

Generic name	activated charcoal
Trade name	Liqui-Char, Actidose, Insta-Char, SuperChar
Mechanism of action	Activated charcoal acts as an adsorbent and will bind with many (but not all chemicals) and slow down or block the absorption of the chemical by the body.
Indications	Poisoning by mouth
Dosage	Adults and children: 1 gram activated charcoal per kilogram of body weight Usual adult dose: 25 to 50 grams Usual infant/child dose: 12.5 to 25 grams
Adverse effects	• Abdominal cramping • Constipation • Black stools • Vomiting (particularly patients who have ingested poisons that cause nausea) • If patient vomits, consider repeating dose once (check with medical direction)
Contraindications	• No permission from medical direction • Altered mental status • Ingestion of acids or alkalis • Inability to swallow
Special considerations	• Obtain an order from medical direction either on-line or off-line to give the medication. • Grasp the container in your hand and shake thoroughly. Since charcoal looks like mud, the patient may need to be persuaded to drink it. Place a straw in the container, or pour the activated charcoal into a glass, and ask the patient to drink it. • If the patient does not drink all the medication in the first drink, shake the container before the second dose because the activated charcoal will settle to the bottom of the container or glass.

combustion. It is the most common cause of death from poisonous gas. Every year a story makes national news because someone, or a group of people, died as a result of carbon monoxide exposure when a fuel-burning appliance malfunctioned (such as an oil or gas furnace, gas water heater, gas range or oven, gas dryer, gas or kerosene space heater, or wood stove). Low levels of carbon monoxide exposure can cause shortness of breath, mild nausea, and mild headaches. Because these symptoms resemble symptoms of other illness such as the flu or food poisoning, they can be overlooked as indicators of carbon monoxide exposure. Moderate levels of carbon monoxide can cause severe headaches, dizziness, confusion, nausea, chest pain, and fainting. High levels of carbon monoxide can cause loss of consciousness and death. An individual who is sleeping or intoxicated and exposed to high levels of carbon monoxide can die from CO poisoning before ever experiencing symptoms.

Other sources of inhaled poisons include:

- Designer drugs
- Wells, sewers
- Anesthetic gases
- Chemical warfare
- Water purification
- Fumes from sprays and liquid chemicals
- Cleaners, degreasing agents, fire extinguishers
- Solvents in dry-cleaning fluid, electrical equipment
- Refrigerator and air conditioner gases in the home and in commercial ice-making plants
- Gases produced as by-products from fires, lightning, heating, and fuel exhausts

Inhalants are household and commercial products that can be abused by intentionally breathing the product's gas or vapors for its mind-altering effects. Inhalant use is called *huffing* or *sniffing*. According to the National Institute on Drug Abuse (NIDA), **sudden sniffing death syndrome (SSDS)** can occur when a person sniffs highly concentrated amounts of the chemicals in solvents or aerosol sprays. Death occurs within minutes because of heart failure. This syndrome is particularly associated with the abuse of butane, propane, and chemicals in aerosols.

A thorough scene size-up on arrival at the scene is essential. Resist the temptation to immediately enter the scene and begin patient care. Without some knowledge of the substance involved, you could place yourself and your crew at unnecessary risk for exposure. Assess the situation for potential or actual danger. Precautions against fire and explosion may be necessary for some gases. If the scene is not safe to enter, move to a safe location. If you have been trained to do so (and are properly equipped), identify and establish safety zones. Contact dispatch for additional resources as necessary.

Examples of inhaled poisons are shown in the following *You Should Know* box.

You Should Know

Examples of Inhaled Poisons

- Nitrous oxide (NOS, Whippets)
- Carbon monoxide
- Carbon dioxide
- Chlorine
- Ammonia
- Propane
- Cyanide
- Freon
- Tear gas
- Inhalants and fumes
  —Hair spray
  —Cleaning fluids
  —Nail polish remover
  —Rubber cement
  —Paint, paint thinner
  —Lighter fluid
  —Room deodorizers
  —Felt marker pens

Patient Assessment

Objective 17

Signs and symptoms of an inhalation exposure depend on the substance inhaled, the amount inhaled, and the extent and duration of exposure. A person who experiences a toxic exposure in a confined space, such as a closed room or garage, is more likely to experience more severe signs and symptoms than a person exposed in an open area. In general, the longer and more concentrated the exposure, the more risk of the incident being fatal. Signs and symptoms of inhalation exposure are listed in the following *You Should Know* box.

You Should Know

Assessment Findings and Symptoms of Inhaled Poisons

- History of inhalation of toxic substance
- Altered mental status
- Difficulty breathing
- Chest pain or discomfort
- Cough
- Hoarseness
- Dizziness
- Headache
- Confusion
- Seizures

Emergency Care

Objective 18

To care for a patient who has inhaled poison:

- Have trained rescuers remove the patient from the poisonous environment and into fresh air as quickly as possible.
- After making sure the scene is safe to enter and you are properly equipped, remove the patient's contaminated clothing. Discard contaminated clothing in an appropriate container.
- Establish and maintain an open airway. Be alert for vomiting; have suction ready. When indicated (and if trauma is not suspected), position the patient in the recovery position to reduce the risk of aspiration.
- Apply a pulse oximeter and give oxygen. If the patient's breathing is adequate, apply oxygen by nonrebreather mask at 10 to 15 L/min if not already done. If the patient's breathing is inadequate, provide positive-pressure ventilation with 100% oxygen and assess the adequacy of the ventilations delivered. Because red blood cells pick up CO quicker than they pick up oxygen, pulse oximetry readings are unreliable for determining carbon monoxide exposures.
- Contact medical direction or a poison center to help determine potential toxicity.
- If relevant, bring all containers, bottles, labels, and other evidence of suspected poisons to the receiving facility.
- Transport the patient to the closest appropriate facility. En route to the receiving facility, reassess (including vital signs) as often as indicated.
- Carefully document all patient care information on a PCR.

Injected Poisons

Objective 19

Poisons that can be injected include:

- Bee, wasp, and ant venom
- Spider, tick, and scorpion venom
- Snake venom
- Drugs

Patient Assessment

Objective 19

The patient's signs and symptoms are related to the substance injected, the amount injected, and the length of time since the exposure occurred. Be alert for signs and symptoms of anaphylaxis. Signs and symptoms of injected poisons are listed in the following *You Should Know* box.

> ### You Should Know
>
> **Assessment Findings and Symptoms of Injected Poisons**
>
> - Weakness
> - Dizziness
> - Chills
> - Fever
> - Abnormal heart rate or rhythm
> - Nausea
> - Vomiting

Emergency Care

Objective 20

To care for a patient with injected poison:

- If possible, determine the type of envenomation. Remove the patient (and rescuers) from the environment if repeated stings or bites are likely.
- Establish and maintain an open airway. Be alert for vomiting; have suction ready.
- Give oxygen. If the patient's breathing is adequate, apply oxygen by nonrebreather mask at 10 to 15 L/min if not already done. If the patient's breathing is inadequate, provide positive-pressure ventilation with 100% oxygen and assess the adequacy of the ventilations delivered.
- Contact medical direction or a poison center to help determine potential toxicity.
- If applicable, send all containers, bottles, labels, and other evidence of suspected poisons to the receiving facility. Unless you are specifically directed otherwise, it is not necessary to bring a scorpion, spider, or snake to the hospital. An accurate description is generally all that is necessary.
- Monitor the patient closely for signs and symptoms of anaphylaxis. If the patient has severe respiratory distress or signs of shock and has been prescribed an epinephrine autoinjector (or if you are authorized to carry it), contact medical direction and request an order to give epinephrine or assist the patient in taking it.
- If swelling or redness is present, mark the outer edge of the area and the time with a pen or marker. This allows other healthcare professionals to monitor the progression of the swelling or redness.

- Transport the patient to the closest appropriate facility, or rendezvous with an ALS unit en route. En route to the receiving facility, reassess (including vital signs) as often as indicated.
- Carefully document all patient care information on a PCR.

Absorbed Poisons

Objective 21

Toxins can enter the body by absorption through the eye, skin, or mucous membranes. Examples of poisons that can be absorbed include:

- Toxins from plants, such as poison ivy, poison oak, and poison sumac
- Pesticides
- Fertilizers
- Cocaine
- Chemical warfare agents

Patient Assessment

Absorbed poisons generally cause redness of the affected area. Signs and symptoms of absorbed poisons are listed in the following *You Should Know* box.

You Should Know

Assessment Findings and Symptoms of Absorbed Poisons

- History of exposure
- Liquid or powder on patient's skin
- Burns
- Itching
- Irritation
- Redness

Emergency Care

Objective 22

To care for a patient who has absorbed poison:
- Remove the patient from the source of the poison. Remove any powder or residue from the patient's skin carefully.
- While wearing chemical protective clothing and gloves, remove the patient's contaminated clothing and jewelry. Dispose of contaminated clothing in an appropriate container.

- Establish and maintain an open airway.
- Give oxygen. If the patient's breathing is adequate, apply oxygen by nonrebreather mask at 10 to 15 L/min if not already done. If the patient's breathing is inadequate, provide positive-pressure ventilation with 100% oxygen and assess the adequacy of the ventilations delivered.
- If the exposure involves the patient's skin and the poison is in powder form, brush the powder off the patient, and then continue as for other absorbed poisons. Be careful not to brush the chemical onto unaffected areas. If the poison is in liquid form, irrigate the skin with clean water for at least 20 minutes (and continue doing so while en route to the receiving facility if possible). Pay particular attention to skin creases and fingernails. Do not apply grease or ointments to the affected area.
- If the exposure involves the patient's eye, flush the affected eye with clean water 2 or 3 inches from the eye for at least 20 minutes. Ask the patient to blink often while flushing. If only one eye is involved, be careful not to contaminate the unaffected eye. Do not allow the patient to rub his eyes. Continue flushing while en route to the receiving facility if possible. When flushing is complete, cover both eyes with moistened dressings or eye pads.
- Contact medical direction or a poison center to help determine potential toxicity.
- If applicable, bring all containers, bottles, labels, or other evidence of suspected poisons to the receiving facility.
- Transport the patient to the closest appropriate facility. En route to the receiving facility, reassess (including vital signs) as often as indicated.
- Carefully document all patient care information on a PCR.

On the Scene   Wrap-Up

As you perform your primary and secondary surveys, you notice that the patient's breathing is shallow and slowly decreasing. She no longer responds when you call her name or apply a painful stimulus. A slow, weak pulse is present. Her blood pressure is 92/60. The patient's pupils are constricted. You recognize that these signs and symptoms are consistent with a toxic exposure to narcotics. Your partner inserts an oral airway and begins positive-pressure ventilation using a bag-mask device connected to 100% oxygen.

On arrival at the hospital, you quickly relay the patient's history and vital signs to the emergency department staff. An ED nurse takes over positive-pressure ventilation while another inserts an intravenous line and gives the patient naloxone (Narcan) IV. Naloxone is used to reverse the symptoms of narcotic overdose. Within minutes the patient is awake and alert, and her respiratory rate, heart rate, and blood pressure have returned to normal. ■

Sum It Up

▶ A poison is any substance taken into the body that interferes with normal body function. Poisoning is exposure to a substance that is harmful in any dosage. A toxin is a poisonous substance. An antidote is a substance that neutralizes a poison.

▶ A poison control center is a medical facility that provides free telephone advice to the public and medical professionals about exposure to poisonous substances. Medical professionals at a PCC can help determine the toxicity of a substance and give advice about the emergency care the patient should receive.

▶ A poison may be a solid, liquid, spray, or gas. Toxins enter the body in four ways: ingestion, inhalation, injection, or absorption. Exposure to a toxin may be accidental or intentional.

▶ Signs and symptoms of a toxic exposure can vary depending on the substance involved; route of entry; the amount ingested, inhaled, injected, or absorbed; and the length of the exposure.

▶ Signs, symptoms, and characteristics that often occur together in toxic exposures are called toxidromes. When the cause of a toxic exposure is unknown, knowing the typical signs and symptoms of certain toxic exposures can help you identify the poison and give appropriate care. Toxic exposures that involve more than one substance (such as alcohol and recreational drugs) are often difficult to recognize and treat. In these situations, the patient will most likely not have signs and symptoms specific to only one toxidrome.

▶ A thorough scene size-up on arrival at the scene of a toxic exposure is essential. Resist the temptation to immediately enter the scene and begin patient care. Without some knowledge of the substance involved, you could place yourself and your crew at an unnecessary risk for exposure. Assess the situation for potential or actual danger. Contact dispatch for additional resources as necessary.

▶ Finding out as much information as you can about the circumstances surrounding a toxic exposure is important. In cases involving an intentional exposure, keep in mind that the history obtained from the patient may not be reliable. Relay all information you obtained when transferring care to ALS personnel or the staff at the receiving facility.

▶ When caring for a patient exposed to a toxin, try to find out (and document) the exact name of the substance. If applicable, bring all containers, bottles, labels, and other evidence of poison agents to the receiving facility.

Psychiatric Disorders

By the end of this chapter, you should be able to:

Knowledge Objectives ▶

1. Define behavior, abnormal behavior, psychiatric disorder, behavioral emergencies, delusions, and hallucinations.
2. Discuss the general factors that may cause an alteration in a patient's behavior.
3. Give examples of psychological crises.
4. Briefly discuss anxiety disorders, panic attacks, obsessive-compulsive disorder, phobias, depression, bipolar disorder, paranoia, and schizophrenia.
5. Define suicide gesture, suicide attempt, and completed suicide, and discuss the characteristics of an individual's behavior that suggest that the patient is at risk for suicide.
6. Discuss the special considerations for assessing a patient with a psychiatric disorder.
7. Discuss the general principles of an individual's behavior that suggest that the person is at risk for violence.
8. Discuss methods of calming a patient who has a psychiatric disorder.
9. Discuss special medical and legal considerations for managing behavioral emergencies.

Attitude Objective ▶

10. Explain the rationale for learning how to modify your behavior toward the patient with a psychiatric disorder.

Skill Objectives ▶

11. Demonstrate the assessment and emergency medical care of a patient with a psychiatric disorder.
12. Demonstrate completing a prehospital care report for a patient with a psychiatric disorder.

You and your EMT partner are working an ambulance night shift in a busy section of the city. You are dispatched to a patient who is mildly combative and stating that he wants to commit suicide. The dispatcher advises you to "stage" for law enforcement. After waiting for a brief period, you get the all clear and enter the scene. As you enter, police officers advise that they were called for a person who had told his sister that he wanted to commit suicide by taking a bottle of pills. The officers tell you that they have the pills and it does not appear that the patient took any. While you are assessing him, the patient tells you he did not take any of the pills. He adds that the stresses in his life right now made him feel like he wanted to die. Your assessment reveals that the patient is alert and oriented to person, place, time, and event. His vital signs are within normal limits. The patient repeatedly tells you that he does not want to go to the hospital. ■

THINK ABOUT IT

As you read this chapter, think about the following questions:

- What precautions should be taken at the scene of a behavioral emergency?
- Are the patient's actions considered a suicide attempt or a suicide gesture?
- Can this patient legally refuse transport to the hospital?

Introduction

You will respond to many situations involving behavioral emergencies. Some behavioral emergencies occur because of an injury or sudden illness. Others may be the result of mental illness or the use of mind-altering substances. You must be able to recognize the factors that can cause changes in a patient's behavior. When providing care for a patient experiencing a behavioral emergency, you must remember to ensure your own safety. You must be able to assess the patient and scene for signs of potential violence. You must also know methods to use to calm a patient experiencing a behavioral emergency and how to apply restraints if these methods are unsuccessful.

Behavior

Objective 1

Behavior is the way in which a person acts or performs. It includes any or all of a person's activities, including physical and mental activity. **Abnormal behavior** is an individual's way of acting or conducting himself that:

- Is not consistent with society's norms and expectations
- Interferes with the individual's well-being and ability to function
- May be harmful to the individual or others

Behavioral Change

Objectives 1, 2, 3

A psychiatric disorder is a disorder of behavior or personality without obvious brain damage. A **behavioral emergency** is a situation in which a patient displays abnormal behavior that is unacceptable to the patient, family members, or community. A behavioral emergency can be the result of extremes of emotion that lead to violence or other inappropriate behavior. A behavioral emergency can also be caused by a psychiatric or physical condition such as mental illness, lack of oxygen, or low blood sugar.

Factors that may cause a change in a patient's behavior include mind-altering substances, situational stressors, medical illnesses, or psychological crises (Table 29-1). Psychological crises include panic, agitation, bizarre thinking and behavior, and destructive behavior. The patient who experiences a psychological crisis may be a danger to herself. She may show self-destructive behavior, such as suicidal gestures. She may also be a danger to others, acting in a threatening manner or even committing violence.

Remember This

Do not assume that a patient has a psychiatric illness until you have ruled out possible physical causes for the behavior.

TABLE 29-1 Factors That May Cause Changes in Behavior

Mind-altering substances	• Alcohol, drugs	
Situational stressors	• Rape • Loss of a job • Career change • Death of a loved one • Marital stress or divorce	• Physical or psychological abuse • Natural disasters (tornado, flood, earthquake, hurricane) • Human-made disasters (war, explosion)
Medical illnesses	• Toxic exposure • Central nervous system infection • Head trauma • Seizure disorder • Lack of oxygen (hypoxia)	• Low blood sugar • Inadequate blood flow to the brain • Extremes of temperature (excessive cold or heat) • Drug or alcohol withdrawal
Psychological crises	• Panic • Agitation • Bizarre thinking and behavior	• Self-destructive behavior, suicidal gesture (danger to self) • Threatening behavior, violence (danger to others)

Psychological Crises

Anxiety and Panic

Objective 4

Anxiety and fear are normal responses to a perceived threat. **Anxiety** is a state of worry and agitation that is usually triggered by a real or imagined situation. It is the person's response to the anxiety that determines its degree of impact. A person who is anxious is afraid of "losing control" or may feel that he will not be able to meet another's expectations. Some anxiety is good. To a point, it can increase awareness and performance. However, as one's level of anxiety increases, it drains energy, shortens one's attention span, and interferes with thinking and problem solving.

Fear is usually triggered by a specific object or situation, such as the possibility of losing a job or being unable to pay the bills. Fear and anxiety bring on various symptoms:

- Worry
- Confusion
- Apprehension
- Helplessness
- Negative thoughts

People show anxiety at different levels of intensity, ranging from uneasiness to a panic attack. Anxiety can have a medical cause. Conditions that may cause anxiety are shown in the following *You Should Know* box.

> **You Should Know**
>
> **Conditions Associated with Anxiety**
>
> - Asthma
> - Diabetes
> - Heart problems
> - Thyroid disorder
> - Seizure disorder
> - Inner ear disturbances
> - Premenstrual syndrome
> - Autism spectrum disorders
> - Withdrawal from alcohol, sedatives, or tranquilizers
> - Reaction to cocaine, amphetamines, caffeine, aspartame, or other stimulants

An **anxiety disorder** is more intense than normal anxiety. Anxiety normally goes away after the stressful situation that caused it is over. An anxiety disorder lasts for months and can lead to phobias. Anxiety disorders are the most common mental illness in America. A patient with an anxiety disorder often has physical signs and symptoms that accompany the patient's intense worry. Common signs and symptoms are shown in the following *You Should Know* box.

Assessment Findings and Symptoms Common to Anxiety Disorders

- Tiredness
- Headaches
- Muscle tension
- Muscle aches
- Difficulty swallowing
- Trembling
- Twitching
- Irritability
- Sweating
- Hot flashes

A **panic attack** is an intense fear that occurs for no apparent reason. Panic attacks can build gradually over several minutes or hours or occur suddenly. Most panic attacks do not last longer than a half hour. Signs and symptoms that are often associated with a panic attack are listed in the following *You Should Know* box. The fear that accompanies a panic attack is very real to the patient. It is sometimes difficult for healthcare professionals to relate to that fear because there may be no obvious trigger. Do not minimize the patient's symptoms. Be supportive, calm, and reassuring.

Assessment Findings and Symptoms Common to Panic Attacks

- Numbness or tingling sensations (usually in the fingers, toes, or lips)
- Shortness of breath or a smothering sensation
- Heart palpitations (a rapid or irregular heartbeat)
- A fear of going crazy or being out of control
- Nausea or abdominal distress
- Choking
- Sweating
- Hot flashes or chills
- A feeling of detachment or being out of touch with oneself
- Trembling or shaking
- Dizziness or faintness
- Fear of becoming seriously ill or dying

Obsessive-Compulsive Disorder

Objective 4

Obsessive-compulsive disorder (OCD) is a type of anxiety disorder. **Obsessions** are recurring thoughts, impulses, or images that cause the person anxiety. Examples of common obsessions include a fear of dirt or germs, extreme need for neatness, and doubts about whether an appliance was turned off. **Compulsions** are recurring behaviors or rituals. The behavior is performed with the hope of preventing obsessive thoughts or making them go away. Examples of compulsions include the following:

- Excessive handwashing
- Checking and rechecking to see if a door is locked
- Touching things in a particular order
- Saying a name or phrase repeatedly
- Repeating a behavior several times

People with OCD often worry that something bad is going to happen to them or a loved one if they don't repeat a certain behavior. For example, they may think that a loved one will be hurt if they do not count to a particular number five times or flip a light switch on and off 48 times. Although some rituals are common in healthy people (such as handwashing), the obsessions and/or compulsions of a person with OCD take up at least 1 hour every day and interfere with the person's normal routine.

OCD usually begins gradually during adolescence or early adulthood. An adult who has OCD recognizes that the thoughts or behaviors are excessive or unreasonable but is unable to control them. A person who has OCD often has another condition, such as depression, another anxiety disorder, or an eating disorder.

Phobias

Objective 4

A **phobia** is an irrational and constant fear of a specific activity, object, or situation (other than a social situation). A **social phobia** is an extreme anxiety response in situations in which the individual may be seen by others. A person who has a social phobia fears that she will act in an embarrassing or shameful manner. Examples of common phobias are shown in Table 29-2.

A phobia is a type of anxiety disorder. Some phobias are common and usually do not create a problem because the person simply avoids the activity, object, or situation. For example, a person who is afraid of elevators or escalators usually avoids that situation or endures it with extreme anxiety. Although an adult recognizes that the fear associated with a phobia is excessive or

TABLE 29-2 Common Phobias

Specific Phobias	Social Phobias
• Animals (especially insects or spiders) • Thunder and/or lightning • Doctors or dentists • Germs, bacteria • Being alone • Blood, injection, or injury • Situations (heights, enclosed places, elevators, crossing bridges, driving or riding in vehicles, airplane travel)	• Public speaking • Eating in public • Using public restrooms • Writing while others are looking on • Performing publicly

unreasonable, a child may not recognize it as such. A child exposed to a phobic stimulus may express anxiety through crying, throwing tantrums, freezing, or clinging.

A phobic reaction resembles a panic attack. The signs and symptoms may include panic, sweating, difficulty breathing, and/or an increased heart rate.

Depression

Objective 4

Depression is a state of mind characterized by feelings of sadness, worthlessness, and discouragement. It often occurs in response to a loss, such as the loss of a job, the death of a loved one, or the end of a relationship. Signs of depression vary with age. Depressed children may be sad or irritable, or may cry frequently. They may express anger by acting out toward parents, teachers, or other authority figures. Older children may have no appetite and may experience headaches or skin disorders. Depressed teens may behave unpredictably, run away, or change their physical and social activities. They may have no appetite, show no interest in their appearance, use alcohol or drugs excessively, or attempt suicide.

You Should Know

More Americans suffer from depression than from coronary heart disease, cancer, and AIDS combined.

Depressed adults show a lack of interest in their job, home, or appearance. They focus on the negative aspects of life, past events, and failures. They may attempt suicide. Depression in an older adult is often related to retirement. It may also be connected to the belief that there is no control over life, or it may result from a loss, such as the death of a spouse or another loved one. Older adults may feel that they are useless or a "burden." They may feel lonely as loved ones die or move away.

Depressed older adults often withdraw, refuse to speak to anyone, and confine themselves to bed. The signs and symptoms of depression are shown in the following *You Should Know* box.

You Should Know

Assessment Findings and Symptoms of Depression

- Loss of appetite
- Diarrhea or constipation
- Tiredness
- Difficulty sleeping or sleeping too much
- Muscle aches
- Vague pains
- Constant feelings of sadness, irritability, or tension
- Significant weight loss or gain
- A loss of interest in usual activities or hobbies
- Crying spells
- An inability to make decisions or concentrate
- Feelings of anger, helplessness, guilt, worthlessness, hopelessness, or loneliness
- Thoughts of suicide or death

Bipolar Disorder

Objective 4

Bipolar disorder (also known as *manic-depressive illness*) is a brain disorder that causes unusual shifts in a person's mood, energy, and ability to function. A person with bipolar disorder has alternating episodes of mood elevation (mania) and depression. When manic, the person often appears restless. He may be extremely energetic and enthusiastic. Typically, a manic person is easily distracted, requires little sleep, and develops unrealistic plans. A person with bipolar disorder will also usually experience periods of depression in which he feels worthless. He may consider suicide. The person's mood is often normal in between the periods of mania and depression.

Paranoia

Objective 4

Paranoia is a mental disorder characterized by excessive suspiciousness or delusions. **Delusions** are false beliefs that the person believes are true, despite facts to the contrary. Common delusions of a paranoid patient include the following:

- Believing that people are following her, harassing her, plotting against her, reading her mind, or controlling her thoughts
- Believing that she possesses great power or special abilities
- Believing that she is a famous person

Remember This

Hallucinations involve the senses. Delusions involve beliefs.

Paranoid patients may experience hallucinations. **Hallucinations** are false sensory perceptions. In other words, the patient sees, hears, or feels things others cannot. For example, a patient with visual hallucinations may think he sees worms or snakes crawling on the floor. An example of an auditory hallucination is hearing voices. An example of a tactile hallucination is feeling insects crawling on the skin.

Paranoid patients are suspicious, distrustful, and prone to conflict. They often feel as if they are being mistreated and misjudged. These patients tend to carry grudges, recalling wrongs done to them years earlier. They are excitable and unpredictable, with outbursts of bizarre or aggressive behavior.

Schizophrenia

Objective 4

Schizophrenia is a group of mental disorders. It is not the same as multiple personality disorder. Symptoms include hallucinations, delusions, disordered thinking, rambling speech, and bizarre or disorganized behavior. Schizophrenic patients are often reserved, withdrawn, and indifferent to the feelings of others. They prefer to be alone and have few, if any, close friends. They can become combative and are at high risk for suicidal and homicidal behavior. Your interpersonal interactions with the schizophrenic patient can either calm or escalate the situation, simply through eye contact and lines of questioning.

Suicide

Objective 5

A **suicide gesture** is self-destructive behavior that is unlikely to have any possibility of being fatal, for instance, threatening to kill oneself and then taking 10 aspirin tablets. A suicide gesture is a conscious or subconscious attempt to call attention to distress rather than to end life. A **suicide attempt** is self-destructive behavior for the purpose of ending one's life that, for unanticipated reasons, fails. For instance, an individual may have taken a sufficient number of aspirin tablets to cause death but was found by a family member before death occurred. A **completed suicide** is death by a self-inflicted, consciously intended action.

Most people who commit suicide express their intentions beforehand. You should take every expression of suicide seriously and arrange for patient transport for evaluation.

You Should Know

Risk Factors for Suicide

- Previous suicide attempt(s)
- History of mental disorders, particularly depression
- History of alcohol and/or substance abuse
- Family history of suicide
- Family history of child maltreatment
- Feelings of hopelessness
- Feeling trapped, no way out
- Impulsive or aggressive tendencies
- Barriers to accessing mental health treatment
- Loss (relational, social, work, or financial)
- Physical illness (cancer, heart failure)
- Easy access to lethal methods
- Ideation or defined lethal plan of action that has been verbalized and/or written
- Unwillingness to seek help because of the stigma attached to mental health and substance abuse disorders or suicidal thoughts
- Cultural and religious beliefs; for example, the belief that suicide is a noble resolution of a personal problem
- Local epidemics of suicide
- Isolation, a feeling of being cut off from other people

Depression is a factor that contributes to suicide. Arrest, imprisonment, or the loss of a job may be a source of depression. The risk of suicide is greatest in persons who have previously attempted suicide. The probability of successful suicide may increase with successive attempts, increasing the patient's risk. For example, a patient who ingested pills on her first attempt may slash her wrists on a second attempt.

Remember This

Men commit suicide more frequently than women do, although women *attempt* suicide more frequently than men do.

The more well thought out the plan, the more serious the suicide risk. A patient who has chosen a lethal plan of action and told others about it is at an increased risk. An unusual gathering of items that could be used to commit suicide increases the risk (such as the purchase of a gun or a large volume of pills). If you've been told that the patient is suicidal, ask him. For example, ask the patient, "Your family says you've thought about killing yourself. Can you tell me about it?" If the patient says he has had suicidal thoughts, ask if he has planned how he would carry it out. Then determine if he has the means to do it.

Excited Delirium

Excited delirium, also called *agitated delirium,* is a term used to describe abnormal behavior characterized by elevated temperature, agitation, aggression, and "superhuman" strength, especially during attempts to restrain the patient. Possible underlying causes include bipolar psychosis, schizophrenia, stimulant abuse, cocaine intoxication, alcohol withdrawal, and head trauma. Excited delirium begins suddenly and may be accompanied by combativeness, hyperactivity, incoherent shouting, and hallucinations.

Research indicates that fatal excited delirium consists of four separate phases that occur in the following order: (1) elevated temperature, (2) agitated delirium, (3) respiratory arrest, and (4) death. Although the patient initially appears agitated, the patient stops struggling shortly after being restrained. Assessment of the patient typically reveals a rapid decrease in mental status and labored or shallow breathing. The patient is often found dead or near dead moments later.

When you are called to provide emergency care for a patient with excited delirium, it is essential to first ensure your safety and that of your crew. Request the assistance of law enforcement personnel, if they are not already present on the scene. In addition, request

that advanced life support personnel be sent to the scene, as it is likely that they will need to administer medications to sedate the patient. When it is safe to do so, approach the patient calmly and cautiously. If it is necessary to restrain the patient, do not restrain the patient in a prone position. The procedure for restraining a patient is discussed in Chapter 2. While the patient is in your care, and especially if the patient is restrained, continuously monitor the patient's mental status, airway, breathing, and circulation. Monitor the patient's vital signs and oxygen saturation.

Remember This

The cessation of struggling or the development of shallow or labored breathing in a patient with excited delirium is a red flag indicating that the patient may be near death and requires *immediate* reassessment.

Assessment and Emergency Care for Patients with Psychiatric Disorders

Objectives 6, 7

Calls to a scene involving a behavioral emergency cause healthcare professionals anxiety because the scene is often unpredictable. Take steps to ensure your safety and that of other healthcare professionals responding to the scene. Start by considering the dispatch information you are given. Have you responded to this location in the past? If so, how many times? Were those calls violent in nature? Find out from your dispatcher if law enforcement personnel are already on the scene. If they are not, ask that they respond to the scene. Remember, your safety comes first.

Remember This

If you suspect a dangerous situation, do *not* enter the scene until law enforcement personnel are present and the safety of the scene is ensured.

When you arrive on the scene, complete a scene size-up before beginning emergency medical care. Carefully assess the scene for possible dangers. Start by visually locating the patient. Visually scan the area for possible weapons (Figure 29-1). Look for signs of violence and evidence of substance abuse. Does the patient have a method or the means of committing suicide? Is this a domestic violence situation? Are there multiple patients? Also, note the general condition of the environment. Look for signs of possible underlying

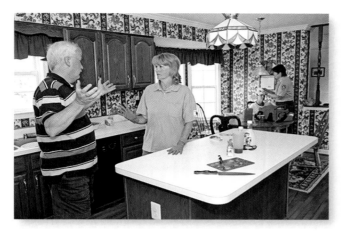

FIGURE 29-1 ▲ When you arrive on the scene of a possible behavioral emergency, carefully assess the scene for possible dangers, including the presence of weapons.

medical problems, such as medications, home oxygen, or other medical equipment.

Check with the family and bystanders to see if the patient has threatened violence or has a history of violence, aggression, or combativeness.

Patient postures that may indicate potential violence include:

- Standing or sitting position that threatens oneself or others
- Inability to sit still, nervous pacing
- Clenched fists or jaw
- Wielding of an unsafe object
- Eyes darting from one object to another

Speech patterns may indicate potential violence. Examples include erratic speech, yelling, shouting, cursing, or threats of harm to oneself or others. Watch the patient's movements closely.

Movements that may indicate potential violence include:

- Movement toward rescuers
- Wielding of heavy or threatening objects
- Tense muscles
- Quick, irregular movements

Other signs of potential violence include a flushed face, agitation, turning away when spoken to, and avoidance of eye contact.

When you are called to the scene of a behavioral emergency, be prepared to spend time at the scene. Limit the number of people around the patient. Take time to calm the patient. Start by approaching the patient slowly and purposefully. Do *not* make any quick movements. If the patient is lying down, it is safest to approach her from the head.

Remember This

Throughout your assessment and care of the patient, maintain alertness to danger. *Never* turn your back on a violent or potentially violent patient, and always ensure easy access to an exit from the room or area. Do *not* place the patient between yourself and an exit.

Clearly identify yourself, and try to build a connection with the patient. Explain who you are and what you are trying to do for him. As you talk with him, begin your assessment of the patient's mental status, airway, breathing, and circulation (ABCs). Is the patient alert and oriented to person, place, time, and event? If the patient is confused, you will probably need to state more than once who you are and what you are doing. Respect the patient's personal space by limiting physical touch. Keep in mind that treating any life-threatening illness or injury that you find takes priority over the patient's behavioral problem.

Be aware of your position and posture when talking to your patient. Standing over her will immediately put her on the defensive. Face the patient and sit or stand at or below the patient's level while maintaining a comfortable distance from her. Maintain eye contact with the patient. Let her know what you expect and what she can expect from you. As you assess and provide care for your patient, keep her informed about what you are doing.

Note the patient's appearance, speech, and mood. Is he speaking normally or is his speech garbled? Does the patient seem anxious, depressed, excited, agitated, angry, hostile, or fearful? If the patient appears disturbed or agitated, try to provide a safe, nonthreatening environment in which you can assess him. Pay attention to the patient's thought process. Does it appear disordered? Is the patient hearing or seeing things that are not there? Does he have unusual worries or fears?

Methods of Calming the Patient Who Has a Psychiatric Disorder

Objective 8

Do not assume that you cannot talk with a patient who has a behavioral problem; always try talking with such patients. Be polite and respectful when talking with the patient. Be careful not to talk down to her. Ask the patient open-ended questions, using a calm, reassuring voice. Open-ended questions require more than a yes or no answer. For example, "Why were we called here today?" After asking a question, give the patient time to answer you. Allow her to tell you her story without you being judgmental. Show you are listening by rephrasing or repeating part of what she said.

Be aware of your own reactions to the situation and to what the patient is saying. For example, an anxious patient may make you anxious. A hostile patient may make you angry. Be careful not to allow your personal feelings to get in the way of your professional judgment. Do not threaten, challenge, or argue with disturbed patients. Keeping your emotions in check when caring for these patients can be difficult. Monitor yourself. If your feelings and actions escalate, it is likely that the patient's feelings and actions will also escalate.

Give your patient honest reassurance. Answer her questions honestly—do not lie to her. However, do not make promises you cannot keep. If the patient is hearing or seeing things, do not "play along." In other words, do not tell the patient you are seeing or hearing the same things she is in an attempt to win her trust. Instead, let the patient know that you do not hear what she is hearing but are interested in knowing what it is that she is hearing.

If possible, involve trusted family members or friends in the patient's care. However, if family members or bystanders are disruptive as you attempt to assess the patient, or if they interfere with your care of the patient, ask law enforcement personnel to remove them from the area.

Stop and Think!

Never leave alone a patient who is experiencing a behavioral emergency.

Medical and Legal Considerations

Objective 9

Emotionally disturbed patients may falsely accuse EMS and law enforcement personnel of unprofessional conduct, including sexual misconduct. To protect yourself against false accusations, it is very important that you document the patient's abnormal behavior. If possible, have witnesses present when you provide patient care. This is especially important during transport. When possible, use attendants of the same gender and involve third-party witnesses.

Emotionally disturbed patients will often resist treatment. To provide care against the patient's will, you must have a reasonable belief that the patient could harm you, himself, or others. If the patient is a threat to you, himself, or others, the patient may be transported without consent after you contact medical direction and receive approval to do so. Law enforcement personnel are usually required.

The patient stated that he wanted to commit suicide but did not actually take any pills. However, because he made the statement that he intentionally wanted to harm himself, it became necessary for the patient to be transported and evaluated by a physician. In this case, the patient went to the hospital without incident. ■

Sum It Up

▶ Behavior is the way in which a person acts or performs. It includes any or all of a person's activities, including physical and mental activity. Abnormal behavior is an individual's way of acting or conducting himself that is not consistent with society's norms and expectations, interferes with the individual's well-being and ability to function, or may be harmful to the individual or others. A psychiatric disorder is a disorder of behavior or personality without obvious brain damage.

▶ As an EMT, you will likely encounter various behavioral emergencies. A behavioral emergency is a situation in which a patient displays abnormal behavior that is unacceptable to the patient, family members, or community. A behavioral emergency can be caused by extremes of emotion or by psychological or physical conditions. A number of factors can result in such emergencies, including mental illness, a lack of oxygen, low blood sugar, alcohol or drugs, situational stressors, medical illnesses, or psychological crises.

▶ Anxiety is a state of worry and agitation that is usually triggered by a real or imagined situation. An anxiety disorder is more intense than normal anxiety.

▶ A panic attack is an intense fear that occurs for no apparent reason.

▶ Obsessive-compulsive disorder is a type of anxiety disorder. Obsessions are recurring thoughts, impulses, or images that cause the person anxiety. Compulsions are recurring behaviors or rituals that are performed with the hope of preventing obsessive thoughts or making them go away.

▶ A phobia is an irrational and constant fear of a specific activity, object, or situation (other than a social situation). A social phobia is an extreme anxiety response in situations in which the individual may be seen by others. A phobic reaction resembles a panic attack.

▶ Depression is a state of mind characterized by feelings of sadness, worthlessness, and discouragement.

It often occurs in response to a loss, such as the loss of a job, the death of a loved one, or the end of a relationship.

▶ Bipolar disorder is a brain disorder that causes unusual shifts in a person's mood, energy, and ability to function. A person with bipolar disorder has alternating episodes of mood elevation (mania) and depression. The person's mood is often normal between the periods of mania and depression.

▶ Paranoia is a mental disorder characterized by excessive suspiciousness or delusions. Paranoid patients are suspicious, distrustful, and prone to argument. They are excitable and unpredictable, with outbursts of bizarre or aggressive behavior.

  ● Delusions are false beliefs that the patient believes are true, despite facts to the contrary.

  ● Hallucinations are false sensory perceptions. The patient sees, hears, or feels things that others cannot.

▶ Schizophrenia is a group of mental disorders. Symptoms include hallucinations, delusions, disordered thinking, rambling speech, and bizarre or disorganized behavior. Schizophrenic patients can become combative and are at high risk for suicidal and homicidal behavior.

▶ A suicide gesture is self-destructive behavior that is unlikely to have any possibility of being fatal. A suicide attempt is self-destructive behavior for the purpose of ending one's life that, for unanticipated reasons, fails. A completed suicide is death by a self-inflicted, consciously intended action.

▶ Most people who commit suicide express their intentions beforehand. You should take every expression of suicide seriously and arrange for patient transport for evaluation.

▶ Excited delirium, also called agitated delirium, is a term used to describe abnormal behavior characterized by elevated temperature, agitation, aggression, and "superhuman" strength, especially during attempts to restrain the patient. Possible underlying causes include manic-depressive psychosis, schizophrenia, stimulant abuse, cocaine intoxication, alcohol withdrawal, and head trauma.

▶ When called to a scene that involves a behavioral emergency, remember that the scene may be unpredictable. Take steps to ensure your safety and that of other healthcare professionals responding to the scene. Complete a scene size-up before beginning emergency medical care. Carefully assess the scene for possible dangers. Start by visually locating the patient. Visually scan the area for possible weapons. Be prepared to spend time at the scene. Limit the number of people around the patient. Take time to calm the patient.

▶ Avoid restraining a patient unless the patient is a danger to you, himself, or others. When using restraints, have police present, if possible, and get approval from medical direction. If you must use restraints, apply them with the help of law enforcement and other EMS personnel.

Diseases of the Nose

By the end of this chapter, you should be able to:

Knowledge Objectives ▶
1. Define epistaxis, and describe common causes of this condition.
2. Identify common assessment findings and symptoms associated with epistaxis.
3. Discuss the emergency care for epistaxis.

Attitude Objectives ▶
No attitude objectives are identified for this lesson.

Skill Objectives ▶
4. Demonstrate the assessment and emergency medical care of a patient with epistaxis.
5. Demonstrate completing a prehospital care report for a patient with epistaxis.

On the Scene

You are dispatched to a local park where you find a small group of people clustered around an 8-year-old girl, who is your patient. She is seated upright on the bench of a picnic table with her head tipped back. Her father is holding his index finger tightly against her upper lip. The patient's father reports that his daughter "bumped" into another child while playing in the park and began bleeding from her nose. Her dad continues by telling you that he has placed a large piece of tissue against the gum under her upper lip and that he is holding it in place to "help stop the bleeding." ■

THINK ABOUT IT

As you read this chapter, think about the following questions:

- Is the care being rendered by the patient's father appropriate?
- How can you best treat this patient and educate the family?

Introduction

A nosebleed is a common occurrence. Although many nosebleeds are treated at home, some patients will call 9-1-1 for assistance. You must be able to assess the patient, provide prompt emergency care, and recognize when the patient will require transport to the hospital for further care. In this chapter we discuss possible causes, common assessment findings and symptoms, and general emergency care for epistaxis.

Causes of Epistaxis

Objective 1

Air enters the body through the nose or the mouth. The nose warms, moistens, and filters the air that we breathe in. The nasal mucosa is supplied with many blood vessels that lie close to the surface where they can be injured and bleed (Figure 30-1). A nosebleed, also called **epistaxis,** can be caused by trauma or medical conditions (see Table 30-1). Although the most common cause of epistaxis is nose picking, in many cases the cause of the bleeding is unknown.

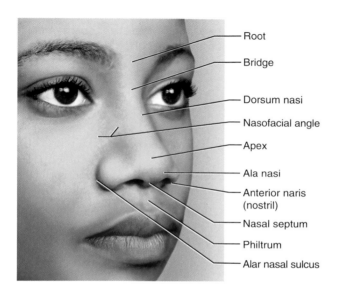

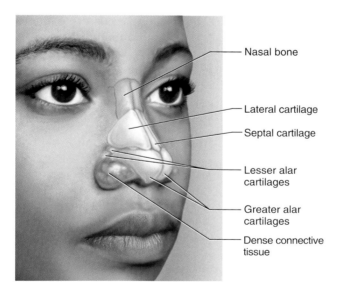

FIGURE 30-1 ▲ Anatomy of the nose: **(a)** external; **(b)** internal.

TABLE 30-1 Causes of Epistaxis	
Traumatic Causes	**Medical Causes**
• Foreign body • Nose picking • Facial and nasal surgery • Facial trauma (usually a sharp blow to the nose or face)	• Dry, heated, indoor air • Dry, hot, low-humidity climates • Allergies • Sinusitis • Hypertension • Bleeding disorders • Upper respiratory infection • Chemical irritants (such as cocaine, industrial chemicals) • Vitamin K deficiency • Use of drugs that thin the blood (aspirin and other nonsteroidal anti-inflammatory medications; warfarin [Coumadin])

Assessment Findings and Symptoms

Objective 2

Typical assessment findings and symptoms associated with epistaxis include bleeding from the nose, which can range from a trickle to a strong flow of blood. Significant bleeding can result in an airway obstruction if the patient is unresponsive. Vomiting may be present if the patient swallowed blood. Localized pain or tenderness may be present, particularly if nasal bleeding was caused by trauma.

Emergency Care

Objective 3

Most nosebleeds come from a bleeding blood vessel in the front of the nose. This type of nosebleed is called an *anterior nosebleed*. It is usually easy to control. Tell the patient with a nosebleed not to blow her nose or sniffle. Doing so can prevent clots from forming or can break clots that have already developed. Do not put anything in the nose to try to control bleeding. If the patient can help you (and there is no risk of spinal injury), have her sit up and lean her head forward. This position helps keep blood from draining into the back of the patient's throat. Blood that is swallowed often makes a person feel sick to

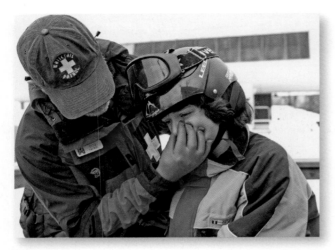

FIGURE 30-2 ▲ To stop a nosebleed, have the patient sit up, with the patient's head tilted forward. Pinch the fleshy part of the patient's nostrils together with your thumb and two fingers for 15 minutes.

the stomach (nauseous), increasing the chance of vomiting. If the patient cannot sit up, place her in the recovery (lateral recumbent) position to enable blood to flow out of her nose/mouth. Tell the patient to breathe through the mouth. Pinch the fleshy part of the patient's nostrils together with your thumb and two fingers for 15 minutes (Figure 30-2).

Remember This

Remember to take appropriate standard precautions when caring for a patient with epistaxis.

Some nosebleeds come from a bleeding blood vessel in the back of the nose. This type of nosebleed is called a *posterior nosebleed*. A posterior nosebleed occurs most often in older adults. This type of nosebleed is difficult to control, and the patient can develop shock. A patient with a posterior nosebleed needs rapid transport to the hospital. Treat for shock if present.

On the Scene | **Wrap-Up**

You politely ask the patient's father if you can help his daughter, and he gives you permission to proceed. Suspecting that the patient has an anterior nosebleed, you begin care by removing the tissue from the patient's mouth and asking her to tilt her head slightly forward. You know that, while there are a large number of "folk remedies" that are used to stop a nosebleed, tipping the head back increases the possibility that the patient will swallow some of the blood, increasing the likelihood of vomiting. You pinch the fleshy part of the patient's nostrils together for about 15 minutes and find that the bleeding has stopped. You explain your treatment to the patient's father, and he agrees to follow your suggestions for treating this problem in the future. After contacting medical direction, you and your partner clear the scene with a refusal of transport. ■

Sum It Up

▶ The nasal mucosa is supplied with many blood vessels that lie close to the surface where they can be injured and bleed. A nosebleed, also called epistaxis, can be caused by trauma or medical conditions.

▶ Typical assessment findings and symptoms associated with epistaxis include bleeding from the nose, which can range from a trickle to a strong flow of blood.

▶ An anterior nosebleed is usually easy to control. If there is no risk of spinal injury, have the patient lean his head forward. Tell the patient to breathe through the mouth. Pinch the fleshy part of the patient's nostrils together with your thumb and two fingers for 15 minutes.

▶ A posterior nosebleed is difficult to control, and the patient can develop shock. A patient with a posterior nosebleed needs rapid transport to the hospital. Treat for shock if present.

CHAPTER

3·1

Hematology

By the end of this chapter, you should be able to:

Knowledge Objectives ▶

1. Define sickle cell disease, and discuss causes of this condition.
2. Identify common assessment findings and symptoms associated with sickle cell disease.
3. Discuss the emergency care for sickle cell disease.
4. Define hemophilia, and discuss causes of this condition.
5. Identify common assessment findings and symptoms associated with hemophilia.
6. Discuss the emergency care for hemophilia.

Attitude Objectives ▶

No attitude objectives are identified for this lesson.

Skill Objectives ▶

7. Demonstrate compassion for patients with nontraumatic pain.
8. Demonstrate the assessment and emergency medical care of a patient with sickle cell disease.
9. Demonstrate completing a prehospital care report for a patient with sickle cell disease.
10. Demonstrate the assessment and emergency medical care of a patient with hemophilia.
11. Demonstrate completing a prehospital care report for a patient with hemophilia.

On the Scene

You are called to a private residence for an "ill woman." You arrive to find a 20-year-old African-American woman sitting in a chair in her living room and crying. She is complaining of extreme pain, primarily in her joints, that she rates 10/10. The patient has a history of sickle cell disease. Your physical examination reveals swollen, painful extremities. ■

THINK ABOUT IT

As you read this chapter, think about the following questions:

• What is sickle cell disease?
• What do you suspect is wrong with this patient?
• What emergency care should you provide to this patient?

Hematology is the study of diseases of the blood and blood-forming organs. In this chapter we discuss possible causes, assessment findings and symptoms, and general emergency care for sickle cell disease and hemophilia.

Sickle Cell Disease

Objective 1

Sickle cell disease is an inherited disorder that affects red blood cells. Individuals who have sickle cell disease inherit two copies of the sickle cell gene—one from each parent. An individual who inherits a sickle cell gene from one parent and a normal gene from the other parent has *sickle cell trait*. An individual who has sickle cell trait does not have sickle cell disease, but has one of the genes that cause the disease. Sickle cell disease mainly affects African Americans and Hispanic Americans. In the United States, the average life expectancy for an individual with sickle cell disease is about 45 years.

The body produces red blood cells in the spongy marrow inside the large bones of the body. Normal red blood cells are smooth and round, move easily through blood vessels, and live about 120 days. In sickle cell disease, the body produces a defective hemoglobin molecule that causes red blood cells to become stiff and shaped like a sickle, or C (see Figure 31-1). Unlike

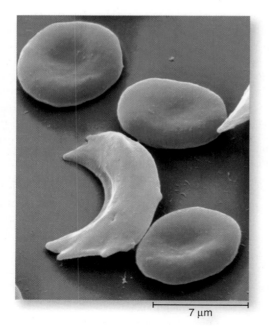

7 µm

FIGURE 31-1 ▲ Sickle-shaped cells found in sickle cell disease.

normal red blood cells, sickled red blood cells usually die after about 10 to 40 days. Because the bone marrow is unable to produce new red blood cells fast enough to replace the dying ones, a lower-than-normal number of red blood cells are present in the body, resulting in **sickle cell anemia.** Anemia is a condition in which the blood has less than the normal number of red blood cells or less than the normal quantity of hemoglobin in the blood. In either case, the oxygen-carrying capacity of the blood is decreased.

Sickled red blood cells carry less hemoglobin than normal red blood cells and do not move easily through blood vessels. They are stiff and have a tendency to stick together and form clumps, subsequently getting stuck in the blood vessels. A **sickle cell crisis** occurs when clumps of sickled cells build up in the blood vessels, blocking blood flow to organs and limbs. Impaired circulation causes pain, swelling, infection, and organ damage and death. There is no cure for sickle cell disease at this time.

Assessment Findings and Symptoms

Objective 2

Although sickle cell anemia is present at birth, signs and symptoms of the disease usually do not develop until after age 4 months. This is because an infant's blood has a large amount of fetal hemoglobin, and therefore a higher oxygen concentration, that protects the infant during this time and inhibits sickling.

Symptoms in patients with sickle cell disease vary from mild to severe. The most common symptom of patients who have sickle cell anemia is fatigue. They may also complain of shortness of breath, dizziness, headache, coldness in the hands and feet, or chest pain. The pain associated with sickle cell disease (sickle cell crisis) may be acute (sudden) or chronic (long term). Acute pain ranges in intensity from mild to severe and usually lasts hours to several days. Chronic pain typically lasts for weeks to months. Sickle cell crises often affect the lungs, abdomen, and bones and joints of the arms and legs.

Remember This

The most common symptoms of individuals with sickle cell disease are fatigue and pain.

Hand-foot syndrome is one of earliest changes of sickle cell disease and results from the blockage of blood vessels in the hands or feet by sickle cells. It usually starts with painful swelling, affecting one or both hands and/or feet at the same time. Swelling typically

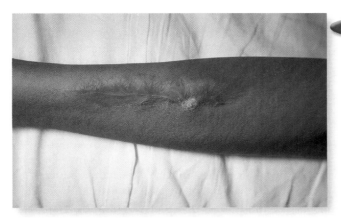

FIGURE 31-2 ▲ Leg ulcer found in a patient with sickle cell disease.

Assessment Findings and Symptoms of Sickle Cell Disease

Patients who have sickle cell disease will typically seek medical assistance when any of the following signs and symptoms is present:

- Fever over 101°F
- Severe pain anywhere
- Sudden change in vision
- Increasing fatigue
- Sudden weakness or loss of feeling in an extremity
- Abdominal swelling
- Headache that is different from usual
- Chest pain
- Difficulty breathing

occurs on the back of the hands and tops of the feet and moves into the fingers and toes.

Ulcers (sores) develop on the lower third of the leg in some patients with sickle cell disease (Figure 31-2). The cause of leg ulcers is unknown.

Acute chest syndrome is a complication of sickle cell disease that can occur because of an infection or blockage of the blood vessels in the lungs by blood clots or sickled red blood cells. Assessment findings and symptoms are similar to those of pneumonia and include fever, chest pain, coughing, and difficulty breathing.

An important function of the spleen is to fight infection by removing bacteria from the blood. The patient who has sickle cell disease is prone to infections because damage to the spleen (caused by sickled red blood cells) results in the inefficient removal of bacteria from the blood. **Splenic crisis** is a condition in which sickled red blood cells become trapped in the spleen, causing a significant fall in the amount of red blood cells and hemoglobin circulating in the bloodstream. This condition is a leading cause of death in children with sickle cell disease. Infants and young children with sickle cell anemia who are between the ages of 2 months and 4 years are at greatest risk of splenic crisis and severe infection, such as pneumonia or meningitis. Pneumonia is the most common cause of death in young children who have sickle cell anemia. Signs and symptoms of splenic crisis include weakness, irritability, unusual sleepiness, tachycardia, pale skin, and pain in the left side of the abdomen.

Individuals who have sickle cell disease are at increased risk of stroke. Most strokes in individuals with sickle cell disease occur in children. Repeat strokes are common, usually occurring within 3 years of the first stroke.

Emergency Care

Objective 3

To care for a patient experiencing a sickle cell crisis:

- Conduct a scene size-up and ensure your safety. Put on appropriate PPE.
- Prehospital care for a patient experiencing a sickle cell crisis is supportive. Request advanced life support personnel to the scene as soon as possible. If the patient's vital signs are stable, ALS personnel will be able to administer medications to help ease the patient's discomfort en route to the hospital.
- Perform a primary survey to identify and treat any life-threatening conditions. Manage the patient's airway and breathing. Allow the patient to assume a position of comfort. Administer oxygen. If the patient's breathing is inadequate, give positive-pressure ventilation with 100% oxygen. Assess the adequacy of the ventilations delivered.
- Perform a physical examination. Take the patient's vital signs, and gather the patient's medical history.
- En route to the hospital, make the patient as comfortable as possible, provide reassurance, and keep him warm.
- Reassess as often as indicated until patient care is turned over to ALS personnel or medical personnel at the receiving facility.
- Record all patient care information, including the patient's medical history and the emergency care provided, on a PCR.

Hemophilia

Objective 4

The normal blood-clotting process involves a number of different clotting factors that work with platelets to stop bleeding. **Hemophilia** is an inherited bleeding disorder caused by an abnormality of a blood-clotting factor. Hemophilia also can be acquired if an individual forms antibodies to the clotting factors in his bloodstream. Hemophilia usually occurs in males, only rarely occurring in females.

Assessment Findings and Symptoms

Objective 5

Signs and symptoms of hemophilia vary depending on the severity of clotting factor deficiency. The primary signs and symptoms of hemophilia are easy bruising and excessive bleeding. Bleeding may be external or internal. External bleeding can be seen. Possible causes of excessive external bleeding in the patient who has hemophilia include a nosebleed with no obvious cause; unexplained bleeding or bruising; or prolonged bleeding from a tooth extraction or cut, or after surgery.

Internal bleeding is not visible because it occurs inside body tissues and cavities. Signs and symptoms of internal bleeding can include chest or abdominal pain, hematuria, hematemesis, or tarry stools. Bleeding in the brain is a complication of hemophilia. Signs and symptoms can include altered mental status, neck pain or stiffness, seizures, extreme fatigue, double vision, long-lasting headache, repeated vomiting, difficulty walking, or arm or leg weakness. Because bleeding into the knees, elbows, hips and shoulders, and muscles of the arms and legs can also occur, be sure to assess each extremity carefully. Initially, bleeding into a joint may cause complaints of "tightness" in the joint, but no pain. As bleeding continues or when sudden bleeding occurs, the joint feels warm to the touch, swelling is present, and joint movement is impaired.

Emergency Care

Objective 6

To care for a patient with hemophilia:

- Conduct a scene size-up and ensure your safety. Put on appropriate PPE.
- Perform a primary survey to identify and treat any life-threatening conditions. Manage the patient's airway and breathing. Allow the patient to assume a position of comfort, and provide calm reassurance. Administer oxygen. If the patient's breathing is inadequate, give positive-pressure ventilation with 100% oxygen. Assess the adequacy of the ventilations delivered. A patient with internal bleeding may vomit. Watch the patient closely to make sure his airway remains clear. Make sure that you have suction within arm's reach at all times. Suction as needed.
- Perform a physical examination. Take the patient's vital signs, and gather the patient's medical history. Assess the patient carefully looking for signs of bruising, obvious bleeding, and signs that suggest internal bleeding. Control external bleeding, if present. Be alert for signs of recurring bleeding if bleeding has been controlled. If signs of shock develop, place the patient in a supine position and transport as soon as possible to the closest appropriate facility.
- En route to the hospital, make the patient as comfortable as possible, provide reassurance, and keep her warm.
- Reassess as often as indicated until patient care is turned over to ALS personnel or medical personnel at the receiving facility.
- Record all patient care information, including the patient's medical history and the emergency care provided, on a PCR.

On the Scene   Wrap-Up

You administer oxygen and continue gathering the medical history while your partner obtains the patient's vital signs. You learn that the patient was admitted to the hospital 2 months ago for an upper respiratory tract infection. Yesterday the patient developed pain in her legs, back, and arms, which has steadily increased in intensity. The patient's vital signs are BP 116/80, P 96, R 24. Based on the patient's past medical history, current complaint, and physical exam findings, you suspect she is experiencing a sickle cell crisis. You and your partner carefully move her to the stretcher and begin transport to the closest appropriate facility while providing supportive care en route. ■

Sum It Up

▶ Sickle cell disease is an inherited disorder that affects red blood cells.

▶ Individuals who have sickle cell disease inherit two copies of the sickle cell gene—one from each parent. An individual who inherits a sickle cell gene from one parent and a normal gene from the other parent has sickle cell trait. An individual who has sickle cell trait does not have sickle cell disease, but has one of the genes that cause the disease.

▶ Sickle cell disease mainly affects African Americans and Hispanic Americans.

▶ In sickle cell disease, the body produces a defective hemoglobin molecule that causes red blood cells to become stiff and shaped like a sickle, or C. Unlike normal red blood cells, sickled red blood cells usually die after about 10 to 40 days. Sickled red blood cells carry less hemoglobin than normal red blood cells.

▶ A sickle cell crisis occurs when clumps of sickled cells build up in the blood vessels, blocking blood flow to organs and limbs.

▶ The most common symptom of the patient who has sickle cell anemia is fatigue. The most common symptoms of individuals with sickle cell disease are fatigue and pain.

▶ Splenic crisis is a condition in which sickled red blood cells become trapped in the spleen, causing a significant fall in the amount of red blood cells and hemoglobin circulating in the bloodstream. This condition is a leading cause of death in children with sickle cell disease.

▶ Hemophilia is an inherited bleeding disorder caused by an abnormality of a blood-clotting factor. Hemophilia also can be acquired if an individual forms antibodies to the clotting factors in the bloodstream. Hemophilia usually occurs in males, only rarely occurring in females.

▶ The primary signs and symptoms of hemophilia are easy bruising and excessive bleeding.

Module 7

Shock

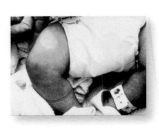

► CHAPTER **32**
Shock 539

Shock

By the end of this chapter, you should be able to:

Knowledge Objectives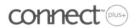

1. Describe possible causes of cardiogenic shock.
2. Differentiate between hemorrhagic and hypovolemic shock, and describe possible causes of each.
3. Describe possible causes of obstructive shock.
4. Describe possible causes of distributive shock.
5. Discuss the stages of shock.
6. Describe common assessment findings and symptoms of shock.
7. Describe the emergency medical care of the patient with signs and symptoms of shock.

Attitude Objective ▶

8. Explain the sense of urgency for transporting patients that are showing signs of shock.

Skill Objectives ▶

9. Demonstrate the care of the patient exhibiting signs and symptoms of shock.
10. Demonstrate completing a prehospital care report for a patient exhibiting signs and symptoms of shock.

connect (plus+)

On the Scene

It is 7:30 p.m. when you and your partner are dispatched for an "ill woman." On arrival at the scene, you find an 85-year-old woman sitting outside a local restaurant. As you approach, you note that the patient is awake and breathing at a rate slightly faster than normal. Her skin looks pale. The patient states she feels weak and dizzy, and is slightly short of breath. She also complains of a dull pain in the middle of her abdomen that radiates to her back. As you count the patient's radial pulse, you notice that her skin is cold and clammy. The patient's initial vital signs reveal the following: blood pressure 70/46, pulse 138, respirations 24. The patient states that she has not eaten since lunch earlier today. A focused physical examination reveals that the patient's abdomen is distended, rigid, and tender. She denies any recent trauma. ■

THINK ABOUT IT

As you read this chapter, think about the following questions:

- What findings suggest that you need to move quickly and begin providing emergency care for this patient?
- What emergency care will you provide?

Introduction

Shock, also called **hypoperfusion,** is the inadequate flow of blood through an organ or a part of the body. If shock is not corrected, it will lead to inadequate tissue perfusion and eventual cell and organ death. Treatment of shock is performed immediately after the primary survey and before patient transport.

In this chapter we discuss the types, stages, and emergency care of shock. It is important that you promptly recognize the signs and symptoms of shock and its possible causes. Promptly recognizing and treating shock is critical to your patient's survival.

Types of Shock

Objectives 1, 2, 3, 4

The structure and function of the cardiovascular system were presented in Chapters 6 and 7. Recall that perfusion is the circulation of blood through an organ or a part of the body. To have adequate perfusion, the heart, vessels, and the flow of blood must function properly. When the body's tissues are adequately perfused, oxygen and other nutrients are carried to the cells of all organ systems, and waste products are removed.

Shock is a life-threatening condition that requires *immediate* emergency care.

Disruptions in circulatory function that can cause shock include the following:

- *Pump failure.* The amount of blood the heart pumps throughout the body depends on how many times the heart beats and the force of the contractions. **Cardiogenic shock** can result if the heart beats too quickly or too slowly or if the heart muscle does not have enough force to pump blood effectively to all parts of the body. This type of shock can occur because of a heart attack, a heart rhythm that is too fast or too slow, an injury to the heart, or other conditions that affect the heart's ability to pump.

- *Fluid loss.* Shock can result if there is not enough blood for the heart to pump through the cardiovascular system. Shock caused by severe bleeding is called **hemorrhagic shock.** The bleeding may be internal, external, or both. However, blood is not the only type of fluid that may be lost from the body. For example, body fluid may be lost because of vomiting or diarrhea. Plasma may be lost as a result of a burn.

Fluid also may be lost because of excessive sweating or urination. Shock caused by a loss of blood, plasma, or other body fluid is called **hypovolemic shock**.

- *Blood flow is slowed or stopped by an obstruction.* Shock that occurs when blood flow is slowed or stopped by a mechanical or physical obstruction is called **obstructive shock.** This type of shock may occur when blood collects in the sac surrounding the heart, preventing efficient cardiac contraction, or when air is present in the chest due to a lung injury, putting pressure on the great vessels in the chest and limiting blood flow.

- *Container failure.* Normally, blood vessels work with the nervous system to increase or decrease the amount of blood sent to different areas of the body. When an area needs more blood, the vessels expand to provide it with more blood and constrict in areas that do not need it. When shock caused by container failure occurs, the blood vessels lose their ability to adjust the flow of blood. Instead of expanding and constricting as needed, the blood vessels remain enlarged. The amount of fluid in the body remains constant (there is no actual loss of fluid), but blood pools in the outer areas of the body. As a result, there is an inadequate amount of blood to fill the enlarged vessels, and the vital organs are not perfused. The four major causes of this type of **distributive shock** are:

1. Injury to the spinal cord (**neurogenic shock**)
2. Severe infection (**septic shock**)
3. Severe allergic reaction (**anaphylactic shock**)
4. Psychological causes (**psychogenic shock**)

Regardless of the type of shock, cells are starved for enough oxygen-rich blood. When the body's cells and organs are not supplied with oxygen and nutrients, they begin to break down, and waste products build up. Unless adequate perfusion is quickly restored, death may soon follow.

You Should Know

Without an adequate supply of oxygen-rich blood:

- The brain, heart, and lungs will suffer damage after 4 to 6 minutes.
- The kidneys and liver will suffer damage after 45 to 90 minutes.
- The skin and muscles will suffer damage after 4 to 6 hours.

The Stages of Shock

Objectives 5, 6

Shock occurs in three stages: early (compensated), late (decompensated), and irreversible (terminal).

Early Shock

Early (compensated) shock is sometimes called *shock with a normal blood pressure*. In early shock, the body's defense mechanisms attempt to protect the vital organs (the brain, heart, and lungs) (Figure 32-1).

You can recognize signs of early shock by assessing the patient for the following:

- *Mental status.* Some of the earliest signs of shock can be seen as changes in the patient's mental status. A patient in early shock will appear anxious and restless. Some patients are combative. These changes occur because the brain is not receiving an adequate supply of oxygenated blood.
- *Breathing.* As the body attempts to draw in more oxygen, the bronchioles expand to draw in more air and the patient's breathing rate increases.
- *Skin color, temperature, and moisture.* As blood is shunted from the skin and muscles to the patient's vital organs, the patient's skin will look pale and feel cool and moist. You may notice that the patient's face appears pale, especially around the mouth and nose. During shock, the body diverts blood to the areas that are most dependent on a continuous, rich supply of oxygen. The patient's skin appears pale because the body diverts blood from the skin first. You may see beads of sweat on the patient's skin. Sweating is usually first visible on the upper lip and around the hairline.

- *Heart rate.* The patient's pulse will feel slightly faster than normal because the heart picks up its pace to pump oxygenated blood throughout the body.
- *The strength of the peripheral pulses.* Pulses in the arms and legs often feel weak because blood is being shunted away from them to protect the body's vital organs.
- *Capillary refill.* In children younger than 6 years of age, delayed capillary refill (3 to 5 seconds) may indicate poor perfusion or exposure to cool temperatures. A capillary refill time longer than 5 seconds is markedly delayed and suggests shock.

Remember This

It may be difficult to determine pale skin color in a dark-skinned person. In these situations, look at the patient's nail beds, the mucous membranes of the eyes, or inside the mouth. If these areas are pale, consider possible shock.

Early shock is often difficult to recognize. Remember to look for it and to consider the patient's mechanism of injury or the nature of the illness when assessing your patient. For example, an increased heart rate may be caused by many things. Fever, fear, pain, anxiety, stress, and exercise can all increase a person's heart rate. However, an increased heart rate accompanied by pale, cool skin and anxiety in a victim of a motorcycle crash should make you immediately think of shock. The sooner shock is recognized and appropriate treatment is begun, the better your patient's chance for survival. Early shock is usually reversible if it is recognized and the patient receives

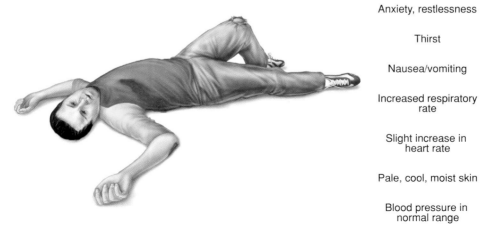

Anxiety, restlessness

Thirst

Nausea/vomiting

Increased respiratory rate

Slight increase in heart rate

Pale, cool, moist skin

Blood pressure in normal range

FIGURE 32-1 ▲ The signs and symptoms of early (compensated) hypovolemic shock.

emergency care to correct the cause of the shock. If early shock is not recognized or corrected, it will progress to the next stage.

Late Shock

When an ill or injured adult patient's systolic blood pressure drops to less than 90 mm Hg, **late (decompensated) shock** is present. The presence of a low blood pressure is the main difference between early (compensated) shock and late (decompensated) shock. In late shock, the body's defense mechanisms lose their ability to make up for the lack of oxygenated blood. A patient in late shock looks very sick (Figure 32-2). He is usually slow to respond or confused, or may even be unresponsive. His breathing is shallow, labored, and irregular. The patient's skin is cool and moist and may be pale, blue, or mottled. His pulse is fast and hard to feel (thready) or may be absent in his arms and legs. The signs of late shock are more obvious than those of early shock, but late shock is more difficult to treat. It is still reversible if the cause of the problem is quickly corrected.

Irreversible Shock

Irreversible shock is also called *terminal shock*. At this stage, the body's defense mechanisms have failed. You will feel an irregular pulse as the patient's heart becomes irritable and begins to beat irregularly. As shock continues, the patient's heart rhythm becomes more chaotic, and the heart can no longer effectively pump blood. Permanent damage occurs to the vital organs because the cells and organs have been without oxygenated blood for too long. Eventually, the heart stops, breathing stops, and death results.

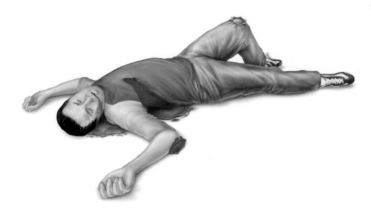

Slow to respond, confused or unresponsive

If awake, extreme thirst

Nausea/vomiting

Shallow, labored, irregular breathing

Rapid heart rate

Cool, moist skin that is pale, blue, or mottled

Low blood pressure

FIGURE 32-2 ▲ The signs and symptoms of late (decompensated) hypovolemic shock.

Shock in Infants and Children

Blood pressure is an unreliable indicator of shock in the pediatric patient. Infants and children can maintain a normal blood pressure until more than half their blood volume is gone. By the time their blood pressure drops, they are close to death. Although children in shock tend to compensate longer than do adults, they also get worse faster when their compensatory mechanisms fail.

Common causes of shock in children are listed in the following *You Should Know* box. Indicators of shock can include altered mental status, tachycardia, weak distal pulses, delayed capillary refill time (Figure 32-3), and cool, mottled extremities (Figure 32-4). Suspect shock in an infant or child who is very listless and whose muscle tone appears floppy.

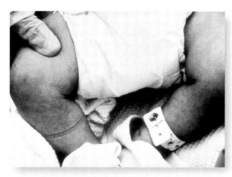
(a)

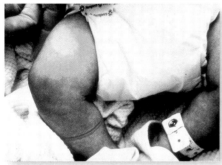
(b)

FIGURE 32-3 ▲ **(a)** Assess capillary refill in children younger than 6 years of age. **(b)** Delayed capillary refill in an infant.

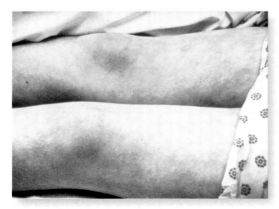

FIGURE 32-4 ▲ Mottled skin in a child.

Common Causes of Shock in Children

- Trauma
- Fluid loss
- Infection
- Anaphylaxis
- Congenital heart disease
- Chest wall injury

Shock in Older Adults

Suspect septic shock in an older adult who is tachycardiac and hypotensive if other causes of shock (such as hemorrhage) are not obvious. Sepsis can occur in older adults due to pneumonia or an infection from an indwelling catheter, among other causes. Fever may or may not be present in septic shock.

Older adults have difficulty tolerating hypotension caused by hemorrhage due, in part, to inefficient blood vessel constriction. In addition, medications that the patient may be taking can prevent the patient's heart rate from increasing, which is the body's normal compensatory response to hemorrhage. For example, the patient may not be tachycardiac if she is taking drugs such as beta-blockers and calcium channel blockers.

When caring for an older adult, keep in mind that opening the airway can be complicated by arthritis of the cervical vertebrae. Look for dentures, and remove them if they are loose or do not fit well. Coughing is often ineffective because of weakened expiratory muscles. An older adult is more likely to have a higher resting respiratory rate, lower tidal volume, and less elasticity and compliance of the chest wall than a younger adult has. In addition, an older adult is likely to have a higher resting heart rate and may have an irregular pulse.

Emergency Care of Shock

Objective 7

To treat a patient in shock, take the following steps:

- Conduct a scene size-up and ensure your safety. Evaluate the mechanism of injury or the nature of the illness before approaching the patient. Put on appropriate PPE.
- Perform a primary survey to identify and treat any life-threatening conditions. Stabilize the cervical spine if needed. Manage the patient's airway and breathing. A patient in shock often has an altered mental status. Many patients are also nauseated and may vomit. Watch the patient closely to make sure his airway remains clear. Suction as needed.

- Give oxygen. If the patient's breathing is adequate, apply oxygen by nonrebreather mask at 10 to 15 L/min if not already done. If the patient's breathing is inadequate, provide positive-pressure ventilation with 100% oxygen and assess the adequacy of the ventilations delivered.

- Control all obvious external bleeding, if present.

- The heart can pump only the blood that it receives. Therefore, there must be an adequate volume of blood in the system and a steady volume of blood returning to the right side of the heart. If you suspect shock, place the patient in the supine position. A woman in late pregnancy should be positioned on her left side instead of on her back. When a woman in late pregnancy is placed on her back, the weight of the fetus compresses major blood vessels, such as the inferior vena cava and aorta. This compression decreases the amount of blood returning to the mother's heart and lowers her blood pressure. Positioning the patient on her left side shifts the weight of her uterus off the abdominal vessels.

- Do not give the patient anything to eat or drink.

- Prevent heat loss by placing blankets under and over the patient. When providing emergency care for older adults, remember that they have less subcutaneous tissue and have diminished shivering and sweating ability, both of which can contribute to hypothermia.

- Perform a physical exam. Take the patient's vital signs, and gather the patient's medical history.

- A patient in shock is a priority patient and needs rapid transport to the closest appropriate hospital. Request the assistance of advanced life support personnel early. Splint any bone or joint injuries en route (see Chapter 37).

- En route to the hospital, comfort, calm, and reassure the patient. Reassess at least every 5 minutes.

- Record all patient care information, including the patient's medical history and the emergency care provided, on a PCR.

On the Scene Wrap-Up

The patient's complaint of abdominal pain, her vital signs, and her rigid, distended abdomen suggest that internal bleeding may be present. Her vital signs and cold, clammy skin are consistent with decompensated shock. Place the patient in a supine position, give 100% oxygen by nonrebreather mask, and begin transport to the closest appropriate facility. En route to the hospital, make the patient as comfortable as possible, provide reassurance, and keep her warm. Reassess at least every 5 minutes. ■

Sum It Up

▶ Perfusion is the circulation of blood through an organ or a part of the body. Shock is the inadequate flow of blood through an organ or a part of the body.

▶ Cardiogenic shock can result if the heart beats too quickly or too slowly or if the heart muscle does not have enough force to pump blood effectively to all parts of the body.

▶ Shock caused by severe bleeding is called hemorrhagic shock. The bleeding may be internal, external, or both. Shock caused by a loss of blood, plasma, or other body fluid is called hypovolemic shock.

▶ Obstructive shock occurs when blood flow is slowed or stopped by a mechanical or physical obstruction. This type of shock may occur when blood collects in the sac surrounding the heart, preventing efficient cardiac contraction, or when air is present in the chest due to a lung injury, putting pressure on the great vessels in the chest and limiting blood flow.

▶ When shock caused by container failure occurs (distributive shock), the blood vessels lose their ability to adjust the flow of blood. Instead of expanding and constricting as needed, the blood vessels remain enlarged. The amount of fluid in the body remains constant (there is no actual loss of fluid), but blood pools in the outer areas of the body. As a result, there is an inadequate amount of blood to fill the enlarged vessels, and the vital organs are not perfused. The four major causes of this type of shock are injury to the spinal cord (neurogenic shock), severe infection (septic shock), severe allergic reaction (anaphylactic shock), and psychological causes (psychogenic shock).

▶ Early (compensated) shock is often difficult to recognize. Remember to look for it and to consider the patient's mechanism of injury or the nature of the illness when assessing your patient. Early shock is usually reversible if it is recognized and the patient receives emergency care to correct the cause of the shock.

▶ Late (decompensated) shock results when the patient's systolic blood pressure drops to less than 90 mm Hg. In this phase of shock, the body's defense mechanisms lose their ability to make up for the lack of oxygenated blood. The signs of late shock are more obvious than those of early shock, but late shock is more difficult to treat.

▶ Irreversible shock is also called terminal shock. You will feel an irregular pulse as the patient's heart becomes irritable and begins to beat irregularly. Permanent damage occurs to the vital organs because the cells and organs have been without oxygenated blood for too long. Eventually, the heart stops, breathing stops, and death results.

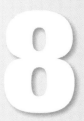

Module 8

Trauma

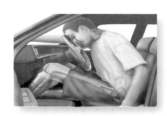

▶ CHAPTER 33

Trauma Overview   547

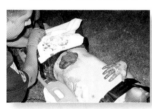

▶ CHAPTER 34

Bleeding and Soft Tissue Trauma   554

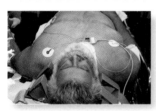

▶ CHAPTER 35   590

Chest Trauma

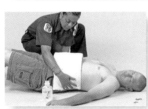

▶ CHAPTER 36

Abdominal and Genitourinary Trauma   605

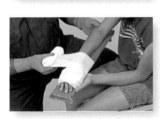

▶ CHAPTER 37

Orthopedic Trauma   612

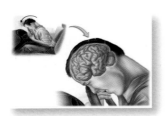

► CHAPTER **38**

Head, Face, Neck, and Spine Trauma   643

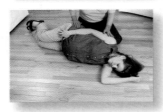

► CHAPTER **39**

Special Considerations in Trauma   683

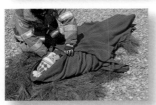

► CHAPTER **40**

Environmental Emergencies   698

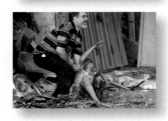

► CHAPTER **41**

Multisystem Trauma   728

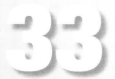
Trauma Overview

By the end of this chapter, you should be able to:

Knowledge Objectives ▶

1. Discuss the reasons for reconsideration of the mechanism of injury.
2. State the reasons for performing a rapid trauma assessment.
3. Recite examples of and explain why patients should receive a rapid trauma assessment.
4. Describe the areas included in the rapid trauma assessment, and discuss what should be evaluated.
5. Discuss the purpose and components of the Revised Trauma Score.
6. Discuss the reason for performing a focused history and physical exam.

Attitude Objective ▶

7. Attend to the feelings that the trauma patient might be experiencing.

Skill Objectives ▶

8. Demonstrate the ability to prioritize patients.
9. Demonstrate the techniques for performing a trauma patient assessment.

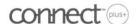

On the Scene

"Respond to a report of possible motor vehicle crash on State Route 40. Be advised, possible involvement of law enforcement officer. Time out: 0210." You and your partner try to ignore the apprehension that you feel as you approach the scene. As you round a curve in the road, you see a sheriff's office vehicle with heavy damage to the right front bumper and "starring" of the windshield on the driver's side just above the hood. You cannot see the officer. You notify dispatch of your arrival on scene and cautiously approach the vehicle as your partner begins to get equipment from the back of your vehicle. ■

THINK ABOUT IT

As you read this chapter, think about the following questions:

- What is the mechanism of injury (MOI) at this scene?
- What does the MOI tell you about the possible injuries that the patient may have suffered?
- What additional resources may be needed in this situation?

Introduction

In this chapter we focus on assessment of the trauma patient, which begins with a scene size-up and evaluation of the mechanism of injury. By evaluating the MOI, you can often predict the types of injuries the patient is most likely to experience. If the MOI is significant, time is of the essence, and you will perform a rapid trauma assessment. If you determine the MOI is not significant, you will perform a focused physical exam. Specific mechanisms of injury were discussed in Chapter 16 and should be reviewed as needed before exploring this chapter.

Remember This

Mechanism of injury is the first important factor when determining whether a trauma patient needs a rapid trauma assessment or a focused physical exam.

Reconsidering the Mechanism of Injury

Objectives 1, 2

At a scene that involves trauma, perform a scene size-up and primary survey, and then reconsider the mechanism of injury. In Chapter 16, we defined *mechanism of injury* as the way in which an injury occurs, as well as the forces involved in producing the injury. Reevaluating the MOI is necessary to rule out the possibility of a more significant MOI than initially suspected or identified during the scene size-up.

Suppose you and your EMT partner are called to the scene of a motor vehicle crash. You arrive to find a 16-year-old male lying on the side of the road. He was the restrained driver of an older model vehicle (no airbags) that struck a bridge abutment at a high rate of speed. There is intrusion of about 12 inches to the front of the vehicle. The steering wheel is bent. The windshield is starred, but not broken. According to bystanders, the patient was initially walking around at the scene and then stumbled and lost consciousness. They estimate he was "out" for about 3 to 5 minutes. Now, the patient is awake and can tell you his name. He is not certain of the place or time. He remembers the crash, but does not remember the loss of consciousness.

This situation involves a significant MOI. Any visible deformity of the steering wheel is an indicator of potentially serious internal injury. The patient needs a rapid trauma assessment. Some injuries may be obvious, while other injuries may be hidden. As you prepare to examine the patient, you must be suspicious of potentially serious internal injuries. This is called having an **index of suspicion.** By evaluating the MOI, you can often predict the types of injuries the patient is most likely to experience.

You Should Know

Hospitals define the age of a pediatric patient in different ways. For example, some hospitals define a pediatric patient as 14 years or younger; others consider a patient less than 16 years of age to be a pediatric patient; and still others consider a pediatric patient to be a person up to the age of 21. From your instructor or EMS agency, find out what the definition of a pediatric patient is in your local area.

Remember This

Factors to Consider in a Motor Vehicle Crash

- Rate of speed
- Seat belt use
- Impact site
- Amount of intrusion
- Airbag deployment
- Vehicle size
- Condition of steering wheel (Figure 33-1)
- Condition of windshield (Figure 33-2)
- Number of passengers in the vehicle
- Position of passengers
- Rollover? Ejection from vehicle?

If the MOI is significant, time is of the essence. It is widely believed that a severely injured patient has the greatest chance of survival if she reaches definitive care within 1 hour of the injury. This is commonly referred to as the **golden hour.** Definitive care for a severely injured trauma patient is surgery. Since the golden hour starts at the time the patient is injured, every action you take ticks away minutes until the patient reaches the operating room. The goal for prehospital trauma care is to limit scene time to 10 minutes. Therefore, your decision regarding the significance of the MOI must be made quickly, using your best judgment. If the MOI is significant, you need to perform a primary survey and follow with a rapid trauma assessment (Figure 33-3). This means that you must move quickly and efficiently, examining the patient from head to toe for obvious and potential injuries. You will also need to consider the need for ALS personnel and immediate transport for all

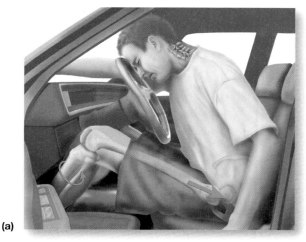

(a)

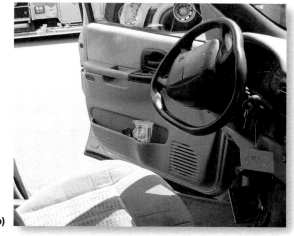

(b)

FIGURE 33-1 ▲ Assessment of steering wheel condition in a motor vehicle crash to discern MOI. **(a)** Injuries from a down-and-under path. **(b)** Bent steering wheel from a down-and-under path.

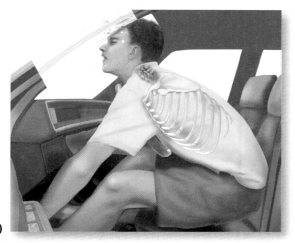

(a)

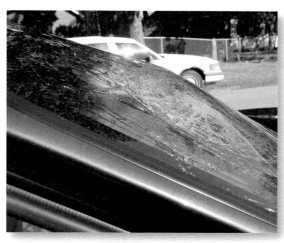

(b)

FIGURE 33-2 ▲ Assessment of windshield condition in an MVC to discern MOI. **(a)** Injuries from an up-and-over path. **(b)** The passenger in this car sustained head, neck, and scalp injuries. Note the indentation of his head in the windshield.

patients who have sustained a significant MOI. EMTs give important emergency care during the golden hour. This care includes making sure the patient has an open airway, giving oxygen, controlling bleeding, and rapidly transporting the patient to the closest appropriate facility.

It is worth noting that some medical professionals question the validity of the golden-hour concept, stating that there is little evidence to either support or refute the concept. However, most medical professionals agree that delays in the definitive care of a trauma patient are undesirable.

If you determine the MOI is not significant, perform a primary survey and then begin the secondary survey with an assessment of the injured body part. This is called a *focused physical exam*. Examine other areas of the body as needed.

Remember This

All healthcare professionals who are involved in trauma care know about the importance of time when caring for a trauma patient. If your trauma patient is a priority patient and your scene time is more than 10 minutes, be prepared to answer questions about your extended scene time to medical personnel at the receiving facility. Sometimes there are logical reasons for an extended scene time. For example, a patient may require special tools and trained personnel before removal from a wrecked vehicle. Or time may be spent trying to convince a patient who initially refuses care to allow treatment and transport. In these situations, it may be helpful to notify medical direction by phone or radio to give them a "heads up" about the delay. Be sure to note the reasons for the delay on your PCR.

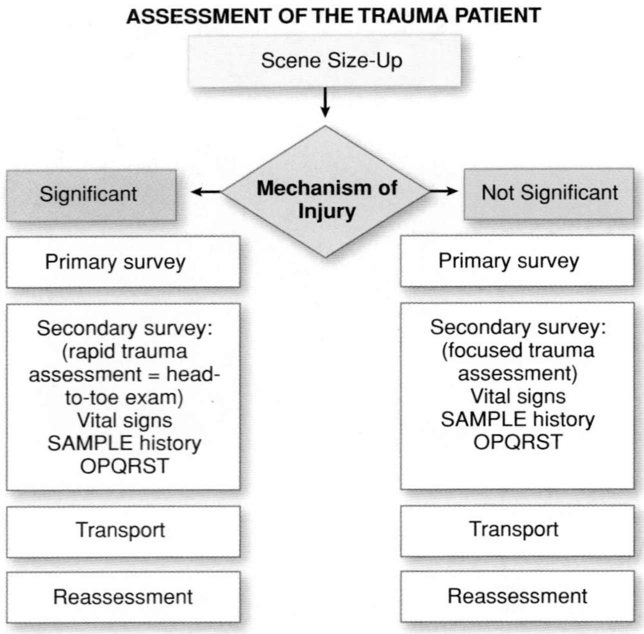

ASSESSMENT OF THE TRAUMA PATIENT

Scene Size-Up

↓

Mechanism of Injury

Significant ← → **Not Significant**

Significant:
- Primary survey
- Secondary survey: (rapid trauma assessment = head-to-toe exam) Vital signs SAMPLE history OPQRST
- Transport
- Reassessment

Not Significant:
- Primary survey
- Secondary survey: (focused trauma assessment) Vital signs SAMPLE history OPQRST
- Transport
- Reassessment

FIGURE 33-3 ▲ Assessment of the trauma patient flowchart.

Making a Difference

Significant Injuries

If the patient has any of the following injuries, transport the patient to a trauma center:

- Penetrating injury to the head, neck, or torso (excluding superficial wounds in which the depth of the wound can be easily determined)
- Penetrating injury to the extremities above the elbow or knee
- Flail chest
- Crushed, degloved, or mangled extremity
- Two or more proximal long bone fractures
- Pelvic fractures
- Open or depressed skull fracture
- Paralysis
- Amputation above the wrist or ankle
- Major burns

Consider transport to a trauma center if the MOI is from any of the following causes:

- Falls
  - —Adult: greater than 20 feet (one story = 10 feet)
  - —Child: greater than 10 feet or 2–3 times the height of the child
- High-risk auto crash
  - —Intrusion of more than 12 inches in occupant site; more than 18 inches at any site
  - —Ejection (partial or complete) from automobile
  - —Death in same passenger compartment

- —Vehicle telemetry data consistent with high risk of injury
- Auto versus pedestrian/bicyclist thrown, run over, or with significant (more than 20 miles per hour) impact
- Motorcycle crash of more than 20 miles per hour

Also consider transport to a trauma center

- Age
  - —Older adults—risk of injury death increases after age 55
  - —Children—should be triaged preferentially to pediatric-capable trauma centers
- Anticoagulation and bleeding disorders
- Burns
  - —Without other trauma mechanism—triage to burn facility
  - —With trauma mechanism—triage to trauma center
- Time-sensitive extremity injury
- End-stage renal disease requiring dialysis
- Pregnancy greater than 20 weeks
- EMS provider judgment

Trauma Patient with Significant Mechanism of Injury

Objectives 2, 3, 4

Rapid Trauma Assessment

A rapid trauma assessment should be performed when:

- A significant MOI exists.
- Additional injuries are suspected.
- A critical injury is found during the focused physical examination.
- A previously stable patient with no significant MOI becomes unstable during the focused physical examination.
- Any emergency intervention has been provided.

Assessment of a trauma patient requires a consistent, organized approach. If a patient has experienced a significant MOI, follow the primary survey with a rapid trauma assessment.

When performing the primary survey, remember that spinal precautions must be initiated as soon as practical, based on the MOI. When assessing the airway of an unresponsive trauma patient, open the airway using a jaw thrust. Clear the airway with suction as needed. Assess ventilation, and administer high-concentration oxygen. Check the thorax and neck. Feel for a deviated trachea, neck and chest crepitation, multiple broken ribs, or a fractured sternum. Listen for breath sounds, and assess for signs and symptoms of a tension pneumothorax. Look for jugular venous distention and chest wounds, and assess chest wall motion. Assess circulation, and look for obvious bleeding. Note the presence or absence of radial and carotid pulses. Apply pressure to sites of external bleeding. Perform a brief neurological exam, and assess pupil size and reactivity. Expose the patient, logrolling him as necessary, to examine for further injuries.

Because life-threatening injuries should have been identified during the primary survey, a **rapid trauma assessment** is a head-to-toe exam performed to detect the presence of additional injuries. If you found life-threatening injuries in the primary survey, it is possible that you may never get to perform the rapid trauma assessment. In situations like this, ask another EMT to perform a rapid trauma assessment while you manage the life-threatening injuries already identified.

You Should Know

Performing a Rapid Trauma Assessment

- Begin the rapid trauma assessment by reassessing the patient's mental status and using the Glasgow Coma Scale (see Table 33-1).
- Assess the patient's head.
- Then examine the neck, chest, abdomen, pelvis, lower extremities, upper extremities, and the back.
- Compare one side of the body to the other. For example, if an injury involves one side of the body, use the uninjured side as the normal finding for comparison.

TABLE 33-1 Revised Trauma Score

	Value	Points	Score
Systolic blood pressure	>89 mm Hg	4	
	76–89 mm Hg	3	
	50–75 mm Hg	2	A _____
	1–49 mm Hg	1	
	0 mm Hg	0	
Respiratory rate	10–29 per minute	4	
	>29 per minute	3	
	6–9 per minute	2	B _____
	1–5 per minute	1	
	0 spontaneous per minute	0	
Glasgow Coma Scale *Eye opening* Spontaneous: 4 To voice: 3 To pain: 2 None: 1 *Verbal response* Oriented: 5 Confused: 4 Inappropriate words: 3 Incomprehensible words: 2 None: 1 *Motor response* Obeys commands: 6 Purposeful movement (pain): 5 Withdraw: 4 Flexion: 3 Extension: 2 None: 1	(Total GCS points) 13–15 9–12 6–8 4–5 3	 4 3 2 1 0	C _____
		Trauma score	**(A + B + C)**

Although the steps for performing a rapid trauma assessment are presented in this chapter in a specific order, keep in mind that some tasks are usually performed simultaneously. For example, your partner may be taking the patient's vital signs and obtaining the medical history while you perform the physical exam. If you find a serious injury, treat it when you find it. If the patient's condition worsens during the physical exam, go back and repeat the primary survey.

Remember This

If the patient is unstable, a rapid trauma assessment should be done en route to the hospital.

Revised Trauma Score

Objective 5

The **Revised Trauma Score (RTS)** is a scoring system used to predict the likelihood of serious injury or death following trauma. It is calculated from a combination of results from three categories: respiratory rate, systolic blood pressure, and Glasgow Coma Scale. The lower the RTS, the higher the risk for the trauma patient. The RTS is scored from the first set of data obtained on the patient and repeated to show trends in the patient's condition. If the RTS is used in your area, remember to relay (and document) this important information when transferring patient care to ALS personnel arriving on the scene or to the staff at the receiving facility.

Transport of the Priority Trauma Patient

If the patient's physical exam findings and MOI (and other factors) indicate you have a priority patient, determine the timeliest method to get the patient to definitive care. To make the best decision for your patient, you will need to consider the distance to the nearest trauma center, availability of ground versus air ambulances, time of day (traffic conditions), and weather. Contact the receiving facility as soon as possible so its personnel can prepare for the patient's arrival. Let them know the patient's condition, the treatment you have given, the patient's estimated time of arrival, and the patient's revised trauma score. Be sure to notify the receiving facility of significant changes in the patient's condition while she is in your care.

Trauma Patient with No Significant Mechanism of Injury

Objective 6

If a trauma patient has no significant MOI, perform a **focused physical examination.** A focused physical exam performed on an injured patient is also called a **focused trauma assessment.** The focused physical examination concentrates on the specific injury site (and related structures) based on what the patient states is wrong and your suspicions based on the MOI and primary survey findings. For example, if your patient presents with a possible fracture of the lower arm, you will assess the injured area. You will also assess pulses, movement, and sensation distal to the injury. A focused physical examination also identifies other injuries that could be life-threatening if not cared for quickly.

Assess the injured area for DCAP-BTLS. Be sure to assess for a pulse, movement, and sensation if the injured area involves an extremity. After completion of the focused physical exam, assess vital signs, and obtain a SAMPLE history. Provide emergency care based on the type and severity of the injury. If the patient's injury requires further care, prepare the patient for transport to the most appropriate facility.

You Should Know

Focused History and Physical Examination

Components:
- Focused physical examination
- Baseline vital signs
- SAMPLE history

The focused physical exam is based on:
- Patient's chief complaint
- MOI (such as a cut finger or a swollen ankle)
- Primary survey findings

Making a Difference

If the patient appeared stable at the end of the primary survey but becomes unstable during the secondary survey, expedite patient transport to the closest appropriate medical facility.

On the Scene Wrap-Up

Recognizing that you need additional resources for patient extrication, you immediately contact dispatch and request appropriate personnel to the scene. The "starring" of the windshield increases your awareness of the potential for head, neck, and spinal injuries and is an indicator of the speed of the vehicle before the collision. You prepare for full spinal stabilization before you even access the patient. Resources needed at the scene may change based on what is found when actual contact is made with the patient, and may also change based on the resources in the area (such as advanced life support personnel and helicopter availability). The scene itself may need such additional resources as traffic control. ∎

▶ At a scene that involves trauma, perform a scene size-up and primary survey and then reconsider the mechanism of injury. Mechanism of injury is the way in which an injury occurs, as well as the forces involved in producing the injury. By evaluating the MOI, you can often predict the types of injuries the patient is most likely to experience.

▶ If the MOI is significant, time is of the essence. If a patient has experienced a significant MOI, follow the primary survey with a rapid trauma assessment. Begin the rapid trauma assessment by reassessing the patient's mental status and then checking the patient's head. Then examine the neck, chest, abdomen, pelvis, lower extremities, upper extremities, and the back. Compare one side of the body to the other. For example, if an injury involves one side of the body, use the uninjured side as the normal finding for comparison.

▶ The Revised Trauma Score is a scoring system used to predict the likelihood of serious injury or death following trauma. It is calculated from a combination of results from three categories: respiratory rate, systolic blood pressure, and Glasgow Coma Scale. The RTS is scored from the first set of data obtained on the patient and repeated to show trends in the patient's condition.

▶ If a trauma patient has no significant MOI, perform a focused physical examination. The focused physical exam concentrates on the specific injury site (and related structures) based on what the patient states is wrong and your suspicions based on the MOI and initial assessment findings.

By the end of this chapter, you should be able to:

Knowledge Objectives ▶

1. State the major functions of the skin.
2. List the layers of the skin.
3. Define wound, and differentiate between an open and closed wound.
4. Differentiate among arterial, venous, and capillary bleeding.
5. Establish the relationship between standard precautions and bleeding and soft tissue injuries.
6. Describe methods of controlling external bleeding.
7. Establish the relationship between mechanism of injury and internal bleeding.
8. List the signs of internal bleeding.
9. List the steps in the emergency medical care of the patient with signs and symptoms of internal bleeding.
10. Differentiate between open and closed soft tissue injuries.
11. List the types of closed soft tissue injuries.
12. Discuss the possible causes, signs, and symptoms of compartment syndrome and crush syndrome.
13. Describe the emergency care of the patient with a closed soft tissue injury.
14. State the types of open soft tissue injuries.
15. Describe the emergency medical care of the patient with an open soft tissue injury.
16. Discuss the emergency medical care considerations for a patient with a penetrating chest injury.
17. Describe the emergency medical care of the patient with an evisceration.
18. Describe the emergency medical care of the patient with an impaled object.
19. Describe the emergency medical care of the patient with an amputation.
20. Describe the emergency medical care of the patient with an open neck injury.
21. Describe the emergency medical care of the patient with an eye injury.
22. Describe the emergency medical care of the patient with a mouth injury.
23. Describe the emergency medical care of the patient with an ear laceration.
24. Identify factors that determine the severity of a burn.
25. List the classifications of burns.
26. Define superficial burn.
27. List the characteristics of a superficial burn.
28. Define partial-thickness burn.
29. List the characteristics of a partial-thickness burn.

30. Define full-thickness burn.

31. List the characteristics of a full-thickness burn.

32. Discuss the use of the rule of nines to estimate the total body surface area burned.

33. Describe the emergency medical care of the patient with a superficial burn.

34. Describe the emergency medical care of the patient with a partial-thickness burn.

35. Describe the emergency medical care of the patient with a full-thickness burn.

36. Describe the emergency care for a chemical burn.

37. Describe the emergency care for an electrical burn.

38. List the functions of dressing and bandaging.

39. Describe the purpose of a bandage.

40. Describe the steps in applying a pressure dressing.

Attitude Objective ▷ 41. Attend to the feelings that the patient with bleeding or soft tissue trauma might be experiencing.

Skill Objectives ▷ 42. Demonstrate the care of the patient with assessment findings and symptoms of external bleeding.

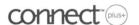

43. Demonstrate the care of the patient with assessment findings and symptoms of internal bleeding.

44. Demonstrate the care of closed soft tissue injuries.

45. Demonstrate the care of open soft tissue injuries.

46. Demonstrate the care of a patient with an open chest wound.

47. Demonstrate the care of a patient with an open abdominal wound.

48. Demonstrate the care of a patient with an impaled object.

49. Demonstrate the care of a patient with an amputation.

50. Demonstrate the care of an amputated part.

51. Demonstrate the care of a patient with superficial burns.

52. Demonstrate the care of a patient with partial-thickness burns.

53. Demonstrate the care of a patient with full-thickness burns.

54. Demonstrate the steps in the emergency medical care of a patient with a chemical burn.

55. Demonstrate completing a prehospital care report for patients with bleeding or soft tissue trauma.

On the Scene

The call went out: "House fire, people trapped." You can see the dark smoke curling up over the hill before you even arrive on the scene. You are on the third unit arriving at the fire; the nearest ambulance will be another 20 minutes. Pulling an elderly man behind him, a firefighter crawls out through the gray smoke belching out of the front door. The incident commander tells you to take the patient. His clothes are smoldering slightly so you roll him on the ground and then quickly remove them. The patient moans as you douse his obvious burns with a bottle of water from your truck. "Call for a helicopter," you order, knowing that he will need to be taken to a burn center. As you apply oxygen, you assess him and can see that he has blistered burns over his face and singed eyebrows. The front of his chest and abdomen are covered with burns. Some burns are yellow, others are waxy white, and scattered charred areas are present. His right arm is burned completely around. ■

As you read this chapter, think about the following questions:

- What depth of burns does this patient have?
- How can you calculate the percentage of his body that has been burned?
- Is there any evidence that he has an inhalation injury?
- Why will he need the specialized resources of a burn center?
- What additional assessment and care will you need to perform?

Introduction

Traumatic injuries and bleeding are some of the most dramatic situations you will encounter. Understanding the mechanism of injury and relevant signs and symptoms of bleeding and shock is important when dealing with the traumatized patient. Your first steps will be to perform a scene size-up and make sure the scene is safe. After assessing and managing the patient's airway and breathing, you must control bleeding from an artery or vein, if it is present. Bleeding that is uncontrolled or excessive will lead to shock.

Soft tissues are the layers of the skin and the fat and muscle beneath them. Soft tissue injuries range from bruises, cuts, and scrapes to amputations and full-thickness burns. Although soft tissue injuries are common and daunting to look at, they are rarely life-threatening. You must be able to recognize the different types of soft tissue injuries and give appropriate emergency care. This care includes controlling bleeding, preventing further injury, and reducing contamination.

Anatomy Review

Functions of the Skin

Objective 1

The skin is the body's largest organ and its first line of defense against bacteria and other organisms, ultraviolet rays from the sun, harmful chemicals, and cuts and tears. The skin is the site where vitamin D is produced. Sweat glands in the skin excrete excess water and some wastes. Remember that the skin has the following functions:

- Helps regulate body temperature
- Senses heat, cold, touch, pressure, and pain
- Helps maintain fluid balance
- Protects underlying tissues from injury

When the skin surface is disrupted, many of these functions are affected. The body loses fluid, and the skin becomes less effective in helping maintain body temperature. Because the skin surface is no longer intact, the body is at an increased risk of infection.

Layers of the Skin

Objective 2

The epidermis is the outermost skin layer and consists of four or five layers. New cells are continuously formed in the deeper layers of the epidermis. Older cells are pushed upward and sloughed off. The epidermis contains keratin, a waterproofing protein. The dermis is the deeper and thicker layer of skin containing sweat and sebaceous glands, hair follicles, blood vessels, and nerve endings. The subcutaneous (fatty) layer helps conserve body heat. Fat can be used as an energy source when adequate food is not available. Accessory structures of the skin include the hair, nails, sweat glands, and oil (sebaceous) glands. Refer to Figure 6-32 in Chapter 6, "The Human Body."

Bleeding

Objective 3

A **wound** is an injury to the soft tissues. A **closed wound** occurs when the soft tissues under the skin are damaged but the surface of the skin is not broken. A bruise is an example of a closed wound. When the skin surface is broken, the injury is called an **open wound.** Cuts and scrapes are examples of open wounds.

If a blood vessel is torn or cut, bleeding occurs. Bleeding can occur from capillaries, veins, or arteries. The larger the blood vessel, the more fluid flows through it. Therefore, the bleeding and blood loss is greater if a larger vessel is injured. **Hemorrhage** (major bleeding) is an extreme loss of blood from a blood vessel. It is a life-threatening condition that requires *immediate* attention. Hemorrhage may be internal or external. If it is not controlled, hemorrhage can lead to shock and, possibly, to death.

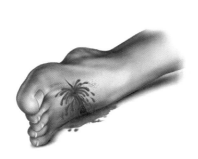 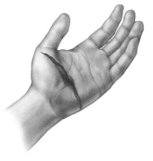 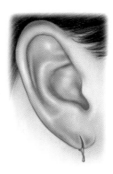

| Arterial bleeding | Venous bleeding | Capillary bleeding |

FIGURE 34-1 ▲ Types of bleeding.

When a blood vessel is cut or torn, the body's normal response is an immediate contraction (spasm) of the wall of the blood vessel. This action slows the flow of blood from the injured vessel by reducing the size of the hole. Next, platelets rush to the area to plug the torn vessel. Layers upon layers of platelets stick to each other like glue to fill the hole. Usually within seconds of the injury, a clot begins to form at the site of the torn vessel. This process is activated by substances from the wall of the injured vessel and from the platelets at the injury site. Clotting is usually complete within 6 to 10 minutes.

Some conditions may affect blood clotting. For example, **hemophilia** is a disorder in which the blood does not clot normally. A person with hemophilia may have major bleeding from minor injuries and may bleed for no apparent reason. Some medications, such as aspirin and Coumadin (a blood thinner), can interfere with blood clotting. A serious injury may also prevent effective clotting.

Types of Bleeding

Objective 4

The three types of bleeding are arterial, venous, and capillary (Figure 34-1). The characteristics of these types of bleeding are noted in Table 34-1.

Arterial Bleeding

Arterial bleeding is the most serious type of bleeding. The blood from an artery is bright red, oxygen-rich blood. When an artery bleeds, blood spurts from the wound because the arteries are under high pressure. Each spurt represents a heartbeat. Because a bleeding artery can quickly lead to the loss of a large amount of blood, arterial bleeding is life-threatening. This type of bleeding can be difficult to control because of high pressure within the artery.

Venous Bleeding

Bleeding occurs more often from veins than from arteries because veins are closer to the skin's surface. Blood lost from a vein flows as a steady stream and is dark red or maroon because it is oxygen-poor blood. Venous bleeding is usually easier to control than arterial bleeding because it is under less pressure. Bleeding from deep veins (such as those in the thigh) can cause major bleeding that is hard to control. Bleeding from a vein is more serious than capillary bleeding.

Capillary Bleeding

Capillary bleeding is common because the walls of the capillaries are fragile and many are close to the skin's surface. When a capillary is torn, blood oozes slowly

	Arterial	**Venous**	**Capillary**
Color	Bright red	Dark red, maroon	Dark red
Blood Flow	Spurts with each heartbeat	Flows steadily	Oozes slowly
Bleeding control	Difficult to control	Usually easier to control than arterial bleeding; bleeding from deep veins may be hard to control	Often clots and stops by itself within a few minutes

TABLE 34-1 Types of Bleeding

from the site of the injury because the pressure within the capillaries is low. Bleeding from capillaries is usually dark red. Capillary bleeding is usually not serious. This type of bleeding often clots and stops by itself within a few minutes.

External Bleeding

External bleeding is bleeding that you can see. You can see this type of bleeding because the blood flows through an open wound, such as a cut, scrape, or puncture. Capillary bleeding is the most common type of external bleeding. Clotting normally occurs within minutes. However, external bleeding must be controlled with your gloved hands and dressings until a clot is formed and the bleeding has stopped.

Remember This

External bleeding may be hidden by clothing.

Emergency Care for External Bleeding

Objectives 5, 6

When you arrive at the scene of an emergency, first consider your personal safety. During the scene size-up, evaluate the mechanism of injury or the nature of the illness before approaching the patient. Personal protective equipment *must* be worn when an exposure to blood or other potentially infectious material can be reasonably anticipated. HIV and the hepatitis virus are examples of diseases to which you may be exposed that can be transmitted by exposure to blood. Remember to put on disposable gloves before physical contact with the patient. Additional PPE, such as eye protection, mask, and gown, should be worn if there is a large amount of blood. PPE should also be worn when the splashing of blood or body fluids into your face or eyes is likely.

After the scene size-up, perform a primary survey. Bleeding may be obvious when you approach the patient. However, remember that making sure the patient has an open airway and adequate breathing takes priority over other care. Stabilize the cervical spine if

Stop and Think!

- *Never* touch blood or body fluids with your bare hands.
- *Always* wear PPE during *every* patient contact.
- If your hands are visibly dirty or soiled with blood or other body fluids, wash your hands with soap and water.
- Use an alcohol-based hand gel if no visible soil or blood is noted after removing gloves.
- Remember to throw away contaminated gloves and other PPE in clearly labeled biohazard bags or containers.
- Report all exposures to your supervisor or risk management department immediately.

needed. During your assessment of the patient's circulation, look for the presence of major (severe) bleeding. If it is present, you will need to control it during the primary survey.

If the patient is bleeding, keep in mind that the sight of blood is frightening for many patients. Conduct your examination professionally and efficiently. Remember to talk with your patient while you are providing care. Because clothing can hide and absorb large amounts of blood, cut or remove your patient's clothing as needed to see where the bleeding is coming from. Remember that your patient will often be anxious about having his clothing removed and having an exam performed by a stranger. Ease your patient's fears by explaining what you are doing and why it must be done. As you remove the patient's clothing, remember to properly drape or shield him from view of others not providing care.

An average adult man has a normal blood volume of about 5 to 6 L (5,000 to 6,000 mL). In a previously healthy patient, a sudden episode of blood loss will usually not produce vital sign changes until the patient has lost 15% to 30% of his blood volume (Table 34-2). Therefore, estimate the severity of blood loss on the

TABLE 34-2	Measures of Severe Blood Loss	
Patient Type	**Normal Blood Volume**	**Severe Blood Loss**
Adult	5,000-6,000 mL	1,000 mL or more
Child (8-year-old)	2,000 mL	500 mL or more
Infant	800 mL	100-200 mL or more

TABLE 34-3 Possible Assessment Findings and Symptoms for Hemorrhagic Shock

Assessment Finding/Symptom	Class of Hemorrhagic Shock			
	Class I	Class II	Class III	Class IV
Estimated blood loss in milliliters	Up to 750	750 to 1,500	1,500 to 2,000	2,000 or more
Estimated percentage of total blood volume	Up to 15%	15–30%	30–40%	40% or more
Mental status	Slightly anxious	Mildly anxious	Anxious, confused	Confused, slow to respond
Ventilatory rate	Within normal limits	20–30 breaths/min	30–40 breaths/min	More than 35 breaths/min
Heart rate	Within normal limits or slightly increased	100–120 beats/min	120–140 beats/min	140 beats/min or more
Systolic blood pressure	Within normal limits	Within normal limits	Decreased	Markedly decreased
Pulse pressure	Within normal limits or increased	Decreased	Decreased	Decreased

Source: Adapted from *Advanced Trauma Life Support for Doctors: ATLS Student Course Manual,* 8th edition. Chicago: American College of Surgeons Committee on Trauma, 2008, Table 3–2, p. 61.

basis of the patient's signs and symptoms. If the patient shows signs and symptoms of shock, consider the bleeding severe. Table 34-3 shows possible patient assessment findings and symptoms for various stages of hemorrhagic shock.

Control bleeding by using direct pressure, splints, or a tourniquet. If bleeding is severe and breathing is adequate, give oxygen by nonrebreather mask. If signs of shock are present, treat the patient for shock. After completing the primary survey, decide whether the patient needs on-scene stabilization or immediate transport with additional emergency care en route to a hospital.

Making a Difference

Although covering a bleeding wound is important for any patient, it is especially important if your patient is a young child. A young child may fear that "all of my blood will leak out" if the wound is not covered quickly.

Controlling External Bleeding

Three methods may be used to control external bleeding:

1. Applying direct pressure to the wound
2. Applying a splint
3. Applying a tourniquet (if the bleeding is severe and cannot be controlled with direct pressure)

Direct Pressure

To control external bleeding, begin by applying **direct pressure** to the bleeding site. Most bleeding can be controlled with direct pressure. Applying direct pressure slows blood flow and allows clotting to take place. Place a sterile **dressing** (such as a gauze pad) or a clean cloth (such as a towel or washcloth) over the wound. If you do not have a dressing or clean cloth available, use your gloved hand to apply firm pressure to the bleeding site until a dressing can be applied (Figure 34-2).

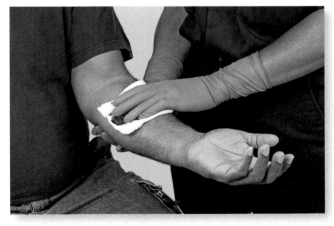

FIGURE 34-2 ▲ Apply direct pressure to a bleeding wound.

Use your gloved fingertips if the bleeding site is small. If the patient has a large, open wound, you may need to apply direct pressure to the site with the palm of your gloved hand. Hold continuous, firm pressure to the bleeding site while the body works to plug the wound with a clot. If the bleeding does not stop within 10 minutes, press more firmly over a wider area.

If the bleeding site is on an extremity, continue direct pressure by applying a pressure bandage. A **pressure bandage** is a bandage with which enough pressure is applied over a wound site to control bleeding. Wrap roller gauze snugly over the dressings to hold them in place on the wound (Figure 34-3). Make sure that the pressure bandage is not so tight that it impedes blood flow past the dressings. For example, if you applied a pressure bandage to a wound on a patient's lower arm, you should be able to feel a pulse at his wrist if the bandage has been applied properly.

Remember This

A pressure bandage that is wrapped too loosely will not be effective in controlling bleeding. A bandage that is applied too tightly can cause tissue damage.

If blood soaks through the dressings, do not remove them. Removing the original dressings could disturb any blood clots that may be forming and cause more bleeding. Add another dressing on top of the first, and continue to apply direct pressure.

Stop and Think!

If PPE is not available and you must provide care for a bleeding patient, use whatever materials are readily available to help protect yourself from disease. For example, use a plastic bag, plastic wrap, or other waterproof material to apply direct pressure to the wound. If the patient is able to help you, ask her to apply direct pressure to the wound with her own hand. When you have finished providing care, be sure to wash your hands with soap and water.

Splints

The sharp ends of broken bones can pierce the skin and cause major bleeding. A broken bone that penetrates the skin is called a **compound (open) fracture.** Unless a broken bone is immobilized, the movement of bone ends or bone fragments can damage soft tissues and blood vessels and this results in more bleeding. Dress and bandage the wound, and then

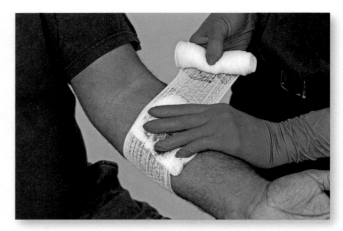

FIGURE 34-3 ▲ Continue direct pressure by applying a pressure bandage.

apply a splint. A **splint** is a device used to limit the movement of an injured arm or leg and reduce bleeding. Dressing and bandaging are discussed in more detail later in this chapter.

A **pressure splint** (also called an *air* or *pneumatic splint*) may help control bleeding associated with soft tissue injuries or broken bones. It can also help stabilize a broken bone. An air splint acts as a pressure bandage, applying even pressure to the entire arm or leg (Figure 34-4). Dress and bandage the wound before applying an air splint. After applying any splint, be sure to check the patient's fingers (or toes) often for color, warmth, and feeling. Direct pressure can be applied with an air splint in place. This may be necessary to control arterial bleeding from an arm or leg. Use a pressure splint only if approved by your local protocol.

The **pneumatic antishock garment (PASG)** is used in some Emergency Medical Services systems. This garment is also called *military antishock trousers (MAST)*. If approved by your local protocol, this device can be used as a pressure splint to help control suspected severe bleeding in the abdomen or pelvis that is

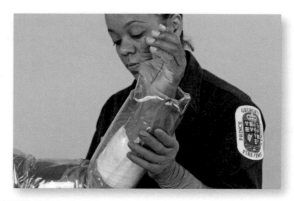

FIGURE 34-4 ▲ An air splint acts as a pressure bandage, applying even pressure to the entire arm or leg.

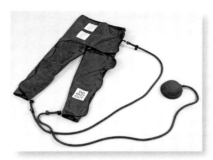

FIGURE 34-5 ▲ The pneumatic antishock garment (PASG).

accompanied by hypotension (Figure 34-5). The PASG has three separate compartments that can be inflated: the abdomen, left leg, and right leg. All three compartments are inflated if there is an injury to the abdomen or pelvis. The abdominal compartment is *never* used without inflating both leg compartments. When the PASG is positioned on the patient, the top edge of the garment must be below the patient's lowest ribs. If the garment is positioned higher on the patient, the pressure caused by inflating the abdominal compartment could hamper the patient's breathing. The PASG is contraindicated in the following situations:

- Pulmonary edema
- Pregnancy
- Traumatic cardiac arrest
- Impaled objects in the abdomen
- Protruding abdominal organs
- Penetrating chest trauma
- Splinting of lower-extremity fractures

Tourniquets

A **tourniquet** is a tight bandage that surrounds an arm or a leg. It is used to stop the flow of blood in an extremity. It may be considered when direct pressure has failed to control hemorrhage.

Stop and Think!

When you apply a tourniquet, you stop arterial and venous blood flow to the affected extremity. Be absolutely sure that you are authorized to apply a tourniquet per local protocol and have exhausted all other methods of bleeding control before considering the use of a tourniquet.

To apply a tourniquet, use the following steps:
- Use a bandage at least 4 inches wide and six to eight layers deep.

- Wrap the bandage around the extremity twice. Choose an area above the bleeding but as close to the wound as possible (Figure 34-6a).
- Tie a single knot in the bandage, and place a stick or rod on top of the knot (Figure 34-6b).
- Tie the ends of the bandage over the stick in a square knot. Twist the stick until the bleeding stops (Figure 34-6c). Note the exact time the tourniquet is applied.
- After the bleeding has stopped, secure the stick or rod in place.
- Write the initials *TK*, for tourniquet, on a piece of adhesive tape and the time the tourniquet was applied. Place the adhesive tape on the patient's forehead. The information must be clearly visible to all who provide care to the patient (Figure 34-6d).
- When transferring patient care, be sure to notify the receiving personnel that you have applied a tourniquet.

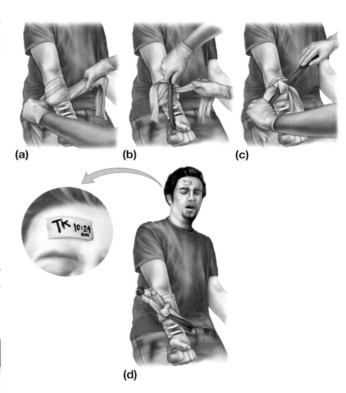

(a)   (b)   (c)

(d)

FIGURE 34-6 ▲ (a) To apply a tourniquet, use a bandage at least 4 inches wide and six to eight layers deep. Wrap the bandage around the extremity twice. Choose an area above the bleeding but as close to the wound as possible. (b) Tie a single knot in the bandage, and place a stick or rod on top of the knot. (c) Tie the ends of the bandage over the stick in a square knot. Twist the stick until the bleeding stops. Note the exact time the tourniquet is applied. (d) Write TK and the time the tourniquet was applied on a piece of adhesive tape. Place the adhesive tape on the patient's forehead.

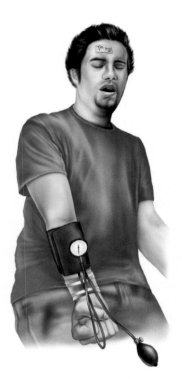

FIGURE 34-7 ▲ A blood pressure cuff may be used as a tourniquet.

Remember This

A blood pressure cuff may be used as a tourniquet, if approved by your local protocol. Place the cuff above the bleeding area. Inflate the cuff just enough to stop the bleeding (Figure 34-7). Check the gauge on the cuff often to make sure there is no drop in pressure in the cuff.

You Should Know

Precautions for Tourniquet Use

Whenever you apply a tourniquet, make sure to take the following precautions:

- Always use a wide bandage. Never use wire, rope, a belt, or any other material that may cut into the skin and underlying tissue.
- Do not remove or loosen the tourniquet once it is applied unless you are directed to do so by a physician.
- Leave the tourniquet in open view so that it is readily seen by others. Do not cover the tourniquet with a bandage, a sheet, or the patient's clothing.
- Never apply a tourniquet directly over a joint. Place the tourniquet as close to the injury as possible.

Internal Bleeding

Objective 7

The body contains hollow and solid organs. Hollow abdominal organs include the stomach, intestines, gallbladder, and urinary bladder. When hollow abdominal organs rupture, they empty their contents into the abdominal cavity. This rupture irritates the abdominal lining and causes pain. Solid abdominal organs include the liver, spleen, and kidneys. These organs are protected by bony structures and do not move around much. Solid organs bleed when injured and can result in a large amount of blood loss. **Internal bleeding** is bleeding that occurs inside body tissues and cavities. It can result in blood loss severe enough to cause shock and death. A **bruise** is a collection of blood under the skin caused by bleeding capillaries. A bruise is an example of internal bleeding that is not life-threatening.

Internal bleeding may result from blunt or penetrating trauma. It can also be caused by medical conditions, such as an ulcer. The two most common causes of internal bleeding are (1) injured or damaged internal organs and (2) fractures, especially fractures of the femur and pelvis. Internal bleeding may occur in any body cavity. However, major bleeding is most likely to occur in the abdominal cavity, chest cavity, digestive tract, or the tissues surrounding broken bones. An injury to the liver or spleen can result in a loss of massive amounts of blood into the abdominal cavity in a short time. A fracture of a long bone can result in a loss of 500–2,000 mL of blood into the surrounding tissues. For example, a femur fracture can produce a blood loss of 1,000–2,000 mL. The only signs of internal bleeding may be localized swelling and bruising.

Internal bleeding can cause blood to pool in a body cavity. This buildup of blood can cause pressure on vital organs. For example, a stab wound to the chest may hit a chamber of the heart. If bleeding escapes from the heart's chamber into the sac around the heart (the pericardial sac), the heart's ability to pump decreases. As blood fills the sac, the pressure in the sac increases and does not allow the heart muscle to expand during relaxation. If a blood vessel in the chest is torn, as much as 1,500 mL of blood can build up in the pleural cavity of each lung. Breathing may be compromised as the blood builds up, crushing the air-filled lung.

Emergency Care for Internal Bleeding

Objectives 8, 9

Internal bleeding is difficult to assess because you cannot see it. However, you should suspect it when the mechanism of injury or the nature of the illness, as well as your patient's signs and symptoms, indicates that it is likely. Suspect internal bleeding when the mechanism

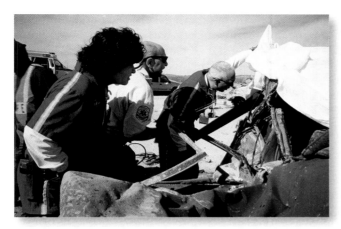

FIGURE 34-8 ▲ When the mechanism of injury suggests that the patient's body was affected by severe force, suspect internal bleeding.

of injury suggests that the patient's body was affected by severe force (Figure 34-8). Examples include penetrating trauma and blunt trauma, such as falls, motorcycle crashes, pedestrian impacts, automobile collisions, and blast injuries.

Trauma is a common cause of internal bleeding. Internal bleeding may also occur in patients with medical emergencies. For example, it may occur because of a problem in the digestive tract, such as an ulcer. A patient with bleeding in the digestive tract may vomit blood or have bloody diarrhea. A patient with bleeding in the urinary tract may have blood in his urine.

Depending on the amount of bleeding, the signs and symptoms of internal bleeding may develop quickly or may take hours or days to develop. Signs and symptoms of internal bleeding are listed in the following *You Should Know* box.

To provide emergency care to a patient with the signs and symptoms of internal bleeding, take the following steps:

- Conduct a scene size-up and ensure your safety. Evaluate the mechanism of injury or the nature of the illness before approaching the patient. Put on appropriate PPE.
- Perform a primary survey to identify and treat any life-threatening conditions. Manage the patient's airway and breathing. Stabilize the cervical spine if needed.
- Perform a physical examination. Identify the signs and symptoms of internal bleeding. Take the patient's vital signs, gather the patient's medical history, and document the information.
- Give oxygen. If the patient's breathing is adequate, apply oxygen by nonrebreather mask at 10 to 15 L/min if not already done. If the patient's breathing is inadequate, provide positive-pressure ventilation with 100% oxygen. Assess the adequacy of the ventilations delivered.
- A patient with internal bleeding may vomit. Watch the patient closely to make sure the airway remains clear. Make sure that you have suction within arm's reach at all times. Suction as needed.
- A patient with internal bleeding is a priority patient and needs rapid transport to the closest appropriate hospital. En route to the hospital, make the patient as comfortable as possible, provide reassurance, and keep her warm. Reassess at least every 5 minutes. Treat the patient for shock if signs of shock develop.
- Record all patient care information, including the patient's medical history and the emergency care provided, on a PCR.

Stop and Think!

Never give a patient who may have internal bleeding or who may be in shock anything to eat or drink. The patient may need surgery and should not have anything in the stomach.

Soft Tissue Injuries

Objective 10

Soft tissue injuries damage the layers of the skin and the fat and muscle beneath them. The skin can be damaged by sharp or blunt objects, falls, or impacts with motionless objects. Chemicals, radiation, electricity, and extreme hot or cold temperatures can also cause injury to the skin.

Soft tissue injuries may be open or closed. A soft tissue injury that is associated with a break in the skin surface is an open wound. A closed wound is one in which the skin surface remains intact. The signs of a soft tissue injury are usually obvious. Do not allow the appearance of a soft tissue injury to distract you from performing a primary survey and treating any life-threatening injuries. These injuries may be imposing to look at. However, you must remember that soft tissue injuries are usually not the patient's most serious injuries—unless they compromise the airway or are associated with severe bleeding. Because of the risk of exposure to blood and body fluids, personal protective equipment must always be worn when dealing with soft tissue injuries.

Closed Wounds

Objective 11

A **closed soft tissue injury** occurs when the body is struck by a blunt object. There is no break in the skin, but the tissues and vessels beneath the skin surface are crushed or ruptured. Because there is no break in the skin, there is no external bleeding.

When assessing a closed wound, look carefully at the surface damage on the patient's skin and consider the mechanism of injury. With your knowledge of anatomy and how the injury occurred, try to visualize the possible damage to the organs and blood vessels beneath the area that was struck. For example, injuries to the upper abdomen can injure the liver, spleen, or pancreas. An injury to the lower abdomen can injure the bladder. An injury to the middle of the back can damage the kidneys. An injury to the neck can damage large blood vessels, the windpipe (trachea), and the spinal cord.

A contusion (bruise) is the most common type of closed wound (Figure 34-9). A contusion results when

an area of the body experiences blunt trauma. In blunt trauma, a forceful impact occurs to the body, but there is no break in the skin. Examples of blunt force include a kick, fall, or blow. The outer skin layer, the epidermis, remains intact. However, the tissue layers and small blood vessels beneath it are damaged. The blunt force causes a small amount of internal bleeding in the area that was struck. Swelling, pain, and discoloration of the skin (ecchymosis) occur as blood leaks from the torn vessels into the surrounding tissue. At first, a contusion usually appears as a red area or as tiny red dots or splotches on the skin. The color changes to purple or blue within 2 to 5 days. After 5 to 10 days, the color changes to green and then yellow. It becomes brownish-yellow in color 10 to 14 days after the injury and then gradually disappears. Most contusions heal and disappear within 2 to 3 weeks.

You Should Know

Knowing the "age" of bruises can be important if you suspect abuse. Does the age of the bruises match the story about the person's injuries? If not, make sure to pass that information along to appropriate personnel when transferring patient care.

If large blood vessels are torn beneath a bruised (contused) area, a **hematoma** forms (see Figure 34-9). A hematoma is a localized collection of blood beneath the skin caused by a tear in a blood vessel. Hematomas often occur with trauma of enough force to break bones. Although similar to a contusion, a hematoma involves a larger amount of tissue damage. The patient may lose 1 or more liters of blood under the skin.

Crush injuries are caused by a compressing force applied to the body (see Figure 34-9). Crush injuries are also called *compression injuries*. Crush injuries may be open or closed injuries. An example of a minor crush injury occurs when a hammer strikes a thumb. Localized swelling and bruising are often present. In a severe crush injury, such as a car running over the chest and abdomen of a toddler, the extent of the injury may be hidden. You may see only minimal bruising, yet the force of the injury may have caused internal organ rupture. Internal bleeding may be severe and lead to shock. Crush injuries can result in compartment syndrome or crush syndrome.

Compartment Syndrome

Objective 12

Muscles of the body are covered by a tough sheet of fibrous tissue called **fascia** (Figure 34-10). Muscles in the arms and legs are separated from each other by fascia,

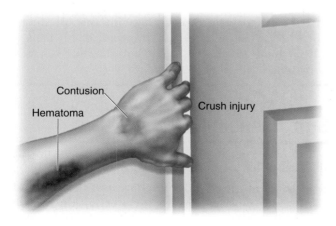

FIGURE 34-9 ▲ A contusion, a hematoma, and a crush injury without a break in the skin are examples of closed wounds.

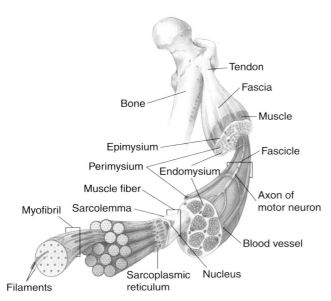

FIGURE 34-10 ▲ Fascia is a tough sheet of fibrous tissue that covers muscles and some organs of the body.

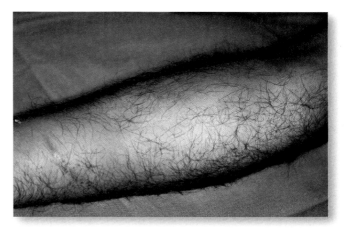

FIGURE 34-11 ▲ Compartment syndrome of the left leg.

forming compartments. Each compartment contains muscle cells and fibers, nerves, and blood vessels. When a compression injury occurs, the muscle is damaged, and swelling and/or bleeding results. Since fascia does not expand, swelling or bleeding causes an increase in pressure within the compartment. Increasing pressure compresses the muscle cells and fibers, nerves, and capillaries. When the pressure in the compartment becomes greater than the blood pressure within the capillaries, the capillaries collapse. This results in a decreased flow of blood (which contains oxygen and nutrients) to muscle and nerve cells. If the pressure in the compartment gets too high, blood flow stops. Without an adequate blood supply, the tissue within the compartment begins to die.

Compartment syndrome develops when the pressure within a compartment causes compression and abnormal function of nerves and blood vessels. Unless the pressure is relieved within 6 to 8 hours, permanent nerve and muscle damage can result, leading to paralysis, loss of the limb, or even death. To relieve the pressure within the compartment and attempt to save the affected limb, a physician will perform a fasciotomy. A **fasciotomy** is a surgical procedure in which the fascia is cut. By cutting the fascia, the pressure within the affected compartment is relieved.

Possible causes of compartment syndrome include:
- Compression injury
- Circumferential burns
- Frostbite
- Constrictive bandages, splints (including the pneumatic antishock garment), casts

- Animal or insect bites
- Bleeding disorders
- Arterial bleeding
- Soft tissue injury
- Fracture

Locations where compartment syndrome can occur include the arms, hands, legs, feet, and buttocks. The most common areas affected by compartment syndrome are the lower leg secondary to tibial fractures and the forearm secondary to fracture of the ulna or radius (see Figure 34-11).

Signs and symptoms of compartment syndrome can be remembered by five Ps shown in the following *You Should Know* box.

You Should Know

Assessment Findings and Symptoms of Compartment Syndrome

Five Ps
1. Pain
2. Paralysis (or weakness)
3. Paresthesias
4. Increased Pressure
5. Diminished peripheral Pulses

The earliest and most common symptom is severe, intense pain. The pain may seem out of proportion to the injury. The pain is worsened with passive stretching of the muscle. Weakness or paralysis of the affected extremity will be present. **Paresthesias** are abnormal sensations, such as tingling, burning, numbness, or a "pins-and-needles" feeling. Paresthesias are an early sign of nerve damage. **Anesthesia** means without sensation and refers to a loss of feeling in the affected limb.

The affected area is usually swollen. It feels tight or full when touched because of increased pressure. Diminished peripheral pulses are a late sign of compartment syndrome.

Crush Syndrome

Objective 12

Crush syndrome can occur when a large amount of skeletal muscle is compressed for a long period. Examples of situations in which this type of injury occurs are listed in the following *You Should Know* box.

> **You Should Know**
>
> **Possible Mechanisms of Injury of Crush Syndrome**
> - Mine cave-ins
> - Trench collapse
> - Motor vehicle crashes
> - Landslide, avalanche, rock slide
> - Rubble from war, earthquake
> - Pinning under heavy objects (such as a tractor)
> - Severe beatings

Crush syndrome should be considered when three criteria exist:
1. Involvement of a large amount of muscle
2. Compression of the muscle mass for a long period (usually 4 to 6 hours, although it may be as little as 1 hour)
3. Compromised local blood flow

Compression of the muscles causes damage to the muscle cells. Blood flow to the nerves, muscles, and tissues in the affected area(s) is compromised, resulting in muscle ischemia. Movement and sensation in the affected areas are also compromised. Damaged cells begin to leak toxic substances into the bloodstream. At the same time, large amounts of fluid build up in the compressed limbs. Hypovolemic shock develops because there is an inadequate volume of circulating blood. (Hypovolemic shock is the most common cause of death during the first few days after a crush injury.) Compartment syndrome develops because of increased pressure within the compressed limbs.

When the compressive force is removed, blood flow is restored to the muscles that were ischemic. Crush syndrome is called a *reperfusion injury* because although blood flow is restored to the muscles when the compressive force is removed, the toxic substances contained within the crushed areas are released into the circulation. The release of these toxins has many damaging effects. Kidney failure may occur within the first 60 hours of removal of the compressive force. Electrolyte abnormalities can cause irregular heart rhythms.

Emergency Care for Closed Wounds

Objective 13

To treat a patient with a closed wound, perform the following steps:

- Conduct a scene size-up and ensure your safety. Evaluate the mechanism of injury before approaching the patient. Put on appropriate PPE. If the mechanism of injury suggests a crushing injury, take extra care to evaluate the scene for hazards.
- Perform a primary survey to identify and treat any life-threatening conditions. Stabilize the cervical spine if needed. If signs of shock are present or if internal bleeding is suspected, treat for shock.
- Perform a physical exam. Take the patient's vital signs, and gather the patient's medical history.
- Splint any bone or joint injuries (see Chapter 37).
- If an extremity is injured, raise it above the level of the heart unless there are signs or symptoms of a possible fracture, such as pain, swelling, or deformity. Apply an ice bag or cold pack. Place a cloth or bandage between the patient's skin and the cold source. Applying cold to the wound helps to reduce pain, constrict injured blood vessels (thereby reducing bleeding), and reduce swelling.
- Comfort, calm, and reassure the patient. En route to the hospital, reassess as often as indicated.
- Record all patient care information, including the patient's medical history and all emergency care given, on a prehospital care report.

Remember This

- Never apply ice, an ice bag, or a cold pack directly to the skin. Doing so can cause tissue damage by freezing the tissue. Always use an insulating material such as a towel between the cold source and the skin.
- When applying ice, an ice bag, or a cold pack to a soft tissue injury, limit the application of the cold source to 20 minutes or less to prevent cold injury.

Special Situations

- If signs of compartment syndrome are present, do not apply ice or elevate the extremity. Applying ice increases blood vessel constriction in an already compromised limb. Stabilize the extremity in the position found, or place it in a position of comfort.

- If signs of compartment syndrome are present, splint the affected extremity for comfort and protection only when necessary, such as for a long transport.

- If the patient is trapped, try to find out how long the patient has been trapped. This information is very important. After finding out this information, contact medical direction for instructions. In general, if the patient has been trapped for less than an hour (and adequate personnel and equipment are on the scene), the patient can be removed from the area and treatment begun. However, if the patient has been trapped for an hour or more, you should suspect crush syndrome. Contact dispatch and request advanced life support (ALS) personnel to the scene. Before removing the patient from the area, ALS personnel will insert intravenous lines and begin infusing fluids. In situations like this, your time on the scene is likely to be much longer than usual. When ALS personnel have infused an adequate amount of IV fluid, they will most likely need your assistance in safely removing the patient from the area.

Open Wounds

Objective 14

In an **open soft tissue injury,** a break occurs in the skin. Because of the break in the skin, open wounds are at risk of external bleeding and infection. Properly dressing the wound helps protect against infection and will help control bleeding.

An **abrasion** is a scrape. It is the most common type of open wound. An abrasion occurs when the outermost layer of skin (epidermis) is damaged by rubbing or scraping (Figure 34-12). Little or no oozing of blood (capillary bleeding) occurs. Although an abrasion is superficial, it can be very painful. Because the pain associated with the injury is like that of a second-degree burn, an abrasion is often called a *rug burn, friction burn,* or *road rash.* Dirt and other foreign material can become ground into the skin with this type of injury. This greatly increases possible infection in a wound that is not properly cleansed with warm, soapy water or a fluid such as normal saline.

A **laceration** is a cut or tear in the skin of any length, shape, and depth (Figure 34-13). A laceration may

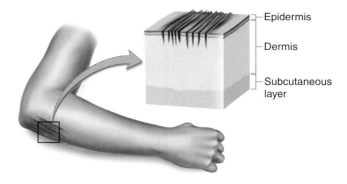

FIGURE 34-12 ▲ An abrasion results when the outermost layer of skin (epidermis) is damaged by rubbing or scraping.

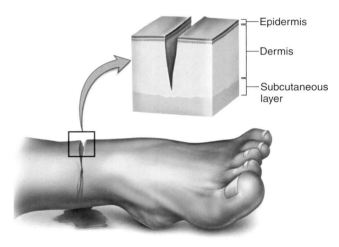

FIGURE 34-13 ▲ Any cut or tear in the skin is called a laceration.

occur by itself or with other types of soft tissue injury. This type of injury can be made by a blunt object tearing the skin. It can also be made by a sharp instrument cutting through the skin, such as a knife, razor blade, or broken glass. This type of laceration is said to be linear, or regular. A stellate laceration is irregularly shaped. It is usually caused by forceful impact with a blunt object. Bleeding may be severe if a laceration is in an area of the body where large arteries lie close to the skin surface, such as in the wrists (Figure 34-14). You must control bleeding from a laceration and cover the wound with a dressing to reduce the risk of infection.

A penetration, or **puncture wound,** results when the skin is pierced with a sharp, pointed object (Figures 34-15 and 34-16). Common objects that cause puncture wounds include nails, needles, pencils, splinters, darts, ice picks, pieces of glass, bullets, or knives. Some animal bites, such as those from cats, typically leave a deep puncture wound. An object that remains embedded in an open wound is called an **impaled**

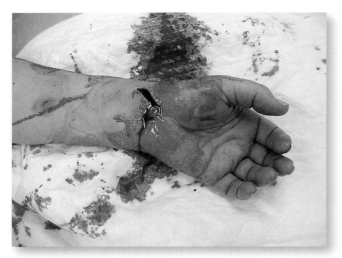

FIGURE 34-14 ▲ Laceration of the radial artery.

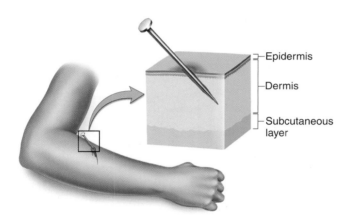

FIGURE 34-15 ▲ A penetration or puncture wound results when the skin is pierced with a sharp, pointed object.

Epidermis

Dermis

Subcutaneous layer

object (Figure 34-17). The severity of a puncture wound depends on where the injury is located. It also depends on how deep the wound is, the size of the penetrating object, and the forces involved in creating the injury. There is an increased risk of infection with this type of injury because the penetrating object may carry dirt and germs deep into the tissues. There may be little or no external bleeding with a puncture wound. However, internal bleeding may be severe. Assess the patient closely for signs and symptoms of shock if the puncture wound is in the chest or abdomen.

Stab and gunshot wounds are types of puncture wounds that can go completely through the body or body part. This creates both an entrance and an exit wound. An entrance wound from a bullet usually looks like many other puncture wounds, while the exit wound is typically larger and more irregular. If a bullet breaks apart, it may create several exit wounds or none at all. Carefully examine your patient to find all wounds.

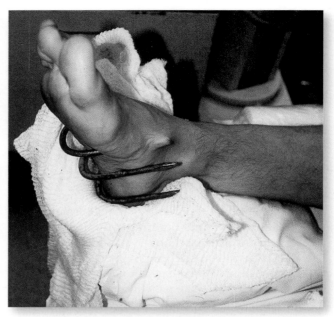

FIGURE 34-16 ▲ This patient has a puncture wound to the foot caused by a gardening tool. Foot x-rays revealed no associated bony injuries.

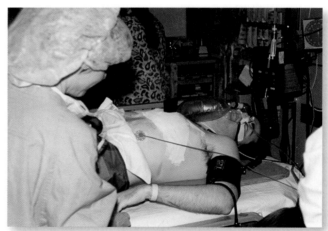

FIGURE 34-17 ▲ An object that remains embedded in an open wound is called an impaled object.

Stop and Think!

- Assume that any penetrating injury to the chest has involved the abdomen. Assume that a penetrating abdominal wound has involved the chest.
- A bullet that enters the body can travel in many directions. Suspect a possible spinal injury in every patient who has suffered a gunshot wound to the head, neck, chest, or abdomen.

Remember This

At a crime scene, disturb the patient and his clothing as little as possible while performing your assessment and during treatment. Cut around rather than through the areas penetrated by the weapon.

An **avulsion** is an injury in which a piece of skin or tissue is torn loose or pulled completely off (Figure 34-18). If the tissue is not totally torn from the body, it often hangs loose, like a flap. The amount of bleeding varies with the extent and depth of the injury. A common avulsion injury is an avulsion of the forehead. This type of injury can occur when an unrestrained motor vehicle occupant is thrown through the windshield. In a **degloving**

avulsion injury, the skin and fatty tissue are stripped away from an extremity like a glove (Figure 34-19).

A crush injury occurs when a part of the body is caught between two compressing surfaces. In an **open crush injury,** broken bone ends may stick out through the skin (Figure 34-20). Internal bleeding may be present and can be severe enough to cause shock. An example of an open crush injury is shown in Figure 34-21.

An **amputation** is the separation of a body part from the rest of the body. If the body part is forcefully separated from the body, the edges of the wound are usually ragged (Figure 34-22). The remaining tissue may look shredded, with bones or tendons exposed. Massive bleeding may be present. Alternatively, bleeding may be limited because blood vessels normally constrict and pull in at the point of injury when damaged. Bleeding can usually be controlled with direct pressure applied to the stump. Be sure to send the severed body part to the hospital with the patient.

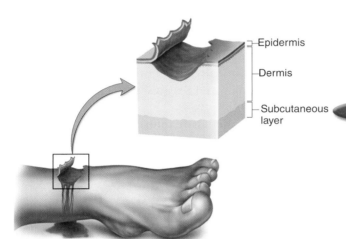

FIGURE 34-18 ▲ In an avulsion, a flap of skin or tissue is torn loose or pulled completely off. If the tissue is not totally torn from the body, it often hangs loose, like a flap. Care for completely avulsed tissue like an amputated part.

You Should Know

Types of Open Wounds

- Abrasion
- Laceration
- Penetration, puncture wound
- Avulsion
- Open crush injury
- Amputation

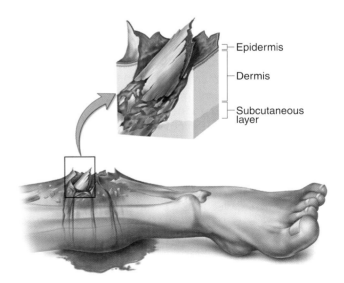

FIGURE 34-20 ▲ In an open crush injury, fractured bone ends may stick out through the skin.

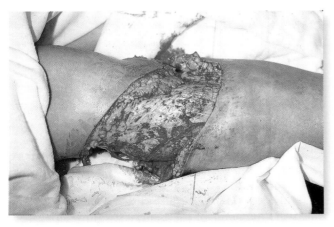

FIGURE 34-19 ▲ This degloving injury occurred after the patient's lower leg became tangled in a rope while she was waterskiing.

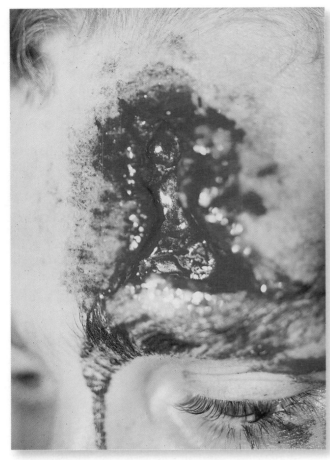

FIGURE 34-21 ▲ A fall from a bicycle resulted in this open crush injury.

Emergency Care for Open Wounds

Objective 15

To treat a patient with an open wound, perform the following steps:

- Conduct a scene size-up and ensure your safety. Evaluate the mechanism of injury before approaching the patient. Put on appropriate PPE.
- Perform a primary survey to identify and treat any life-threatening conditions. Stabilize the cervical spine if needed. If major bleeding is present from an open wound, expose the wound to assess the injury. You may need to remove and cut away clothing. Control bleeding. As with any significant or potentially significant injury, treat for shock.
- Once major bleeding is controlled, apply a sterile dressing to prevent further contamination of the wound. An incomplete avulsion should be covered with an appropriate dressing. Regardless of its size, incomplete avulsions should never be removed. The skin flap may be replaced in correct anatomic position before applying a dressing. Bandage the dressing securely in place.

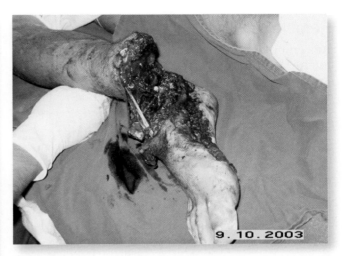

FIGURE 34-22 ▲ A 22-year-old with a traumatic amputation caused by a gear.

- Perform a physical exam. Take the patient's vital signs, and gather the patient's medical history.
- Splint any bone or joint injuries.
- Comfort, calm, and reassure the patient. Reassess as often as indicated.
- Record all patient care information, including the patient's medical history and all emergency care given, on a PCR.

Special Considerations

The following soft tissue injuries require special consideration:

- Penetrating chest injuries
- Eviscerations
- Impaled objects
- Amputations
- Neck injuries
- Eye injuries
- Mouth injuries
- Ear injuries

Penetrating Chest Injuries

Objective 16

A **penetrating** (open) **chest injury** is a break in the skin over the chest wall (Figure 34-23). This type of injury results from penetrating trauma, such as gunshot wounds, stabbings, blast injuries, or an impaled object. The severity of an open chest injury depends on the size of the wound. If the chest wound is more than two-thirds the diameter of the patient's windpipe, air will enter the chest wound rather than move through the trachea with each breath. You may hear a sucking or gurgling sound escaping from the wound when the

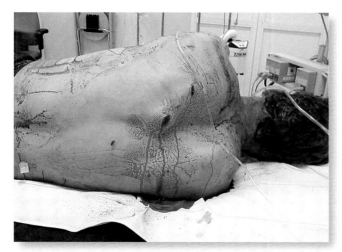

FIGURE 34-23 ▲ The front of this patient's chest showed visible bleeding, but no obvious injury. When the patient's back is examined, multiple wounds are found. Remember, the back is part of the chest. Always remember to check the back.

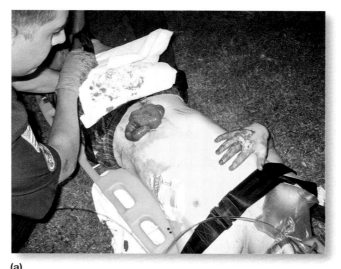

(a)

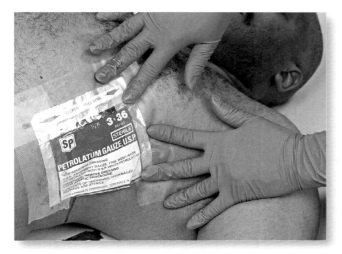

FIGURE 34-24 ▲ Cover an open chest wound with an airtight dressing taped on three sides.

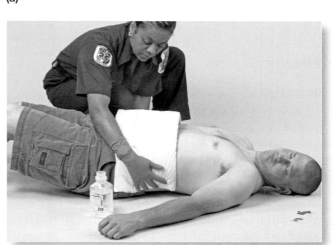

(b)

FIGURE 34-25 ▲ **(a)** Handle exposed organs as little as possible. **(b)** Cover the exposed organs and wound by applying a thick, moist dressing lightly over the organs and wound. Secure the dressing in place with a large bandage to retain moisture and prevent heat loss.

patient breathes in. This sound occurs as air moves into the pleural cavity through the open chest wound. This type of injury is called a **sucking chest wound.** It is a life-threatening injury because the open wound can cause the lung on the injured side to collapse, affecting the patient's breathing.

You should consider *any* open chest wound a sucking chest wound. If an open chest wound is present, apply an occlusive (airtight) dressing to the wound. Examples of occlusive dressings include petroleum gauze, aluminum foil, or a piece of plastic wrap. Tape the dressing on three sides (Figure 34-24). The dressing will be sucked over the wound as the patient

breathes in, preventing air from entering the chest. The open end of the dressing allows air that is trapped in the chest to escape as the patient breathes out. After covering the wound, give oxygen. Place the patient in a position of comfort if no spinal injury is suspected. If spinal injury is suspected, the patient should be placed on a long backboard and secured to the board.

Eviscerations

Objective 17

An **evisceration** occurs when an organ sticks out through an open wound. In an abdominal evisceration, abdominal organs stick out through an open wound in the wall of the abdomen (Figure 34-25a). Do not touch the exposed organ or try to place it back into the body. Carefully remove clothing from around the wound. Lightly cover the exposed organ and wound with a thick, moist dressing. Secure the dressing in place with a large bandage to keep moisture in and prevent heat loss (Figure 34-25b). Place the patient in a position of comfort if no spinal injury is suspected. Keep the patient warm. Assess for signs of shock and treat if present.

Remember This

Never cover exposed organs with a dressing that will stick to them. The use of aluminum foil was recommended years ago. This is no longer recommended because exposure to the sun may literally bake the organs.

Impaled Objects

Objective 18

An impaled object is an object that remains embedded in an open wound. An impaled object is also called an *embedded object*. Do not remove an impaled object unless it interferes with cardiopulmonary resuscitation (CPR) or is impaled through the cheek and interferes with care of the patient's airway. After removing an object from the cheek, apply direct pressure to the bleeding by reaching inside the patient's mouth with gloved fingers.

Leave the object in the wound, and manually secure it to prevent movement. Shorten the object only if necessary. Any movement of the object can cause further damage to nerves, blood vessels, and other surrounding tissues. Expose the wound area and control bleeding. Stabilize the object with bulky dressings and bandage them in place. Assess the patient for signs of shock and treat if present.

Amputations

Objective 19

In the case of an amputated body part, control bleeding at the stump. In most cases, direct pressure will be enough to control the bleeding. While providing care for the patient, ask an assistant to find the amputated part. At the hospital, a surgeon may be able to reattach the amputated part. Because reattaching an amputated part is attempted only in very limited situations, do not suggest to the patient that it will be done.

Care for an amputated part or completely avulsed tissue by gently rinsing the amputated part with lactated Ringer's (LR) solution. Wrap the part in sterile

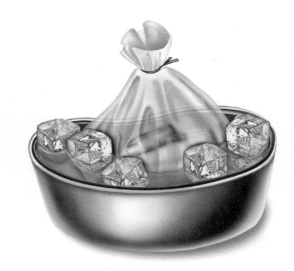

FIGURE 34-26 ▲ Place an amputated part, moistened in sterile gauze, in a dry plastic bag or waterproof container. Seal the bag or container, label it, and place it in water that contains a few ice cubes or crushed ice.

gauze moistened with LR solution and place it in a dry plastic bag or waterproof container. Carefully seal the bag or container, label it, and place it in water that contains a few ice cubes or crushed ice (Figure 34-26). Immobilize the injured area to prevent further injury. Treat the patient for shock and keep her warm. Comfort, calm, and reassure the patient. Reassess every 5 minutes. Transport the amputated part with the patient to an appropriate facility.

Remember This

When faced with a situation involving an amputated part, remember the following:

- Never use dry ice to keep an amputated part cool.
- Do not allow an amputated part to freeze.
- Never place an unwrapped or unpackaged amputated part directly on ice or in water.

Neck Injuries

Objective 20

The neck contains many important blood vessels and airway structures. Swelling can cause an airway obstruction. A penetrating injury to the neck can result in severe bleeding (Figure 34-27). The signs and symptoms of a neck injury include shortness of breath, difficulty breathing, and a hoarse voice. Possible causes of a neck injury are listed in the next *You Should Know* box.

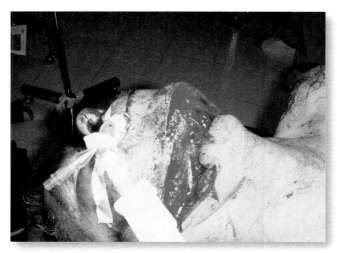

FIGURE 34-27 ▲ This patient is a 33-year-old man involved in a motor vehicle crash. He wore no seat belt and hit the windshield of the car he was driving. Despite the appearance of the injury, there were no injuries to the major blood vessels, trachea, or esophagus. The patient underwent surgery and was sent home 72 hours later.

You Should Know

Possible Causes of Neck Injuries

- A hanging
- Impact with a steering wheel
- "Clothesline" injuries, in which a person runs into a stretched wire or cord that strikes the throat
- Knife or gunshot wounds

If a blood vessel is torn and exposed to the air, air can be sucked into the vessel and travel to the heart, the lungs, the brain, or other organs. This condition is called an **air embolism.** The air displaces blood and prevents tissue perfusion. Sometimes if a neck injury has damaged the airway, air will leak into the tissues. If this happens, there may be obvious swelling. When you palpate the skin, you will feel a "popping" as if there were crisped rice cereal trapped beneath it. This is called **subcutaneous emphysema** and is a very important finding to report to other healthcare professionals.

To care for an open neck wound:
- Immediately place a gloved hand over the wound to control bleeding.
- Cover the wound with an airtight (occlusive) dressing.

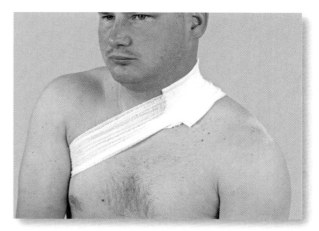

FIGURE 34-28 ▲ To care for an open neck wound, control bleeding and cover the wound with an airtight dressing. Apply a pressure bandage. Wrap it across the injured side of the neck and under the opposite armpit.

- Apply a bulky dressing over the occlusive dressing. To control bleeding, apply pressure over the dressing with a gloved hand. Compress the carotid artery only if absolutely necessary to control bleeding. When applying pressure, make sure not to press on the trachea; pressing on it may cause an airway obstruction. Do not press on both carotid arteries at the same time. Doing so can slow blood flow to the brain. It can also slow the patient's heart rate.
- Apply a pressure bandage. Wrap it across the injured side of the neck and under the opposite armpit (Figure 34-28). *Never apply a circular bandage around a patient's neck.* Strangulation can occur.
- Treat the patient for shock.

Remember This

Consider an injury to the neck an injury to the spine. Immobilize the patient accordingly.

Eye Injuries

Objective 21

Eye injuries are common and often result from blunt and penetrating trauma. Causes of eye injuries are shown in the next *You Should Know* box. Swelling, bleeding, and the presence of a foreign object in the eye are common signs of an eye injury and are easily seen. A foreign body, such as dirt, sand, and metal or wood slivers, may enter the eye and cause severe pain.

Causes of Eye Injuries

- Motor vehicle crashes
- Sports and recreational activities
- Violence
- Chemical exposure from household and industrial accidents
- Foreign bodies
- Animal bites and scratches

If a foreign body is in the eye, try flushing it out of the affected eye. Do not exert any pressure on the eye. Hold the patient's eyelid open, and gently flush the eye with warm water. Flush from the nose side of the affected eye toward the ear, away from the unaffected eye. It is important to flush *away* from the uninjured eye so that foreign bodies or chemicals are not transferred into the uninjured eye. Make sure to use a gentle flow of water when flushing the eye. A bulb or irrigation syringe, nasal cannula, or a bottle can be used for this purpose (Figure 34-29). Alternatively, IV tubing connected to an IV bag of normal saline can be used. If none of these devices is available, try placing the patient's head under a gently running faucet and rinse the eye. Flush the eye for at least 5 minutes. If you are unable to remove the foreign body, cover both

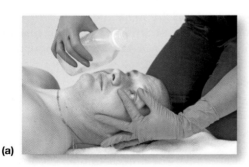

(a)

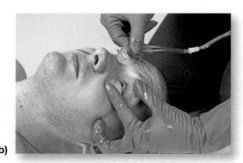

(b)

FIGURE 34-29 ▲ **(a)** To flush a foreign body from the eye, hold the patient's eyelid open and gently flush the eye with warm water. **(b)** Flush from the nose side of the affected eye toward the ear, away from the unaffected eye.

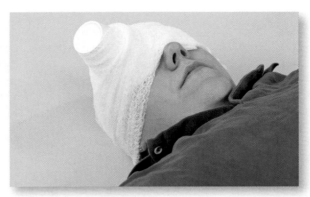

FIGURE 34-30 ▲ If a foreign body is protruding from the eye, stabilize it with bulky gauze. Then cover the eye with a paper or Styrofoam cup secured with tape to keep the object from moving. Cover the unaffected eye to limit movement of the affected eye.

eyes and transport to the nearest appropriate medical facility.

If a foreign body is protruding from the eye, stabilize the object and transport as quickly as possible. Do not attempt to remove the object. If the object is long, stabilize it with bulky gauze. Then cover the eye with a paper or Styrofoam cup secured with tape to keep the object from moving (Figure 34-30). If the object is short, make a doughnut-shaped base from roller gauze or a triangular bandage and place it around the eye. Be careful not to bump the object. Because both eyes normally move together, you will also need to cover the unaffected eye with a dressing. If you cover both eyes, be sure to tell the patient everything that you are doing. The patient may be frightened when she cannot anticipate movements and other procedures.

A chemical burn is the most urgent eye injury. The damage to the eye depends on the type and concentration of the chemical. The length of exposure and the elapsed time until treatment also affect the extent of damage. Early signs and symptoms of a chemical burn to the eye are shown in the following *You Should Know* box.

Early Signs and Symptoms of a Chemical Burn to the Eye

- Pain
- Redness
- Irritation
- Tearing
- An inability to keep the eye open
- A sensation of "something in my eye"
- Swelling of the eyelids
- Blurred vision (usually caused by pain or tearing of the eye) or loss of vision

Alkali burns are more dangerous than acid burns because they penetrate more deeply and rapidly. Common household substances that contain alkalies include lye, cement, lime, and ammonia. One of the most common chemicals associated with acid burns to the eye is sulfuric acid. The exposure usually occurs because of automobile battery explosions, as batteries contain sulfuric acid.

Ask the patient if he is wearing contact lenses. If so, have him remove them as soon as possible. If the lenses are left in, the irrigating solution will not be able to reach parts of the eye. If the patient does not wear contact lenses or if the lenses have been removed, immediately flush the eye with water or normal saline. Continue flushing the eye for at least 20 minutes. Flush away from the unaffected eye (as previously described). Transport immediately. Irrigation should be continued throughout transport.

You Should Know

Pepper spray is an irritant that causes significant pain when sprayed into the eyes. Vision is not usually affected, and the spray rarely causes eye damage. Flushing the affected eye for 5 minutes with warm water will generally stop further irritation.

A nonchemical burn to the eye can be caused by heat, radiation, lasers, infrared rays, and ultraviolet light (such as sunlight, arc welding, and bright snow). The patient will complain of severe pain in the eyes 1 to 6 hours after the exposure. Emergency care for a nonchemical burn to the eye includes covering both eyes with moist pads. Darken the room to protect the patient from further exposure to light. Transport the patient for further care.

Mouth Injuries

Objective 22

An injury to the mouth can result in severe swelling or bleeding that causes an airway obstruction. Because the tongue is attached to the lower jaw (mandible), a lower-jaw fracture may allow the tongue to fall against the back of the throat, blocking the airway. The signs and symptoms depend on the area of the jaw affected. Tenderness, bruising, and swelling are common (Figure 34-31).

You Should Know

If a patient is unable to open her mouth or move her lower jaw side to side without pain, suspect a fracture.

The upper jawbone (maxilla) is often fractured in high-speed crashes. The patient's face is thrown forward into the windshield, steering wheel, and dash-

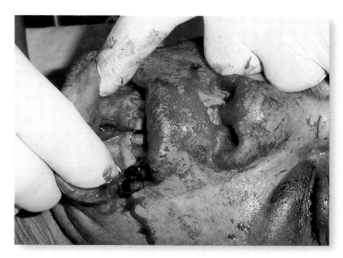

FIGURE 34-31 ▲ Jaw fracture resulting from direct frontal trauma.

board. A fracture of the maxilla is often accompanied by a black eye. The patient's face may appear unusually long. Swelling and pain are usually present.

Ear Injuries

Objective 23

A blow to the ear can result in bruising of the outer (external) portion of the ear. A severe blow can result in damage to the eardrum, with pain, bleeding, or both. Suspect a possible skull fracture if you see blood or fluid draining from a patient's ear. Place a sterile dressing loosely over the ear to absorb the drainage, and bandage it in place. Never put anything into the ear to control bleeding. If the ear is avulsed, collect the avulsed part and care for it as you would an amputated part. Make sure that the avulsed part is transported with the patient to the hospital. An ear laceration is treated like any other soft tissue injury (Figure 34-32).

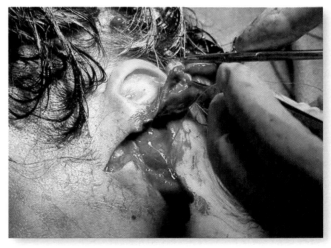

FIGURE 34-32 ▲ Ear laceration.

Burns

Burns may occur because of exposure to heat (thermal burn), chemicals, electricity, or radiation. Most burns are thermal burns that result from flames, scalds, or contact with hot substances. Chemical burns are caused by substances that produce chemical changes in the skin, resulting in tissue damage on contact. Acids and alkalies are substances that are commonly associated with a chemical burn. An electrical burn occurs when a person comes into contact with a source of electricity, including lightning. Body organs may be injured from the heat generated as the electrical current enters the body and travels through the tissues. Burns may also result from a high level of radiation exposure. Radiation burns are the least common type of burn.

The skin is the body's largest organ. Remember that the skin helps regulate body temperature; senses heat, cold, touch, pressure, and pain; helps maintain fluid balance; and protects underlying tissues from injury. When the skin is disrupted because of a burn, many of these functions are affected. The body loses fluid, and the skin becomes less effective in helping maintain body temperature. Because the skin surface is no longer intact, the body is at an increased risk of infection.

Determining the Severity of a Burn

Objective 24

The severity of a burn is determined by a number of factors:

- The depth of the burn (how deeply the burn penetrates the skin)
- The extent of the burn (how much of the body surface is burned)
- The location of the burn
- Medical or surgical conditions present before the burn
- The patient's age
- Associated factors (such as the mechanism of injury)

The Depth of the Burn

Objective 25

Burns are classified by how deeply the body's skin layers are affected. There are three categories of burns: superficial (first degree), partial thickness (second degree), and full thickness (third degree).

> **You Should Know**
>
> A burn wound continues to change up to 24 hours after the injury.

Superficial Burns

Objectives 26, 27

A **superficial burn,** also called a *first-degree burn,* affects only the epidermis. It results in only minor tissue damage (Figure 34-33). A sunburn is an example of a superficial burn. The skin is red, tender, and very painful (Figure 34-34). Blistering does not occur with a superficial burn. This type of burn does not usually require medical care and heals in 2 to 5 days with no scarring.

Partial-Thickness Burns

Objectives 28, 29

A **partial-thickness burn,** also called a *second-degree burn,* involves the epidermis and dermis. The hair follicles and sweat glands are spared in this degree of burn

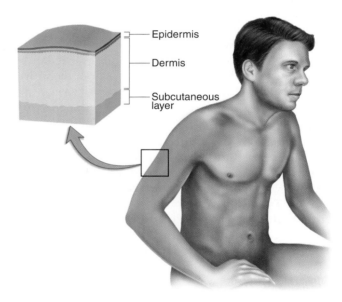

FIGURE 34-33 ▲ A superficial (first-degree) burn affects only the epidermis.

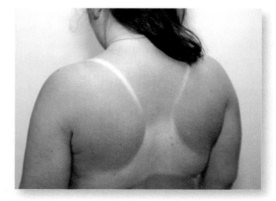

FIGURE 34-34 ▲ Superficial (first-degree) burn.

(Figure 34-35). These burns commonly result from contact with hot liquids or flash burns from gasoline flames. A partial-thickness burn produces intense pain and some swelling. Blistering may be present (Figure 34-36). The skin appears pink, red, or mottled, and is sensitive to air current and pressure. This type of burn usually heals within 5 to 34 days. Scarring may or may not occur, depending on the depth of the burn.

You Should Know

Not all partial-thickness burns blister. However, if blistering is present, it is a partial-thickness burn.

Full-Thickness Burns

Objectives 30, 31

A **full-thickness burn,** also called a *third-degree burn*, destroys both the epidermis and dermis and may include subcutaneous tissue, muscle, and bone (Figure 34-37). The color of the patient's skin may vary from yellow or pale to black. The skin has a dry, waxy, or leathery appearance (Figure 34-38). A full-thickness burn is numb because the burn destroys nerve endings in the skin. However, many full-thickness burns are surrounded by areas of superficial and partial-thickness burns, which are painful. A large full-thickness burn requires skin grafting. Small areas may heal from the edges of the burn after weeks. Because the skin is so severely damaged in this type of burn, it cannot perform its usual protective functions. Rapid fluid loss often occurs. Be ready to treat the patient for shock.

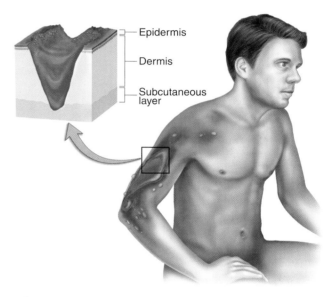

FIGURE 34-37 ▲ A full-thickness (third-degree) burn causes damage to all layers of the epidermis and dermis and may include subcutaneous tissue, muscle, and bone.

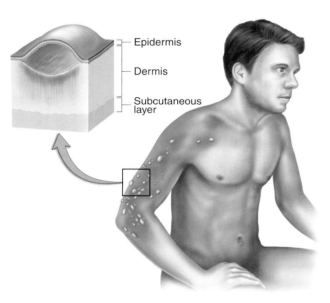

FIGURE 34-35 ▲ A partial-thickness (second-degree) burn affects the epidermis and dermis.

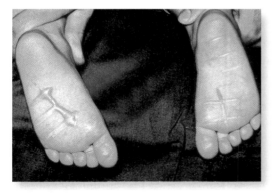

FIGURE 34-36 ▲ Partial-thickness (second-degree) burn.

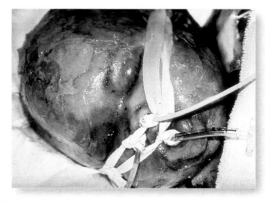

FIGURE 34-38 ▲ Full-thickness (third-degree) burn.

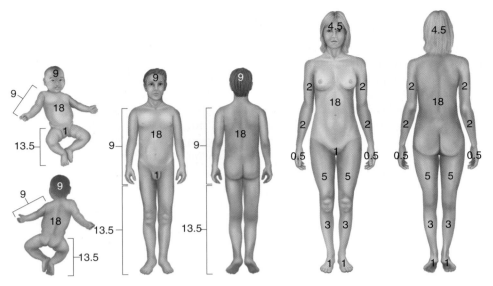

FIGURE 34-39 ▲ The rule of nines for an infant, a child, and an adult.

The Extent of the Burn

Objective 32

When determining the seriousness of a burn, the extent of the burned area is important to determine. The depth of the burn must also be considered, although superficial burns are not included in the calculation of the extent a burn. The **rule of nines** is a guide used to estimate the total body surface area (BSA) burned. The rule of nines divides the adult body into sections that are 9% or are multiples of 9% (Figure 34-39). The rule of nines has been modified for children and infants (Table 34-4). To use the rule of nines to estimate the extent of a burn, add the percentages of the areas burned. For example, if an adult burned the front of the trunk (18%), the front and back of one arm (9%), and the front and back of one leg (18%), 45% of her BSA is burned.

TABLE 34-4	The Rule of Nines		
Body Area	**Adult**	**Child**	**Infant**
Head and neck	9%	18%	18%
Front of trunk	18%	18%	18%
Back of trunk	18%	18%	18%
Each arm (shoulder to fingertips)	9%	9%	9%
Each leg (groin to toe)	18%	13.5%	13.5%
Genitals	1%	1%	1%

You Should Know

Only partial-thickness (second-degree) and full-thickness (third-degree) burns are included when calculating the extent of a burn.

Remember This

The **rule of palms** can be used for small or irregularly shaped burns or for burns that are scattered over the patient's body. The palm of the *patient's* hand equals 1% of the patient's BSA. If the patient's palm would fit over the burned area eight times, the extent of the burn is 8% of the BSA.

Other Factors Related to Burn Severity

The Location of the Burn

The location of a burn is an important factor when determining burn severity. Burns to the face can cause breathing difficulty. Burns of the face and neck can interfere with the ability to eat or drink. Burns of the hands and feet can interfere with the patient's ability to walk, work, eat, and perform other daily activities. Burns of the genitalia are prone to infection.

Preexisting Medical Conditions

A preexisting medical problem may increase a patient's risk of death or complications following a burn injury. Examples of preexisting conditions include diabetes, asthma, and malnutrition.

Age as a Factor in Burns

A burn is considered severe if the patient is younger than 5 years of age or older than 55 years of age. The skin of infants, young children, and elderly people is thin. Burns in these patients may be more severe than they initially appear. See the following *Remember This* box for specifics about burns in infants, children, and older adults.

Remember This

Burn Considerations for Infants and Children

- Though the rule of nines offers an easy way to estimate the amount of BSA affect, in reality, children have a greater BSA in proportion to adults. This larger surface area results in greater fluid and heat loss.
- Children who are burned are more likely than adults to develop shock or airway problems.
- Consider the possibility of child abuse when treating a burned child. A common burn associated with child abuse is caused by dipping the child in scalding water. "Stockinglike" burns with no associated splash marks are often present on the buttocks, genitalia, or extremities (Figure 34-40). Report all suspected cases of abuse to law enforcement and emergency department personnel in accordance with your state's regulations.

Burn Considerations for Older Adults

- Many older adults have thin skin and poor circulation. These factors affect the depth of a burn and slow the healing process.
- In older adults, the mechanisms and severity of burn injury are related to living alone. Older adults also tend to wear loose-fitting clothing while cooking and fall asleep while smoking. In addition, these patients tend to have declining vision, hearing, and sense of smell. Older adults may have a slowed reaction time and problems with balance and/or memory.
- Burns in older adults most often occur in the home. Scalds and flame burns are the most common type of burns in this age group.
- Older adults are more likely to have a preexisting medical condition, which increases their risk of complications after a burn. In some cases, the preexisting condition may be the cause of the burn. For example, an older adult may collapse because of a stroke while smoking or cooking.

Burns Best Treated in a Burn Center

Although most burns are minor, some types of burns are best treated in a burn center. A burn center offers

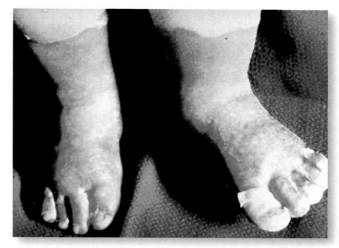

FIGURE 34-40 ▲ "Stockinglike" burns with no associated splash marks are caused by dipping a child in scalding water. This type of injury is usually seen in children younger than 2 years of age. The child's caregiver punishes the child, for example, for an "accident" when he is being potty trained.

specialized care—including services, equipment, and trained staff for treating serious burn injuries.

A patient with any of the following types of burns should be transported to a burn center:

- Partial-thickness (second-degree) burns involving more than 10% of the total BSA in adults or 5% of the total BSA in children
- Chemical burns
- All burns involving the hands, face, eyes, ears, feet, or genitalia
- **Circumferential burns** of the torso or extremities
- Any full-thickness (third-degree) burn in a child
- All inhalation injuries
- Electrical burns, including lightning injuries
- All burns complicated by fractures or other trauma
- All burns in high-risk patients, including older adults; the very young; and those with preexisting conditions, such as diabetes, asthma, and epilepsy

Emergency Care for Thermal Burns

Objectives 33, 34, 35

To treat a patient with a thermal burn, perform the following steps:

- Conduct a scene size-up and ensure your safety. Evaluate the mechanism of injury before approaching the patient. Put on appropriate PPE.
  —If the patient is still in the area of the heat source, remove the patient from the area. If the patient's clothing is in flames, "stop, drop, and

roll." Place the patient on the floor or ground. Roll her in a blanket to smother the flames.

—Remove smoldering clothing and jewelry. If the patient's clothing is stuck to the burned area, do not attempt to remove it. Instead, cut around the clothing, leaving the burn untouched.

- Perform a primary survey to identify and treat any life-threatening conditions. Manage the patient's airway and breathing. Stabilize the cervical spine if needed.

- If the patient was in a confined space and was exposed to smoke, flames, or steam, you should be alert for potential airway problems. Examples of confined spaces include a room, vehicle, silo, pit, vessel, or vault. The signs and symptoms that suggest a possible airway problem are shown in the following *You Should Know* box. Patients who have signs of an inhalation injury will likely have inhaled poisonous gases such as carbon monoxide or cyanide. These gases are produced as a by-product of the substances that burn. High-flow oxygen is always indicated in these situations.

- Check the pulses in all extremities. Burn swelling that encircles an extremity can act as a tourniquet.

- After all immediate life threats have been managed, care for the burn itself. Perform a physical exam. Quickly determine the severity of the burn. Take the patient's vital signs, and gather the patient's medical history. Consider the following questions about the burn:

—How long ago did the burn occur?

—How did it occur?

—What was done to treat the burn before you arrived?

- Keep in mind that even after being removed from the heat source, burned tissue will continue to burn. You can help limit the progression of a surface burn injury if you can rapidly cool the burn shortly after it happens. Stop the burning process with clean, room temperature water applied for no more than 1 to 2 minutes. *Cooling the burn for more than 2 minutes can cause a critical loss of body heat and shock.*

- Cover the burned area with a dry dressing or sheet. If blisters are present, leave them intact and cover them loosely with a sterile dressing. Cover the patient with clean, dry sheets and blankets to keep him warm. Because burned tissue loses its ability to regulate temperature, cover the patient even when the outside temperature is warm. The sheet does not have to be sterile.

- Remove all jewelry as soon as possible. Swelling of the hands and fingers may occur soon after a burn. Wrap gauze around each digit to keep skin from touching.

- Look for other injuries and signs of shock. Treat and immobilize possible fractures. Treat soft tissue injuries if present. Treat shock if present.

- Keep burned extremities elevated above the level of the heart.

- Transport to the closest appropriate facility. Comfort, calm, and reassure the patient. Perform ongoing assessments as often as indicated.

- Record all patient care information, including the patient's medical history and all emergency care given, on a PCR.

You Should Know

Assessment Findings and Symptoms of Possible Inhalation Injury

- Facial burns
- Soot in the nose or mouth
- Singed facial or nasal hair
- Swelling of the lips or the inside of the mouth
- Coughing
- An inability to swallow secretions
- A hoarse voice

Remember This

- Do not apply butter, oils, sprays, lotions, or ointments to a burn.
- If a blister has formed, do not break it.
- Do not place ice or wet sheets on a burn.
- Do not transport a burn patient on wet sheets, wet towels, or wet clothing.

Chemical Burns

It has been estimated that more than 25,000 chemicals currently in use are capable of burning the skin or mucous membranes. Chemical burns can result from contact with wet or dry chemicals. The degree of injury in a chemical burn is based on the following:

- The mechanism of action of the chemical
- The strength of the chemical
- The concentration and amount of the chemical
- How long the patient was in contact with the chemical
- The body part in contact with the chemical
- The extent of tissue penetration

In some cases, the damage caused by the chemicals is not limited to the skin. Some chemicals, such as hydrofluoric acid, can be absorbed into the body and cause damage to internal organs.

Emergency Care for Chemical Burns

Objective 36

To treat a patient with a chemical burn, take the following steps:

- Conduct a scene size-up. As in all situations, your personal safety must be your primary concern. Evaluate the mechanism of injury before approaching the patient. Take the necessary scene safety precautions to protect yourself from exposure to hazardous materials. Wear gloves, eye protection, and other PPE as necessary. Additional resources, such as law enforcement, the fire service, the state or local hazardous materials team, and special rescue personnel, may be needed to secure the scene before you can safely enter the area.

- Perform a primary survey to identify and treat any life-threatening conditions.

    —Manage the patient's airway and breathing. Stabilize the cervical spine if needed.

    —Remove the patient's jewelry and clothing, including shoes and socks, which can trap concentrated chemicals. Do not remove clothing over the patient's head. Instead, cut the clothing as needed. Place the items in plastic bags to limit the exposure of others to the chemical.

- Perform a physical exam. Take the patient's vital signs, and gather the patient's medical history.

- Stop the burning process by removing the chemical. Wet chemicals can be flushed with large amounts of water. Brush away dry chemicals before flushing.

    —Brush off a dry chemical from the patient's skin with towels, sheets, or your gloved hands. Brush the chemical *away* from the patient.

    —Flush the burn with large amounts of room temperature water at low pressure. If the burn covers a large area, put the patient in the shower or use a garden hose, if available. Chemical burns should be flushed for at least 20 minutes.

- Treat other injuries, if present.

- The patient should be decontaminated before transport to the hospital. If the patient is not fully decontaminated before transport, the receiving facility should be notified as soon as possible. This notification will allow them time to prepare to decontaminate the patient on arrival at the facility.

- Comfort, calm, and reassure the patient. Reassess as often as indicated.

- Record all patient care information, including the patient's medical history and all emergency care given, on a PCR. Constantly check for status of scene safety, as it can change rapidly in a contamination scene.

Stop and Think!

The severity of a chemical burn can be misleading. The skin may not appear to be significantly damaged, yet a severe injury may be present. You may be contaminated by the chemical if you do not use appropriate precautions.

Electrical Burns

The severity of an electrical injury is related to the following:

- Amperage (the flow of the current)
- Voltage (the current's force)
- The type of current (alternating current or direct current)
- The current's pathway through the body
- The resistance of tissues to the current
- The duration of contact with the current

Normally, the skin is a resistor to the flow of electrical current into the body. When electricity enters the body, it is converted to heat. Inside the body, the current follows the paths of blood vessels, nerves, and muscles. This results in major damage to the body's internal organs. The skin may show no signs or only minimal signs of injury despite massive internal damage.

Emergency Care for Electrical Burns

Objective 37

To treat a patient with an electrical burn, perform the following steps:

- Conduct a scene size-up, and make sure the scene is safe before entering. Evaluate the mechanism of injury before approaching the patient. Take the necessary scene safety precautions to protect yourself from exposure to electrical hazards. Wear gloves, eye protection, and other PPE as necessary. If the patient is still in contact with the electrical source, you may need to contact appropriate resources before approaching the

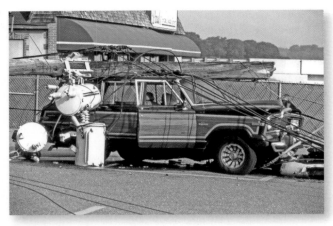

FIGURE 34-41 ▲ In situations involving electricity, additional resources, such as law enforcement, fire service, and utility company personnel, may be needed to secure the scene before you can safely enter the area.

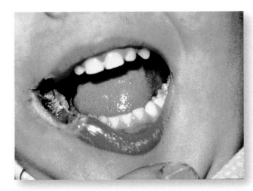

FIGURE 34-42 ▲ Electrical burn.

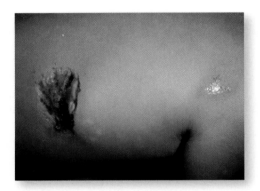

FIGURE 34-43 ▲ Electrical burn showing typical entrance and exit wounds.

patient. These resources may include law enforcement, fire service, and utility company personnel (Figure 34-41). Do not attempt to remove the patient from the electrical source unless you have been trained to do so. If the patient is still in contact with the electrical source or you are unsure, do not touch the patient.

- Perform a primary survey to identify and treat any life-threatening conditions. Manage the patient's airway and breathing. Stabilize the cervical spine if needed. Monitor the patient closely for respiratory and cardiac arrest. Make sure an automated external defibrillator is immediately available to you. Cardiac arrest caused by an electrical injury usually responds to treatment if defibrillation is performed quickly.

- Perform a physical exam (Figure 34-42). Take the patient's vital signs and gather the patient's medical history. Provide oxygen.

- Look for and treat other injuries if present. The patient may have fallen or been thrown from the electrical source. Treat the soft tissue injuries associated with the burn.

- Look for both an entrance and an exit wound. The entrance wound may look dry and leathery. The exit wound is usually much larger (Figure 34-43).

- *All* electrical burns should be evaluated by a physician. Transport the patient to the hospital.

- Comfort, calm, and reassure the patient. Reassess as often as indicated.

- Record all patient care information, including the patient's medical history and all emergency care given, on a PCR.

Remember This

Because electrical burns do more damage on the inside of the body than they do on the outside, it will be impossible for you to tell how bad an electrical burn really is. All electrical burns need to be evaluated at a hospital.

Emotional Support

Bleeding and soft tissue injuries are dramatic injuries. The emergency care that you provide for bleeding and soft tissue injuries is very important. It is also important to consider the psychological impact of these injuries. The patient and/or his family may experience many different emotions because of the injury. Remember that although grief is most often associated with death, *any* change of circumstance can cause a person to experience grief. A patient who has suffered a massive soft tissue injury or major burn often goes through the stages of the grief process. You may see the emotions of fear, anger, guilt, and depression. Provide emotional support for the patient and family.

Some of the injuries you will care for will be the result of a suicide attempt. After an unsuccessful suicide attempt, the patient may want to talk with you about it or may deny the attempt. Other injuries you will care for may be the result of abuse involving a child, spouse, or older adult. If you suspect abuse, share your concerns privately with the healthcare professional to whom you transfer patient care. Follow your local protocol regarding reporting suspected cases of abuse. In addition to notifying the person to whom you transfer care, you may also be required to notify law enforcement or emergency department personnel. Although these situations may be difficult, you must not be confrontational with the patient, family members, or others at the scene.

When providing care for bleeding and soft tissue injuries, you may experience anger, anxiety, frustration, fear, grief, and feelings of helplessness, especially if you are unable to relieve a patient's suffering or if a patient dies despite your care. You may feel sick at the sight of these injuries. These emotions are common and expected. You should not feel embarrassed or ashamed when these situations affect you. Seek the help of a peer counselor, mental health professional, social worker, or member of the clergy when you need assistance coping with these situations.

Making a Difference

The physical care you provide for a patient's illness or injury is very important. Good emergency care involves attending to the patient's physical *and* emotional needs in a professional, caring, concerned, and sensitive way. Always place the interests of the patient first when making patient care decisions.

Dressing and Bandaging

Objective 38

A **dressing** is an absorbent material placed directly over a wound. A **bandage** is material used to secure a dressing in place. The functions of dressing and bandaging wounds include:

- Helping to stop bleeding
- Absorbing blood and other drainage from the wound
- Protecting the wound from further injury
- Reducing contamination and the risk of infection

Dressings

When choosing a dressing, select one that is lint-free and large enough to cover the wound. A dressing of the right size should extend beyond the edges of the wound. If it is available, use a sterile dressing whenever possible because the dressing will be in direct contact with the open wound. When applying the dressing to the wound, wear gloves and hold the dressing by a corner. Place the dressing right over the wound—do not slide it in place.

Types of Dressings

The types of dressings commonly used in emergency care are sterile gauze pads, trauma dressings, occlusive dressings, and nonadherent pads.

Sterile Gauze Pads

Sterile gauze pads are the most common dressing used (Figure 34-44). They come in different shapes and sizes and are made of loosely woven material. This woven material allows blood and fluids to pass through the material and be absorbed.

Small gauze pads are classified by their size in inches. For example, a "2 by 2" refers to a small dressing that is 2 inches long and 2 inches wide.

Remember This

If blood soaks through a dressing, do not remove it. Apply more dressings and another bandage.

Trauma Dressings

Trauma dressings are thick dressings available in various sizes (Figure 34-45). This type of dressing is made of two layers of gauze with absorbent cotton in the center. A

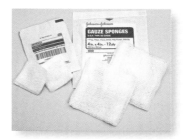

FIGURE 34-44 ▲ Sterile gauze pads come in different shapes and sizes.

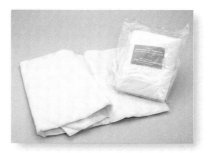

FIGURE 34-45 ▲ Trauma dressings are thick dressings that are used for large wounds. They are available in different sizes.

trauma dressing is used for large wounds. It can also be used to pad an injured arm or leg inside a splint.

Occlusive Dressings

An occlusive dressing is a special type of dressing made of nonporous material. This type of dressing is used to cover an open wound of the chest or neck and create an airtight seal. Although commercially made occlusive dressings are available, plastic wrap or aluminum foil may also be used (Figure 34-46).

Nonadherent Pads

Nonadherent pads are gauze pads that have a special coating. They are used to cover an open wound that is leaking fluid, such as a scrape or burn, but not stick to it (Figure 34-47). Eye pads are nonadherent pads that are used to cover the eyes after a minor eye injury (Figure 34-48). They may also be used to cover a small wound, such as a puncture. Adhesive strips, such as Band-Aids, are a combination of a nonadherent sterile dressing and a bandage.

Bandages

Objective 39

A bandage is applied to keep a dressing in place. Because a dressing separates the wound and the bandage, the bandage does not have to be sterile. Before applying a bandage on an extremity, remove the patient's jewelry and check the pulse distal to the wound. Tape is used to secure most dressings in place. Most tape used in first aid and EMS kits today is made of silk, paper, or plastic because some patients are allergic to adhesive tape.

Types of Bandages

Objective 40

Fingertip and knuckle bandages are adhesive strips that are a sterile dressing and bandage combination. A knuckle bandage is made of cloth and shaped like an H. This type of bandage is useful for covering minor cuts or abrasions on a knuckle, elbow, heel, or chin.

Roller gauze (often called by the brand name *Kling*) is wrapped around and around a dressing to secure it in place. This type of bandage comes in different widths and lengths (Figure 34-49). Pick a roller bandage width that is appropriate for the body part to be bandaged. A 1-inch roll is used to bandage fingers, and a 2-inch roll is used for wrists, hands, and feet. A 3-inch roll can be used for elbows and upper arms. A 4- to 6-inch roll is used for ankles, knees, and legs.

A roller bandage (often called by the brand name *Kerlix*) is made of soft, slightly elastic material and is available in various widths (Figure 34-50). Elastic bandages (such as an Ace bandage or elastic wrap) should not be used to secure a dressing in place (Figure 34-51). If the injured area swells, the elastic bandage may act as a

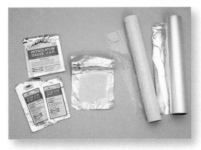

FIGURE 34-46 ▲ An occlusive dressing is used to cover an open wound and create an airtight seal. This type of dressing is made of nonporous material. Although commercially made occlusive dressings are available, plastic wrap or aluminum foil may also be used.

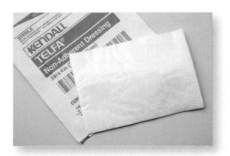

FIGURE 34-47 ▲ Nonadherent pads are used to cover an open wound but not stick to it.

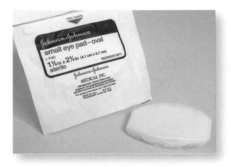

FIGURE 34-48 ▲ Eye pads are used to cover the eyes after a minor eye injury.

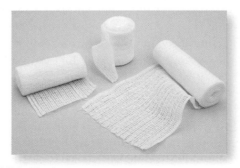

FIGURE 34-49 ▲ Roller gauze.

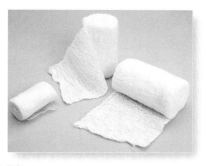

FIGURE 34-50 ▲ Roller bandage.

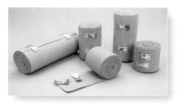

FIGURE 34-51 ▲ Elastic bandage.

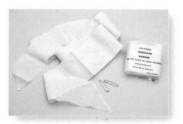

FIGURE 34-52 ▲ Triangular bandage.

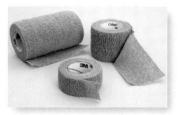

FIGURE 34-53 ▲ Coban is a self-adherent elastic wrap.

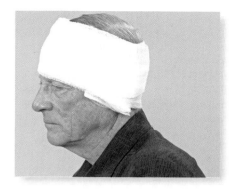

FIGURE 34-54 ▲ Head or ear bandage.

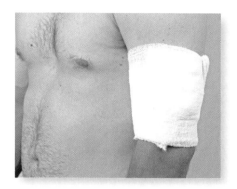

FIGURE 34-55 ▲ Upper arm bandage.

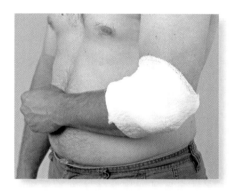

FIGURE 34-56 ▲ Elbow bandage.

tourniquet. A triangular bandage is a large piece of muslin that can be folded and used as a bandage or sling (Figure 34-52). A triangular bandage that has been folded is called a *cravat*.

Coban and Kimberly-Clark self-adherent wrap are elastic wraps coated with a self-adhering material that functions like tape (Figure 34-53). No pins or clips are required to hold the bandage in place. This type of bandage is often used as a pressure bandage.

A pressure bandage is a bandage with which enough pressure is applied over a wound site to control bleeding.

To apply a pressure bandage:
- Cover the wound with several sterile gauze dressings or a bulky dressing.

- Apply direct pressure to the wound until bleeding is controlled.
- Secure the dressing firmly in place with a bandage. Assess the patient's pulse distal to the bandage.
- If possible, do not cover fingers or toes so you can determine if the bandage is too tight. A bandage may be too tight if the fingers or toes become cold to the touch, the fingers or toes begin to turn pale or blue, or the patient complains of numbness in the extremity.

Skill Drill 34-1 shows the steps used to apply a roller bandage. Figures 34-54 through 34-59 show the bandaging techniques for different soft tissue injuries.

Applying a Roller Bandage

STEP 1 ▶ Start below the wound and work upward, applying the bandage directly over the sterile dressing on the wound.

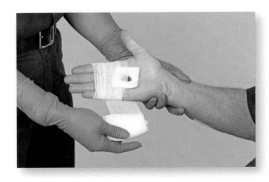

STEP 2 ▶ Using overlapping turns, cover the dressing completely. Unless the fingers are injured, leave them exposed so that you can assess circulation.

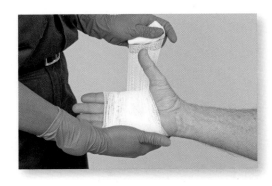

STEP 3 ▶ Tape or tie the bandage in place.

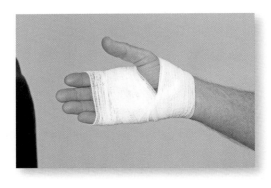

STEP 4 ▶ To make sure the bandage is not too tight, check a pulse distal to the wound site, the color of the fingers, and the temperature of the skin.

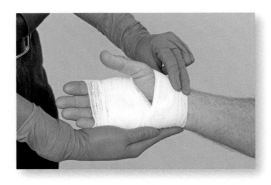

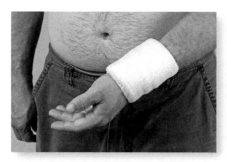

FIGURE 34-57 ▲ Wrist or forearm bandage.

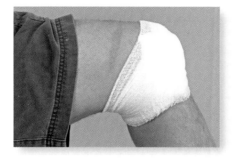

FIGURE 34-58 ▲ Knee bandage.

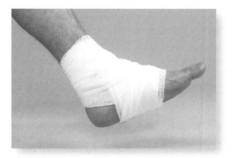

FIGURE 34-59 ▲ Foot or ankle bandage.

On the Scene   Wrap-Up

The estimated time of arrival for the helicopter is 5 minutes. You cover the patient with a clean sheet and then a warm blanket. He is responsive to painful stimulus only. His vital signs are blood pressure 104/70, pulse 128, respirations 24. As you continue your assessment, you can hear wheezing in his lungs. You are worried about his right arm because his fingers are pale and cold and you cannot feel a radial pulse in that arm. As the aircraft lands, the patient's breathing rate increases. He is using neck muscles to breathe, and he is making a high-pitched noise with each inhalation. The flight crew springs into action. They start an IV, give him some drugs, and place a breathing tube before they move him to the helicopter. As they lift off, your partner shakes his head, commenting, "When will people learn that they can't smoke in bed?" ■

Sum It Up

▶ The skin is the body's first line of defense against bacteria and other organisms, ultraviolet rays from the sun, harmful chemicals, and cuts and tears.

▶ A wound is an injury to soft tissues. A closed wound occurs when the soft tissues under the skin are damaged but the surface of the skin is not broken (for example, a bruise). An open wound results when the skin surface is broken (for example, a cut or scrape).

▶ Hemorrhage (also called major bleeding) is an extreme loss of blood from a blood vessel. It is a life-threatening condition that requires *immediate* attention. If it is not controlled, hemorrhage can lead to shock and potentially to death.

▶ Hemophilia is a disorder in which the blood does not clot normally. A person with hemophilia may have major bleeding from minor injuries and may bleed for no apparent reason. Some medications or a serious injury may also prevent effective clotting.

▶ Arterial bleeding is the most serious type of bleeding. The blood from an artery is bright red, oxygen-rich blood. A bleeding artery can quickly lead to the loss of a large amount of blood.

▶ Venous bleeding is usually easier to control than arterial bleeding because it is under less pressure. Blood lost from a vein flows as a steady stream and is dark red or maroon because it is oxygen-poor blood.

▶ Capillary bleeding is common because the walls of the capillaries are fragile and many are close to the skin's surface. Bleeding from capillaries is usually dark red. When a capillary is torn, blood oozes slowly from the site of the injury because the pressure within the capillaries is low. Capillary bleeding often clots and stops by itself within a few minutes.

▶ External bleeding is bleeding that you can see. Clotting normally occurs within minutes. However, external bleeding must be controlled with your gloved hands and dressings until a clot is formed and the bleeding has stopped.

▶ You *must* wear PPE when you anticipate exposure to blood or other potentially infectious material. HIV and the hepatitis virus are examples of diseases to which you may be exposed that can be transmitted by exposure to blood.

▶ Three methods may be used to control external bleeding. You must know the methods of external bleeding control that are approved by medical direction and your local protocol.

- Applying direct pressure slows blood flow and allows clotting to take place.
- A splint is a device used to limit the movement of an injured arm or leg and reduce bleeding. After applying the splint, make sure to check the patient's fingers (or toes) often for color, warmth, and feeling. A pressure splint (also called an air or pneumatic splint) can help control bleeding from soft tissue injuries or broken bones. It can also help stabilize a broken bone.
- A tourniquet is a tight bandage that surrounds an arm or a leg. It is used to stop the flow of blood in an extremity. A tourniquet should be used to control life-threatening bleeding in an arm or a leg when you cannot control the bleeding with direct pressure.

▶ Internal bleeding is bleeding that occurs inside body tissues and cavities. A bruise is a collection of blood under the skin caused by bleeding capillaries. A bruise is an example of internal bleeding that is not life-threatening.

▶ Closed soft tissue injuries occur because of blunt trauma. In blunt trauma, a forceful impact occurs to the body, but there is no break in the skin. In a closed soft tissue injury, there is no actual break in the skin, but the tissues and vessels may be crushed or ruptured. When assessing a closed soft tissue injury, it is important to evaluate surface damage and consider possible damage to the organs and major vessels beneath the area of impact.

▶ Closed soft tissue injuries include contusions, hematomas, and crush injuries. A contusion is a bruise. In a contusion, the epidermis remains intact. Cells are damaged, and blood vessels are torn in the dermis. Localized swelling and pain are typically present. A buildup of blood causes discoloration (ecchymosis). A hematoma is the collection of blood beneath the skin. A larger amount of tissue is damaged compared with a contusion. Larger blood vessels are damaged. Hematomas frequently occur with trauma sufficient to break bones. Crush injuries are caused by a crushing force applied to the body. These injuries can cause internal organ rupture. Internal bleeding may be severe and lead to shock.

▶ Compartment syndrome is a compression injury. It develops when the pressure within a compartment causes compression and abnormal function of nerves and blood vessels. Unless the pressure is relieved within 6 to 8 hours, permanent nerve and muscle damage can result, leading to paralysis, loss of the limb, or even death.

▶ Crush syndrome can occur when a large amount of skeletal muscle is compressed for a long period.

Crush syndrome should be considered when three criteria exist:

1. Involvement of a large amount of muscle
2. Compression of the muscle mass for a long period (usually 4 to 6 hours, although it may be as little as 1 hour)
3. Compromised local blood flow

▶ In open soft tissue injuries, a break occurs in the continuity of the skin. Because of the break in the skin, open injuries are susceptible to external hemorrhage and infection. In an abrasion, the outermost layer of skin (epidermis) is damaged by shearing forces (e.g., rubbing or scraping). A laceration is a break in the skin of varying depth. A laceration may be linear (regular) or stellate (irregular). Lacerations may occur in isolation or with other types of soft tissue injury. A puncture results when the skin is pierced with a pointed object, such as a nail, pencil, ice pick, splinter, piece of glass, bullet, or knife. An object that remains embedded in the open wound is called an impaled object. In an avulsion, a flap of skin or tissue is torn loose or pulled completely off. In a degloving avulsion injury, the skin and fatty tissue are stripped away. In an amputation, extremities or other body parts are severed from the body. In an open crush injury, soft tissue and internal organs are damaged. These injuries may cause painful, swollen, deformed extremities. Internal bleeding may be severe.

▶ An evisceration occurs when an organ sticks out through an open wound. In providing care, do not touch the exposed organ or try to place it back into the body. Carefully remove clothing from around the wound. Lightly cover the exposed organ and wound with a thick, moist dressing. Secure the dressing in place with a large bandage to keep moisture in and prevent heat loss.

▶ An impaled object is an object that remains embedded in an open wound. Do not remove an impaled object unless it interferes with CPR or is impaled through the cheek and interferes with care of the patient's airway. Control bleeding and stabilize the object with bulky dressings, bandaging them in place. Assess the patient for signs of shock, and treat if present.

▶ In the case of an amputated body part, control bleeding at the stump. In most cases, direct pressure will be enough to control the bleeding. Ask an assistant to find the amputated part, as it may be possible to reattach it at the hospital. Put the amputated part in a dry plastic bag or waterproof container. Carefully seal the bag or container, and place it in water that contains a few ice cubes.

- There are three categories of burns:
  - A superficial (first-degree) burn affects only the epidermis. It results in only minor tissue damage (such as sunburn). The skin is red, tender, and very painful. This type of burn does not usually require medical care and heals in 2 to 5 days with no scarring.
  - A partial-thickness (second-degree) burn involves the epidermis and dermis. The hair follicles and sweat glands are spared in this degree of burn. A partial-thickness burn produces intense pain and some swelling. Blistering may be present. The skin appears pink, red, or mottled and is sensitive to air current and pressure. This type of burn usually heals within 5 to 34 days. Scarring may or may not occur, depending on the depth of the burn.
  - A full-thickness (third-degree) burn destroys both the epidermis and dermis and may include subcutaneous tissue, muscle, and bone. The color of the patient's skin may vary from yellow or pale to black. The skin has a dry, waxy, or leathery appearance. Because the skin is so severely damaged in this type of burn, it cannot perform its usual protective functions. Rapid fluid loss often occurs. Be ready to treat the patient for shock.
- The rule of nines is a guide used to estimate the total body surface area burned. The rule of nines divides the adult body into sections that are 9% or are multiples of 9%. This guideline has also been modified for children and infants. To estimate the extent of a burn by using the rule of nines, add the percentages of the areas burned.
- A dressing is an absorbent material placed directly over a wound. A bandage is used to secure a dressing in place. A pressure bandage is a bandage applied with enough pressure over a wound site to control bleeding. Dressings and bandages serve the following functions:
  - Help to stop bleeding
  - Absorb blood and other drainage from the wound
  - Protect the wound from further injury
  - Reduce contamination and the risk of infection

Chest Trauma

By the end of this chapter, you should be able to:

Knowledge Objectives ▶

1. List the contents of the chest cavity.
2. List five deadly chest injuries and two potentially deadly chest injuries.
3. List two classifications of chest injuries.
4. Describe the causes, assessment findings, symptoms, and emergency care for rib fractures.
5. Describe the causes, assessment findings, symptoms, and emergency care for flail chest.
6. Describe the causes, assessment findings, symptoms, and emergency care for simple pneumothorax.
7. Describe the causes, assessment findings, symptoms, and emergency care for tension pneumothorax.
8. Describe the causes, assessment findings, symptoms, and emergency care for hemothorax.
9. Describe the causes, assessment findings, symptoms, and emergency care for cardiac tamponade.
10. Describe the causes, assessment findings, symptoms, and emergency care for traumatic asphyxia.
11. Describe the causes, assessment findings, symptoms, and emergency care for pulmonary contusion.
12. Describe the causes, assessment findings, symptoms, and emergency care for myocardial contusion.
13. Describe commotio cordis, including common causes and signs and symptoms of this condition.
14. Describe the causes, assessment findings, symptoms, and emergency care for open pneumothorax.

Attitude Objective ▶

15. Understand the importance of quickly assessing and treating chest injuries.

Skill Objectives ▶

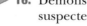

16. Demonstrate assessment and appropriate emergency care of a patient with a suspected chest injury.
17. Demonstrate completing a prehospital care report for patients with injuries to the chest.

You and your emergency medical technician partner are called to a private residence for a "fall injury." You arrive to find an 81-year-old man lying on the floor in his living room. The patient's wife tells you that she was helping her husband to the bathroom when he suddenly felt weak and fell to the floor, hitting the left side of his chest on the tile floor. The patient is awake, alert, and oriented to person, place, time, and event. You note that his left arm is in a cast. He explains that the cast is the result of a fall 2 days ago. The patient and his wife assure you that he did not hit his head today or lose consciousness. However, the patient did hit his head when he fell 2 days ago.

Using your stethoscope, you hear wheezes on the right side of the chest. Breath sounds are clear on the left side. Palpation of his left rib cage elicits pain, but no instability. The patient says he has had a "terrible headache" all day. He mentions that he had a heart attack 10 years ago, and now takes a "heart pill" daily. His blood pressure is 192/78, pulse 58 (strong and regular). His skin is pink, warm, and dry. His respiratory rate is 36. ∎

THINK ABOUT IT

As you read this chapter, think about the following questions:

- What type of chest injury has this patient sustained?
- After carefully evaluating the patient's vital signs and the historical information he provided, what are possible causes of his headache?
- What additional assessment and care will you need to perform?

Introduction

In this chapter we discuss the types of injuries that may result from trauma to the chest. You must know when to suspect these injuries and how to provide appropriate care.

Anatomy of the Chest Cavity

Objective 1

The chest is the upper part of the trunk between the diaphragm and the neck. It contains the mediastinum and pleural cavities. The mediastinum is the area between the lungs that extends from the sternum to the vertebral column. The mediastinum includes all the contents of the chest cavity (except the lungs), including the esophagus, trachea, heart, and large blood vessels. The right lung is in the right pleural cavity; the left lung is in the left pleural cavity.

The organs of the chest are protected by the rib cage and the upper portion of the spine (Figure 35-1). The rib cage includes the ribs, thoracic vertebrae, and the sternum. The ribs are connected to the vertebrae in back. All but two pairs of ribs are connected by cartilage to the sternum in the front. The rib cage encloses the lungs and heart. Damage to the ribs can result in damage to these organs.

Categories of Chest Injuries

Objectives 2, 3

Some injuries to the chest are immediately life-threatening and must be identified in the primary survey (Table 35-1). Others are potentially life-threatening and need to be identified during the secondary survey.

Chest injuries are categorized as closed or open injuries. In closed chest injuries, no break occurs in the skin over the chest wall. These injuries are usually the result of blunt trauma, such as the chest hitting the steering wheel during a motor vehicle crash. Underlying structures, such as the heart, lungs, and great vessels, may sustain significant injury. In open

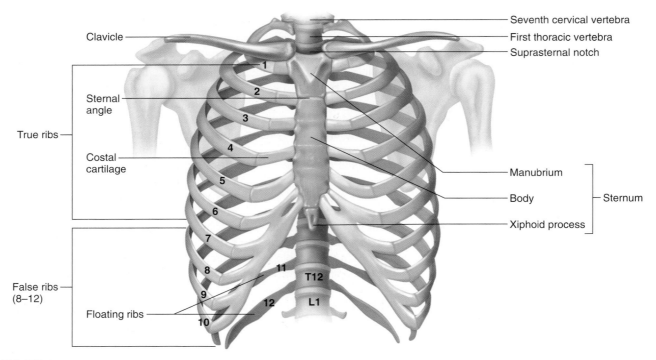

FIGURE 35-1 ▲ The rib cage and upper portion of the spine provide protection for the organs of the chest.

TABLE 35-1 Deadly and Potentially Deadly Chest Injuries	
Deadly Chest Injuries	**Potentially Deadly Chest Injuries**
Tension pneumothorax	Pulmonary contusion
Open pneumothorax	Myocardial contusion
Massive hemothorax	
Cardiac tamponade	
Flail chest	

chest injuries, a break occurs in the skin over the chest wall. These injuries result from penetrating trauma, such as a gunshot wound, a stabbing, or an impaled object.

Closed Chest Injuries

Rib Fractures

Objective 4

Rib fractures are a common injury resulting from blunt trauma to the chest. The presence of a rib fracture suggests significant force caused the injury. Rib fractures may be associated with injury to the underlying lung or the heart.

Although seat belts have reduced the number of deaths and the severity of injuries resulting from motor vehicle crashes (MVCs), they occasionally cause injury. For example, a properly worn three-point restraint harness can result in rib fractures (Figure 35-2). Lap belts can cause lumbar fractures and abdominal injuries, such as bruising or rupture of the intestines.

The seriousness of a rib fracture increases with age, the number of fractures, and the location of the fracture. Children are less likely to sustain rib fractures than adults are because a child's chest wall is more flexible than that of an adult. Rib fractures most commonly occur in older adults because the ribs of an older adult are more brittle and rigid.

Ribs 1–3 are protected by the shoulder girdle. Fractures of ribs 1 and 2 are associated with significant trauma. These fractures are often associated

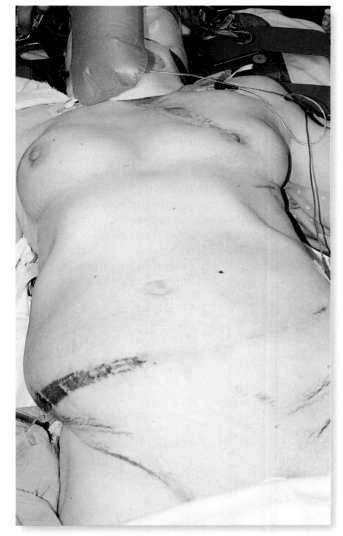

FIGURE 35-2 ▲ This patient experienced multiple rib fractures and bruising of the small intestine from a three-point seat belt injury.

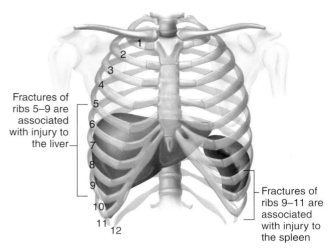

Fractures of ribs 5–9 are associated with injury to the liver

Fractures of ribs 9–11 are associated with injury to the spleen

FIGURE 35-3 ▲ Consider the possibility of injury to underlying structures with lower rib fractures. For example, fractures of ribs 9–11 on the left are associated with rupture of the spleen. Fractures of ribs 5–9 on the right are associated with injury to the liver.

finding is the patient's attempt to "splint" the injury because of pain. The patient's pain is usually localized to the injured area and increases when she breathes deeply, coughs, or moves. The patient may breathe shallowly to decrease the pain associated with breathing. You may notice a crackling sensation under your fingers while assessing the patient's chest. This finding is called *subcutaneous emphysema* and represents trapped air between layers of skin. You may hear and feel **crepitus,** a grating sound produced by bone fragments rubbing together. Other signs and symptoms of a rib fracture are listed in the following *You Should Know* box.

with injury to the head, neck, spinal cord, lungs, and the major blood vessels. Ribs 4–9 are the most commonly fractured because these ribs are long, thin, and poorly protected. Fractures of ribs 5–9 on the right are associated with injury to the liver (Figure 35-3). Also consider the possibility of injury to underlying structures with lower rib fractures. For example, fractures of ribs 9–11 on the left are associated with rupture of the spleen. Multiple rib fractures may result in inadequate breathing and pneumonia. Posterior rib fractures are usually the result of deceleration accidents.

When assessing the chest of a responsive patient who has a rib fracture, you may notice that the patient holds her arm close to her chest. This common

You Should Know

Assessment Findings and Symptoms of Rib Fracture

- Localized pain at the fracture site that worsens with deep breathing, coughing, or moving
- Self-splinting of the injury by holding the arm close to the chest
- Pain on inspiration
- Shallow breathing
- Tenderness on palpation
- Deformity of the chest wall
- Crepitus
- Swelling and/or bruising at the fracture site
- Possible subcutaneous emphysema

To treat a patient with a rib fracture, perform the following steps:

- Put on appropriate personal protective equipment.
- If spinal injury is suspected, maintain manual in-line stabilization until the patient is secured to a long backboard. Establish and maintain an open airway.
- Assess the adequacy of ventilation and the presence of hypoxemia. Because inadequate ventilation can result in the collapse of alveoli, which can lead to pneumonia, encourage the patient to cough and breathe deeply while recognizing that the patient will experience discomfort when doing so. Reassess breath sounds often while the patient is in your care.
- Give oxygen. If the patient's breathing is adequate, apply oxygen by nonrebreather mask at 10 to 15 L/min if not already done. If the patient's breathing is inadequate, provide positive-pressure ventilation with 100% oxygen. Assess the adequacy of the ventilations delivered.
- Do not apply tape or straps to the ribs or chest wall. Applying tape or straps limits chest wall motion and reduces the effectiveness of ventilation.
- Allow the patient to hold a pillow for comfort, if appropriate. Self-splinting will reduce pain, and a pillow will not provide excessive pressure to reduce ventilatory effectiveness. It also encourages deeper breathing, since the chest wall expands into the soft, padded surface.
- Reassess as often as indicated.
- Record all patient care information, including the patient's medical history and all emergency care given, on a prehospital care report.

Flail Chest

Objective 5

A **flail chest** occurs when two or more adjacent ribs are fractured in two or more places or when the sternum is detached (Figure 35-4). The section of the chest wall between the fractured ribs becomes free-floating because it is no longer in continuity with the thorax. This free-floating section of the chest wall is called the **flail segment.** The flail segment does not move with the rest of the rib cage when the patient attempts to breathe **(paradoxical chest movement).** When the patient inhales, the flail segment is drawn inward instead of moving outward (Figure 35-5). When the patient exhales, the flail segment moves outward instead of moving inward.

A flail chest is a life-threatening injury. Flail chest most commonly occurs in MVCs (especially crushing rollover crashes) but may also occur because of:

- Falls from a height
- Assault
- Industrial accidents
- Neonatal trauma during childbirth

The forces necessary to produce a flail chest cause bruising of the underlying lung (pulmonary contusion). Although instability of the chest wall results in paradoxical movement of the chest wall during breathing, it is the bruising of the underlying lung and pain associated with breathing that contributes to hypoxia.

Respiratory failure may occur because of:

- Bruising of the underlying lung and associated hemorrhage of the alveoli, reducing the amount of lung tissue available for gas exchange

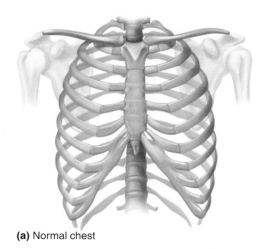

(a) Normal chest

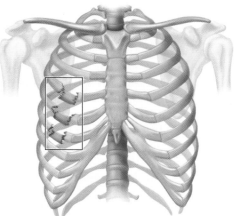

(b) Flail chest occurs when two or more adjacent ribs fracture in two or more places

FIGURE 35-4 ▲ **(a)** Normal chest; **(b)** flail segment.

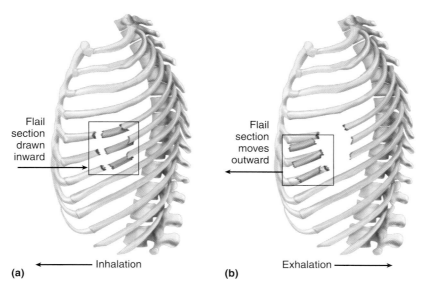

FIGURE 35-5 ▲ Paradoxical chest movement. **(a)** When the patient inhales, the flail segment is drawn inward instead of moving outward. **(b)** When the patient exhales, the flail segment moves outward instead of moving inward.

- Instability of the chest wall and pain associated with breathing, leading to decreased ventilation and hypoxia
- Interference with the normal bellows action of the chest, resulting in inadequate gas exchange

A flail chest may be associated with other injuries, including:

- Bruising of the underlying lung (pulmonary contusion)
- Bruising of the heart muscle (myocardial contusion)
- Hemothorax
- Pneumothorax

You Should Know

Assessment Findings and Symptoms of Flail Chest

- Crepitus
- Breathing difficulty
- Bruising of the chest wall
- Increased heart rate (tachycardia)
- Decreased or absent breath sounds on the affected side
- Pain and self-splinting of the affected side
- Increased respiratory rate (tachypnea)
- Pain in the chest associated with breathing
- Paradoxical chest wall movement

To treat a patient with a flail chest, perform the following steps:

- Put on appropriate PPE. Keep on-scene time to a minimum. Request an early response of advanced life support (ALS) personnel to the scene, or consider an ALS intercept while en route to the receiving facility. Do not delay transport for ALS arrival.
- Suspect associated spinal injuries. Maintain manual in-line stabilization until the patient is secured to a long backboard.
- Establish and maintain an open airway.
- Give oxygen. If the patient's breathing is adequate, apply oxygen by nonrebreather mask at 10 to 15 L/min if not already done. If the patient's breathing is inadequate, provide positive-pressure ventilation with 100% oxygen. Assess the adequacy of the ventilations delivered. Monitor closely for development of a tension pneumothorax (discussed later in this chapter).
- Continually monitor and reassess breath sounds, respiratory rate, rhythm, depth, and effort; vital signs (including pulse oximetry); degree of paradoxical chest movement; and skin temperature, color, and condition (moisture).
- Treat for shock if indicated.
- Transport promptly to the closest appropriate facility. Reassess, including vital signs, at least every 5 minutes en route.
- Record all patient care information, including the patient's medical history and all emergency care given, on a PCR.

- Paradoxical chest movement is probably most readily seen in an unresponsive patient. In patients with thick or muscular chest walls, it may be difficult to observe paradoxical movement. In some conscious patients, spasm and self-splinting of the chest muscles may cause paradoxical motion to go unnoticed.
- Studies show that many patients who have a flail chest injury have long-term problems, including ongoing chest wall pain, deformity, and difficulty breathing with exertion.

Simple Pneumothorax

Objective 6

A pneumothorax is a collection of air or gas outside the lung and between the lung and the chest wall. In a **simple pneumothorax,** air enters the chest cavity, causing a loss of negative pressure (vacuum) and a partial or total collapse of the lung (Figure 35-6). A simple pneumothorax may occur because of blunt or penetrating chest trauma. For instance, a simple pneumothorax may occur because of a blast injury or diving accident. Air may also enter the chest cavity through a hole in the chest wall (sucking chest wound) or a hole in the lung tissue, bronchus, or trachea. As air enters and fills the pleural space, lung tissue is compressed. This reduces the amount of lung tissue available for gas exchange.

The patient's signs and symptoms depend on the size of the pneumothorax and the patient's general health. Small tears may self-seal, resolving by themselves. The patient may not experience difficulty breathing or other signs of respiratory distress. Larger tears may progress, resulting in signs and symptoms of respiratory distress. Signs and symptoms of a simple pneumothorax are shown in the following *You Should Know* box.

Assessment Findings and Symptoms of Simple Pneumothorax

- Sudden onset of sharp pain in the chest associated with breathing
- Shortness of breath
- Difficulty breathing
- Decreased or absent breath sounds on the affected side
- Increased respiratory rate (tachypnea)
- Increased heart rate (tachycardia)
- Subcutaneous emphysema (may not be present)

A **spontaneous pneumothorax** is a type of pneumothorax that does not involve trauma to the lung. There are two types of spontaneous pneumothorax. A **primary spontaneous pneumothorax** occurs in people with no history of lung disease. This condition most commonly occurs in tall, thin men between the ages of 20 and 40. It rarely occurs in persons older than 40 years. A **secondary spontaneous pneumothorax** most often occurs as a complication of lung disease. Chronic obstructive pulmonary disease (COPD) is the most common underlying disorder. Other lung diseases associated with this condition include asthma, pneumonia, tuberculosis, and lung cancer. A secondary spontaneous pneumothorax usually occurs in older persons. A spontaneous pneumothorax typically occurs while the patient is at rest or during sleep. It is usually caused by the rupture of a **bleb** (a small air- or fluid-filled sac) in the lung. Although they depend on the size of the pneumothorax, common signs and symptoms include a sudden onset of chest pain on the affected side, shortness of breath, an increased respiratory rate, and a cough. The patient's chest pain may be described as dull, sharp, or stabbing.

To treat a patient with a pneumothorax, perform the following steps:
- Put on appropriate PPE.
- If spinal injury is suspected, maintain manual in-line stabilization until the patient is secured to a long backboard. If spinal injury is not suspected, place the patient in a position of comfort. Most patients will be more comfortable sitting up.
- Establish and maintain an open airway.

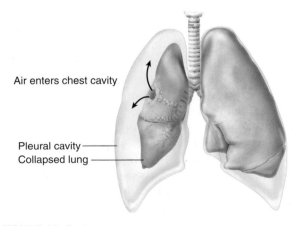

Air enters chest cavity

Pleural cavity

Collapsed lung

FIGURE 35-6 ▲ In a simple pneumothorax, air enters the chest cavity, causing a loss of negative pressure and a partial or total collapse of the lung.

- Give oxygen. If the patient's breathing is adequate, apply oxygen by nonrebreather mask at 10 to 15 L/min if not already done. If the patient's breathing is inadequate, provide positive-pressure ventilation with 100% oxygen. Assess the adequacy of the ventilations delivered.
- Transport promptly to the closest appropriate facility. Reassess breath sounds, respiratory rate, rhythm, depth, and effort, and vital signs as often as indicated. Reassess frequently for signs of a tension pneumothorax (explained in the next section).
- Record all patient care information, including the patient's medical history and all emergency care given, on a PCR.

Tension Pneumothorax

Objective 7

Tension pneumothorax is a life-threatening injury. It can occur because of blunt or penetrating trauma or as a complication of treatment of an open pneumothorax. In an *open pneumothorax*, there is an open wound in the chest wall into the pleural cavity. In a tension pneumothorax, air enters the pleural cavity during inspiration and progressively builds up under pressure. The flap of injured lung acts as a one-way valve, allowing air to enter the pleural space during inspiration but trapping it during expiration. The injured lung collapses completely. Pressure rises, forcing the trachea, heart, and major blood vessels to be pushed toward the opposite side (Figure 35-7). Shifting of the trachea from its normal midline position is called *tracheal deviation*

(or *tracheal shift*). In a tension pneumothorax, the trachea shifts to the uninjured lung (the side opposite the injury). To effectively assess tracheal deviation, examine the trachea by feeling for the tubular shape of the trachea between your thumb and index finger just above the sternum in the suprasternal notch. Assessing above this area for tracheal deviation may not reveal a shift of the trachea even if it does exist. Because significant pressure must build up to cause tracheal deviation, it is a late physical examination finding. Shifting of the heart and major blood vessels from their normal position is called **mediastinal shift.** Shifting of the major blood vessels causes them to kink, resulting in a backup of blood into the venous system. The backup of blood into the venous system results in jugular venous distention (JVD), decreased blood return to the heart, and signs of shock. Signs and symptoms of a tension pneumothorax are listed in the following *You Should Know* box.

You Should Know

Assessment Findings and Symptoms of Tension Pneumothorax

- Cool, clammy skin
- Increased pulse rate
- Cyanosis (late sign)
- JVD
- Decreased blood pressure
- Severe respiratory distress
- Agitation, restlessness, anxiety
- Possible visible chest wall trauma
- Bulging of intercostal muscles on the affected side
- Decreased or absent breath sounds on the affected side
- Tracheal deviation toward the unaffected side (late sign)
- Possible subcutaneous emphysema in the face, neck, or chest wall

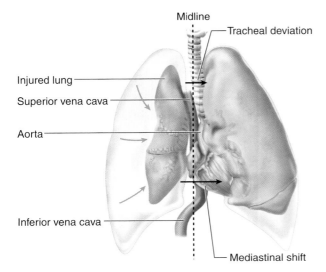

FIGURE 35-7 ▲ In a tension pneumothorax, air enters the pleural cavity during inspiration and progressively builds up under pressure.

Follow these steps when providing emergency care for a possible tension pneumothorax:
- Put on appropriate PPE. Keep on-scene time to a minimum. Request an early response of ALS personnel to the scene, or consider an ALS intercept while en route to the receiving facility. Do not delay transport for ALS arrival.
- If spinal injury is suspected, maintain manual in-line stabilization until the patient is secured to a long backboard.
- Establish and maintain an open airway.

- Give oxygen. If the patient's breathing is adequate, apply oxygen by nonrebreather mask at 10 to 15 L/min if not already done. If the patient's breathing is inadequate, provide positive-pressure ventilation with 100% oxygen and assess the adequacy of the ventilations delivered.

- Treat for shock if indicated.

- If an open chest wound was bandaged with an occlusive dressing, release the dressing. If air is present under tension, air will rush out of the wound. Once the air is released, reseal the wound again with a dressing taped on three sides.

- Transport promptly to the closest appropriate facility, reassessing breath sounds, respiratory rate, rhythm, depth, and effort, and vital signs at least every 5 minutes en route.

- Record all patient care information, including the patient's medical history and all emergency care given, on a PCR.

Hemothorax

Objective 8

A **hemothorax** is a collection of blood in the pleural cavity that may result from injury to the chest wall, the major blood vessels, or the lung because of penetrating or blunt trauma (Figure 35-8). Rib fractures are a common cause of a hemothorax. A hemothorax is often seen with a simple or tension pneumothorax.

The chest cavity can hold 2,000–3,000 mL of blood. The term **massive hemothorax** is used to describe blood loss of more than 1,500 mL in the chest cavity. A massive hemothorax is a life-threatening injury. Signs and symptoms of hemothorax are listed in the following *You Should Know* box.

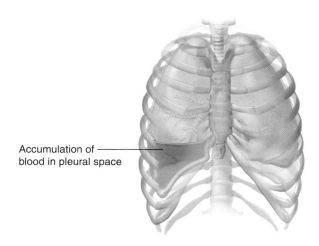

Accumulation of blood in pleural space

FIGURE 35-8 ▲ A hemothorax is a collection of blood in the pleural cavity.

Follow these steps when providing emergency care to a patient with a possible hemothorax:

- Put on appropriate PPE. Keep on-scene time to a minimum. Request an early response of ALS personnel to the scene, or consider an ALS intercept while en route to the receiving facility. Do not delay transport for ALS arrival.

- If spinal injury is suspected, maintain manual in-line stabilization until the patient is secured to a long backboard.

- Establish and maintain an open airway.

- Give oxygen. If the patient's breathing is adequate, apply oxygen by nonrebreather mask at 10 to 15 L/min if not already done. If the patient's breathing is inadequate, provide positive-pressure ventilation with 100% oxygen and assess the adequacy of the ventilations delivered.

- Treat for shock if indicated.

- Reassess frequently for development of a tension pneumothorax.

- Transport promptly to the closest appropriate facility, reassessing breath sounds, respiratory rate, rhythm, depth, and effort, and vital signs at least every 5 minutes en route.

- Record all patient care information, including the patient's medical history and all emergency care given, on a PCR.

Cardiac (Pericardial) Tamponade

Objective 9

Cardiac tamponade is a life-threatening injury. It most frequently occurs because of penetrating chest trauma, but it can occur because of blunt trauma to the chest.

You Should Know

Assessment Findings and Symptoms of Hemothorax

- Cool, clammy skin
- Weak, thready pulse
- Restlessness, agitation, anxiety
- Coughing up of blood (**hemoptysis**) (may not occur)
- Rapid, shallow breathing (tachypnea)
- Flat neck veins (caused by hypovolemia)
- Decreasing blood pressure (hypotension)
- Decreased or absent breath sounds on the affected side

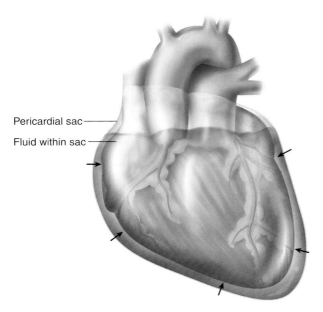

Pericardial sac
Fluid within sac

FIGURE 35-9 ▲ Cardiac tamponade occurs when blood enters the pericardial sac and compresses the heart. This decreases the amount of blood the heart can pump out with each contraction.

Cardiac tamponade occurs when blood enters the pericardial sac because of:

- Laceration of a coronary blood vessel
- Ruptured coronary artery
- Laceration of a chamber of the heart
- Significant bruising of the heart (myocardial contusion)

The blood in the pericardial sac compresses the heart, decreasing the amount of blood the heart can pump out with each contraction (Figure 35-9). The patient's signs and symptoms depend on how quickly blood collects in the pericardial sac. Signs and symptoms of cardiac tamponade are listed in the following *You Should Know* box.

You Should Know

Assessment Findings and Symptoms of Cardiac Tamponade

- Cool, clammy skin
- Normal breath sounds
- Narrowing pulse pressure
- Trachea in midline position
- Increased heart rate (tachycardia)
- Cyanosis of head, neck, and upper extremities
- Muffled heart sounds (often difficult to assess in the field)
- Distended neck veins (may not be present in hypovolemia)

Perform the following steps to treat a patient with suspected cardiac tamponade:

- Put on appropriate PPE. Keep on-scene time to a minimum. Request an early response of ALS personnel to the scene, or consider an ALS intercept while en route to the receiving facility. Do not delay transport for ALS arrival.
- If spinal injury is suspected, maintain manual in-line stabilization until the patient is secured to a long backboard.
- Establish and maintain an open airway.
- Give oxygen. If the patient's breathing is adequate, apply oxygen by nonrebreather mask at 10 to 15 L/min if not already done. If the patient's breathing is inadequate, provide positive-pressure ventilation with 100% oxygen and assess the adequacy of the ventilations delivered.
- Treat for shock if indicated.
- Transport promptly to the closest appropriate facility, reassessing breath sounds, respiratory rate, rhythm, depth, and effort, and vital signs at least every 5 minutes en route.
- Record all patient care information, including the patient's medical history and all emergency care given, on a PCR.

Traumatic Asphyxia

Objective 10

Traumatic asphyxia occurs because of a severe compression injury to the chest, such as compression of the chest under a heavy object or between a vehicle's seat and steering wheel. Blood backs up into the veins, venules, and capillaries of the head, neck, extremities, and upper torso, resulting in capillary rupture (Figure 35-10). The skin of the head and neck becomes deep red, purple, or blue. This characteristic finding is called *hooding* or a *purple cape* by EMS professionals. Signs and symptoms of traumatic asphyxia are shown in the following *You Should Know* box.

You Should Know

Assessment Findings and Symptoms of Traumatic Asphyxia

- JVD
- Swelling of the tongue and lips
- Eyes that appear bloodshot and bulging
- Deep red, purple, or blue discoloration of the head and neck (hooding, or purple cape)
- Low blood pressure once the compression is released
- Normal-looking pink skin below the level of the crush injury (unless other injuries are present)

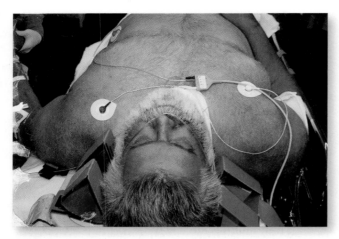

FIGURE 35-10 ▲ Traumatic asphyxia. This 45-year-old man was working under a truck when it fell on his chest. He was pinned under the truck and unable to breathe for 3 to 4 minutes until his coworkers rescued him. Note the discoloration of his upper body. The patient was observed in the hospital overnight and recovered with no complications.

To treat a patient with traumatic asphyxia, perform the following steps:

- Put on appropriate PPE. Keep on-scene time to a minimum. Request an early response of ALS personnel to the scene, or consider an ALS intercept while en route to the receiving facility. Do not delay transport for ALS arrival.
- Suspect spinal injuries and multiple organ damage. Maintain manual in-line stabilization until the patient is secured to a long backboard.
- Establish and maintain an open airway.
- Give oxygen. If the patient's breathing is adequate, apply oxygen by nonrebreather mask at 10 to 15 L/min if not already done. If the

patient's breathing is inadequate, provide positive-pressure ventilation with 100% oxygen. Assess the adequacy of the ventilations delivered.

- Control any bleeding, if present. If indicated, treat for shock.
- Transport promptly to the closest appropriate facility, reassessing breath sounds, respiratory rate, rhythm, depth, and effort, and vital signs at least every 5 minutes en route. Monitor closely for development of a tension pneumothorax and/or cardiac tamponade.
- Record all patient care information, including the patient's medical history and all emergency care given, on a PCR.

Pulmonary Contusion

Objective 11

A **pulmonary contusion** (bruising of the lung) is a potentially life-threatening injury. A pulmonary contusion occurs in about 75% of patients with flail chest. Most pulmonary contusions occur because of a rapid deceleration injury, such as a fall, high-speed MVC, or other blunt trauma. It can also occur as a result of blunt trauma without rib fracture. A pulmonary contusion is often missed because of the presence of other associated injuries.

In a pulmonary contusion, the alveoli fill with blood and fluid because of bruising of the lung tissue (Figure 35-11). As a result, the area of the lung available for gas exchange is decreased. The severity of the patient's signs and symptoms depends on the amount of lung tissue injured. Bleeding from a pulmonary contusion may result in a blood loss of 1,000–1,500 mL. Signs and symptoms of pulmonary contusion are shown in the next *You Should Know* box.

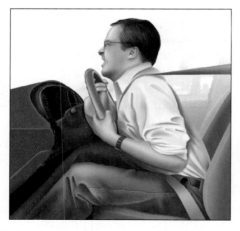

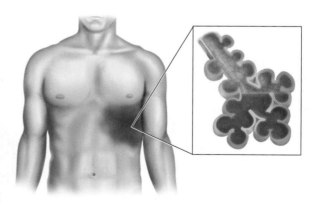

FIGURE 35-11 ▲ In a pulmonary contusion, the alveoli fill with blood and fluid because of bruising of the lung tissue.

Assessment Findings and Symptoms of Pulmonary Contusion

- Signs of blunt chest trauma
- Restlessness, anxiety
- Increased respiratory rate
- Increased heart rate
- Cough
- Coughing up of blood (hemoptysis)
- Chest pain
- Difficulty breathing
- Cyanosis

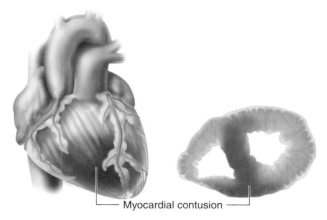

FIGURE 35-12 ▲ A myocardial contusion is a bruise of the heart.

To treat a patient with a suspected pulmonary contusion, perform the following steps:

- Put on appropriate PPE. Keep on-scene time to a minimum. Request an early response of ALS personnel to the scene, or consider an ALS intercept while en route to the receiving facility. Do not delay transport for ALS arrival.

- Suspect spinal injuries. Maintain manual in-line stabilization until the patient is secured to a long backboard.

- Establish and maintain an open airway.

- Give oxygen. If the patient's breathing is adequate, apply oxygen by nonrebreather mask at 10 to 15 L/min if not already done. If the patient's breathing is inadequate, provide positive-pressure ventilation with 100% oxygen. Assess the adequacy of the ventilations delivered.

- Treat for shock if indicated.

- Transport promptly to the closest appropriate facility, reassessing breath sounds, respiratory rate, rhythm, depth, and effort, and vital signs at least every 5 minutes en route.

- Record all patient care information, including the patient's medical history and all emergency care given, on a PCR.

Myocardial (Cardiac) Contusion

Objective 12

A **myocardial contusion** is bruising of the heart (Figure 35-12). It occurs because of blunt chest trauma, such as:

- Chest compressions during cardiopulmonary resuscitation (CPR)
- Acceleration or deceleration injuries
- Fractures of the sternum
- Fractures of ribs 1–3

A myocardial contusion is a potentially life-threatening injury. Signs and symptoms of a myocardial contusion include chest pain or discomfort, increased or slowed heart rate, and (possibly) an irregular heart rhythm.

To treat a patient with a suspected myocardial contusion, perform the following steps:

- Put on appropriate PPE. Keep on-scene time to a minimum. Request an early response of ALS personnel to the scene, or consider an ALS intercept while en route to the receiving facility. Do not delay transport for ALS arrival.

- Suspect spinal injuries. Maintain manual in-line stabilization until the patient is secured to a long backboard.

- Establish and maintain an open airway.

- Give oxygen. If the patient's breathing is adequate, apply oxygen by nonrebreather mask at 10 to 15 L/min if not already done. If the patient's breathing is inadequate, provide positive-pressure ventilation with 100% oxygen and assess the adequacy of the ventilations delivered.

- Treat for shock if indicated.

- Transport promptly to the closest appropriate facility, reassessing breath sounds, respiratory rate, rhythm, depth, and effort, and vital signs at least every 5 minutes en route.

- Record all patient care information, including the patient's medical history and all emergency care given, on a PCR.

Commotio Cordis

Objective 13

Commotio cordis (which means "disturbed or agitated heart motion") is sudden cardiac death due to a blunt force injury to the chest (directly over the left ventricle of the heart) without causing any significant structural injury to the heart. The blow to the chest occurs at a certain point of a person's heartbeat, causing ventricular fibrillation and sudden cardiac death. The speed of the blow typically ranges from 30 to 50 mph. Although cases of commotio cordis have been reported in individuals ranging from 3 months to 50 years of age, it occurs most frequently in males between 4 and 16 years of age, with an average age of 14 years.

Since 1996, more than 180 cases of commotio cordis have been reported in the United States. The impact to the chest is most often from a baseball, but it has also been reported during hockey, softball, lacrosse, karate, and other sports activities in which a relatively hard projectile or bodily contact caused impact to the individual's anterior chest. Infrequent cases have been associated with basketball, cricket, martial arts, boxing, and motor vehicle crashes. Interestingly, rare incidents of commotio cordis have been associated with playful shadow boxing, parent-to-child discipline, gang rituals, a snowball, a pet dog (collie) head, a plastic (hollow) toy bat, a hiccups remedy by a friend, and a fall on monkey bars.

Once the individual sustains a blow to the center of the chest, he may collapse immediately or walk a couple of steps and then collapse. The patient is typically found to be unresponsive, apneic, and pulseless. Many patients are cyanotic. Seizures have been observed in some individuals at the time of collapse. Bruising of the chest wall at the site of impact is present in about one-third of patients.

Survival is uncommon and is most dependent on early resuscitation (within 1 to 3 minutes of the event), including cardiopulmonary resuscitation and defibrillation. Delays in starting CPR generally occur because observers underestimate the severity of the blow or believe that the wind has been knocked out of the person. Widespread access to automated external defibrillators during organized sporting events and education of athletic trainers and coaches in their use are recommended by many sports-related organizations.

Open Chest Injuries

Open Pneumothorax

Objective 14

An **open pneumothorax** is also called a *sucking chest wound*. It is a life-threatening injury that is caused by penetrating trauma.

Possible causes of open pneumothorax include:
- Blast injuries
- Knife wounds

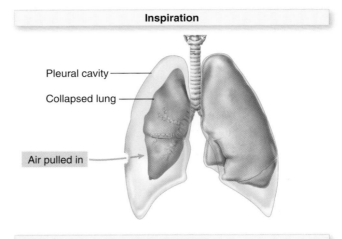

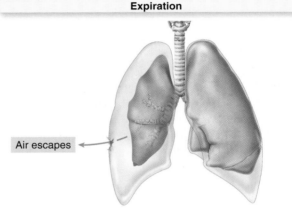

FIGURE 35-13 ▲ An open pneumothorax is a life-threatening injury that is caused by penetrating trauma.

- Impaled objects
- Gunshot wounds
- MVCs

Air enters the chest cavity through an open wound in the chest wall into the pleural cavity (Figure 35-13). The severity of an open pneumothorax depends on the size of the wound. If the diameter of the chest wound is more than two-thirds the diameter of the patient's trachea, air will enter the chest wound rather than through the trachea with each breath. A sucking or gurgling sound is heard as air moves in and out of the pleural space through the open chest wound. If the flap of chest wall closes during expiration, air will become trapped inside the pleural cavity. As air collects in the pleural cavity, pressure builds with each inspiration. This eventually results in a tension pneumothorax. Signs and symptoms of open pneumothorax are listed in the following *You Should Know* box.

Assessment Findings and Symptoms of Open Pneumothorax

- Shortness of breath
- Increased heart rate
- Pain at the site of injury
- Increased respiratory rate
- Subcutaneous emphysema
- Sucking sound on inhalation
- Open wound in the chest wall
- Decreased breath sounds on the affected side

To treat a patient with an open pneumothorax, perform the following steps:

- Put on appropriate PPE. Keep on-scene time to a minimum. Request an early response of ALS personnel to the scene, or consider an ALS intercept while en route to the receiving facility. Do not delay transport for ALS arrival.
- Suspect spinal injuries. Maintain manual in-line stabilization until the patient is secured to a long backboard.
- Establish and maintain an open airway.
- Promptly close the chest wound with an airtight (occlusive) dressing. Plastic wrap and petroleum gauze are examples of dressings that may be used. Make sure that the dressing is large enough so that it is not pulled into the wound during inspiration. Tape the dressing on three sides (one-way valve). The dressing will be sucked over the wound as the patient inhales, preventing air from entering. The open end of the dressing allows air to escape as the patient exhales. If signs and symptoms of a tension pneumothorax develop after an airtight dressing has been applied, release the dressing. Reassess the patient's airway, breathing, circulation, and mental status. If the patient's breathing returns to normal, replace the airtight dressing and again secure it in place over the wound by taping it in place on three sides.
- Give oxygen. If the patient's breathing is adequate, apply oxygen by nonrebreather mask at 10 to 15 L/min if not already done. If the patient's breathing is inadequate, provide positive-pressure ventilation with 100% oxygen. Assess the adequacy of the ventilations delivered. Watch closely for development of a tension pneumothorax.
- Control any external bleeding. Treat for shock if indicated.

- Transport promptly to the closest appropriate facility. Reassess breath sounds, respiratory rate, rhythm, depth, and effort, and vital signs at least every 5 minutes.
- Record all patient care information, including the patient's medical history and all emergency care given, on a PCR.

On the Scene   Wrap-Up

A repeat set of vital signs reveals the following: blood pressure 196/70, pulse 56, and respiration 32. You suspect the patient's chest injury is probably a bruised muscle over a rib or rib fracture. However, on the basis of your physical examination findings, the patient's complaint of a severe headache, and his vital signs, you suspect the patient may have a bigger problem—bleeding in his brain. The patient's vital signs are consistent with signs of increasing intracranial pressure. Possible causes include a subdural hematoma (most likely from the fall 2 days ago) or a stroke. Remember that a patient who has a subdural hematoma may appear as if he is having a stroke or is under the influence of drugs or alcohol. Using the Cincinnati Prehospital Stroke Scale, you note that the patient has no facial droop, his speech is clear, and he is able to hold his arms in front of him with no arm drift. You give oxygen, place the patient in a position of comfort, and transport him to the hospital. A few hours later, an emergency department nurse calls to compliment you for taking the time to look at the big picture and not only the patient's chest trauma. The patient was admitted to the hospital for a subdural hematoma. By recognizing the significance of the patient's abnormal vital signs, you definitely made a difference in his emergency care. ■

Sum It Up

► Chest injuries are categorized as closed or open injuries. In closed chest injuries, no break occurs in the skin over the chest wall. These injuries are usually the result of blunt trauma. Underlying structures, such as the heart, lungs, and great vessels, may sustain significant injury. In open chest injuries, a break occurs in the skin over the chest wall. These injuries result from penetrating trauma, such as a gunshot wound, stabbing, or an impaled object.

► Rib fractures are a common injury. Fractures of ribs 1 and 2 are associated with significant trauma. Fractures of ribs 9–11 on the left are associated with rupture of the spleen. Fractures of ribs 5–9 on the right are associated with injury to the liver.

- Flail chest occurs when two or more adjacent ribs are fractured in two or more places or when the sternum is detached. The section of the chest wall between the fractured ribs becomes free-floating because it is no longer in continuity with the thorax. This free-floating section of the chest wall is called a *flail segment*. The flail segment does not move with the rest of the rib cage when the patient attempts to breathe *(paradoxical movement)*.

- A pneumothorax is a collection of air or gas outside the lung, between the lung and the chest wall. In a simple pneumothorax, air enters the chest cavity, causing a loss of negative pressure and a partial or total collapse of the lung.

- A spontaneous pneumothorax is a type of pneumothorax that does not involve trauma to the lung. It is usually caused by the rupture of a bleb (a small air- or fluid-filled sac) in the lung. A primary spontaneous pneumothorax occurs in people with no history of lung disease. A secondary spontaneous pneumothorax most often occurs as a complication of lung disease, such as COPD, asthma, pneumonia, tuberculosis, or lung cancer.

- An open pneumothorax is also called a *sucking chest wound*.

- A tension pneumothorax is a life-threatening condition in which air enters the pleural cavity during inspiration and progressively builds up under pressure. The flap of injured lung acts as a one-way valve, allowing air to enter the pleural space during inspiration but trapping it during expiration. The injured lung collapses completely. Pressure rises, forcing the trachea, heart, and major blood vessels to be pushed toward the opposite side. Shifting of the major blood vessels causes them to kink, resulting in a backup of blood into the venous system. The backup of blood into the venous system results in JVD, decreased blood return to the heart, and signs of shock.

- A hemothorax is a collection of blood in the pleural cavity that may result from injury to the chest wall, the major blood vessels, or the lung because of penetrating or blunt trauma. A hemothorax is often seen with a simple or tension pneumothorax. A massive hemothorax is blood loss of more than 1,500 mL in the chest cavity.

- Cardiac tamponade usually occurs because of penetrating chest trauma, but it can also occur because of blunt trauma to the chest. Cardiac tamponade occurs when blood enters the pericardial sac. The blood in the pericardial sac compresses the heart, decreasing the amount of blood the heart can pump out with each contraction. The patient's signs and symptoms depend on how quickly blood collects in the pericardial sac.

- Traumatic asphyxia occurs because of a severe compression injury to the chest, such as compression of the chest under a heavy object or between a vehicle's seat and steering wheel. Blood backs up into the veins, venules, and capillaries of the head, neck, extremities, and upper torso, resulting in capillary rupture.

- A pulmonary contusion is bruising of the lung. In a pulmonary contusion, the alveoli fill with blood and fluid because of bruising of the lung tissue. As a result, the area of the lung available for gas exchange is decreased.

- A myocardial contusion is bruising of the heart muscle. Signs and symptoms of a myocardial contusion include chest pain or discomfort, increased heart rate, and (possibly) an irregular heart rhythm.

- Commotio cordis is sudden cardiac death due to a blunt force injury to the chest (directly over the left ventricle of the heart) without causing any significant structural injury to the heart. The impact to the chest is most often from a baseball, but it has also been reported during hockey, softball, lacrosse, karate, and other sports activities in which a relatively hard projectile or bodily contact caused impact to the individual's anterior chest. The patient is typically found to be unresponsive, apneic, and pulseless. Survival is most dependent on early resuscitation, including CPR and defibrillation.

- The severity of an open pneumothorax depends on the size of the wound. If the diameter of the chest wound is more than two-thirds the diameter of the patient's trachea, air will enter the chest wound rather than through the trachea with each breath. Promptly close the chest wound with an airtight (occlusive) dressing. Plastic wrap and petroleum gauze are examples of dressings that may be used. Make sure that the dressing is large enough so that it is not pulled into the wound during inspiration. Tape the dressing on three sides. If signs and symptoms of a tension pneumothorax develop after an airtight dressing has been applied, release the dressing.

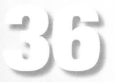
Abdominal and Genitourinary Trauma

By the end of this chapter, you should be able to:

Knowledge Objectives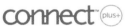

1. State the possible causes, signs, and symptoms of an abdominal injury.
2. Differentiate between closed and open abdominal injuries.
3. State the possible causes, signs, and symptoms of a genitourinary injury.
4. Describe the assessment and emergency care for a patient with a possible abdominal injury.
5. Describe the assessment and emergency care for a patient with injuries to the external male genitalia.
6. Describe the assessment and emergency care for a patient with injuries to the external female genitalia.

Attitude Objective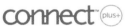

7. Understand the importance of quickly assessing and treating abdominal and genitourinary injuries.

Skill Objectives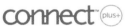

connect plus+

8. Demonstrate assessment of a patient with a suspected abdominal injury.
9. Demonstrate assessment of a patient with a suspected genitourinary injury.
10. Demonstrate assessment of a male patient with a suspected injury to the external genitalia.
11. Demonstrate assessment of a female patient with a suspected injury to the external genitalia.
12. Demonstrate completing a prehospital care report for patients with injuries to the gastrointestinal or genitourinary system.

On the Scene

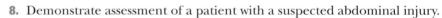

You respond to a report of an all-terrain vehicle (ATV) crash on one of the county roads in your first due area. After just 3 minutes, you are approaching the area where the accident occurred. Your partner is the first to notice skid marks in the dust of the roadway that lead right off the road on the edge of a steep embankment. After safely parking your vehicle, you and your partner approach the edge of the road. You are looking down a 20-foot embankment and can see a four-wheel ATV lying on one side in the area below. At the base of a large pine tree, you see a young man about 20 years of age sitting upright looking back at you. You and your partner scramble down the embankment with your equipment. As you get closer, you note that your patient appears to be holding his groin. As you kneel next to him, he tells you that he hit the tree with his "crotch." ■

THINK ABOUT IT

As you read this chapter, think about the following questions:

- Does this mechanism of injury involve blunt or penetrating trauma?
- What organs or organ systems may have been injured?
- What is the proper method to use to assess this patient's injuries?
- What additional resources are needed to properly care for this patient?

Introduction

Injuries to the abdomen and pelvis can result from blunt or penetrating trauma. Examples of common blunt-force mechanisms include motor vehicle crashes, falls, and assaults. Examples of penetrating forces include the use of guns and knives. Deaths from abdominal trauma result mainly from hemorrhage or infection. Trauma to the genitourinary system seldom occurs separately from trauma to other body systems and is most often associated with abdominal trauma. In this chapter we discuss common mechanisms of injury, assessment, and initial emergency care for the patient with abdominal or genitourinary trauma.

Abdominal Trauma

Objective 1

You should maintain an index of suspicion for abdominal trauma on the basis of the mechanism of injury (MOI).

Important information to consider regarding the MOI includes the following:
- Type of trauma (motor vehicle crash, fall injury, assault)
- Object involved during impact (bullet, knife, car, motorcycle, handlebars, tree)
- Energy exchanged (estimated speed of the vehicle at impact, size or caliber of gun, length of knife, distance of a fall)
- Restraints used (seat belts, airbags); protective gear used

In some situations, it will not always be clear if an injury to a patient's torso involves only the chest, only the abdomen, or both. For instance, suppose your patient has a stab wound in the area of the ninth rib on the right side of his body. Can you be sure that the damage inflicted by the knife blade is limited to the chest? No, for a couple of reasons. First, remember that the diaphragm divides the chest and abdominal cavities. However, the position of the diaphragm changes with respiration (Figure 36-1). When a person takes a deep breath in, the diaphragm may be well below the lower edge of the rib cage (costal margin). This increases the likelihood of injury to the organs in the chest cavity. With full exhalation, the diaphragm may be at the level of the nipple line. This increases the likelihood of injury to the abdominal organs. Second, the forces involved in producing the injury and the course a penetrating object takes in the body cannot be determined with 100% accuracy by simply looking at the point of impact or penetration. For these reasons, it is best to assume that an injury to the chest or abdomen involves both body cavities. In this way, injuries are less likely to be overlooked.

Recall from Chapter 6 that the abdomen is divided into four quadrants to make things easier when identifying the abdominal organs and the location of pain or injury (Figure 36-2). These quadrants are created by drawing two imaginary lines that intersect with the

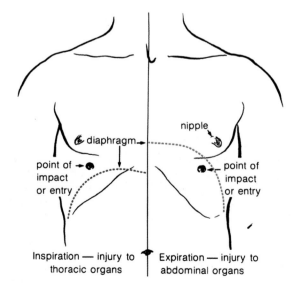

FIGURE 36-1 ▲ The position of the diaphragm changes with respiration.

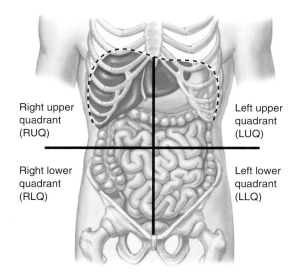

FIGURE 36-2 ▲ The abdominal area is divided into four quadrants.

midline through the navel. Knowing the organs found within each of the four quadrants will help you describe the location of a patient's injury and anticipate possible complications of the injury (Table 36-1).

The abdomen contains both hollow and solid organs (Table 36-2). If hollow organs are cut or ruptured, their contents spill into the abdominal cavity, causing inflammation. Open wounds of hollow organs, such as the stomach or small intestine, may be accompanied by intense pain. Infection is a delayed complication that may be fatal.

Severe bleeding may result if a solid organ is cut or ruptured. However, abdominal pain from solid organ penetration or rupture typically is of slow onset and generally does not occur immediately.

Types of abdominal injuries include open injuries, in which the skin is broken, and closed injuries, in which the skin is not broken. Closed or open wounds to the abdomen may involve multiple organs and major blood vessels, including the abdominal

aorta and inferior vena cava. Signs and symptoms of abdominal injuries are listed in the following *You Should Know* box.

Closed Abdominal Injuries

Objective 2

Trauma sustained from a motor vehicle crash, fall, or assault produces compression and deceleration injuries. A **compression injury of the abdomen** occurs when abdominal contents are squeezed between the vertebral column and the impacting object. In a **deceleration injury,** the individual's body stops its forward movement on impact but the organs continue to move forward until structural impact, tear, or rupture occurs. Other common mechanisms of injury involving blunt trauma to the abdomen are listed in the next *You Should Know* box.

TABLE 36-1 Abdominal Organs by Quadrant	
Abdominal Quadrant	**Organs**
Right upper quadrant	Liver, gallbladder, portions of the stomach, ascending colon, transverse colon, major blood vessels
Right lower quadrant	Appendix, ascending colon, right ovary (female), right fallopian tube (female)
Left upper quadrant	Stomach, spleen, pancreas, transverse colon, descending colon
Left lower quadrant	Descending colon, sigmoid colon, left ovary (female), left fallopian tube (female)

TABLE 36-2 Hollow and Solid Abdominal Organs

Hollow Organs	Solid Organs
Stomach	Liver
Small intestine	Spleen
Large intestine	Pancreas
Gallbladder	Kidneys
Urinary bladder	Adrenal glands
Uterus (female)	Ovaries (female)

You Should Know

Common MOIs of Blunt Trauma to the Abdomen

- Compression
- Deceleration
- Motor vehicle crash
- Motorcycle collision
- Pedestrian injury
- Fall
- Assault
- Blast injury

Open Abdominal Injuries

Objective 2

Penetrating trauma to the abdomen can result from low-, medium-, or high-energy weapons. A knife or ice pick is an example of a low-energy weapon. Medium-energy weapons include handguns and shotguns. High-energy weapons include military and hunting rifles. Most patients with a penetrating abdominal injury have underlying solid and hollow organ injuries.

You Should Know

Blunt trauma to the abdomen results in injury to the spleen (40–55%), liver (35–45%), and small intestine (5–10%). As many as 67% to 75% of stab wounds to the anterior abdomen penetrate the peritoneum. In order of frequency, stab wounds to the abdomen most commonly involve the following organs:

- Liver
- Small intestine
- Diaphragm
- Large intestine

Specific Injuries

The liver is the largest abdominal organ and is very vascular. It has been estimated that the liver holds about 200 to 400 mL of blood. Damage to the liver can result in hemorrhage, leading to shock. Suspect an injury to the liver with lower right rib fractures or penetrating trauma to the right upper quadrant of the abdomen.

The spleen is a vascular organ in the left upper quadrant that is susceptible to injury since it is protected only by the rib cage. Common mechanisms of injury involving splenic injury include auto crashes, falls, bicycle accidents, and motorcycle crashes. Suspect an injury to the spleen with lower left rib fractures or penetrating trauma to the left upper quadrant of the abdomen. Left upper quadrant pain that radiates to the left shoulder is called **Kehr's sign.** The presence of Kehr's sign suggests injury or rupture of the spleen or injury to the diaphragm.

Injury to the pancreas is uncommon, but it can occur from both blunt trauma and penetrating trauma. Blunt trauma to the pancreas typically involves a crushing injury, such as handlebar pressure to the abdomen, a fall, or a direct blow. Initial signs and symptoms of pancreatic injury can include upper abdominal pain or flank tenderness. Later signs and symptoms can include abdominal distention and shock.

Both blunt and penetrating traumas can cause injury to the diaphragm. Diaphragmatic injury more commonly occurs on the left side because the liver protects the diaphragm on the right. The patient with an injury to the diaphragm may complain of shortness of breath and have abnormal respiratory sounds.

Injury to the stomach and intestines can result in leakage of organ contents into the peritoneum, resulting in peritonitis and shock. The duodenum can be injured because of penetrating or blunt trauma. Rupture of the duodenum has been associated with the lap portion of seat belts, unrestrained drivers involved in frontal-impact motor vehicle crashes, and direct blows to the abdomen. The patient with a duodenal injury generally complains of abdominal pain and/or vomiting. Injuries to the large intestine are usually the result of gunshot wounds and stabbings. Evisceration is more common from stab wounds than gunshot wounds.

The abdominal cavity contains many vascular structures, including the abdominal aorta and inferior vena cava. A penetrating injury to vascular structures in the abdomen is also associated with injury to surrounding organs and can result in significant hemorrhage, peritoneal irritation, abdominal distention, and shock.

You Should Know

Signs and symptoms of peritonitis can take hours to develop and may not be apparent during the period in which the patient is in your care.

Genitourinary Trauma

Objective 3

The genitourinary system consists of the kidneys, ureters, bladder, urethra, and external genitalia. Injury to the kidney is usually caused by blunt trauma from motor vehicle crashes, falls, or contact sports. Penetrating injury to the kidney can result from gunshot or stab wounds. Injury to a ureter is uncommon because the ureters are protected by the spinal column, large intestine, pelvic organs, and abdominal wall. Penetrating trauma to a ureter is more common than blunt trauma. Blunt trauma may be caused by severe compression of the abdomen, such as occurs when a child is run over by an automobile.

The urinary bladder lies in the pelvis when empty, but may distend and rise above the umbilicus when full. Most bladder injuries are the result of blunt trauma caused by motor vehicle crashes, falls, direct blows, and sports injuries. Injury to the urethra should be suspected in cases of trauma to the perineum, pelvic fractures, and straddle injuries. An injury of the kidneys, ureters, bladder, or urethra can result in hematuria.

Injuries to the external male genitalia include cuts, bruises, penetrating objects, amputations, and avulsions. The scrotum can hold a large volume of blood or fluid. Injuries to the scrotum can be caused by an animal attack, self-mutilation, sports injury, straddle injury, assault, automobile crash, or blow or kick to the area. Signs and symptoms include pain, swelling, bruising, abdominal pain, nausea, vomiting, and difficulty urinating. Soft tissue injury to the penis can result through multiple mechanisms, including infections, burns, human or animal bites, and degloving injuries that involve machinery, such as the power takeoff of a farm tractor. A fractured penis, caused by the sudden bending of an erect penis, can occur during intercourse, resulting in immediate loss of the erection, tenderness, bruising, swelling, and the onset of severe pain. Penetrating trauma to the penis can result from gunshot or stab wounds. Complete or partial amputation of the penis is usually self-inflicted. In most cases, the patient is believed to be mentally ill. An injury to the penis may also involve an injury to the urethra.

The internal female genitalia are rarely injured except in the pregnant patient or in cases of sexual assault with penetration. Blunt injuries may rupture the uterus, causing loss of life of the fetus and severe hemorrhage. Injuries to the external female genitalia usually result from straddle injuries or lacerations produced by sexual activity, such as foreign objects in the vagina, or sexual assault.

Patient Assessment

Objectives 4, 5, 6

Begin your assessment by ensuring scene safety. Assess the patient's level of responsiveness, airway status, breathing effort, and circulatory status. If the mechanism of injury suggests a head or spinal injury, ask your partner to maintain manual stabilization of the patient's head and neck until the patient has been completely immobilized on a long backboard.

To properly assess the abdomen, you will need to remove the patient's clothing and make sure that the patient is supine. Assess the abdomen for DCAP-BTLS. Look to see if abdominal distention is present, which can be caused by blood, fluid, or air. Look for entrance and exit wounds, logrolling the patient as needed to assess the posterior body.

If the patient is responsive, ask her to point to the area that hurts (point tenderness). Assess the area that hurts last. Place one hand on top of the other, and using the pads of the fingers of the lower hand, gently feel the upper and lower areas of the abdomen. Watch the patient's face while you palpate the abdomen. A grimace may indicate tenderness over a particular abdominal area. Ask the patient to rate her pain on a 0 to 10 scale. Determine if the abdomen feels soft or hard (rigid). Document your findings.

The abdomen can hold a large volume of blood due to injuries of solid organs and major blood vessels. Large amounts of intra-abdominal bleeding may occur without much external evidence. During your patient assessment and evaluation of the patient's vital signs, look for signs of impending shock that can include restlessness, anxiety, decreasing level of responsiveness, pallor, tachycardia, and narrowing pulse pressure.

If the male patient with a genitourinary injury is responsive, explain to him that you will need to view the area and then obtain permission from him to proceed. Be aware that he will most likely be anxious and may be embarrassed. Offer emotional support, maintain the patient's privacy, and protect his modesty.

Looking at the external female genitalia is necessary if the patient complains of bleeding from the vaginal or rectal area. Before viewing the area, tactfully explain that you will need to view the area and obtain permission from the patient to do so. If possible, it is advisable to have a female EMS professional in attendance during the assessment. Your assessment of the female genitalia is limited to *looking* at the area, while maintaining the patient's privacy and protecting her modesty. You must *never* insert anything into the vagina or attempt to examine the internal female genitalia. These actions are outside the emergency medical technician's scope of practice.

Emergency Care

Objectives 4, 5, 6

To treat a patient with an abdominal or genitourinary injury, perform the following steps:

- Put on appropriate PPE. Keep on-scene time to a minimum.
- If spinal injury is suspected, maintain manual in-line stabilization until the patient is secured to a long backboard. If a spinal injury is not suspected, place the patient in a position of comfort. For example, the patient may prefer to flex his hips and knees to decrease tension on the abdominal and groin muscles.
- Establish and maintain an open airway. If the patient is unresponsive, insert an oral airway. Suction if needed.
- Give oxygen. If the patient's breathing is adequate, apply oxygen by nonrebreather mask at 10 to 15 L/min if not already done. If the patient's breathing is inadequate, provide positive-pressure ventilation with 100% oxygen and assess the adequacy of the ventilations delivered.
- Expose the wound site. Control external bleeding by applying direct pressure to the wound with a sterile dressing. Control severe vaginal bleeding with external padding using sanitary pads or trauma dressings. Nothing should be placed in the vagina, including dressings or tampons. If blood soaks through the dressing, apply additional dressings and reapply pressure. If signs of shock are present or if internal bleeding is suspected, treat for shock.
- Do not remove penetrating objects; rather, stabilize in place with bulky dressings. (Refer back to Figure 34-17 in Chapter 34, "Bleeding and Soft Tissue Trauma.")
- Manage avulsed or amputated parts as you would other soft tissue injuries. Every effort should be made to locate the amputated part. (Refer to Figure 34-18 in Chapter 34.)
- Do not touch protruding organs. Carefully remove clothing from around the wound. Apply a large sterile dressing, moistened with sterile water or saline, over the organs and wound. Secure the dressing in place with a large bandage to retain moisture and prevent heat loss. (Refer to Figure 34-25 in Chapter 34.)
- Protect the patient's modesty and provide emotional support.
- Transport promptly. Reassess at least every 5 minutes en route.
- Record all patient care information, including the patient's medical history and all emergency care given, on a PCR.

On the Scene   Wrap-Up

On the basis of the mechanism of injury, you suspect the possibility of spinal injury and ask your partner to perform manual cervical spine stabilization as you begin your assessment. You note no injuries to the patient's head, neck, or chest. When you lift his shirt to assess the abdomen, you note an abrasion and discoloration in the midline of the abdomen that begins at the umbilicus and extends down into the patient's shorts. Assessing the patient's external genitalia, you note that significant swelling and bruising are present. A laceration to the scrotal sac exhibits light bleeding. The additional support you requested earlier has arrived and assists you in moving the patient to the stretcher and then up the hill. Having completed your assessment and discovered the extent of the patient's injuries, you determine that the patient should be flown to a trauma center. Your patient begins to exhibit the signs and symptoms of shock as the helicopter touches down. You describe the scene and the care given to the patient and transfer care to the flight crew. ■

Sum It Up

▶ Injuries to the abdomen and pelvis can result from blunt or penetrating trauma. Deaths from abdominal trauma result mainly from hemorrhage or infection. Trauma to the genitourinary system seldom occurs separately from trauma to other body systems and is most often associated with abdominal trauma.

▶ It is best to assume that an injury to the chest or abdomen involves both body cavities. In this way, injuries are less likely to be overlooked.

▶ Knowing the organs found within each of the four abdominal quadrants will help you describe the location of a patient's injury and anticipate possible complications of the injury.

▶ The abdomen contains both hollow and solid organs. If hollow organs are cut or ruptured, their contents spill into the abdominal cavity, causing inflammation. Open wounds of hollow organs, such as the stomach or small intestine, may be accompanied by intense pain. Infection is a delayed complication that may be fatal. Severe bleeding may result if a solid organ is cut or ruptured. However, abdominal pain from solid organ penetration or rupture typically is of slow onset and generally does not occur immediately.

▶ Types of abdominal injuries include open injuries, in which the skin is broken, and closed injuries, in which the skin is not broken.

▶ Trauma sustained from a motor vehicle crash, fall, or assault produces compression and deceleration injuries. A compression injury occurs when abdominal contents are squeezed between the vertebral column and the impacting object. In a deceleration injury, the individual's body stops its forward movement on impact but the abdominal organs continue to move forward until structural impact, tear, or rupture occurs.

▶ Penetrating trauma to the abdomen can result from low-, medium-, or high-energy weapons. A knife or ice pick is an example of a low-energy weapon. Medium-energy weapons include handguns and shotguns. High-energy weapons include military and hunting rifles.

▶ The genitourinary system consists of the kidneys, ureters, bladder, urethra, and external genitalia. An injury of the kidneys, ureters, bladder, or urethra can result in hematuria. Injuries to the external male genitalia include cuts, bruises, penetrating objects, amputations, and avulsions. The internal female genitalia are rarely injured except in the pregnant patient or in cases of sexual assault with penetration. Injuries to the external female genitalia usually result from straddle injuries or lacerations produced by sexual activity, such as foreign objects in the vagina, or sexual assault.

Orthopedic Trauma

By the end of this chapter, you should be able to:

Knowledge Objectives ▶

1. Describe the anatomy and physiology of the musculoskeletal system.
2. List the major bones or bone groupings of the spinal column, the thorax, the upper extremities, and the lower extremities.
3. Discuss orthopedic trauma caused by direct and indirect forces.
4. Differentiate between open and closed orthopedic injuries.
5. Discuss and differentiate among the following types of fractures: greenstick, comminuted, linear, transverse, oblique, and spiral.
6. Define and discuss dislocations, subluxations, and luxations.
7. Differentiate between sprains and strains.
8. Discuss the assessment findings and symptoms associated with musculoskeletal injuries.
9. List the six Ps of musculoskeletal injury assessment.
10. Describe the emergency medical care for a patient with orthopedic trauma.
11. Define splint, and state the reasons for splinting.
12. List possible hazards of improper splinting.
13. List the general rules of splinting.
14. Discuss types of splints, and give examples of situations in which each type might be used.
15. List warning signs of a splint that is too tight.

Attitude Objective ▶

16. Explain the rationale for immobilization of a painful, swollen, deformed extremity.

Skill Objectives ▶

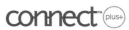

17. Demonstrate the emergency medical care of a patient with orthopedic trauma.
18. Demonstrate completing a prehospital care report for a patient with a musculoskeletal injury.

The dispatch speaker crackles, "Respond to 22 St. Louis Lane. Person has fallen." When you get there, your 80-year-old patient is lying in a crumpled heap at the bottom of 10 steps. Her husband says she was carrying a load of laundry, lost her footing, and fell from the top step. She is alert but moaning. She says she has pain in her arms and leg. Your partner maintains in-line stabilization of her head as you continue your exam. Her skin is pink and warm, but she is grimacing, and there are beads of sweat on her forehead. Her vital signs are blood pressure 168/100, pulse 116, and respirations 20. When you touch the back of her neck, she says that it hurts. She has no pain or obvious injury in her chest, abdomen, or pelvis. Her left leg has obvious swelling between the knee and hip. That leg seems to be rotated slightly. Her left upper arm is very tender and swollen between her shoulder and her elbow. Her right wrist is angled strangely, and she groans loudly when you touch the area. "We're going to do a few things to help your pain, Mrs. Brown," you tell your patient as your partner heads back to your rescue truck for supplies. ■

THINK ABOUT IT

As you read this chapter, think about the following questions:

- Why did your partner maintain in-line stabilization of the patient's head before you knew that the patient had neck pain?
- What bones are likely to be injured as evidenced by the information that you have now?
- How will you splint her injuries?
- What additional assessments should you perform?
- Which injuries could cause the patient to develop shock?

Introduction

Injuries to the musculoskeletal system are some of the most common traumatic injuries you will encounter. Most of these injuries are not life-threatening, but they may be very dramatic. Although an injury may not be life-threatening, it may have a sudden impact on a patient physically, as well as emotionally and socially. You must be able to recognize a musculoskeletal injury and provide appropriate emergency care. This care includes preventing further injury, reducing pain, and decreasing the likelihood of permanent damage.

The Musculoskeletal System

Objective 1

The musculoskeletal system has the following attributes:

- Gives the body its shape
- Provides a rigid framework that supports and protects internal organs

- Provides body movement
- Maintains posture
- Helps stabilize joints
- Produces body heat

The human skeleton provides the support for the body, much like the internal framework of a house. The skeleton provides a frame for other parts of the musculoskeletal system to attach to, including ligaments, tendons, and muscles. All parts of the musculoskeletal system work together to enable movement.

The Skeletal System

Objectives 1, 2

The skeletal system has the following attributes:

- Gives the body shape, support, and form
- Works with muscles to provide body movement
- Stores minerals such as calcium and phosphorus

- Produces red blood cells
- Protects vital internal organs:
  —The skull protects the brain.
  —The rib cage protects the heart and lungs.
  —The lower ribs protect most of the liver and spleen.
  —The spinal canal protects the spinal cord.

The skeletal system is divided into the axial and appendicular skeletons (Figure 37-1). The axial skeleton includes the skull, spinal column, sternum, and ribs (Table 37-1). The appendicular skeleton is made up of the upper and lower extremities (arms and legs), the shoulder girdle, and the pelvic girdle (Table 37-2). The axial skeleton is made up of 80 bones. The appendicular skeleton consists of 126 bones.

The shoulder girdle is the bony arch formed by the collarbones (clavicles) and shoulder blades (scapulae). The pelvic girdle is made up of the ilium, ischium, and pubis, which enclose and protect the organs of the pelvic cavity. It provides a point of attachment for the lower extremities and the major muscles of the trunk. It also supports the weight of the upper body.

The skull is made up of the cranial bones, which house and protect the brain, and the facial bones, including the upper jaw (the maxilla), the lower jaw (the mandible), and the cheekbones (zygomatic bones). The skull is supported by the neck, which receives its strength from the vertebrae.

The vertebral column is made up of 7 cervical (neck) vertebrae, 12 thoracic vertebrae, 5 lumbar vertebrae, 5 fused vertebrae that form the sacrum, and 3 to 4 fused vertebrae that form the coccyx (tailbone). The vertebral column gives rigidity to the body while allowing movement. It also encloses the spinal cord. It extends from the base of the skull to the coccyx.

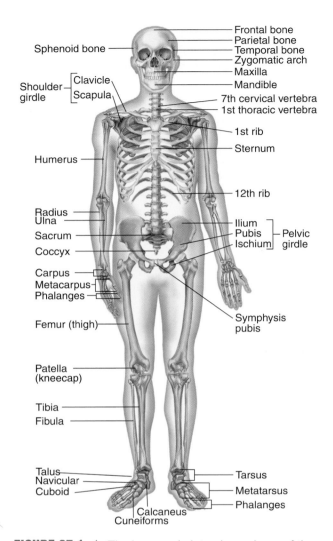

FIGURE 37-1 ▲ The human skeleton is made up of the axial skeleton, which consists of the skull, vertebral column, sternum, and ribs. The appendicular skeleton (blue) is attached and includes the shoulder and pelvic girdles as well as the limb bones.

TABLE 37-1	The Axial Skeleton
Bone	**Purpose**
Skull (cranium)	Houses and protects the brain Serves as a rigid container
Facial bones (eye sockets, cheeks, upper nose, and upper and lower jaw)	Houses and protects the brain and sensory organs (the structures that provide sight, smell, and taste) Provides shape and unique features
Spinal column	Protects the spinal cord Provides a center axis of support
Sternum (breastbone) and ribs	Protects the heart, lungs, and major blood vessels in the chest

TABLE 37-2   The Appendicular Skeleton

Bone	Purpose
Upper Extremities	
Shoulder girdle (collarbone and shoulder blade)	Provide structural support, movement, and leverage
Upper arm bone (humerus)	
Forearm bones (radius and ulna)	
Wrist bones (carpals)	
Hand bones (metacarpals)	
Fingers (phalanges)	
Lower Extremities	
Pelvic girdle (ilium, ischium, pubis)	Protects the bladder, female reproductive organs, and major blood vessels Provides a point of attachment for the legs and major muscles of the trunk Supports the weight of the upper body
Thigh (femur)	Provides structural support
Kneecap (patella)	Provides joint protection and support
Shin (tibia and fibula)	Provides structural support
Ankle (tarsals)	Provides structural support, movement, and leverage
Foot (metatarsals)	Provides structural support, movement, and leverage
Toes (phalanges)	Provides structural support, movement, and leverage

The chest (thorax) is made up of the 12 thoracic vertebrae, 12 pairs of ribs, and the breastbone (sternum). These structures form the thoracic cage, which protects the organs within the thoracic cavity (for example, the heart, lungs, and major blood vessels). All the ribs are attached posteriorly by ligaments to the thoracic vertebrae.

The sternum (breastbone) consists of three sections:

1. The manubrium is the uppermost (superior) portion; it connects with the clavicle and the first rib.
2. The body is the middle portion.
3. The xiphoid process is a piece of cartilage that makes up the lowermost (inferior) portion.

The uppermost portion of the sternum is attached to the clavicles, which joins the axial skeleton to the appendicular skeleton.

The upper extremities are made up of the bones of the shoulder girdle, the arms, the forearms, and the hands. The humerus is the upper arm bone. The biceps and triceps muscles are attached here, allowing the shoulder to flex and extend. The forearm contains two bones: the radius (lateral or thumb side) and the ulna (medial side). The elbow is the joint where the humerus connects with the radius and the ulna. The forearm is connected to the wrist (carpals) and then to the hand (metacarpals) and fingers (phalanges).

The lower extremities are made up of the bones of the pelvis, the upper legs, the lower legs, and the feet. The pelvis is a bony ring formed by three separate bones (the ilium, ischium, and pubis) that fuse to become one bone in an adult. The lower extremities are attached to the pelvis at the hip joint. The hip joint is a ball-and-socket joint formed by a cup-shaped hollow in the pelvis (the acetabulum) into which the upper end of the femur fits.

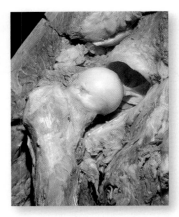

FIGURE 37-2 ▲ The hip joint is an example of a ball-and-socket joint.

The knee is protected anteriorly by the kneecap (patella) and attaches the femur to the two lower leg bones, the tibia (shinbone) and fibula. The lower leg attaches to the foot by the ankle, which is made up of seven tarsal bones. The largest tarsal bone, the calcaneus, makes up the heel. The metatarsals make up the main part of the foot. The toes (phalanges) are the foot's equivalent to the fingers.

The skeletal system includes many joints. A **joint** is a place where two bones come together. Fibrous joints, such as those found on the bone edges of the skull, do not move. Cartilaginous joints, found in the spine and ribs, allow for only a little movement. Synovial joints, such as those found at the hip, shoulders, elbows, knees, wrists, and ankles, allow movement in many directions. Synovial joints are broken down into groups according to their shape and movement. Examples include ball-and-socket joints and hinge joints. Ball-and-socket joints allow movement in all directions (Figure 37-2). The only ball-and-socket joints in the body are the hip joint (pelvic bone and femur) and shoulder joint (scapula and humerus). A hinge joint allows only flexion and extension. Examples include the elbow (humerus and ulna) and knee (femur and tibia) (Figure 37-3).

The Muscular System

Objective 1

The human body has over 600 muscles (Figure 37-4). Muscles are bundles of tiny fibers that expand and contract. Muscle fibers shorten (contract) when stimulated. They shorten by converting energy obtained from food (chemical energy) into movement (mechanical energy).

Skeletal muscles produce movement of the bones to which they are attached. Skeletal muscles

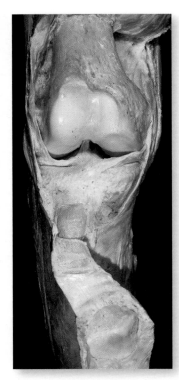

FIGURE 37-3 ▲ The knee joint is an example of a hinge joint.

also produce heat, which helps maintain a constant body temperature and maintain posture. Skeletal muscles have a rich supply of blood vessels and nerves. In most cases, an artery and at least one vein accompany each nerve in a skeletal muscle. Skeletal muscle fibers are surrounded by connective tissue. The connective tissue covering supports and protects the delicate fibers. It also provides a pathway through which blood vessels and nerves can pass. A skeletal muscle fiber must receive a signal from a nerve before it can contract. When the signal is received, skeletal muscles produce rapid, forceful contractions.

Most skeletal muscles are attached to bones by means of tendons. Tendons create a pull between bones when muscles contract. The tendons of many muscles cross over joints, which contributes to the stability of the joint. Tendons can be damaged from overextension or overuse. Ligaments connect bone to bone.

A skeletal muscle has three main parts (Figure 37-5):

- The **origin** is the stationary attachment of the muscle to a bone.
- The **insertion** is the movable attachment to a bone.
- The **body** is the main part of the muscle.

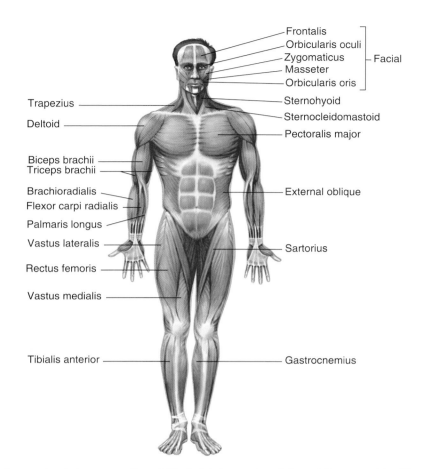

FIGURE 37-4 ▲ The human body has more than 600 skeletal muscles. A few of them are identified here.

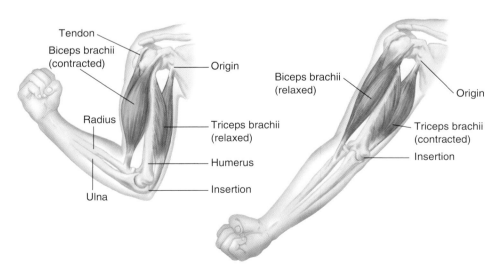

FIGURE 37-5 ▲ The origin of a skeletal muscle is the stationary attachment of the muscle to a bone. The insertion is the movable attachment to a bone. The body is the main part of the muscle.

Musculoskeletal Injuries

Mechanism of Injury

Objective 3

Injuries to bones and joints can be caused by direct forces, indirect forces, and twisting forces (Figure 37-6). A direct force causes injury at the point of impact, such as being struck in the face by a fist. Indirect forces cause injury at a site other than the point of impact. For example, if your hand strikes the ground (direct force) during a fall, the energy travels up your arm and may result in an injury near your elbow, shoulder, or clavicle (indirect force). A twisting force causes one part of an extremity to remain in place while the rest twists, such as an ankle twisted while a person is playing basketball. Twisting injuries commonly affect the joints, such as ankles, knees, and wrists. Twisting forces cause ligaments to stretch and tear.

Types of Musculoskeletal Injuries

Objectives 4, 5, 6, 7

Injuries to bones and joints may be open or closed. In an open injury, the skin surface is broken. The bone may protrude through the wound or may pull back inside the body from muscle contraction. Such injuries can result in serious blood loss. An open injury also increases the risk of contamination and infection. In closed bone and joint injuries, the skin surface is not broken. In any case, an open or closed bone or joint injury is often painful, swollen, and deformed. When caring for the patient you must try to ensure that a closed injury does not become an open injury.

A **fracture** is a break in a bone. If a bone is broken, chipped, cracked, or splintered, it is said to be fractured. Figure 37-7 shows some types of fractures. The bones of a child are more flexible than those of an adult and tend to bend more without breaking. This characteristic

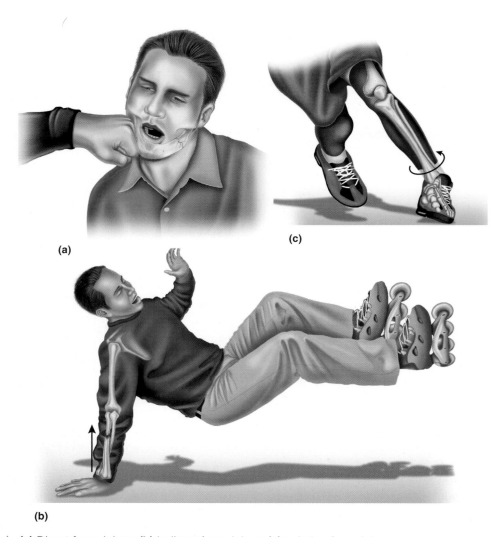

(a)

(c)

(b)

FIGURE 37-6 ▲ **(a)** Direct force injury; **(b)** indirect force injury; **(c)** twisting force injury.

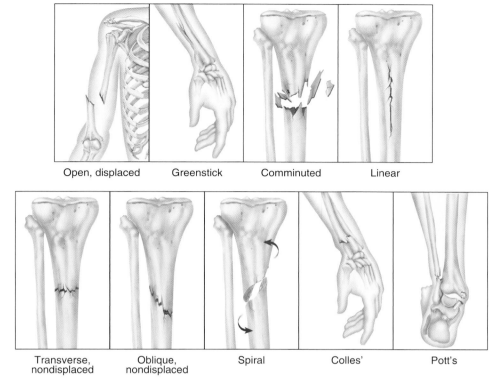

Open, displaced   Greenstick   Comminuted   Linear

Transverse,   Oblique,   Spiral   Colles'   Pott's
nondisplaced   nondisplaced

FIGURE 37-7 ▲ Some types of fractures.

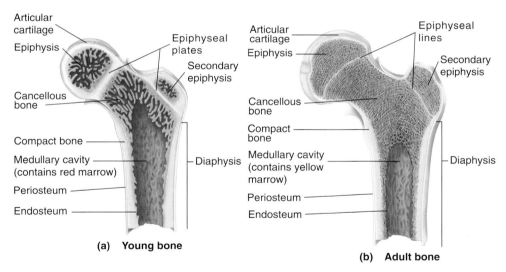

Articular cartilage
Epiphysis
Epiphyseal plates
Secondary epiphysis
Cancellous bone
Compact bone
Medullary cavity (contains red marrow)
Diaphysis
Periosteum
Endosteum

(a) Young bone

Articular cartilage
Epiphysis
Epiphyseal lines
Secondary epiphysis
Cancellous bone
Compact bone
Medullary cavity (contains yellow marrow)
Diaphysis
Periosteum
Endosteum

(b) Adult bone

FIGURE 37-8 ▲ **(a)** The femur (thigh bone) of a child showing the growth plate (epiphyseal plate); **(b)** adult long bone.

explains the greenstick fracture that is seen in children. A **greenstick fracture** occurs when the bone breaks on one side but not the other, like bending a green tree branch. In children and adolescents, an area of growing tissue called the **growth plate (epiphyseal plate)** can be found near each end of a long bone (Figure 37-8). During adolescence, the growth plates are replaced by solid bone when growth is complete. In a child, the growth plate is the weakest part of the skeleton. The growth plate is even weaker than the surrounding ligaments and tendons. An injury to the growth plate is a fracture. Most growth plate injuries are caused by falls. Growth of the bone can be affected if a fracture in or around the growth plate causes the blood supply to the bone to be cut off. The healing of this type of injury is watched closely by the child's doctor.

A **comminuted fracture** is one in which the bone is splintered or crushed, resulting in several breaks in the bone and multiple bone fragments. A **linear fracture** is one in which the break runs parallel to the long axis of the bone. A **transverse fracture** is one in which the break is at about a 90-degree angle to the bone, whereas an **oblique fracture** is one in which the break is at about a 45-degree angle to the bone. A **spiral fracture** is a bone break caused by a twisting motion and usually occurs in the long bones of the body, such as the humerus and femur. In this type of fracture, the break crosses the bone at an oblique angle, creating a spiral pattern. **Colles' fracture** is a break in the distal radius that is usually caused by falling on an outstretched hand in an attempt to break a fall. The patient's body weight on the hand may cause the radius to fracture just above the wrist. Individuals at greatest risk for this type of fracture include women of middle age and older who have **osteoporosis,** a condition that develops when the rate of old bone removal occurs too quickly or new bone growth occurs too slowly. **Pott's fracture** is a fracture of the lower part of the fibula with displacement of the foot. There are varying degrees of Pott's fractures. In the most severe type, the tibia is also fractured. The direction of foot displacement varies with the severity of the fracture. Pott's fracture is most common in young adults and often associated with sports injuries and falls.

An open fracture may result from bone ends or fragments tearing out through the skin (Figure 37-9). It may also be caused by a penetrating injury that has damaged a bone and the surrounding soft tissues, such as a gunshot wound. Closed fractures have no opening through the skin but can result in nerve damage and serious internal bleeding. For example, typical blood loss in an uncomplicated fracture of the tibia or fibula during the first 2 hours can be as much as 550 mL. A broken femur can result in the loss of up to 1 L of blood, and a fractured pelvis can result in the loss of 2 L. If the fracture is closed, the blood will have no place to go except to the surrounding tissue. As bleeding continues, the blood vessels and tissues of the thigh become compressed, reducing blood flow throughout the leg. Whether a fracture is open or closed, the movement of sharp bone ends can cause damage to arteries, muscles, and nerves. A suspected fracture should be immobilized to prevent further injury and pain. Fracture complications are listed in the following *You Should Know* box.

> ### You Should Know
>
> **Possible Complications of Fractures**
> - Hemorrhage
> - Instability
> - Loss of tissue
> - Contamination
> - Long-term disability
> - Interruption of blood supply
> - Pregnancy complications with pelvic fracture

A **dislocation** occurs when the end of a bone is forced from its normal position in a joint (Figure 37-10). A partial dislocation **(subluxation)** means the bone is partially out of the joint. **Luxation,** a complete dislocation, means it is all the way out. Dislocations and subluxations usually result in temporary deformity of the affected joints, loss of limb function, immediate swelling, and point tenderness, and they may result in sudden and severe pain. The surrounding muscles often spasm from the disruption, and this worsens the pain. The pain stops almost immediately once the bone is back in place.

Dislocations most often occur in major joints such as the shoulder, hip, knee, elbow, or ankle (Figure 37-11). They can occur in smaller joints such as the finger, thumb or toe. Dislocations are usually caused by trauma, such as a fall. They can also be caused by an underlying disease, such as rheumatoid arthritis.

Dislocations and subluxations are dangerous because the change of position of the bone or bones involved can compress or damage the joint and its surrounding muscles, ligaments, nerves, or blood vessels. Severe damage to nerves and blood vessels can occur if a joint is not put back into place properly. For this reason, you should not try to reduce (put back into place) a dislocation. A dislocation or subluxation may go back into place by itself. Be sure to let the healthcare professional to whom you are transferring patient care know if this occurs.

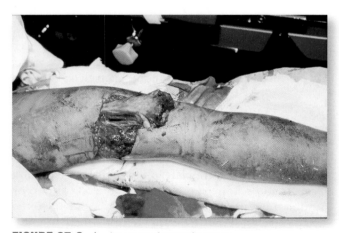

FIGURE 37-9 ▲ An open femur fracture.

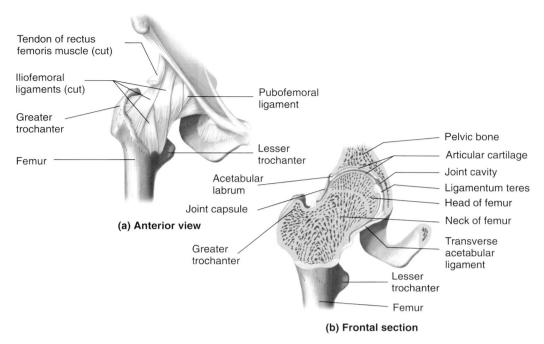

(a) Anterior view

(b) Frontal section

FIGURE 37-10 ▲ Dislocation of the right hip joint. **(a)** Anterior view; **(b)** frontal section.

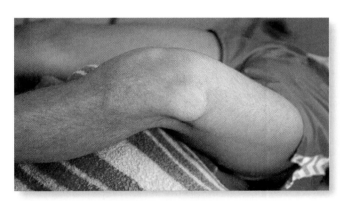

FIGURE 37-11 ▲ Knee dislocation.

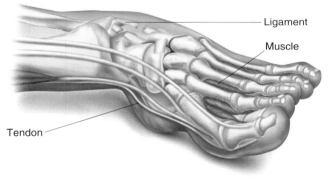

FIGURE 37-12 ▲ A sprain is a stretching or tearing of a ligament. Pain and bruising are usually present with all types of sprains.

Remember This

Remember: Ligaments "sprain"; muscles "strain."

A **sprain** is a stretching or tearing of a ligament, the connective tissue that joins the end of one bone with another (Figure 37-12). Sprains are classified as mild, moderate, and severe. Pain and bruising are usually present with all categories of sprains. When a sprain occurs, the patient usually feels a tear or pop in the joint. A severe sprain produces excruciating pain at the moment of injury as the ligaments tear completely or separate from the bone. Tearing or separation loosens the joint and makes it nonfunctional. A moderate sprain partially tears the ligament, loosens the joint, and produces some swelling. A ligament is stretched in a mild sprain, but there is no joint loosening.

A **strain** is a twisting, pulling, or tearing of a muscle (Figure 37-13). Muscle injuries are more common than bone injuries. A muscle strain usually occurs when a muscle is stretched beyond its limit. A strain often occurs near the point where the muscle joins the tough connective tissue of the tendon. For example, muscles of the lower back may be strained when improper lifting or moving techniques are used. The signs and symptoms of a strain include pain with movement, little or no swelling, and a limited ability to bear weight on

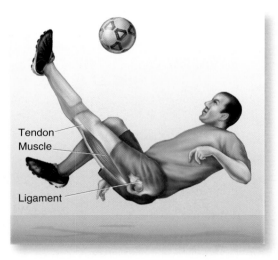

Tendon
Muscle
Ligament

FIGURE 37-13 ▲ A strain is a twist, pull, or tear of a muscle or tendon.

the affected extremity. The area around the injury may be tender to the touch. Bruising may be present if blood vessels are broken.

Remember This

Because they are treated in the same way, it is not important for you to know if an injury is a particular type of fracture or if the injury involves a muscle or bone. Treat any injury to an arm or leg as if a fracture exists.

Patient Assessment

Objectives 8, 9

Begin your assessment by ensuring scene safety. Assess the mechanism of injury before approaching the patient. Put on appropriate PPE. Perform a primary survey to identify and treat any life-threatening conditions. Assess the patient's level of responsiveness, airway status, breathing effort, and circulatory status. If the mechanism of injury suggests a head or spinal injury, ask your partner to maintain manual stabilization of the patient's head and neck until the patient has been completely immobilized on a long backboard.

Quickly determine if the patient's injury is life- or limb-threatening. In general, there are four classes of patients with musculoskeletal trauma:

1. Patients with life- or limb-threatening injuries or conditions, including life- or limb-threatening musculoskeletal trauma

2. Patients with other life- or limb-threatening injuries and only simple musculoskeletal trauma

3. Patients with life- or limb-threatening musculoskeletal trauma and no other life- or limb-threatening injuries

5. Patients with only isolated, non-life- or non-limb-threatening injuries

Treat all life-threatening conditions first, and then address limb-threatening injuries. If signs of shock are present or if internal bleeding is suspected, treat for shock. Provide care for non-life- and non-limb-threatening injuries as time permits. Do not allow a horrible-looking but noncritical musculoskeletal injury distract you.

When assessing a patient with orthopedic trauma, remember the six Ps of musculoskeletal assessment:
1. **Pain** or tenderness (on palpation or movement)
2. **Pallor**
3. **Paresthesia** (pins-and-needles sensation)
4. **Pulses** (present, diminished, or absent)
5. **Paralysis** (inability to move)
6. **Pressure**

Perform a physical examination, take the patient's vital signs, and gather the patient's medical history. Remember the DCAP-BTLS memory aid to recall what to look and feel for during the physical exam. The assessment findings and symptoms of musculoskeletal injuries vary depending upon the severity and type of injury. The three most common signs and symptoms of a musculoskeletal injury are pain, deformity, and swelling. Signs and symptoms of musculoskeletal injuries are shown in the following *You Should Know* box.

You Should Know

Assessment Findings and Symptoms of Musculoskeletal Injuries

- Pain or tenderness over the injury site
- Swelling
- Deformity, angulation (abnormal position of an extremity)
- Crepitation (grating sensation or sound)
- Limited movement
- Joint locked into position
- Exposed bone ends
- Bruising
- Bleeding
- Difference in length, shape, or size of one extremity compared with the other
- Loss of pulse or sensation below the injury site

Look for deformities, open injuries, and swelling. Note if signs of compartment syndrome are present (see Chapter 34). Feel along the length of the extremity for deformities, tenderness, and swelling. Feel and listen for crepitus, which is the grating of broken bone ends against each other. Check the **p**ulse, **m**ovement, and **s**ensation (PMS) in each extremity. Compare each extremity to the opposite extremity. Assess the dorsalis pedis pulse (on top of the foot) in each lower extremity. Assess the radial pulse in each upper extremity. If the patient is awake, assess movement of the lower extremities by asking if she can push her feet into your hands. Assess movement of the upper extremities by asking the patient to squeeze your fingers. Compare the strength of her grips and note if they are equal or if one side appears weaker. If the patient is awake, assess sensation by touching the fingers and toes of each extremity and asking her to tell you where you are touching. Assess the patient's thumb or pinky (or great toe or baby toe) to avoid the confusion of having to describe which "middle" digit is being touched. If the patient is unresponsive, assess movement and sensation by gently pinching each foot and hand. See if the patient responds to pain with facial movements or movement of the extremity being pinched.

Emergency Care

Objective 10

To treat a patient with orthopedic trauma, perform the following steps:

- Put on appropriate PPE.
- Keep on-scene time to a minimum.
- If spinal injury is suspected, maintain manual in-line stabilization until the patient is secured to a long backboard. If a spinal injury is not suspected, place the patient in a position of comfort.
- Establish and maintain an open airway. If the patient is unresponsive, insert an oral airway. Suction if needed.
- Give oxygen. If the patient's breathing is adequate, apply oxygen by nonrebreather mask at 10 to 15 L/min if not already done. If the patient's breathing is inadequate, provide positive-pressure ventilation with 100% oxygen and assess the adequacy of the ventilations delivered.
- Apply a cold pack to the area of a painful, swollen, deformed extremity to reduce swelling and pain. Generally, cold is used in the first 48 hours of the injury to reduce swelling, and heat is used after 48 hours to increase circulation to the injured area.

- Cover open wounds with a sterile dressing. If bone ends are visible, do not intentionally reposition or replace them.
- Splint any bone or joint injuries. This technique is explained in detail in the next section.
  - Before applying a splint, you should manually stabilize the injured extremity. This will require another person, who will use his hands to gently support the extremity. To stabilize an injured bone, support the joints above and below the injury. For example, if a bone in the lower leg is broken, your assistant should use his hands to stabilize both the ankle and the knee. When a splint is applied, the splint must be long enough to stabilize both these joints. To stabilize an injured joint, support the bones above and below it. Additional support may be needed underneath the injured area so that it does not sag. Do not release manual stabilization until the injured area has been properly immobilized.
  - Pad a rigid or semirigid splint before applying it. Padding helps lessen patient discomfort caused by pressure, especially around bony areas. After the extremity is splinted, apply an ice bag or cold pack. Place a cloth or bandage between the patient's skin and the cold source.
  - If the patient is in critical condition, fractures can be temporarily stabilized using a long board. The goal is to reduce the time it takes to get the patient to definitive care.
- Most sprains and strains can be treated with rest, ice, and elevation.
  - *Rest.* Using a body part increases blood flow to that area and can increase swelling. Tell the patient to avoid using the injured area while it heals. The length of rest is determined by how severe the injury is.
  - *Ice.* Use a cold pack or place ice in a plastic bag and remove the excess air. Do not apply ice or a cold pack directly to the skin. Wrap the cold source in a cloth. Apply the ice to the injured area for 20 minutes and then remove it for 40 minutes. Follow this rotation hourly. Ice reduces blood flow into the affected area, which in turn reduces swelling.
  - *Elevation.* To reduce swelling, keep the injured extremity higher than the patient's heart. This also helps remove waste products from the injured area.
- Comfort, calm, and reassure the patient, family members, and friends of the patient. Reassess as often as needed.

- Record all patient care information, including the patient's medical history and all emergency care given, on a prehospital care report.

Stop and Think!

- If you are not sure whether a musculoskeletal injury is present, manually stabilize the injured area and then apply a splint. If no life-threatening conditions are present, splint an injured extremity before moving the patient.
- *Always* assess pulses, movement, and sensation in an extremity before and after care of the injury. Compare your assessment with an assessment of the opposite extremity. Be sure to document your findings.
- Make sure to remove any jewelry or tight clothing distal to an extremity injury. Doing so will allow for easy removal without cutting. It will also prevent injury from tissue compression once swelling increases.

Splinting

Objectives 11, 12

A splint is a device used to immobilize (limit movement of) a body part to prevent pain and further injury. The next *You Should Know* box lists the reasons for splinting. It also lists the hazards associated with improper splinting.

In some situations, the patient will have already splinted the injury by holding the injured part close to his body in a comfortable position. For example, you may find a patient with an injured wrist holding his arm close to his chest. With this type of injury, the patient will usually support the injured arm with his uninjured arm. The use of the body as a splint is called an **anatomic splint,** also known as a *self-splint.*

Many types of ready-made splints are available. If a ready-made splint is not available, a splint can be made. Materials commonly used include rolled-up magazines, branches, newspapers, umbrellas, boards, canes, cardboard, broom handles, wooden spoons, or a foam sleeping pad. An injured body part is usually secured to a splint with wide bandages or straps. If these materials are not available, you can substitute bandannas, climbing webbing, or torn pieces of clothing. Do not use narrow pieces of material because they can act like a tourniquet. A bandage or strap should never be tight enough to impede blood flow.

You Should Know

Reasons for Splinting

- Limit the motion of bone fragments, bone ends, or dislocated joints.
- Lessen the damage to muscles, nerves, or blood vessels caused by broken bones.
- Help prevent a closed injury from becoming an open injury.
- Lessen the restriction of blood flow caused by bone ends or dislocations compressing blood vessels.
- Reduce bleeding resulting from tissue damage caused by bone ends.
- Reduce pain associated with the movement of the bone and the joint.
- Reduce the risk of paralysis caused by a damaged spine.

Hazards of Improper Splinting

- The compression of nerves, tissues, and blood vessels from the splint
- A delay in transport of a patient with a life-threatening injury
- Distal circulation that is reduced as a result of the splint being applied too tightly to the extremity
- Aggravation of the musculoskeletal injury
- Cause or aggravation of tissue, nerve, vessel, or muscle damage from excessive bone or joint movement

General Rules of Splinting

Objective 13

Follow these general guidelines when splinting a musculoskeletal injury:

- Wear appropriate PPE. In most situations, the patient should not be moved before splinting unless she is in danger.
- If possible, remove or cut away clothing to expose the injury. Remove jewelry from the injured area.
- Assess pulses, movement, and sensation distal to the injury before and after applying a splint. You may find it helpful to lightly mark the pulse location with a pen to save time when rechecking pulses. Assess pulses, movement, and sensation every 15 minutes, and document your findings.
- Cover open wounds with a sterile dressing.
- Before applying a rigid or semirigid splint, pad it to reduce patient discomfort caused by pressure, especially around bony areas.

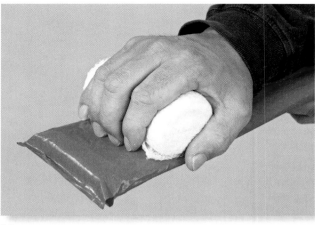

(a)

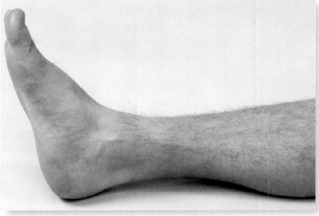

(b)

FIGURE 37-14 ▲ Position of function for **(a)** the hand and **(b)** the foot.

- Splint the area above and below the injury. If a bone is injured, immobilize the joint above and below the injury. If a joint is injured, immobilize the bones above and below the injury.
- Before splinting an injured hand or foot, place it in the **position of function** (Figure 37-14). The natural position of the hand at rest looks as if the hand were gently grasping a small object, such as a baseball. Use a roll of tape, roller gauze, or a rolled-up sock or glove as the "ball," and place it in the patient's palm before splinting his hand. Do not place the hand or foot in a position of function if you find it in an abnormal position and meet resistance or cause pain when you attempt to place it in the position of function.
- Pad the hollow areas (voids) between the splint and the extremity.
- Do not intentionally replace protruding bones. During the splinting process, bone ends may be

drawn back into the wound. This is to be expected and is acceptable.
- Avoid excessive movement of the injured area when applying a splint.
- When securing the splint to the injured area, avoid placing ties or straps directly over the injury.
- Splint the injury before moving the patient unless she is in danger or life-threatening conditions exist.
- When in doubt about whether a musculoskeletal injury is present, splint the injury.
- If the patient shows signs of shock, align him in the anatomical position on a long backboard. Treat the patient for shock and arrange for transport.

Stop and Think!

If your patient does not have a pulse in an extremity or has lost sensation or the ability to move the fingers or toes of the injured extremity after you applied a splint, the splint is too tight. Manually immobilize the injured area, loosen the splint, and adjust it. Reassess often, and be sure to notify the healthcare professional who assumes responsibility for the patient when you transfer care.

Remember This

Warning Signs That a Splint Is Too Tight

- The patient's fingers or toes become cold to the touch in the splinted extremity.
- The patient's fingers or toes begin to turn pale or blue in the splinted extremity.
- The patient is unable to move fingers or toes in the splinted extremity.
- The patient experiences increased pain in the splinted extremity.
- The patient experiences increased swelling below the splint.
- The patient complains of numbness or tingling in the extremity.
- The patient complains of burning or stinging in the splinted extremity.

Types of Splints

Objectives 14, 15

A variety of materials and techniques can be used for splinting. You may have to improvise because of the limited availability of splinting materials and/or the patient's position. Remember: The splint must be long enough to immobilize the area above and below the injury.

Rigid Splints

Rigid splints are made of hard material, such as wood, strong cardboard, or plastic (Figure 37-15). They are available in different sizes. Some are preformed to fit certain body areas. Some rigid splints are padded, but others must be padded before they are applied to the patient. This type of splint is useful for immobilizing injuries that occur to the middle portion (midshaft) of a bone. The SAM Splint and aluminum ladder splints are examples of semirigid (flexible) splints. These splints can be molded to the shape of the extremity and are very useful for immobilizing joint injuries (Figure 37-16). They can be used in combination with other splints, such as a sling and swathe.

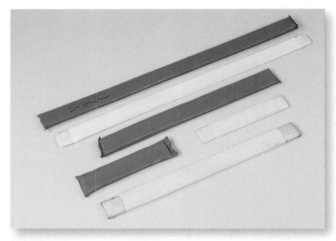

FIGURE 37-15 ▲ Rigid splints.

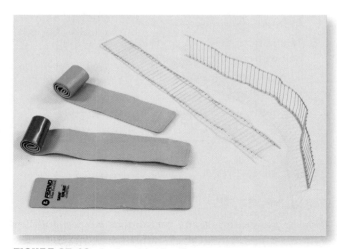

FIGURE 37-16 ▲ Semirigid splints.

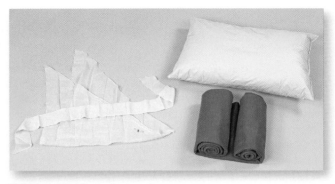

FIGURE 37-17 ▲ Soft splints.

Soft Splints

Soft splints are flexible and useful for immobilizing injuries of the lower leg or forearm. Examples of soft splints include sling and swathe combinations, blanket rolls, pillows, and towels (Figure 37-17). A sling and swathe are used to immobilize injuries to the shoulder (scapula), collarbone (clavicle), or upper arm bone (humerus). A triangular bandage is often used to make a sling. A **swathe** is a piece of soft material used to secure the injured extremity to the body. Roller gauze can also be used as a swathe.

- To make a swathe, unwrap a triangular bandage and place it on a flat surface. Grab the point of the shorter end of the triangle, and fold it toward the longer end, like a bandanna.
- The swathe must be tight enough to limit movement of the arm but not so tight that chest movement is restricted. The patient may have difficulty breathing if chest movement is restricted. Make sure the patient's fingers remain exposed so that you can assess the pulse, movement, and sensation.

Making a Difference

When a triangular bandage is used to apply a sling, place the knot to either side of the patient's neck. It will be very uncomfortable for the patient if the knot is tied behind the cervical spine.

Traction Splints

A **traction splint** is a device used to immobilize a midshaft fracture of the femur (Figure 37-18). When applied, this type of splint maintains a steady pull (traction) on the femur. A traction splint decreases muscle spasm and pain. It also keeps broken bone ends in a near-normal position. A unipolar traction splint has

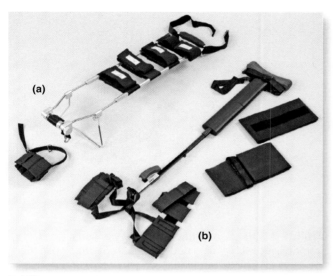

FIGURE 37-18 ▲ Traction splints. **(a)** Bipolar traction splint; **(b)** unipolar traction splint.

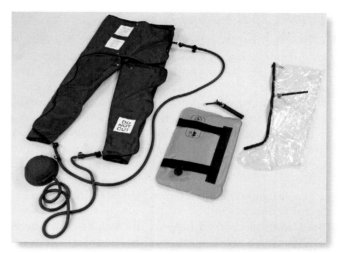

FIGURE 37-19 ▲ Pneumatic splints.

one pole that provides external support for the injured leg. A bipolar traction splint uses two external poles, one on each side of the injured leg, to provide external support. Two emergency care professionals are needed to apply a bipolar traction splint. Contraindications to the use of a traction splint are shown in the following *You Should Know* box. It is important to note that controversy exists regarding whether or not a traction splint can or should be used to immobilize an open fracture of the femur. Be sure to ask your instructor, EMS agency coordinator, or medical director regarding the use of a traction splint for this type of injury in your area.

Pneumatic Splints

A **pneumatic splint** requires that air be pumped in or suctioned out. The pressure within a pneumatic splint can vary with temperature and altitude. The air splint, vacuum splint, and the pneumatic antishock garment (PASG) are examples of pneumatic splints (Figure 37-19). A pneumatic splint is placed around the injured area and is inflated (air splint or PASG) or deflated (vacuum splint) until it becomes firm. When using an air splint, inflate it until you can make a slight dent in the splint with your fingers.

If permitted by local protocol, a PASG may be used to help control suspected severe bleeding in the abdomen or pelvis that is accompanied by hypotension. Remember that the PASG has three separate compartments that can be inflated: the abdomen, left leg, and right leg. All three compartments are inflated if there is an injury to the abdomen or pelvis. The abdominal compartment is *never* used without inflating both leg compartments. When the PASG is positioned on the patient, the top edge of the garment must be below the patient's lowest ribs. If the garment is positioned higher on the patient, the pressure caused by inflating the abdominal compartment can hamper the patient's breathing.

Remember This

Apply padding to any splint that is hard or does not precisely fit the area to which it will be applied. *Before* placing the splint against the patient, secure the padding to the splint to keep it from bunching up.

Care of Specific Musculoskeletal Injuries

Upper-Extremity Injuries

Upper-extremity injuries include injuries to the shoulder (clavicle, scapula, and humerus), upper arm (humerus), elbow, forearm (radius and ulna), wrist, and hand.

Injuries to the Shoulder

A shoulder injury typically involves three bones: the collarbone (clavicle), shoulder blade (scapula), and the upper arm bone (humerus). The patient will usually hold her arm in a position of comfort. The patient who has an anterior shoulder dislocation will usually hold her arm close to her chest. The patient who has a posterior shoulder dislocation may prefer to hold her arm over her head. When splinting, you may need to be creative. Improvise as needed to hold the injury in place.

A sling and swathe are often used for an upper-extremity injury (Skill Drill 37-1). The sling forms a pouch and is used to support the weight of the arm. The swathe is used to immobilize the injury by securing the patient's arm to her chest.

If ready-made materials are not available, fold up the bottom of the patient's shirt and pin or tape it in place for a sling. The arms of a long-sleeved shirt can be tied to one side of the patient's neck and the rest of the shirt used as a sling. A jacket that is zipped closed or wide strips cut from a sheet (or from the bottom of the patient's shirt) can be used as a swathe.

If the patient is holding her arm away from her body, provide support for the injured area, using a pillow, rolled towels, or similar material to fill the gap between the patient's arm and her chest. Secure the patient's arm and any support material to the patient's chest with a swathe. Ask the patient to hold her uninjured arm out to the side. Wrap the swathe around her chest and the injured extremity. Secure the swathe in place with a knot.

Injuries to the Upper Arm (Humerus)

The upper arm bone (humerus) extends from the shoulder to the elbow. It is most often fractured at its upper end near the shoulder or in the middle of the bone. Fractures of the upper end of the bone typically occur in older adults who fall on an outstretched hand. The middle of the bone is more often fractured in young adults. An upper arm injury should be immobilized from the shoulder (the joint above) to the elbow (the joint below). This type of injury is usually best immobilized with a sling and swathe. The swathe should not be placed directly on top of the injury. It should be positioned either above or below the fracture site. A padded splint or a SAM Splint formed around the upper arm and held in place with roller gauze can be used to provide additional support (Figure 37-20).

Follow these steps to immobilize a closed, nonangulated fracture of the humerus, radius, ulna, femur, tibia, or fibula:

- Wear appropriate PPE. Remove or cut away clothing to expose the injury. Remove jewelry from the injured limb.

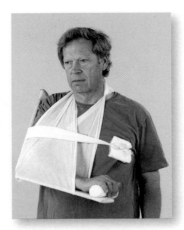

FIGURE 37-20 ▲ An upper arm injury is usually best immobilized with a sling and swathe. A padded splint can be used to provide additional support. Here, a humerus injury is immobilized with the elbow bent.

- Ask an assistant to manually support the injured extremity, using one hand above the injury and one hand below the injury.
- Assess pulses, movement, and sensation below the injured area.
- Select a splint, and measure it for proper length against the uninjured extremity. Make sure that the joint above and below the injured area will be immobilized. Pad a rigid or semirigid splint.
- Apply the splint, immobilizing the injured bone as well as the joint above and below the injury. When possible, immobilize the injured hand or foot in a position of function. Avoid excessive movement of the injured area when applying the splint.
- Pad the hollow areas between the extremity and the splint. Avoid placing ties or straps directly over the injury. Secure the entire injured extremity.
- Assess pulses, movement, and sensation every 15 minutes, and document your findings.

Injuries to the Elbow

The elbow is formed by the joining of the upper arm bone (humerus) and the two forearm bones (radius and ulna). Because there are many nerves and blood vessels in the elbow area, consider an elbow injury a serious injury. Splinting an elbow injury requires immobilizing the humerus (the bone above the injury) and the radius and ulna (the bones below the injury). Many patients will not allow an injured elbow to be moved.

If you find the patient with his elbow in a bent position, consider using a semirigid or vacuum splint to immobilize the injury. These splints will conform to the shape of the arm, despite its odd position. You might also use a padded splint. After you have applied a splint, use a sling and swathe to further limit movement if the

Immobilizing a Shoulder Injury

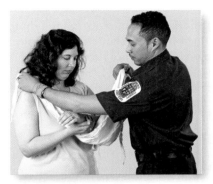

STEP 1 ▲ • A sling and swathe are typically used to immobilize a shoulder injury. After assessing for pulse, movement, and sensation in the injured arm, drape one end of a triangular bandage under the injured arm.
• Drape the other end over the opposite shoulder and around the patient's neck.

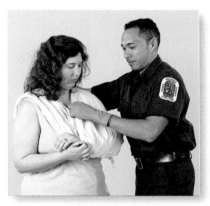

STEP 2 ▲ Pull the end of the bandage that is under the injured arm up to the patient's neck.

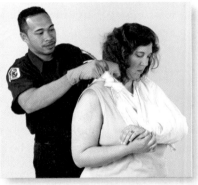

STEP 3 ▲ • Tie the two ends of the bandage to one side of the patient's neck.
• Twist and tuck the corner of the sling at the elbow.

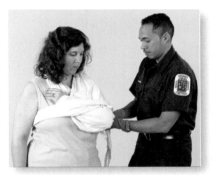

STEP 4 ▲ Use another bandage as a swathe, and secure the arm to the chest.

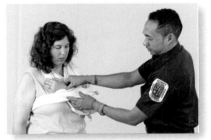

STEP 5 ▲ Reassess pulse, movement, and sensation in the injured arm.

patient's condition allows him to be placed in a sitting or semisitting position.

If the arm is straight, use a soft or rigid splint that extends from the armpit to the wrist. Secure the injured arm to the body to prevent movement (Figure 37-21). Prepare for immediate transport.

Follow these steps to immobilize a closed, nonangulated injury to the elbow or knee:

- Wear appropriate PPE. Remove or cut away clothing to expose the injury. Remove jewelry from the injured limb.
- Ask an assistant to manually support the injured extremity with one hand above and one hand below the injury.

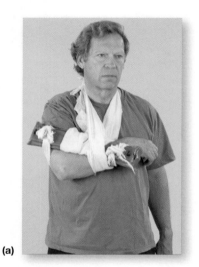

(a)

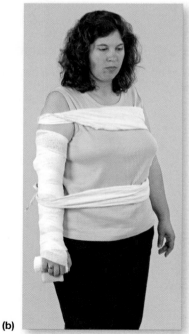

(b)

FIGURE 37-21 ▲ Elbow injury immobilized **(a)** with the elbow bent and **(b)** in a straight position.

- Assess pulses, movement, and sensation below the injured area.
- Select a splint, and measure it for proper length against the uninjured extremity. Make sure that the bones above and below the injured area will be immobilized. Pad a rigid or semirigid splint.
- Apply the splint, immobilizing the injured joint and the bones above and below the injury. When possible, immobilize an injured hand or foot in a position of function. Avoid excessive movement of the injured area when applying the splint.
- Pad the hollow areas between the extremity and the splint. Secure the entire injured extremity.
- Assess pulses, movement, and sensation every 15 minutes, and document your findings.

Injuries to the Forearm, Wrist, and Hand

The forearm, wrist, and hand contain many bones and are commonly injured. These areas can sustain serious injury with or without any visible deformity. The forearm extends from the elbow to the wrist. Some wrist fractures may present with gross deformity and hand displacement. Immobilize the extremity in the position found with a soft, rigid, or pneumatic splint.

When immobilizing an injury of the forearm, wrist, or hand with a rigid, semirigid, or soft splint:

- Place the splint underneath the forearm. Remember that the joints above and below the injury site must be immobilized. Therefore, the splint must extend from the elbow (the joint above) to beyond the hand (the joint below).
- An injured forearm or wrist should be placed in a sling and secured to the body with a swathe (Figure 37-22).

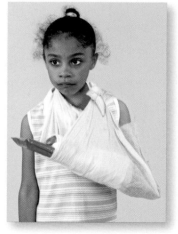

FIGURE 37-22 ▲ Immobilization of an injury to the forearm or wrist.

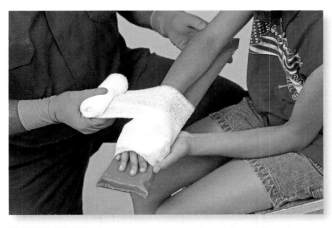

FIGURE 37-23 ▲ Immobilization of an injured hand.

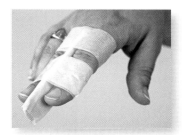

FIGURE 37-24 ▲ Immobilization of a finger injury.

- A hand injury can be immobilized by using a variety of materials. Before applying the splint, place the hand in a position of function unless there is gross deformity or displacement (Figure 37-23). When possible, remember to leave the fingers exposed to check color, movement, and sensation.

- If a finger is injured, you can use an anatomic splint by taping the injured finger to an uninjured finger next to it. Taping fingers (or toes) together is also called **buddy taping.** Provide additional support for the injured finger by placing padding between it and the finger next to it (Figure 37-24). If more than one finger is injured, immobilize the entire hand.

Making a Difference

The patient who has an isolated arm injury is often most comfortable in a sitting or semisitting position. If the patient's condition requires that he be positioned on his back, the weight of the patient's arm and splint on his chest and upper abdomen can hamper chest movement. If the patient *must* be positioned on his back and the arm must be immobilized with the elbow bent, try to splint the patient's arm so that the weight of the arm and splint will be supported on the patient's upper legs, rather than on his chest or abdomen. Using a soft pillow under the injured extremity will help alleviate pain and distribute the weight more evenly across the chest and allow better lung expansion if the patient must absolutely be transported flat on his back.

The Sager Emergency Fracture Response System (SEFRS) includes the SX405 compact traction splint and SEFRS Adaptor. The SEFRS compact kit treats any limb fracture in the body without traction and immobilizes the fracture "as found." The ability of this device to treat any fracture is attributable to the use of the adaptor, which is manipulated free of the patient and exactly simulates the disfigurement of the fracture. This is accomplished by holding and adjusting the device next to the patient's injury or, in some cases, lightly placing the device on the limb and allowing it to precisely mimic the shape and the angle of the fracture. When the adaptor is locked, it is then assembled with its padded arms and applied. The fracture is then secured with special cravats (Skill Drill 37-2).

Lower-Extremity Injuries

Lower-extremity injuries involve the pelvis, hip, thigh (femur), knee, lower leg (tibia and fibula), ankle, foot, and toes.

Injuries to the Pelvis and Hip

An injury to the pelvis can result in massive, life-threatening internal bleeding. Swelling and obvious deformity may not be easy to see because the pelvis is protected by many muscles and soft tissues. Call for advanced life support (ALS) personnel immediately. Keep in mind that a force strong enough to cause an injury to the pelvis demands spinal stabilization as well. Treat the patient for shock if an injury to the pelvis is present.

Remember that the hip joint is a ball-and-socket joint formed by a cup-shaped hollow in the pelvis (the acetabulum) into which the upper end of the femur fits. In a hip dislocation, the upper end of the femur is popped out of its socket. As the bone is pushed out of its socket, blood vessels and nerves can be damaged. The patient usually complains of severe pain and is unable to move the affected leg. If nerve damage is present, the patient may not have any feeling in the foot or ankle area. You may see that one leg is shorter than the other, and the affected leg may be turned inward or outward. When present, these signs suggest a hip fracture; however, they are not always present. About 50% of patients with a hip dislocation have other injuries, such as injuries to the pelvis, legs, back, or head.

Applying the SEFRS Adaptor

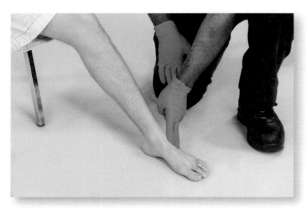

STEP 1 ▲ Assess distal pulses, movement, and sensation in the injured limb.

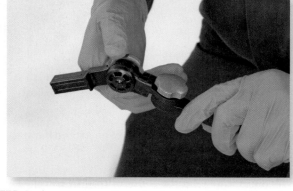

STEP 2 ▲ Remove the adaptor from the pack and unlock the knobs.

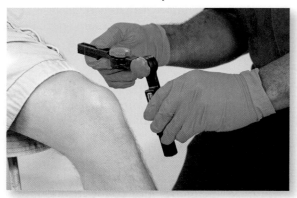

STEP 3 ▲ Using a "no touch" assessment, determine the fracture configuration and "mimic" the angle of the fracture by adjusting the adaptor.

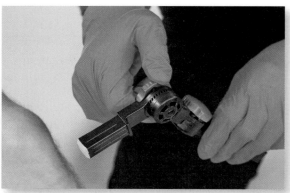

STEP 4 ▲ Tighten both adaptor adjusting knobs to fix the angle.

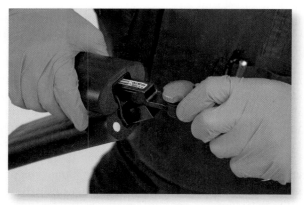

STEP 5 ▲ Pull the two halves of the outer tube apart about 8 inches. Then insert the longest arm of the adaptor into the largest hole.

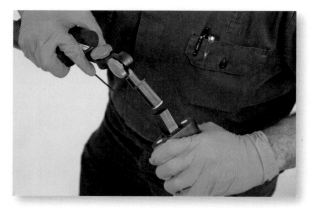

STEP 6 ▲ Insert the other end of the adaptor into the hole on the other arm.

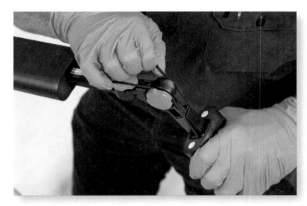

STEP 7 ▲ Pull the bungee cords looped over the adaptor knobs. Depending on the size of the limb, the extender shaft can be added to the splint.

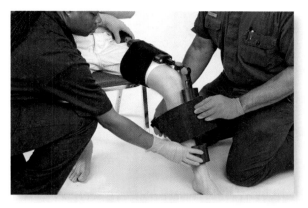

STEP 8 ▲ Gently place the fully assembled splint on the injured limb.

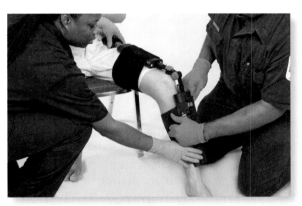

STEP 9 ▲ Securely apply the cravats to complete immobilization of the limb.

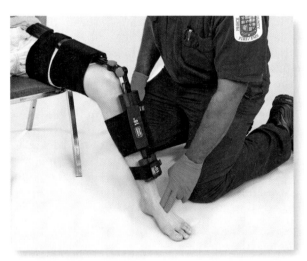

STEP 10 ▲ Reassess distal pulses, movement, and sensation in the injured limb.

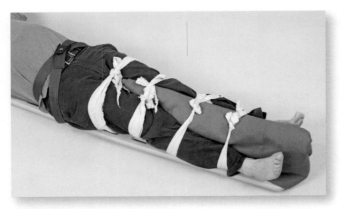

FIGURE 37-25 ▲ Immobilization of an injury to the pelvis or hips.

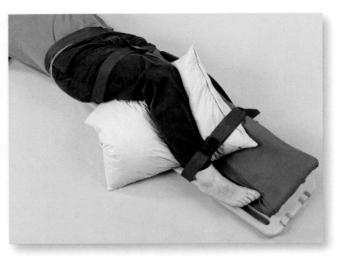

FIGURE 37-26 ▲ Immobilization of a hip injury.

In most hip dislocations, the head of the femur is pushed out and back (a posterior dislocation). This most often occurs during a motor vehicle crash (MVC) when a front seat occupant strikes the dashboard with her knees. The energy from the impact is transmitted along the femur to the hip joint. In a posterior dislocation, the hip is in a fixed position, bent and twisted in toward the middle of the body.

In an anterior hip dislocation, the upper end of the femur slips out of its socket and moves forward. With this type of injury, the hip is usually only slightly bent, and the leg twists out and away from the middle of the body. An anterior dislocation is much less common than a posterior dislocation.

Immobilizing the pelvis or hip requires the use of a splint that extends from the level of the lower back to past the knee on the affected side. A long backboard is usually used for this purpose. A blanket or similar padding is placed between the patient's legs. The injured leg is secured to the uninjured leg, and the patient's entire body is secured to the backboard (Figure 37-25).

When splinting the legs together:

- Move the good leg to the injured leg. If possible, *do not move the injured leg to the good leg.*

- Secure the legs together with straps, triangular bandages, or roller gauze secured in four places on the legs—two above the knee and two below. Ties are usually placed just above the ankles, at the calves, just above the knees, and at the thighs. Make sure the knots are secured over the padded material between the patient's legs so that they do not rub against the patient.

- Additional straps or triangular bandages should be used around the pelvis to secure it to the backboard and limit movement.

In many cases, a patient with a hip injury will not be able to move the affected leg into a straight position. In these situations, support the affected leg with pillows and rolled blankets between and under the legs. Secure the patient's hips and legs to a long backboard with straps, triangular bandages, or roller gauze to limit movement (Figure 37-26). An injury to the pelvis can also be immobilized with a PASG or pelvic sling. These devices may be used *only* if medical direction allows you to do so. Check with your instructor or medical director.

Injuries to the Upper Thigh (Femur)

Because the femur is protected by large muscles, a great deal of force is required to break it. Most femur fractures involve the middle or upper end of the bone. A broken femur can occur in activities such as skiing, and cycling, in falls from a great height, and in MVCs. It can also occur as a result of child abuse. The injured leg will often appear shorter than the other leg. In addition, the injured leg is often externally rotated. A broken femur is a true emergency because a patient can easily lose more than a liter of blood internally. Call for ALS personnel immediately. Bone fragments can cause damage to blood vessels, nerves, and soft tissues. Life-threatening bleeding may be present if both femurs are broken.

A fracture of the upper third of the femur is treated as a hip fracture (Figure 37-27).

Most femur fractures can be adequately immobilized by using two long boards:

- Use a board on the outside of the leg that extends from the patient's armpit to below the bottom of the foot.

- Use a board on the inside of the leg that extends from the patient's groin to below the bottom of the foot.

- Be sure to pad any hollow areas, and then secure the boards to the patient with straps, triangular

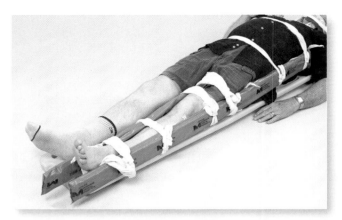

FIGURE 37-27 ▲ Immobilization of a femur fracture.

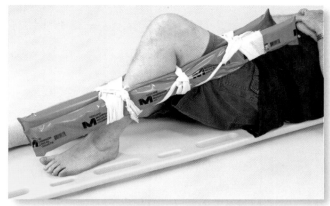

FIGURE 37-28 ▲ Immobilization of the knee in a bent position.

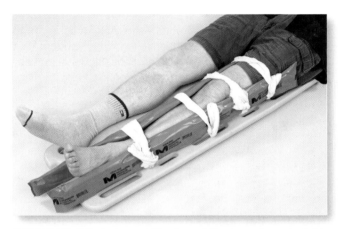

FIGURE 37-29 ▲ Immobilization of the knee in a straight position.

bandages, or roller gauze. Secure the boards under the patient's arms, at the hips, just above the knees, at the calves, and just above the ankles. Be sure the knots are secured on the outside of the boards.

- Additional straps or triangular bandages must be used when you are securing the patient to a long backboard.

- Alternately, a vacuum splint or mattress or a traction splint can be used to immobilize a closed midshaft femur fracture.

Applying traction to a fractured femur helps stabilize the bone ends and reduces pain. It also reduces the likelihood of a closed fracture becoming an open one and reduces further soft tissue damage (Skill Drills 37-3 and 37-4).

Injuries to the Knee

The knee joint is formed by the lower end of the femur, the upper end of the tibia, and the patella. The patella is frequently dislocated from injuries, such as a fall. This type of injury usually appears as a lump on the lateral side of the knee. You will often find the patient complaining of pain with one leg in a bent position at the knee. Distal pulses are usually present.

A knee dislocation may result from violent direct force, such as the knee hitting the dashboard during an MVC. This type of injury is serious because the popliteal artery behind the knee can be cut or compressed. The patient is often unable to move the leg. The affected leg is usually grossly deformed around the knee. Extensive swelling is usually present, and distal pulses may be absent. Check distal pulses frequently. Call for ALS personnel immediately.

If you find the patient with a knee in a bent position:
- Support the affected knee with a pillow, if available.
- To limit movement, place a padded board splint on each side of the knee from the thigh to the calf (Figure 37-28).

- Secure the boards in place with triangular bandages or roller gauze above and below the knee.

If the knee is straight:
- Place a long, padded board splint on each side of the knee (Figure 37-29). The board on the outside of the leg should extend from the patient's hip to the ankle. The board on the inside of the leg should extend from the groin to the ankle.
- Tie triangular bandages or roller gauze above and below the knee, at the uppermost part of the thigh, and just above the ankle. Be sure the ties are positioned on the outside of the splint.

Injuries to the Lower Leg

The tibia and fibula are the bones of the lower leg. A fracture of the tibia is the most common type of long bone fracture. Fractures of the lower leg usually occur as a result of a direct force injury, such as a fall, an

Applying the Sager SX 405 Unipolar Traction Splint

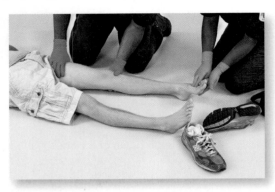

STEP 1 ▲ Expose the fracture site. Ask an assistant to stabilize the patient's leg while you remove the patient's shoe and assess distal pulses, movement, and sensation in the injured leg.

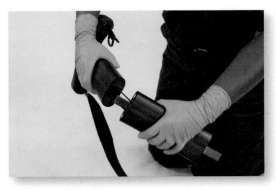

STEP 2 ▲ Remove and unfold the outer shaft assembly.

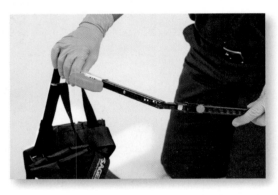

STEP 3 ▲ Remove, unfold, and lock the inner shaft assembly.

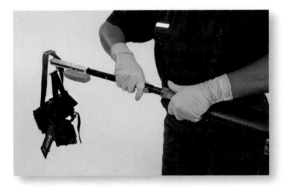

STEP 4 ▲ Insert the inner shaft assembly into the outer shaft assembly. The splint is now ready to be applied.

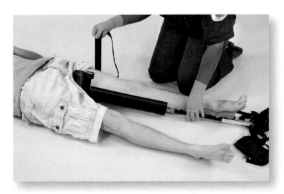

STEP 5 ▲ Position the splint between the patient's legs: Rest the ischial perineal cushion (the saddle) against the ischial tuberosity, with the shortest end of the articulating base toward the ground.

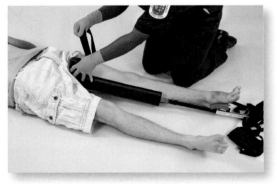

STEP 6 ▲ Press down on the (saddle) cushion while pulling the thigh strap laterally under the thigh to seat the saddle against the ischial tuberosity.

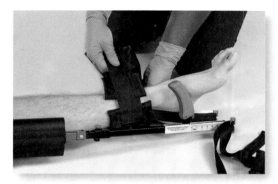

STEP 7 ▲ Using the attached hook and loop straps, wrap the ankle harness around the ankle to secure snugly.

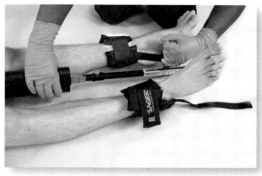

STEP 8 ▲ Pull the control tabs to engage the ankle harness tightly against the crossbar. Apply traction by grasping the padded shaft of the splint with one hand and the red traction handle with the other. Gently extend the inner shaft until the desired amount of traction is recorded on the traction scale.

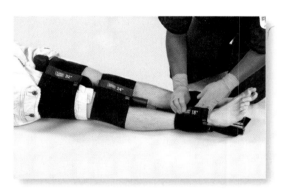

STEP 9 ▲ Adjust the thigh strap at the upper thigh, and make sure that it is not too tight, but snug and secure. Then firmly secure the tensor cravats.

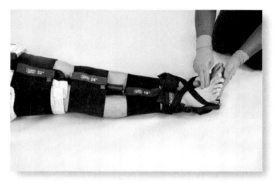

STEP 10 ▲ Apply the figure-eight strap around the feet to prevent rotation. Reassess distal pulses, movement, and sensation in the injured limb.

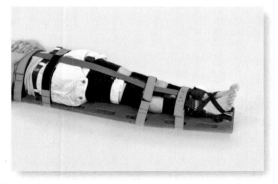

STEP 11 ▲ Place the patient on a long backboard, and secure the patient to the board.

Applying a Bipolar Traction Splint

STEP 1 ▶
- Adjust the traction splint to the proper length. Position the splint next to the patient's uninjured leg, and use the bony prominence of the buttock (ischial tuberosity) as a landmark. Extend the splint 6–12 inches beyond the patient's uninjured heel. Lock the splint in position.
- Position the support straps at the midthigh, above the knee, below the knee, and above the ankle. Do not position a strap over the fracture. Open the straps and fasten them under the splint.

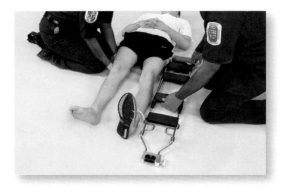

STEP 2 ▶
- Stabilize the injured leg so that it does not move while an assistant fastens the ankle hitch around the patient's foot and ankle.
- Support the leg under the injured area while your assistant applies gentle in-line traction to the injured leg by using the ankle hitch and foot.

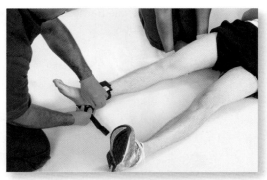

STEP 3 ▶
- While your assistant continues to apply gentle manual traction, position the splint under the injured leg. The ischial pad should rest against the ischial tuberosity.
- Raise the heel stand after the splint is in position.

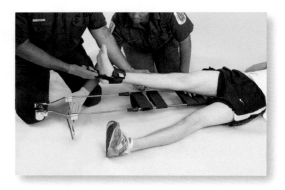

STEP 4 ▶
- Pad the groin area.
- Attach the ischial strap. Secure the strap over the groin and thigh.

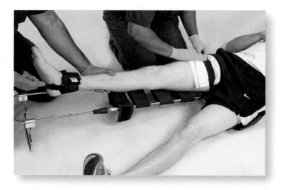

STEP 5 ▶ While your assistant continues to apply gentle manual traction, attach the S hook of the splint to the D ring of the ankle hitch.

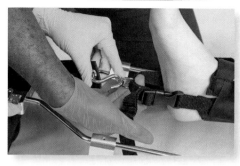

STEP 6 ▶ • While manual traction continues, begin tightening the ratchet on the splint to apply mechanical traction.
• Continue tightening until mechanical traction is equal to the manual traction and the patient's pain and muscle spasms are reduced. If the patient is unconscious, continue tightening until the length of the injured leg equals that of the uninjured leg.

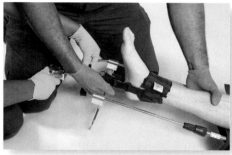

STEP 7 ▶ • Fasten the leg support straps over the injured leg.
• Recheck the ischial strap and ankle hitch. Make sure both are fastened securely. The assistant maintaining manual traction can slowly release traction after all straps are securely in place.

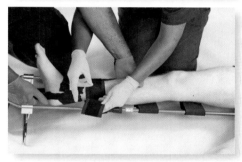

STEP 8 ▶ Reassess distal pulses, movement, and sensation in the injured limb.

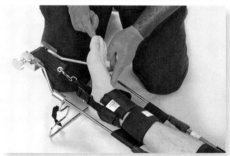

STEP 9 ▶ • Place the patient on a long backboard.
• Secure the leg and splint in place. Place padding between the splint and the uninjured leg.

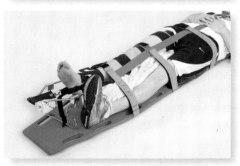

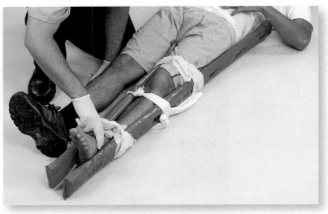

(a)

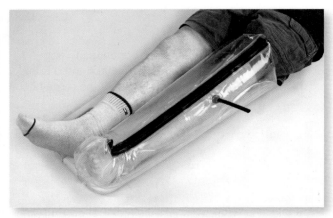

(b)

FIGURE 37-30 ▲ Immobilization of the lower leg by means of **(a)** padded boards and **(b)** an air splint.

MVC, or a twisting force. A fracture of either the tibia or the fibula can occur by itself. However, a tibia fracture is usually associated with a fibula fracture because the force that causes the tibia fracture is transmitted to the fibula. Bruising, swelling, and tenderness are usually present over the fracture site. When the tibia is broken, the patient will complain of pain when he puts weight on it. Because the tibia lies very close to the skin surface, a large number of fractures involving these bones are open fractures.

Immobilize a fracture of the tibia and fibula with a splint that extends from the hip to the foot:
- Place a padded board splint on each side of the leg (Figure 37-30). The board on the outside of the leg should extend from the patient's hip to the foot. The board on the inside of the leg should extend from the groin to the foot.
- Make sure to pad behind the knee to keep it in a position of comfort.
- Use triangular bandages or roller gauze to secure the boards in place.
- For a closed injury, an air splint that extends above the knee and covers the entire foot may be used instead of padded boards.

Injuries to the Ankle and Foot

The ankle is formed by the lower ends of the tibia and the fibula (the shinbones) and the many smaller bones of the foot. It is difficult to tell when an ankle or foot injury is a fracture or a sprain because both are very painful and swell a great deal. An ankle or foot injury is best immobilized with a preformed lower leg splint, a soft splint such as a pillow or blanket (Figure 37-31), or an air splint.

Splints that can be used for various bone and joint injuries are listed in Table 37-3.

FIGURE 37-31 ▲ Immobilization of an ankle or foot injury.

On the Scene **Wrap-Up**

You have applied a cervical collar before the paramedics arrive. The crew chief listens as you give your report. You tell her there are good pulses, movement, and sensation distal to each of the patient's injuries. You and your partner apply a traction splint to care for the suspected femur fracture. The paramedic fashions a rigid splint to support the patient's upper arm injury. "Pad a formable splint, and put it on her right lower arm," the

TABLE 37-3 Possible Splints for Bone and Joint Injuries

Site of Injury	Possible Splints
Shoulder	Sling and swathe, Sager Emergency Fracture Response System (SEFRS), Sentry Tactical Orthopedic Response Matrix (STORM)
Upper arm (humerus)	Padded board splint, padded wire ladder splint, sling and swathe, SAM Splint, SEFRS, STORM
Elbow	Padded board splint, padded wire ladder splint, air splint, vacuum splint, sling and swathe, SAM Splint, SEFRS, STORM
Forearm (radius, ulna)	Padded board splint, padded wire ladder splint, air splint, vacuum splint, sling and swathe, SAM Splint, SEFRS, STORM
Wrist, hand	Padded board splint, padded wire ladder splint, air splint, vacuum splint, sling and swathe, SAM Splint, SEFRS, STORM
Pelvis	Long backboard, scoop stretcher, PASG, pelvic sling, STORM wrap and cravats
Hip	Long backboard with blanket or pillow between the legs, scoop stretcher, PASG
Thigh (femur)	Traction splint, long padded board splints, other leg used as a splint, SEFRS, STORM
Knee	Pillow, padded board splint, SAM Splint, air splint, vacuum splint, other leg used as a splint, SEFRS, STORM
Lower leg (tibia, fibula)	Padded board splint, SAM Splint, air splint, vacuum splint, other leg used as a splint, SEFRS padded arm, STORM padded arm
Ankle, foot	Preformed lower leg splint, pillow or blanket, air splint, vacuum splint, SEFRS, STORM

paramedic instructs you. Your crew carefully reassesses each extremity after the splints are applied to ensure that pulses, movement, and sensation are still present. You apply ice packs to each injured area and move the patient to the ambulance. En route to the hospital, you reassess her vital signs while the paramedic starts an IV. The paramedic contacts medical direction and receives an order to give the injured woman some medicine to relieve her pain. As you get ready to step off the ambulance, you notice that your patient's eyes close and her face visibly relaxes. ∎

Sum It Up

▶ The skeletal system is divided into the axial and appendicular skeletons. The axial skeleton includes the skull, spinal column, sternum, and ribs. The appendicular skeleton is made up of the upper and lower extremities (arms and legs), the shoulder girdle, and the pelvic girdle.

▶ Skeletal muscles produce movement of the bones to which they are attached. Most skeletal muscles are attached to bones by means of tendons. Tendons create a pull between bones when muscles contract. The tendons of many muscles cross over joints, which contributes to the stability of the joint. Tendons can be damaged from overextension or overuse. Ligaments connect bone to bone.

▶ A skeletal muscle has three main parts: The origin is the stationary attachment of the muscle to a bone, the insertion is the movable attachment to a bone, and the body is the main part of the muscle.

▶ The mechanism of injury to bones and joints can be caused by direct forces, indirect forces, and twisting forces:

- A direct force causes injury at the point of impact.
- An indirect force causes injury at a site other than the point of impact.
- A twisting force causes one part of an extremity to remain in place while the rest twists. Twisting injuries commonly affect the joints such as ankles, knees, and wrists. Twisting forces cause ligaments to stretch and tear.

▶ Injuries to bones and joints may be open or closed. In an open injury, the skin surface is broken. An open injury increases the risk of contamination and infection. These injuries can also result in serious blood loss. In closed injuries of bones and joints, the skin surface is not broken. The injury is often painful, swollen, and deformed.

▶ A fracture is a break in a bone. If a bone is broken, chipped, cracked, or splintered, it is said to be fractured.

▶ A greenstick fracture occurs when the bone breaks on one side but not the other, like bending a green tree branch.

▶ A comminuted fracture is one in which the bone is splintered or crushed, resulting in several breaks in the bone and multiple bone fragments.

▶ A linear fracture is one in which the break runs parallel to the long axis of the bone.

▶ A transverse fracture is one in which the break is at about a 90-degree angle to the bone, whereas an oblique fracture is one in which the break is at about a 45-degree angle to the bone.

▶ A spiral fracture is a bone break caused by a twisting motion and usually occurs in the long bones of the body, such as the humerus and femur.

▶ Colles' fracture is a break in the distal radius that is usually caused by falling on an outstretched hand in an attempt to break a fall.

▶ Pott's fracture is a fracture of the lower part of the fibula with displacement of the foot.

▶ Typical blood loss in an uncomplicated fracture of the tibia or fibula during the first 2 hours can be as much as 550 mL. A broken femur can result in the loss of up to 1 L of blood, and a fractured pelvis can result in the loss of 2 L.

▶ A dislocation occurs when the end of a bone is forced from its normal position in a joint. A partial dislocation (subluxation) means the bone is partially out of the joint. Luxation, a complete dislocation, means it is all the way out. Dislocations and subluxations usually result in temporary deformity of the affected joints, loss of limb function, immediate swelling, and point tenderness, and they may result in sudden and severe pain.

▶ A sprain is a stretching or tearing of a ligament, the connective tissue that joins the end of one bone with another. Sprains are classified as mild, moderate, and severe.

▶ A strain is a twisting, pulling, or tearing of a muscle or tendon. A muscle strain usually occurs when a muscle is stretched beyond its limit. A strain often occurs near the point where the muscle joins the tough connective tissue of the tendon.

▶ Most sprains and strains can be treated with rest, ice, and elevation.

▶ In assessing extremity injuries, check the **p**ulse, **m**ovement, and **s**ensation (PMS) in each extremity.

▶ A splint is a device used to immobilize (limit movement of) a body part to prevent pain and further injury.

  • In some situations, the patient will have already splinted the injury by holding the injured part close to her body in a comfortable position. Using the body as a splint is called a self-splint or anatomic splint.

  • Before splinting an injured hand or foot, place it in the position of function. The natural position of the hand at rest looks as if you were gently grasping a small object, such as a baseball.

▶ Rigid splints are made of hard material, such as wood, strong cardboard, or plastic. This type of splint is useful for immobilizing injuries that occur to the middle portion (midshaft) of a bone. Some rigid splints are padded, but others must be padded before they are applied to the patient.

▶ Semirigid (flexible) splints are very useful for immobilizing joint injuries. These splints can be molded to the shape of the extremity. Examples include the SAM Splint and aluminum ladder splints. Semirigid splints can be used in combination with other splints, such as a sling and swathe.

▶ Soft splints are flexible and useful for immobilizing injuries of the lower leg or forearm. Examples of soft splints include a sling and swathe, blanket rolls, pillows, and towels. A sling and swathe are used to immobilize injuries to the shoulder, collarbone, or upper arm bone. A triangular bandage is often used to make a sling. A swathe is a piece of soft material used to secure the injured extremity to the body.

▶ A traction splint is a device used to immobilize a femur fracture. This type of splint maintains a steady pull on the bone. A traction splint keeps broken bone ends in a near-normal position. Controversy exists regarding whether or not a traction splint can or should be used to immobilize an open fracture of the femur. Be sure to ask your instructor, EMS agency coordinator, or medical director regarding the use of a traction splint for this type of injury in your area.

▶ A pneumatic splint requires air to be pumped in or suctioned out of it. An air splint, vacuum splint, and the pneumatic antishock garment are examples of pneumatic splints. A pneumatic splint is placed around the injured area and is inflated (air splint or PASG) or deflated (vacuum splint) until it becomes firm.

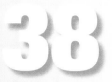

CHAPTER

38

Head, Face, Neck, and Spine Trauma

By the end of this chapter, you should be able to:

Knowledge Objectives ▶

1. Describe the components, anatomy, and physiology of the nervous system.
2. Define the structure of the skeletal system as it relates to the nervous system.
3. Distinguish between head injury and brain injury.
4. Relate mechanism of injury to potential injuries of the head and spine.
5. Differentiate between closed and open head injuries.
6. Discuss types of skull fractures.
7. Describe the possible causes, signs, and symptoms of a head injury.
8. Describe the emergency care of the patient with a head injury.
9. Describe the anatomy and physiology of the structures of the face.
10. Relate mechanism of injury to potential injuries of the face.
11. Describe the assessment findings and symptoms of an injury to the face.
12. Describe the emergency care of the patient with an injury to the face.
13. Describe the anatomy and physiology of the structures of the neck.
14. Relate mechanism of injury to potential injuries of the neck.
15. Describe the assessment findings and symptoms of an injury to the neck.
16. Describe the emergency care of the patient with an injury to the neck.
17. Describe the possible causes, signs, and symptoms of a concussion.
18. Describe the possible causes, signs, and symptoms of a cerebral contusion.
19. Explain the concept of increasing intracranial pressure (ICP).
20. Describe the possible causes, signs, and symptoms of a subdural hematoma.
21. Describe the possible causes, signs, and symptoms of an epidural hematoma.
22. Describe the possible causes, signs, and symptoms of an intracerebral hematoma.
23. Describe the emergency care of the patient with a possible brain injury.
24. Differentiate between a spinal cord injury and a spinal column injury.
25. State the assessment findings and symptoms of a potential spine injury.
26. Describe the method of determining whether a responsive patient may have a spine injury.
27. Relate the airway emergency medical care techniques to the patient with a suspected spine injury.
28. Describe the emergency care of the patient with a possible spine injury.
29. Describe how to stabilize the cervical spine.
30. Discuss indications for sizing and using a cervical spine immobilization device.
31. Describe a method for sizing a cervical spine immobilization device.

32. Discuss possible complications of a cervical collar that does not fit properly.
33. Describe how to logroll a patient with a suspected spine injury.
34. Describe how to secure a patient to a long spine board.
35. List instances when a short spine board or vest-type device should be used.
36. Describe how to stabilize the spine of a seated patient.
37. Describe how to stabilize the spine of a standing patient.
38. Describe the indications for the use of rapid extrication.
39. State the circumstances in which a helmet should be left on the patient.
40. Discuss the circumstances in which a helmet should be removed.
41. Describe how the patient's head is stabilized to remove a helmet.
42. Discuss methods of helmet removal.

Attitude Objectives ▶ 43. Explain the rationale for stabilization of the entire spine when a cervical spine injury is suspected.
44. Explain the rationale for using a short spine stabilization device when moving a patient from the sitting to the supine position.
45. Defend the reasons for leaving a helmet in place for transport of a patient.
46. Defend the reasons for removal of a helmet before transport of a patient.

Skill Objectives ▶ 47. Demonstrate opening the airway in a patient with an injury to the head, face, neck, or spine.

connect(plus+)
48. Demonstrate the care of a patient with an injury to the head, face, neck, or spine.
49. Demonstrate completing a prehospital care report for a patient with an injury to the head, face, neck, or spine.
50. Demonstrate stabilization of the cervical spine.
51. Demonstrate the three-person logroll for a patient with a suspected spinal cord injury.
52. Demonstrate securing a patient to a long spine board.
53. Demonstrate using the short board or vest-type immobilization device.
54. Demonstrate methods for stabilization of a helmet.
55. Demonstrate helmet removal techniques.

On the Scene

You and your partner are dispatched to a construction site for a head injury. Upon arrival, you find a 28-year-old man lying on the floor in the construction site office. Your first impression reveals the patient is awake and aware of your approach. He appears to be breathing normally and his skin color is pink. A coworker is holding a bloodied towel to the side of the patient's head.

The patient states that, while he was working, an 8-pound sledgehammer fell from about 8–10 feet above him onto his head. He then walked about 80 feet to his supervisor's office where they laid him down and controlled the bleeding from his head wound. Your partner finds an approximately 1-inch full-thickness laceration to the patient's right temporal area. The patient's initial vital signs are as follows: pulse 110, strong and regular; respirations 16, unlabored; blood pressure 138/60. The patient denies any loss of consciousness and states that he feels dizzy and nauseated. ■

Introduction

According to the Brain Trauma Foundation, an estimated 1.5 million head injuries occur every year in the United States. The National Spinal Cord Injury Statistical Center indicates that there are about 12,000 new cases of spinal cord injury (SCI) each year in the United States. Motor vehicle crashes account for 42% of reported SCI cases. The next most common cause of SCI is falls, followed by acts of violence (primarily gunshot wounds), and recreational sporting activities. Since 2005, the average age at the time of a spinal cord injury is 39.5 years.

If a head or spine injury is missed or improperly treated, permanent disability or death may result. Your initial treatment of a patient with a possible injury to the head or spine can prevent further injury. You must know when to suspect these types of injuries and how to provide appropriate care.

Anatomy and Physiology Review

Central Nervous System

Objectives 1, 2

The nervous system controls the voluntary and involuntary activities of the body. The central nervous system (CNS) is made up of the brain and spinal cord. The brain occupies the entire space within the cranium. Meninges (literally, "membranes") are three layers of connective tissue coverings that surround the brain and spinal cord (Figure 38-1). The **pia mater** (literally, "gentle mother") forms the delicate inner layer that clings gently to the brain and spinal cord. It contains many blood vessels that supply the nervous tissue. The **arachnoid** (literally, "resembling a spider's web") layer is the middle meningeal layer with delicate fibers resembling a spider's web. It con-

tains few blood vessels. The **dura mater** (literally, "hard" or "tough mother") is the tough, durable, outermost layer that clings to the inner surface of the cranium.

Cerebrospinal fluid (CSF) surrounds the brain and spinal cord. It acts as a shock absorber. It also provides a means for exchange of nutrients and wastes between the blood, brain, and spinal cord.

The cerebrum is the largest part of the human brain (Figure 38-2). It consists of two cerebral hemispheres. The corpus callosum joins the two hemispheres. Each cerebral hemisphere has four lobes:

1. The frontal lobe, which controls motor function
2. The parietal lobe, which receives and interprets nerve impulses from sensory receptors
3. The occipital lobe, which controls eyesight
4. The temporal lobe, which controls hearing and smell

The cerebellum is the second-largest part of the human brain. It is responsible for precise control of muscle movements, maintenance of posture, and maintaining balance. The brainstem includes the **midbrain, pons,** and **medulla oblongata.** The midbrain connects the pons and cerebellum with the cerebrum. It acts as a relay for auditory and visual impulses. The pons (literally, "bridge") connects parts of the brain with one another by means of tracts. It influences respiration. The medulla oblongata extends from the pons and is continuous with the upper portion of the spinal cord. It is involved in the regulation of heart rate, blood vessel diameter, respiration, coughing, swallowing, and vomiting.

The spinal column consists of 33 bones. The spinal cord extends from the medulla of the brainstem to the level of the upper border of the second lumbar vertebra in an adult. An adult's spinal cord is about 16–18 inches in length. The spinal cord is well protected by the spinal column in the back. Injuries associated with a lot of force are usually necessary to cause damage to the spinal cord.

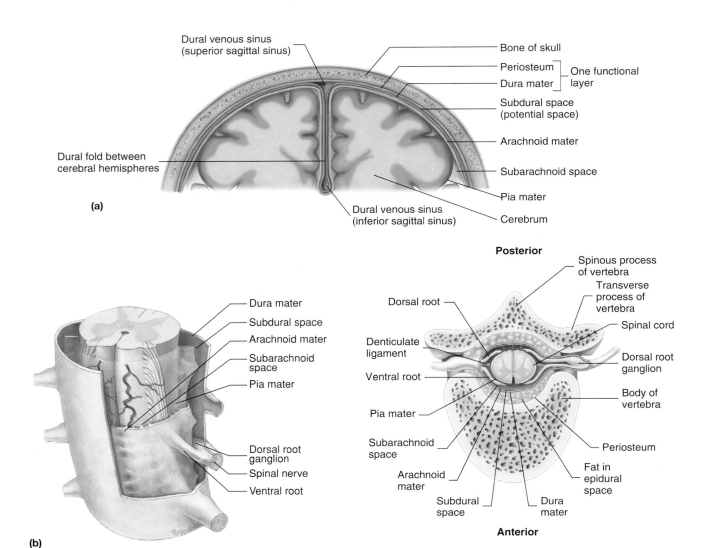

FIGURE 38-1 ▲ Meningeal coverings of **(a)** the brain and **(b)** the spinal cord.

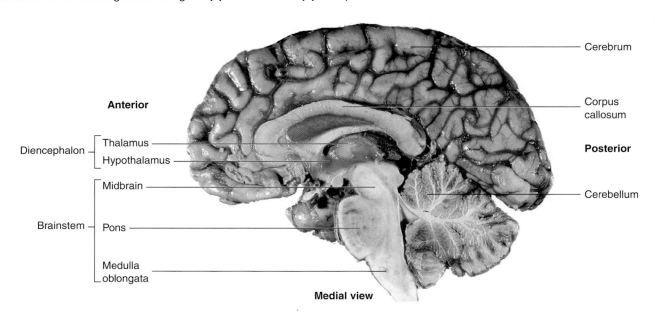

FIGURE 38-2 ▲ Areas of the brain.

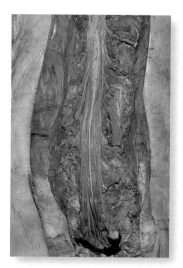

FIGURE 38-3 ▲ A dissected spinal cord and roots of the spinal nerves.

The spinal cord is made up of long tracts of nerves that join the brain with all body organs and parts (Figure 38-3). It is the center for many reflex activities of the body. **Motor nerves** carry responses from the brain and spinal cord, stimulating a muscle or organ. **Sensory nerves** send signals to the brain about the activities of the different parts of the body relative to their surroundings. For example, when you want a finger to move, the message, "Attention, finger! Move!" is sent down the spinal cord and through the nerve of the finger, and your finger moves. At about the same time, the finger sends a reply to the brain saying, "Mission complete." If the spinal cord is severely damaged, nerve signals cannot get from the brain to the parts of the body below the injury. The patient's signs and symptoms will depend on the type and location of the injury (Figure 38-4).

Peripheral Nervous System

The peripheral nervous system (PNS) consists of all nervous tissue found outside the brain and spinal cord. There are 12 pairs of cranial nerves. They connect the brain with the neck and structures in the thorax and abdomen. The oculomotor nerve originates in the midbrain and controls pupil size. Pressure on this nerve causes nerve paralysis. If the oculomotor nerve is paralyzed, the affected pupil will not react to light. The vagus nerve originates in the medulla. Pressure on this nerve causes slowing of the heart rate.

There are 31 pairs of spinal nerves. Sensory nerves transmit messages to the brain and spinal cord *from* the body. Motor nerves transmit messages from the brain and spinal cord *to* the body.

The PNS has two divisions; both divisions contain sensory (afferent) and motor (efferent) nerves. The somatic (voluntary) division has receptors and nerves

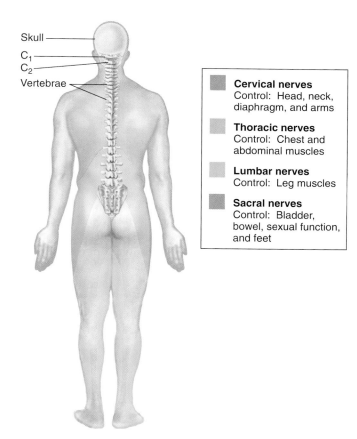

FIGURE 38-4 ▲ If the patient has a spinal cord injury, signs and symptoms will depend on the location of the injury.

concerned with the external environment. It influences the activity of the musculoskeletal system. The autonomic (involuntary) division, also called the *autonomic nervous system (ANS)*, has receptors and nerves concerned with the internal environment. The ANS controls the involuntary system of glands and smooth muscle and functions to maintain a steady state in the body. The autonomic division is further divided into the sympathetic division and parasympathetic division. The sympathetic division mobilizes energy, particularly in stressful situations (the "fight-or-flight" response). Its effects are widespread throughout the body. The parasympathetic division conserves and restores energy. Its effects are localized in the body.

Injuries to the Head

Objective 3

A **head injury** is a traumatic insult to the head that may result in injury to soft tissue, bony structures, and/or brain injury. A **traumatic brain injury (TBI)** occurs when an external force to the head causes the brain to move within the skull or the force causes the skull to break and directly injures the brain. Head injuries are discussed in this section. Injuries to the brain are discussed later in this chapter.

Mechanism of Injury

Objective 4

Blunt trauma to the head usually is caused by motor vehicle crashes, falls, sports, and assaults with blunt weapons. Gunshot and stab wounds are the usual mechanisms of penetrating trauma to the head. Head injuries generally result in pain, swelling, bleeding, and deformity. Motor vehicle crashes and falls often cause the patient to become unresponsive. When a patient loses consciousness, he loses the ability to protect his own airway. Appropriate airway management and breathing support are critical when treating a patient with a head injury.

Injuries to the Scalp

The outermost part of the head is called the **scalp.** An injury to the scalp may occur because of blunt or penetrating trauma. The scalp consists of five layers containing tissue, hair follicles, sweat glands, oil glands, and a rich supply of blood vessels. Because the brain is protected by a rigid container, the skull, a scalp injury may or may not cause an injury to the brain. When injured, the scalp may bleed heavily. In children, the amount of blood loss from a scalp wound may be enough to produce shock. In adults, shock is usually not caused by a scalp wound or internal skull injuries. More often, in adults, shock results from an injury elsewhere.

Assess the scalp carefully for cuts because some are not easy to detect. Control bleeding with direct pressure. Do not apply excessive pressure to the open wound if you suspect a skull fracture. Doing so can push bone fragments into the brain. Dressings and bandages applied to control bleeding from the scalp should not close the patient's mouth.

Injuries to the Skull

Objectives 5, 6

The skull is made up of two main groups of bones, the bones of the cranium and the bones of the face. The cranium contains eight bones that house and protect the brain:

- Frontal (forehead) bone
- Two parietal (top sides of cranium) bones
- Two temporal (lower sides of cranium) bones
- Occipital (back of skull) bone

- Sphenoid (central part of floor of cranium) bone
- Ethmoid (floor of cranium, nasal septum) bone

The bones of the face are discussed later in this chapter. A head injury may be closed or open. In a closed head injury, the skull remains intact. However, the brain can still be injured by the forces or objects that strike the skull. The forces that impact the skull cause the brain to move within the skull. The brain strikes the inside of the skull, which causes injuries to the brain tissue. The impact and shearing forces that affect the brain can cause direct damage to the brain tissue. These forces can also injure the surrounding blood vessels. The skull is a rigid, closed container (Figure 38-5). If bleeding occurs within the skull, the pressure within the skull increases as the blood takes up more space within the closed container. If the bleeding continues and the pressure continues to rise, the patient can suffer severe brain damage and even death.

In an open head injury, the skull is not intact, and the risk of infection is increased. It is important to emphasize that the phrase "open head injury" refers to the condition of the skull and not the brain. Broken bones or foreign objects forced through the skull can cut, tear, or bruise the brain tissue itself. If the skull is cracked, the blood and CSF that normally surround the brain and spinal cord can leak through the crack in the skull and into the surrounding tissues. If the forces are strong enough to cause an open head injury, then the brain will most likely sustain an injury as well.

Significant force, such as a severe impact or blow, can result in a skull fracture. There are several types of skull fractures. A depressed skull fracture exists when the broken portion of the skull moves in toward the brain. In a compound skull fracture, the scalp is cut and the skull is fractured. A fracture at the base of the skull (near the neck) is called a *basilar skull fracture.* The skull bones fractured are usually the temporal bone, occipital bone, sphenoid bone, or ethmoid bone, and sometimes the foramen magnum (the opening at the base of the skull) (Figure 38-6). A basilar skull fracture can compress, entrap, and damage nerves and blood vessels that pass through the foramen magnum. If the area of the temporal bone near the ear is fractured, blood or cerebrospinal fluid may leak from the ear. Cerebrospinal fluid is normally clear, but may appear pink if it contains blood. *Battle's sign* (bruising behind the ear) is a delayed finding, generally taking hours to develop. If the break in the skull occurs in the anterior cranial fossa, the patient typically develops bruising around the eyes, commonly called "raccoon eyes." If the ethmoid bones are disrupted, cerebrospinal fluid may leak from the nose. The signs of a skull fracture are shown in Figure 38-7.

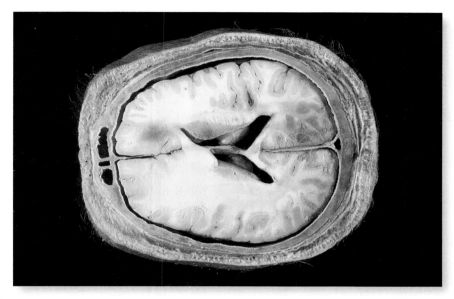

FIGURE 38-5 ▲ The skull is a rigid, closed container. If bleeding occurs within the skull, the pressure within the skull increases as the blood takes up more space within the closed container.

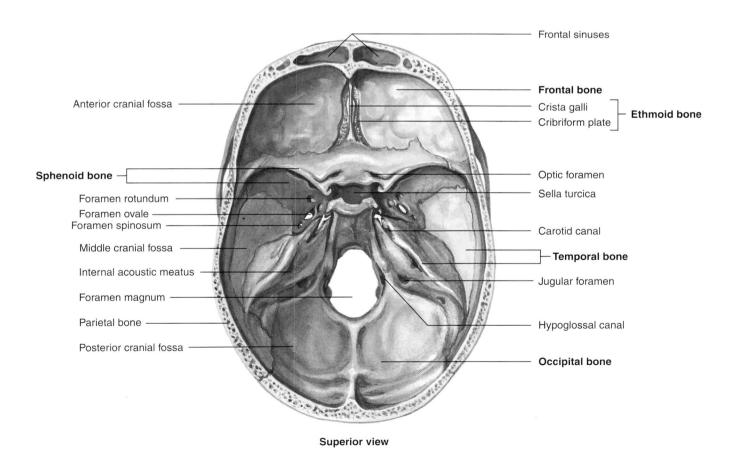

Superior view

FIGURE 38-6 ▲ Floor of the cranial vault.

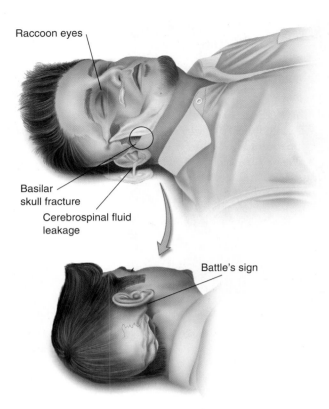

Raccoon eyes

Basilar
skull fracture

Cerebrospinal fluid
leakage

Battle's sign

FIGURE 38-7 ▲ Signs of a skull fracture.

You Should Know

Assessment Findings and Symptoms of a Skull Fracture

- Bruises or cuts to the scalp
- Deformity to the skull
- Discoloration around the eyes (raccoon eyes)
- Discoloration behind the ears (Battle's sign)
- Loss of consciousness
- Confusion
- Convulsions
- Restlessness, irritability
- Drowsiness
- Blood or clear, watery fluid (cerebrospinal fluid) leaking from the ears or nose
- Visual disturbances
- Changes in pupils (unequal pupil size or pupils that are not reactive to light)
- Slurred speech
- Difficulties with balance
- Stiff neck
- Vomiting

Patient Assessment

Objective 7

Conduct a scene size-up and ensure your safety. Evaluate the mechanism of injury before approaching the patient. Put on appropriate PPE. Carefully assess the patient's airway while maintaining spinal stabilization. The head trauma patient is prone to an airway obstruction caused by blood, avulsed teeth, vomitus, or the tongue. Suction as needed to keep the airway open. Give 100% oxygen, assisting ventilation as needed. Even if the airway is open, gas exchange may be impaired due to a decreased respiratory effort, CNS depression due to drugs or alcohol, or other injuries, such as a flail chest, open pneumothorax, or tension pneumothorax. Assess the patient's circulatory status and control hemorrhage with direct pressure, if present. Initially, assess the patient's level of consciousness using the AVPU scale. Follow this assessment with a more accurate one using the Glasgow Coma Scale (GCS) and assessment of the pupils. (Review the GCS in Chapter 33, "Trauma Overview," Table 33-1.) Healthcare professionals use the GCS score to determine the severity of an injury to the head or brain (see Table 38-1). It is important to determine the GCS score as early as possible to establish a baseline and then periodically repeat the assessment. Treat any life-threatening injuries before proceeding to the secondary survey. A short on-scene time and rapid transport to an appropriate trauma center are critical when caring for a head-injured patient.

Hypoxia can cause further damage in already injured tissue. Monitor the patient's blood oxygenation continuously using a pulse oximeter, and obtain the patient's vital signs. Maintain the patient's oxygen saturation at 90% or above. Monitor the patient's heart rate, respiratory rate and regularity, and blood pressure closely for signs of increasing intracranial pressure (discussed later in this chapter). The signs and symptoms of a head injury appear in the next *You Should Know* box.

Emergency Care

Objective 8

To treat a patient with a head injury, use the following steps:

- Head trauma patients with impaired airway or ventilation, open wounds, or abnormal vital signs or who do not respond to painful stimuli may need rapid extrication. Ask your partner to manually stabilize the patient's head and neck until the patient has been completely stabilized on a long backboard.

TABLE 38-1 Head or Brain Injury Severity

Classification	Glasgow Coma Scale Score	Notes
Minor	13 to 15	• Patient conscious and talking with a history of disorientation, amnesia for events immediately before and after the injury, or brief loss of consciousness • May experience temporary vision loss or a seizure • Excellent prognosis
Moderate	9 to 12	• Typically confused but able to follow simple commands • Good prognosis
Severe	3 to 8	• Unable to follow commands • Unequal pupil size • Most survivors have significant disabilities

You Should Know

Assessment Findings and Symptoms of a Head Injury

- Changes in mental status that range from confusion and repetitive questioning to unresponsiveness
- Deep cuts or tears to the scalp or face
- Exposed brain tissue (a very bad sign)
- Penetrating injuries such as gunshot wounds and impaled objects
- Swelling ("goose eggs"), bruising of the skin
- Edges or fragments of bone seen or felt through the skin
- A deformity of the skull such as "sunken" areas (depressions)
- Swelling or discoloration behind the ears (Battle's sign; may not be seen until hours after the injury)
- Swelling or discoloration around the eyes (raccoon eyes; may not be seen until hours after the injury)
- Pupils that are unequal in size, irregular in shape, or do not react to light equally; dilation of both pupils
- Elevated blood pressure
- An irregular breathing pattern
- Slow heart rate
- Nausea and/or vomiting
- Seizures
- Blood or clear, watery fluid from the ears or nose
- Weakness or numbness of one side of the body
- A loss of bladder or bowel control

- Establish and maintain an open airway. Adequate airway, ventilation, and oxygenation are critical to the outcome of head trauma patients. If you must open the patient's airway, use a modified jaw thrust. Head trauma patients frequently vomit—keep suction within arm's reach and monitor the patient's airway closely.
- Give oxygen by nonrebreather mask. If the patient's breathing is inadequate, assist the breathing with a bag-mask device connected to 100% oxygen.
- Control bleeding. If bleeding is present from an open head wound, apply firm pressure with a trauma pad to control blood loss over a broad area. If blood soaks through the dressing, apply additional dressings on top and continue to apply pressure. If signs of shock are present, treat for shock.
- If the patient has an adequate or elevated blood pressure, raise the head of the backboard 30 degrees to help minimize increases in intracranial pressure.
- Head trauma patients frequently have seizures; protect the patient from harm if a seizure occurs.
- Transport head trauma patients to an appropriate trauma center.
- Note that a head trauma patient may deteriorate rapidly and need air medical transport.
- Comfort, calm, and reassure the patient and family members. En route to the receiving facility, reassess as often as indicated. Closely monitor the patient's airway, breathing, pulse, and mental status for deterioration. Be alert for slowing of the heart rate, a change in breathing pattern, and/or rising blood pressure. Redetermine the

patient's Glasgow Coma Scale score when reassessing the patient. Report your findings when transferring patient care.

- Record all patient care information, including the patient's medical history and all emergency care given, on a PCR.

Injuries to the Face

Anatomy and Physiology Review

Objective 9

The face receives its arterial blood supply from branches of the common carotid artery. The common carotid artery branches into the internal and external carotid arteries (Figure 38-8). The internal carotid arteries supply blood to the brain. Branches of the external carotid arteries supply blood to the face, nose, mouth, and neck. The internal and external jugular veins are the major veins that drain blood from the head and neck. The muscles of facial expression are stimulated by the facial nerve. Branches of the trigeminal nerve supply sensation to the face.

The bones of the face protect the brain and the sensory organs: the eyes, ears, nose, and mouth. Seven bones form the cone-shaped openings into the skull that are called the *orbits* (eye sockets). The orbit possesses four walls: a roof, lateral wall, floor, and medial wall. The medial walls of the orbit are paper-thin. Because the floor and medial walls of the orbits are weak, the orbit can be fractured by blunt forces, such as a direct blow to the globe of the eye or rim of the orbit. The orbits contain several openings through which the optic nerve and blood vessels pass.

The external part of the nose is made up mostly of cartilage. A pair of nasal bones forms the bridge of the nose, which is the area between the eyes. The nasal bones are the most commonly fractured bones of the face. The area called the *midface* is made up of the maxilla (upper jaw), zygomatic bones (cheekbones), bones of the orbit, and the nasal bones. The zygomatic arch is a bridge across the side of the face that is formed by the

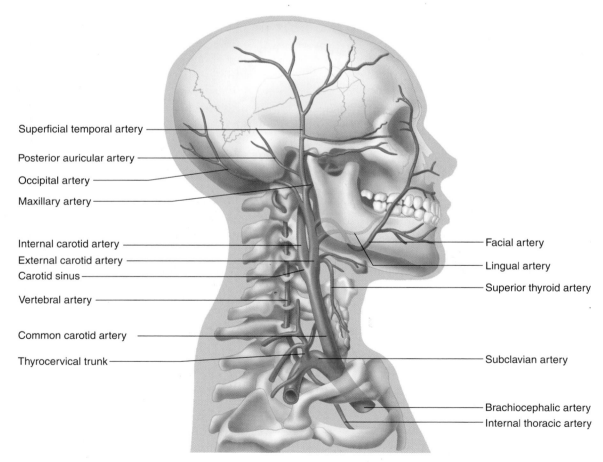

Lateral view

FIGURE 38-8 ▲ Arteries of the head and neck.

temporal and zygomatic bones. Muscles attached to the zygomatic arch enable movement of the mandible (lower jaw). The maxilla houses the upper teeth and the mandible houses the lower teeth. Facial trauma, including fractures of the facial bones, can cause airway obstruction, impaired gas exchange, and death if airway and breathing are not adequately established.

The eye receives its blood supply via the retinal artery and retinal vein. The conjunctiva is the mucous membrane that lines the posterior surface of the eyelids and the anterior portion of the globe. It is normally colorless, except when its vessels are dilated because of inflammation (conjunctivitis).

The eye contains three layers called *tunics* (Figure 38-9). The outer layer of the eye, called the fibrous tunic, contains the sclera and cornea. The sclera is the white of the eye, providing eye protection and points of attachment for some of the eye muscles, and helping to maintain the shape of the eye. The cornea is located on the anterior portion of the eye and is transparent. It allows light to enter the eye. In fact, most of the refraction (bending) of light by the eye takes place not in the lens but at the surface of the cornea. Because of its location, the cornea is prone to injury from chemicals, abrasions, and foreign bodies. The eyelids, which protect the eyes from foreign objects, close on stimulation of the cornea (corneal reflex).

The middle layer of the eye is called the vascular tunic. It is made up of the iris, ciliary body, and choroid. The iris is the colored part of the eye. It contains smooth muscles that surround the opening of the eye, called the *pupil*. Light passes through the pupil, and the iris controls the diameter of the pupil, which affects the amount of light entering the eye. The outer edge of the iris attaches to the ciliary body, which connects the choroid with the iris. The ciliary body contains smooth muscles called *ciliary muscles* that attach to the lens of the eye by suspensory ligaments. The muscles of the ciliary body continually expand and contract, pulling on the suspensory ligaments, which changes the shape of the lens. By altering its form and thickness, the lens adjusts the focus of light from different distances on the retina. This function is called *accommodation*. With age, the lens becomes increasingly yellow, hard, and less elastic, which can affect vision. The ciliary body produces a watery fluid called *aqueous humor*, which helps maintain pressure within the eye, refracts light, and provides nutrients to the inner surface of the eye. The choroid consists of a vascular network that delivers oxygen and nutrients to the retina.

The innermost layer of the eye is called the *nervous tunic*, or *retina*. It contains two layers: an outer pigmented retina and an inner sensory retina. In conjunction with the choroid, the pigmented retina keeps light from reflecting back into the eye. Photoreceptor cells called *rods* and *cones* are located in the sensory retina. These photoreceptor cells convert light rays into electrical impulses, which are then carried to the brain via the optic nerves. These impulses are processed in the occipital lobe of the cerebrum of the brain and interpreted as images.

The inside of the eye contains two compartments that are separated by the lens. The anterior chamber, located at the front of the eye, is filled with aqueous humor. The posterior chamber contains a transparent jellylike substance called the vitreous humor, which serves to hold the lens and retina in place, help maintain pressure within the eye, and hold the shape of the posterior chamber.

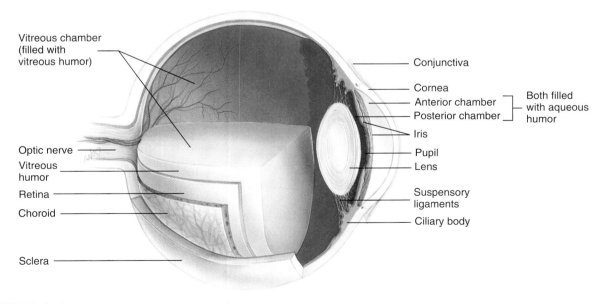

FIGURE 38-9 ▲ Layers and compartments of the eye.

Mechanism of Injury

Objective 10

Trauma to the face is usually the result of blunt trauma, most commonly from fists and clubs; falls; and windshields, dashboards, and steering wheels in motor vehicle crashes. Penetrating trauma may result from gunshot wounds, stabbings, dog bites, human bites, or biting of the tongue. An increasing number of patients (adults and children) with facial trauma are victims of intimate partner violence. Be particularly observant when assessing the scene involving a patient with facial trauma. Be alert for subtle signs of intimate partner violence throughout your patient assessment and when obtaining the patient's medical history.

Injuries to the Mouth

An injury to the mouth can result in severe swelling or bleeding that causes an airway obstruction. The skin of the lips is very thin, and lacerations of this area can result in significant bleeding that can be controlled with direct pressure. Lacerations of the tongue can cause significant bleeding, requiring frequent suctioning to maintain an open airway. Because the tongue is attached to the lower jaw (mandible), a lower-jaw fracture may allow the tongue to fall against the back of the throat, blocking the airway. The signs and symptoms depend on the area of the jaw affected. Tenderness, bruising, and swelling are common (Figure 38-10).

You Should Know

If a patient is unable to open her mouth or move her lower jaw side to side without pain, suspect a fracture.

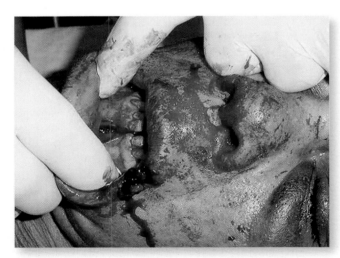

FIGURE 38-10 ▲ Jaw fracture resulting from direct frontal trauma.

The upper jawbone (maxilla) is often fractured in high-speed crashes. The patient's face is thrown forward into the windshield, steering wheel, and dashboard. A fracture of the maxilla is often accompanied by a black eye. The patient's face may appear unusually long. Swelling and pain are usually present.

A patient with a jaw fracture should receive spinal stabilization because of the mechanism of injury. Carefully look in the patient's mouth for teeth, blood, vomitus, and other potential obstructions. Suction as necessary. Look in the mouth for broken or missing teeth. If dentures or missing teeth are found, they should be transported with the patient. If a knocked-out (avulsed) tooth is found, handle the tooth by the crown. Do not handle the tooth by the root (the part that was embedded in the gum). Rinse the tooth (do not scrub it) in water. Place the tooth in milk or in a Save-a-Tooth kit (or similar product) if it is available. Control bleeding and treat for shock if indicated. Transport the tooth with the patient to the hospital.

Injuries to the Nose

An injury to the nose can result in significant bleeding and a possible airway obstruction. Palpate the nose for tenderness or crepitus. Assume that a patient who presents with bruising or tenderness over the bridge of the nose has a nasal bone fracture. Assume that clear fluid draining from the nose is cerebrospinal fluid until proved otherwise. Bleeding from lacerations to the nose and anterior epistaxis should be controlled with direct pressure.

Injuries to the Ear

Injuries to the ear include abrasions, contusions, lacerations, avulsions, and hematomas, which are treated like any other soft tissue injury. Never put anything into the ear to control bleeding.

You should assume that clear fluid draining from the ear is cerebrospinal fluid until proved otherwise. Place a sterile dressing loosely over the ear to absorb the drainage, and bandage it in place.

Injuries to the Eyes

A buildup of blood in the anterior chamber of the eye is called a **hyphema**, a sight-threatening injury (Figure 38-11). Although typically caused by blunt trauma, it can develop spontaneously in people with sickle cell disease. Unless contraindicated, elevate the patient's head to maintain low pressure within the eye. Keep the patient calm to reduce the risk of additional bleeding.

A **blowout fracture** refers to cracks or breaks in the facial bones that make up the orbit of the eye. Significant blunt trauma to the eye, such as getting hit by a

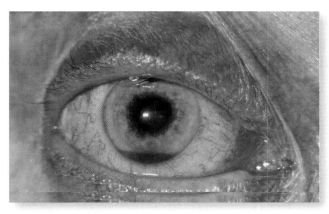

FIGURE 38-11 ▲ A hyphema. Note the pooled blood at the bottom of the iris.

bat, baseball, hockey stick, or puck, or getting kicked in the face may not injure the eye itself, but may fracture an orbital bone. The sudden rise in pressure generated by the trauma is transmitted to the orbit, where the thinnest portion of the orbit (usually the floor or medial wall) ruptures. Typical assessment findings and symptoms of a severe blowout fracture include recession of the eyeball within the orbit (enophthalmos), numbness over the cheek, epistaxis on the same side as the impact, and an inability to move one eye upward. Paralysis of upward gaze occurs because muscles in the eye become entrapped in the fracture.

Chemical burns to the eye were discussed in Chapter 34. Ultraviolet keratitis is a radiation injury to the eye. Sources of ultraviolet light include the sun as well as artificial sources such as a welder's arc, suntanning beds, photographic flood lamps, lightning, electric sparks, and halogen desk lamps. Ultraviolet keratitis is also called *welder's flash, arc eye,* and *snow blindness.* Although the cornea absorbs most ultraviolet radiation, damage to the surface of the cornea is cumulative. This process has been compared to the effects of the sun on the skin surface, resulting in a sunburn. Usually within 12 hours of overexposure to ultraviolet light, the patient complains of blurry vision and sensitivity to light. Generally, the patient complains of mild to severe pain in both eyes, but symptoms may be worse in the eye that received more ultraviolet radiation. Covering both eyes with eye pads may provide temporary relief until the patient can be evaluated at the hospital by a physician.

Injuries to the Midface

Injuries to the midface are most often caused by blunt trauma from an assault or a motor vehicle crash. Although most of the midface is formed by the maxilla, gentle palpation of the orbital rims, nose, zygoma, and maxilla is necessary to assess bone integrity of the midface. Suspect a fracture of the zygoma or maxilla if bruising of the cheek is present. A fracture of the maxilla is often accompanied by a black eye. The patient's face may appear unusually long. Swelling and pain are usually present. Assessment findings of a zygomatic fracture can include an eye droop, bruising in and around the eye, and a nosebleed on the injured side. Fractures involving multiple bones of the midface are often associated with significant bleeding into the nose or mouth. These patients will require constant airway monitoring and frequent suctioning to maintain an open airway.

Injuries to the Mandible

Injuries to the mandible are common and most often caused by blunt trauma from an assault or a motor vehicle crash (MVC). After nasal fractures, the mandible is the next most common fracture of the face. Bruising, swelling, and pain are usually present at the site of impact. Diminished or absent sensation of the lower lip may be present. The patient who has a mandible fracture or a combined fracture of the nose, maxilla, and mandible is at risk of an airway obstruction. Remember that the tongue is attached by muscles to the mandible. Therefore, a fractured mandible can affect the patient's ability to maintain an airway. This is particularly true when the patient is placed in a supine position and the tongue falls posteriorly, blocking the airway. Dentures, avulsed teeth, and blood are also possible causes of airway obstruction. Frequent reassessment is important to ensure that the airway remains open.

A patient with a jaw fracture should receive spinal stabilization because of the mechanism of injury. Carefully look in the patient's mouth for teeth, blood, vomitus, and other potential obstructions. Suction as necessary. Look in the mouth for broken or missing teeth.

Patient Assessment

Objective 11

After performing a scene size-up and ensuring your safety, put on appropriate PPE. Ask an assistant to maintain in-line stabilization of the patient's head and neck while you care for the patient, if consistent with your local protocols.

The patient with trauma to the face is at risk of airway obstruction. Inspect the mouth for loose or avulsed teeth, blood, vomitus, or other fluids, and suction as needed to keep the airway open. Assess the patient's breathing and circulation. Apply direct pressure to control hemorrhage, if needed. Look for life-threatening injuries to other areas of the body, such as the chest, and treat them before performing a secondary survey.

Perform a physical exam looking for open wounds, swelling, bruising, deformity of bones, and symmetry of the face and eyes. Palpate the facial bones. Without putting pressure on the eyeball, pull down the lower eyelid to assess the color of the conjunctiva and sclera. The conjunctiva should be pink. The sclera should be white. Assess the size, shape, and symmetry of the pupils. Remember that some patients normally have unequal pupils, a condition called *anisocoria*. Assess the eye muscles by asking the patient to follow your fingers up, down, and from side to side in the shape of an H. Both eyes should follow your fingers. Note if the patient can see letters on a card, pen, or shirt, and document your findings. Eye injuries require patching of both eyes.

Facial trauma can be accompanied by severe psychological trauma. Provide calm reassurance to the patient and family members as often as necessary while the patient is in your care.

You Should Know

Because some studies have shown that cervical spine injury associated with facial fractures is rare, some medical directors and EMS agencies feel that cervical spine stabilization is unnecessary in patients with isolated facial injuries. However, significant force is necessary to fracture bones of the face. As a result, cervical spine stabilization has conventionally been considered the standard of care for these patients. Research your local protocols to learn what is practiced in your area.

Emergency Care

Objective 12

To treat a patient with an injury to the face, perform the following steps:

- If the mechanism of injury suggests a head or spinal injury, continue manual stabilization of the patient's head and neck until the patient has been completely stabilized on a long backboard, if this procedure is consistent with your local protocols. The patient with a nasal fracture and significant bleeding may need to be transported in a sitting position or on his left side with spinal stabilization as needed.

- Establish and maintain an open airway. If you must open the patient's airway, use a modified jaw thrust. Monitor the patient's airway closely while the patient is in your care. Avoid the use of a nasal airway in the patient with facial trauma. Frequent suctioning may be necessary to maintain an open airway.

- Give oxygen by nonrebreather mask. If the patient's breathing is inadequate, assist her breathing with a bag-mask device connected to 100% oxygen. Providing positive-pressure ventilation to a patient with severe soft tissue or bony trauma to the midface may present a difficult challenge if the injuries prevent establishment of an adequate seal between the face and the mask.

- Control bleeding from a wound by applying a dressing and then direct pressure over the dressing with a gloved hand. If blood soaks through the dressing, apply additional dressings on top and continue to apply pressure. If signs of shock are present or if internal bleeding is suspected, treat for shock. Control bleeding from the nose by applying direct pressure to the nostrils.

- Dress and bandage any open wounds.

- If dentures or missing teeth are found, they should be transported with the patient. If a knocked-out (avulsed) tooth is found, handle the tooth by the crown. Do not handle the tooth by the root (the part that was embedded in the gum). Rinse the tooth in water. Place the tooth in milk or in a Save-a-Tooth kit (or similar product) if it is available. Transport the tooth with the patient to the hospital.

- A foreign body in the eye can be flushed out of the affected eye (see Chapter 34). Do not exert any pressure on the eye. Hold the patient's eyelid open, and gently flush the eye with warm water. Flush from the nose side of the affected eye toward the ear, away from the unaffected eye. It is important to flush away from the uninjured eye so that foreign bodies or chemicals are not transferred into the uninjured eye. Flush the eye for at least 5 minutes. If you are unable to remove the foreign body, cover both eyes and transport to the nearest appropriate medical facility.

- A chemical burn to the eye should be immediately flushed with copious amounts of water or normal saline. Continue flushing the eye for at least 20 minutes. Flush away from the unaffected eye (as previously described). Transport immediately. Irrigation should be continued throughout transport. Monitor where the runoff goes so that another part of the body is not contaminated.

- Emergency care for a nonchemical burn to the eye includes covering both eyes with moist pads. When possible, darken the back of the ambulance to protect the patient from further exposure to light. Transport the patient for further care.

- Eyelid lacerations should be treated as other soft tissue injures. If the eye is exposed, cover it with an eye pad moistened in sterile saline and bandage it in place. Cover the other eye to prevent sympathetic movement.

- If a foreign body is protruding from the eye, stabilize the object in place with bulky dressings and transport as quickly as possible. Do not attempt to remove the object.

- Although uncommon, handle an eviscerated eye gently. Do not attempt to replace the eye. Place a sterile 4×4 dressing moistened with sterile saline on the eye, and then cover the eye with a cup. Secure the cup in place with a bandage.

- An impaled object in the cheek may be removed if bleeding obstructs the airway. After removing an object from the cheek, apply direct pressure to the bleeding site by reaching inside the patient's mouth with gloved fingers. A patient with an impaled object in the check may be more comfortable sitting up, if there is no risk of spinal injury.

- Comfort, calm, and reassure the patient and family members. En route to the receiving facility, reassess as often as indicated. Closely monitor the patient's airway, breathing, pulse, and mental status for deterioration.

- Record all patient care information, including the patient's medical history and all emergency care given, on a PCR.

Injuries to the Neck

Anatomy and Physiology Review

Objective 13

A blunt or penetrating neck injury can rapidly become a life-threatening emergency because the neck houses many critical structures. The neck is bordered by the head superiorly and the sternal notch and clavicles inferiorly (Figure 38-12). The anterior area of the neck contains the pharynx and trachea. The trachea is kept open by a series of cartilages, including the thyroid and cricoid cartilages. The larynx lies behind the thyroid cartilage. The thyroid gland lies just below the larynx and in front of the upper part of the trachea. The esophagus lies behind the trachea. Posteriorly, the neck is bordered by the cervical spine.

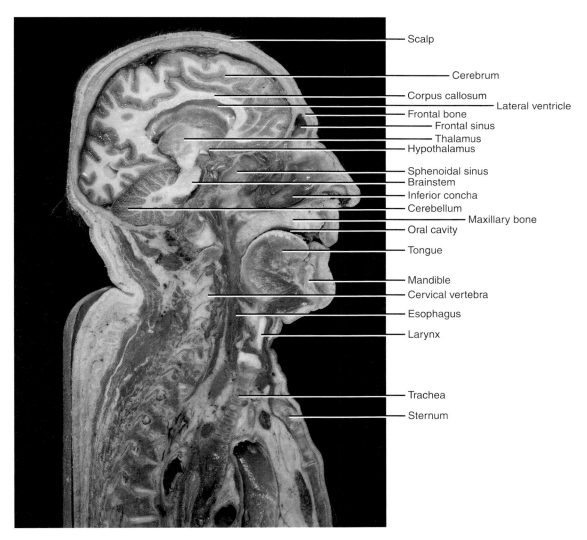

Scalp
Cerebrum
Corpus callosum
Lateral ventricle
Frontal bone
Frontal sinus
Thalamus
Hypothalamus
Sphenoidal sinus
Brainstem
Inferior concha
Cerebellum
Maxillary bone
Oral cavity
Tongue
Mandible
Cervical vertebra
Esophagus
Larynx
Trachea
Sternum

FIGURE 38-12 ▲ Sagittal section of the head and neck.

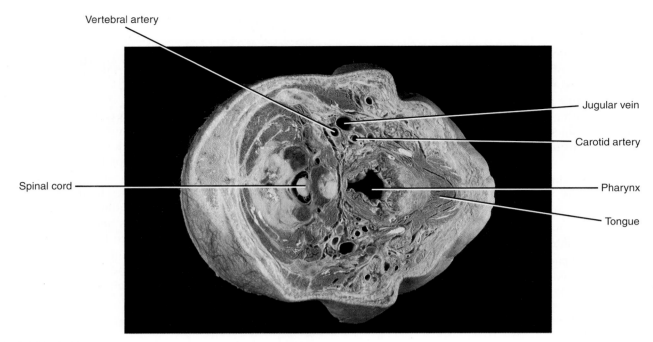

Vertebral artery

Jugular vein

Carotid artery

Spinal cord

Pharynx

Tongue

FIGURE 38-13 ▲ Transverse section of the neck, inferior view.

The neck contains several large muscles that provide support and enable movement of the head. The carotid, vertebral, and subclavian arteries are the major arteries of the neck. Injury to any of these vessels can result in massive bleeding or the formation of a hematoma that can compromise the airway. About one-half of patients with blunt trauma to the neck involving the carotid artery will have no external signs of neck injury. The internal jugular veins can be found lateral to the carotid arteries (Figure 38-13). Air may enter the circulatory system if there is penetrating injury to a large blood vessel in the neck.

Mechanism of Injury

Objective 14

A neck injury can be caused by a hanging, impact with a steering wheel, a knife or gunshot wound, strangulation, a sports injury, or a "clothesline" injury, in which a person runs into a stretched wire or cord that strikes the throat. The patient with a neck injury may also have an underlying spinal injury.

Patient Assessment

Objective 15

Conduct a scene size-up and ensure your safety. Evaluate the mechanism of injury before approaching the patient. Put on appropriate PPE. Assess the patient's

airway, breathing, and circulation while maintaining spinal stabilization. Work quickly, keeping in mind that an open wound to the neck may bleed profusely and cause death. Bubbling from a neck wound suggests involvement of the respiratory tract, such as injury to the larynx or trachea. Swelling of the structures in the neck can cause an airway obstruction. The patient may experience shortness of breath, difficulty breathing, and/or a hoarse voice.

Examine the neck for DCAP-BTLS. Assessment findings and symptoms of blunt trauma to the neck include hoarseness, bruising, deformity, and subcutaneous emphysema. The presence of subcutaneous emphysema suggests involvement of the respiratory tract. Stridor may be present, suggesting an upper airway obstruction. Look for handprints from a blow or possible choking and rope marks on the neck that may be caused by hanging. Palpate the trachea to determine if it is in its normal midline position. While making sure that the head and neck remain in a neutral, in-line position, gently palpate the cervical spine for tenderness and deformity.

Laryngeal injuries may be accompanied by hematomas, swelling, or hemorrhaging, increasing the risk of airway obstruction. Crepitus in the laryngeal area, subcutaneous emphysema, stridor, hoarseness, or an inability to speak may indicate a fracture of the larynx. Remember that the cricoid cartilage is the only complete ring of cartilage in the larynx. A fracture of the cricoid cartilage can result in death due to an airway obstruction.

Injuries to the esophagus are rare. Assessment findings and symptoms can include blood in the saliva, hematemesis, hoarseness, stridor, neck tenderness, and difficulty swallowing. Frequent suctioning may be needed to maintain an open airway. Monitor the patient's airway throughout your care.

Emergency Care

Objective 16

To treat a patient with a neck injury, perform the following steps:

- Patients with a neck injury should be transported to a trauma center. An ALS intercept or air medical transport may be necessary in severe cases of airway compromise.
- If the mechanism of injury suggests a head or spinal injury, continue manual stabilization of the patient's head and neck until the patient has been completely stabilized on a long backboard. When trauma to the neck is present, avoid rigid cervical collars or other devices that obstruct your view of the area. In this situation, it is likely that you will need to improvise to provide adequate stabilization of the patient's head and neck. If a cervical collar is applied, do not apply tape to the anterior hole in the collar. Doing so will impede your ability to adequately reassess the patient's neck.
- Establish and maintain an open airway. If you must open the patient's airway, use a modified jaw thrust maneuver. Monitor the patient's airway closely while the patient is in your care. Suction as necessary. If the entire patient has been secured to a long backboard, the backboard may need to be tilted to adequately clear the airway.
- Give oxygen. If the patient's breathing is inadequate, assist her breathing with a bag-mask device connected to 100% oxygen.
- Control bleeding. To care for an open neck wound, immediately place a gloved hand over the wound to control bleeding. Cover the wound with an airtight (occlusive) dressing, and apply a bulky dressing over the occlusive dressing. If blood soaks through the dressing, apply additional dressings on top and continue to apply pressure. The application of pressure using one gloved finger to control bleeding from a carotid artery or jugular vein may be necessary. Do not apply pressure to both carotid arteries at the same time. Doing so can compromise blood flow to the brain. If signs of shock are present or if internal bleeding is suspected, treat for shock.

- Do not remove a penetrating object. Instead, stabilize it in place with bulky dressings.
- Dress and bandage any open wounds.
- Comfort, calm, and reassure the patient and family members. En route to the receiving facility, reassess as often as indicated. Closely monitor the patient's airway, breathing, pulse, and mental status for deterioration.
- Record all patient care information, including the patient's medical history and all emergency care given, on a PCR.

Injuries to the Brain and Spinal Cord

Injuries to the Brain

Concussion

Objective 17

A **concussion** is a traumatic brain injury that results in a temporary loss of function in some or all of the brain. A concussion occurs when the head strikes an object or is struck by an object (Figure 38-14). The injury may or may not cause a loss of consciousness. A headache, loss of appetite, vomiting, and pale skin are common soon after the injury. A patient who experiences a concussion often appears confused and may not remember what happened. The patient may ask the same questions over and over, such as, "What happened? What happened?" This action is called *repetitive questioning*. If memory loss occurs, maximum memory loss usually

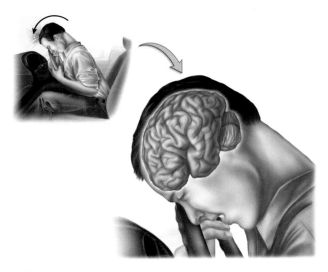

FIGURE 38-14 ▲ A concussion occurs when the head strikes an object or is struck by an object.

happens immediately after the injury and memory returns as time passes. The signs and symptoms of a concussion are an indication of a brain injury. Although the symptoms of a concussion usually disappear within 48 hours, the patient needs to be evaluated by a physician. Worsening symptoms suggest a more serious injury.

Cerebral Contusion

Objective 18

A **cerebral contusion** is a brain injury in which brain tissue is bruised and damaged in a local area. Bruising may occur at both the area of direct impact (coup) and/or on the side opposite the impact (contrecoup). Bruising of the brain is usually present when the forces involved in the injury were sufficient to cause prolonged unconsciousness. The patient's signs and symptoms depend on the location and size of the bruise. For example, a large bruise in the area of the brain's temporal lobe can cause aggressive or combative behavior.

Remember This

An altered or decreasing mental status is the best indicator of a brain injury. Always consider hypoxia as a cause of altered mental status.

Hematomas

Objectives 19, 20, 21, 22

Bleeding beneath the dura (subdural) or between the dura and skull (epidural) may be associated with bruising of the brain and other injuries (Figure 38-15). When bleeding occurs in the skull, the pressure within the skull (intracranial pressure, or ICP) increases as the blood takes up more space within the closed container.

As the pressure within the skull increases, blood flow to the brain decreases. When the brain senses a decrease in blood flow, it signals the cardiovascular system to increase blood pressure, thereby increasing blood flow. At the same time, signals are sent to the respiratory system to increase the rate of breathing to increase oxygen. If intracranial pressure continues to rise, the patient's breathing pattern becomes irregular and his heart rate decreases. In a head-injured patient, these three findings (increased systolic blood pressure, abnormal breathing pattern, and decreased heart rate) are called **Cushing's triad.** It is very important to recognize these signs. When they are present, you must move quickly and transport rapidly to the closest appropriate facility.

You Should Know

Cushing's Triad

1. Increased systolic blood pressure
2. Abnormal breathing pattern
3. Decreased heart rate

A **subdural hematoma** usually results from tearing of veins located between the dura and the cerebral cortex after an injury to the head. Blood builds up in the space between the dura and the arachnoid layer of the meninges (Figure 38-16). In an acute subdural hematoma, most patients develop signs and symptoms within minutes or hours after the injury because the blood builds up quickly. An example of a situation in which an acute subdural hematoma may occur is a sports-related head injury. In a chronic subdural hematoma, the buildup of blood occurs gradually. This makes signs and symptoms more difficult to recognize. Examples of patients in whom a chronic subdural hematoma may occur include infants who have been subjected to

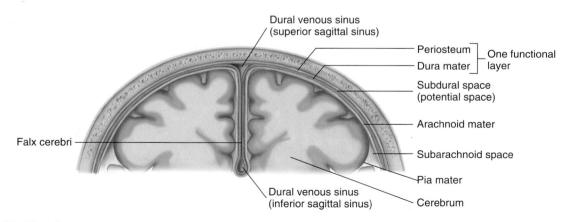

Dural venous sinus
(superior sagittal sinus)

Periosteum ⎤ One functional
Dura mater ⎦ layer

Subdural space
(potential space)

Arachnoid mater

Falx cerebri

Subarachnoid space

Pia mater

Dural venous sinus
(inferior sagittal sinus)

Cerebrum

FIGURE 38-15 ▲ A view of the head from the front to show the meninges.

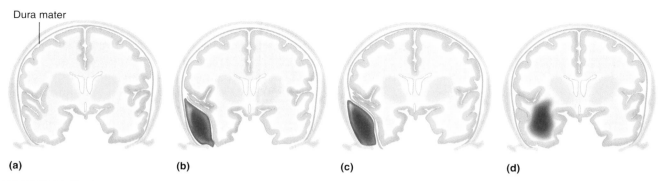

Dura mater

FIGURE 38-16 ▲ **(a)** Normal brain; **(b)** subdural hematoma; **(c)** epidural hematoma; **(d)** intracerebral hematoma.

shaken baby syndrome, patients who are alcoholics (because of frequent falls), and older adults. Signs and symptoms of a subdural hematoma depend on the amount of bleeding within the subdural space and the location of the injury. The patient may appear as if she were having a stroke or were under the influence of drugs or alcohol. Other signs and symptoms are listed in the following *You Should Know* box.

You Should Know

Assessment Findings and Symptoms of Subdural Hematoma

- Restlessness
- Headache
- Altered mental status
- Difficulty concentrating
- Slurred speech
- Vomiting
- Seizures

An **epidural hematoma** involves a rapid buildup of blood between the dura and the skull. Most epidural hematomas are associated with an overlying skull fracture. Whereas a subdural hematoma usually involves tearing of veins, an epidural hematoma often involves the tearing of an artery, usually the middle meningeal artery. As blood builds up between the skull and the dura and intracranial pressure increases, most patients will complain of a severe headache. Some patients (less than 30%) experience a loss of consciousness that is followed by a "lucid interval." This means that the patient regains consciousness for a short period (minutes to hours). This is followed by a steady decline in mental status. An early sign of an epidural hematoma is a fixed and dilated pupil on the same side as the injury. A fixed pupil means that the pupil does not react to light. Other signs and symptoms include nausea, vomiting, and sei-

zures. Epidural hematomas occur most often in young adults. This type of brain injury is less common than a subdural hematoma. A patient who has an epidural hematoma must be transported rapidly to the closest appropriate facility with neurosurgical capabilities.

An **intracerebral hematoma** is a collection of blood within the brain. Many intracerebral hematomas are associated with other brain injuries, such as a cerebral contusion. Signs and symptoms depend on the area of the brain involved, the amount of bleeding, and associated injuries.

Brain injuries can occur for reasons other than trauma. For example, a nontraumatic injury may result from clots or hemorrhaging. This type of injury occurs when a patient has a stroke. Nontraumatic brain injuries can cause an altered mental status. Their signs and symptoms are similar to those of traumatic brain injuries.

Making a Difference

ALS Assist

When caring for a head- or brain-injured patient, obtaining a baseline Glasgow Coma Scale score is important. Be alert for changes in the patient's condition that reflect signs of increasing intracranial pressure. These signs include a headache that becomes increasingly severe, confusion, decreasing level of consciousness, vomiting, pupil changes, a slow or irregular pulse, irregular breathing, increasing blood pressure, and seizures. If you note any of these signs and symptoms, be sure to relay this information to the ALS personnel who assume responsibility for patient care. This information can help the ALS personnel decide if a tube needs to be placed in the patient's airway, determine the medications that may need to be given, and decide the most appropriate facility to which the patient should be transported.

Emergency Care

Objective 23

To treat a patient with a suspected brain injury, take the following steps:

- Remember to put on appropriate PPE. The patient with an impaired airway or ventilation, open wounds, or abnormal vital signs or who does not respond to painful stimuli may need rapid extrication. Ask your partner to manually stabilize the patient's head and neck until the patient has been completely stabilized on a long backboard.

- A short on-scene time and rapid transport to an appropriate trauma center are critical when caring for a brain-injured patient. An ALS intercept or air medical transport may be necessary.

- Adequate airway, ventilation, and oxygenation are critical to a good patient outcome. Establish and maintain an open airway. If you must open the patient's airway, use a modified jaw thrust maneuver. For an unresponsive patient without a gag reflex, insert an oral airway. Avoid using a nasal airway in a brain-injured patient. Be prepared for vomiting by keeping suction within arm's reach. Monitor the patient's airway closely.

- Give 100% oxygen by nonrebreather mask. Apply a pulse oximeter, and maintain the patient's oxygen saturation at 90% or more. If the patient's breathing is inadequate, assist his breathing with a bag-mask device connected to 100% oxygen.

- Control bleeding. If bleeding is present from an open head wound, apply firm pressure with a trauma dressing to control blood loss over a broad area. If blood soaks through the dressing, apply additional dressings on top and continue to apply pressure. If signs of shock are present or if internal bleeding is suspected, treat for shock. Do not attempt to stop the flow of blood or cerebrospinal fluid from the ears or nose. Cover the area with a loose sterile dressing to absorb the drainage.

- If the patient has an adequate or elevated blood pressure, raise the head of the backboard 30 degrees to help minimize increases in intracranial pressure.

- Do not remove a penetrating object. Instead, stabilize it in place with bulky dressings.

- Dress and bandage any open wounds.

- Comfort, calm, and reassure the patient and family members. En route to the receiving facility, reassess as often as indicated. Remember that the patient may ask the same questions over and over because of the injury. Closely monitor the patient's airway, breathing, pulse, and mental status for deterioration and/or the development of seizures. Be alert for slowing of the heart rate, a change in breathing pattern, and/or rising blood pressure. Repeat the patient's Glasgow Coma Scale score when reassessing the patient. Report your findings when transferring patient care.

- Record all patient care information, including the patient's medical history and all emergency care given, on a PCR.

Injuries to the Spinal Cord

Mechanism of Injury

Objectives 4, 24

Most spinal injuries occur to the cervical spine. The next most commonly injured areas are the thoracic and lumbar spine. The spinal column normally allows a limited amount of movement in a forward, backward, and side-to-side direction. Movement beyond this normal range can result in damage to the spinal column and possibly to the spinal cord. A spinal *column* injury (bony injury) can occur with or without a spinal *cord* injury. A spinal *cord* injury can also occur with or without an injury to the spinal *column*. The spinal cord does not have to be severed in order for a loss of function to occur. In most people with a spinal cord injury, the spinal cord is intact, but the damage to it results in a loss of function. Children and the elderly are most likely to suffer an injury to the spinal cord without damage to the vertebrae.

A compression injury of the spine can drive the weight of the head into the neck, or the pelvis into the torso (Figure 38-17). Compression fractures of the spine result in weakened vertebrae. A compression fracture can occur with or without a spinal cord injury. Compression injuries can result from any of the following:

- Contact sports
- MVCs with unrestrained occupants
- Diving into shallow water
- Falls from moving vehicles
- Falls from a significant height onto the head or legs

Severe backward movement (extension) of the head can result from diving into shallow water, banging the face into the windshield in a MVC (Figure 38-18), or falling and striking the face or chin (usually seen in elderly people). Severe forward movement (flexion) of the head onto the chest can result from diving into shallow water (Figure 38-19), riding in a motor vehicle that suddenly slows, or being thrown from a horse or motorcycle. Severe rotation of the torso or head and neck can move one side of the spinal column against the other. A rotation injury can result from a motorcycle

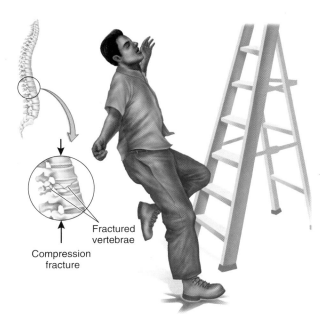

FIGURE 38-17 ▲ A compression injury of the spine can result from a fall from a significant height onto the head or legs. The force of the injury can drive the weight of the head into the neck, or the pelvis into the torso.

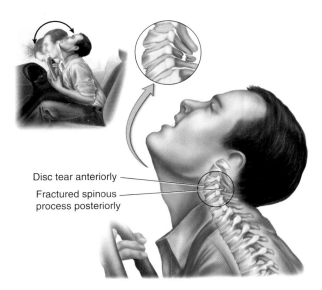

FIGURE 38-18 ▲ Severe backward movement of the head can result if the face hits the windshield in a motor vehicle crash.

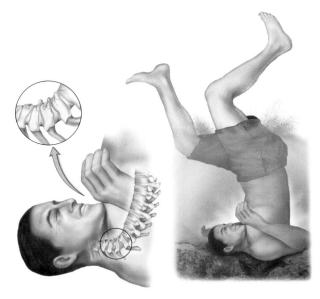

FIGURE 38-19 ▲ Severe forward movement of the head onto the chest can result from diving into shallow water.

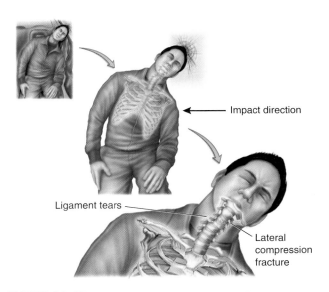

FIGURE 38-20 ▲ T-bone motor vehicle crashes can cause a sudden side impact that moves the torso sideways. The head remains in place until it is moved along by its attachments to the cervical spine.

crash or rollover MVC. Injuries caused by flexion, extension, or rotation can dislocate the discs between the vertebrae, compress the spinal cord, and stretch or tear ligaments in the neck or spine.

Contact sports or "T-bone" MVCs can cause a sudden side impact that moves the torso sideways (lateral bending). The head remains in place until it is moved along by its attachments to the cervical spine. Lateral bending can compress and displace the vertebrae and stretch ligaments (Figure 38-20).

The spine can also be pulled apart (distraction). When the spine is distracted, ligaments and muscles are overstretched or torn and the vertebrae are pulled apart (Figure 38-21). This type of injury occurs in hangings, or schoolyard or playground accidents, or when a snowmobile or motorcycle is ridden under rope or wire. The spine may also be injured because of a penetrating wound to the head, neck, or torso.

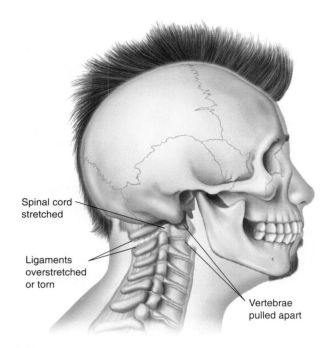

FIGURE 38-21 ▲ Ligaments and muscles are over-stretched or torn and the vertebrae are pulled apart when the spine is distracted.

As is evident from the mechanisms of injury mentioned here, a spinal injury is often seen in a patient with injuries to other areas of the body, such as the head, chest, or abdomen. For this reason, it is important to treat every patient with a significant mechanism of injury as if she has a spinal injury until it is proved otherwise.

You should have a high index of suspicion for a spinal injury in situations involving any of the following mechanisms of injury:

- MVCs
- Blunt trauma (such as an assault)
- Ejection or fall from a transportation device (such as a bicycle, motorcycle, motorized scooter, snowmobile, skateboard, in-line skates)
- Electrical injuries, lightning strike
- Involvement in an explosion
- Unresponsive trauma patients
- Hangings
- Any fall, particularly in an older adult
- Any shallow-water diving incident
- Any injury in which a helmet is broken (including a sports helmet, motorcycle helmet, and industrial hardhat)
- Any injury that penetrates the head, neck, or torso
- Any pedestrian-vehicle crash
- Any high-impact, high-force, or high-speed collision involving the head, spine, or torso

Signs and Symptoms of a Spinal Injury

Objective 25

The most common and devastating spinal injuries occur in the area of the neck (cervical spine). An injury to the spinal cord may be complete or incomplete. A complete injury occurs when the spinal cord is severed. The patient has no voluntary movement or sensation below the level of the injury. Both sides of the body are equally affected. **Paraplegia** is the loss of movement and sensation of the lower half of the body from the waist down. Paraplegia results from a spinal cord injury at the level of the thoracic or lumbar vertebrae (Figure 38-22).

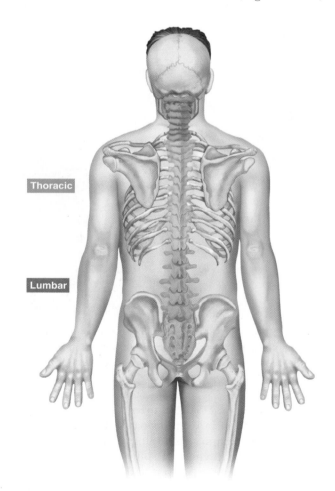

FIGURE 38-22 ▲ Paraplegia results from a spinal cord injury at the level of the thoracic or lumbar vertebrae.

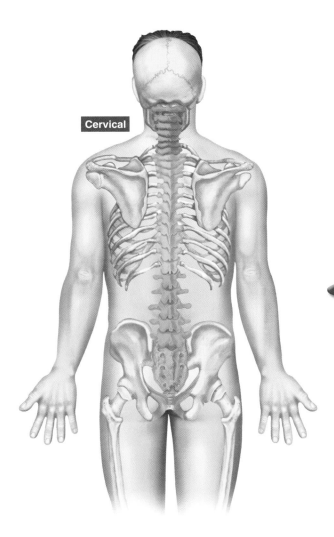

Cervical

FIGURE 38-23 ▲ Quadriplegia (also called tetraplegia) results from a spinal cord injury at the level of the cervical vertebrae.

Quadriplegia (also called *tetraplegia*) is a loss of movement and sensation in both arms, both legs, and the parts of the body below an area of injury to the spinal cord. Quadriplegia results from a spinal cord injury at the level of the cervical vertebrae (Figure 38-23). In paraplegia and quadriplegia, the spinal cord is damaged so severely that nerve signals cannot be sent to areas below the damaged area or back again. About 3% of patients with a complete spinal cord injury will show some improvement over the first 38 hours after being injured. After 38 hours, improvement is almost never seen.

With an incomplete spinal cord injury, some parts of the spinal cord remain intact. Therefore, the patient has some function below the level of the injury. The patient may be able to move one extremity more than another, may be able to feel parts of the body that cannot be moved, or may have more function on one side of the body than the other. With an incomplete injury,

there is potential for recovery because function may be lost only temporarily.

Signs and symptoms of possible spinal cord injury are listed in the following *You Should Know* box.

The amount of weakness or loss of sensation your patient has will depend on the extent of the injury. It will also depend on the amount of pressure on the spinal cord or spinal nerves. Be prepared for breathing problems if your patient has an injury to the cervical or thoracic spine. An important nerve that stimulates the diaphragm exits the spinal cord between the third and fifth vertebrae in the neck. "C3, 4, and 5 keep the diaphragm alive." (This saying refers to cervical vertebrae 3, 4, and 5). If this nerve is severed or compressed, the patient's diaphragm is usually paralyzed. If the diaphragm is paralyzed, you will see shallow abdominal breathing. A spinal cord injury involving the lower neck or upper chest may result in paralysis of the muscles between the ribs. Patients with these injuries will usually need help breathing with a bag-mask device connected to 100% oxygen.

Making a Difference

Managing a patient with a suspected spinal injury can directly affect the patient's outcome. The early recognition of a spinal injury can help reduce permanent disability and even prevent death. It is *critical* that you have a high index of suspicion for a spinal injury based on the mechanism of injury, even when there are no outward signs of trauma. If the mechanism of injury suggests it, suspect a spinal injury and treat your patient accordingly.

Assessing the Potential Spine-Injured Patient

Objective 26

Conduct a scene size-up and ensure your safety. Evaluate the mechanism of injury before approaching the patient. Put on appropriate PPE.

Perform a primary survey, and determine the urgency of further assessment and care. If the mechanism of injury suggests the possibility of spinal injury, ask the patient not to move his head while answering questions. Face the patient so that he does not have to turn his head to talk with you. Quickly assess the patient's mental status, airway, breathing, and circulation. Observe if the patient has normal chest wall movement or an abdominal breathing pattern, the latter of which may indicate a cervical spine injury. Identify and treat any life-threatening conditions. If the possibility of a spinal injury exists, ask an assistant to manually stabilize the patient's cervical spine while you assess the patient's airway (Figure 38-24). (Refer to the *Remember This!* box, "Manually Stabilizing the Head and Neck," that follows this section.) Maintain manual stabilization of the patient's cervical spine until the patient has been completely immobilized on a long backboard. Long backboards help stabilize the head, neck and torso, pelvis, and extremities. They are used to immobilize patients found in a lying, standing, or sitting position.

Priority patients are those who:
- Give a poor general impression
- Have severe pain anywhere
- Have uncontrolled bleeding
- Are experiencing difficulty breathing
- Have signs and symptoms of shock
- Are unresponsive, with no gag reflex or cough
- Are responsive and unable to follow commands
- Have paralysis or altered sensation distal to the site of injury

In these situations, request advanced life support (ALS) personnel as soon as possible. If ALS personnel are not available, the patient should be transported promptly to the closest appropriate facility.

Perform a physical examination. If a significant mechanism of injury exists, continue in-line spinal stabilization throughout the examination. In the responsive patient, symptoms should be sought before and during the physical exam. If the patient is awake, instruct her not to move during the examination. Look closely at the patient's head, neck, chest, abdomen, pelvis, extremities, and posterior body for cuts (lacerations), scrapes (abrasions), bruises (contusions), deformities, penetrations, and swelling. Feel each area for tenderness, deformity, swelling, and instability. The patient will generally complain of pain and tenderness at the site of injury. Feel and listen for crepitus, the grating of broken bone ends against each other. Check distal pulses, movement, and sensation in each extremity. Compare each extremity to the opposite extremity. To assess sensation, touch the fingers and toes of each extremity and ask the patient to tell you where you are touching. If sensation is present and the patient has experienced a spinal injury, sensation may be altered distal to the injury. The patient may complain of numbness, tingling, or "electric shocks." If sensation is absent, note the specific area of impairment and document your findings.

To assess movement, ask the patient if she can:
- Shrug her shoulders
- Spread the fingers of both hands
- Squeeze your fingers and release them
- Wiggle her toes
- Push down with each foot against your hand ("gas pedal") and then pull the foot up

Stop if the patient experiences pain. Note if movement is normal, absent, or weak. Note the level of impairment. If the patient is unresponsive, assess movement and sensation by gently pinching each foot and hand. See if the patient responds to pain with facial movements or movement of the pinched extremity.

After assessing the front and back of the patient's neck, apply a rigid cervical collar (also called a *C-collar*). The technique for applying a cervical collar is discussed

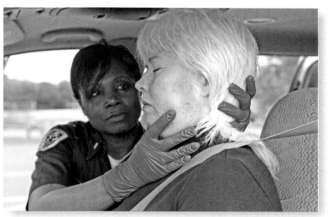
(c)

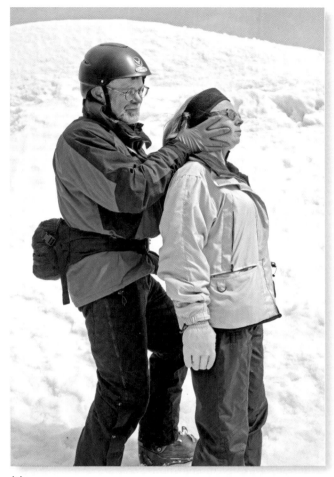
(a)

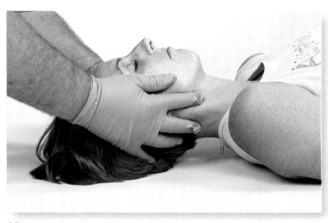
(d)

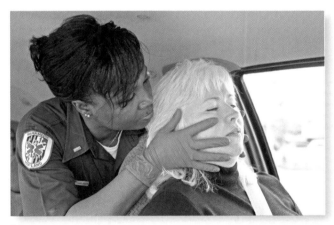
(b)

FIGURE 38-24 ▲ To manually stabilize the patient's head and neck, position yourself so you can place the patient's head between your hands. Place your palms over the patient's ears. Keep her head in a neutral position—eyes facing forward and level—and support the weight of her head. Manual stabilization of the head and neck **(a)** with the patient standing, **(b)** from behind the patient, **(c)** from the patient's side, and **(d)** with the patient supine.

in the next section. If a cervical collar is applied, the patient will need to be immobilized on a backboard.

Other signs or symptoms associated with spinal cord trauma include the inability to maintain body temperature, loss of bowel or bladder control, and priapism. Priapism is a sustained erection of the penis that is painful and can last several hours.

Take the patient's vital signs, and gather the patient's medical history. Hypotension may be present with cervical or high thoracic spine injuries. The patient's heart rate may be slow or fail to increase in response to hypotension.

Determine the events leading to the present situation by asking the following questions:

- What happened?
- When did the injury occur?
- Where does it hurt?
- Does your neck or back hurt?
- Were you wearing a seat belt?
- Did you pass out before the accident?
- Did you move or did someone move you before we arrived?
- Have your symptoms changed from the time of the injury until the time we arrived?

If the spine-injured patient is a child, you will probably find it useful to have the child's caregiver present during your assessment. It may also be helpful to begin your assessment at the child's feet and move upward, assessing his head last. Doing so may decrease the child's anxiety and reduce the risk of worsening any injuries. Remember to remove clothing, assess the child, and then quickly replace clothing. Ideally, the caregiver should be present when removing the clothing of a minor.

Emergency Care of a Spinal Injury

Objectives 27, 28, 29

To treat a patient with a spinal injury, perform the following steps:

- Maintain manual stabilization of the patient's cervical spine until the patient has been completely immobilized on a long backboard.

- Establish and maintain an open airway. If the patient is unresponsive, remember that a modified jaw thrust maneuver is the preferred method for opening the airway in a patient with a suspected spinal injury. However, use a head tilt–chin lift maneuver if the modified jaw thrust does not open the airway. Insert an oral airway if needed. Suction as necessary. Since an unresponsive patient cannot protect his own airway, it will be important for you to make sure that the patient's airway remains open and free of secretions.

- Remember that injuries to the cervical and thoracic spine may affect the patient's ability to breathe. An injury involving the lower cervical or upper thoracic portion of the spinal cord may result in paralysis of the intercostal muscles. If the patient's breathing is adequate, give oxygen by nonrebreather mask. If it is inadequate, assist breathing with a bag-mask device connected to 100% oxygen. Whenever possible, positive-pressure ventilation must be performed while the patient's spine is stabilized in an in-line position. Reassess the adequacy of the patient's breathing often while he is in your care.

- Control bleeding, if present. If signs of shock are present or if internal bleeding is suspected, treat for shock.

- Cover open wounds with a sterile dressing.

- Splint any bone or joint injuries. If the mechanism of injury suggests the patient has experienced an injury to the spine, the spine must be immobilized. Spinal stabilization techniques are discussed in the next section.

- Comfort, calm, and reassure the patient. Keep in mind that injuries to muscles and bones are painful. Your patient may be worried about a permanent loss of function of the injured area or possible disfigurement. Listen to your patient, and do your best to comfort him. Reassess at least every 5 minutes if the patient is unstable and every 15 minutes if the patient is stable.

- Record all patient care information, including the patient's medical history and all emergency care given, on a PCR.

Remember This

Manually Stabilizing the Head and Neck

Manual stabilization of the head and neck is also called *in-line stabilization*. Manual stabilization of the head and neck helps prevent further injury to the spine.

- To manually stabilize the patient's head and neck, position yourself so that you can place the patient's head between your hands. You must be able to hold that position comfortably for a significant length of time. Place your palms over the patient's ears. Spread your fingers on each side of the patient's head for added stability. Keep her head in a neutral position and support the weight of her head.
  —When the head and neck are in a neutral ("in-line") position, they are in an anatomically correct position. The eyes are facing forward and level, and the patient's nose is in line with the navel.

- Do *not* excessively move the head forward, backward, or from side to side. Do *not* pull on the patient's head or neck. If the patient is lying on her back, place your forearms on the ground for support.

- If an attempt to move the patient's head and neck into a neutral position results in any of the following, *stop* any movement and stabilize the head in the position in which it was found:
  —Airway obstruction
  —Difficulty breathing

—Neck muscle spasm

—Increased pain

—An onset or worsening of numbness or tingling, or a loss of movement

—Resistance that is felt when moving the head to a neutral position

A cervical collar cannot be applied to the patient in these situations. Use rolled towels or blanket rolls secured with tape or triangular bandages to stabilize the head and neck in the position in which it was found.

- In all other cases, continue manual stabilization of the patient's cervical spine until either a cervical collar has been applied and the patient is fully immobilized on a long backboard or additional EMS resources have arrived and have assumed patient care.

Spinal Stabilization Techniques

You may be expected to immobilize or assist with immobilizing a patient with a suspected spinal injury. Equipment used for spinal stabilization includes:

- A cervical collar, large towels, a blanket, or a commercial device to secure the head (such as a head block)
- A long backboard
- Straps, tape, triangular bandages, or 4-inch roller gauze

When stabilizing the patient's spine, remember that the joint above and the joint below the injured area must be immobilized. For example, if an injury to the cervical spine or thoracic spine is suspected, stabilize the patient's spine from the head to the pelvis. Since sideways movement of the patient's legs can cause movement of the pelvis, the patient's legs must also be secured to the board. Some of the more common techniques used for spinal stabilization are discussed in the following sections.

Remember This

In cases of a potential spinal cord injury at any point along the vertebral column, defer to your company policy or consult with medical direction if you are considering not immobilizing the whole patient.

Cervical Collars

Objectives 30, 31, 32

After assessing the front and back of the patient's neck, apply a rigid cervical collar. When used alone, a rigid C-collar does not immobilize the cervical spine. For effective stabilization, a rigid collar must be used with manual stabilization or a spinal stabilization device, such as a backboard. A rigid collar is used to:

- Temporarily splint the head and neck in a neutral position.
- Limit movement of the cervical spine.
- Support the weight of the patient's head while he is in a sitting position.
- Help maintain the cervical spine in a neutral position when the patient is lying on his back.
- Remind the patient and other healthcare professionals that the mechanism of injury suggests a possible spinal injury.

The technique for applying a cervical collar is shown in Skill Drill 38-1.

If a cervical collar is not available or does not fit the patient, the patient's head and neck can be stabilized by using a long backboard and rolled towels or a blanket (Figure 38-25).

You should apply a rigid cervical collar *only* if it fits properly:

- If the collar is too tight, it can apply pressure on the blood vessels in the patient's neck and reduce blood flow.
- If the collar is too loose, it can cover the patient's chin and mouth, causing an airway obstruction. If it is too loose, it will also not adequately stabilize the head and neck.
- A collar that is too short will not provide adequate stabilization because the patient's head can move forward.
- A collar that is too tall will not provide adequate stabilization because the patient's head will be moved backward by the collar. The collar can also force the jaw closed, limiting access to the airway.

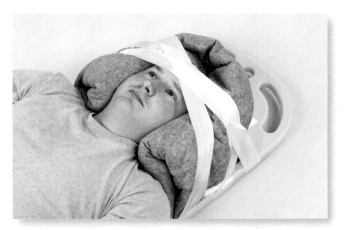

FIGURE 38-25 ▲ If a cervical collar is not available or does not fit the patient, the patient's head and neck can be stabilized by using a long backboard and rolled towels or a blanket.

Applying a Cervical Collar

STEP 1 ▶
- Put on appropriate personal protective equipment. Ask an assistant to maintain manual stabilization of the patient's head and neck in a neutral position.
- Assess distal pulses, movement, and sensation.
- Measure the width of the patient's neck by placing your fingers between the patient's lower jaw and shoulder.

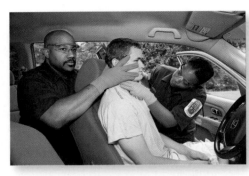

STEP 2 ▶ Select a rigid cervical collar and measure the device. Adjust the size of the collar to fit the patient's measurements as necessary.

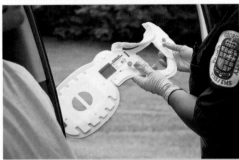

STEP 3 ▶
- Apply the cervical collar to the patient.
- Check to make sure the collar fits according to the manufacturer's instructions.
- Continue manual stabilization of the patient's head and neck until the patient is fully immobilized on a long backboard.
- Do not obscure your view of the patient's neck by placing tape over the anterior hole in the collar.
- Remember to check distal pulses, movement, and sensation after applying the collar.

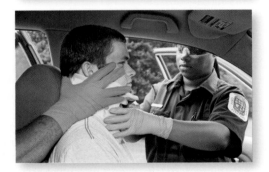

Three-Person Logroll

Objective 33

You may encounter situations in which you find an unresponsive patient who is lying facedown. If the scene suggests that the patient may have experienced some type of trauma such as a fall or a blow to the body, you should assume a spinal injury exists. A logroll is a technique used to move a patient from a facedown or side-lying position to a face-up position while keeping the head and neck in line with the rest of the body. This technique is also used to place a patient with a suspected spinal injury on a backboard. The steps to perform a three-person logroll are shown in Skill Drill 38-2.

Making a Difference ∼∼∼∼

Remember: Once immobilized on the long backboard, a patient will have limited sight. Explain all movements to the patient before starting the move so that she will not be frightened.

∼∼∼∼∼∼∼∼∼∼

Immobilization of a Supine Patient on a Long Backboard

Objective 34

After a patient has been logrolled onto a long backboard, she must be secured to it. To maintain an adult's head and

Three-Person Logroll

STEP 1 ▶
- Put on appropriate personal protective equipment.
- Rescuer 1 kneels at the patient's head and maintains manual in-line immobilization of the patient's head and neck. This rescuer will direct the move.

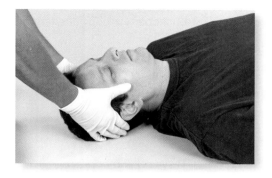

STEP 2 ▶ Rescuer 2 sizes and applies a rigid cervical collar.

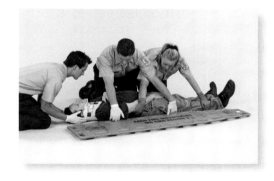

STEP 3 ▶
- Rescuers 2 and 3 position a long backboard at one side of the patient.
- Rescuer 2 is positioned at the patient's mid-chest with his hands placed on the patient's far shoulder and hip.
- Rescuer 3 is positioned at the patient's upper legs with her hands placed on the patient's hip and hand as well as his lower leg.
- If the patient has an injury to his chest or abdomen, he should be rolled onto his uninjured side if possible.

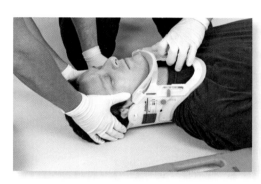

STEP 4 ▶
- When everyone is ready, Rescuer 1 gives the order to roll the patient.
- Rescuer 1 maintains manual stabilization of the patient's head and neck.
- Rescuers 2 and 3 roll the patient on his side toward them. The patient's head, shoulders, and pelvis are kept in line during the roll.

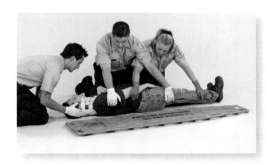

Continued

Three-Person Logroll *Continued*

STEP 5 ▶ The patient's back is quickly assessed. A long backboard is positioned under the patient.

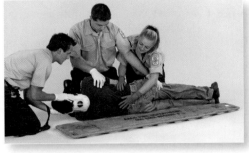

STEP 6 ▶
- When everyone is ready, Rescuer 1 gives the order to roll the patient onto the backboard. If the backboard was angled, the patient and the backboard are lowered to the ground together.
- Manual stabilization of the patient's head and neck is continued until the patient is fully immobilized on the backboard.

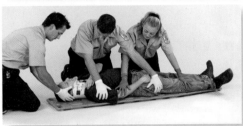

neck in a neutral position, place 1–2 inches of padding on the board under the patient's head (Figure 38-26). Be careful to avoid extra movement. Special modifications of spinal stabilization techniques may be necessary for older adults because of age-related changes in spinal anatomy.

To maintain the head of an infant or a child younger than age 3 in a neutral position, you may need to place padding under the infant's or child's torso. The padding should extend from the shoulders to the pelvis. It should be thick enough for the child's shoulders to be in line with his ear canal (Figure 38-27). An older child may not require padding to obtain a neutral position. Pediatric immobilization devices are available

that accommodate the unique anatomy of children. For example, a pediatric pad is available that can be placed on a long backboard to help with proper head and neck positioning. Pediatric backboards are also available. They are smaller in length and width than a standard backboard. Some have a recessed area built into the board to compensate for the patient's larger head.

Pad any hollow areas (spaces) between the patient and the board as necessary. These spaces include the small of the back and under the patient's knees. Immobilize the patient's torso to the board. Immobilize the upper torso to the board with one strap over the chest or, preferably, with two straps placed in an X fashion. Make

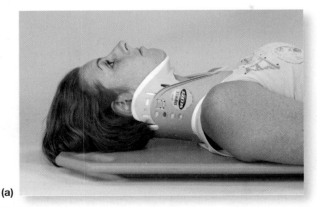

(a)

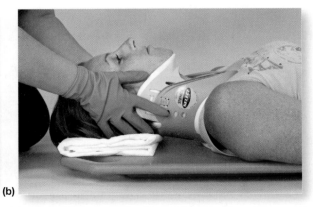

(b)

FIGURE 38-26 ▲ Head and neck stabilization of an adult **(a)** without padding and **(b)** with 1–2 inches of padding on the board under the patient's head.

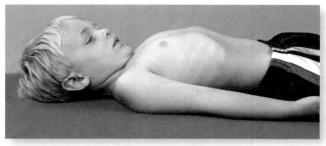

(a)

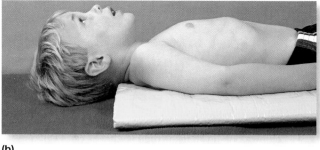

(b)

FIGURE 38-27 ▲ **(a)** Infants and young children have large heads. The size of the head causes it to tip forward when placed on a flat surface. **(b)** To maintain the head in a neutral position, you may need to place padding under the child's torso. The padding should extend from the shoulders to the pelvis and be thick enough so that the child's shoulders are in line with the ear canal.

sure that the straps are tight enough to limit patient movement but not so tight that they restrict breathing. If your patient is a woman, place the chest strap above her breasts and under her arms, not across the breasts.

Immobilize the pelvis to the board with a strap centered over the patient's hips. Secure the patient's upper legs to the board with a strap across the legs above the knees. Secure the lower legs with a strap across the legs below the knees. Secure the patient's arms to the board. The head is secured to the board *last.* You must maintain manual stabilization of the head and neck until the head and the rest of the body are secured to the board. Secure the patient's head to the board with a ready-made head immobilizer, rolled towels, or blanket rolls. Place a strap or tape snugly across the patient's lower forehead. Place another strap or tape snugly across the front portion of the cervical collar. Reassess the security of the straps. Reassess pulses, movement, and sensation in all extremities (Figure 38-28).

Stop and Think!

Once a patient has been fully immobilized on a backboard, a healthcare professional must remain with the patient *at all times.* Because immobilization will restrict the patient's ability to keep his airway open, a healthcare professional must assume this responsibility. If the patient vomits, turn the board and patient together as a unit and clear the airway.

Spinal Stabilization of a Seated Patient

Objectives 35, 36

If a patient with a possible spinal injury is found in a seated position, stabilize the patient's spine by using a short-backboard immobilization device. However, if the patient must be moved urgently because of injuries, the need to gain access to others, or dangers at the scene,

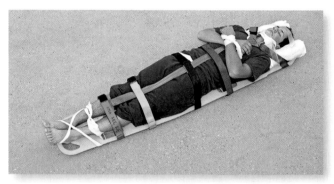

FIGURE 38-28 ▲ A patient fully immobilized on a long backboard.

carefully lower the patient directly onto a long backboard while providing manual spinal stabilization.

There are several types of short-backboard immobilization devices, including vest-type devices and a rigid short backboard. Short backboards help immobilize a patient's head, neck, and torso. A short backboard is used for the following purposes:

- To immobilize a seated patient who has a suspected spinal injury and stable vital signs
- To immobilize a patient in a confined space
- As a long backboard for a small child

In most areas, vest-type devices are used primarily for extrication. They feature straps to secure the patient's head, chest, and legs. Once extricated, the patient should remain in the device and be secured to a long backboard. The steps used to apply a vest-type device are shown in Skill Drill 38-3.

Spinal Stabilization of a Standing Patient

Objective 37

If the patient with a possible spinal injury is found in a standing position, stabilize the patient's spine by using a long backboard. Skill Drill 38-4 shows the steps for spinal stabilization of a standing patient.

Spinal Stabilization of a Seated Patient

STEP 1 ▶
- Put on appropriate personal protective equipment. Rescuer 1 manually stabilizes the patient's head and neck.
- Rescuer 2 assesses the patient's pulses, movement, and sensation in all extremities.
- After assessing the front and back of the patient's neck, a rigid cervical collar is applied.

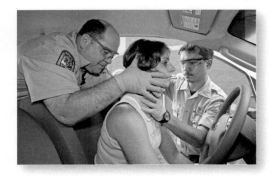

STEP 2 ▶ Rescuer 2 positions the vest-type device behind the patient.

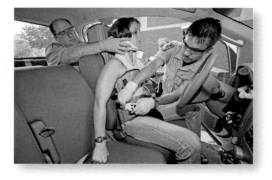

STEP 3 ▶
- Rescuer 2 positions the chest panels snugly into the patient's armpits.
- The device is then secured to the patient's torso. Rescuer 2 fastens the middle and bottom chest straps and makes sure that the straps are snug but do not interfere with breathing. The top chest strap will be fastened just before moving the patient. Alternately, the top chest strap can be fastened at this point but not pulled taut until just before the patient is moved.

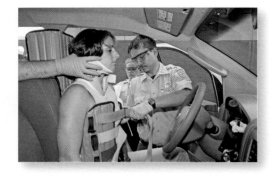

STEP 4 ▶
- Rescuer 2 secures the patient's legs next. The leg straps are loosened and wrapped around the leg on the same side. The straps are then fastened and tightened.
- Rescuer 2 evaluates the position of the device and makes sure all straps are secure.

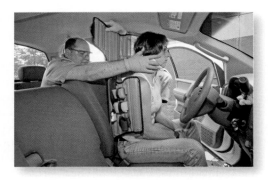

STEP 5 ▶ • To keep the patient's head in a neutral position, Rescuer 2 applies firm padding to any hollow areas between the patient's head and the headpiece of the device.
• Rescuer 2 then positions the head flaps on the side of the patient's head, coordinating with Rescuer 1 to maintain manual stabilization of the head and neck.
• Rescuer 2 then secures the head flaps by using elastic straps or wide tape.

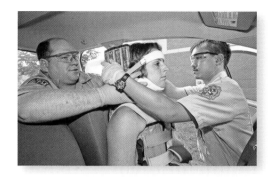

STEP 6 ▶ • After the patient's head is secured to the device, Rescuer 1 releases manual stabilization of the head.
• Rescuer 2 reassesses distal pulses, movement, and sensation in each extremity. The top chest strap should now be securely fastened; make sure that the strap is snug but does not interfere with breathing.

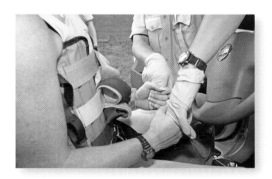

STEP 7 ▶ • The patient is rotated so that her back is to the opening through which she will be removed. A long backboard is positioned through the opening and placed under the patient.
• The patient is lowered onto the long backboard and slid into position on the board.

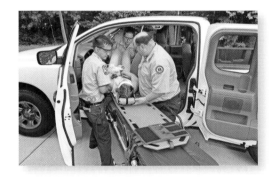

STEP 8 ▶ • The top chest strap is loosened immediately upon moving the patient to the long backboard. The leg straps on the vest-type device are loosened so that the patient can extend her legs out straight. The leg straps are then retightened.
• The patient is then secured to a long backboard.
• Pulses, movement, and sensation are reassessed in all extremities.

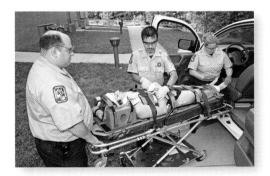

Skill Drill 38-4

Spinal Stabilization of a Standing Patient

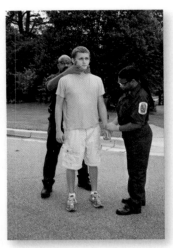

STEP 1 ▲ • Put on appropriate personal protective equipment. Rescuer 1 positions himself behind the patient and manually stabilizes the patient's head and neck. This rescuer will direct the move.
• Rescuer 2 assesses the patient's pulses, movement, and sensation in all extremities.

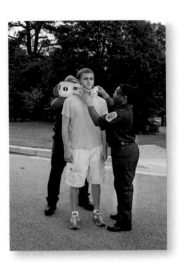

STEP 2 ▲ After assessing the front and back of the patient's neck, size and apply a rigid cervical collar. Rescuer 1 continues manual stabilization of the head and neck.

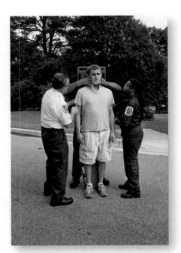

STEP 3 ▲ • Rescuer 2 and Rescuer 3 position a long backboard behind patient and make sure the board is centered behind the patient.
• While maintaining manual stabilization of the patient's head and neck, Rescuer 1 adjusts the position of his elbows to make room for positioning the backboard.

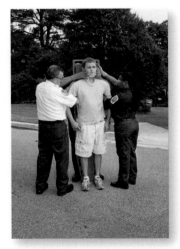

STEP 4 ▲ While Rescuer 1 continues manual stabilization from behind the patient, Rescuer 2 and Rescuer 3 position themselves on either side of the patient. Using the hand that is closest to the patient, Rescuers 2 and 3 reach under the patient's armpits and grasp the board. The board is grasped at the same level as the patient's armpit or higher.

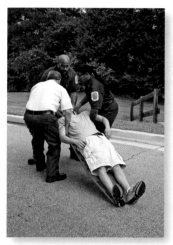

STEP 5 ▲ • While Rescuer 1 continues manual stabilization from behind the patient, he explains to the patient that he must not move as the rescuers begin lowering the patient and board to the ground.
• Rescuer 1 directs the move, walking backward as the patient and board are slowly lowered to the ground. At the same time, Rescuers 2 and 3 begin walking forward.
• At the direction of Rescuer 1, Rescuers 2 and 3 pause as needed to allow Rescuer 1 to adjust his body position.

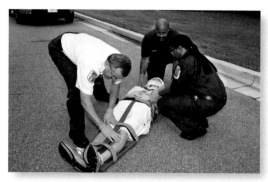

STEP 6 ▲ Once the board is on the ground, Rescuer 1 maintains manual stabilization of the patient's head and neck while the patient is assessed by the other rescuers. The patient is then secured to the board.

Rapid Extrication

Objective 38

Rapid extrication is an example of an urgent move (see Chapter 2). Rapid extrication should be performed when there is an immediate threat to life, such as in the following situations:

• Altered mental status
• Inadequate breathing
• Shock

Other indications for rapid extrication include an unsafe scene and situations in which a patient blocks your access to another, more seriously injured patient.

Rapid extrication must be accomplished quickly, without compromise or injury to the patient's spine. The steps for rapid extrication are shown in Chapter 2, Skill Drill 2-3.

You Should Know

Indications for Rapid Extrication
• Unsafe scene
• Altered mental status
• Inadequate breathing
• Shock
• Patient blocking access to another, more seriously injured patient

Helmet Removal

Objectives 39, 40, 41, 42

It can be a challenge to properly assess a patient wearing a helmet. There are two main types of helmets: sports helmets and motorcycle helmets. Sports helmets usually open in the front and provide easy access to the patient's airway once the face guard is removed. The face guard can be unclipped, unsnapped, removed with a screwdriver, or cut off with rescue scissors. Some sports helmets, such as those used in football and ice hockey, are custom-fitted to the individual. Motorcycle helmets usually have a shield that covers the entire face. The face shield can be unbuckled or snapped off to access the patient's airway.

Do not assume that a helmet must be removed. If your patient has a spinal injury, removing the helmet could worsen the injury. To determine whether a helmet should be left in place or removed, you should first ask yourself the following questions:

- Can I access the patient's airway?
- Is the patient's airway clear?
- Is the patient breathing adequately?
- Is there room to apply a face mask if it is necessary to assist the patient's breathing?
- How well does the helmet fit?
- Can the patient's head move within the helmet?
- Can the patient's spine be stabilized in a neutral position if the helmet is left in place?

You should *leave a helmet in place* in the following circumstances:

- There are no impending airway or breathing problems.
- The helmet fits well, with little or no movement of the patient's head within the helmet.
- Helmet removal would cause further injury to the patient.
- Proper spinal stabilization can be performed with the helmet in place.
- The presence of the helmet does not interfere with your ability to assess and reassess airway and breathing.

You should *remove a helmet* in these circumstances:

- You are unable to assess and/or reassess the patient's airway and breathing.
- The helmet limits your ability to adequately manage the patient's airway or breathing.
- The helmet does not fit properly, allowing excessive head movement within the helmet.
- You cannot properly stabilize the patient's spine with the helmet in place.
- The patient is in cardiac arrest.

At least two rescuers are needed to remove a helmet. The method used for helmet removal depends on the type of helmet worn by the patient. Skill Drill 38-5 shows the steps for removing a motorcycle helmet from a patient with a possible spinal injury.

On the Scene   Wrap-Up

Remember that a significant mechanism of injury is one that is likely to produce serious injury. Because this patient experienced a significant mechanism of injury, a rapid trauma assessment should be performed. Provide manual stabilization of the patient's head and neck until the patient has been completely immobilized on a long backboard. Because the patient has experienced a blow to the head and is complaining of nausea, be alert for vomiting and have suction ready. Give 100% oxygen by nonrebreather mask. Dress and bandage the patient's head wound, and then prepare the patient for transport to the closest appropriate facility. En route to the receiving facility, reassess at least every 5 minutes. Closely monitor the patient's airway, breathing, pulse, and mental status for deterioration. ■

Sum It Up

- A head injury is a traumatic insult to the head that may result in injury to soft tissue, bony structures, and/or brain injury. A traumatic brain injury occurs when an external force to the head causes the brain to move within the skull or the force causes the skull to break and directly injures the brain. A short on-scene time and rapid transport to an appropriate trauma center are critical when caring for a head-injured patient.

- Blunt trauma to the head usually is caused by motor vehicle crashes, falls, sports, and assaults with blunt weapons. Gunshot and stab wounds are the usual mechanisms of penetrating trauma to the head. Appropriate airway management and breathing support are critical when treating a patient with a head injury.

- A scalp injury may or may not cause an injury to the brain. When injured, the scalp may bleed heavily. In children, the amount of blood loss from a scalp wound may be enough to produce shock. In adults, shock is usually not caused by a scalp wound or internal skull injuries. More often, in adults, shock results from an injury elsewhere.

- A head injury may be closed or open. In a closed head injury, the skull remains intact. However, the brain can still be injured by the forces or objects that strike the skull. The forces that impact the skull

Helmet Removal

STEP 1 ▶ Rescuer 1 positions himself at the patient's head and removes the face shield from the helmet to assess airway and breathing. If the patient is wearing eyeglasses, they should be removed.

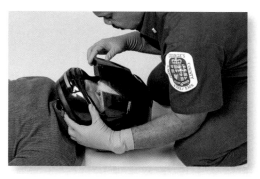

STEP 2 ▶
- Rescuer 1 stabilizes the helmet by placing his hands on each side of the helmet. His fingers should be on the patient's lower jaw to prevent movement.
- Rescuer 2 loosens the helmet strap.

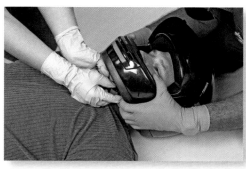

STEP 3 ▶ Rescuer 2 assumes manual stabilization by placing one hand on the patient's lower jaw at the angle of the jaw. The rescuer's other hand goes under the neck and behind the patient's head at the back of the head.

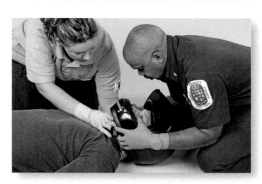

STEP 4 ▶ Rescuer 1 pulls out on the sides of the helmet to clear the patient's ears, gently slips the helmet halfway off the patient's head, and then stops.

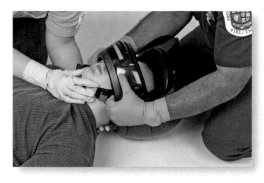

Continued

Helmet Removal   *Continued*

STEP 5 ▶   • Rescuer 2 slides the hand supporting the occiput (the back of the patient's head) toward the top of the patient's head to prevent the head from falling back after complete helmet removal.
   • Rescuer 1 tilts the helmet backward to clear the nose and removes the helmet completely.

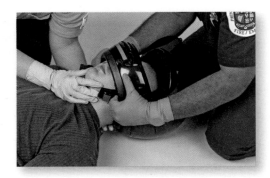

STEP 6 ▶   Manual stabilization is continued until the patient is fully immobilized to a long backboard.

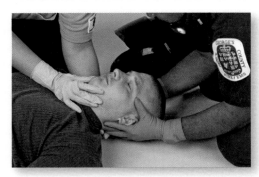

cause the brain to move within the skull. The brain strikes the inside of the skull, which causes injuries to the brain tissue. The impact and shearing forces that affect the brain can cause direct damage to the brain tissue. If bleeding occurs within the skull, the pressure within the skull increases as the blood takes up more space within the closed container. If the bleeding continues and the pressure continues to rise, the patient can suffer severe brain damage and even death.

▶ In an open head injury, the skull is not intact and the risk of infection is increased. It is important to emphasize that the phrase "open head injury" refers to the condition of the skull and not the brain. Broken bones or foreign objects forced through the skull can cut, tear, or bruise the brain tissue itself. If the skull is cracked, the blood and CSF that normally surround the brain and spinal cord can leak through the crack in the skull and into the surrounding tissues. If the forces are strong enough to cause an open head injury, then the brain will most likely sustain an injury as well.

▶ A depressed skull fracture exists when the broken portion of the skull moves in toward the brain. In a compound skull fracture, the scalp is cut and the skull is fractured. A fracture at the base of the skull is called a basilar skull fracture. The skull bones usually fractured are the temporal bone, occipital bone, sphenoid bone, or ethmoid bone, and sometimes the foramen magnum. If the area of the temporal bone near the ear is fractured, blood or cerebrospinal fluid may leak from the ear. Battle's sign (bruising behind the ear) is a delayed finding, generally taking hours to develop. If the break in the skull occurs in the anterior cranial fossa, the patient typically develops bruising around the eyes, commonly called raccoon eyes. If the ethmoid bones are disrupted, cerebrospinal fluid may leak from the nose.

▶ The Glasgow Coma Scale score is used to determine the severity of an injury to the head or brain. It is important to determine the GCS score as early as possible to establish a baseline and then periodically repeat the assessment.

- Hypoxia can cause further damage in already injured tissue. Monitor the patient's blood oxygenation continuously using a pulse oximeter, and obtain the patient's vital signs. Maintain the patient's oxygen saturation at 90% or above. Monitor the patient's heart rate, respiratory rate and regularity, and blood pressure closely for signs of increasing intracranial pressure.

- Trauma to the face is usually the result of blunt trauma, most commonly from fists and clubs; falls; and windshields, dashboards, and steering wheels in motor vehicle crashes. Penetrating trauma may result from gunshot wounds, stabbings, dog bites, human bites, or biting of the tongue. An increasing number of patients (adults and children) with facial trauma are victims of intimate partner violence.

- An injury to the nose can result in significant bleeding and a possible airway obstruction. Injuries to the ear include abrasions, contusions, lacerations, avulsions, and hematomas, which are treated like any other soft tissue injury. Never put anything into the ear to control bleeding.

- A buildup of blood in the anterior chamber of the eye is called a hyphema, a sight-threatening injury. Unless contraindicated, elevate the patient's head to maintain low pressure within the eye.

- A blowout fracture refers to cracks or breaks in the facial bones that make up the orbit of the eye. Typical assessment findings and symptoms of a severe blowout fracture include recession of the eyeball within the orbit, numbness over the cheek, epistaxis on the same side as the impact, and an inability to move one eye upward. Paralysis of upward gaze occurs because muscles in the eye become entrapped in the fracture.

- Ultraviolet keratitis is a radiation injury to the eye. Generally, the patient complains of mild to severe pain in both eyes, but symptoms may be worse in the eye that received more ultraviolet radiation.

- Injuries to the midface are most often caused by blunt trauma from an assault or a motor vehicle crash. Although most of the midface is formed by the maxilla, gentle palpation of the orbital rims, nose, zygoma, and maxilla is necessary to assess bone integrity of the midface. Fractures involving multiple bones of the midface are often associated with significant bleeding into the nose or mouth. These patients will require constant airway monitoring and frequent suctioning to maintain an open airway. Avoid the use of a nasal airway in the patient with facial trauma.

- Injuries to the mandible are common and most often caused by blunt trauma from an assault or a motor vehicle crash. The patient who has a mandible fracture or a combined fracture of the nose, maxilla, and mandible is at risk of an airway obstruction.

- An impaled object in the cheek may be removed if bleeding obstructs the airway. After removing an object from the cheek, apply direct pressure to the bleeding site by reaching inside the patient's mouth with gloved fingers. A patient with an impaled object in the check may be more comfortable sitting up, if there is no risk of spinal injury.

- A blunt or penetrating neck injury can rapidly become a life-threatening emergency because the neck houses many critical structures. A neck injury can be caused by a hanging, impact with a steering wheel, knife or gunshot wounds, strangulation, sports injuries, and "clothesline" injuries, in which a person runs into a stretched wire or cord that strikes her throat. The patient with a neck injury may also have an underlying spinal injury. Patients with a neck injury should be transported to a trauma center. An ALS intercept or air medical transport may be necessary in severe cases of airway compromise.

- When trauma to the neck is present, avoid rigid cervical collars or other devices that obstruct your view of the area. In this situation, it is likely that you will need to improvise to provide adequate stabilization of the patient's head and neck.

- A concussion is a traumatic brain injury that results in a temporary loss of function in some or all of the brain. A concussion occurs when the head strikes an object or is struck by an object. The injury may or may not cause a loss of consciousness. A headache, loss of appetite, vomiting, and pale skin are common soon after the injury.

- A cerebral contusion is a brain injury in which brain tissue is bruised and damaged in a local area. Bruising may occur at both the area of direct impact (coup) and on the side opposite the impact (contrecoup).

- A subdural hematoma usually results from tearing of veins located between the dura and the cerebral cortex after an injury to the head. Blood builds up in the space between the dura and the arachnoid layer of the meninges.

- An epidural hematoma involves a rapid buildup of blood between the dura and the skull. An epidural hematoma often involves the tearing of an artery, usually the middle meningeal artery.

- An intracerebral hematoma is a collection of blood within the brain. Signs and symptoms depend on the area of the brain involved, the amount of bleeding, and associated injuries.

- An altered or decreasing mental status is the best indicator of a brain injury. Always consider hypoxia as a cause of altered mental status.

- Most spinal injuries occur to the cervical spine. The next most commonly injured areas are the thoracic and lumbar spine. A spinal column injury (bony injury) can occur with or without a spinal cord injury. A spinal cord injury can also occur with or without an injury to the spinal column. The spinal cord does not have to be severed in order for a loss of function to occur.

▶ Compression fractures of the spine result in weakened vertebrae. A compression fracture can occur with or without a spinal cord injury.

▶ Distraction occurs when the spine is pulled apart. When the spine is distracted, ligaments and muscles are overstretched or torn and the vertebrae are pulled apart.

▶ An injury to the spinal cord may be complete or incomplete. A complete spinal cord injury occurs when the spinal cord is severed. The patient has no voluntary movement or sensation below the level of the injury. Both sides of the body are equally affected. Paraplegia is the loss of movement and sensation of the lower half of the body from the waist down. Paraplegia results from a spinal cord injury at the level of the thoracic or lumbar vertebrae. Quadriplegia (also called *tetraplegia*) is a loss of movement and sensation in both arms, both legs, and the parts of the body below the area of injury to the spinal cord. Quadriplegia results from a spinal cord injury at the level of the cervical vertebrae. With an incomplete spinal cord injury, some parts of the spinal cord remain intact. The patient has some function below the level of the injury. With this type of injury, there is a potential for recovery because function may be only temporarily lost.

▶ Manual stabilization of the head and neck is also called in-line stabilization. Manual stabilization of the head and neck helps prevent further injury to the spine.

▶ As an EMT, you may need to apply a rigid cervical collar (also called a C-collar) in treating a spinal injury. When used alone, a rigid cervical collar does not immobilize. For effective immobilization, a rigid collar must be used with manual stabilization or a spinal immobilization device, such as a backboard.

▶ A logroll is a technique used to move a patient from a facedown or side-lying position to a face-up position while maintaining the head and neck in line with the rest of the body. This technique is also used to place a patient with a suspected spinal injury on a backboard.

▶ A long backboard helps stabilize the head, neck, torso, pelvis, and extremities. It is used to immobilize patients found in a lying, standing, or sitting position.

▶ A short backboard helps immobilize a patient's head, neck, and torso. It can also be used as a long backboard for a small child. Examples include vest-type devices and rigid short backboards. A short backboard should not be used when rapid extrication is indicated.

▶ Rapid extrication should be performed when there is an immediate threat to life, such as in the following situations: altered mental status, inadequate breathing, and shock. Other indications for rapid extrication include an unsafe scene and situations in which a patient blocks your access to another, more seriously injured patient.

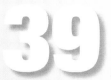

CHAPTER

39

Special Considerations in Trauma

By the end of this chapter, you should be able to:

Knowledge Objectives ▶
1. Discuss mechanisms of injury associated with trauma in pregnancy.
2. Discuss the unique anatomy, physiology, and pathophysiology considerations of the pregnant trauma patient.
3. Discuss the assessment findings associated with trauma in the pregnant patient.
4. Describe the emergency care of the pregnant trauma patient.
5. Discuss mechanisms of injury associated with pediatric trauma.
6. Discuss the unique anatomy, physiology, and pathophysiology considerations of the pediatric trauma patient.
7. Discuss the assessment findings associated with trauma in infants and children.
8. Describe the emergency care of the pediatric trauma patient.
9. Discuss mechanisms of injury associated with trauma in older adults.
10. Discuss the unique anatomy, physiology, and pathophysiology considerations of the older adult trauma patient.
11. Discuss the assessment findings associated with trauma in older adults.
12. Describe the emergency care of the older adult trauma patient.
13. Define cognitive impairment, and discuss challenges in assessing the cognitively impaired patient.

Attitude Objective ▶
14. Value the importance of maintaining a trauma patient's modesty during assessment and management.

Skill Objectives ▶
15. Demonstrate assessment and appropriate emergency care of a pregnant trauma patient.
16. Demonstrate completing a prehospital care report for a pregnant trauma patient.
17. Demonstrate assessment and appropriate emergency care of a pediatric trauma patient.
18. Demonstrate completing a prehospital care report for a pediatric trauma patient.
19. Demonstrate assessment and appropriate emergency care of an older adult trauma patient.
20. Demonstrate completing a prehospital care report for an older adult trauma patient.
21. Demonstrate assessment and appropriate emergency care of a cognitively impaired trauma patient.

683

You and your partner are dispatched for a report of a motor vehicle crash near one of the local malls. You arrive to find a two-car collision. The first vehicle is a late model sports utility vehicle with heavy damage to the front. The occupants of vehicle 1 are already out of the vehicle walking around and denying any injuries. The second vehicle has about 12 inches of intrusion on the driver's door. The driver of vehicle 2 is an unconscious, unrestrained woman who is still seated in the car. A passenger of vehicle 2 is a 30-year-old man who reports no injuries and informs you that the driver is 6 months pregnant. ■

THINK ABOUT IT

As you read this chapter, think about the following questions:

- Does the use or nonuse of restraint systems make a difference in the injuries sustained by a pregnant trauma patient in a motor vehicle crash?
- How does the assessment of the pregnant trauma patient differ from any other trauma patient?
- In what position should this patient be transported? Why?

Introduction

In previous chapters, we have discussed the effects of trauma on various areas of the body, such as the head, face, neck, chest, abdomen, extremities, soft tissues, and spine. In this chapter we discuss specific groups of trauma patients and their unique types of injuries, assessment considerations, and management considerations.

Trauma in Pregnancy

Mechanism of Injury

Objective 1

Trauma is the leading cause of death in pregnant patients and the leading cause of death in women of childbearing age. Although pregnant patients can sustain all types of trauma, motor vehicle crashes are the most frequent cause of injury, followed by falls and intimate partner violence. Direct or indirect trauma to a pregnant uterus can cause injury to the uterine muscle. This can cause the release of chemicals that cause uterine contractions, perhaps inducing premature labor. The effects of trauma on the fetus depend on:

- The length of the pregnancy (the age of the fetus)
- The type and severity of the trauma
- The severity of blood flow and oxygen disruption to the uterus

You Should Know

Causes of Trauma in Pregnancy
- Motor vehicle crashes (MVCs)
- Falls
- Intimate partner violence
- Gunshot wounds
- Stabbings
- Burns

Motor vehicle crashes are the most common cause of serious blunt trauma in pregnancy (Figure 39-1). Gunshot wounds and stab wounds to the abdomen of a pregnant patient do not usually result in the mother's death. However, the likelihood of fetal death is high.

One in four pregnant women experiences a fall during pregnancy, and falls become more common after the 20th week of pregnancy. A woman's center of gravity shifts as the size of her abdomen increases during pregnancy and her pelvic ligaments loosen. As a result, a pregnant woman must readjust her body alignment and balance, and this increases her risk for falls and injury. Some of these falls are a result of walking on slippery floors, hurrying, or carrying of objects.

For some women, pregnancy is a time when intimate partner violence starts. Physical abuse can result in the following conditions:

- Blunt trauma to the abdomen
- Severe bleeding

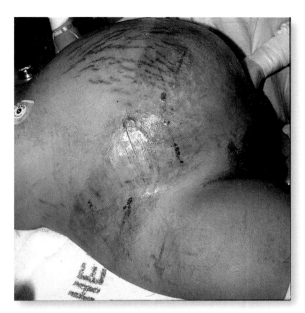

FIGURE 39-1 ▲ This woman experienced significant blunt trauma to the abdomen during her third trimester of pregnancy.

- Uterine rupture
- Miscarriage
- Premature labor
- Premature rupture of the amniotic sac

A thermal burn of more than 20% of the mother's body surface area increases the risk of fetal death. In cases of electrical burns, the likelihood of fetal death is high, even with a rather low electrical current. This is most likely because the fetus is floating in amniotic fluid and has a low resistance to the current.

Special Considerations

Objective 2

Anatomic changes occur during pregnancy that affect nearly every organ system. In the respiratory system, the diaphragm becomes elevated, and the mother's resting respiratory rate increases because of the enlarging uterus. During pregnancy, the speed with which food and liquids move through the gastrointestinal tract decreases, increasing the risk of vomiting and aspiration after trauma.

The mother's blood volume circulates through the uterus every 8 to 11 minutes at term. As a result, the uterus can be a source of significant blood loss if injured. Before the 12th week of pregnancy, the uterus is protected by the bones of the pelvis. After the 12th week of pregnancy, the uterus begins to rise out of the pelvis and becomes susceptible to injury. By the 20th week, the uterus is at the level of the umbilicus, and at 34 to 36 weeks it reaches the costal margin. Thus the risk of

trauma to the mother and fetus increases as pregnancy progresses. As the uterus increases in size, the mother's abdominal organs are displaced superiorly (Figure 39-2). This displacement decreases the likelihood of injury to the mother's liver, spleen, and intestines but increases the likelihood of uterine and fetal injury.

Early in the pregnancy, the mother's body begins to produce more blood to carry oxygen and nutrients to the fetus, resulting in an increased plasma volume and an increased volume of red blood cells. Her heart rate gradually increases by as much as 10 to 15 beats/min during pregnancy. During the first 6 months of pregnancy, the mother's systolic blood pressure may drop by 5–10 mm Hg. Her diastolic blood pressure may drop by 10–15 mm Hg. During the last 3 months of pregnancy, her blood pressure gradually returns to near normal. You will recall that an increase in heart rate is one of the earliest signs of shock. The changes in vital signs that typically occur during pregnancy can make it difficult to detect shock, particularly in late pregnancy. When shock occurs, the mother's blood pressure is preserved by the shunting of blood from nonvital organs, such as the uterus, to vital organs. Constriction of the uterine arteries decreases perfusion to the uterus, potentially compromising the fetus to save the mother. The fetus will often show signs of distress before any change in maternal vital signs. In fact, the healthy pregnant patient can lose 30% to 35% of her blood volume with no change in vital signs. However, her condition will rapidly worsen when blood loss exceeds this amount.

The uterus grows from a prepregnancy size of 70 g to a term pregnancy size of about 1,000 g. When a woman in late pregnancy is placed on her back, the weight of the fetus compresses major blood vessels, such as the inferior vena cava and the aorta (Figure 39-3). This compression decreases the amount of blood returning to the mother's heart and lowers her blood pressure (supine hypotensive syndrome). As a result, the amount of oxygen and nutrients delivered to the fetus is decreased.

A woman who is 20 weeks pregnant or more should be positioned on her left side. Positioning the patient on her left side shifts the weight of her uterus off the abdominal vessels. If the patient is immobilized to a backboard, tilt the board slightly to the left by placing a rolled towel, small pillow, blanket, or other padding under the right side of the board. Doing so will shift the weight of the patient's uterus and decrease the pressure on the abdominal blood vessels.

Fetal death may occur because of death of the mother, separation of the placenta, maternal shock, uterine rupture, or fetal head injury. Of these, maternal death is the number one cause of fetal death. The second most common cause of fetal death is abruptio placentae. **Abruptio placentae** (also called *placental abruption*) occurs when a normally implanted placenta separates prematurely from the wall of the uterus

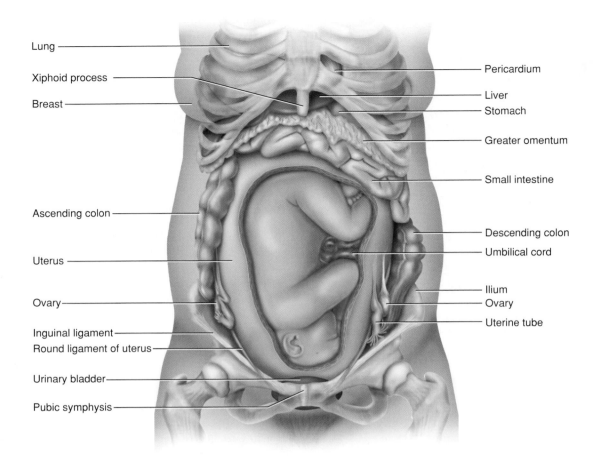

FIGURE 39-2 ▲ At term, the average fetus weighs 7–8 pounds, and the average mother has gained 30 pounds. Note that the mother's abdominal organs are displaced superiorly.

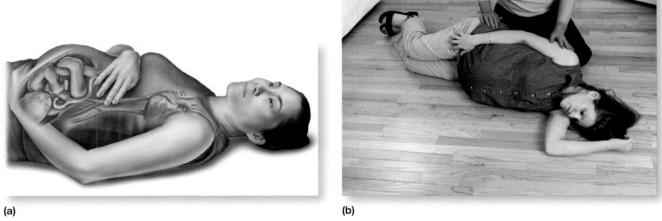

(a)   (b)

FIGURE 39-3 ▲ **(a)** When a woman 20 weeks pregnant or more is placed on her back, the weight of the fetus compresses major blood vessels in the abdomen, such as the inferior vena cava and aorta. This decreases the amount of blood returning to the mother's heart and lowers her blood pressure. **(b)** To relieve pressure on the abdominal blood vessels, place the pregnant patient on her left side.

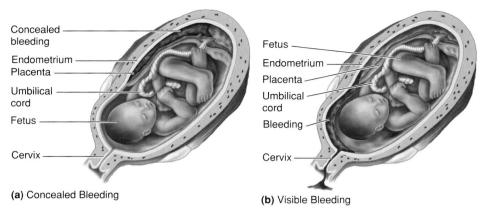

Concealed bleeding
Endometrium
Placenta
Umbilical cord
Fetus
Cervix

(a) Concealed Bleeding

Fetus
Endometrium
Placenta
Umbilical cord
Bleeding
Cervix

(b) Visible Bleeding

FIGURE 39-4 ▲ **(a)** Abruptio placentae occurs when a normally implanted placenta separates prematurely from the wall of the uterus (endometrium) during the last trimester of pregnancy. Vaginal bleeding may be absent (concealed or hidden bleeding). **(b)** Vaginal bleeding that is visible may be moderate to severe and is usually dark red.

(endometrium) during the last trimester of pregnancy. If the placenta begins to peel away from the wall of the uterus, bleeding occurs from the blood vessels that transfer nutrients to the fetus from the mother. The larger the area that peels away, the greater the amount of bleeding. The placenta may separate partially or completely (Figure 39-4). Partial separation may allow time for treatment of the mother and fetus. Separation of more than 50% of the placental surface often results in death of the fetus. Classic signs of placental abruption include abdominal pain, vaginal bleeding, and preterm labor. However, vaginal bleeding may be absent in 30% of abruptions following trauma.

A **ruptured uterus** is the actual tearing of the uterus. Uterine rupture can occur when the patient has been in strong labor for a long period; this is the most common cause. It can also occur when the patient has sustained abdominal trauma, such as a severe fall or a sudden stop in a motor vehicle collision. Signs and symptoms of uterine rupture include abdominal pain, vaginal bleeding, and shock.

You Should Know

Assessment Findings and Symptoms of Pregnancy Complications

Abruptio Placentae
- Abdominal pain
- Vaginal bleeding
- Preterm labor

Ruptured Uterus
- Abdominal pain
- Vaginal bleeding
- Shock

Women should use automobile restraints while pregnant, whether driving or riding as a passenger. Correct seat belt use can significantly reduce both maternal and fetal injury following motor vehicle crashes. Studies have shown that unbelted pregnant women are twice as likely to experience vaginal bleeding and two times more likely to give birth within 48 hours of a crash than properly belted pregnant women are. Fetal death is three to four times more likely to occur when pregnant women are unbelted. Injuries can occur if restraints are improperly worn. In a motor vehicle crash, uterine rupture can occur if a lap belt is worn too high over the pregnant uterus. Wearing a lap belt without a shoulder strap can result in compression of the uterus with possible uterine rupture or abruptio placentae. During pregnancy, correct positioning of the lap belt is underneath the pregnant abdomen across the hips and high on the thighs. The shoulder strap should be positioned snugly between the breasts and off to the side of the pregnant abdomen.

Penetrating trauma in pregnancy is usually the result of gunshot or knife wounds, of which gunshot wounds are more common. Abdominal stab wounds during pregnancy usually occur in the upper abdomen above the umbilicus. Stab wounds to the lower abdomen are more likely to injure the uterus. Although the maternal outcome of penetrating trauma in pregnancy is usually favorable, the fetal death rate is high.

Cardiac arrest in the pregnant trauma patient poses some unique challenges. Because the pregnant patient's diaphragm is elevated during pregnancy, it may be necessary to ventilate using less volume. Chest compressions should be performed higher on the sternum, slightly above the center of the sternum. If the patient is 20 weeks pregnant or more, it will be necessary to perform chest compressions with the patient on a backboard tilted 15 to 30 degrees to the left to offset the problems associated with supine hypotension.

Patient Assessment

Objective 3

Conduct a scene size-up and ensure your safety. Evaluate the mechanism of injury before approaching the patient. Put on appropriate PPE. As you begin your assessment, remember that you have two patients to consider—the mother and the fetus. Carefully assess the patient's airway while maintaining spinal stabilization. The pregnant trauma patient is at greater risk for vomiting and subsequent aspiration. Suction as needed to keep the airway open, and reassess the airway often. When suctioning, do not suction for more than 15 seconds at a time. Never withhold oxygen from a pregnant trauma patient. Give 100% oxygen, assisting ventilation as needed. Continuously monitor oxygenation using a pulse oximeter. Assess the patient's circulatory status, and control external hemorrhage with direct pressure, if present. Assess the patient's level of consciousness using the AVPU scale. Treat any life-threatening injuries before proceeding to the secondary survey. A short on-scene time and rapid transport to an appropriate trauma center are important when caring for the pregnant trauma patient. In situations involving major trauma, an ALS intercept or air medical resources may be needed.

Obtain the patient's vital signs, and gather the patient's medical history. Remember that the mother's vital signs may be within normal limits despite significant internal bleeding. In addition to the usual questions asked with obtaining a SAMPLE history, additional key questions include the following:

- (If the mechanism of injury involved a motor vehicle crash:) Were you wearing a seat belt? Lap belt and shoulder strap?
- Did you feel the baby move before the trauma? After the trauma?
- Did you experience any direct trauma to your abdomen?
- Are you experiencing any contractions?
- Are you experiencing any vaginal bleeding?
- Did your water break? If yes, what color was it?
- When was your last menstrual period?
- What is your due date?
- Have you received any prenatal care?
- Is this your first pregnancy? How many babies are expected?
- Do you have any medical problems (diabetes, high blood pressure)?

Emergency Care

Objective 4

To treat an injured pregnant woman:

- Put on appropriate PPE. Keep on-scene time to a minimum.
- If spinal injury is suspected, immobilize the patient to a long backboard and tilt the board to the left if the patient is 20 weeks pregnant or more.
- Establish and maintain an open airway. Have suction equipment within arm's reach.
- Administer 100% oxygen. If the patient's breathing is adequate, apply oxygen by nonrebreather mask at 10 to 15 L/min. If the patient's breathing is inadequate, provide positive-pressure ventilation with 100% oxygen and assess the adequacy of the ventilations delivered. Continue monitoring oxygenation using pulse oximetry.
- Control external bleeding by applying direct pressure to the wound with a sterile dressing. If blood soaks through the dressing, apply additional dressings and reapply pressure. If signs of shock are present or if internal bleeding is suspected, treat for shock.
- Protect the patient's modesty and provide emotional support. Keep the patient warm.
- Transport promptly. Generally, the pregnant trauma patient who has a heart rate of more than 110 beats/min, chest or abdominal pain, or loss of consciousness or who is in her third trimester of pregnancy should be transported to a trauma center. Follow your local protocols.
- Reassess at least every 5 minutes en route. En route, relay the patient's due date, injuries, vital signs, and care provided to the receiving facility. Doing so allows time for appropriate healthcare professionals and equipment to be mobilized and ready for the patient's arrival.
- Record all patient care information, including the patient's medical history and all emergency care given, on a PCR.

Pediatric Trauma

Mechanism of Injury

Objective 5

Injuries are the leading cause of death in infants and children. Blunt trauma is the most common mechanism of serious injury in the pediatric patient. Examples of causes of common blunt trauma injuries are shown in the following *You Should Know* box.

Causes of Common Blunt Trauma Injuries in Children

- Falls
- Bicycle-related injuries
- Motor vehicle–related injuries (restrained and unrestrained passengers)
- Car-pedestrian incidents
- Drowning
- Sports-related injuries
- Abuse and neglect

The injury pattern seen in a child may be different from that seen in an adult. For example, an adult about to be struck by an oncoming vehicle will typically turn away from the vehicle. This results in injuries to the side or back of the body. In contrast, a child will usually face an oncoming vehicle, resulting in injuries to the front of the body.

In a motor vehicle crash, an unrestrained infant or child will often have head and neck injuries. Restrained passengers often have abdominal and lower spine injuries. Child safety seats are often improperly secured, resulting in head and neck injuries. Contributing factors to pediatric motor vehicle–related injuries include failure to use (or improper use of) passenger restraints, inexperienced adolescent drivers, and alcohol abuse.

Deaths resulting from pedestrian injuries are common among children 5 to 9 years of age. The child is unable to judge the speed of the traffic and typically bolts out into the street. Children are often injured while chasing a toy, friend, or pet into the path of an oncoming vehicle. A child struck by a car is likely to sustain injury to the head, the chest or abdomen, and an extremity (Waddell's triad). The vehicle first strikes the left side of the child. The bumper contacts the left femur, and the fender strikes the left side of the child's abdomen. The child is thrown against the vehicle's hood or windshield. The child is thrown to the ground, striking his head on the pavement as the vehicle comes to a stop. The child is then often run over by the vehicle.

Bicycle-related injuries often involve head trauma, abdominal injuries (from striking the handlebars), and trauma to the face and extremities. Sports injuries often involve injuries to the head and neck.

Drowning is a significant cause of death and disability in children younger than 4 years of age. Alcohol appears to be a significant risk factor in adolescent drowning.

Most fire-related deaths occur in private residences, usually in homes without working smoke detectors.

Smoke inhalation, scalds, and contact and electrical burns are especially likely to affect children younger than 4 years of age.

Injuries caused by a firearm include an entrance wound, exit wound, and an internal wound. Most guns used in unintentional shootings are found in the home and often found loaded in readily accessible places. The presence of a gun in the home has been linked to an increased likelihood of adolescent suicide.

Falls are a common cause of injury in infants and children. Infants and young children have large heads in comparison to their body size, making them more prone to falls. Note the distance of the fall, the surface on which the child landed, and the body area(s) struck. Any fall more than 10 feet or more than two to three times the child's height should be considered serious. Concrete and asphalt are associated with more severe injuries than are other surfaces. Children who land on hard ground or concrete sustain a more severe injury than those who hit grass, even when the heights of the falls are similar. If the child fell from a height or was diving into shallow water, suspect injuries to the head and neck.

Special Considerations

Objective 6

Children are prone to head injuries because their heads are large and heavy when compared with their body size. The younger the child, the softer and thinner the skull. The force of injury is more likely to be transferred to the underlying brain instead of fracturing the skull. The blood vessels of the face and scalp bleed easily. Even a small wound can lead to major blood loss. Striking the head jars the brain. The brain bounces back and forth, causing multiple bruised and injured areas.

Shaken baby syndrome (also called abusive head trauma) may cause brain trauma. The National Center on Shaken Baby Syndrome defines shaken baby syndrome as a term used to describe the group of signs and symptoms resulting from violent shaking or shaking and impacting of the head of an infant or small child. Shaken baby syndrome occurs when an infant or child is shaken by the arms, legs, or shoulders with enough force to cause the baby's brain to bounce against her skull. Just 2 to 3 seconds of shaking can cause bruising, swelling, and bleeding in and around the brain. It can lead to severe brain damage or death. *Never shake or jiggle an infant or child.*

Signs and symptoms of a head injury vary according to the location and severity of the injury. Possible signs and symptoms are listed in the following *You Should Know* box.

You Should Know

Possible Assessment Findings and Symptoms of Head Injury in Children

- Altered mental status (usually the first sign of head injury)
- Headache
- Nausea and vomiting
- Abnormal behavior
- Seizures
- Dilation of one pupil
- Dilation of both pupils, unresponsive to light (late sign, suggests severe brain injury)

Airway and breathing problems are common with head injuries. The most common cause of hypoxia in the unresponsive head injury patient is the tongue obstructing the airway. You must make sure that the child's airway is open and that his breathing is adequate.

Signs of blunt trauma to the chest and abdomen may be hard to see on the body surface. The younger the patient, the softer and more flexible the ribs. Therefore, rib fractures are less common in children than in adults. However, the force of the injury can be transferred to the internal organs of the chest, resulting in major damage. The presence of a rib fracture in a child suggests that major force caused the injury. Bruising of the lung (pulmonary contusion) is one of the most frequently observed chest injuries in children. This injury is potentially life-threatening.

The abdomen is a more common site of injury in children than in adults. The abdomen is often a source of hidden injury. In fact, abdominal trauma is the most common cause of unrecognized fatal injury in children. The abdominal organs of an infant or child are prone to injury because the organs are large and the abdominal wall is thin. As a result, the organs are closer to the surface of the abdomen and less protected. In infants and young children, the liver and spleen extend below the lower ribs (Figure 39-5). The organs' location gives them less protection and makes them more susceptible to injury. A swollen, tender abdomen is a cause for concern.

Remember This

Abdominal trauma is the most common cause of unrecognized fatal injury in children. A swollen, tender abdomen is a cause for concern.

Pelvic fractures are uncommon in children. However, when such fractures do occur, they are often the

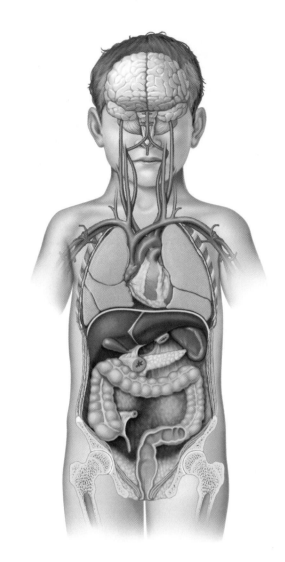

FIGURE 39-5 ▲ Because the diaphragm in a child is relatively flat, all the abdominal organs are extremely close together. (The stomach has been removed in this illustration to allow you to see the spleen and pancreas.)

result of the child's being struck by a moving vehicle. Because the pelvis contains major blood vessels, you must be alert for signs of internal bleeding and shock.

Extremity trauma is common in children. The younger the child, the more flexible the bones. When a child has multiple injuries, fractures are often missed. Assessing nondisplaced fractures in young children can be difficult because these patients cannot verbalize well. If a child is not walking on an injured extremity or using an upper extremity during normal activity, suspect a fracture until proved otherwise. Fractures of both thighs can cause a major blood loss, resulting in shock. Extremity injuries in children are managed in the same way as are those in adults.

Patient Assessment

Objective 7

When arriving on the scene, complete a scene size-up before beginning emergency medical care. Evaluate the mechanism of injury before approaching the patient and put on appropriate PPE. Be sure to comfort, calm, and reassure the patient throughout your assessment. Find out the child's name, and use it when providing care.

Keep on-scene time to a minimum. In situations involving major trauma, request an early response of ALS personnel to the scene, or consider an ALS intercept while en route to the receiving facility. Do not delay transport for ALS arrival.

As you approach the patient, form a general impression and assess the child's appearance, work of breathing, and skin color. Perform a primary survey to determine the presence of life-threatening injuries. If the child is not alert or the mechanism of injury suggests that the child experienced trauma to the head or neck, stabilize the child's spine. Assume that any patient who has an injury above the collarbones has a spinal injury and immobilize accordingly. An unresponsive infant or child should always be immobilized, especially when the cause is unknown. Remember that you may need to place padding under the torso of infants and young children to maintain the cervical spine in a neutral position.

Making sure the child's airway is open and clear of secretions is the most important step in managing a trauma patient. Gurgling or stridor may indicate an upper airway obstruction. Vomiting is common in the pediatric trauma patient. Make sure suction is within arm's reach. Suction the mouth as needed with a rigid suction catheter. Because a young infant breathes primarily through her nose and not her mouth, be sure to keep the nasal passages clear. If the patient is unresponsive, use the jaw thrust maneuver to open the airway. Insert an oral airway to help keep the airway open.

Because inadequate breathing is common in the pediatric trauma patient, carefully assess the rate and depth of the patient's breathing. The respiratory rate of an infant and a child is faster than that of an adult. Rates that are too fast or slow can indicate respiratory failure. Look for signs of increased work of breathing, such as retractions and accessory muscle use. If the child's breathing is inadequate or there is no air movement, assist breathing with bag-mask or mouth-to-mask ventilation. Remember to ventilate with just enough force to produce gentle chest rise to reduce the risk of gastric distention. Give supplemental oxygen to all pediatric trauma patients, even if there is no apparent breathing difficulty. A pulse oximeter should be routinely used and continuously monitored in any trauma patient.

Control obvious bleeding if present. Check for signs of shock by assessing the child's mental status, heart rate, peripheral versus central pulses, and skin color. In an injured child, delayed capillary refill time (if the child is 6 years of age or younger), cool distal extremities, and decreases in peripheral versus central pulse quality are generally more reliable signs of shock than is blood pressure. This is because a healthy child can maintain a normal blood pressure until he has lost 25% to 30% of his total blood volume. The extremities of a young child may appear mottled in response to cold. Remember to keep the child warm. If signs and symptoms of shock are present with a closed head injury, look for signs of other injuries (such as internal bleeding) that may be the cause of the shock.

Assess the child's mental status using the AVPU scale, and follow with a repeat assessment using the Glasgow Coma Scale. Repeat your mental status assessment each time you repeat the patient's vital signs. Obtain the patient's vital signs, recognizing that respiratory rates, pulse rates, and blood pressures vary by age. A blood pressure in children younger than 3 years of age is unreliable. Remember to assess a brachial pulse in infants. Regardless of age, a slow pulse rate in an infant or child indicates hypoxia until proved otherwise. Normal vital signs in an injured child can be deceiving. It is essential to obtain vital signs frequently and look closely for changes in the child's respiratory rate, heart rate, and blood pressure that may indicate impending respiratory failure or shock.

Obtain a SAMPLE history from the patient or family members. Throughout your assessment and delivery of emergency care to the patient, remember to talk to your patient. Keep the family informed of what you are doing and where the patient will be transported for further care.

Emergency Care

Objective 8

To treat an injured child, use the following steps:

- Put on appropriate PPE. Keep on-scene time to a minimum. Request an early response of ALS personnel to the scene, or consider an ALS intercept while en route to the receiving facility. Do not delay transport for ALS arrival.

- If spinal injury is suspected, maintain manual in-line stabilization until the patient is secured to a long backboard. Provide padding beneath an infant and young child from the shoulders to the hips during immobilization to prevent flexion of the neck.

- Establish and maintain an open airway. Suction as needed. When suctioning an infant or a child, do not apply suction for more than 10 seconds at a time.
- Give oxygen by nonrebreather mask. If the patient's breathing is inadequate, assist her breathing with a bag-mask device connected to 100% oxygen. Monitor oxygenation with a pulse oximeter. Consider the cause of a slow heart rate in a pediatric patient a sign of hypoxia, and assist ventilation as needed.
- Promptly seal an open chest wound with an airtight dressing. Tape the dressing on three sides. If signs and symptoms of a tension pneumothorax develop after an airtight dressing has been applied, release the dressing. Reassess the patient's airway, breathing, circulation, and mental status. If the patient's breathing returns to normal, replace the airtight dressing and again secure it in place over the wound by taping it in place on three sides.
- Control external bleeding by applying direct pressure to the wound with a sterile dressing. If blood soaks through the dressing, apply additional dressings and reapply pressure.
- If signs of shock are present or if internal bleeding is suspected, treat for shock. Keep the patient warm.
- Do not remove penetrating objects; rather, stabilize them in place with bulky dressings.
- Manage avulsed or amputated parts as you would other soft tissue injuries.
- Extremity injuries should be stabilized by immobilizing the joint above and below the fracture site. In the critical patient, this should be done en route to a trauma center as time permits. Remember to assess pulses, motor function, and sensation in the affected extremity before and after immobilization.
- Reassess at least every 5 minutes during transport. Record all patient care information, including the patient's medical history and all emergency care given, on a PCR.

Trauma in Older Adults

Mechanism of Injury

Objective 9

Falls are the most common cause of injury in older adults, followed by motor vehicle crashes, pedestrian versus vehicle incidents, and assaults. Factors that increase an older adult's risk of falling are shown in the following *You Should Know* box. Most falls involving older adults occur at home and are low-level falls (falls from a standing height). Injuries to the head, pelvis, and lower extremities are common. Fractures sustained during a fall usually involve the hip, femur, and wrist.

You Should Know

Risk Factors for Falls in Older Adults
- Older age
- Female gender
- Sedative use
- Impaired vision
- Syncope
- Arthritis
- Lower-extremity weakness
- Balance difficulties
- History of stroke, previous fall
- Environmental hazards (rug, stairs, lighting, uneven ground)

Motor vehicle crashes involving older adults often occur during the daytime, close to home, and at an intersection. Factors increasing the risk of MVCs in older adults include decreased hearing and vision and slower reaction time. Injuries sustained by older adults in MVCs are similar to those of younger patients except that adults over 65 years of age have an increased incidence of sternal fractures from seat belts.

Pedestrian versus vehicle incidents involving older adults are associated with a high death rate, usually from a severe head or major vascular injury. The older adult is frequently struck within a marked crosswalk or walks directly into the path of an oncoming vehicle. Factors increasing the risk of pedestrian versus vehicle incidents include poor eyesight and hearing, decreased mobility, and longer reaction times.

Most burn injuries in older adults occur at home. Although the frequency of burn injuries is lower in older adult than in younger patients, the death rate from burn injuries in older adults is high. Any older adult who has experienced a burn injury should be triaged to a burn center, if available in your area.

Consider the possibility of elder abuse if your assessment reveals any of the signs shown in the following *You Should Know* box. Elder neglect should be suspected if the patient has signs of dehydration, malnutrition, untreated bedsores, or poor personal hygiene.

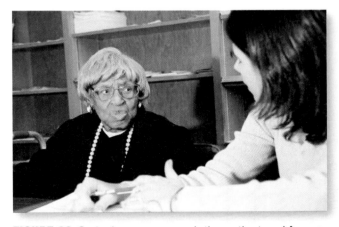

You Should Know

Possible Signs of Elder Abuse

- Bruises, black eyes, welts, lacerations, rope marks
- Bone fractures, skull fractures
- Open wounds, cuts, punctures, untreated injuries in various stages of healing
- Older adult's report of being hit, slapped, kicked, or mistreated
- Physical signs of being subjected to punishment
- Signs of being restrained
- Older adult's sudden change in behavior
- Caregiver's refusal to allow visitors to see an older adult alone

Special Considerations

Objective 10

The physiologic changes associated with aging were discussed in detail in Chapter 8. Changes associated with aging in the pulmonary, cardiovascular, neurological, and musculoskeletal systems make older adults susceptible to trauma. As the brain shrinks with age, there is a higher risk of cerebral bleeding following head trauma. Loss of strength, sensory impairment, and medical illnesses increase the risk of falls. Skeletal changes cause curvature of the upper spine that may require padding when stabilizing the spine. Cardiovascular system changes associated with aging include thickening of the blood vessels, decreased vessel elasticity, and increased peripheral vascular resistance, which contribute to reduced blood flow to organs. There is often a marked increase in the systolic blood pressure and a slight increase in the diastolic blood pressure because of increased peripheral vascular resistance. In some situations, a "normal" blood pressure in an older adult who is usually hypertensive may actually represent hypotension.

Older adults often take multiple medications including cardiac drugs, diuretics ("water pills"), sedatives, antidepressants, and medications that affect blood clotting. Tachycardia, an early indicator of shock, may not be evident in the older adult taking cardiac medications such as beta-blockers and calcium channel blockers. The patient who is taking a diuretic may have a decreased blood volume even before an injury occurs. Sedatives and antidepressants can alter mental status, increasing the older adult's risk of injury. Many older adults who have a history of stroke or an irregular heart rhythm or have had a heart valve replaced are prescribed anticoagulants (such as aspirin, Coumadin, Plavix), which affect the blood's ability to clot. Anticoagulants can worsen bleeding, such as in situations involving internal and external hemorrhage and intracranial bleeding.

Patient Assessment

Objective 11

Conduct a scene size-up and ensure your safety. Evaluate the mechanism of injury, and put on appropriate PPE before approaching the patient. If you have been called to the patient's residence, take a moment to scan your surroundings. Is the home well kept or littered with trash? An untidy home may be a symptom of decreased mobility, depression, or lack of interest in self-care. Falls leading to trauma must be investigated as to the reason for the fall and the information relayed to healthcare professionals at the receiving facility. Is the temperature in the room reasonable for the time of year, or is it too hot or too cold? A cold home in winter or very warm home in the summer may be a symptom of a fixed income and rising electric bills.

As you approach the patient and form a general impression, note the patient's appearance, work of breathing, and skin color (Figure 39-6). Fractures of the spinal column are common in older adults. If trauma is suspected, carefully assess the patient's airway while maintaining spinal stabilization. Keep in mind that the older adult may wear dentures, which, if ill-fitting, may cause an airway obstruction. If they do not fit well, remove them. An older adult's cough reflex may be diminished, so suction as needed to keep the airway open. Assess the patient's rate, depth, and rhythm of breathing. Give 100% oxygen, assisting ventilation as needed. Use a pulse oximeter to monitor oxygenation. Assess the patient's circulatory status, and control hemorrhage with

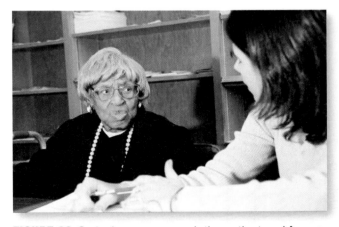

FIGURE 39-6 ▲ As you approach the patient and form a general impression, note the patient's appearance, work of breathing, and skin color.

direct pressure, if present. When assessing the patient's pulse, note its rate, rhythm, and quality. Bear in mind that an older adult's pulse may be irregular, and that a slower than expected heart rate may be caused by prescribed cardiac medications.

Initially, assess the patient's level of consciousness using the AVPU scale. Assessing the mental status of an older adult trauma patient can be challenging, particularly if the patient has a medical condition such as Alzheimer's disease. In situations like this, it will be difficult to determine if the patient has an altered mental status that is "new" as opposed to what is "normal" for that patient. If a family member or caregiver is available, ask what is normal for the patient and compare the response with your assessment findings. Follow the AVPU assessment with one using the Glasgow Coma Scale (GCS). Obtain a Revised Trauma Score, and document your findings.

Expose the patient as necessary, remembering to respect his modesty. Because the older adult's ability to regulate body heat production and heat loss is altered, it is important to minimize the areas of the body exposed, keeping the patient covered as much as possible to maintain warmth. Treat any life-threatening injuries before proceeding to the secondary survey.

Generally, it is a good idea to do a head-to-toe examination of any older adult who has been injured, including repeated vital sign assessments. A thorough examination is important because even minor injuries in an older adult can be significant. Carefully assess the patient using the DCAP-BTLS memory aid to ensure injuries are not missed. Remember to look for medical jewelry that can provide valuable information regarding the patient's history. If time permits, it is appropriate to ask the patient or a family member if an advance directive exists.

Emergency Care

Objective 12

To treat an injured elderly patient, perform the following steps:
- Put on appropriate PPE. Keep on-scene time to a minimum.
- If spinal injury is suspected, maintain manual in-line stabilization until the patient is secured to a long backboard. The musculoskeletal system is the most commonly injured organ system in older adult trauma patients. Nontraditional immobilization techniques and extra padding may be necessary to adapt to musculoskeletal changes, such as curvature of the upper spine.
- Establish and maintain an open airway. Because respiratory difficulty can develop quickly, make

sure that airway adjuncts and suction equipment are readily available.
- Administer supplemental oxygen to all older adult trauma patients. If the patient's breathing is adequate, apply oxygen by nonrebreather mask at 10 to 15 L/min. If the patient's breathing is inadequate, provide positive-pressure ventilation with 100% oxygen and assess the adequacy of the ventilations delivered. Continue monitoring oxygenation using pulse oximetry.
- Control external bleeding by applying direct pressure to the wound with a sterile dressing. If blood soaks through the dressing, apply additional dressings and reapply pressure. If signs of shock are present or if internal bleeding is suspected, treat for shock.
- Do not remove penetrating objects; rather, stabilize in place with bulky dressings.
- Manage avulsed or amputated parts as you would other soft tissue injuries. Every effort should be made to locate the amputated part.
- Do not touch protruding organs. Carefully remove clothing from around the wound. Apply a large sterile dressing, moistened with sterile water or saline, over the organs and wound. Secure the dressing in place with a large bandage to retain moisture and prevent heat loss.
- Protect the patient's modesty and provide emotional support. Keep the patient warm.
- Transport promptly. Reassess at least every 5 minutes en route.
- Record all patient care information, including the patient's medical history and all emergency care given, on a PCR.

Trauma in the Cognitively Impaired Patient

Objective 13

Cognition refers to mental functions, including memory, learning, awareness, reasoning, judgment, and the ability to think, plan, form and comprehend speech, process information, and understand and solve problems. A **cognitive impairment** is a change in a person's mental functioning caused by an injury or a disease process. A cognitive impairment affects a person's ability to process, plan, reason, learn, understand, and remember information. Individuals who are cognitively impaired may have a condition such as Alzheimer's disease, vascular dementia, Down syndrome, an autistic disorder, or a traumatic brain injury, or may have a history of stroke.

Although signs and symptoms vary, a patient with a cognitive impairment may be confused or easily agitated. Some patients bang their heads. Others injure themselves or are unafraid of danger, and this makes them more susceptible to trauma. Some patients have difficulty communicating and interacting with other people. The patient may seem withdrawn, may not make eye contact with you, and may become agitated if touched. The degree of cognitive impairment varies. Many patients attend school, maintain a job, and are cared for at home. Others may be bedridden or under nursing home care.

The patient's inability to communicate any complaints can pose significant challenges to healthcare professionals. Depending on the degree of impairment, the patient may be an unreliable historian regarding past medical history or events of trauma. The adult patient may not be legally able to consent to treatment.

Family members and caregivers often are important resources that should be tapped when you are called to provide care to a cognitively impaired patient. They will know the patient's medical history. They will also know if the patient's vital signs, assessment findings, or capabilities are different from normal. This information can help you assess the urgency of the patient's condition. Examples of questions to ask are listed in the following *You Should Know* box.

You Should Know

Questions to Ask the Family of the Cognitively Impaired Patient

- Can you tell me why you called us today?
- What is the patient's name?
- How does the patient normally communicate?
- How aware is she of the environment?
- What are his usual motor skills and level of activity?
- What is her usual sleep pattern and appetite?
- Does he have any problems with his sight?
- Does she have any problems with her hearing?

Generally, it is helpful to have a caregiver present during the physical exam. Ask for the patient's name, and use it when providing patient care. Ask the patient's family or caregiver to describe the patient's normal mental status. Then ask if the patient's behavior today is different from usual and, if so, how the behavior is different. The AVPU and Glasgow Coma Scales may not be accurate for such patients. While enlisting the help of the family, attempt to take the patient's vital signs when he is calm. Patients with mild to moderate cognitive impairment can often communicate the presence of pain through verbal or nonverbal communication and rate the intensity of their pain. Careful observation of the patient's posture and facial expressions can be helpful when determining the presence or absence of pain. Family members or caregivers can also provide important information about changes in the patient's behavior that might indicate the presence of pain. Attempt to make the patient as comfortable as possible during transport.

On the Scene   Wrap-Up

You are extremely concerned that this patient is unconscious and recognize that your assessment and treatment of the mother will also affect the fetus. You quickly contact dispatch and request that advanced life support personnel be sent to the scene. You find that your patient has a weak, rapid radial pulse and low blood pressure. Within 2 minutes, the ALS unit is on the scene, and the patient is rapidly extricated from the vehicle and placed on a long backboard for movement to the ALS ambulance. As the ambulance prepares to leave for the closest trauma center, the paramedic thanks you for remembering to place a small pillow under the right side of the backboard to improve venous return to the patient's heart. ■

Sum It Up

▶ Trauma is the leading cause of death in pregnant patients and the leading cause of death in women of childbearing age. Although pregnant patients can sustain all types of trauma, motor vehicle crashes are the most frequent cause of injury, followed by falls and intimate partner violence. Direct or indirect trauma to a pregnant uterus can cause injury to the uterine muscle. This can cause the release of chemicals that cause uterine contractions, perhaps inducing premature labor. The effects of trauma on the fetus depend on the length of the pregnancy (the age of the fetus), the type and severity of the trauma, and the severity of blood flow and oxygen disruption to the uterus.

▶ The frequency of falls during pregnancy becomes more common after the 20th week of pregnancy. A woman's center of gravity shifts as the size of her abdomen increases during pregnancy and her pelvic ligaments loosen. As a result, a pregnant patient must readjust her body alignment and balance, and this increases her risk for falls and injury.

- Anatomic changes occur during pregnancy that affect nearly every organ system. In the respiratory system, the diaphragm becomes elevated, and the mother's resting respiratory rate increases because of the enlarging uterus. The mother's blood volume circulates through the uterus every 8 to 11 minutes at term. As a result, the uterus can be a source of significant blood loss if injured. After the 12th week of pregnancy, the uterus begins to rise out of the pelvis and becomes susceptible to injury. As the uterus increases in size, the mother's abdominal organs are displaced superiorly. This displacement increases the likelihood of uterine and fetal injury.

- Early in the pregnancy, the mother's body begins to produce more blood to carry oxygen and nutrients to the fetus, resulting in an increased plasma volume and an increased volume of red blood cells. Her heart rate gradually increases by as much as 10 to 15 beats/min during pregnancy. During the first 6 months of pregnancy, the mother's systolic blood pressure may drop by 5–10 mm Hg. Her diastolic blood pressure may drop by 10–15 mm Hg. During the last 3 months of pregnancy, her blood pressure gradually returns to near normal. The changes in vital signs that typically occur during pregnancy can make it difficult to detect shock, particularly in late pregnancy.

- When shock occurs, the mother's blood pressure is preserved by the shunting of blood from nonvital organs, such as the uterus, to vital organs. Constriction of the uterine arteries decreases perfusion to the uterus, potentially compromising the fetus to save the mother. The fetus will often show signs of distress before any change in maternal vital signs. The healthy pregnant patient can lose 30% to 35% of her blood volume with no change in vital signs.

- A woman who is 20 weeks pregnant or more should be positioned on her left side. Positioning the patient on her left side shifts the weight of her uterus off the abdominal vessels. If the patient is immobilized on a backboard, tilt the board slightly to the left by placing a rolled towel, small pillow, blanket, or other padding under the right side of the board.

- Fetal death may occur because of death of the mother, separation of the placenta, maternal shock, uterine rupture, or a fetal head injury. Of these, maternal death is the number one cause of fetal death. The second most common cause of fetal death is abruptio placentae. Abruptio placentae (also called placental abruption) occurs when a normally implanted placenta separates prematurely from the wall of the uterus (endometrium) during the last trimester of pregnancy. Partial separation may allow time for treatment of the mother and fetus. Separation of more than 50% of the placental surface often results in death of the fetus.

- A ruptured uterus is the actual tearing of the uterus. Uterine rupture can occur when the patient has been in strong labor for a long period; this is the most common cause. It can also occur when the patient has sustained abdominal trauma, such as a severe fall or a sudden stop in a motor vehicle collision.

- Correct seat belt use can significantly reduce both maternal and fetal injury following motor vehicle crashes. Injuries can occur if restraints are improperly worn. In a motor vehicle crash, uterine rupture can occur if a lap belt is worn too high over the pregnant uterus. Wearing a lap belt without a shoulder strap can result in compression of the uterus with possible uterine rupture or abruptio placentae.

- Penetrating trauma in pregnancy is usually the result of gunshot or knife wounds, of which gunshot wounds are more common. Although the maternal outcome of penetrating trauma in pregnancy is usually favorable, the fetal death rate is high.

- Cardiac arrest in the pregnant trauma patient poses some unique challenges. Because the pregnant patient's diaphragm is elevated during pregnancy, it may be necessary to ventilate using less volume. Chest compressions should be performed higher on the sternum, slightly above the center of the sternum. If the patient is 20 weeks pregnant or more, it will be necessary to perform chest compressions with the patient on a backboard tilted 15 to 30 degrees to the left to offset the problems associated with supine hypotension.

- A short on-scene time and rapid transport to an appropriate trauma center are important when caring for the pregnant trauma patient. In situations involving major trauma, an ALS intercept or air medical resources may be needed. Generally, the pregnant trauma patient who has a heart rate of more than 110 beats/min, chest or abdominal pain, or loss of consciousness or who is in her third trimester of pregnancy should be transported to a trauma center. Follow your local protocols.

- Injuries are the leading cause of death in infants and children. Blunt trauma is the most common mechanism of serious injury in the pediatric patient. The injury pattern seen in a child may be different from that seen in an adult. For example, an adult about to be struck by an oncoming vehicle will typically turn away from the vehicle. This results in injuries to the side or back of the body. In contrast, a child will usually face an oncoming vehicle, resulting in injuries to the front of the body.

- Falls are a common cause of injury in infants and children. Infants and young children have large heads in comparison to their body size, making them more prone to falls. Note the distance of the

- fall, the surface on which the child landed, and the body area(s) struck. Any fall more than 10 feet or more than two to three times the child's height should be considered serious.

- Children are prone to head injuries because their heads are large and heavy when compared with their body size. Shaken baby syndrome is a group of signs and symptoms resulting from violent shaking or shaking and impacting of the head of an infant or small child. Shaken baby syndrome occurs when an infant or child is shaken by the arms, legs, or shoulders with enough force to cause the baby's brain to bounce against the skull.

- The younger the patient, the softer and more flexible the ribs. Therefore, rib fractures are less common in children than in adults. However, the force of the injury can be transferred to the internal organs of the chest, resulting in major damage.

- Bruising of the lung (pulmonary contusion) is one of the most frequently observed chest injuries in children. This injury is potentially life-threatening.

- Abdominal trauma is the most common cause of unrecognized fatal injury in children. The abdominal organs of an infant or a child are prone to injury because the organs are large and the abdominal wall is thin. As a result, the organs are closer to the surface of the abdomen and less protected.

- Extremity trauma is common in children. Fractures of both thighs can cause a major blood loss, resulting in shock. Extremity injuries in children are managed in the same way as are those for adults.

- In an injured child, delayed capillary refill time (if the child is 6 years of age or younger), cool distal extremities, and decreases in peripheral versus central pulse quality are generally more reliable signs of shock than blood pressure. This is because a healthy child can maintain a normal blood pressure until she has lost 25% to 30% of her total blood volume.

- Falls are the most common cause of injury in older adults, followed by motor vehicle crashes, pedestrian versus vehicle incidents, and assaults. Most falls involving older adults occur at home and are low-level falls (falls from a standing height).

- Injuries sustained by older adults in MVCs are similar to those of younger patients except that adults over 65 years of age have an increased incidence of sternal fractures from seat belts.

- Any older adult who has experienced a burn injury should be triaged to a burn center, if available in your area.

- As the brain shrinks with age, there is a higher risk of cerebral bleeding following head trauma. Loss of strength, sensory impairment, and medical illnesses increase the risk of falls. Skeletal changes cause curvature of the upper spine that may require padding when stabilizing the spine.

- In some situations, a "normal" blood pressure in an older adult who is usually hypertensive may actually represent hypotension.

- Because the older adult's ability to regulate body heat production and heat loss is altered, it is important to minimize the areas of the body exposed, keeping the patient covered as much as possible to maintain warmth.

- Bear in mind that an older adult's pulse may be irregular, and that a slower than expected heart rate may be caused by prescribed cardiac medications.

- Generally, it is a good idea to do a head-to-toe examination of any older adult who has been injured, including repeated vital sign assessments. A thorough examination is important because even minor injuries in an older adult can be significant. Carefully assess the patient using the DCAP-BTLS memory aid to ensure injuries are not missed.

- The musculoskeletal system is the most commonly injured organ system in older adult trauma patients. Nontraditional immobilization techniques and extra padding may be necessary to adapt to musculoskeletal changes, such as curvature of the upper spine.

- Cognition refers to mental functions, including memory, learning, awareness, reasoning, judgment, and the ability to think, plan, form and comprehend speech, process information, and understand and solve problems. A cognitive impairment refers to a change in a person's mental functioning caused by an injury or disease process. Individuals who are cognitively impaired may have a condition such as Alzheimer's disease, vascular dementia, Down syndrome, autistic disorders, traumatic brain injury, or history of stroke. Family members and caregivers often are important resources that should be tapped when you are called to provide care to a cognitively impaired patient.

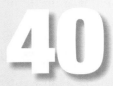
Environmental Emergencies

By the end of this chapter, you should be able to:

Knowledge Objectives ▶

1. Describe the various ways that the body loses heat.
2. List the assessment findings and symptoms of exposure to cold.
3. Explain the steps in providing emergency medical care to a patient exposed to cold.
4. List the assessment findings and symptoms of exposure to heat.
5. Explain the steps in providing emergency care to a patient exposed to heat.
6. Recognize the signs and symptoms of water-related emergencies.
7. Describe the complications of drowning.
8. Discuss the emergency medical care of bites and stings.

Attitude Objectives ▶

There are no attitude objectives identified for this lesson.

Skill Objectives ▶

connect™ (plus+)

9. Demonstrate the assessment and emergency medical care of a patient with exposure to cold.
10. Demonstrate the assessment and emergency medical care of a patient with exposure to heat.
11. Demonstrate the assessment and emergency medical care of a drowning patient.
12. Demonstrate completing a prehospital care report for patients with environmental emergencies.

On the Scene

You and your partner are called for a 45-year-old woman who was bitten by a rattlesnake. Upon arrival at the scene, you find the patient sitting at her kitchen table. She points to her right index finger, which you notice is swollen. The patient states she was trying to kill a baby rattlesnake with a garbage can lid when it bit her. The patient is alert and oriented to person, place, time, and event and denies any other injuries. ■

THINK ABOUT IT

As you read this chapter, think about the following questions:

- What additional information should you try to obtain from the patient?
- What treatment measures would be appropriate for this patient?
- How should the patient's injured extremity be positioned?

Introduction

Environmental emergencies include exposure to heat and cold, water-related emergencies, and bites and stings. Medical conditions can be caused or worsened by the weather, terrain, atmospheric pressure, or other local factors. The keys to appropriate management of any environmental emergency are recognizing signs and symptoms of the emergency as early as possible and providing prompt, efficient emergency medical care.

You must be aware of the ways in which the body loses heat in order to effectively manage patients with temperature-related emergencies. Cold-related emergencies occur in many groups of individuals, including hunters, sailors, skiers, climbers, swimmers, and military personnel. A cold emergency may occur in the wilderness, as well as in rural and urban settings. It can also occur in the summer at night, in a cold building, or after a water exposure. Heat-related emergencies occur in many different settings and may occur during any season of the year. Heat emergencies range from minor effects to life-threatening conditions. Drowning is the most common type of water-related emergency you will encounter.

Because of differences in climates and terrain, not all species of spiders, snakes, insects, scorpions, or marine animals are present in all areas of the United States. Recognizing the signs and symptoms of poisonous bites and stings may help minimize the patient's risk of loss of life or limb.

Body Temperature

Body temperature is the balance between the heat produced by the body and the heat lost from the body. Body temperature is measured in heat units called degrees (°). The body is divided into two areas for temperature control: core temperature and peripheral (surface) temperature. The body core (the deep tissues of the body) includes the contents of the skull, vertebral column, chest, abdomen, and pelvis. Core temperature is the temperature that is essential for the body to convert food to energy (metabolism). The temperature of the periphery is not critical. The body core is normally maintained at a fairly constant temperature, usually within 1°F (approximately 0.6°C) of normal, unless a person develops a fever.

Body temperature remains constant if the heat produced by the body equals the heat lost. When the body produces too much heat, the temperature can temporarily rise to as high as 101°F to 104°F (38.3°C to 40.0°C). This type of temporary rise in temperature

can occur, for example, during strenuous exercise. When the body is exposed to cold, its temperature can often fall to below 96°F (35.6°C).

You Should Know

A rectal temperature is considered a measurement of the body's core temperature. When measured orally, the average normal temperature is between 98.0°F (Fahrenheit) and 98.6°F, which is about 37°C (Celsius). The temperature measured in the armpit (the axillary temperature) or orally is about 1°F (about 0.6°C) less than the rectal (core) temperature.

The peripheral area of the body includes the skin, subcutaneous tissue, and fat. The temperature of the body's extremities rises and falls in response to the environment. At room temperature, the temperature in the peripheral areas of the body is slightly below that of the body core.

Temperature Regulation

The skin plays a very important role in temperature regulation. Cold and warmth sensors (receptors) in the skin detect changes in temperature. These receptors relay the information to the hypothalamus. The hypothalamus (located in the brain) functions as the body's thermostat. It coordinates the body's response to temperature.

The cardiovascular system regulates blood flow to the skin. Blood vessels widen (dilate) and narrow (constrict) in response to messages from the hypothalamus. When high temperatures are sensed, blood vessels in the skin dilate. When low temperatures are sensed, blood vessels in the skin constrict. When these vessels narrow, sweating stops and the major body muscles shiver to increase heat.

You Should Know

The body regulates core temperature through vasodilation, vasoconstriction, sweating (which cools the body through evaporation), shivering, an increase or decrease in activity, and behavioral responses (such as applying or removing layers of clothing, which ultimately results in heat regulation).

Heat Production

Body heat is produced mainly by **metabolism** (the conversion of food to energy). Most of the heat produced in the body is made by the liver, brain, heart, and the skeletal muscles during exercise. The heat made by skeletal muscle is important in temperature control. This is because muscle activity can be increased to produce heat when needed.

The body begins a series of actions when its cold sensors are stimulated. These actions are designed to conserve heat and increase heat production. One action is to produce more epinephrine and other hormones, which increase the rate at which the body converts food to energy, which increases heat production. Another action is to constrict peripheral blood vessels. This constriction decreases blood flow and heat loss through the skin and keeps warm blood in the body's core. Muscle activity also increases; it may be voluntary (such as walking, running, or moving about) or involuntary (such as shivering).

Heat Loss

Objective 1

Knowing how the body loses heat will allow you to prevent further heat loss when treating patients with a cold-related emergency. The body loses heat to the environment in five ways (Figure 40-1):

1. Radiation
2. Convection
3. Conduction
4. Evaporation
5. Respiration

Most heat loss occurs when heat is transferred from the deeper body organs and tissues to the skin. From there it is lost to the air and other surroundings. Some heat loss occurs through the mucous membranes of the respiratory, digestive, and urinary systems.

More than half the heat lost from the body occurs by radiation. **Radiation** is the transfer of heat, as infrared heat rays, from the surface of one object to the surface of another without contact between the two objects. The heat from the sun is an example of radiation. When the temperature of the body is more than the temperature of the surroundings, the body will lose heat. **Convection** is the transfer of heat by the movement of air current. Wind speed affects heat loss by convection (wind-chill factor). **Conduction** is the

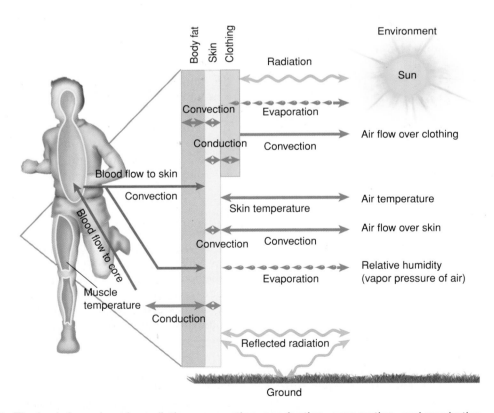

FIGURE 40-1 ▲ The body loses heat by radiation, convection, conduction, evaporation, and respiration.

transfer of heat between objects that are in direct contact. Heat flows from warmer areas to cooler ones. The amount of heat lost from the body by conduction depends on the following:

- The temperature difference between the body and the object
- The amount of time the body and the object are in contact
- The amount (surface area) of the body in contact with the object

Evaporation is a loss of heat by vaporization of moisture on the body surface. The body will lose heat by evaporation if the skin temperature is higher than the temperature of the surroundings. The body gains heat when the temperature of the surrounding air is higher than body temperature. As relative humidity rises, the effectiveness of body cooling by evaporation decreases.

Through **respiration,** The body also loses heat by breathing in cool air and exhaling the air that has become heated in the lungs. Additionally, the body continuously loses a relatively small amount of heat through the evaporation of moisture from within the lungs.

When the body's warmth sensors are stimulated, the body takes action to increase heat loss. Peripheral blood vessels dilate. Blood flow to the body surface increases. Heat escapes from the skin surface by radiation and conduction. When air currents pass across the skin, additional heat is lost by convection. This heat loss cools the body's core. The body's sweat gland secretion also increases. The sweat travels to the skin's surface. When air currents pass across the skin, heat is lost through evaporation.

Making a Difference

Consider a situation in which a patient is found lying on the ground or roadway after a motor vehicle crash. In cold climates, the patient may experience a cold-related emergency after lying on a cold surface. Taking a long time to assess the patient increases the amount of time she is exposed to the environment. In warm climates, patients have experienced severe burns from prolonged exposure to the hot ground or pavement. Even after being placed on a long backboard, patients have experienced burns on the back surfaces of their arms because they were left in contact with the pavement. Do not assume that a patient's complaints are related only to injuries from the crash. The complaints may also be related to the environment in which you found her. Be sensitive to these types of situations.

Exposure to Cold

There are two main types of cold emergencies: a generalized cold emergency (generalized hypothermia) and a local cold injury. A local cold injury is damage to a specific area of the body, such as fingers or toes. Local cold injury is discussed later in this chapter.

Hypothermia

Hypothermia is a core body temperature of less than 95°F (35°C). This condition results when the body loses more heat than it gains or produces. Hypothermia can be broken down into three stages: mild, moderate, and severe.

- Mild hypothermia (core body temperature 93.2°F to 96.8°F, or 34.0°C to 37.0°C)
- Moderate hypothermia (86.0°F to 93.1°F, or 30.0°C to 33.9°C)
- Severe hypothermia (less than 86.0°F or 30.0°C)

It is important to realize that the stages of hypothermia are not a hard-and-fast rule for everyone. Some patients may show signs and symptoms at different temperatures. It is also important to understand that the temperatures shown here are core body temperatures. The usual methods for measuring temperature (oral and tympanic) may not accurately reflect the core temperature. A rectal temperature gives the most accurate measure of core temperature. However, obtaining a rectal temperature in the field often raises issues of patient sensitivity and welfare, such as exposure to cold by removing clothing. In most cases, you will need to make judgments about hypothermia based on your patient's signs and symptoms.

Remember This

Temperatures below 95°F (35°C) are significant because at or below this temperature, the body typically does not generate enough heat to restore normal body temperature or maintain proper organ function.

Hypothermia may occur from exposure to conditions that result in excessive heat loss. Hypothermia can occur even in warm weather. For example, a person who remains in a cool environment, such as a swimming pool, can experience hypothermia. Hypothermia can also occur when the body loses its ability to maintain a normal body temperature. This situation can occur in patients who are in shock.

Some factors increase a person's risk of experiencing hypothermia (see the following *You Should Know* box). A person's age is one factor. Many hypothermia cases occur in urban settings and involve older adults.

Factors That Contribute to Hypothermia

- Ambient temperature, wind speed, moisture
- Prolonged exposure to a cool environment
- Activity level of the victim
- Immersion in water
- Improper, inadequate, or wet clothing
- Low body weight, low body fat
- Poor physical condition
- Low blood sugar
- Alcohol or medication ingestion
- Extremes in age (very young children, older adults)
- Impaired judgment resulting from mental illness or Alzheimer's disease
- Preexisting illness or injury
- Suicide attempt
- Previous cold exposure
- Medications that interfere with internal heat regulation

Older adults are at risk of hypothermia because of the following:

- Lack of heat in the home
- Poor diet or appetite
- Loss of subcutaneous fat for body insulation
- Lack of activity
- Delayed circulation
- Decreased efficiency of temperature control mechanisms

Young children are at risk of hypothermia because they have less subcutaneous fat for body insulation. Their large surface area in relation to their overall size also results in a more rapid heat loss. Newborns are unable to shiver. Infants and very young children are unable to protect themselves from the cold. They cannot put on clothes and cannot move to warm surroundings without help.

Some illnesses and injuries increase a person's risk of hypothermia. These conditions include shock, head or spinal injuries, burns, generalized infection, and low blood sugar. The use of drugs or alcohol can affect a person's judgment, preventing him from taking proper safety measures. These safety measures might include wearing more clothing, increasing the room temperature, or coming in from the cold. Alcohol dilates the body's peripheral vessels and depresses the central nervous system. Heat loss may occur quickly because of dilated vessels. Sedation from alcohol can cause the sedation that comes from cold exposure to go unrecognized.

Assessment of the Patient with a Cold-Related Injury

Objective 2

When you are called for a patient with a possible cold-related injury, make sure that you are dressed appropriately for the environment and carefully size up the scene on arrival. A cold environment requires special safety considerations because of the presence of ice, snow, or wind. You may need to wait on the scene until the necessary equipment or rescue personnel arrive.

Look at the patient's environment for signs of cold exposure. The signs of exposure may be very obvious or very subtle.

Subtle indicators of exposure include:

- Alcohol ingestion
- Underlying illness
- Overdose or poisoning
- Major trauma
- Outdoor recreation
- Decreased room temperature (such as in the home of an older adult)

Removing the patient from the environment must be your main concern. Use trained rescuers for this purpose when necessary. While you assess the need for additional resources, think about what your department or agency can handle safely. For example, can your department safely remove a person who is trapped in a freezing lake? In all cases of cold-related emergencies, you should request advanced life support (ALS) personnel as soon as possible.

Stop and Think!

What equipment do you have in place right now to help you treat a cold-related emergency? Your answer to this question should be a reminder to check your seasonal equipment for use in an emergency setting, including personal clothing.

After ensuring your safety, perform a primary survey. Approach the patient and form a general impression. Notice the clothing the patient is wearing. Is it adequate for your climate? What are the surroundings like? As you continue your assessment, keep in mind that you need to move the patient to a warm location as quickly and as safely as possible. Remove any cold or wet clothing. Protect the patient from the environment. This may include shielding the patient from the wind. Cover the patient to help preserve body heat. A lot of body heat is lost through the head. Covering the patient's head can help reduce heat loss. Stabilize the spine if needed.

Assess the patient's mental status, airway, breathing, and circulation. Remember that mental status decreases as the patient's body temperature drops. However, as the patient's body temperature drops, there may be no clear difference between the stages of hypothermia.

The patient may show the following signs of hypothermia:

- Difficult (slow, slurred) speech
- Confusion
- Memory lapse (amnesia)
- Mood changes
- Combativeness
- Unresponsiveness
- Loss of motor skills and coordination
- Uncontrollable shivering; later, a lack of shivering

Remember This

A patient who has severe hypothermia may be alive but may have such a weak pulse or shallow breathing that you are unable to feel it. Do not assume a patient is dead until he is warm and has no pulse. Take longer than usual to assess the breathing and heart rate of a patient who has been exposed to cold before starting cardiopulmonary resuscitation (CPR). Assess breathing for 30 to 45 seconds. Also, assess for a pulse for 30 to 45 seconds.

The patient's vital signs will also change as hypothermia worsens. The patient's breathing rate is initially increased, then slow and shallow, and finally absent. The heart rate is initially increased, then slow and irregular, and finally absent. Blood pressure may be normal at first and then low to absent. The pupils dilate and are slow to respond. The skin is initially red; then pale; then blue; and finally gray, hard, and cold to the touch. To assess the patient's general temperature, place the back of your hand between the patient's clothing and her abdomen. The patient experiencing a generalized cold emergency will have a cool or cold abdominal skin temperature.

The patient's motor and sensory functions also change with the degree of hypothermia. The patient may initially complain of joint aches or muscle stiffness. He may show a lack of coordination and a staggering walk. Shivering is usually present initially. As hypothermia worsens, shivering gradually decreases until it is absent. Shivering stops below 86.0°F to 89.6°F (30.0°C to 32.0°C). The patient loses sensation and the muscles become rigid. Be certain to assess the patient for other injuries. Identify any life-threatening conditions, and provide care based on your findings. The signs and symptoms of hypothermia are listed in Table 40-1.

If the patient is responsive, or if family members or bystanders are available, try to obtain a SAMPLE history. Keep in mind that some illnesses or injuries increase a person's risk of hypothermia. Find out if the patient has a history of alcohol abuse; thyroid disorder; diabetes; stroke; or trauma to the head, neck, or spine.

TABLE 40-1 Assessment Findings and Symptoms of Hypothermia

Mild	Moderate	Severe
• Increased heart rate • Increased respiratory rate • Cool skin (to preserve core temperature) • Shivering • Difficulty talking, slurred speech • Difficulty moving • Memory lapse (amnesia), mood changes, combative attitude • Joint aches, muscle stiffness • Altered mental status, confusion, or poor judgment (patient may actually remove clothing)	• Shivering that may gradually decrease and become absent; shivering replaced with rigid muscles • Decreasing heart rate and respiratory rate • Irregular heart rate • Pale, blue (cyanotic), or mottled skin • Progressive loss of responsiveness • Dilated pupils • Blood pressure that is difficult to obtain	• Irrational attitude that changes to unresponsiveness • Rigid muscles • Cold skin • Blue or mottled skin • Slow or absent breathing • Slowly responding pupils • A heart rate that is slow, irregular, or absent • A pulse that is hard to feel or absent • Low-to-absent blood pressure • Cardiopulmonary arrest

When finding out what events led to the patient's present situation, ask the following questions:

- How long has the patient been exposed to the cold?
- What was the source of the cold (for example, water or snow)? If the patient was exposed to water, what was the approximate water temperature?
- What was the patient doing when his symptoms began?

Remember This

Moving water robs the body of heat faster than still water.

Emergency Care of Patients with Hypothermia

Objective 3

The basic principles of rewarming a hypothermic patient involve conserving the heat she has and replacing the body fuel she is burning up to generate that heat. Remove the patient from the cold environment as quickly and as safely as possible to protect her from further heat loss. When moving the patient, keep in mind known or suspected injuries. Cut away cold or wet clothing rather than tugging and pulling at the patient's clothes. Protect the patient from the cold with available materials, such as blankets, a sleeping bag, newspapers, or plastic garbage bags (Figure 40-2).

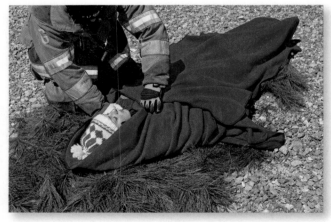

FIGURE 40-2 ▲ Protect the patient from the cold with available materials. Make sure to cover the patient's head, leaving her face exposed so that you can watch her airway. Place insulating material between the patient and the surface on which she is lying.

Make sure to cover the patient's head. However, leave her face exposed so that you can watch her airway. Place insulating material between the patient and the surface on which she is lying. Protect the patient from drafts.

Handle the patient gently. Avoid rough handling. Do not allow the patient to walk or exert herself. Rough handling or exertion may force cold blood in the periphery to the body's core. Make sure the patient's airway is open and that suction is within arm's reach. As the body cools, the cough reflex is depressed and respiratory secretions increase. Frequent suctioning may be necessary.

Give oxygen. If the patient's breathing is adequate, apply oxygen by nonrebreather mask at 10 to 15 L/min. If the patient's breathing is inadequate, assist her breathing with a bag-mask or mouth-to-mask device. Assess pulses for 30 to 45 seconds. If the patient has no pulse, begin CPR.

Stop and Think!

The decision to rewarm a hypothermic patient depends on your local protocol and the degree of hypothermia. Be sure to consult with medical direction before rewarming the patient.

There are two main types of rewarming: passive and active. **Passive rewarming** is the warming of a patient with minimal or no use of heat sources other than the patient's own heat production. Passive rewarming methods include placing the patient in a warm environment, applying clothing and blankets, and preventing drafts. Passive external rewarming is appropriate for all hypothermic patients.

Active rewarming involves adding heat directly to the surface of the patient's body. Active rewarming should not delay definitive care and may be used if the patient is alert and responding appropriately (follow local protocol).

Steps for active rewarming:

- If the patient shows signs of mild hypothermia, apply warm blankets. Apply heat packs or hot water bottles to the groin, armpits, and the back of the neck. To prevent burns, place a towel or dressings between the heat pack or hot water bottle and the patient's skin.
- If the patient shows signs of moderate hypothermia, apply warm blankets. Apply heat packs or hot water bottles to the torso only. Take care to avoid burning the underlying tissue.
- If the patient shows signs of severe hypothermia, apply warm blankets. Active rewarming will need

to be done at the hospital. Alert the receiving facility of the patient's condition and your estimated time of arrival.

- Do not allow a patient to eat or drink stimulants (such as coffee, tea, or chocolate) or to drink alcohol. Do not rub or massage the patient's extremities. Doing so can cause cold blood to move from the extremities to the body core, causing a further decrease in temperature.

- During transport, turn the heat up in the patient area of the ambulance. En route to the receiving facility, reassess (including vital signs) as often as indicated. Carefully document all patient care information on a prehospital care report.

Remember This

In general, chemical heat packs can provide 100°F (37.8°C) heat for about 6 to 10 hours. Hot water bottles and warm rocks or towels are also good sources of heat. However, remember that a patient who has an altered mental status may not recognize when a heat source is too hot. No matter what heat source is used, careful monitoring is essential.

Local Cold Injury

When the body is exposed to cold, blood is forced away from the extremities to the body core. This puts the arms and legs at risk of local cold injury. **Local cold injury** (also called *frostbite*) involves tissue damage to a specific area of the body. It occurs when a body part, such as the nose, ears, cheeks, chin, hands, or feet, is exposed to prolonged or intense cold. Local tissue injury usually occurs when these areas are wet, poorly protected, or unprotected. Cold causes the blood vessels to narrow in the affected part. This narrowing decreases circulation to the involved area. Ice crystals form within the cells, which damages them. Hypothermia is often accompanied by frostbite.

Patients at risk of local cold injury include those with circulation problems, such as diabetics. Patients with a history of heart or blood vessel disease are also at risk. Alcohol, nicotine, and some medications decrease blood flow to the skin, increasing the risk of a local cold injury. Patients who have experienced a soft tissue injury such as a burn or a previous cold injury are also at risk. Other factors that affect the risk of local cold injury include the following:

- Ambient temperature
- Wind-chill factor
- The length of exposure

- The type and number of clothing layers worn, including tight gloves and tight or tightly laced footwear
- Whether or not the patient is wet
- Whether or not the patient has had direct contact with cold objects

A local cold injury may be early (superficial frostbite) or late (deep frostbite). A superficial cold injury involves the uppermost skin layers. Early (superficial) local cold injury is also called *frostnip*. In a superficial cold injury, the skin of the exposed area first appears red and inflamed. With continued cooling, the area then becomes gray or white. When you press on the skin, normal color does not return (blanching). You may see a clear demarcation (a visible line of color change), although this sign may not be present at the scene. The patient may complain of a loss of feeling in the injured area. The skin beneath the affected area remains soft. If the area is rewarmed, the patient experiences tingling or burning. This is followed by a pins-and-needles sensation as the area thaws and circulation improves.

A deep cold injury involves more tissue layers. This type of injury is more serious than superficial frostbite. In a deep cold injury, the whitish skin color is followed by a waxy appearance. The affected area becomes frozen. It will feel stiff and solid when you touch it. The patient may complain of slight burning pain followed by a feeling of warmth and then numbness. Swelling may be present. Blisters may be present, usually appearing in 1 to 7 days. If the affected area has thawed or partially thawed, the skin may appear flushed, with areas that are blue, purple, pale, or mottled.

Emergency Care of Patients with Local Cold Injury

Complete a scene size-up before beginning emergency medical care. After making sure that the scene is safe, remove the patient from the cold environment. Protect the affected area from further injury. Give oxygen. If the patient's breathing is adequate, apply oxygen by nonrebreather mask at 10 to 15 L/min if not already done. If the patient's breathing is inadequate, provide positive-pressure ventilation with 100% oxygen and assess the adequacy of the ventilations delivered.

If the injury is *early* or *superficial,* gently remove any jewelry or wet or restrictive clothing. If clothing is frozen to the skin, leave it in place. Rewarm the affected part by placing it against a warm part of the body such as the stomach or armpit (Figure 40-3). Splint the affected extremity and apply soft padding. (Avoid pressure when applying the soft padding.) Loosely cover the affected area with dry sterile dressings or clothing. Do not rub or massage the affected area or reexpose

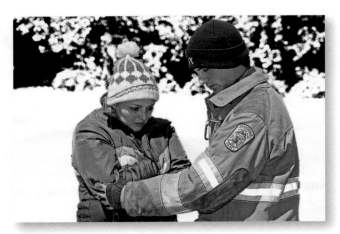

FIGURE 40-3 ▲ To care for an early (superficial) local cold injury, warm the affected part by placing it against a warm part of the body, such as the stomach or armpit.

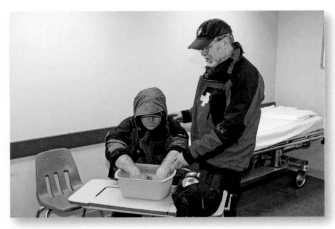

FIGURE 40-4 ▲ If you are instructed to do so, care for a late or deep local cold injury by placing the affected part in a warm (not hot) water bath.

the affected area to the cold. Doing so can cause damage to the skin and surrounding tissue.

If the injury is *late* or *deep*, gently remove any jewelry or wet or restrictive clothing. If clothing is frozen to the skin, leave it in place. Loosely cover the affected area with dry, sterile dressings or clothing.

Take care to avoid doing any of the following:
- Breaking blisters
- Rubbing or massaging the affected area
- Applying heat to or rewarming the affected area
- Allowing the patient to walk on an affected extremity

Remember This

Check your local protocol about care for local cold injuries. Do not use dry sources of heat (such as heat packs, a heating pad, fire, or a radiator) for rewarming. These heat sources are difficult to control. The skin of the affected area will be numb and insensitive to the heat. Therefore, these heat sources can result in skin burns.

When an extremely long or delayed transport is certain, contact medical direction for instructions or follow your local protocol. Do not begin rewarming if there is a risk that the affected part will be exposed to the cold again. If you are instructed to begin active, rapid rewarming, be aware that the patient will complain of intense pain during thawing. Handle the affected area gently. Submerge the affected area in a warm water bath (100°F to 105°F, or 37.8°C to 40.6°C) (Figure 40-4.) Do *not* use hot water. If a thermometer is not available, test the water by pouring some of it over

FIGURE 40-5 ▲ Thawed frostbite. This picture shows the typical appearance of frostbite soon after rewarming. The patient experienced deep frostbite as a result of wearing mountaineering boots that were too tight in extreme cold at high altitude.

the inside of your arm. Check the temperature of the water often, adding more warm water as needed. Continuously stir the water around the affected part to keep heat evenly distributed. Continue rewarming until the affected part is soft and color and sensation return (Figure 40-5). Gently dry the area after rewarming. Dress the area with dry, sterile dressings. If the affected area is a hand or foot, place dry sterile dressings between the fingers or toes. Elevate the affected extremity to decrease swelling. Protect against refreezing of the warmed part. En route to the receiving facility, reassess (including vital signs) as often as indicated. Carefully document all patient care information on a PCR.

Exposure to Heat

According to the Centers for Disease Control and Prevention (CDC), more than 300 people die of heat-related illnesses every year. Many others require medical attention because of heat-related illnesses.

Hyperthermia (a high core body temperature) results when the body gains or produces more heat than it loses. There are three main types of heat emergencies: heat cramps, heat exhaustion, and heat stroke. Heat cramps are the mildest form of heat-related emergencies. Heat stroke is the most severe.

Predisposing Factors

Although everyone is susceptible to heat illness, it affects people differently. The human body can adjust to heat stress if it is given several weeks to adapt to changes in temperature and humidity. This process is called *acclimation* or *acclimatization*. Physically fit, acclimatized, well-hydrated people are more likely to tolerate extremes of heat. Less physically fit people, older adults, and children are less likely to tolerate extremes of heat.

The climate can increase a person's risk of hyperthermia. High ambient temperature reduces the body's ability to lose heat by radiation. High relative humidity reduces the body's ability to lose heat by the evaporation of sweat. Cooling of the body through the evaporation of sweat becomes ineffective as humidity rises, particularly if the humidity is above 50%. Exercise and strenuous activity can cause the loss of more than 1 L of sweat per hour. However, dehydration does not occur only when a person is exercising in the heat. A person can become dehydrated when doing other activities involving prolonged exposure to heat, such as spending a day at the beach, working in the yard, or visiting a theme park.

Older adults are at higher risk for heat emergencies for many reasons, including the following:
- Medications
- Lack of mobility (the patient cannot escape the hot environment)
- Impaired ability to maintain a normal temperature
- Impaired ability to adapt to temperature changes
- Impaired sense of thirst

Newborns and infants are at a higher risk for heat-related emergencies. This higher risk results from their impaired ability to maintain a normal temperature and their inability to remove their own clothing.

Some medications can increase the risk of hyperthermia. For example, amphetamines and cocaine increase muscle activity, which increases heat production. Alcohol impairs the body's ability to regulate heat.

Tricyclic antidepressants and antihistamines weaken the body's ability to lose heat. Factors that increase the risk of a heat-related emergency are shown in the following *You Should Know* box.

Types of Heat-Related Emergencies

Objective 4

Heat cramps usually affect people who sweat a lot during strenuous activity in a warm environment. Water and electrolytes are lost from the body during sweating. This loss leads to dehydration. The loss of water and electrolytes causes painful muscle spasms that usually occur in the shoulders, arms, abdomen, and muscles at the back of the lower legs. The cramps usually improve when the patient is moved to a cool environment, drinks water, and rests.

Heat exhaustion is also a result of too much heat and dehydration. It is the most common heat-related illness. The signs and symptoms of heat exhaustion are shown in the next *You Should Know* box. A patient who has heat exhaustion usually sweats heavily. His oral body temperature is usually normal or slightly elevated (up to 101–102°F, or 38.3–38.9°C). The patient's symptoms usually improve with a move to a cool environment, the removal of excess clothing, and rest. The patient may drink water if he is awake and alert and is not nauseated (and if approved by medical direction). Severe heat exhaustion often requires intravenous fluids, so call for ALS backup if you suspect severe heat exhaustion. Heat exhaustion may progress to heat stroke if it is not treated.

Heat stroke is the least common but most serious form of heat-related illness. Heat stroke is a medical emergency. It occurs when the body can no longer regulate its temperature. In other words, the body's cooling system has completely shut down. Most patients have hot, flushed skin, and many do not sweat. Athletes and firefighters who wear heavy uniforms and perform strenuous activity for long periods in a hot environment are at risk for heat stroke. Military recruits, athletes, construction workers, and foundry and laundry workers are also at risk.

A patient with heat stroke has a very high body temperature. She also has an altered mental status. She may have a seizure or become unresponsive. Fifty to eighty percent of patients who experience heat stroke die. You must act quickly to lower the patient's body temperature and increase her chances of survival. Prompt treatment may lower the death rate to between 15% and 20%. Call for ALS personnel as soon as possible. The patient will need IV fluids and further care at the hospital.

Emergency Care of Patients with Heat-Related Emergencies

Objective 5

The first step in the emergency care of a patient suffering from a heat-related illness is to remove him from the hot environment. Move the patient to a cool (air-conditioned) location.

If the patient has moist, pale skin that is normal to cool in temperature, follow these guidelines:

- Consult medical direction or follow local protocol.
- Give oxygen. If the patient's breathing is adequate, apply oxygen by nonrebreather mask at 10 to 15 L/min. If the patient's breathing is inadequate, assist his breathing with a bag-mask or mouth-to-mask device.
- Remove as much of the patient's outer clothing as possible. Loosen clothing that cannot be easily removed. Cool the patient by fanning (Figure 40-6). Do not cool the patient to the point of shivering because shivering generates heat. *Do not delay transport to cool the patient!*
- Place the patient in a supine position. If the patient's mental status worsens and you do not suspect trauma, place him in the recovery position.
- If the patient is awake and alert and is not nauseated, have him slowly drink water. (Consult medical direction or follow local protocol.) If the patient has an altered mental status, is nauseated,

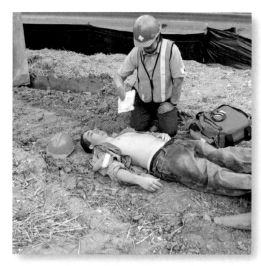

FIGURE 40-6 ▲ Place the patient on his back and cool him by fanning.

or is vomiting, do *not* give fluids. Place the patient in the recovery position.

- Comfort, calm, and reassure the patient. En route to the receiving facility, reassess (including vital signs) as often as indicated.
- Carefully document all patient care information on a PCR.

If the patient has hot and dry or moist skin, follow these guidelines:

- Consult medical direction or follow local protocol.
- Call for ALS personnel as soon as possible. If ALS personnel are not available, transport *immediately* to the closest appropriate facility. Alert the receiving facility of the patient's condition and your estimated time of arrival.
- Give oxygen. If the patient's breathing is adequate, apply oxygen by nonrebreather mask at 10 to 15 L/min. If the patient's breathing is inadequate, assist her breathing with a bag-mask or mouth-to-mask device.
- Start cooling the patient. Remove as much of the patient's outer clothing as possible. Apply cool packs to the back of the neck, armpits, and groin. Make sure to place a towel or dressings between the cool pack and the patient's skin to prevent local cold injury. Wet the patient's skin and keep it wet by applying water with a sponge, wet towels, or spray bottle (Figure 40-7). Alternately, you can cover the patient with a sheet and keep the sheet wet. Fan the patient aggressively to promote evaporation and convective cooling. Note that fanning may not be effective if the humidity is high. *Never* try to cool a patient by placing her in an ice water bath.

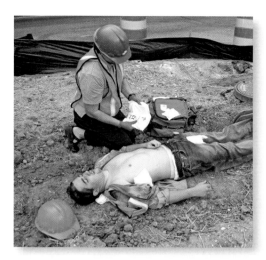

FIGURE 40-7 ▲ Place the patient on his back. Remove as much of the patient's outer clothing as possible. Cool the patient by applying cool packs to the back of the neck, armpits, and groin. Wet the patient's skin, and keep it wet by applying water with a sponge or wet towels.

- Comfort, calm, and reassure the patient. En route to the receiving facility, reassess (including vital signs) every 5 minutes.
- Carefully document all patient care information on a PCR.

Remember This

Spray bottles filled with water are an excellent resource when trying to cool a patient who has been exposed to the heat.

Water-Related Emergencies

Drowning

Drowning is a process that results in harm to the respiratory system from submersion or immersion in a liquid. **Delayed drowning** (also called *secondary drowning*) occurs when a victim appears to have survived an immersion or submersion episode but later dies from respiratory failure or an infection. **Immersion** refers to covering of the face and airway in water or other fluid. In a **submersion** incident, the victim's entire body, including his airway, is under the water or other fluid.

Risk Factors

Drowning is associated with risk factors (see the next *You Should Know* box). The highest drowning rate occurs in children under 1 year of age. Drowning in this age group occurs most often in bathtubs, buckets, or toilets. Among children 1 to 4 years of age, most drowning occurs in residential swimming pools. Drowning involving older children tends to occur in open water areas, such as ponds, lakes, and rivers. In the United States, drowning is second only to motor vehicle crashes as the most common cause of injury and death in children between the ages of 1 month and 14 years.

Drowning involves males more often than females. Studies suggest that males may be more at risk for drowning because of higher exposure rates to water-related activities, higher alcohol consumption while in or around water, and more risk-taking behavior.

There are racial differences in drowning rates between African-Americans and white Americans, particularly in children. During 2002–2003, African-American children ages 5 to 19 years fatally drowned at more than twice the rate of white children in this age group. Environmental factors may be a reason. Research shows that white children usually drown in a backyard swimming pool. African-American children tend to drown in lakes (unsupervised swimming) and unattended canals or quarries (accidental falls).

The children of parents who can swim are more likely to be strong swimmers than are children of parents who cannot swim. Reportedly, men of all ages, races, and educational levels are stronger swimmers than women are. However, as noted previously, white males have a higher incidence of drowning than white females.

The use of alcohol or drugs near water increases a person's risk of drowning. According to the National Center for Injury Prevention and Control, alcohol use is involved in about 25% to 50% of adolescent and adult deaths associated with water recreation. Alcohol affects judgment, balance, and coordination. Alcohol's effects are intensified with exposure to the sun and heat. Drugs such as phencyclidine (PCP), lysergic acid diethylamide (LSD), and marijuana alter the senses and affect judgment.

Consider the presence of an underlying illness or associated injury in all drowning incidents. For example, a person who has low blood sugar, heart disease, irregular heart rhythm, seizures, fainting, depression, anxiety or panic disorder, or severe arthritis is at increased risk of drowning. Because drowning is the most common cause of unintentional injury for persons with seizure disorders, a person with a seizure history should always be supervised when swimming or boating. Possible injuries that may be associated with drowning include head or spinal cord injury (from diving, falls, horseplay, surfing, waterskiing, or jet skiing), cuts, bites, and stings. Child abuse, suicide, or homicide may be a factor in some drowning incidents. Carefully assess the patient for other signs of injury.

Drowning victims are at risk of hypothermia because water conducts heat 25 to 30 times more than air. Water colder than 91.4°F (33°C) will lead to ongoing heat loss. Children are at increased risk for hypothermia because they have less subcutaneous fat and a relatively greater body surface area than adults.

Effects of Drowning

The sequence of events that leads to drowning, particularly in cold water, begins with an initial period of panic as the victim realizes that he cannot make it to safety. Temperature receptors in the skin stimulate the conscious victim to take several deep breaths (hyperventilation) in an attempt to store oxygen before breath holding. The victim may swallow large amounts of water, causing the stomach to swell (distend). This increases the risk of vomiting. The victim holds his breath until breathing reflexes override the breath-holding effort. How long the victim is voluntarily able to hold his breath until breathing reflexes take over is determined by the levels of oxygen and carbon dioxide in the blood.

In some individuals, cold water stimulation of the temperature receptors in the skin triggers the **mammalian diving reflex.** This reflex is present in seals and other diving mammals. In humans, the diving reflex is strongest in infants less than 6 months old, and the effects decrease with age. The diving reflex triggers the shunting of blood to the brain and heart from the skin and extremities. The victim's heart rate slows in response to the increased volume of blood in the body's core. These actions help the body conserve oxygen and may help the victim survive.

As carbon dioxide builds up as a result of breath holding, a decreased supply of oxygen is delivered to the body's tissues (hypoxia). The victim begins struggling violently and gasping for air. Without adequate oxygen, acid builds up in the blood and tissues. The buildup of acid is called **acidosis.** In about 85% of drowning incidents, large amounts of water enter the trachea and lungs (aspiration). The entry of water into the trachea and lungs is commonly called a *wet drowning.* The patient's chances of survival are affected by the amount and type of material taken into the lungs. Aspirating cold water may hasten the onset of hypothermia.

In about 15% of drowning incidents, little water is aspirated. This occurs because the sensitive tissue near the vocal cords begins to spasm **(laryngospasm).** This protective reflex causes closing of the larynx to prevent the passage of water into the lungs. This is commonly called a *dry drowning.* Although laryngospasm causes little fluid to enter the lungs, it also prevents the entry of air. As a result, hypoxia worsens and the victim suffocates. There is little difference in the patient's lungs regardless of which type of water submersion occurred (freshwater versus saltwater).

You Should Know

The American Heart Association's 2005 Resuscitation Guidelines recommend that the following terms related to drowning should no longer be used: near-drowning, dry and wet drowning, active and passive drowning, silent drowning, secondary drowning, and drowned versus near-drowned.

Although many factors influence a drowning victim's chances for survival (see the following *You*

Should Know box), the most important are the length of the immersion or submersion and the severity of the hypoxia.

You Should Know

Factors That Influence a Drowning Victim's Chances for Survival

- Length of immersion or submersion
- Duration of hypoxia
- Ability to swim
- Age of the victim
- Cleanliness of the water
- Temperature of the water
- Duration and degree of hypothermia
- Preexisting medical conditions
- Presence of drugs and/or alcohol
- Presence of associated injuries (especially to the cervical spine and head)
- Response to initial resuscitation efforts

Assessment of the Drowning Victim

Objectives 6, 7

Study the scene, and determine whether approaching the patient is safe. Evaluate the mechanism of injury. Obtain additional help *before* contact with the patient(s). A cold environment requires special safety considerations because of the presence of ice, snow, or wind. Call for specially trained personnel as needed to remove the patient from the environment. Do not enter a body of water unless you have been trained in water rescue and have the proper safety equipment and personnel with you. Do not enter fast-moving water or venture out on ice unless you have been trained in this type of rescue.

Remember This

Professionals trained in water rescue are generally called for incidents that involve the removal of the victim(s) from any body of water other than a swimming pool. This includes lakes, ponds, canals, washes, rivers, or any other body of water, whether still or moving.

Perform a primary survey. Stabilize the patient's spine as needed (see the following *You Should Know* box). If the patient is in the water and spinal injury is suspected, place the patient on a long backboard before removing the patient from the water.

Signs and symptoms of drowning vary. The most common signs and symptoms are reflected in changes in the nervous and respiratory systems. While assessing the patient, protect her from environmental temperature extremes.

Assess the patient's mental status. A drowning victim's mental status may range from awake and alert to confused, combative, difficult to arouse, or unresponsive. Some patients have seizures. These variations in mental status may be caused by an associated injury or by a lack of oxygen from immersion or submersion.

Hypoxia can result from fluid in the lungs and contaminants from the water and/or laryngospasm. Coughing, vomiting, choking, or signs of airway obstruction may be present. The drowning victim may have difficulty breathing or absent or inadequate breathing. Gastric distention may be present. The victim may cough up pink, frothy fluid. Respiratory failure and pneumonia are possible complications that can occur in victims who survive a drowning incident. The onset of symptoms can be delayed for as long as 24 to 36 hours after the incident. If water was inhaled into the lungs (aspirated), it may take days for normal lung function to return.

Hypoxia and acidosis can cause irregular heart rhythms. If the heart muscle is deprived of an adequate oxygen supply, damage to the heart muscle can occur. This can result in cardiogenic shock. In **cardiogenic shock,** the heart muscle fails to pump blood effectively to all parts of the body. Effects of an inadequate oxygen supply and acidosis on the cardiovascular system may include a fast or slow heart rate, an irregular heart rhythm, or even an absent pulse. The patient's skin is often cool, clammy, and pale or cyanotic. Possible signs and symptoms of drowning are listed in the following *You Should Know* box.

Identify any life-threatening conditions, and provide care based on these findings. Establish patient priorities.

Priority patients include:

- Patients who give a poor general impression
- Patients experiencing difficulty breathing
- Patients with signs and symptoms of shock
- Unresponsive patients with no gag reflex or cough
- Responsive patients who are unable to follow commands

Request ALS assistance as soon as possible. If ALS personnel are not available, transport the patient promptly to the closest appropriate facility.

Perform a secondary survey. If the patient is unresponsive, perform a rapid physical examination. Follow with evaluation of baseline vital signs and gathering of the patient's medical history. If the patient is responsive, gather information about the patient's medical history before performing a focused physical exam. When performing a physical examination, carefully assess the patient for other injuries.

When gathering a SAMPLE history, attempt to find out the following:

- When did the incident occur (length of submersion)?
- Where did the incident occur (such as near rocks, pool, bathtub)? Note the cleanliness of the water. Try to find out the temperature of the water.
- How did the incident occur?
- Did the patient experience any loss of responsiveness?

- Was the incident witnessed? This information is useful in determining possible head or spinal injury. Look for signs of abuse or neglect in infants, children, and older adults.

Emergency Care of the Drowning Victim

Steps for caring for a drowning victim:
- Ensure the safety of all rescue personnel. Remove the patient from the water as quickly and safely as possible.
- If spinal injury is suspected and the patient is still in the water, stabilize the head and spine. Move and secure the patient onto a long backboard, and then remove the patient from the water. If spine injury is not suspected, place the patient on the left side (recovery position) to allow water, vomitus, and secretions to drain from the upper airway. Suction as needed to remove debris, vomitus, or other foreign material from the upper airway.
- Rescue breathing is the most important initial care you can provide for a drowning victim. After making sure the scene is safe, start rescue breathing as soon as you can open the victim's airway. In most cases, rescue breathing is started when the victim is in shallow water or has been removed from the water. Do not use abdominal thrusts in an attempt to clear water from the patient's airway. This can cause injury, vomiting, and aspiration and delay CPR.

Remember This

Most drowning victims who require rescue breathing or chest compressions vomit. Be sure to always have suction equipment within arm's reach when caring for a drowning victim.

- Give oxygen. If the patient's breathing is adequate, apply oxygen by nonrebreather mask at 10 to 15 L/min if not already done. If the patient's breathing is inadequate, provide positive-pressure ventilation with 100% oxygen. Assess the adequacy of the ventilations delivered.
- It may be difficult to feel a pulse in a drowning victim, particularly if the victim is cold. If you cannot feel a central pulse, begin CPR after the patient has been removed from the water. After ensuring you, other assisting EMTs, and the patient are dry and on dry surfaces, attach an automated external defibrillator (AED), and follow the AED prompts.
- After the patient has been removed from the water and is in a safe location, quickly remove wet clothing and dry the patient to prevent heat loss. Treat for hypothermia if indicated. The hypothermic drowning victim must be handled gently. As with all other hypothermic patients, remove wet clothing. Then dry and wrap the patient in blankets to maintain body heat.
- Transport promptly. Keep the patient warm during transport. En route to the hospital, reassess every 15 minutes if the patient is stable. If the patient is unstable, reassess every 5 minutes.
- Record all patient care information, including the patient's medical history and the emergency care provided, on a PCR.

Making a Difference

Because of the possibility of delayed complications, *all* victims of an immersion or submersion incident should be transported for physician evaluation.

You Should Know

Drowning Prevention
- Take swimming lessons that include instruction in general water safety and emergency water survival training.
- Use properly fitted U.S. Coast Guard–approved personal flotation devices when on boats or participating in water sports.
- Avoid alcohol use around water.
- Obey warning signs in dangerous areas.
- Swim in areas with lifeguard coverage, when possible.
- Ask a lifeguard about water depth and conditions before entering the water. Be aware that weather conditions can change quickly.
- Make sure an adult is constantly watching children swimming or playing in or around water.
- Never swim alone or in unsupervised places. Always swim with a buddy.
- Know local weather conditions and the forecast before swimming or boating. Strong winds and thunderstorms with lightning strikes are dangerous to swimmers and boaters.
- Watch for dangerous waves and signs of rip currents (water that is discolored and unusually choppy, foamy, or filled with debris). If you are caught in a rip current, swim parallel to the shore. Once out of the current, swim toward the shore.

Diving Emergencies

Barotrauma

Barotrauma is a diving-related injury caused by pressure. It can occur on ascent or descent. Barotrauma occurring on ascent is called *pulmonary overpressurization syndrome (POPS)* or *burst lung*. Barotrauma occurring on descent is called *lung squeeze* or the *squeeze*. Air pressure in the body's air-filled cavities increases, causing damage to the tissues within the cavity (such as the ears, sinuses, lungs, and GI tract). The signs and symptoms of barotraumas are listed in the following *You Should Know* box.

You Should Know

Assessment Findings and Symptoms of Barotrauma

- Ears: Bloody drainage from the ears; mild to severe pain in the ears; nausea, dizziness, disorientation
- Sinuses: Mild to severe pain over the sinuses; bleeding from the nose
- Lungs: Difficulty breathing, chest pain, cough, pulmonary edema
- GI tract: Mild to severe abdominal pain

Emergency Care for Barotrauma

Steps for caring for patients with barotrauma:
- Establish and maintain an open airway.
- Give oxygen at 10 to 15 L/min by nonrebreather mask. Some authorities do not recommend positive-pressure ventilation because of the risk of further injury. Consult with medical direction and check local protocol.
- Transport promptly.

Air Embolism

An **air embolism** may occur when divers ascend too rapidly or hold their breath during ascent. Onset is usually rapid and dramatic, often occurring within minutes of surfacing. As the diver ascends, air trapped in the lungs expands. If the air is not exhaled, the alveoli rupture, damaging adjacent blood vessels. Air bubbles are forced into the circulatory system through ruptured pulmonary veins. The air bubbles become lodged in small arteries, cutting off circulation. The size and location of the bubbles determines the patient's signs and symptoms. Signs and symptoms of an air embolism are listed in the following *You Should Know* box.

You Should Know

Assessment Findings and Symptoms of an Air Embolism

- Dizziness
- Confusion
- Shortness of breath
- Visual disturbances
- Weakness or paralysis in extremities
- Sudden unresponsiveness after surfacing (can occur before surfacing)
- Pink, frothy sputum
- Respiratory arrest
- Cardiac arrest

Emergency Care for an Air Embolism

Steps for caring for a patient with an air embolism:
- Establish and maintain an open airway.
- Give oxygen. If the patient's breathing is adequate, apply oxygen by nonrebreather mask at 10 to 15 L/min if not already done. If the patient's breathing is inadequate, provide positive-pressure ventilation with 100% oxygen and assess the adequacy of the ventilations delivered.
- If neck or spine injury is not suspected, the patient should be placed on the left side with the head and chest tilted downward. Some authorities recommend placing the patient in a supine position because of the difficulty of maintaining the position described previously. Consult medical direction or follow local protocol regarding patient positioning.
- Maintain body temperature. Remove wet clothing. Dry the patient, and cover with blankets, towels, or dry clothing.
- If possible, obtain all relevant information regarding the patient's dive and relay to the receiving facility.
- Consult medical direction about transport to a recompression facility.

Decompression Sickness

Decompression sickness (also called the *bends*) is a diving-related injury that results from dissolved nitrogen in the blood and tissues. As a diver descends, nitrogen and oxygen are dissolved in the blood. If the diver ascends rapidly, there is not enough time for the nitrogen to be reabsorbed from the blood. Nitrogen bubbles form in the bloodstream, interfering with tissue perfusion. The size and location of the bubbles determine the patient's signs and symptoms. Signs and symptoms of decompression sickness are listed in the following *You Should Know* box.

You Should Know

Assessment Findings and Symptoms of Decompression Sickness

- Fatigue
- Weakness
- Shortness of breath
- Skin rash
- Itching
- Joint soreness
- Dizziness
- Headache
- Paralysis
- Seizures
- Unresponsiveness

Emergency Care for Decompression Sickness

Steps for caring for a patient with decompression sickness:

- Establish and maintain an open airway.
- Give oxygen. If the patient's breathing is adequate, apply oxygen by nonrebreather mask at 10 to 15 L/min if not already done. If the patient's breathing is inadequate, provide positive-pressure ventilation with 100% oxygen and assess the adequacy of the ventilations delivered.
- If neck or spine injury is not suspected, the patient should be placed on the left side with the head and chest tilted downward. Some authorities recommend placing the patient in a supine position because of the difficulty of maintaining the position described previously. Consult medical direction or follow local protocol regarding patient positioning.
- Maintain body temperature. Remove wet clothing. Dry the patient, and cover with blankets, towels, or dry clothing.
- If possible, obtain all relevant information regarding the patient's dive and relay to the receiving facility.
- Consult medical direction about transport to a recompression facility.

Bites and Stings

Snakebites

Venomous snakes in the United States include pit vipers and coral snakes (see Table 40-2). Pit vipers—which include rattlesnakes, cottonmouths (water moccasins), and copperheads—are responsible for 98% of all venomous snakebites in the United States. In about 20% of snakebites, venom is not injected ("dry bites"). Most snakebites have the following attributes:

- Occur in men between the ages of 17 and 27 years
- Occur on an arm (67%) or leg (33%)
- Occur between April and October
- Are associated with alcohol intoxication

Pit vipers have the following features:
- Infrared pit (heat sensor) between eye and nostril (used to determine the position of its prey by the relative intensity of heat noted by its heat sensors; also used to guide the direction of the strike)
- Catlike elliptical pupils
- Triangular head
- Two long fangs (each fang having a least three pairs of alternate fangs behind it)

Rattlesnakes may strike without warning (Figure 40-8). They do not always "rattle" before striking. Most deaths from rattlesnake bites are a result of envenomation by the eastern and western diamondback rattlesnakes. A cottonmouth can strike while under water (Figure 40-9). The inside of its mouth is pale white, thus, the reason for its name. The copperhead is often found in wooded mountains, abandoned buildings, and damp, grassy areas. Its head is reddish brown to copper in color (Figure 40-10). A copperhead can climb low bushes and trees in search of food. The bites of copperheads are not as toxic as a rattlesnake or cottonmouth bite.

Signs and symptoms of most pit viper bites usually appear within 30 to 60 minutes. Common characteristics of pit viper bites include one or more fang marks, swelling, and burning pain in the area of the bite. Pain usually begins within 5 minutes and swelling within 10 minutes of a bite, but these can be delayed for several hours. Discoloration is common, appearing over the bite site within 3 to 6 hours (Figures 40-11 and 40-12). Signs and symptoms are listed in the next *You Should Know* box and depend on the following:

- Location of the bite
- Amount and properties of the venom injected
- Victim's general health
- Size of the victim

TABLE 40-2 Poisonous North American Snakes

Species	Common Name
Viperidae	
Large rattlesnakes	Eastern diamondback rattlesnake
	Western diamondback rattlesnake
	Mojave Desert sidewinder
	Timber or canebrake rattlesnake
	Rock rattlesnake
	Speckled rattlesnake
	Black-tailed rattlesnake
	Twin-spotted rattlesnake
	Mojave rattlesnake
	Tiger rattlesnake
	Western rattlesnake
	Prairie rattlesnake
	Grand Canyon rattlesnake
	Southern Pacific rattlesnake
	Great Basin rattlesnake
	Northern Pacific rattlesnake
	Ridge-nosed rattlesnake
Smaller rattlesnakes	Massasauga
	Pygmy
Water moccasins	Copperhead
	Eastern and western cottonmouths
Elapidae	
Coral snakes	Sonoran (Arizona) coral snake
	Eastern coral snake
	Texas coral snake

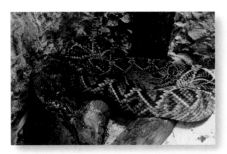

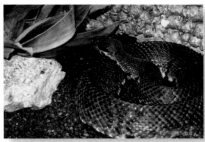

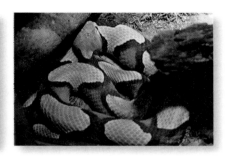

FIGURE 40-8 ▲ Rattlesnakes do not always rattle before striking. The eastern diamondback, the largest U.S. rattlesnake, is shown here.

FIGURE 40-9 ▲ A cottonmouth.

FIGURE 40-10 ▲ The head of a copperhead is reddish brown to copper in color, thus, the reason for its name.

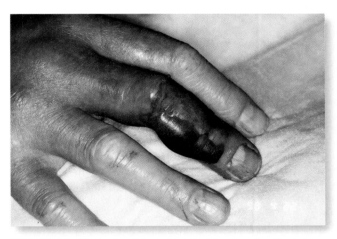

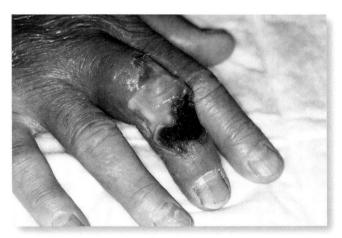

FIGURE 40-11 ▲ A rattlesnake bite 6 hours after the injury.

FIGURE 40-12 ▲ The same patient as in Figure 40-11, 7 weeks after the rattlesnake bite.

You Should Know

Assessment Findings and Symptoms of Pit Viper Bites

Local Signs and Symptoms
- Fang marks or semicircle of teeth marks
- Burning pain
- Red and swollen area around the fang or teeth marks
- Discoloration and blisters common

Systemic Signs and Symptoms
- Weakness
- Sweating
- Nausea and vomiting
- Shock

Coral snakes are shy and nocturnal and seldom bite. The Sonoran (Arizona) coral snake is about 15 to 20 inches long. The eastern coral snake and Texas coral snake average 20 to 45 inches in length. Coral snakes have the following features:

- Black, red, and yellow (or cream) bands that completely encircle the snake's body (Figure 40-13)
- Black head
- Short, small fangs
- Round, black eyes
- No facial pits

Whereas pit vipers tend to strike and release their venom, coral snakes tend to hang on and inject their venom with a series of chewing movements. The venom of a coral snake primarily affects the nervous system. Signs and symptoms may be delayed up to 12 hours after the bite. Because of the snake's small mouth, scratch marks or tiny puncture marks may be visible at the injection site with little or no pain at the site. There is usually minimal to moderate swelling. Early signs and symptoms include slurred speech, difficulty swallowing, and dilated pupils. If the bite is not treated, paralysis can occur within 8 to 24 hours. Death occurs because

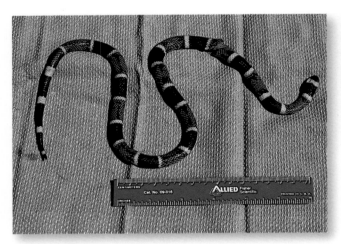

FIGURE 40-13 ▲ The bite of a coral snake is poisonous. A coral snake has black and red-on-yellow (or cream) bands that completely encircle the snake's body.

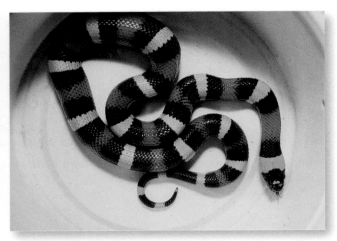

FIGURE 40-14 ▲ This is a picture of a Mexican milk snake. Its red-on-black rings indicate a nonvenomous snake. Unfortunately this "rule" applies only to snakes native to the United States.

of respiratory failure secondary to paralysis of the respiratory muscles. Signs and symptoms of coral snake bites are shown in the *You Should Know* box.

You Should Know

Assessment Findings and Symptoms of Coral Snake Bites

Early Signs and Symptoms
- Scratch marks or tiny puncture marks
- Little or no pain at the site
- Minimal to moderate swelling
- Slurred speech
- Muscle weakness
- Difficulty swallowing
- Dilated pupils

Late Signs and Symptoms (may be delayed for up to 12 hours)
- Nausea or vomiting
- Difficulty breathing
- Seizures
- Paralysis
- Respiratory failure

Remember This

Coral snakes can be differentiated from other striped snakes by remembering, "Red on yellow, kill a fellow; red on black, venom lack" or "Red on black is a friend of Jack's; red on yellow can kill a fellow." See Figure 40-14.

Emergency Care for Snakebites

To care for victims of snakebite:
- Ensure the safety of all rescuers. Make sure that the patient and rescuers are beyond the snake's striking distance, which is about the same as its body length. *It is not necessary to capture the snake for identification.* If the snake is dead, transport it in a closed container to the hospital with the patient (if required by your local protocol).
- Establish and maintain an open airway.
- Give oxygen. If the patient's breathing is adequate, apply oxygen by nonrebreather mask at 10 to 15 L/min if not already done. If the patient's breathing is inadequate, provide positive-pressure ventilation with 100% oxygen and assess the adequacy of the ventilations delivered.
- Keep the patient calm. Limit the patient's physical activity to minimize circulation of venom.
- Remove rings, watches, and tight clothing from the injured area before swelling begins.
- The pressure immobilization technique should be used for situations involving a coral snake bite. This technique involves immediately wrapping the entire bitten extremity with an elastic bandage or article of clothing as you would for a sprain (Figure 40-15). Wrapping the extremity slows lymph flow from the bite site, delaying toxicity. After the arm or leg is wrapped, the bandage should be snug, but loose enough to fit a finger under. After wrapping the extremity, follow by splinting with any available object. Position the splinted arm or leg slightly below the level of the patient's heart.

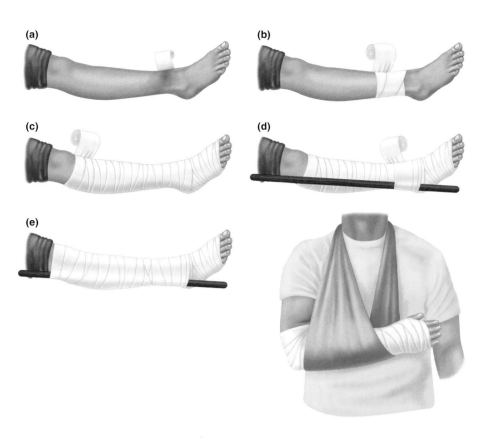

(a)

(b)

(c)

(d)

(e)

FIGURE 40-15 ◀ Pressure immobilization technique for coral snake bite, steps **(a)** through **(e)**.

—Pit viper bites cause more local tissue injury and pain than coral snake bites. Since the pressure immobilization technique causes an increase in pressure within the wrapped area, this technique is not currently recommended for pit viper bites. Position the affected arm or leg slightly below the level of the patient's heart.

- Frequently reassess the presence of distal pulses in the affected extremity. If swelling is present, mark the outer edge of the swelling and the time with a pen or marker (Figure 40-16). This allows other healthcare professionals to monitor the swelling progression.

- Some authorities recommend washing the wound, and some do not. Those who do not recommend washing say that not washing the wound allows for identification of venom from the wound. Be sure to check your local protocol.

Remember This

When caring for snakebites:

- Do not apply heat or cold to the bite site.
- Do not cut the wound.
- Do not attempt to suck out the venom.
- Do not apply a constricting band or tourniquet.

- If a tourniquet or constricting band was applied to the affected arm or leg before your arrival, and pulses are present in the extremity, leave it in place until the victim is evaluated at the hospital. If a tourniquet or constricting band was applied and pulses are absent in the extremity, consult medical direction for instructions.

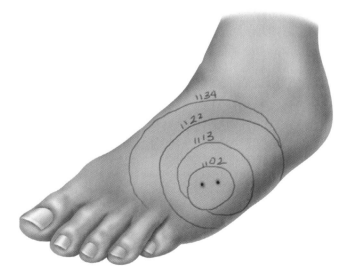

FIGURE 40-16 ▲ If swelling is present as a result of a bite or sting, mark the outer edge of the swelling and note the time with a pen or marker.

- Observe the patient closely for the development of signs and symptoms of an allergic reaction; treat as needed.
- Because the onset of signs and symptoms can be delayed, all snakebite victims should be transported for physician evaluation. En route to the hospital, reassess as often as indicated.
- Carefully document all patient care information on a PCR.

You Should Know

Typical signs and symptoms of an injection-related poisoning include the history of a bite (spider or snake) or sting (insect, scorpion, or marine animal), pain, redness, swelling, weakness, dizziness, chills, fever, nausea, vomiting, bite marks, or the presence of a stinger.

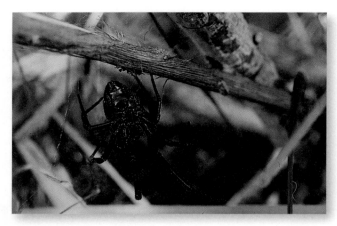

FIGURE 40-17 ▲ A black widow spider has a shiny, black body with a red hourglass figure on the abdomen.

Spider Bites

Arthropods are animals that have a segmented body, jointed legs, a digestive tract, and, in most cases, a hard outer shell. They have no backbone. Examples of arthropods include:

- Spiders
- Insects
- Crustaceans
- Scorpions
- Lice
- Fleas
- Ticks
- Bed bugs
- Horseshoe crabs
- Centipedes
- Millipedes
- Mites

A black widow spider has a shiny, black body with a red hourglass figure on the abdomen (Figure 40-17). The male is approximately half the size of the female and brown, and its venomous bite tends to be milder than envenomation by a female. The red or yellow-orange hourglass figure on the abdomen may be absent or hard to see in young female spiders. Black widow spiders spin irregular webs under rocks, logs, and vegetation and in woodpiles, barns, garages, trash piles, and outdoor structures.

The venom of a black widow spider primarily affects nerves and muscles. Signs and symptoms of a black widow spider bite are shown in the *You Should Know* box. See also Figure 40-18.

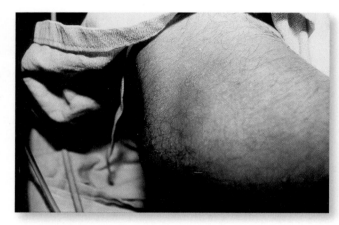

FIGURE 40-18 ▲ Black widow spider bite.

You Should Know

Assessment Findings and Symptoms of a Black Widow Spider Bite

- Vague history of sharp pinprick followed by dull, numbing pain
- Tiny red marks at the point of entry of the venom
- Localized swelling initially
- Difficulty breathing
- Severe pain beginning 15 to 60 minutes after bite and increasing for 12 to 48 hours
- Lower-extremity bite: localized pain followed by abdominal pain and rigidity
- Upper-extremity bite: pain and rigidity in chest, back, and shoulders

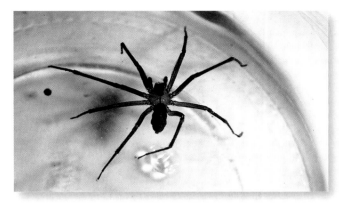

FIGURE 40-19 ▲ Brown recluse spider.

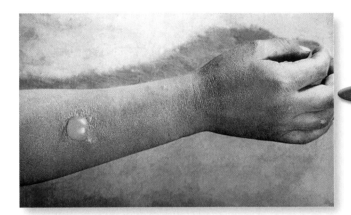

FIGURE 40-20 ▲ A brown recluse spider bite about 8 hours after the bite.

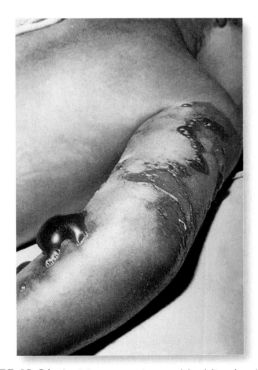

FIGURE 40-21 ▲ A brown recluse spider bite about 24 hours after the bite.

Brown recluse spiders are small and brown or tan in color and have a dark band shaped like a violin on the head and thorax (Figure 40-19). Many victims of a brown recluse spider bite do not recall being bitten. However, shortly after the bite, the victim experiences a mild stinging sensation. This soon changes to an aching feeling that is accompanied by itching. Swelling soon follows. Large blisters may form within 8 hours to 2 days after the bite (Figures 40-20, 40-21). The area often becomes larger over the next 24 to 72 hours. The tissue may die, resulting in a purple or black dry scab in the center of the area. Over a period of 2 to 5 weeks, the scab separates, leaving a deep, poorly healing ulcer (Figure 40-22). Signs and symptoms of a brown recluse spider bite are listed in the following *You Should Know* box.

You Should Know

Assessment Findings and Symptoms of a Brown Recluse Spider Bite

- Mild stinging sensation at the site of bite
- Local swelling
- Reddish ring appears around the bite within 2 to 8 hours after the bite
- Fever, chills
- Weakness
- Rash
- Nausea or vomiting
- Joint pain
- Redness and blister formation at site
- Open sore formation at site in 7 to 14 days

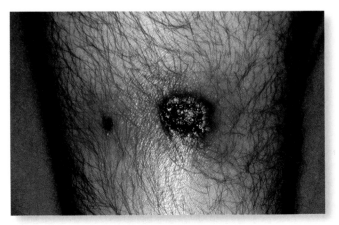

FIGURE 40-22 ▲ A deep, poorly healing sore from a brown recluse spider bite about 2 to 5 weeks after the bite.

Emergency Care for Spider Bites

Objective 8

To care for victims of spider bites:

- Establish and maintain an open airway.
- Give oxygen. If the patient's breathing is adequate, apply oxygen by nonrebreather mask at 10 to 15 L/min if not already done. If the patient's breathing is inadequate, provide positive-pressure ventilation with 100% oxygen and assess the adequacy of the ventilations delivered.
- Gently wash the area.
- If possible, remove jewelry from the injured area before swelling begins.
- If swelling is present, mark the outer edge of the swelling and note the time with a pen or marker.
- If the bite is on an arm or leg, position the limb slightly below the level of the patient's heart.
- Observe the patient closely for the development of signs and symptoms of an allergic reaction; treat as needed.
- Transport promptly. En route to the hospital, reassess as often as indicated.
- Carefully document all patient care information on a PCR.

Scorpion Stings

In North America, the sculptured or bark scorpion is the only species of scorpion that injects venom that is dangerous to humans (Figure 40-23). The scorpion injects venom by means of a stinger located on its tail. Scorpion venom is very rapidly absorbed. It can be lethal in very young children and in older adults who have chronic illnesses. Signs and symptoms of a scorpion sting are shown in the following *You Should Know* box. They usually peak in about 5 hours. Numbness, tingling, and pain can last up to 2 weeks after the sting.

Emergency Care for Scorpion Stings

Objective 8

To care for victims of scorpion stings:

- Establish and maintain an open airway. Excessive oral secretions may require frequent suctioning.
- Give oxygen. If the patient's breathing is adequate, apply oxygen by nonrebreather mask at 10 to 15 L/min if not already done. If the patient's breathing is inadequate, provide positive-pressure ventilation with 100% oxygen and assess the adequacy of the ventilations delivered.
- Gently wash the area.
- If possible, remove jewelry from the injured area before swelling begins.
- If swelling is present, mark the outer edge of the swelling and note the time with a pen or marker.

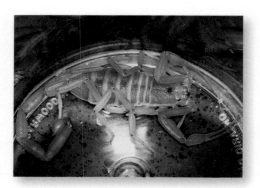

FIGURE 40-23 ▲ A bark scorpion is yellow to brown and usually less than 5 cm long.

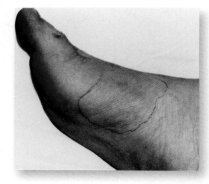

FIGURE 40-24 ▲ The bite of a bark scorpion typically produces pain, numbness or tingling, swelling, and redness at the sting site.

- If the bite is on an arm or leg, position the limb slightly below the level of the patient's heart.
- Watch the patient closely for the development of signs and symptoms of an allergic reaction; treat as needed.
- Transport promptly. En route to the hospital, reassess as often as indicated.
- Carefully document all patient care information on a PCR.

Hymenoptera Stings (Bees, Wasps, and Ants)

Stings from bees, hornets, wasps, and fire ants usually result in local pain, mild redness, swelling, and itching. When a honeybee stings, the barb on its stinger serves to anchor it in its victim (Figures 40-25 and 40-26). A honeybee stings only once and then dies when the sac detaches from its body. The sac then rhythmically continues to squeeze while anchored in its victim. The stingers of wasps, yellow jackets, hornets, and ants are not barbed. As a result, these insects are capable of repeatedly stinging their victim.

Africanized honeybees (also known as *Africanized bees* or *killer bees*) have been present in the United States since the early 1990s. To date, they are present in Florida, Texas, New Mexico, Arizona, Nevada, and California. It is anticipated that they may eventually be distributed as far north and east as North Carolina. Although their venom is not known to be more toxic than typical honeybees, they are much more aggressive. Africanized bees may be agitated by everyday occurrences, such as vibrations from passing vehicles, power equipment, and even people walking by on foot. Perceiving a threat to their nests, they have been known to attack in swarms of hundreds and chase their victims for long distances from the hive.

Signs and symptoms of hymenoptera stings vary. In many cases, the victim feels a stinging sensation at the site of the sting that is followed by local pain, redness, swelling, and itching. In sensitized individuals, anaphylaxis may occur within minutes in response to an insect sting and may cause death.

Emergency Care for Hymenoptera Stings

Objective 8

To care for victims of hymenoptera stings:
- Establish and maintain an open airway. Excessive oral secretions may require frequent suctioning.
- Give oxygen. If the patient's breathing is adequate, apply oxygen by nonrebreather mask at 10 to 15 L/min if not already done. If the patient's breathing is inadequate, provide positive-pressure ventilation with 100% oxygen and assess the adequacy of the ventilations delivered.
- If a stinger is present, remove it by scraping with a credit card or other flat, straight edge. Avoid using tweezers or forceps as these can squeeze venom from the venom sac into the wound.
- Gently wash the area.
- If possible, remove jewelry from the injured area before swelling begins. If swelling is present, mark the outer edge of the swelling and note the time with a pen or marker.
- Watch the patient closely for the development of signs and symptoms of an allergic reaction; treat as needed.
- Transport promptly. En route to the hospital, reassess as often as indicated.
- Carefully document all patient care information on a PCR.

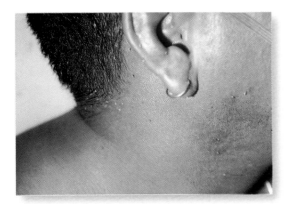

FIGURE 40-25 ▲ This patient's cheek, ear, and hairline show numerous stingers (barbs and venom sacs) from honeybees.

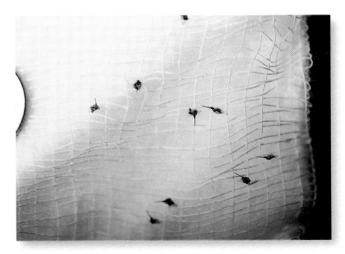

FIGURE 40-26 ▲ The barbs and attached venom sacs after removal from the patient.

Marine Life Stings

Marine life envenomations usually occur when the creature is stepped on, swum into, or intentionally or accidentally picked up. In the United States, most marine life envenomations are caused by the stingray. Stingrays are found in the waters off coastal areas. They usually lie partially hidden in the sand and strike with their tail when disturbed. A stingray's tail can produce one to four venomous stings. The injury produced by the stingray's tail is a puncture wound (Figure 40-27). The lower extremities are the most common sites of injury, followed by the upper extremities, abdomen, and chest. Although the puncture wound is small, the sting is followed by immediate, excruciating localized pain. The pain usually reaches maximum intensity in about 90 minutes and takes several hours to resolve. Other signs and symptoms of stingray envenomation are listed in the following *You Should Know* box. Although a stingray injury is rarely fatal, wounds to the chest and abdomen are associated with an increased risk of death.

You Should Know

Assessment Findings and Symptoms of Stingray Envenomation

- Immediate, excruciating pain
- Swelling
- Nausea, vomiting
- Diarrhea
- Sweating
- Muscle cramps
- Weakness
- Headache
- Dizziness
- Fainting
- Paralysis
- Seizures
- Respiratory depression
- Low blood pressure
- Irregular heart rhythm

Emergency Care for Venomous Marine Injuries

Objective 8

To care for victims of venomous marine injuries:
- Establish and maintain an open airway. Excessive oral secretions may require frequent suctioning.
- Give oxygen. If the patient's breathing is adequate, apply oxygen by nonrebreather mask at 10 to

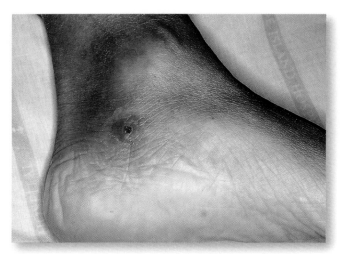

FIGURE 40-27 ▲ Puncture wound from a stingray.

15 L/min if not already done. If the patient's breathing is inadequate, provide positive-pressure ventilation with 100% oxygen and assess the adequacy of the ventilations delivered.
- In the case of a stingray injury, flush the wound *immediately* and then immerse the injured part in hot water to patient tolerance (109–113°F, or 43–45°C) for 30 to 90 minutes to inactivate the venom and provide pain control. Do *not* apply cool compresses or ice. Cover the wound with a sterile dressing.
- If possible, remove jewelry from the injured area before swelling begins. If swelling is present, mark the outer edge of the swelling and note the time with a pen or marker.
- Transport promptly. En route to the hospital, reassess as often as indicated.
- Carefully document all patient care information on a PCR.

Dog and Cat Bites

Dog and cat bites are common. In fact, someone in the United States seeks medical attention for a dog bite–related injury every 40 seconds. Dog bites are more common than cat bites. Because a dog's jaw can exert more than 450 pounds of pressure per square inch, dog bites usually result in crushing-type injuries, cuts, scrapes, and puncture wounds (Figure 40-28). Injuries may involve bones, vessels, tendons, muscles, and nerves.

In adults, most dog bites occur on the extremities. In children 4 years of age and younger, most dog bites occur on the face, neck, and scalp. Children are at greater risk of injury and death from dog bites than adults are. This may be because of a child's small size and inability to fend off an attack and because many

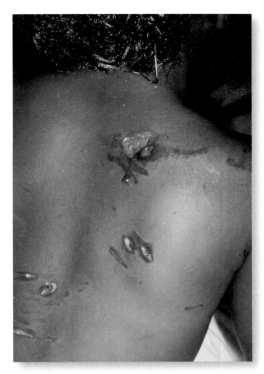

FIGURE 40-28 ▲ The dog bites occurred when an 8-year-old girl was attacked by several dogs.

Emergency Care for Dog and Cat Bites

Objective 8

To care for patients with dog and cat bites:

- When obtaining a SAMPLE history, find out the type of animal involved and time elapsed since the injury. Find out when the patient last had a tetanus shot. Also, find out if the animal's shots are current. Be sure to relay this information to the receiving facility staff. Knowing this information helps the staff decide on an appropriate treatment plan for the patient.

- Establish and maintain an open airway.

- Give oxygen. If the patient's breathing is adequate, apply oxygen by nonrebreather mask at 10 to 15 L/min if not already done. If the patient's breathing is inadequate, provide positive-pressure ventilation with 100% oxygen and assess the adequacy of the ventilations delivered.

- Control bleeding, if present, with direct pressure and cover the wound with a sterile dressing. If there is no bleeding, gently wash the wound and then cover it with a sterile dressing.

- If possible, remove jewelry from the injured area before swelling begins. If swelling is present, mark the outer edge of the swelling and note the time with a pen or marker.

- Because of the high risk of wound infection, the patient should be transported for physician evaluation. En route to the hospital, reassess as often as indicated.

- Carefully document all patient care information on a PCR.

Human Bites

Human bites in children usually occur while playing or fighting. In adults, bites are associated with alcohol use and clenched-fist injuries that occur during fights. Human bites can occur with child, elder, or spousal abuse. A human bite may or may not break the skin.

A **clenched-fist injury** (also called a *fight bite*) is the most serious human bite. In this type of injury, the fist of an individual strikes the teeth of another. The skin on the hand may or may not be broken. The underlying tissue and joints may be injured, even if the skin is not broken. If the skin is broken, tissue and joints may be injured, and the likelihood of infection is increased. When a bite is inflicted by an adult, infection is common because the human mouth contains many types of bacteria. Bites inflicted by children rarely become infected because they are usually superficial.

children do not know how to behave around a dog. Dog bite–related injuries are highest for children 5 to 9 years of age. Males are bitten more often than females.

In the United States, most dog bites occur at home. The victim is often the dog's owner or a friend of the owner. In most cases, the attack involves an unrestrained dog on the owner's property. Deaths involving neonates (less than 30 days of age) usually occur on the dog owner's property and involve one dog and a sleeping child. Unneutered male dogs are more likely to bite than are female and spayed or neutered dogs.

According to the CDC, data pertaining to deadly dog attacks that occurred during the period 1979–1998 revealed that at least 25 breeds of dogs were involved in the fatal attacks. Pit bull–type dogs and Rottweilers were involved in more than half the deaths for which the breed was known. However, since 1975, dogs belonging to more than 30 breeds have been responsible for fatal attacks on people, including Dachshunds, a Yorkshire terrier, and a Labrador retriever.

Cat bites occur more often to females. They usually happen in or near the victim's home. Because cats have narrower, sharper teeth than dogs, a cat bite is usually a puncture wound. Since infectious material is deposited deep in the tissue, most cat bites become infected.

Emergency Care for Human Bites

Objective 8

To care for patients with a human bite:

- Establish and maintain an open airway.
- Give oxygen. If the patient's breathing is adequate, apply oxygen by nonrebreather mask at 10 to 15 L/min if not already done. If the patient's breathing is inadequate, provide positive-pressure ventilation with 100% oxygen and assess the adequacy of the ventilations delivered.
- Control bleeding, if present, with direct pressure and cover it with a sterile dressing. If there is no bleeding, gently wash the wound and then cover it with a sterile dressing.
- If possible, remove jewelry from the injured area before swelling begins. If swelling is present, mark the outer edge of the swelling and note the time with a pen or marker.
- Because of the high risk of wound infection, the patient should be transported for physician evaluation. Reassess as often as indicated.
- Carefully document all patient care information on a PCR.

On the Scene Wrap-Up

The patient assures you that the snake is dead out on the back porch. You quickly remove the patient's rings and watch from the injured hand and then position the affected arm slightly below the level of her heart. You use a pen to mark the outer edge of the swelling in her finger with the time. While your partner performs a focused physical examination, you obtain the patient's vital signs. Her blood pressure is 140/90, pulse 92 (strong and regular), and respirations 16. Lung sounds are clear bilaterally. The patient's skin is pink, warm, and dry. The patient states that she has a history of depression for which she takes Prozac, she is allergic to lithium, and she last ate about 2 hours before your arrival. She denies any respiratory difficulty, chest discomfort, or other symptoms. Other than the swollen index finger, your partner did not find any other abnormal findings during his examination. Distal pulses in the affected extremity are strong and regular.

You apply oxygen by nonrebreather mask at 15 L/min and contact your poison control center. The PCC asks you to provide a description of the snake and then transport the patient to the closest appropriate facility for physician evaluation. En route to the hospital, you reassess the patient's vital signs and the injured finger. Although distal pulses in the affected extremity remain strong and regular, the patient's index finger is swelling rapidly, and she is becoming increasingly anxious. Once again, you mark the outer edge of the swelling in her finger with the time. After contacting medical direction with a brief report, you focus your attention on calmly reassuring the patient during the remainder of the short ride to the hospital. ■

Sum It Up

▶ The skin plays a very important role in temperature regulation. Cold and warmth sensors (receptors) in the skin detect changes in temperature. These receptors relay the information to the hypothalamus. The hypothalamus (located in the brain) functions as the body's thermostat. It coordinates the body's response to temperature.

▶ The body loses heat to the environment in five ways:

1. *Radiation:* Radiation is the transfer of heat from the surface of one object to the surface of another without contact between the two objects. When the temperature of the body is more than the temperature of the surroundings, the body will lose heat.

2. *Convection:* Convection is the transfer of heat by the movement of air current. Wind speed affects heat loss by convection (wind-chill factor).

3. *Conduction:* Conduction is the transfer of heat between objects that are in direct contact. Heat flows from warmer areas to cooler ones.

4. *Evaporation:* Evaporation is a loss of heat by vaporization of moisture on the body surface. The body will lose heat by evaporation if the skin temperature is higher than the temperature of the surroundings.

5. *Respiration:* The body loses heat through breathing. With normal breathing, the body continuously loses a relatively small amount of heat through the evaporation of moisture.

▶ Hypothermia is a core body temperature of less than 95°F (35°C). This condition results when the body loses more heat than it gains or produces.

- A rectal temperature gives the most accurate measure of core temperature. However, obtaining a rectal temperature in the field often raises issues of patient sensitivity and welfare, such as exposure to cold by removal of clothing.

- Your main concern in providing care should be to remove the patient from the environment. Use trained rescuers for this purpose when necessary. Perform a primary survey, keeping in mind that you need to move the patient to a warm location as quickly and as safely as possible. Remove any cold or wet clothing. Protect the patient from the environment. Assess the patient's mental status, airway, breathing, and circulation. Keep in mind that mental status decreases as the patient's body temperature drops.

- You may need to rewarm the patient. The two main types of rewarming are passive and active.

    —Passive rewarming is the warming of a patient with minimal or no use of heat sources other than the patient's own heat production. Passive rewarming methods include placing the patient in a warm environment, applying warm clothing and blankets, and preventing drafts.

    —Active rewarming should be used only if sustained warmth can be ensured. Active rewarming involves adding heat directly to the surface of the patient's body. Warm blankets, heat packs, and/or hot water bottles may be used, depending on how severe the hypothermia is.

▶ Local cold injury (also called frostbite) involves tissue damage to a specific area of the body. It occurs when a body part, such as the nose, ears, cheeks, chin, hands, or feet, is exposed to prolonged or intense cold. When the body is exposed to cold, blood is forced away from the extremities to the body's core. A local cold injury may be early (superficial frostbite) or late (deep frostbite).

▶ When the body gains or produces more heat than it loses, hyperthermia (a high core body temperature) results. The three main types of heat emergencies are heat cramps, heat exhaustion, and heat stroke.

1. Heat cramps usually affect people who sweat a lot during strenuous activity in a warm environment. Water and electrolytes are lost from the body during sweating. This loss leads to dehydration and causes painful muscle spasms.

2. Heat exhaustion is also a result of too much heat and dehydration. A patient with heat exhaustion usually sweats heavily. The body temperature is usually normal or slightly elevated. Severe heat exhaustion often requires IV fluids. Heat exhaustion may progress to heat stroke if it is not treated.

3. Heat stroke is the most severe form of heat-related illness. It occurs when the body can no longer regulate its temperature. Most patients have hot, flushed skin and do not sweat. Individuals who wear heavy uniforms and perform strenuous activity for long periods in a hot environment are at risk for heat stroke.

▶ The first step in the emergency care of a patient suffering from a heat-related illness is to remove him from the hot environment. Move the patient to a cool (air-conditioned) location, and follow treatment guidelines recommended for the patient's degree of heat-related illness.

▶ When providing emergency care for a drowning victim, ensure the safety of the rescue personnel. Suspect a possible spine injury if a diving accident is involved or unknown.

▶ Any breathless, pulseless patient who has been submerged in cold water should be resuscitated.

▶ Signs and symptoms of bites and stings typically include a history of a bite (spider, snake) or sting (insect, scorpion, marine animal), pain, redness, swelling, weakness, dizziness, chills, fever, nausea, and vomiting. Bite marks may be present.

▶ If a stinger is present, remove it by scraping the stinger out with the edge of a card. Avoid using tweezers or forceps as these can squeeze venom from the venom sac into the wound.

▶ When caring for a victim of a bite or sting, watch closely for development of signs and symptoms of an allergic reaction; treat as needed.

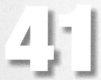
Multisystem Trauma

By the end of this chapter, you should be able to:

Knowledge Objectives ▶
1. Define multisystem trauma.
2. Discuss the principles of prehospital trauma care.
3. Define blast injury and the categories of blast injuries.
4. Discuss the types of injuries that may result from each category of blast injury.

Attitude Objective ▶
5. Explain the rationale for rapid transport of the multisystem trauma patient to the closest appropriate facility.

Skill Objectives ▶
6. Demonstrate the assessment and emergency care of the patient with multisystem trauma.
7. Demonstrate completing a prehospital care report for patients with multisystem trauma.

On the Scene

You and your partner are dispatched to a report of an explosion in the local quarry. You are familiar with the quarry operation and know that blasting is used as a means of loosening the gravel that is mined and processed. En route, you are notified that there are two patients that may have been injured by a mistimed explosion, and you notify your dispatch to send an additional unit. You are met at the front gate to the quarry by a security guard who then escorts you to the scene. You verify that the scene is safe before approaching the patients and are given assurances that there are no additional blasts scheduled to occur. ■

THINK ABOUT IT

As you read this chapter, think about the following questions:

- What predictable sequence of events occurs during a blast injury?
- What are the categories of blast injuries?
- What organs are injured by a blast wave?

Introduction

During your EMS career, it is likely that you will respond to many calls involving multisystem trauma. In previous chapters, we have discussed the effects of injuries on specific areas of the body. We have also discussed various mechanisms of injury, including blunt and penetrating trauma. In this chapter we discuss assessment and treatment of the trauma patient who has experienced injury to more than one body area. We also discuss blast injuries, which can result in multisystem trauma.

Multisystem Trauma

Objectives 1, 2

An individual who has been subjected to significant forces that affect more than one area of the body at the same time is a victim of **multisystem trauma** (also called *polytrauma*). Typically, a patient who has multisystem trauma has more than one major body system or organ involved. For example, a patient may experience head and spinal trauma, chest and abdominal trauma, or burns and extremity trauma. Multisystem trauma should be suspected in any patient subjected to significant external forces.

Stop and Think!

Sometimes an obvious injury does not have the most potential for harm. For example, a fracture of an upper extremity has less potential for harm than a severe blow to the head.

Patients who experience multisystem trauma are at a greater risk of developing shock and have a high frequency of serious injury and death. Definitive care for multisystem trauma may include surgery, which cannot be done in the field. Short scene times and rapid transport to the closest appropriate facility, such as a trauma center, are essential to help ensure a positive patient outcome. Hospital care for the multisystem trauma patient involves a team of physicians that may include specialists, such as neurosurgeons, thoracic surgeons, and orthopedic surgeons. You must know your local trauma system capabilities in advance to determine the appropriate destination for the multisystem trauma patient.

As with all emergency calls, conduct a scene size-up as you approach the scene to ensure your safety as well as that of your crew, bystanders, and the patient. It

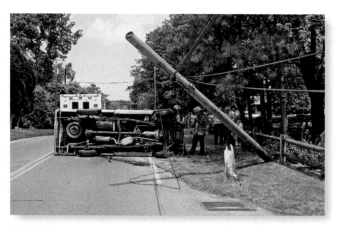

FIGURE 41-1 ▲ Remember: No matter the circumstances, scene safety must always be your primary concern.

is essential to ensure your own safety because if you are injured, you cannot provide needed care. Remember that a scene size-up is an ongoing process and continues throughout any emergency scene. Evaluate the mechanism of injury, such as a motorcycle crash, motor vehicle collision, vehicle rollover, fall, shooting, or stabbing (Figure 41-1). Be sure to assess the environment for hazards or potential hazards such as passing automobiles, hazardous materials, a hostile environment, an unsecured crime scene, or a suicidal patient who may become homicidal. Call for additional resources early. When performing a scene size-up and recognizing that the mechanism of injury probably resulted in multisystem trauma, call for advanced life support personnel right away. In some situations, air medical transport may be necessary.

After ensuring that the scene is safe, begin assessment and treatment of the patient using the principles of prehospital trauma care shown in the *Remember This* box on the next page. Put on appropriate PPE, and perform a primary survey to find and treat any life-threatening injuries. Rapid extrication should be considered for critically injured (unstable) patients involved in a motor vehicle crash. Backboards serve as entire body splints when an unstable patient is appropriately secured. If the mechanism of injury suggests a head or spinal injury, ask an assistant to provide manual stabilization of the patient's head and neck until the patient has been completely stabilized on a long backboard while you assess the patient's airway. An open airway and adequate ventilation and oxygenation are essential to a positive patient outcome following an injury. The airway must remain open and clear of fluids, loose teeth, and foreign objects while the patient is in your care. Frequent suctioning may be necessary to maintain an open airway. Remember to avoid the use of a nasal airway in the patient with facial trauma.

Adequate ventilation is critical. Administer high concentration oxygen to all trauma patients, and maintain the oxygen saturation at 95% or more. If the patient's breathing is adequate, apply oxygen by nonrebreather mask at 10 to 15 L/min. A patient who has an inadequate rate or depth of breathing should receive assisted ventilation. If an open chest wound is present, promptly cover the wound with an airtight dressing taped on three sides. Continuously monitor oxygenation with a pulse oximeter.

Adequate oxygenation cannot occur if a patient is bleeding profusely and losing red blood cells. Arterial bleeding must be stopped as quickly as possible with direct pressure. Consider the use of a tourniquet if severe extremity bleeding cannot be controlled with direct pressure. If signs of internal bleeding are present, place the patient in a supine position and keep her warm.

Determine the patient's level of consciousness using the AVPU scale, and repeat using the Glasgow Coma Scale as soon as possible. Obtain a Revised Trauma Score. Because rapid transport to definitive care is essential, a head-to-toe physical exam should be performed en route to the receiving facility. En route, notify the receiving facility of the patient's impending arrival. Doing so allows time for appropriate healthcare professionals and equipment to be mobilized and ready. Obtain a complete set of vitals. Monitor and reassess vital signs continuously.

Manage avulsed or amputated parts as other soft tissue injuries. Protruding organs should be covered with a large sterile dressing, moistened with sterile water or saline. Secure the dressing in place with a large bandage to retain moisture and prevent heat loss. Extremity injuries should be splinted as time permits.

EMS professionals are typically the only healthcare professionals at the scene with multisystem trauma patients. You are the eyes and ears of the physicians who will be assuming care of the patient. You will need to re-create the scene and relay information about the mechanism of injury, which is important to the trauma team. Changes in the patient's vital signs or assessment findings while en route are critical to report and document.

Blast Injuries

Objectives 3, 4

Blast injuries are one mechanism of injury that can produce multisystem trauma. Blast injuries result from pressure waves generated by an explosion. When the explosion occurs, there is an immediate rise in pressure over the atmospheric pressure. This creates a blast (overpressurization) wave. Blast waves cause disruption of major blood vessels, rupture of major organs, and lethal cardiac disturbances in a victim. Blast winds (forced, superheated airflow) and ground shock can collapse buildings and cause trauma.

Blast injuries are divided into five categories: primary, secondary, tertiary, quaternary, and quinary injuries.

1. A primary blast injury occurs from the blast wave impacting the body surface. Individuals closest to the explosion are at the greatest risk of injury. Organs filled with air (such as the middle ear, lungs, and gastrointestinal tract) are particularly susceptible to primary blast injury. The ear is the organ most sensitive to the effects of the primary blast. The patient may report hearing loss, ear pain, or dizziness. Bleeding from the external ear canal may be present. Injury to a lung is the cause of greatest serious injury and death following a primary blast. Suspect a lung injury in anyone complaining of dyspnea, cough, hemoptysis, or chest pain following a blast. An abdominal injury should be suspected in anyone who complains of abdominal pain, nausea, vomiting, hematemesis, rectal pain, or testicular pain or who has unexplained hypovolemia. Consider the possibility of a traumatic brain injury if the victim complains of a headache, fatigue, poor concentration, lethargy, depression, anxiety, or insomnia.

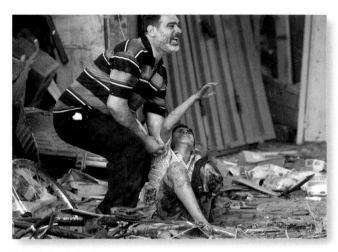

FIGURE 41-2 ▲ A secondary blast injury occurs from projectiles, such as bomb fragments, flying debris, and materials attached to the explosive device.

2. A secondary blast injury occurs from projectiles, such as bomb fragments, flying debris, and materials attached to the explosive device (such as screws, nails, bolts, ball bearings, or other small metal objects), resulting in blunt and/or penetrating trauma (Figure 41-2). The closer the person is to the site of the blast, the greater the injury. Most deaths in an explosion are due to secondary blast injuries. Injuries include open and closed brain injury, extremity fractures, bleeding, and shock. Lacerations of the heart and great vessels may also occur. A patient with a secondary blast injury also may have primary blast injuries.

3. A tertiary blast injury is caused by an individual flying through the air because of displacement from the blast wind. The victim may be thrown to the ground or through the air into other objects. Injuries include blunt and penetrating trauma, fractures, and traumatic amputations. A patient with a tertiary blast injury also may have primary and secondary blast injuries.

4. A quaternary blast injury is any other injury from the blast not categorized as a primary, secondary, or tertiary blast injury. Quaternary injuries include burns, crushing injuries, open and closed brain injuries, and respiratory illnesses related to dust, fumes, toxic smoke, and worsening of a chronic illness, such as asthma or chronic obstructive pulmonary disease.

5. A quinary blast injury results from absorption of toxic materials associated with the blast, which can include bacteria and radiation.

Scene safety is a concern at the site of any explosion and will likely require many additional resources.

If an incident management system has been established at the scene, report to the command post and follow the directions given (see Chapter 48). If you are assigned to perform patient care, it is important to remember that a blast victim should be reassessed often and transported as soon as possible to the closest appropriate facility.

Remember This

Do not develop tunnel vision and focus on a patient who is complaining of pain and screaming for your help while a patient who is hypoxic and bleeding internally is quiet and cannot call to you for help because of a decreased level of consciousness.

On the Scene Wrap-Up

Your partner and the security guard move to the patient on the left and find that he is unresponsive but breathing. He has a weak pulse. Your patient is conscious and breathing, and has a pulse with a blood pressure of 104/70. Upon the arrival of the second unit, each patient is rapidly secured to a long backboard and transported to the local trauma center. ■

Sum It Up

▶ An individual who has been subjected to significant forces that affect more than one area of the body at the same time is a victim of multisystem trauma (also called polytrauma). Multisystem trauma should be suspected in any patient subjected to significant external forces.

▶ Patients who experience multisystem trauma are at a greater risk of developing shock and have a high frequency of serious injury and death. Short scene times and rapid transport to the closest appropriate facility, such as a trauma center, are essential to help ensure a positive patient outcome. You must know your local trauma system capabilities in advance to determine the appropriate destination for the multisystem trauma patient.

▶ When performing a scene size-up and recognizing that the mechanism of injury probably resulted in multisystem trauma, call for advanced life support personnel right away. In some situations, air medical transport may be necessary. Assess and treat the patient using the principles of prehospital trauma care.

- Blast injuries are one mechanism of injury that can produce multisystem trauma. Blast injuries result from pressure waves generated by an explosion. Blast waves cause disruption of major blood vessels, rupture of major organs, and lethal cardiac disturbances in a victim. Blast winds and ground shock can collapse buildings and cause trauma.

- Blast injuries are divided into five categories: primary, secondary, tertiary, quaternary, and quinary injuries. A primary blast injury occurs from the blast wave impacting the body surface. A secondary blast injury occurs from projectiles, such as bomb fragments, flying debris, and materials attached to the explosive device. A tertiary blast injury is caused by an individual flying through the air because of displacement from the blast wind. A quaternary blast injury includes all other injuries from the blast not categorized as a primary, secondary, or tertiary blast injury. A quinary blast injury results from absorption of toxic materials associated with the blast, which can include bacteria and radiation. A blast victim should be reassessed often and transported as soon as possible to the closest appropriate facility.

Module 9

Special Patient Populations

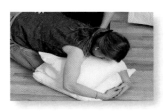

▶ CHAPTER 42

Obstetrics   734

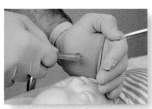

▶ CHAPTER 43

Neonatal Care   763

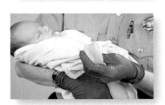

▶ CHAPTER 44

Pediatrics   769

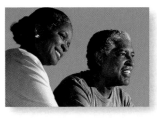

▶ CHAPTER 45

Older Adults   791

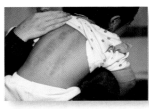

▶ CHAPTER 46

Patients with Special Challenges   803

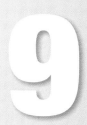

Obstetrics

By the end of this chapter, you should be able to:

Knowledge Objectives ▶

1. Identify the following structures: uterus, vagina, fetus, placenta, umbilical cord, amniotic sac, and perineum.

2. Discuss the physiologic changes that normally occur during each trimester of pregnancy.

3. Discuss assessment of the pregnant patent.

4. Discuss obtaining a SAMPLE history from a pregnant patient.

5. Define the following terms: labor, delivery, presenting part, crowning, and Braxton-Hicks contractions.

6. Describe each of the stages of labor.

7. Differentiate between true and false labor contractions.

8. State indications of an imminent delivery.

9. Establish the relationship between standard precautions and childbirth.

10. Identify and explain the use of the contents of an obstetrics kit.

11. State the steps in the predelivery preparation of the mother.

12. State the steps in assisting in a delivery.

13. Describe care of the baby as the head appears.

14. Describe how and when to cut the umbilical cord.

15. Discuss the steps in the delivery of the placenta.

16. List the steps in the emergency medical care of the mother after delivery.

17. Explain the purpose of uterine massage, and describe how to perform this procedure.

18. Discuss abuse and substance abuse as complications of pregnancy.

19. Discuss diabetes as a complication of pregnancy.

20. Discuss abortion and ectopic pregnancy as bleeding complications of pregnancy.

21. Discuss placenta previa, abruptio placentae, and uterine rupture as complications of pregnancy.

22. Discuss the possible causes, assessment findings, symptoms, and emergency care for hypertensive disorders of pregnancy.

23. Discuss the following conditions of high-risk pregnancy: precipitous labor, postterm pregnancy, meconium staining, multiple gestation, and intrauterine fetal death.

24. Discuss complications of labor, including premature rupture of membranes and preterm labor.

25. Discuss complications of delivery, including abnormal presentations and prolapsed cord.

26. Discuss postpartum complications, including hemorrhage and amniotic fluid embolism.

Attitude Objective ▶ 27. Explain the rationale for understanding the implications of treating two patients (mother and baby).

Skill Objectives ▶ 28. Demonstrate the steps to assist in a normal cephalic delivery.

connect™ (plus+)

29. Demonstrate necessary care of the baby as the head appears.
30. Demonstrate how and when to cut the umbilical cord.
31. Attend to the steps in the delivery of the placenta.
32. Demonstrate the postdelivery care of the mother.
33. Demonstrate emergency care procedures for excessive vaginal bleeding, breech presentation, and prolapsed cord.
34. Demonstrate completing a prehospital care report for patients with obstetrical emergencies.

On the Scene

It is late in your shift at a manufacturing plant when the emergency page goes out: "Emergency response teams, report to the warehouse." It's clear when you arrive, as one of your company's employees cross-trained in EMS, that this is no ordinary emergency. A woman is squatting on the floor and grunting and screaming, "The baby's coming; the baby's coming!"

You can tell by the dark stain on her jeans that her bag of waters has broken. The plant supervisor tells you that the paramedics are en route, but about 20 minutes away. You put on your goggles, mask, and gloves; ask your partner to get the obstetrics kit; and prepare to deliver a baby. ■

THINK ABOUT IT

As you read this chapter, think about the following questions:

- What questions should you ask the mother to determine if this will be a complicated delivery?
- What equipment will you need?
- How will you assist with the delivery of the baby?
- How will you assess the baby?

Introduction

You may be called to care for a woman in labor. Although childbirth is a natural process and most deliveries occur with no complications, these situations are often stressful for the patient, the patient's family, and emergency care professionals. Once the mother delivers, you will be responsible for her care and for that of her baby. To provide the best possible care for both patients, you must know how to assist during childbirth and how to provide care for both mother and baby after delivery. In this chapter we discuss care of the mother. Care of the newborn is discussed in the next chapter.

Anatomy and Physiology Review

Objective 1

The female reproductive organs are found in the pelvic cavity (Figure 42-1). The **ovaries** are paired, almond-shaped organs located on either side of the uterus. The ovaries perform two main functions: producing eggs and secreting hormones, such as estrogen and progesterone. Each ovary contains thousands of follicles. About once a month during a woman's reproductive years, a follicle matures to release an egg **(ovulation).** The fallopian tubes (also called *uterine tubes*) extend from each ovary to the uterus. They receive and transport the egg to the uterus after ovulation. Fertilization normally takes place in the upper third of the fallopian tube.

The **uterus** (womb) is a pear-shaped, hollow, muscular organ located in the pelvic cavity. It prepares for pregnancy each month of a woman's reproductive life. If pregnancy does not occur, the inner lining of the uterus sloughs off and is discarded. This discharge of blood and tissue from the uterus is called **menstruation.** It is often referred to as a woman's *period.* If pregnancy does occur, the developing embryo implants in the uterine wall and develops there. The uterus stretches throughout pregnancy to adjust to the increasing size of the fetus. During **labor,** the uterus contracts powerfully and rhythmically to expel the infant from the mother's body. After delivery of the infant, the uterus quickly clamps down to stop bleeding.

The **cervix** is the narrow opening at the distal end of the uterus. It connects the uterus to the vagina. During pregnancy, it contains a plug of mucus. The mucus plug seals the opening to the uterus, keeping bacteria from entering. When the cervix begins to widen during early labor, the mucus plug, sometimes mixed with blood **(bloody show),** is expelled from the vagina. The **vagina** is also called the *birth canal.* It is a muscular tube that serves as a passageway between the uterus and the outside of the body (see Figures 42-1 and 42-2). It receives the penis during intercourse. It also serves as the passageway for menstrual flow and the delivery of an infant. The

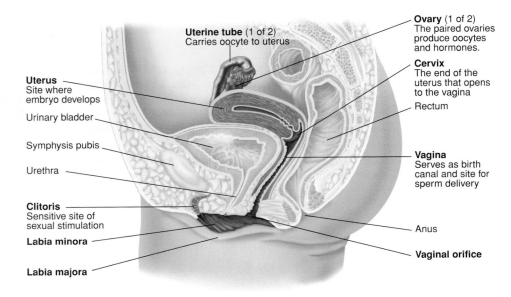

FIGURE 42-1 ▲ The structures of the female reproductive system.

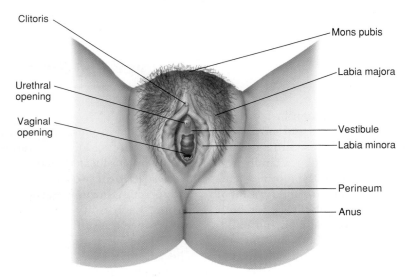

FIGURE 42-2 ▲ External female reproductive structures.

perineum is the area between the vaginal opening and anus. It is commonly torn during **childbirth.**

The Structures of Pregnancy

Pregnancy begins when an egg (ovum) joins with a sperm cell (fertilization). The **zygote** (fertilized egg) passes from the fallopian tube into the uterus. The zygote implants in the wall of the uterus (implantation) (Figure 42-3). During the first 3 weeks after fertilization, the developing structure is called a **blastocyst.** From the 3rd to the 8th week, the developing structure is called an **embryo.** From the 8th week until birth, the developing structure is called a **fetus.**

The **placenta** is a specialized organ through which the fetus exchanges nourishment and waste products during pregnancy (Figure 42-4). It is also called the *afterbirth* because it is expelled after the baby is born.

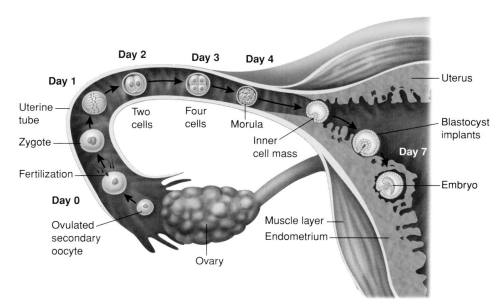

FIGURE 42-3 ▲ Pregnancy begins when an egg joins with a sperm cell (fertilization). The fertilized egg passes from the fallopian tube into the uterus. The egg implants in the wall of the uterus around day 7.

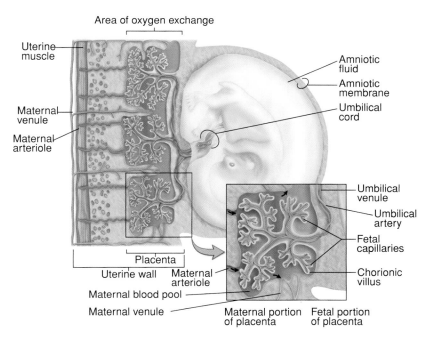

FIGURE 42-4 ▲ In the placenta, nutrients and oxygen pass from the maternal blood to the embryo while wastes pass in the opposite direction.

The placenta begins to develop about 2 weeks after fertilization occurs. It attaches to the mother at the inner wall of the uterus and to the fetus by the umbilical cord. The placenta is responsible for:

- The exchange of oxygen and carbon dioxide between the blood of the mother and fetus (the placenta serves the function of the lungs for the developing fetus)
- The removal of waste products from the fetus
- The transport of nutrients from the mother to the fetus
- The production of a special pregnancy hormone that maintains the pregnancy and stimulates changes in the mother's breasts, cervix, and vagina in preparation for delivery
- The maintenance of a barrier against harmful substances
- The transfer of heat from the mother to the fetus

The **umbilical cord** is the lifeline that connects the placenta to the fetus. It contains two arteries and one vein. The umbilical arteries carry blood low in oxygen from the fetus to the placenta. The umbilical vein carries oxygenated blood to the fetus. This is the opposite of normal circulation. The umbilical cord attaches to the umbilicus (navel) of the fetus.

The **amniotic sac** (also called the *bag of waters*) is a membranous bag that surrounds the fetus inside the uterus. It contains fluid (amniotic fluid) that helps protect the fetus from injury. The amniotic fluid provides an environment that is at a constant temperature. It also allows the fetus to move and functions much like a shock absorber. The amniotic sac contains about 1 L of fluid at term.

You Should Know

Although the placenta is an effective protective barrier between the mother and fetus, it does not protect the baby from everything. Some medications and toxic substances (such as alcohol) pass easily from the mother's blood to the baby. It is very important for a pregnant woman to consult with her doctor before taking any medicine or herbal supplement.

Normal Pregnancy

Objective 2

Pregnancy usually takes 40 weeks and is divided into three 90-day intervals called *trimesters*.

The First Trimester

During the first trimester (months 1–3, weeks 1–12), the mother stops menstruating (missed period). Her breasts become swollen and tender. She urinates more frequently and may sleep more than usual. Nausea and vomiting (usually called *morning sickness*) are usually at their worst during the second month. Despite its name, morning sickness can occur at *any* time of day. During the first weeks after conception, the mother's body begins to produce more blood to carry oxygen and nutrients to the fetus. Her heart rate increases by as much as 10 to 15 beats/min because her heart must work harder to pump this increased amount of blood. Normal weight gain during the first trimester is only about 2 pounds (about 907 grams, or 0.907 kilogram).

During the first 13 weeks of pregnancy, the fetus is developing rapidly. Cells differentiate into tissues and organs. The arms, legs, heart, lungs, and brain begin to form. By the end of the first trimester, the fetus is about 3 inches long and weighs about half an ounce.

The Second Trimester

In the second trimester (months 4–6, weeks 13–27), the signs of pregnancy become more obvious. The uterus expands to make room for the fetus and can be felt above the pubic bone. The mother's abdomen also enlarges, and her center of gravity often changes. As a result, she will often walk and move differently. The mother begins to feel the fetus move at about the 4th or 5th month. Her circulatory system continues to expand and this lowers her blood pressure. During the first 6 months of pregnancy, her systolic blood pressure may drop by 5–10 mm Hg. Her diastolic blood pressure may drop by 10–15 mm Hg. In her third trimester, her blood pressure gradually returns to its prepregnancy level. The mother may feel dizzy or faint when taking a hot bath or shower or in hot weather. This occurs because heat causes the capillaries in her skin to dilate, temporarily reducing the amount of blood returning to her heart and, thus, reducing the amount of blood pumped to her brain.

During the second trimester (between the 13th and 24th week of pregnancy), the fingers, toes, eyelashes, and eyebrows of the fetus are formed. About the 5th month, the heartbeat of the fetus can be heard with a stethoscope. By the end of this trimester, the heart, lungs, and kidneys are formed. The fetus weighs about 1.75 pounds (about 794 grams, or 0.794 kilogram) and is about 13 inches (about 33 centimeters) long.

The Third Trimester

During the third trimester (months 7–9, weeks 28–40), the mother may complain of a backache because of

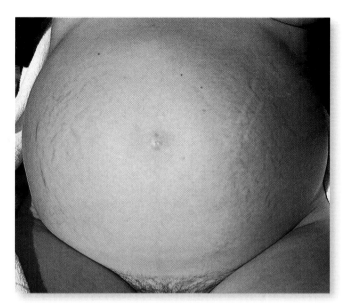

FIGURE 42-5 ▲ This woman is 39 weeks pregnant. Stretch marks are common in the third trimester of pregnancy.

muscle strain. Stretch marks may appear (Figure 42-5). The mother urinates frequently because the weight of the uterus presses on the bladder. She may be short of breath as her uterus expands beneath the diaphragm.

During the third trimester, the fetus continues to grow rapidly, gaining about one-half pound a week and reaching a length of about 20 inches. Fetal movement occurs often and is stronger.

The uterus and presenting part of the fetus descend into the pelvis in preparation for delivery about 10 days (average) before the onset of labor. This is called *lightening*. The **presenting part** is the part of the infant that comes out of the birth canal first. When lightening occurs, increased pressure from the presenting part leads to urinary frequency, backache and leg pain, increased vaginal discharge, and easier breathing. **Preterm labor** (also called *premature labor*) occurs when a woman has labor before her 37th week of pregnancy.

Assessing the Pregnant Patient

Objective 3

Assessment of the pregnant patient is the same as that of other patients. However, because of the normal changes in vital signs that occur with pregnancy, the patient's vital signs may not be as diagnostically helpful as they are in a nonpregnant patient. For example, the pregnant patient's heart rate is normally slightly faster than usual. Her breathing rate is also slightly faster and more shallow than normal. Her blood pressure is often slightly lower than normal until the third trimester. It is important to take vital signs in all patients. However, you will need to pay special attention to the pregnant patient's history and look for other signs that may suggest a potential problem. For example, a patient with a history of vaginal bleeding for 3 hours who has cold, pale, clammy skin is probably in shock—even if her vital signs appear normal.

Despite a significant amount of internal or external bleeding, young, healthy pregnant patients can maintain relatively normal vital signs for a significant time and then develop signs of shock very quickly. For example, the pregnant patient may lose as much as 1.5 L of blood before you will see a decrease in blood pressure. Blood flow to the fetus may be significantly decreased before signs of shock are obvious in the mother.

The signs of early shock are difficult to detect in the pregnant patient. As blood is lost because of trauma or complications of pregnancy, available blood is shunted away from the uterus and to the mother's heart and brain. This change compromises blood flow to the fetus. You can increase blood flow to the fetus by placing the pregnant patient on her left side.

Obtaining a SAMPLE History

Objective 4

Obtain a SAMPLE history to gather information about the pregnant patient's medical history.

- **Signs and symptoms.** The signs and symptoms that may indicate a possible complication of pregnancy include:
  —Seizures
  —Weakness
  —Dizziness
  —Faintness
  —Signs of shock
  —Lightheadedness
  —Vaginal bleeding
  —Altered mental status
  —Passage of clots or tissue
  —Swelling of the face and/or extremities
  —Abdominal cramping or pain (may be constant or may come and go)
- **Allergies.** Ask if the patient has any allergies to medications or other materials, such as latex.
- **Medications.** If childbirth is likely while the patient is in your care, the patient's answers to your questions about drugs are *very* important. For example, if the patient admits to heroin use within the last 4 hours, you must anticipate that her baby will need resuscitation when it is

delivered. Examples of questions to ask about medications include the following:

—Do you take any prescription medications? What is the medication for? When did you last take it? Are you taking prenatal vitamins? Have you taken fertility medications?

—Do you take any over-the-counter medications, such as aspirin, allergy medications, cough syrup, or vitamins? Do you take any herbs?

—Have you recently started taking any new medications? Have you recently stopped taking any medications?

—Do you use alcohol or any recreational drugs (crack, heroin, methadone, cocaine, marijuana)?

- **Past medical history.** Ask the patient the following questions:

—Have you been seeing a doctor during your pregnancy?

—Do you have a history of heart problems, respiratory problems, high blood pressure, diabetes, epilepsy, or any other ongoing medical conditions?

—Do you smoke? Do you use alcohol?

- **Last oral intake.** When did you last have something to eat or drink?

- **Events leading to the injury or illness.** Find out about the events leading to the present situation by asking specific questions. Ask the following questions:

—Do you know your due date?

—Is this your first pregnancy? Is there only one fetus, or are there multiples? If so, how many?

—How many children do you have? Were your children delivered vaginally? Did you have any problems with any of those pregnancies (such as premature labor, large babies, hemorrhage, cesarean section, miscarriage, abortion)?

—Have you had any prenatal care?

—Have you had any problems with this pregnancy?

—Do you know if the baby is head first or breech? (Has the baby turned?)

If the patient is having contractions, ask specific questions to determine if delivery is about to happen. These questions are covered later in this chapter. If the patient is complaining of abdominal pain, remember to use OPQRST to help identify the type and location of the patient's pain. Examples of additional questions to ask include the following:

- When was your last menstrual period? Was it a normal period? Are your periods usually regular? Did you have any bleeding after that period?

- Where is your pain exactly? (Ask the patient to point to the location.) What is it like (constant, comes and goes, dull, sharp, cramping)?

- Have you had any vaginal bleeding or discharge? What color was it?

Perform a physical exam. Conduct the examination professionally and efficiently, and talk with your patient throughout the procedure.

As an EMT, you must not visually inspect the vaginal area unless major bleeding is present or you anticipate that childbirth is about to occur. In these situations, it is best to have another healthcare professional or law enforcement officer present. If possible, include a female attendant or rescuer in your examination. Keep in mind that your patient may be anxious about having her clothing removed and having an examination performed by a stranger. Be certain to explain what you are about to do and why it must be done. Remember to properly drape or shield an unclothed patient to maintain her privacy.

Do not insert your fingers into the vagina when performing a vaginal examination. The vaginal area is touched *only* during delivery and (ideally) when another healthcare professional or law enforcement officer is present.

Remember This

When caring for a pregnant patient, keep in mind that the well-being of the fetus is entirely dependent on the well-being of the mother.

Normal Labor

Objectives 5, 6, 7

Labor is the process in which the uterus repeatedly contracts to push the fetus and placenta out of the mother's body. It begins with the first uterine muscle contraction and ends with delivery of the placenta. **Delivery** is the actual birth of the baby at the end of the second stage of labor.

Stages of Labor

In the days or weeks leading up to the birth, the presenting part of the fetus normally settles in the pelvis. The mother may feel she can "breathe easier," but she will also feel the need to urinate frequently. The cervix begins to open (dilate) and thin out (efface) in response to hormone changes. The mucus plug may be expelled (bloody show) after the beginning of cervical changes and increased pressure of the presenting part. The amniotic sac may rupture spontaneously producing leakage of clear or cloudy amniotic fluid. Some women experience a burst of energy 24 to 48 hours before the onset of labor.

The First Stage of Labor

The first stage of labor begins with the first uterine contraction. This stage ends with a complete thinning and opening (dilation) of the cervix (Figure 42-6). Contractions usually begin as regular cramplike pains that gradually increase in strength. They usually last from 30 to 60 seconds and occur every 5 to 15 minutes. In a woman who has not previously given birth, this stage of labor lasts about 8 to 16 hours. It lasts about 6 to 8 hours in a woman who has previously given birth. The bag of waters (amniotic sac) often bursts during this stage.

You Should Know

Timing Contractions

You will need to know how far apart your patient's contractions are and how long each contraction lasts. Place the fingertips of one hand high on the patient's uterus. When you feel the patient's abdomen become hard under your fingers, the contraction has started. When the hardness is gone, the contraction has ended.

Using a watch that shows seconds, begin timing at the start of a contraction. End timing at the beginning of the next contraction. This measure tells you how far apart the contractions are. You will need to time a series of contractions, such as four or five contractions in a row, to see if they are regular or irregular.

To determine how long a contraction is, begin timing at the start of a contraction and end timing when the same contraction is over.

The Second Stage of Labor

The second stage of labor begins with the opening of the cervix and ends with delivery of the infant. Contractions during this stage are stronger. They last from 45 to 60 seconds and occur every 2 to 3 minutes.

During this stage, the fetus begins its descent into the birth canal. Normally, the first part of the infant that descends into the birth canal is the head. This is called a **cephalic (head) delivery** or presentation. If the buttocks or feet descend first, it is called a **breech delivery** or presentation.

Toward the end of this stage of labor, the mother experiences an urge to bear down or push with each contraction. The presenting part will appear and disappear at the vaginal opening between contractions. As the presenting part presses on the rectum, the mother will feel an urge to move her bowels. Eventually, the presenting part will remain visible at the vaginal opening between contractions. This is called **crowning.** This stage of labor averages 1 to 2 hours in a woman who has not previously given birth. In a woman who has given birth in the past, this stage of labor lasts 20 to 30 minutes.

The Third Stage of Labor

The third stage of labor begins with delivery of the infant and ends with delivery of the placenta. This stage of labor normally lasts 5 minutes to an hour. During this stage of labor, the placenta peels away from the wall of the uterus, leaving tiny blood vessels exposed. The uterus normally contracts to close these blood

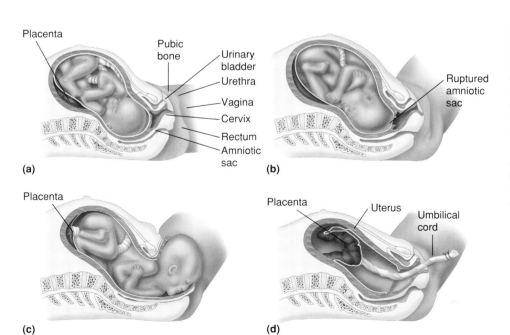

(a) Placenta — Pubic bone — Urinary bladder — Urethra — Vagina — Cervix — Rectum — Amniotic sac

(b) Ruptured amniotic sac

(c) Placenta

(d) Placenta — Uterus — Umbilical cord

FIGURE 42-6 ◀ The stages of labor. **(a)** The relationship of the fetus to the mother. **(b)** Stage 1 begins with the onset of uterine contractions and ends with complete thinning out and opening of the cervix. **(c)** Stage 2 begins with full dilation of the cervix and ends with delivery of the baby. **(d)** Stage 3 begins with delivery of the baby and ends with delivery of the placenta.

vessels. The placenta usually delivers within 15 to 30 minutes of the infant's birth.

Remember This

The Stages of Labor

Stage 1. Begins with the onset of uterine contractions; ends with complete thinning and opening of the cervix

Stage 2. Begins with opening of the cervix; ends with delivery of the infant

Stage 3. Begins with delivery of the infant; ends with delivery of the placenta

You Should Know

False Labor

Women often have false labor pains about 2 to 4 weeks before delivery. False labor pains are called *Braxton-Hicks contractions.* These contractions help prepare the woman's body for delivery by softening and thinning her cervix. It is sometimes difficult to tell the difference between false labor and true labor. Table 42-1 lists the differences between the contractions of true and false labor.

Normal Delivery

Predelivery Considerations

Generally, you should transport a woman in labor to the hospital unless delivery of the baby is expected within a few minutes. You must determine if there is time for the mother to reach the hospital or if preparations should be made for delivery at the scene.

To make this decision, ask the patient the following questions:

- Is this your first pregnancy?
  —Labor with a first pregnancy is usually longer than that of subsequent deliveries.
- When is your due date?
  —Knowing the due date will help you determine if the baby is premature or full term.
- Has your bag of waters broken? When? What was the color of the water?
  —Labor usually begins shortly after the bag of waters breaks. The greater the length of time since the bag of waters has broken until the start of labor, the greater the risk of fetal infection. The fetus usually needs to be delivered within 18 to 24 hours after the bag of waters has ruptured. Some women may not be sure if their water has broken or not. Some will tell you there was a "big gush of water." Others will describe a steady trickle of water when their water breaks. In others, the bag of waters may not break until well into the labor process. The fluid from the amniotic sac should be clear. If the mother tells you that the color of the water was brownish-yellow or green (like pea soup), expect that the baby's airway may need special care after delivery. The discolored water is the result of **meconium,** which is material that collects in the intestines of a fetus and forms the first stools of a newborn.
- Have you experienced any vaginal bleeding or discharge? How long ago? Did you have any pain with the bleeding?
  —A discharge of mucus mixed with blood (bloody show) is a sign that labor has begun. If excessive bleeding is present, the mother is at risk for shock, and the baby's well-being is also at risk.
- Are you having any contractions? When did they start? How close are they now?

TABLE 42-1 True and False Labor Contractions	
True Labor Contractions	**False Labor Contractions**
• Occur regularly	• Are usually weak, irregular
• Get closer together	• Do not get closer together over time
• Become stronger as time passes, each lasting about 30 to 60 seconds	• Do not get stronger
• Continue despite the patient's activity	• May stop or slow down when the patient walks, lies down, or changes position

—Contractions that are strong and regular, last 45 to 60 seconds, and are 1 to 2 minutes apart indicate the delivery will happen soon.

- Do you feel the need to push or bear down?
  —The urge to push, bear down, or have a bowel movement occurs as the baby moves down the birth canal and presses on the bladder and rectum. Delivery will occur soon.

- How many babies are there?
  —If delivery is to occur at the scene, this information will help you determine the additional resources you may need to call to help you. It will also help you determine the equipment you need to gather to assist with the delivery.

Additional questions that are important to ask include:
- Have you taken any medications or drugs?
  —Some medications or drugs taken by the mother will affect her baby. If the mother has taken narcotics within 4 hours of delivery, the baby's breathing may be very slow at delivery.

- Has your doctor told you if the baby is coming head first or feet first?
  —Normally, the baby's head presents first in the birth canal. If the mother has been told that her baby is coming feet first (breech delivery) and the baby will be delivered on the scene, call for additional help.

Signs of Imminent Delivery

Objective 8

Consider delivering at the scene in the following three circumstances:

1. Delivery can be expected in a few minutes.

   - A woman in late pregnancy feels the urge to push, bear down, or have a bowel movement.
   - Crowning is present. To determine if crowning is present, you will need to look at the patient's perineum (Figure 42-7). Take appropriate standard precautions, such as gloves, mask, gown, and eye protection. Position the patient on her back, and remove her undergarments. Place padding under the hips to elevate them. Ask the patient to bend her knees and spread her thighs apart. Look at the patient's perineum while the patient is having a contraction. If you see bulging or the baby's head beginning to emerge from the birth canal, prepare for immediate delivery. After visually examining the perineum, remember to cover the area with a towel or sheet to protect the patient's modesty.
   - Contractions are regular, last 45 to 60 seconds, and are 1 to 2 minutes apart.

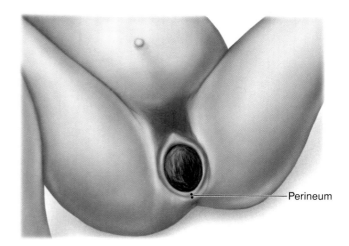

FIGURE 42-7 ▲ Delivery is imminent when crowning is present.

2. No suitable transportation is available.
3. The hospital cannot be reached because of heavy traffic, bad weather, a disaster, or a similar situation.

If there is time to transport the patient to the hospital, remove any undergarments that might obstruct delivery. Place the patient on her left side. Arrange for prompt transport.

Preparing for Delivery

Objective 9, 10, 11

If you make the decision that the delivery will occur on the scene, you will need to prepare yourself and the patient. As you make preparations for the delivery, keep in mind that the mother-to-be is doing all the work. Your job is to help the mother and newborn. For most women, the pain of labor and delivery is one of the things that worries them the most about having a baby. Although some women have labor with relatively little pain, most women experience considerable pain that worsens as labor progresses. The amount of pain experienced varies from woman to woman. Even if your patient has previously given birth, the pain she experiences may be different with each delivery.

Although you may be nervous about helping with the delivery, it is important that you appear calm and confident. Reassure the mother-to-be that you will not leave her alone and that you are there to help her. Because labor and delivery are very hard work, she may become tired and quite cranky. If she is irritable, do not take any comments she makes personally. Help her through her labor by offering words of support such as, "You're doing

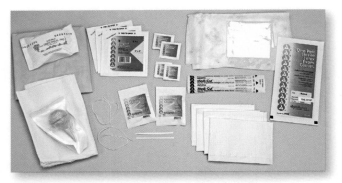

FIGURE 42-8 ▲ Contents of a ready-made childbirth delivery kit.

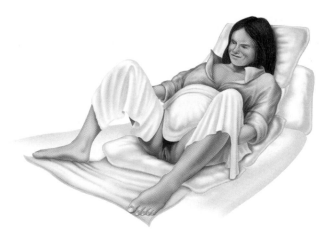

FIGURE 42-9 ▲ To prepare the mother for delivery, position her on her back with her head and back supported with pillows.

great!" Coach her to breathe slowly in through her nose and out through her mouth. As she tires, she may become less and less receptive to your instructions. You may need to repeat these instructions often. Repeat them as often as needed without appearing frustrated. As you prepare the patient and surroundings for the baby's arrival, remember to explain what you are doing to the patient and any family members that may be present.

Because blood and amniotic fluid are expected during childbirth and may splash, you must use standard precautions, including gloves, mask, eye protection, and a gown. You will need a ready-made childbirth delivery kit (also called an *obstetrics* or *OB kit*) (Figure 42-8). If a ready-made kit is not available, substitute the items in the list below with similar items that will serve the same purpose:

- Scissors or scalpel (used to cut the umbilical cord)
- Hemostats or cord clamps (used to clamp the umbilical cord) or umbilical tape (used to tie the umbilical cord instead of clamping it)
  —If these items are not available, you can use thick string, gauze, or clean shoelaces to tie off the umbilical cord.
- A bulb syringe (used to clear secretions from the infant's mouth and nose)
- Gauze sponges or towels (used to wipe and dry the infant)
- Sterile gloves (for protection from infection during delivery)
- A baby blanket (used to wrap and warm the infant)
- Sanitary pads (used to absorb vaginal drainage after delivery)
- A plastic bag or large plastic container with a lid (used to transport the placenta to the hospital)
- A sterile sheet, sterile towels, or barrier drapes (to create a sterile field around the vaginal opening).
  —If these items are not available, you can use clean towels or clothing, a plastic sheet, or newspapers to provide a clean surface.

Position your patient on her back with her head and back raised (Figure 42-9). Support her head and back with pillows. This position allows gravity to help when she pushes. Remove the patient's clothing and undergarments from the waist down. Gather clean, absorbent materials such as towels, sheets, blankets, clean clothing, or paper barriers. Place some of the absorbent material under the patient's buttocks. Make sure there is enough room in front of the mother's buttocks to provide a firm surface to support the infant after delivery. Have the patient bend her knees and spread her thighs apart. Place a towel, folded sheet, or paper barrier over the patient's abdomen and another across the inside of the patient's thighs. Remember not to touch the patient's vaginal area except during delivery and when another healthcare professional or law enforcement officer is present.

Your patient may tell you she feels as if she needs to have a bowel movement. Do not let her go to the bathroom. This sensation is caused by the presenting part of the infant in the birth canal pressing against the walls of the patient's rectum. If the mother urinates or has a bowel movement during a contraction, remove the material completely with a pad or washcloth and replace the soiled absorbent materials with clean ones. Do not hold the mother's legs together or attempt to delay or restrain delivery in any way.

Remember This

Positioning the mother flat on her back compresses major blood vessels. This can lower her blood pressure and decrease blood flow to the uterus. It is also very hard for the patient to push well when lying flat.

Delivery Procedure

Objectives 12, 13, 14, 15, 16, 17

When the mother's cervix is completely open, she will feel an almost involuntary need to push. Pushing is done only with uterine contractions. When a contraction begins, tell the mother to take in a deep breath and blow it out. Have her take another deep breath, hold it while you or a family member quickly counts to 10, and bear down as if she is straining to have a bowel movement. Your patient will be holding her breath for about 6 seconds (not 10), but a quick count of 10 will be helpful to her. At the end of the count of 10, tell her to breathe out and quickly take another breath in, holding for another count of 10. Most contractions are long enough to permit two or three attempts at this. Once the contraction is over, she should blow out any remaining air and begin restful breathing. Encourage her to relax completely to conserve energy and recover for the next contraction.

At this point, it is common for your patient to say, "I just can't do this anymore." Offer her words of encouragement. Praise her on the progress she is making. You may notice more bloody show during this stage of labor. This is normal as the patient's cervix stretches open and some of the tiny blood vessels break.

When the infant's head appears, cup your gloved fingers over the bony part of the infant's crowning head. Although many variations are possible, the infant's head most commonly presents facedown. Apply very gentle pressure to prevent the baby's head from coming out too fast and tearing the perineum (an explosive delivery) (Figure 42-10). Do not apply pressure to the infant's face or the soft spots on the baby's head (fontanelles). If the bag of waters does not break or has not broken, use your gloved fingertips in a pinching motion to break the bag. Push the sac away from the infant's head and mouth as they appear.

As the baby's head is being delivered, check the infant's neck to see if a loop of the umbilical cord is wrapped around the neck. If the cord is around the neck, gently loosen the cord and try to slip it over the baby's shoulder or head. If the umbilical cord is wrapped tightly around the baby's neck and cannot be loosened or is wrapped around the neck more than once, the cord must be removed. To do this, place two umbilical clamps or ties on the cord about 3 inches apart (Figure 42-11). Carefully cut the cord between the two clamps. Remove the cord from the baby's neck. Immediately notify dispatch and request an ALS intercept (if not already done).

As the baby's head is delivered and before delivery of the shoulders, support the head with one hand and clear the infant's airway (Figure 42-12). Squeeze the bulb of a bulb syringe, and then gently insert the narrow end of the syringe into the baby's mouth. Babies breathe mostly through their nose. Suction the baby's mouth first to be sure there is nothing for the baby to suck into its lungs if the baby should gasp when you suction its nose. To apply suction, slowly release pressure on the bulb. Remove the syringe from the baby's mouth, and squeeze it several times to remove secretions from the syringe. Suction the mouth two to three times. Do not apply suction for more than 3 to 5 seconds per attempt. Be careful not to touch the back of the baby's throat with the bulb syringe. This can cause severe slowing of the baby's heart rate. After clearing the mouth, suction each

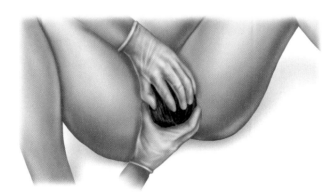

FIGURE 42-10 ▲ When the infant's head appears during crowning, cup your gloved fingers over the bony part of the infant's skull. Exert very gentle pressure to prevent the baby's head from coming out too fast and tearing the perineum.

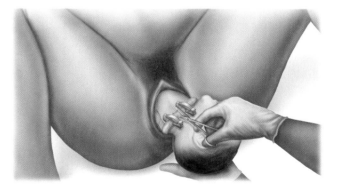

FIGURE 42-11 ▲ If the umbilical cord is wrapped tightly around the baby's neck and cannot be loosened, you will need to remove it. To do this, place two umbilical clamps or ties on the cord, approximately 3 inches apart. Carefully cut the cord between the two clamps. Remove the cord from the baby's neck.

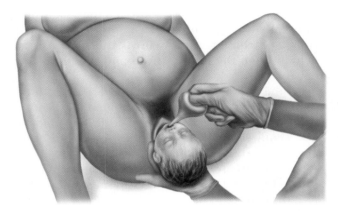

FIGURE 42-12 ▲ As the baby's head is delivered and before delivery of the shoulders, support the baby's head with one hand and clear the airway with a bulb syringe.

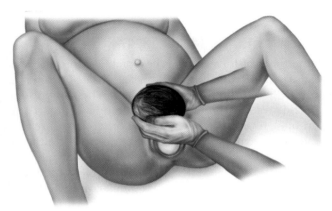

FIGURE 42-13 ▲ Gently guide the head upward to deliver the bottom shoulder.

nostril. If a bulb syringe is not available, use a clean gauze pad or a cloth to wipe secretions from the baby's mouth and nose.

Once the baby's head is delivered, its head will usually turn to line up with its shoulders. This allows the baby's shoulders and the rest of the body to pass through the birth canal. Gently guide the head downward to deliver the top shoulder. Gently guide the head upward to deliver the bottom shoulder (Figure 42-13). Do not pull on the baby's head! Tell the mother not to push during this time.

After the shoulders are delivered, the rest of the baby's body should slip right out. Because the baby will be covered with blood and amniotic fluid, the baby will be wet and very slippery. You may find it helpful to use a clean towel to hold onto the baby. As the baby's chest and abdomen are born, support the newborn with both hands. As the feet are born, grasp the feet. Try to remember to note the time the baby was born. Keep the baby at or around the same level as the mother's vaginal opening until it is time to clamp the umbilical cord (Figure 42-14).

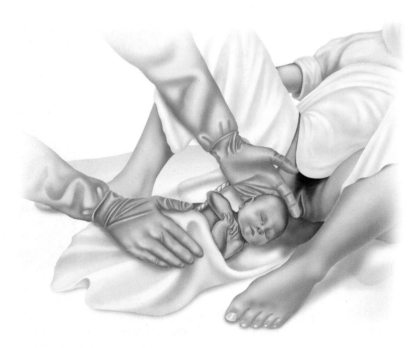

FIGURE 42-14 ▲ Keep the baby at or around the same level as the mother's vaginal opening until it is time to clamp the umbilical cord. Quickly dry the baby's body and head to remove blood and amniotic fluid.

Remember This

It is important to keep the baby at or around the same level as the mother's vaginal opening until the umbilical cord has been clamped. This is because blood can continue to flow between the newborn and the placenta. If you position the baby above the level of the mother's vaginal opening, such as on the mother's abdomen or chest, blood may drain from the baby's circulation into the placenta. This will decrease the amount of blood in the baby's circulation. If you place the baby below the level of the mother's vaginal opening, blood may drain from the placenta into the baby's circulation. The increased blood volume may overload the baby's circulatory system.

Once the baby is born, you will have two patients—the newborn and the mother. Care of the newborn is discussed in Chapter 43. After drying, suctioning, and stimulating the baby, clamp or tie the umbilical cord in two places between the mother and the baby. Place the first clamp or tie approximately 4 to 6 inches from the baby's belly. Place the second clamp or tie about 2 to 3 inches distal to the first clamp (further away from the baby). If the clamps or ties are firmly in place, cut the cord between the two clamps with scissors or a scalpel (Figure 42-15). After the cord is cut, periodically check the cut ends for bleeding. If the cut end of the cord attached to the

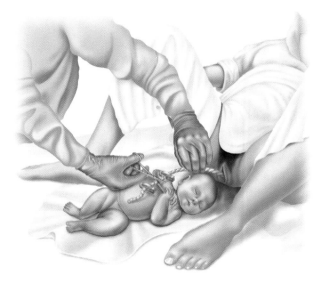

FIGURE 42-15 ▲ Clamping and cutting the umbilical cord.

baby is bleeding, clamp (or tie) the cord proximal to the existing clamps or ties. Do not remove the first clamp or tie.

Remember This

Because it will tear easily, always handle the umbilical cord very gently.

Gently wipe away any blood and amniotic fluid from the mother's perineum. Watch for delivery of the placenta. The placenta is usually delivered within 30 minutes of the baby. It is not necessary to wait for the placenta to deliver before transporting the mother and infant.

The signs that indicate separation of the placenta from the uterus include:

- A gush of blood
- Lengthening of the umbilical cord
- Contraction of the uterus
- An urge to push

Encourage the mother to push to help deliver the placenta. Wrap the placenta in a towel. If the cord was cut, place the placenta in an appropriate biohazard container. If you clamped but did not cut the cord, place the wrapped placenta next to the baby.

Stop and Think!

Never pull on the umbilical cord to speed delivery of the placenta. Pulling or tugging on the cord can cause the uterus to turn inside out. Uncontrollable bleeding and shock often follow.

After delivery of the placenta, check the mother's perineum for bleeding. When looking at the mother's vaginal area for bleeding, keep in mind that it is normal for the mother to lose up to 500 mL (0.5 L) of blood during childbirth. This amount of blood loss will not negatively affect most healthy young women. If the mother appears alarmed or concerned about the amount of blood, reassure her that this is normal. Place a sanitary pad over the vaginal opening, lower the mother's legs, and help her hold them together. While the patient is in your care, reassess her often to be sure she does not lose too much blood.

During delivery, the perineum can tear as it stretches to make room for the baby's head and body. Although most tears are usually small, they can be very large and extend from the vaginal opening to the rectum. Use a sanitary pad or pads to apply pressure to any bleeding tears. Be careful not to touch the side of the pad that will be placed against the patient. Do not place anything inside the vagina.

If vaginal bleeding appears excessive, give oxygen to the mother at 10 to 15 L/min by nonrebreather mask. Stimulate the uterus to contract by performing uterine massage.

Steps for performing uterine massage:
- With your fingers fully extended, place one hand horizontally across the abdomen, just above the pubic bone (Figure 42-16). This positioning is very important. It helps prevent downward shifting of the uterus during the massage.
- Cup your other hand around the uterus. Massage the area using a kneading motion.
- Continue massaging until the uterus feels firm, like a ball. Bleeding should lessen as the uterus becomes firm.
- Recheck the patient every 5 minutes.

If bleeding continues to appear excessive, reassess your massage technique and treat the patient for shock. If you have not already done so, record the time of delivery.

Making a Difference

Uterine massage is painful. Try to understand your patient's complaints of pain if you must perform this procedure. Explain what you are doing and why.

Encourage the mother to breastfeed her baby. Breastfeeding stimulates the uterus to contract.

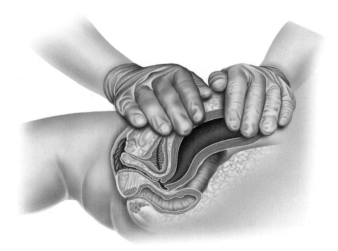

FIGURE 42-16 ▲ Performing uterine massage.

When the uterus contracts, blood vessels within the walls of the uterus constrict, decreasing bleeding. Make sure that the placenta is transported to the hospital with the mother. Hospital staff will look closely at the placenta for completeness. If pieces of the placenta stay in the uterus, the mother will have ongoing bleeding.

En route to the hospital, continue to provide supportive care.

Supportive care includes the following:
- Taking the patient's vital signs often
- Helping the mother to a position of comfort
- Keeping her warm
- Rechecking the amount of vaginal bleeding; replacing sanitary pads with clean ones as needed
- Replacing any soiled sheets and blankets with fresh ones
- Carefully placing all soiled items in an appropriate biohazard container

Pregnancy and Birth—Cultural Considerations

It is important to recognize that an individual's culture affects beliefs and practices regarding pregnancy and childbirth. For example:

- A common belief among African Americans, Anglo-Americans, Asians, and Hispanics is that the arms of the mother-to-be should not be raised above her head during pregnancy. Doing so is thought to increase the risk of the umbilical cord being wrapped around the baby's neck.
- Some African-American women believe that unsatisfied food cravings during pregnancy can cause birthmarks on the baby.
- Some Hispanic women believe that unsatisfied food cravings can cause injuries or birth defects in the baby. A pregnant Cuban woman is kept away from loud noises and from looking at people with deformities.
- Some Ethiopian women believe that sorcery is the cause of miscarriages, premature delivery, and birth defects.
- Some Chinese Americans believe that certain activities will affect the baby during pregnancy. For example, going to the zoo will cause the baby to look like one of the animals.
- A Filipino woman is encouraged to eat slippery foods, such as eggs, as the time of delivery nears

to enable the baby to "slip" through the birth canal.

- Many Samoans consider pregnancy an illness. A pregnant Samoan cannot be left unattended, especially at night, and is not permitted to eat specific foods, such as octopus. Garlands, jewelry, and garments fastened under the arms are also forbidden during pregnancy.

It is not important that you agree or disagree with the patient's belief and/or custom. What is important is that you respect the patient's beliefs and provide compassionate care to her and her family throughout labor and delivery. Although it is not possible to elaborate on every culture and its corresponding beliefs pertaining to pregnancy and children, some examples are provided in the following paragraphs.

Anglo-Americans

Anglo-American women typically seek prenatal care. The patient's husband is generally the preferred labor partner and a hospital setting is usually preferred for delivery.

Native Americans

Although labor practices vary by tribe, the patient's mother or other female relative is traditionally in attendance during a normal delivery. During childbirth, the patient generally endures labor without complaining or getting upset. After delivery, the mother and newborn are encouraged to rest and remain indoors for 20 days postpartum, or until the umbilical cord falls off, depending upon custom. In some tribes, the remnants of the umbilical cord are saved because it is believed to have spiritual value.

African Americans

More than half of African-American women seek prenatal care after their first trimester of pregnancy. Traditionally, only females are in attendance during labor and delivery, although this practice varies. Many African-American women express pain openly and publicly. After delivery, the patient's family members care for the new mother and baby. Generally, the new mother will avoid bathing and washing her hair until postpartum bleeding has stopped.

Arab Americans

Some Arab-American women delay seeking prenatal care because pregnancy is viewed as a normal condition and not an illness requiring medical attention. Because labor pains are greatly feared, the Arab-American woman is likely to be anxious, moan and groan loudly, and may scream during labor and delivery. The patient's mother, sister, or mother-in-law is expected to be present and provide emotional support during delivery. The patient's husband is not expected to be present. After delivery, the new mother and newborn are encouraged to rest while the patient's mother or sister looks after the household.

Hispanic Americans

A Hispanic-American woman may not seek prenatal care because pregnancy is viewed as a normal condition. She is likely to engage in practices that she believes will protect her infant during pregnancy such as sleeping on her back, keeping active to ensure a small infant and easy delivery, and satisfying food cravings. The patient's husband is not expected to be present during labor and delivery, and he generally does not see his wife and newborn after delivery until both have been cleaned and dressed. The patient's mother, sister, or both may be present during delivery. Most Hispanic-American women prefer to give birth in a hospital. Many laboring Hispanic-American women will yell "ay ay ay " during labor and delivery. This phrase is actually a form of controlled breathing that is used to relieve pain. After delivery, a coin or marble that has been cleaned with alcohol is sometimes strapped to the newborn's navel to make it attractive. Traditionally, the new mother rests, stays warm, and avoids bathing and exercise for 40 days after delivery.

Chinese Americans

Most Chinese women are stoic during labor and delivery, but some will express pain by moaning. The patient's female family members are usually present during the birth process. The patient's husband and other male family members do not normally play an active role. The patient is usually fully clothed during labor and prefers to deliver her baby while in a sitting position. For the first 30 days after delivery, the Chinese believe that the mother's pores remain open, allowing the entry of cold air into the body. As a result, a new mother traditionally avoids exposure to cold, going outdoors, taking a shower or bath, and exercising during this time. The new parents may avoid naming the baby for up to 30 days. A celebratory feast takes place 1 month after the baby's birth.

Japanese Americans

Japanese-American women readily seek prenatal care early in pregnancy. The patient's husband is usually present during labor and delivery. The patient's mother may also be present. After delivery, the new mother is expected to rest for several weeks. A Japanese-American woman views hygiene as extremely important and will bathe and shower frequently. Because the new mother is expected to rest for several weeks, the patient's mother typically remains with the family to assist with childcare and household responsibilities.

Complications of Pregnancy

Abuse

Objective 18

According to the Centers for Disease Control and Prevention, intimate partner violence (IPV) affects as many as 324,000 pregnant women each year. IPV during pregnancy can lead to blunt trauma to the abdomen, hemorrhage (including placental separation), uterine rupture, miscarriage or stillbirth, preterm labor, premature rupture of the membranes, premature delivery, or even death of the mother.

Increased violence may be brought on by jealousy where the woman's partner feels that he is receiving less attention or by stress associated with the pregnancy, such as anxiety over finances. Because the pregnant patient must leave her home for routine checkups, an abuser may feel threatened because signs of his abuse may become known during an examination. According to the National Coalition Against Domestic Violence, 50% to 70% of women abused before pregnancy are abused during pregnancy. Battery may also begin or intensify during pregnancy. A man who was previously emotionally or verbally abusive may turn to physical abuse. Physical violence may include slapping, scratching, pushing, choking, shaking, burning, biting, or hitting; using a knife, gun, or other weapon; or persuading others to commit such acts. Once a woman is pregnant, a man who was a physical abuser may change his target area from general body blows to the face and abdomen. Psychological and emotional abuse often occurs along with physical or sexual violence.

According to the National Coalition Against Domestic Violence, 77% of pregnant homicide victims are killed during their first trimester of pregnancy. In 2005, the CDC reported that homicide is a leading cause of traumatic death among new and expectant mothers, with higher risks for women who are younger than 20 or African American. In this study, married women were found at less risk than unmarried women; women who received no prenatal care had a higher risk of homicide than those who did; and most maternal homicides were caused by gunfire, with stabbings ranked second.

Be aware of warning signs of possible intimate partner violence and mandatory reporting laws in your state. An abused woman may appear frightened, depressed, or anxious. Although most pregnant patients have many questions, an abused woman may simply obey your instructions and not appear to question your authority. The abused woman may be distrustful of healthcare professionals. Behaviors of the abuser in the presence of healthcare professionals may include the following:

- Being overly caring
- Answering questions for the patient
- Being hostile or demanding
- Never leaving the patient's side
- Monitoring the woman's responses to questions

When obtaining a medical history from the patient, ask questions of her apart from her partner and away from family or friends. If signs of abuse are evident, do *not* ask questions such as, "Why don't you just leave?" or "What did you do to make him so angry?" Although signs of violence may be evident, the abused woman may not truthfully answer questions about her injuries. According to the CDC, reasons for not disclosing violence to healthcare professionals include the following:

- Embarrassment and shame
- Fear of retaliation by the violent partner
- Lack of trust in others
- Economic dependence
- Desire to keep the family together
- Lack of awareness of alternatives
- Lack of a support system

Accurate documentation of your findings is essential. Whenever possible, use the patient's own words to describe the violence. Be certain to privately relay your findings when transferring patient care.

Substance Abuse

Objective 18

Smoking during pregnancy increases the risk of stillbirth or premature birth. The amount of alcohol that a woman can "safely" drink during pregnancy is not known. Because the fetal brain is developing during the first trimester of pregnancy, mothers who drink during this period have children with the most severe problems. Drinking alcohol during pregnancy can cause physical and behavioral problems in children, including fetal alcohol syndrome. There is no cure for fetal alcohol syndrome. Conditions associated with fetal alcohol syndrome are shown in the following *You Should Know* box. Alcohol-related neurodevelopmental disorder is a condition that refers to children who display only the behavioral and emotional problems of fetal alcohol syndrome without any signs of developmental delay or physical growth deficiencies.

Conditions Associated with Fetal Alcohol Syndrome

- Low birth weight
- Epilepsy
- Mental retardation
- Birth defects
- Abnormal facial features
- Growth problems
- Problems with the central nervous system
- Trouble remembering and/or learning
- Vision or hearing problems
- Behavior problems

Studies suggest that the use of methamphetamine (also known as speed, ice, crank, and crystal meth) during pregnancy increases the risk of pregnancy complications, such as premature delivery and placental problems. Infants exposed to amphetamines before birth appear to undergo withdrawal-like symptoms after delivery.

Risks associated with heroin use during pregnancy include poor fetal growth, premature rupture of the membranes, premature delivery, and stillbirth. Infants exposed to heroin before birth go through withdrawal after delivery.

Cocaine use during early pregnancy may increase the risk of miscarriage. Use later in pregnancy may prompt preterm labor or cause placental problems, including placental abruption. According to the March of Dimes, cocaine use during pregnancy may cause an unborn baby to have a stroke, which can result in irreversible brain damage.

Diabetes Mellitus

Objective 19

Diabetes that exists before pregnancy is called *pregestational diabetes*. Diabetes that develops during pregnancy is called *gestational diabetes*. The pregnant diabetic patient must closely monitor and control her blood sugar levels throughout her pregnancy. The patient is at increased risk of hypoglycemia, particularly during the first trimester, and hyperglycemia, particularly in the second trimester.

Diabetes in a pregnant patient can cause a variety of problems, particularly if the diabetes is not controlled. The pregnant diabetic patient is at increased risk of premature birth and giving birth to an infant with serious birth defects, such as heart defects; defects of the brain or spinal cord; and kidney, gastrointesti-

nal, and limb defects. The pregnant diabetic patient with poorly controlled diabetes is at increased risk for having a very large baby (10 pounds or more). It is sometimes difficult to deliver the infant vaginally. These infants are at increased risk for injuries during birth and intrauterine death.

Bleeding

Abortion

Objective 20

An **abortion** is the termination of pregnancy before the fetus is able to live on its own outside the uterus. A **therapeutic abortion** is an abortion performed for medical reasons, often because the pregnancy poses a threat to the mother's health. An **elective abortion** is an abortion performed at the request of the mother. A **threatened abortion** is a condition in which the cervix remains closed and the fetus remains in the uterus but the patient experiences vaginal spotting or bleeding and/or pain resembling menstrual cramps. A threatened abortion may progress to a complete abortion or may subside, and the pregnancy may continue to term. An **incomplete abortion** is one in which part of the products of conception have been passed but some remain in the uterus. The cervix is open, and the patient will bleed heavily until all the products of conception are removed from the uterus.

A **spontaneous abortion,** also called a *miscarriage*, is the loss of a fetus because of natural causes. It usually occurs before the 20th week of pregnancy, most often between the 7th and 12th weeks of pregnancy. In most miscarriages, the fetus dies because of a genetic abnormality that is usually unrelated to the mother. During a miscarriage, the mother often experiences lower back pain or cramping abdominal pain, vaginal bleeding, and the passage of tissue or clotlike material from the vagina.

Not all abdominal pain or bleeding that occurs during the early weeks of pregnancy indicates a miscarriage. Bleeding sometimes occurs during early pregnancy, and the mother is still able to carry the fetus to full term. The patient needs to be evaluated by a physician. Prepare the patient for transport to the hospital. Give oxygen, and treat the patient for shock if signs are present. Place bulky dressings against the vaginal opening if necessary, but do not pack any material into the vagina. Keep the patient warm. Collect any tissue or clotlike material passed from the vagina. A clean plastic container with a lid or a biohazard bag can be used for this purpose. Be sure the collected tissue accompanies the patient to the hospital. Reassess as often as indicated during transport. Record all patient care information, including the patient's medical history and all emergency care given, on a prehospital care report.

Any situation that involves bleeding during pregnancy is likely to be a very emotional one. Most women associate bleeding during pregnancy with "losing the baby." This may or may not be the case and cannot be accurately determined in the field. Grief is a very normal reaction to the threatened loss of the pregnancy. While treating your patient's physical condition, remember to provide her with emotional support as well.

Ectopic Pregnancy

Objective 20

An **ectopic pregnancy** occurs when a fertilized egg implants outside the uterus. An ectopic pregnancy is a medical emergency. The most common site where this occurs is inside a fallopian tube (Figure 42-17). Less commonly, the egg implants in the abdomen, cervix, or an ovary. In an ectopic pregnancy, the growing fetus bursts through the tissue in which it has implanted. Severe bleeding can occur as a result of ruptured blood vessels.

If rupture occurs, the patient often complains of a sudden onset of severe pain on one side of the lower abdomen. Vaginal bleeding may or may not be present. The patient may feel faint or may actually faint. In addition, the patient may complain of severe pain in the back of the shoulder (referred pain). Severe internal bleeding may be present. The patient may have signs of shock, such as decreasing blood pressure, an increased heart rate, and cool, clammy skin.

Prepare for immediate transport to the closest appropriate facility. Keep on-scene time to a minimum. Consider an ALS intercept while en route to the receiv-ing facility. Do not delay transport for ALS arrival. Give oxygen by nonrebreather mask at 10 to 15 L/min. Treat the patient for shock if signs are present. Keep the patient warm. Remember to provide emotional support for the patient and family. Reassess as often as indicated during transport. Record all patient care information, including the patient's medical history and all emergency care given, on a PCR.

Although there are many causes of abdominal pain, you must consider lower abdominal pain in any woman of childbearing age to be caused by an ectopic pregnancy until proved otherwise. An ectopic pregnancy is a medical emergency.

Placental and Uterine Problems

Objective 21

Vaginal bleeding may occur late in pregnancy (third trimester). It may or may not be accompanied by pain. The possible causes of vaginal bleeding in late pregnancy include placenta previa, abruptio placentae, and a ruptured uterus. All third-trimester bleeding should be considered a life-threatening emergency.

Placenta previa occurs when the placenta attaches low in the wall of the uterus instead of at its top or sides. In this position, the placenta may cover all or part of the cervix (the entrance to the birth canal) (Figure 42-18). If the placenta covers the cervical opening during the early months of pregnancy, it will often shift position as the uterus grows, moving away from the cervical opening. If the placenta does not shift

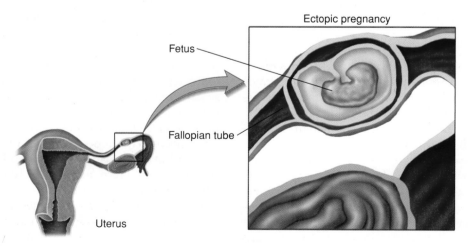

Ectopic pregnancy

Fetus

Fallopian tube

Uterus

FIGURE 42-17 ▲ An ectopic pregnancy occurs when a fertilized egg implants outside the uterus, usually inside a fallopian tube.

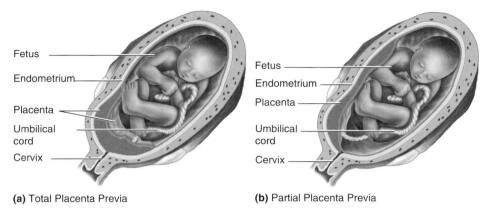

(a) Total Placenta Previa   **(b)** Partial Placenta Previa

FIGURE 42-18 ▲ Placenta previa. **(a)** In a total placenta previa, the placenta completely covers the cervix. **(b)** In a partial placenta previa, the placenta partially covers the cervix.

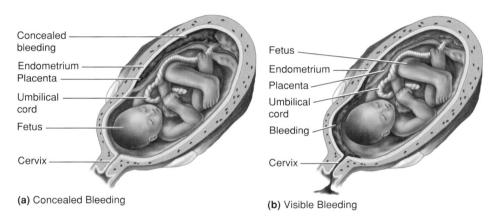

(a) Concealed Bleeding   **(b)** Visible Bleeding

FIGURE 42-19 ▲ **(a)** Abruptio placentae occurs when a normally implanted placenta separates prematurely from the wall of the uterus (endometrium) during the last trimester of pregnancy. Vaginal bleeding may be absent (concealed or hidden bleeding). **(b)** Vaginal bleeding that is visible may be moderate to severe and is usually dark red.

from the cervical opening as the pregnancy progresses, then placenta previa exists.

Normally, the cervix begins to widen and thin out in the latter part of pregnancy. This is the body's way of preparing for labor. If the mother has placenta previa, vaginal bleeding can occur because placental blood vessels that are implanted in the wall of the uterus are torn as the cervix widens and thins out. The more the placenta covers the cervical opening, the greater the risk of bleeding.

Abruptio placentae (also called *placental abruption*) occurs when a normally implanted placenta separates prematurely from the wall of the uterus (endometrium) during the last trimester of pregnancy. The placenta may separate partially or completely (Figure 42-19). Partial separation may allow time for treatment of the mother and fetus. Placental separation of 50% or more often results in death of the fetus.

A **ruptured uterus** is the actual tearing of the uterus. Uterine rupture can occur when the patient has been in strong labor for a long period, which is the most common cause. It can also occur when the patient has sustained abdominal trauma, such as a severe fall or a sudden stop in a motor vehicle collision.

A patient with any of these conditions needs ALS care and immediate transport to the closest appropriate facility. Keep on-scene time to a minimum. Consider an ALS intercept while en route to the receiving facility. Do not delay transport for ALS arrival. Because exposure to blood is possible, be sure to wear appropriate PPE. Give oxygen by nonrebreather mask at 10 to 15 L/min if breathing is adequate, and treat the patient for shock. Keep the patient warm. Reassess at least every 5 minutes during transport. Record all patient care information, including the patient's medical history and all emergency care given, on a PCR.

TABLE 42-2 Causes of Vaginal Bleeding in Late Pregnancy

Assessment Findings and Symptoms	Placenta Previa	Abruptio Placentae	Uterine Rupture
Vaginal bleeding	• Sudden • Bright red	• May be absent (concealed or hidden) • If seen, may be moderate to severe; usually dark red	• May or may not be present
Abdominal pain	• Usually none (**P**ainless = **P**revia)	• Sudden, severe	• Sudden, severe • Abdomen tender, rigid • Possible contractions
Signs of shock	• Likely	• Yes; may seem out of proportion to amount of blood loss seen	• Yes
Fetal movement	• Usually present	• Decreased • May be absent	• Absent

Table 42-2 lists some of the causes, signs, and symptoms of vaginal bleeding in late pregnancy.

You Should Know

Placenta previa is the cause of most cases of severe bleeding in the third trimester of pregnancy.

Hypertensive Disorders

Objective 22

Preeclampsia (also called *pregnancy-induced hypertension* or *toxemia of pregnancy*) is a disorder of pregnancy that causes blood vessels to spasm and constrict. Blood vessel constriction results in high blood pressure. It also decreases blood flow to the mother's organs, including the placenta. Less blood flow to the placenta usually means that less oxygenated blood and nutrients reach the baby. In some cases, the baby may need to be delivered early to protect the health of the mother. Preeclampsia also causes changes in the blood vessels. These changes cause the mother's capillaries to leak fluid into her tissues. This results in swelling.

The cause of preeclampsia is not known. It usually occurs during the third trimester of pregnancy. It tends to occur in young mothers during their first pregnancy and in women whose mothers or sisters had preeclampsia. The risk of preeclampsia is also higher in women older than age 40, in women carrying multiple babies, and in teenage mothers. Women who had high blood pressure, diabetes, or kidney disease before they became pregnant are also at risk of preeclampsia. The signs and symptoms of preeclampsia are listed in the following *You Should Know* box.

You Should Know

Assessment Findings and Symptoms of Preeclampsia

- Weight gain of more than 2 pounds per week or a sudden weight gain over 1 to 2 days
- Visual disturbances, such as blurred vision or the appearance of flashing lights or spots before the eyes
- Swelling of the face and hands that is present on arising from sleep
- Headaches
- Right upper quadrant abdominal pain
- Increased blood pressure (more than 140/90 mm Hg)

Remember This

If your patient complains of blurred vision, nausea, a severe headache, and pain in the right upper quadrant of the abdomen, she may be very close to having a seizure (eclampsia). Because eclampsia is associated with a significant risk of death for the mother and fetus, move quickly and begin patient transport as soon as possible.

If untreated, preeclampsia may progress to eclampsia. **Eclampsia** is the seizure phase of preeclampsia. Eclampsia is associated with a significant risk of death for the mother and fetus. Keep on-scene time to a minimum. Consider an ALS intercept while en route to the receiving facility. Do not delay transport for ALS arrival. Be sure to have suction readily available. Give oxygen. If the patient's breathing is adequate, apply oxygen by nonrebreather mask at 10 to 15 L/min if not already done. If the patient's breathing is inadequate, provide positive-pressure ventilation with 100% oxygen. Assess the adequacy of the ventilations delivered. Keep the patient calm, and position her on her left side. Avoid any stimulus that might trigger a seizure, such as bright lights and siren noise. Dim the lights. Prepare for immediate transport *without* lights or siren. If the patient has a seizure, protect her from injury and watch her breathing closely. When the seizure is over, make sure her airway is clear and give oxygen. Reassess as often as indicated during transport. Record all patient care information, including the patient's medical history and all emergency care given, on a PCR.

Remember This

It is not necessary for you to determine the cause of vaginal bleeding. However, it is important for you to recognize that the patient needs immediate transport and evaluation by a physician.

Emergency Care of Pregnancy Complications

To care for patients with pregnancy complications:

- When you arrive at the scene, first consider your personal safety. During the scene size-up, evaluate the mechanism of injury or the nature of the illness before approaching the patient.
- An **obstetric emergency** (an emergency related to pregnancy or childbirth) is frequently associated with bleeding. Take standard precautions and put on appropriate PPE. In addition to gloves, you should wear eye protection, a mask, and a gown. During childbirth, blood and amniotic fluid are expected and may splash.
- Determine the total number of patients. If a delivery is about to happen, there is going to be another patient. Call for additional help to the scene to assist you in caring for both mother and baby.
- After the scene size-up, form a general impression by pausing a short distance from the patient to determine if the patient appears "sick" or "not sick." Determine the urgency of further assessment and care.
- Perform a primary survey to identify, and treat any life-threatening conditions.
  —As with all patients, your initial attention must be directed at making sure the patient has an open airway, adequate breathing, and adequate circulation.
  —Manually stabilize the patient's head and neck if trauma is suspected.
  —Control obvious external bleeding, if present. If vaginal bleeding is present, apply external vaginal pads as necessary. As the pad becomes blood-soaked, replace it with a new one. Place all blood-soaked clothing and pads in a biohazard container, and send them to the hospital with the patient. These items will be used to estimate the patient's blood loss.
  —Treat for shock if indicated. Give oxygen by nonrebreather mask at 10 to 15 L/min if breathing is adequate, and maintain the patient's body temperature. Use blankets or sheets as needed to prevent heat loss.
- Perform a physical exam. Take the patient's vital signs, and gather the patient's medical history.
- If a spinal injury is suspected, the patient should be immobilized on a long backboard. If the patient is 20 weeks pregnant or more remember to tilt the board slightly to the left by placing a rolled towel, small pillow, blanket, or other padding under the right side of the board to reduce the risk of supine hypotension.
- Prepare for transport to the nearest appropriate hospital. Consider an ALS intercept. Provide emotional support to the patient on the scene and during transport.
- Reassess as often as indicated during transport. Record all patient care information, including the patient's medical history and all emergency care given, on a PCR.

Stop and Think!

If the mother suffers a cardiac arrest, continue cardiopulmonary resuscitation (CPR). If the mother is more than 24 weeks pregnant, the fetus may be able to be delivered and survive. Inform dispatch so that it can notify the hospital that will receive the patient. On arrival at the hospital, special equipment will be used to assess the condition of the fetus.

High-Risk Pregnancy

Precipitous Labor and Birth

Objective 23

Precipitous labor lasts less than 3 hours from the start of contractions to delivery. It occurs more often in a woman who has previously delivered a child than in a woman who is pregnant for the first time. Precipitous labor can result in lacerations of the cervix and vagina, hemorrhage, and fetal distress.

Postterm Pregnancy

Objective 23

Postterm pregnancy, also called prolonged pregnancy, is a pregnancy that lasts longer than 42 weeks. At about 42 weeks gestation, the volume of amniotic fluid decreases significantly, reducing the cushioning effect of the fluid. As the volume of fluid decreases, the risk that the fetus will entrap or compress its own cord increases. If the umbilical cord is entrapped or compressed, blood flow to and from the fetus is compromised and can result in intrauterine fetal death.

As the duration of the pregnancy increases, the likelihood of meconium passage into the amniotic fluid increases. *Meconium* is material that forms the first stools of a newborn. Meconium expelled into the already diminished volume of amniotic fluid causes the meconium to thicken. If inhaled, meconium may cause severe inflammation of the lungs and pneumonia in the newborn.

Postterm pregnancy also poses risks to the mother, including prolonged labor and injury to the perineum. The patient may complain of extreme fatigue and marked physical discomfort. She may be irritable, impatient, and frustrated because her pregnancy has not been completed "like everyone else's." It is important to anticipate the patient's feelings, respect them, and provide emotional support when providing emergency care. Prepare the patient for transport, positioning her on her left side. Reassess as often as indicated.

Meconium Staining

Meconium staining refers to the passage of fetal stool into the amniotic fluid. The color of meconium varies from yellow to light green or dark green (pea soup). The thicker and darker the fluid, the higher the risk of complications if it is aspirated. Meconium staining is seen most often in postterm deliveries. Emergency care includes suctioning of the baby's mouth and nose as soon as the head is delivered.

Multiple Gestation

Objective 23

A woman pregnant with twins (or more babies) usually goes into labor during or before her 37th week of pregnancy. The more babies a woman is expecting, the higher the risk of having a premature delivery. If the mother has been seeing a doctor regularly, she will usually know if she is expecting more than one baby.

Multiple-birth babies are usually smaller than a single full-term baby and, if they are delivered vaginally, are easier for the mother to push out. However, complications can occur during delivery. For example, the umbilical cord may be compressed by one or more of the babies because the uterus is crowded. The first baby is often born head first, but the babies after that may be in a breech, transverse (sideways), or head-first position when they enter the birth canal.

Anticipate multiple births if:

- The mother's abdomen appears unusually large.
- The mother's abdomen remains large after the first infant is delivered.
- Contractions continue after delivery of the first infant.

If multiple births are expected, request an early response of ALS personnel to the scene or consider an ALS intercept while en route to the receiving facility. Be prepared to resuscitate more than one baby. The steps for delivery and care of multiple babies, the mother, and placentas are the same as with the delivery of one baby. Each baby may be attached to its own placenta, or they may all be attached to the same one. Clamp or tie the umbilical cord after the first baby is born, and then cut the cord.

If the second baby is not delivered within 10 minutes of the first, the mother and baby must be transported immediately for delivery of the second baby. If delivery of the second baby begins during transport, the ambulance should be pulled over to the side of the road for the delivery. Remember to note the time of birth for each baby. Clearly label and identify each baby. Reassess as often as indicated during transport. Record all patient care information, including the patient's medical history and all emergency care given, on a PCR.

Intrauterine Fetal Death

Possible causes of intrauterine fetal death include abruptio placentae, infection, genetic abnormalities, preeclampsia, fetal skull fracture, and umbilical cord complications. Complications of maternal medical illnesses such as hypertension, diabetes, obesity, chronic renal disease, and thyroid disorders can also result in fetal death. Sometimes the cause is unknown.

The majority of fetal deaths occur before 32 weeks gestation. Fetal deaths that occur before the onset of labor are called *antepartum deaths*. Those that occur during labor are called *intrapartum stillbirths*. Most fetal deaths occur before the onset of labor.

Complications of Labor

Premature Rupture of the Membranes

Objective 24

Premature rupture of the membranes (PROM) is rupture of the amniotic sac before the onset of labor. Once the protective barrier of the amniotic sac is broken, there is an increased risk of fetal infection because of the proximity to bacteria present in the mother's vagina and rectal area. There is also an increased risk of umbilical cord compression because of the decreased volume of amniotic fluid. The beginning of the onset of labor varies after the membranes rupture. The patient should be transported for physician evaluation and positioned on her left side if 20 weeks pregnant or more.

Preterm Labor

Objective 24

Preterm labor is labor that begins before the 37th week of gestation. Possible causes include uterine or cervical anatomical abnormalities, premature rupture of the membranes, multiple gestation, and intrauterine infection. Complications of preterm labor may result in premature delivery of the infant. A patient who has preterm labor requires transport for evaluation and treatment by an appropriate health care provider.

A **premature infant** is one born before the 37th week of gestation or weighing less than 5.5 pounds (2.5 kilograms). Premature babies (also called *preemies*) can have many health challenges, including serious infections and respiratory distress caused by underdeveloped lungs. They are also at increased risk for hypothermia and low blood sugar. Premature infants often require resuscitation.

Care for a premature infant as you would for a term baby with the following special considerations:

- Keep the infant warm to reduce heat loss. Wrap the infant in dry, warm blankets. Cover the infant's body and head (keep the face exposed). Wrap the bundled baby in aluminum foil or a survival blanket to help preserve body heat. The foil should not be directly against the baby's skin but only around the bundled blankets.

- Keep the mouth and nose clear of fluid and mucus.

- Give blow-by oxygen. Do not allow cold oxygen to blow directly into the infant's face. Provide positive-pressure ventilation if breathing is inadequate.

- Prevent bleeding from the umbilical cord. Frequently check the cut end of the umbilical cord to be sure it is not bleeding. Premature infants cannot tolerate the loss of even small amounts of blood.

- Protect the infant from contamination. Premature infants are highly susceptible to infection. Do not breathe directly into the infant's face.

- Reassess as often as indicated during transport. Record all patient care information, including the patient's medical history and all emergency care given, on a PCR.

Complications of Delivery

Abnormal Presentations

Objective 25

When the back of the fetal head (occiput) appears as the presenting part, it is called an *occiput posterior presentation*. This type of presentation occurs in about 10–25% of deliveries. The patient will usually complain of severe back pain or pain above the pubic bone. Although most fetuses rotate to an anterior position on their own and deliver vaginally, some do not. In a face presentation, the presenting part is the chin. In a brow presentation, the presenting part is the brow. Prolonged labor occurs in nearly half the cases of brow presentations. In a compound presentation one or more fetal extremities accompany the presenting part. The most common combination is the head and an upper extremity. The most common complication of a compound presentation is umbilical cord prolapse. Consult with medical direction, and prepare for immediate transport as soon as you recognize an abnormal presentation. Depending on the circumstances, you may be advised to request ALS personnel to the scene, consider an ALS intercept while en route to the receiving facility, or transport rapidly to the closest appropriate facility. Give oxygen to the mother, and keep the patient on her left side to minimize the risk of supine hypotension unless you are instructed by medical direction to place the mother in an alternate position.

A breech presentation occurs when the baby's buttocks or feet come out of the uterus first. There are three types of breech presentation: frank breech,

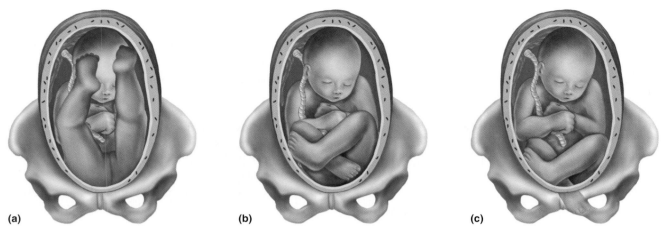

FIGURE 42-20 ▲ Breech presentation. **(a)** Frank breech, **(b)** Full (complete) breech, **(c)** Footling breech.

full or complete breech, and footling breech (Figure 42-20). In a frank breech presentation, the fetal legs are extended across the abdomen toward the shoulders. This is the most common type of breech presentation. In a full (or complete) breech presentation, the head, knees, and hips are flexed, and the buttocks are the presenting part. In a footling breech presentation, the presenting part is one or both feet.

A breech presentation is dangerous for the fetus because of the increased likelihood of delivery trauma or suffocation caused by a prolapsed cord. A breech presentation is best managed in the hospital. As soon as you recognize the presenting part is the baby's buttocks or leg, request an early response of ALS personnel to the scene or consider an ALS intercept while en route to the receiving facility. Give oxygen to the mother by nonrebreather mask at 10 to 15 L/min if breathing is adequate, and place her in the knee-chest position or on her left side with her hips and legs elevated. These positions allow gravity to pull the baby away from the mother's cervix.

If delivery is about to occur, use standard precautions, including gloves, mask, eye protection, and a gown. Prepare the mother in the same way as for a head-first delivery. Position the mother, give her oxygen, and prepare the OB kit. Allow the buttocks and trunk of the baby to deliver on their own. *Do not pull on the baby.* Pulling may cause the mother's cervix to clamp down tighter on the baby's head. Once the legs are clear, support *(do not pull or lift)* the baby's legs and trunk. Support the baby's body on your forearm, or gently grasp the bony part of the baby's pelvis. Be careful not to grasp the baby's abdomen to avoid injury to its internal organs. The head should deliver on its own.

If the head does not deliver within 3 minutes of the time the trunk was delivered, place a gloved hand into the vagina with your palm toward the baby's face. Spread your fingers and form a V with your index and middle finger on either side of the baby's nose (Figure 42-21). Bend your fingers slightly, and push the vaginal wall away from the baby's face. Hold the baby's mouth open slightly with your finger. This may allow air to enter the baby's mouth and nose. You must continue this position until the baby's head is delivered. If possible, give blow-by oxygen to the area near the baby's nose. For transport, place the patient on her left side. Reassess as often as indicated during transport. Record all patient care information, including the patient's medical history and all emergency care given, on a PCR.

Prolapsed Cord

Objective 25

A **prolapsed cord** is a serious emergency that endangers the life of the unborn fetus. A prolapsed cord occurs when a portion of the umbilical cord falls down below the presenting part of the fetus and presents through the birth canal before delivery of the head. When the umbilical cord is wrapped around the baby's neck, it is called a *nuchal cord*. With each contraction of the uterus, the cord is compressed between the presenting part and the mother's bony pelvis (Figure 42-22). Without blood flowing through the cord, the baby will suffocate. The pressure on the cord must be reduced or relieved as quickly as possible.

Prepare for immediate transport, and consider an ALS intercept while en route to the receiving facility. Place the mother in the knee-chest position. To do this, position her on her hands and knees. Then ask her to lower her head and chest to the floor (Figure 42-23).

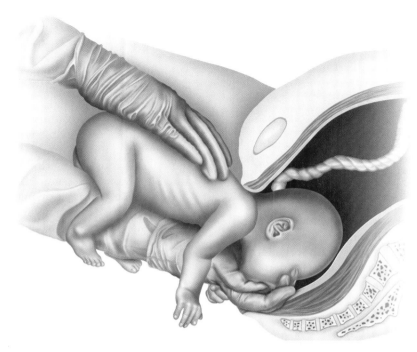

FIGURE 42-21 ▲ Creating an airway with a breech presentation.

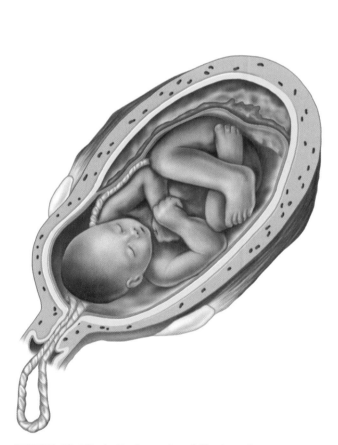

FIGURE 42-22 ▲ Prolapsed umbilical cord.

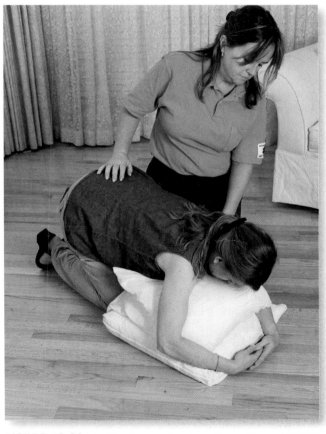

FIGURE 42-23 ▲ The knee-chest position. The mother is positioned on her hands and knees. Her head and chest are then lowered to the floor.

This will help lessen pressure on the cord in the birth canal. Insert a sterile gloved hand into the vagina, and push the presenting part of the fetus away from the cord. Apply only enough pressure to the presenting part so that a pulse returns in the cord. A pulsating umbilical cord indicates the fetus is alive. Once this has been accomplished, leave your hand in place. Do *not* attempt to push the cord back into the vagina. With a wet gauze pad or cloth, cup the cord against the mother's body to keep it moist. Give oxygen to the mother at 10 to 15 L/min by nonrebreather mask if breathing is adequate. Transport rapidly to the closest appropriate medical facility. Keep pressure off the cord, and monitor the cord pulsations during transport. Do not remove your hand until relieved by healthcare staff at the receiving facility. Reassess as often as indicated during transport. Record all patient care information, including the patient's medical history and all emergency care given, on a PCR.

Postpartum Complications

Hemorrhage

Objective 26

Postpartum hemorrhage is hemorrhage greater than 500 mL following delivery. The major causes of postpartum hemorrhage are a lack of uterine tone, vaginal or cervical tears, retained pieces of the placenta, and clotting disorders. Postpartum hemorrhage is the most common complication of labor and delivery and most likely to occur during the first hour after delivery of the placenta. Immediate postpartum hemorrhage is blood loss that occurs within the first 24 hours of delivery. Delayed postpartum hemorrhage is blood loss that occurs 24 hours to 6 weeks after delivery. Delayed postpartum hemorrhage is often caused by retained pieces of the placenta.

When obtaining the patient's history, determine if the patient gave birth to a large infant, if multiple births occurred, if she had prolonged labor, and if she has previously had placenta previa or abruptio placentae.

Administer oxygen by nonrebreather mask at 10 to 15 L/min if breathing is adequate. Place the patient in a supine position, and keep her warm. Place the infant at the mother's breast (if just delivered) to stimulate uterine contractions. If the uterus feels soft on palpation, perform uterine massage. Do not attempt to force delivery of the placenta. Do not pack the vagina. Consult with medical direction. You may be advised to request ALS personnel to the scene, consider an ALS intercept while en route to the receiving facility, or transport rapidly to the closest appropriate facility.

Amniotic Fluid Embolism

Objective 26

Although rare, amniotic fluid embolism is a tragic complication of labor and delivery. During labor and delivery, amniotic fluid leaks into the mother's venous circulation, travels to the pulmonary circulation, and causes sudden, severe obstruction. Generally, there is a history of a rapid, vigorous labor, signs of abruptio placentae, or history of uterine trauma at or around the time of delivery. Assessment findings and symptoms include a sudden onset of dyspnea and tachycardia, often during delivery. These signs are often followed by severe hypotension, severe hypoxia, and loss of consciousness. Heavy uterine bleeding may be present. Respiratory arrest and cardiac arrest soon follow. Consult with medical direction. You may be advised to request ALS personnel to the scene, consider an ALS intercept while en route to the receiving facility, or transport rapidly to the closest appropriate facility. Give oxygen by nonrebreather mask at 10 to 15 L/min if breathing is adequate. If breathing is inadequate, assist ventilations as necessary with a bag-mask device. Perform cardiopulmonary resuscitation if indicated.

On the Scene   **Wrap-Up**

The woman tells you that she already has had seven children and that the previous one came in 30 minutes. You place a hand on her abdomen and can tell that her contractions last about a minute with only 2 minutes between them. As you open the OB kit, she begins to grunt and her eyes bulge as she strains. The supervisor clears the area. When you remove the patient's jeans, you can see the baby's head protruding from her vagina. "Pant," you tell her as you grab a blanket and a bulb syringe. With the next contraction, the baby's head is delivered. You quickly suction its mouth and nose. One more push and the baby's body is guided out, one shoulder at a time into your waiting hands.

You carefully hang on to the slippery little infant and suction the little boy. You smile when you see the baby's face scrunch into a grimace and hear a hearty cry. You note the time as you glance at your watch to check his pulse. The paramedics arrive, and one of them assumes care of the baby while you turn your attention to the mother. You can see the umbilical cord move up and down slightly and hear her moan. A moment later there is a small gush of blood, and the placenta is delivered. Moments later you assist the paramedics in wheeling the patients toward the ambulance. A short time later, the paramedics call to tell you that mom and baby are doing fine and commend both of you for doing a great job. ■

▶ The vagina is also called the birth canal. It is a muscular tube that serves as a passageway between the uterus and the outside of the body.

▶ The placenta is a specialized organ through which the fetus exchanges nourishment and waste products during pregnancy.

▶ The umbilical cord is the lifeline that connects the placenta to the fetus. It contains two arteries and one vein. The umbilical vein carries oxygen-rich blood to the fetus. The umbilical cord attaches to the umbilicus (navel) of the fetus.

▶ The amniotic sac is a membranous bag that surrounds the fetus inside the uterus. It contains fluid (amniotic fluid) that helps protect the fetus from injury.

▶ Pregnancy usually takes 40 weeks and is divided into three 90-day intervals called trimesters.

▶ The uterus and presenting part of the fetus descend into the pelvis in preparation for delivery about 10 days (average) before the onset of labor. This is called lightening. The presenting part is the part of the infant that comes out of the birth canal first. Premature labor (also called preterm labor) occurs when a woman has labor before her 37th week of pregnancy.

▶ Assessment of the pregnant patient is the same as that of other patients. However, because of the normal changes in vital signs that occur with pregnancy, the patient's vital signs may not be as diagnostically helpful as they are in a nonpregnant patient. Despite a significant amount of internal or external bleeding, young, healthy pregnant patients can maintain relatively normal vital signs for a significant time and then develop signs of shock very quickly.

▶ Labor is the process in which the uterus repeatedly contracts to push the fetus and placenta out of the mother's body. It begins with the first uterine muscle contraction and ends with delivery of the placenta. Delivery is the actual birth of the baby at the end of the second stage of labor. The first stage of labor begins with the first uterine contraction. This stage ends with a complete thinning and opening (dilation) of the cervix. The second stage of labor begins with the opening of the cervix and ends with delivery of the infant. During labor, the presenting part will eventually remain visible at the vaginal opening between contractions. This is called crowning. The third stage of labor begins with delivery of the infant and ends with delivery of the placenta.

▶ Consider delivering at the scene in the following three circumstances:

- Delivery can be expected in a few minutes.
- No suitable transportation is available.
- The hospital cannot be reached because of heavy traffic, bad weather, a natural disaster, or a similar situation.

▶ Because blood and amniotic fluid are expected during childbirth and may splash, you must use standard precautions, including gloves, mask, eye protection, and a gown.

▶ Intimate partner violence may begin or intensify during pregnancy. Be aware of possible warning signs of possible intimate partner violence and mandatory reporting laws in your state. Accurate documentation of your findings is essential.

▶ Substance abuse during pregnancy can increase the risk of birth defects and complications during labor and delivery.

▶ Diabetes that exists before pregnancy is called pregestational diabetes. Diabetes that develops during pregnancy is called gestational diabetes. The pregnant diabetic patient must closely monitor and control her blood sugar levels throughout her pregnancy.

▶ An abortion is the termination of pregnancy before the fetus is able to live on its own outside the uterus. A spontaneous abortion, also called a miscarriage, is the loss of a fetus because of natural causes. It usually occurs before the 20th week of pregnancy, most often between the 7th and 12th weeks of pregnancy.

▶ An ectopic pregnancy occurs when a fertilized egg implants outside the uterus. An ectopic pregnancy is a medical emergency. The most common site where this occurs is inside a fallopian tube.

▶ The possible causes of vaginal bleeding in late pregnancy include placenta previa, abruptio placentae, and a ruptured uterus. All third-trimester bleeding should be considered a life-threatening emergency.

▶ Preeclampsia is a condition of high blood pressure and swelling that occurs in some women, usually during the third trimester of pregnancy. Eclampsia is the seizure phase of preeclampsia. Eclampsia is associated with a significant risk of death for the mother and fetus.

▶ Precipitous labor lasts less than 3 hours from the start of contractions to delivery.

▶ Postterm pregnancy, also called prolonged pregnancy, is a pregnancy that lasts longer than 42 weeks.

▶ Meconium staining refers to the passage of fetal stool into the amniotic fluid.

▶ A woman pregnant with twins (or more babies) usually goes into labor during or before her 37th week of pregnancy. The more babies a woman is expecting, the higher the risk of having a premature delivery.

- Possible causes of intrauterine fetal death include abruptio placentae, infection, genetic abnormalities, preeclampsia, fetal skull fracture, and umbilical cord complications. Complications of maternal medical illnesses such as hypertension, diabetes, obesity, chronic renal disease, and thyroid disorders can also result in fetal death. Sometimes the cause is unknown.

- Premature rupture of the membranes is rupture of the amniotic sac before the onset of labor. Once the protective barrier of the amniotic sac is broken, there is an increased risk of fetal infection because of the proximity to bacteria present in the mother's vagina and rectal area.

- Preterm labor is labor that begins before the 37th week of gestation. Possible causes include uterine or cervical anatomical abnormalities, premature rupture of the membranes, multiple gestation, and intrauterine infection. Complications of preterm labor may result in premature delivery of the infant.

- A premature infant is one born before the 37th week of gestation or weighing less than 5.5 pounds (2.5 kilograms). Premature babies (also called preemies) can have many health challenges.

- Consult with medical direction and prepare for immediate transport as soon as you recognize an abnormal presentation. Depending on the circumstances, you may be advised to request ALS personnel to the scene, consider an ALS intercept while en route to the receiving facility, or transport rapidly to the closest appropriate facility. Give oxygen to the mother by nonrebreather mask at 10 to 15 L/min if breathing is adequate, and keep the patient on her left side to minimize the risk of supine hypotension unless you are instructed by medical direction to place the mother in an alternate position.

- A prolapsed cord is a serious emergency that endangers the life of the unborn fetus. A prolapsed cord occurs when a portion of the umbilical cord falls down below the presenting part of the fetus and presents through the birth canal before delivery of the head. When the umbilical cord is wrapped around the baby's neck, it is called a nuchal cord.

- Postpartum hemorrhage is hemorrhage greater than 500 mL following delivery. It is the most common complication of labor and delivery and most likely to occur during the first hour after delivery of the placenta.

- Amniotic fluid embolism is a tragic complication of labor and delivery. During labor and delivery, amniotic fluid leaks into the mother's venous circulation, travels to the pulmonary circulation, and causes sudden, severe obstruction.

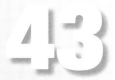

Neonatal Care

By the end of this chapter, you should be able to:

Knowledge Objectives ▶
1. Discuss special considerations of meconium.
2. Explain the importance of keeping a newborn warm.
3. Identify the primary signs used for evaluating a newborn.
4. Give examples of appropriate techniques used to stimulate a newborn.
5. Determine when ventilatory assistance is appropriate for a newborn.
6. Determine when chest compressions are appropriate for a newborn.
7. Assess patient improvement due to chest compressions and ventilations.
8. Discuss central cyanosis and acrocyanosis and their importance when assessing a newborn.
9. Determine when blow-by oxygen delivery is appropriate for a newborn.
10. Discuss use of the Apgar score when caring for a newborn.

Attitude Objective ▶
11. Explain the importance of understanding neonatal resuscitation procedures.

Skill Objectives ▶

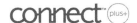

12. Demonstrate postdelivery care of an infant.
13. Demonstrate appropriate assessment technique for examining a newborn.
14. Calculate the Apgar score given various newborn situations.
15. Demonstrate appropriate suctioning of a newborn.
16. Demonstrate blow-by oxygen delivery for a newborn.
17. Demonstrate appropriate assisted ventilations for a newborn.
18. Demonstrate appropriate chest compression and ventilation techniques for a newborn.

On the Scene

You and your partner have been dispatched to a report of "childbirth" at the intersection of a regional highway and a local street about 2 miles from the local hospital. While you are still responding, your dispatcher tells you that there is a state highway patrol officer on scene reporting that the "baby has been delivered." ■

THINK ABOUT IT

As you read this chapter, think about the following questions:

- What initial care should be delivered to the infant?
- What memory aid can be used to help remember the evaluation criteria of a newborn?
- What are the "normal" vital signs for a newborn?

Introduction

Once the baby is born, you will have two patients—the newborn and the mother. If possible, position the baby between you and the mother so that you can periodically observe the mother while providing care for her baby. In this chapter we discuss the initial steps for providing emergency care to a newborn.

Caring for the Newborn

Objectives 1, 2

During labor and delivery, the newborn undergoes many changes during the transition from fetal to neonatal circulation. For example, the airways and alveoli of a fetus are filled with fluid. At birth, the newborn's respiratory system must suddenly begin working and maintain oxygenation. At about the same time, the newborn's blood pressure increases because of constriction of the umbilical vessels. The newborn's cries and deep breaths help move fetal lung fluid out of the airways, which is usually complete within 24 hours of birth. If the newborn does not breathe sufficiently to force fluid from alveoli or if meconium blocks air from entering alveoli, hypoxia will result and permanent brain damage can occur. When the baby is born, look at the baby and ask yourself four questions at the time of birth:

1. Term gestation?
2. Clear of meconium?
3. Breathing or crying?
4. Good muscle tone?

If the answer to all those questions is yes, proceed with providing warmth, clearing the baby's airway, and drying. If the answer to any question is no, you will need to begin the initial steps of resuscitation.

You Should Know

Although relatively few newborns require resuscitation, the need for resuscitation measures usually increases as birth weight decreases.

Meconium forms the first stools of a newborn. It is thick and sticky in consistency and varies in color. Meconium contains swallowed amniotic fluid, mucus, fine hair, blood, and other by-products of growth. In the newborn with a properly functioning gastrointestinal tract, the color and consistency of meconium changes after 3 or 4 days of feedings of breast milk or formula.

Amniotic fluid is normally colorless. Amniotic fluid containing meconium may be thin and watery or thick and may be brownish-yellow or green in color. The presence of meconium in the amniotic fluid is an indication of possible fetal distress. Normally, meconium is not passed from the infant's rectum until after birth. However, during birth, if there is a low oxygen supply, the fetus's anal sphincter may relax and allow the passage of meconium into the amniotic fluid. A low oxygen supply may occur from compression of the umbilical cord, abruptio placentae, or maternal shock, among other causes. If inhaled, meconium may cause severe inflammation of the lungs and pneumonia in the newborn.

If meconium is observed during delivery, be sure to suction the baby's mouth and nose as soon as the head is delivered. By suctioning the baby before the shoulders and chest are delivered and before the baby begins breathing, you reduce the baby's risk of sucking the meconium into the lungs.

Quickly dry the baby's body and head to remove blood and amniotic fluid (Figure 43-1). Immediately remove the wet towel or blanket from the infant, and then quickly wrap the baby in a clean, warm blanket. It is very important to keep a newborn warm. Newborns lose heat very quickly because they are wet and suddenly exposed to an environment that is cooler than that inside the uterus. Because most body heat is lost through the head as a result of evaporation, immediately dry the baby and cover its head as soon as possible. After the infant's head has been dried, heat loss from the head is largely due to radiation. Given the infant's head size (relative to the body) and the degree of perfusion, heat loss from radiation may be pronounced. Wrap the baby's body and head in dry, warm blankets to prevent heat loss, keeping the face exposed.

Place the baby on its back or side with the neck in a neutral position. Wipe blood and mucus from the baby's mouth and nose. Suction the mouth and then the nose again. This suctioning will often cause the baby to begin crying and breathing.

Remember This

Dry the newborn, provide warmth, position the baby, clear the airway as necessary, and stimulate the baby. These actions should take 30 seconds or less to accomplish.

Airway and Breathing

Objectives 3, 4, 5

You should begin to assess the newborn immediately after birth. Focus on the baby's breathing rate and effort, the heart rate, and skin color. Most babies will begin

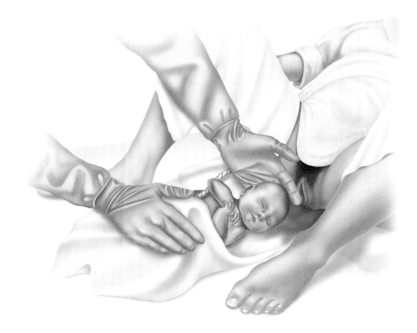

FIGURE 43-1 ▲ Keep the baby at or around the same level as the mother's vaginal opening until it is time to clamp the umbilical cord. Quickly dry the baby's body and head to remove blood and amniotic fluid.

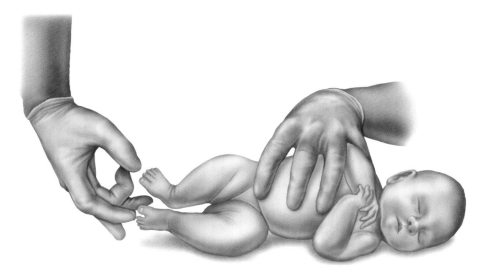

FIGURE 43-2 ▲ If the baby has not begun to breathe or is breathing very slowly, stimulate the baby by rubbing the baby's back, chest, or extremities, or by tapping or flicking the bottom of the feet.

crying and breathing as a result of the stimulation provided during warming, suctioning, and drying. If the baby has not begun to breathe or is breathing very slowly, stimulate the baby. Do this by rubbing its back, chest, or extremities, or by tapping or flicking the bottom of the feet (Figure 43-2). These methods may be tried for 5 to 10 seconds to stimulate breathing.

If the baby's breathing is adequate, assess the heart rate. If the baby's breathing is not adequate and there is no improvement after 5 to 10 seconds, help the baby breathe by using mouth-to-mask breathing or an appropriately sized bag-mask device connected to 100% oxygen. Breathe at a rate of 40 to 60 breaths/min (slightly less than 1 breath per second). Use just enough pressure to see a gentle chest rise. If you use too much pressure, you will force air into the baby's stomach, which will compromise breathing.

Heart Rate

Objectives 6, 7

Assess the baby's pulse by feeling the brachial pulse on the inside of the upper arm. Count the heart rate for 6 seconds, and multiply by 10 to estimate the beats/min. Because a baby's heart rate is usually very fast, it may be helpful to tap out the heart rate as you count it. If the baby's heart rate is less than 100 beats/min, immediately breathe for the baby by using mouth-to-mask breathing or a bag-mask device. Reassess the baby's breathing, heart rate, and color after 30 seconds. If there is no improvement and the baby's heart rate is less than 60 beats/min, begin chest compressions (see Appendix A). If the baby's heart rate is more than 60 beats/min but breathing is inadequate, continue breathing for the baby by using mouth-to-mask breathing or an appropriately sized bag-mask device. Reassess in 30 seconds. If the baby's heart rate is more than 100 beats/min, assess the baby's skin color.

> **You Should Know**
>
> A full-term baby's respiratory rate is normally between 30 and 60 breaths/min and the heart rate is normally 100 to 180 beats/min in the first 12 hours of life. After that, a newborn's normal respiratory rate is 30 to 50 breaths/min and the heart rate is 120 to 160 beats/min.

Skin Color

Objectives 8, 9

Look at the color of the baby's face, chest, or inside the mouth. A bluish tint in these areas is called **central cyanosis.** The skin of a newborn's extremities is often blue **(acrocyanosis)** immediately after delivery. This finding is common and requires no specific intervention. The baby's color should quickly improve if the baby is breathing adequately and is kept warm. If the baby is breathing adequately and has a heart rate of more than 100 beats/min but central cyanosis is present, give blow-by oxygen (Figure 43-3). To do this, cup your hand around the oxygen tubing. Hold the tubing close to the baby's nose and mouth. Do not blow oxygen directly into the baby's face. The oxygen source should be set to deliver at least 5 L/min.

Apgar Score

Objective 10

An **Apgar score** is used to assess an infant's condition at 1 and 5 minutes after birth. The Apgar score is used to as-

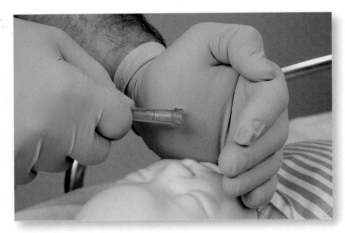

FIGURE 43-3 ▲ Giving blow-by oxygen.

sess five specific signs: *a*ppearance (color), *p*ulse (heart rate), *g*rimace (irritability), *a*ctivity (muscle tone), and *r*espirations. Each sign is assigned a value of either 0, 1, or 2 and added for a total Apgar score (Table 43-1). An Apgar score of 0 to 3 indicates a newborn in severe distress. A score of 4 to 6 indicates a newborn in moderate distress. A score of 7 to 10 indicates a newborn in mild distress or with no distress. If the 5-minute Apgar score is abnormal (less than 7), appropriate resuscitation measures should be started and Apgar scores assigned every 5 minutes until the infant is stabilized. However, do not delay resuscitation of a newborn to obtain an Apgar score.

Recent studies have shown that although the Apgar score has demonstrated usefulness and is of value in assessment of the newborn, there is substantial variability in the scores obtained by healthcare professionals. Of the areas evaluated using the score, appearance (color) has little predictive value of the need for newborn resuscitation. Further, prematurity influences the vigor of the newborn's respiratory effort, muscle tone, and reflex responses, which make up a significant portion of the score.

Making a Difference

Virginia Apgar

The Apgar score is named for an American anesthesiologist, Virginia Apgar (1909–1974), who invented the scoring method in 1952. Having assisted at thousands of deliveries, Dr. Apgar wanted an organized way for delivery room personnel to assess neonates. Dr. Apgar was the first woman to be appointed a full professor at Columbia University's College of Physicians and Surgeons.

After assessment and initial emergency care, prepare the newborn for transport as quickly as possible. Reassess at least every 5 minutes.

TABLE 43-1 Apgar Score

Sign	0	1	2
Appearance (color)	Blue or pale	Body pink Extremities blue	Completely pink
Pulse (heart rate)	Absent	Below 100/min	Above 100/min
Grimace (irritability)	No response	Grimace	Cough, sneeze, cry
Activity (muscle tone)	Limp	Some flexion of extremities	Active motion
Respirations (respiratory effort)	Absent	Slow, irregular	Good, crying
Total each column			

Score	Interpretation
0—3	Newborn in severe distress
4—6	Newborn in moderate distress
7—10	Newborn in mild distress or no distress

You Should Know

One method that may be used to assess grimace is to gently place a soft catheter into the nare of the infant to elicit a grimace response.

On the Scene   Wrap-Up

As you approach the scene, you hear the sounds of a baby crying. You announce your arrival to the officer, who is leaning into the open door of a late model car. The officer raises his head and grins as he says, "It's a girl!" You look into the car and find that the baby is nestled comfortably in her mother's arms. You observe the mother smiling and sitting up in the backseat.

Using the Apgar score, you quickly assess the infant and find that her extremities are blue, she has a pulse rate of about 110, cries loudly, and moves well when stimulated. Minutes after administering blow-by oxygen, the infant is completely pink. You and your partner begin preparing the patients for transport. ■

Sum It Up

▶ During labor and delivery, the newborn undergoes many changes during the transition from fetal to neonatal circulation. The airways and alveoli of a fetus are filled with fluid. At birth, the newborn's respiratory system must suddenly begin and maintain oxygenation. If the newborn does not breathe sufficiently to force fluid from alveoli or if meconium blocks air from entering alveoli, hypoxia will result and permanent brain damage can occur.

▶ When the baby is born, look at the baby and ask yourself four questions at the time of birth:

  1. Term gestation?
  2. Clear of meconium?
  3. Breathing or crying?
  4. Good muscle tone?

If the answer to all those questions is yes, proceed with providing warmth, clearing the baby's airway, and drying. If the answer to any question is no, you will need to begin the initial steps of resuscitation.

▶ Meconium forms the first stools of a newborn. The presence of meconium in the amniotic fluid is an indication of possible fetal distress. If meconium is observed during delivery, be sure to suction the baby's mouth and nose as soon as the head is delivered. By suctioning the baby before the shoulders and chest are delivered and before the baby begins breathing, you reduce the baby's risk of sucking the meconium into the lungs.

▶ It is very important to keep a newborn warm. Newborns lose heat very quickly because they are wet and suddenly exposed to an environment that is cooler than that inside the uterus. Because most body heat is lost through the head as a result of evaporation, immediately dry the baby and cover its head as soon as possible. Wrap the baby's body and head in dry, warm blankets to prevent heat loss, keeping the face exposed.

- Assess the newborn immediately after birth, focusing on the baby's breathing rate and effort, the heart rate, and skin color. If the baby has not begun to breathe or is breathing very slowly, stimulate the baby.

- If the baby's breathing is not adequate and there is no improvement after 5 to 10 seconds, help the baby breathe by using mouth-to-mask breathing or an appropriately sized bag-mask device connected to 100% oxygen.

- Assess the baby's pulse by feeling the brachial pulse on the inside of the upper arm. If the baby's heart rate is less than 100 beats/min, immediately breathe for the baby by using mouth-to-mask breathing or a bag-mask device. Reassess the baby's breathing, heart rate, and color after 30 seconds. If there is no improvement and the baby's heart rate is less than 60 beats/min, begin chest compressions.

- Look at the color of the baby's face or chest or inside of the mouth. A bluish tint in these areas is called central cyanosis. The skin of a newborn's extremities is often blue (acrocyanosis) immediately after delivery. This finding is common and requires no specific intervention. If the baby is breathing adequately and has a heart rate of more than 100 beats/min but central cyanosis is present, give blow-by oxygen.

- An Apgar score is used to assess an infant's condition at 1 and 5 minutes after birth. The Apgar score is used to assess five specific signs: *a*ppearance (color), *p*ulse (heart rate), *g*rimace (irritability), *ac*tivity (muscle tone), and *r*espirations.

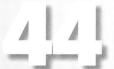

Pediatrics

By the end of this chapter, you should be able to:

Knowledge Objectives ▷ 1. Describe differences in anatomy and physiology of the infant, child, and adult patient.

2. Describe assessment of an infant and child.

3. Describe possible causes, assessment findings, symptoms, and emergency care for an airway obstruction.

4. Describe possible causes, assessment findings, symptoms, and emergency care for respiratory emergencies in an infant and child.

5. Differentiate between respiratory distress and respiratory failure.

6. Describe possible causes, assessment findings, symptoms, and emergency care for cardiopulmonary failure.

7. Describe possible causes, assessment findings, symptoms, and emergency care for altered mental status in an infant and child.

8. Describe possible causes, assessment findings, symptoms, and emergency care for shock in an infant and child.

9. Describe possible causes, assessment findings, symptoms, and emergency care for fever in an infant and child.

10. Describe possible causes, assessment findings, symptoms, and emergency care for seizures in an infant and child.

11. Describe possible causes, assessment findings, symptoms, and emergency care for poisoning in an infant and child.

12. Describe possible causes, assessment findings, symptoms, and emergency care for drowning in an infant and child.

13. Describe possible causes, assessment findings, symptoms, and emergency care for sudden infant death syndrome.

Attitude Objectives ▷ 14. Explain the rationale for having knowledge and skills appropriate for dealing with infant and child patients.

15. Attend to the feelings of the family when dealing with an ill or injured infant or child.

16. Understand the provider's own emotional response to caring for infants or children.

Skill Objectives ▷ 17. Demonstrate the assessment of an infant and child.

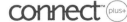

18. Demonstrate bag-mask ventilation for the infant.

19. Demonstrate bag-mask ventilation for the child.

20. Demonstrate oxygen delivery for the infant and child.

21. Demonstrate the care of an infant and child with respiratory distress or respiratory failure.

22. Demonstrate the care of an infant and child with cardiopulmonary failure.
23. Demonstrate the care of an infant and child with altered mental status.
24. Demonstrate the care of an infant and child with shock.
25. Demonstrate the care of an infant and child with a fever.
26. Demonstrate the care of an infant and child with seizures.
27. Demonstrate the care of an infant and child with a toxic exposure.
28. Demonstrate the care of the patient and family for sudden infant death syndrome.

On the Scene

You are dispatched for a "child with difficulty breathing." As you walk into the room, it is obvious that a 4-year-old girl is struggling to catch her breath. She is pale and leaning forward on the edge of her bed, and her nostrils flare open with each breath. A high-pitched whistle is audible even without use of the stethoscope. "She has asthma," her father tells you, "but it seems worse this time." You count her breathing at 40 breaths/min. Her radial pulse is 146. When you lift her shirt, you can see the skin between her ribs pull in with each breath. ■

THINK ABOUT IT

As you read this chapter, think about the following questions:

- Which signs of respiratory distress have you observed in this child?
- Are her vital signs within normal limits?
- What treatment should you consider for this patient?

Introduction

Remember This

The key to working with children is, "Keep it simple." Children respond very well to basic management skills.

Children are not small adults. Children have unique physical, mental, emotional, and developmental characteristics that you must consider when assessing and caring for them. You may be anxious when treating a child because of lack of experience in treating children, fear of failure, or identifying the patient with your own child. If you understand the expected physical and developmental characteristics of infants and children of different ages, you will be able to more accurately assess your patient and provide appropriate care. We discussed the developmental stages of children in Chapter 8 and communication techniques in Chapter 15. In this chapter, we focus on the anatomic differences between children and adults, assessment of a child, and the illnesses and injuries you are most likely to encounter in the pediatric patient.

You Should Know

Age Classifications of Infants and Children

Life Stage	Age
Newly born infant	Birth to several hours after birth
Neonate	Birth to 1 month
Infant	1 to 12 months
	• Young infant: 1 to 6 months
	• Older infant: 6 months to 1 year
Toddler	1 to 3 years
Preschooler	3 to 5 years
School-age child	6 to 12 years
Adolescent	13 to 18 years

Depending on the state that you reside in or the pediatric hospital in your area, the upper-age limit for a pediatric patient may be 14, 18, or 21 years of age. Be sure to check with your instructor to find out the upper-age limit for a pediatric patient in your area.

Anatomical and Physiological Differences in Children

Objective 1

Head

A child's head is proportionately larger and heavier than an adult's until the child is about 4 years of age. It takes several months for a child to develop neck muscles that are strong enough to support his head. Because the back of a child's head (occiput) sticks out and a child's forehead is large, these areas are susceptible to injury. It is not unusual for children to have multiple forehead bruises from hitting their heads on tables and floors. Trauma to the head may result in flexion and extension injuries.

The necks of infants and toddlers are flexed when they are lying flat because the back of the skull is large. The chin is then angled toward the chest (Figure 44-1). Appropriate positioning of an infant's or a toddler's head will be one of the most important techniques that you will use when managing children. Proper positioning is an important factor when managing the airway.

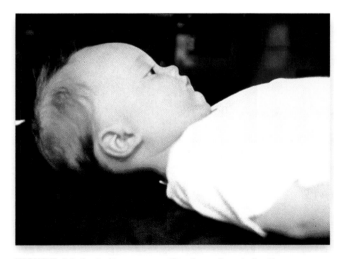

FIGURE 44-1 ▲ Proper positioning of an infant's or a toddler's head is an important consideration during airway management.

The bones of the head of an infant are soft and flexible to allow for growth of the brain. On both the top and the back of the head are small diamond-shaped openings called **fontanels** *(soft spots)*. These areas will not completely close until about 6 months of age for the rear fontanel and 18 months for the top one. You should assess the fontanels of an infant and toddler for bulging or depression. The soft spots of an infant or toddler are normally nearly level with the skull. Coughing, crying, or lying down may cause the soft spots to bulge temporarily. Bulging in an ill-appearing noncrying infant or toddler suggests increased pressure within the skull, such as pressure from fluid or pressure on the brain. A depression in an ill-appearing infant or toddler suggests the patient is dehydrated.

The brain and spinal cord of an infant or child are less well protected than those of an adult's. The pediatric brain requires nearly twice the blood flow that an adult's requires. An infant's or child's brain tissue and vascular system are more fragile and prone to bleeding from injury. The subarachnoid space is relatively smaller, with less cushioning effect for the brain. Hypoxia and hypotension in a child with a head injury can cause ongoing damage. In situations involving trauma, the momentum of the head may result in bruising and damage to the brain. Spinal cord injuries are less common in infants and children. Cervical spine injuries are more commonly ligamentous injuries.

Face

A child's nasal passages are very small, short, and narrow. It is easy for children to develop obstruction of these areas with mucus or foreign objects. Newborns are primarily nose breathers. A newborn will not automatically open her mouth to breathe when her nose becomes obstructed. As a result, any obstruction of the nose will lead to respiratory difficulty. You must make sure the newborn's nose is clear to avoid breathing problems.

Although the opening of the mouth is usually small and the jaw is small, a child's tongue is large in proportion to the mouth. The tongue of an infant or child fills the majority of the space in the mouth. The tongue is the most common cause of upper airway obstruction in an unconscious child because the immature muscles of the lower jaw (mandible) allow the tongue to fall to the back of the throat.

Airway

In children, the opening between the vocal cords (glottic opening) is higher in the neck and more toward the front than it is in an adult. As children grow

TABLE 44-1 Normal Respiratory Rates in Children at Rest

Life Stage	Age	Breaths/Min
Newborn	Birth to 1 month	30 to 50
Infant	1 to 12 months	20 to 40
Toddler	1 to 3 years	20 to 30
Preschooler	3 to 5 years	20 to 30
School-age child	6 to 12 years	16 to 30
Adolescent	13 to 18 years	12 to 20

up, the neck gets longer and the glottic opening drops down. The flap of cartilage that covers this opening, the epiglottis, is long, floppy, and narrow and extends at a 45-degree angle into the airway in children. Therefore, any injury to or swelling of this area can block the airway.

The trachea is the tube through which air passes from the mouth to the lungs. In children, this area is softer and more flexible, smaller in diameter, and shorter in length than it is in adults. The trachea has rings of cartilage that keep the airway open. In children, this cartilage is soft and collapses easily, and this can then obstruct the airway. Extending or flexing the neck too far can result in crimping of the trachea and a blocked airway. To avoid blocking the airway, place the head of an infant or young child in a neutral or "sniffing" position. This position is covered in more detail later in this chapter.

Breathing

A child's ribs are soft and flexible because they are made up mostly of cartilage. Bone growth occurs with time, filling in the cartilaginous areas from the center out to the ends. Because the rib cage is softer than that in an adult, rib fractures are less common in a child. However, when rib fractures are present, they represent significant energy transmission and are often accompanied by multisystem injuries. The lungs are prone to pneumothorax from excessive pressures during bag-mask ventilation.

The muscles between the ribs (intercostal muscles) help lift the chest wall during breathing. Because these muscles are not fully developed until later in childhood, the diaphragm is the primary muscle of breathing. As a result, the abdominal muscles move during breathing. During normal breathing, the abdominal muscles should move in the same direction as the chest wall. The movement of abdominal muscles opposite each other is called *seesaw breathing* and is abnormal. A child's respiratory rate is faster than an adult's and decreases with age (Table 44-1). Because the muscles between the ribs are not well developed, a child cannot keep up a rapid rate of breathing (faster than normal for the patient's age) for very long.

The stomach of an infant or child often fills with air during crying. Air can also build up in the stomach if rescue breathing is performed. As the stomach swells with air, it pushes on the lungs and diaphragm. This action limits movement and prevents good ventilation. Infants' and young children's breathing is dependent on the diaphragm. Breathing difficulty results if movement of the diaphragm is limited.

Infants and children have a higher oxygen demand per kilogram of body weight (about twice that of an adolescent or adult) but have smaller lung oxygen reserves. A higher oxygen demand with less reserve increases the risk of hypoxia with apnea or ineffective bag-mask ventilation. When ventilating with a bag-mask device, use a larger bag for ventilating the pediatric patient. Regardless of the size of the bag used for ventilation, use only enough force to cause gentle chest rise.

Circulation

Children breathe faster than adults, and their hearts beat harder and faster than those of adults. Infants and young children have a relatively smaller blood volume (80 mL/kg). A sudden loss of 0.5 L (500 mL) of the blood volume in a child or 100–200 mL of the blood volume in an infant is considered serious.

A child's heart rate will increase as a result of shock, fever, anxiety, and pain. It will also increase as she loses body fluid (hypovolemia). This condition can occur because of bleeding, vomiting, or diarrhea. Most of an infant's body weight is water, so vomiting and diarrhea can result in dehydration. Blood loss resulting from broken bones and soft tissue injuries may quickly result in shock. The system of an infant or child tries to make up for a loss of blood or fluid through an increase in heart rate and a constriction of the skin's blood vessels. These actions help deliver as much blood and oxygen as possible to the brain, heart, and lungs.

A child's rate and effort of breathing will increase when the amount of oxygen in the blood is decreased (as in late shock). This helps make up for a lack of oxygen. As the child tires and the blood oxygen level becomes very low, the heart muscle begins to pump less effectively. As a result, the child's heart rate slows. If the lack of oxygen is not corrected, the child will stop breathing (respiratory arrest). A child will often survive a respiratory arrest as long as his oxygen level is maintained sufficiently so that the heart does not stop. Normal heart rates for children at rest are shown in Table 44-2.

Remember This

In children, circulatory problems often develop because of respiratory problems.

If you have the necessary equipment, measure the blood pressure in children older than 3 years of age. The blood pressure of a child is normally lower than that of an adult (see Table 44-3). In children 1 to 10 years of age, the following formula may be used to determine the lower limit of a normal systolic blood pressure: 70 + (2 × child's age in years) = systolic blood pressure. The lower limit of normal systolic blood pressure for a child 10 or more years of age is 90 mm Hg. The diastolic blood pressure should be about two-thirds the systolic pressure.

Infants and young children have limited glucose stores. They are also susceptible to changes in temperature. A child has a large body surface area (BSA) compared with her weight. The larger the BSA that is exposed, the greater the area of heat loss.

An infant's skin is thin with few fat deposits under it. This condition contributes to an infant's sensitivity to extremes of heat and cold. Infants have poorly developed temperature-regulating mechanisms. For example, newborns are unable to shiver in cold temperatures. In addition, their sweating mechanism is immature in warm temperatures. Because infants and children are at risk of hypothermia, it is very important

TABLE 44-2 Normal Heart Rates in Children at Rest

Life Stage	Age	Beats/Min
Newborn	Birth to 1 month	120 to 160
Infant	1 to 12 months	80 to 140
Toddler	1 to 3 years	80 to 130
Preschooler	3 to 5 years	80 to 120
School-age child	6 to 12 years	70 to 110
Adolescent	13 to 18 years	60 to 100

TABLE 44-3 Lower Limit of Normal Systolic Blood Pressure by Age

Life Stage	Age	Lower Limit of Normal Systolic Blood Pressure
Term neonate	0 to 28 days	60 mm Hg or strong central pulse
Infant	1 to 12 months	70 mm Hg or strong central pulse
Child or adolescent	1 to 10 years	70 + (2 × age in years)
	10 years and older	90 mm Hg

to keep them warm. Cover the head (but not the face) to minimize heat loss. Newborns should not be overwarmed, as this can worsen their neurologic outcomes.

The skin of an infant or child will show changes related to the amount of oxygen in the blood.

- The tissue in the mouth of a healthy child should be pink and moist, regardless of the child's race.
- Pale (whitish) skin may be seen in shock, fright, or anxiety.
- A bluish (cyanotic) tint, often seen first around the mouth, suggests inadequate breathing or poor perfusion. This is a critical sign that requires immediate treatment.
- The skin may appear blotchy (mottled) in shock, hypothermia, or cardiac arrest.
- Flushed (red) skin may be caused by fever, heat exposure, or an allergic reaction.
- Yellowing of the skin (jaundice) and the sclerae of the eyes suggest a liver problem.

Most children should feel slightly warm to the touch. Their skin should be tight and not dry or flaky.

You Should Know

Most newborns have some degree of jaundice, which is most easily seen immediately after a finger is pressed onto the skin. Jaundice results from having too much bilirubin in the blood. Bilirubin is formed when the body breaks down old red blood cells. Before birth, the placenta removes the bilirubin from the infant, and the liver of the infant's mother processes and removes the bilirubin from the blood. Immediately after birth, the immature liver of the newborn is not as efficient at removing bilirubin from the bloodstream as was the mother's liver. Therefore, bilirubin levels may be a little higher than normal after birth, causing jaundice. Jaundice generally appears 2 to 3 days after birth, peaks between days 2 and 4, and clears within 2 weeks. Because sunlight helps break down bilirubin, thus enabling the liver to process it more easily, mild jaundice is often treated at home by placing the infant in indirect light from a window for 10 minutes twice a day.

Abdomen

The abdominal muscles of an infant and child are less developed than those of adults, and the abdominal

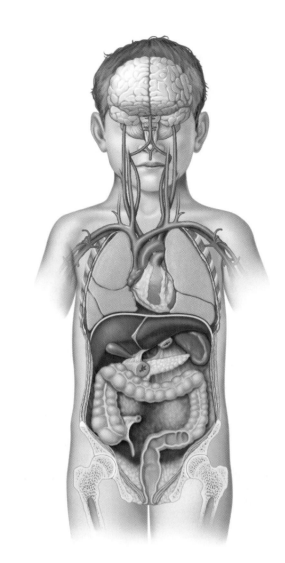

FIGURE 44-2 ▲ A child's anatomy.

muscles and organs are situated more anteriorly. Therefore, they receive less protection from the rib cage. As a result, seemingly insignificant forces can cause serious internal injury. Because the liver and spleen are proportionally larger in an infant and child, they are more frequently injured (Figure 44-2). Multiple organ injury is common.

Extremities

The bones of an infant and child are softer than those of adults. The growth plates of the bones are weaker than ligaments and tendons, so injury to the growth plate can result in differences in bone length (Figure 44-3). When

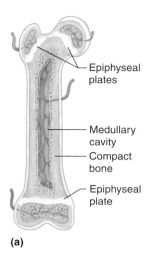

Epiphyseal plates

Medullary cavity

Compact bone

Epiphyseal plate

(a)

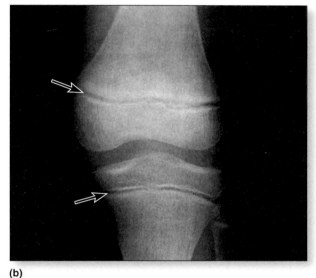

(b)

FIGURE 44-3 ▲ **(a)** Endochondral bone of a child. Note the epiphyseal growth plates. **(b)** Radiograph of a child's bone. Growth plates are indicated by arrows.

you are caring for an extremity injury in an infant or child, a sprain or strain should be immobilized because it is more likely a fracture.

Assessment of the Infant and Child

Scene Size-Up

Objective 2

Before responding to any call involving an infant or child, it is essential to know where pediatric equipment is located in your emergency bags.

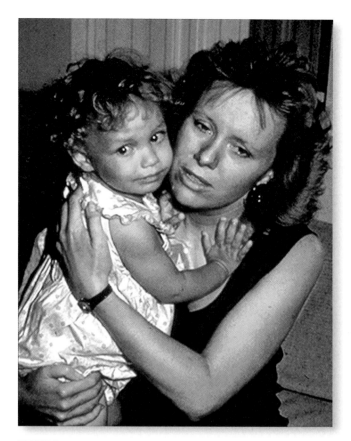

FIGURE 44-4 ▲ Quickly determine if the emergency is the result of trauma or a medical condition. If the emergency is the result of trauma, determine the mechanism of injury.

Making a Difference

It is not appropriate to search for age-appropriate equipment for the first time at an emergency scene. Become familiar with the location of all your equipment—including that used for pediatric patients. While en route to a call involving an infant or child, think about age-appropriate vital signs and anticipated developmental stage based on the dispatch information given. If you have this information stored on a note card or in a pocket guide, locate it en route to the call and have it readily accessible (such as attached to your clipboard).

On arrival at the scene, evaluate the scene for safety threats to yourself, your crew, the patient, and others. Quickly determine if the emergency is a result of trauma or a medical condition. If the emergency is a result of trauma, determine the mechanism of injury (Figure 44-4). If the emergency is the result of a medical condition, determine the nature of the illness. This information can be obtained from the patient, family members, or bystanders, as well as from your observations of the scene.

Survey the patient's environment for clues to the cause of the emergency. Note any hazards or potential hazards. For example, pills, open medicine bottles or bottles of cleaning solution, alcohol, or drug paraphernalia may indicate a possible toxic ingestion or exposure. Make a note of the position and location in which the patient is found.

Look at the child's environment. Does it appear clean and orderly? Do other children appear healthy and well cared for? Determine if you need additional resources, including law enforcement personnel. Remember to wear appropriate personal protective equipment before approaching the patient.

Making a Difference

Communicating with scared, concerned parents and family is an important aspect of your responsibilities at the scene of an ill infant or child. Be professional and compassionate, and remember to include them while providing care to their loved one.

Primary Survey

Objective 2

Any incident that involves children will cause some degree of anxiety and stress among every person present. Your emotional response in such situations will play an important part in how effective you can be. Your emotional response may be related to a limited exposure to children as a healthcare professional and/or caregiver. Alternatively, caring for an ill or injured child who is the same age as a member of your own family may also affect your response.

In most situations, your approach to an ill or injured infant or child should include the patient's caregiver. Watch the interaction between the caregiver and the child. Does the caregiver appear concerned? Or angry or indifferent? Keep in mind that an agitated caregiver results in an agitated child. A calm caregiver results in a calm child. If the child's caregiver is adding to the child's anxiety, give the adult something to do. For example, you might ask the caregiver to locate the child's favorite comfort object. Including the caregiver in the child's care reassures both the child and the caregiver. It also allows the adult a chance to take part in the child's recovery. Although a child's caregiver may not have medical training, she is the expert on what is normal or abnormal for her child. She also knows what measures will have a calming effect on the child.

General Impression

Your assessment of an infant or child should begin "across the room." When forming a general impression of an infant or child, look at his appearance, breathing, and circulation. Quickly determine whether the child appears sick or not sick.

- *Appearance.* A child should be alert and responsive to her surroundings. Is the child awake and alert? Does the child behave appropriately for her age? Does she recognize her caregiver? Is the child playing or moving around, or does she appear drowsy or unaware of her surroundings? Does the child show interest in what is happening? Does the child appear agitated or irritable? Does she appear confused or combative? If the child appears agitated, restless, or limp or if she appears to be asleep, proceed immediately to the ABCDE assessment.

- *(Work of) breathing.* With normal breathing, both sides of the chest rise and fall equally. Breathing is quiet and painless and occurs at a regular rate. Is the child sitting up, lying down, or leaning forward? Can you hear abnormal breathing sounds such as stridor (a high-pitched sound), wheezing, or grunting? Stridor suggests an upper airway obstruction. Wheezing suggests narrowing of the lower airways. Do you see retractions (sinking in around the ribs and collarbones; Figure 44-5), nasal flaring, or shoulder hunching? Is the child's breathing rate faster or slower than expected? Is his head bobbing up and down toward his chest? If the child appears to be struggling to breathe, has noisy breathing, moves his chest abnormally, or has a rate of breathing that is faster or slower than normal, proceed immediately to the ABCDE assessment.

- *Circulation.* Visual signs of circulation relate to skin color, obvious bleeding, and moisture. What color is the child's skin? Is it pink, pale, mottled, flushed, or blue? Do you see any bleeding? If bleeding is present, where is it coming from? How much blood is there? Does the child look sweaty? Or do the child's lips look dry and flaky? If the child's skin looks pale, mottled, flushed, gray, or blue, proceed immediately to the ABCDE assessment.

Once your general impression is complete, your next steps are based on your findings. If the child's condition appears unstable (urgent), perform a hands-on ABCDE assessment. Treat any life threats and transport as quickly as possible. If the child's condition appears stable, proceed with a hands-on ABCDE assessment followed by a focused history and secondary survey. Examples of questions to ask when obtaining a focused history are listed in the next *You Should Know* box.

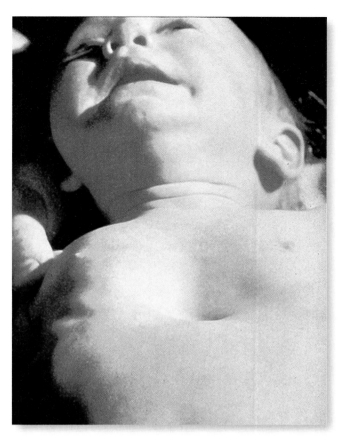

FIGURE 44-5 ▲ Retractions are a sign of an increased work of breathing.

In a responsive infant or child, use a toes-to-head or trunk-to-head approach. This approach should help reduce the infant's or the child's anxiety. Begin transport, starting potential treatments en route.

You Should Know

Focused History Questions

- Symptoms and duration (fever; activity level; recent eating, drinking, and urine output history; history of vomiting, diarrhea, or abdominal pain; rashes)
- Allergies (medications, environmental)
- Medications currently taking
- Past medical problems or chronic illnesses
- Key events leading to the injury or illness

Level of Responsiveness and Cervical Spine Protection

After forming a general impression, assess the patient's level of responsiveness (mental status) and the need for cervical spine protection.

Level of Responsiveness (Mental Status)

Is the child awake and alert? An alert infant or young child (younger than 3 years of age) smiles, orients to sound, follows objects with her eyes, and interacts with those around her. As the infant or young child's mental status decreases, you may see the following changes (in order of decreasing mental status):

- The child may cry but can be comforted.
- The child may show inappropriate, constant crying.
- The child may become irritable and restless.
- The child may be unresponsive.

Assessing the mental status of a child older than 3 years of age is the same as assessing that of an adult. Most children will be agitated or resist your assessment. A child who is limp, allows you to perform any assessment or skill, or does not respond to his caregiver is sick. Unresponsiveness in an infant or child usually indicates a life-threatening condition. If the patient is a child with special healthcare needs, the child's caregiver will probably be your best resource. The caregiver will be able to tell you what normal is for the child, regarding his mental status, vital signs, and level of activity.

Depending on the child's age, you may ask the child or caregiver, "Why did you call 9-1-1 today?" If the child appears to be asleep, gently rub her shoulder and ask, "Are you okay?" or "Can you hear me?" If the child does not respond, ask the family or bystanders to tell you what happened while you continue your assessment.

Remember This

An infant or child who does not recognize your presence is sick.

Cervical Spine Protection

If you suspect trauma to the head, neck, or back or if the child is unresponsive with an unknown nature of illness, take spinal precautions. If the child is awake and you suspect trauma, face him so that he does not have to turn his head to see you. Tell him not to move his head or neck. Use your hands to manually stabilize the child's head and neck in line with his body. Once begun, manual stabilization must be continued until the child has been secured to a backboard with his head stabilized.

Remember This

If the child complains of pain or if you meet resistance when moving the child's head and neck to a neutral position, stop and maintain the head and neck in the position in which they were found.

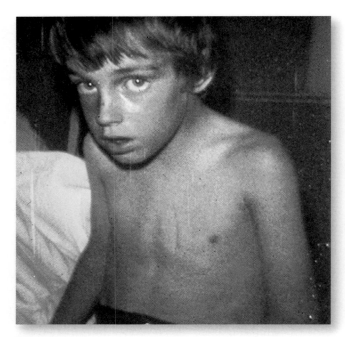

FIGURE 44-6 ▲ In cases of serious upper airway obstruction, the child will instinctively position himself to breathe easier and create his own airway.

A *Is for Airway*

Is the child's airway open? A child who is talking or crying has an open airway. If the child is responsive and the airway is open, assess the child's breathing. If the child is responsive but unable to speak, cry, cough, or make any other sound, her airway is completely obstructed. If the child has noisy breathing, such as snoring or gurgling, she has a partial airway obstruction.

A responsive child may have assumed a position to maintain an open airway. Allow the child to maintain this position as you continue your assessment. For example, in cases of serious upper airway obstruction, the child may instinctively assume a "sniffing" position (Figure 44-6). In this position, the child is seated with his head and chin thrust slightly forward, as if sniffing a flower. In cases of severe respiratory distress, the child may assume a "tripod" position. In this position, the child is seated and leaning forward (Figure 44-7).

If the child is unresponsive and no trauma is suspected, use the head tilt–chin lift maneuver to open the airway. If trauma to the head or neck is suspected, the modified jaw thrust maneuver is the preferred method of opening the airway. Do not hyperextend the neck. Doing so can cause an airway obstruction. To help maintain the proper positioning of the patient's head and neck, you may need to place padding under the torso of an infant or small child. The padding should be firm and evenly shaped and extend from the shoulders to the pelvis. The padding should be thick

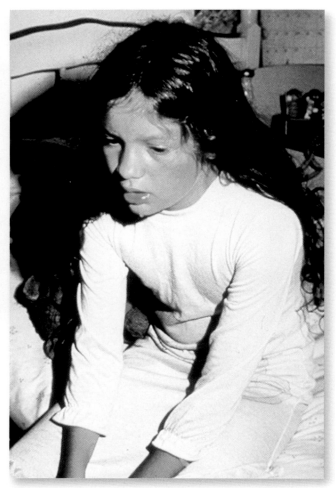

FIGURE 44-7 ▲ In cases of severe respiratory distress, the child may assume a "tripod" position. In this position, the child is seated and leaning forward.

enough so that the child's shoulders are in alignment with the ear canal (Figure 44-8). Using irregularly shaped or insufficient padding or placing padding only under the shoulders can result in movement or misalignment of the spine.

After opening the airway, look in the mouth of every unresponsive child. To do this, open the child's mouth with your gloved hand. Look for an actual or potential airway obstruction, such as a foreign body, blood, vomitus, teeth, or the child's tongue. If you see a foreign body in the child's mouth, attempt to remove it with your gloved fingers. If there is blood, vomitus, or other fluid in the airway, clear it with suctioning.

Clearing the Airway

Depending on the cause of the obstruction, methods you can use to clear the patient's airway include foreign body airway obstruction maneuvers (see Appendix A), the recovery position, finger sweeps, and suctioning.

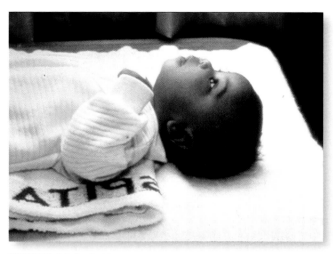

FIGURE 44-8 ▲ To assist in maintaining the proper positioning of the patient's head and neck, it is often necessary to place padding under the torso of an infant or small child.

If the child is unresponsive, uninjured, and breathing adequately, you can place him on his side. In this position, gravity allows fluid to flow from the child's mouth. Do *not* place a child with a known or suspected spinal injury in the recovery position. You must continue to monitor the child until you transfer care to a qualified healthcare professional.

If you *see* foreign material in an unresponsive child's mouth, remove it by using a finger sweep:
- If the child is uninjured, roll her to her side.
- Wipe any liquids from the airway with your index and middle fingers covered with a 4×4-inch gauze pad.
- Remove solid objects that you can see with a gloved finger positioned like a hook. Use your little finger when performing a finger sweep in an infant or child.
- *Remember: Never* perform a blind finger sweep.

Suctioning may be needed to clear the patient's airway. Use a rigid suction catheter to remove secretions from the child's mouth. Remember that the catheter should be inserted into the child's mouth no more deeply than the base of the tongue.

A bulb syringe is used to remove secretions from an infant's mouth or nose (Figure 44-9).

To use a bulb syringe:
- Squeeze the bulb.
- Insert it into the baby's nose.
- Release the bulb.
- Remove the syringe from the infant's nose and empty the contents.

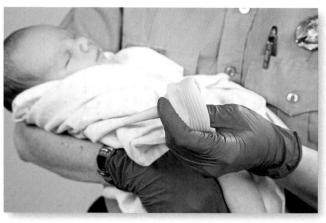

(a)

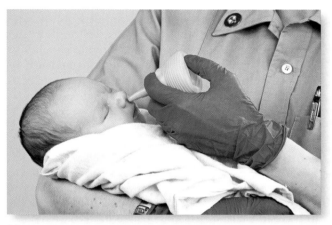

(b)

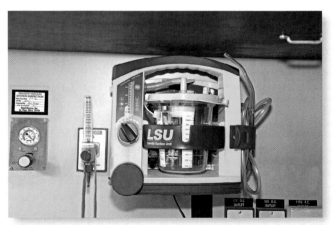

(c)

FIGURE 44-9 ▲ To use a bulb syringe, **(a)** squeeze the bulb. **(b)** Insert it into the baby's nose. Release the bulb. Remove the syringe from the nose and empty the contents. **(c)** A suction unit in the ambulance may be portable so it can be brought to the patient.

If both the mouth and the nose need to be suctioned, always suction the mouth first and then the nose. Gentle suctioning is usually enough to remove secretions.

Do not suction a newborn for more than 3 to 5 seconds per attempt. When suctioning an infant or child, do not apply suction for more than 10 to 15 seconds at a time. The child's heart rate may slow or become irregular because of a lack of oxygen or because the tip of the device stimulates the back of the tongue or throat. If the patient's heart rate slows, stop suctioning and provide ventilation. Give oxygen between each suctioning attempt.

Airway Adjuncts

An oral airway may be used to help keep the airway open in an unresponsive child. Remember that this airway is used only if the patient does not have a gag reflex. If the child gags, coughs, chokes, or spits out the airway, do not use it. A nasal airway may be used to help keep the airway open in an unresponsive or semiresponsive child. Remember to select a device of proper size by aligning the airway on the side of the patient's face and selecting an airway that extends from the tip of the nose to the earlobe. Review the information about oral and nasal airways in Chapter 12 if needed.

B *Is for Breathing*

Is the child breathing? After you have made sure that the child's airway is open, assess her breathing. To do this, you must be able to see her chest or abdomen. Watch and listen to the child as she breathes. Look for the rise and fall of the chest. Does the chest rise and fall equally? Count the child's respiratory rate for 30 seconds. Double this number to determine the breaths per minute. If the breathing is irregular, you should count for a full 60 seconds.

Listen for air movement. To minimize the possibility of sound transmission from one side of the chest to the other, listen under each armpit and in the midclavicular line under each clavicle. Alternate from side to side and compare your findings. Assess breath sounds. Determine if breathing is absent, quiet, or noisy. Stridor is a high-pitched sound that is heard when the upper airway passages are partially blocked. Wheezing is heard when the lower airway passages are narrowed. Wheezing may be present because of swelling, spasm, secretions, or the presence of a foreign body. If air movement is inadequate, wheezing may not be heard. Listen for a change in the child's voice or cry. Hoarseness may be caused by a foreign body or an inflamed upper airway. Look for signs of increased breathing effort, such as nasal flaring (widening of the nostrils), retractions, head bobbing, seesaw respirations, or the use of accessory muscles. Feel for air movement from the child's nose or mouth against your chin, face, or palm.

If breathing is present, quickly determine whether breathing is adequate or inadequate. If the child's breathing is inadequate or absent, you must begin breathing for him immediately. If the chest does not rise, assume the airway is blocked. Depending on the cause of the obstruction, methods you can use to clear the patient's airway include foreign body airway obstruction maneuvers (see Appendix A), the recovery position, finger sweeps, and suctioning. The patient's situation will dictate which technique is most appropriate.

C *Is for Circulation*

Does the child have a pulse? Is severe bleeding present? Note the rate, regularity (rhythm), and quality of the pulse. Pulse regularity normally changes with respirations (increases with inspiration, decreases with expiration). Use the carotid artery to assess the pulse in an unresponsive child older than 1 year of age. Feel for a brachial pulse in an unresponsive infant. Feel for a pulse for about 10 seconds. If there is no pulse, or if a pulse is present but the rate is less than 60 beats/min with signs of shock, you must begin chest compressions.

In infants and children, it is important to compare the pulse of the central blood vessels (such as the femoral artery) with those found in peripheral areas of the body (such as the feet). For example, locate the dorsalis pedis pulse on top of the foot. Then place your other hand in the child's groin area. Compare the strength and rate of the pulses in these areas. They should feel the same. If they do not, a circulatory problem is present. For example, a weak central pulse can be a sign of late shock.

Assess capillary refill in children 6 years of age or younger. To assess capillary refill, firmly press on the child's nail bed until it blanches (turns white) and then release. Observe the time it takes for the tissue to return to its original color. If the temperature of the environment is normal to warm, color should return within 2 seconds. Delayed capillary refill may occur because of shock or hypothermia, among other causes.

Assess blood pressure in children older than 3 years of age. Remember that blood pressure is one of the *least* sensitive indicators of adequate circulation in children. A child may have compromised circulation despite a normal blood pressure. A properly sized cuff must be used to obtain accurate readings. A cuff that is too wide will cause a falsely low reading. A cuff that is too narrow will cause a falsely high reading. The width of the cuff should be about two-thirds the length of the long bone used (such as the upper arm or thigh).

If severe bleeding is present, control it by using direct pressure. Assess the child's skin temperature, color, and moisture. Determine if the skin is warm, hot, or cold; moist or dry; and loose or firm. Hot skin suggests fever or heat exposure. Cool skin suggests inadequate circulation or exposure to cold. Cold skin suggests extreme exposure to cold. Clammy (cool and moist) skin suggests shock, among many other conditions. Wet or moist skin may indicate shock, a heat-related illness, or a diabetic emergency. Excessively dry skin may indicate dehydration. Loose skin over the forehead or sternum may be a sign of dehydration.

Secondary Survey

Objective 2

When performing a secondary survey, remember to assess the patient systematically, placing special emphasis on areas suggested by the chief complaint and present illness. After examining any part of the body, be sure to promptly cover the area to minimize heat loss. Ask a parent or family member to help you lessen the child's anxiety. Assess body areas for DCAP-BTLS. When examining the head, look for bruising and swelling, and assess the fontanels, if present. Use a penlight or flashlight to check the pupils for size, shape, equality, and reactivity. Assess the nose for drainage that might obstruct the patient's ability to breathe through her nose. Examine the ears for drainage suggestive of trauma or infection. Look in the mouth for loose teeth, blood, or other fluids. Note any identifiable odors. Examine the neck for bruising or swelling. If the patient has a fever, note whether she is unable to move her neck and document your findings. Assess the chest and back for bruises, injuries, and rashes. Assess the abdomen for distention, tenderness, seat belt abrasions, or bruising. Examine the extremities for deformity, swelling, or pain on movement. Life-threatening conditions must be managed as soon as they are found. Less critical conditions can be managed as they are found during or after completing the secondary survey.

Common Problems in Infants and Children

Airway Obstruction

Objective 3

There are many causes of an airway obstruction, including:

- Foreign body
- Mucus plug
- Blood or vomitus
- The tongue
- Trauma to the head or neck
- Infection, such as croup or pneumonia

If a child is unable to speak, cry, cough, or make any other sound, his airway is completely obstructed. If the child has noisy breathing, such as snoring or gurgling, he has a partial airway obstruction. A child with a partial airway obstruction and good air exchange is typically alert and sitting up. You may hear stridor or a crowing sound and see retractions when the child breathes in. The child's skin color is usually normal, and a strong pulse is present. You should allow an older child to assume a position of comfort. Assist a younger child in sitting up. Do not allow him to lie down. He may prefer to sit on his caregiver's lap.

Do not agitate the child. If the child has a foreign body in her airway, agitation could cause the object to move into a position that completely blocks the airway. Encourage the child to cough and allow her to continue her efforts to clear her own airway. Continue to watch the child closely.

You will need to intervene if the child has a complete airway obstruction. You will also need to intervene if the child has a partial airway obstruction that is accompanied by any of the following signs of poor air exchange:

- Ineffective cough
- Increased respiratory difficulty accompanied by stridor
- Loss of responsiveness
- Altered mental status

Clear the child's airway by using the techniques described in Appendix A for removal of a foreign body airway obstruction. Reassess as often as indicated. Record all patient care information, including the patient's medical history and all emergency care given, on a prehospital care report.

Respiratory Emergencies

Objectives 4, 5

Respiratory emergencies are the most common medical emergencies encountered in children. There are many causes of respiratory emergencies in children. Some conditions affect the upper airway, some affect the lower airway, and some affect both. Upper airway problems usually occur suddenly. Examples of conditions that affect the upper airway include croup, epiglottitis, and foreign body aspiration. Lower airway problems usually take longer to develop. Examples of conditions that affect the lower airway include asthma, bronchiolitis, pneumonia, and a foreign body obstruction. A patient with an upper airway problem is more likely to worsen during the time you are providing care than one with a lower airway problem. You must watch closely for changes in the patient's condition and adjust your treatment as needed.

There are three levels of severity of respiratory problems: (1) respiratory distress, (2) respiratory failure, and (3) respiratory arrest. Most children will present with either respiratory distress or respiratory failure. *Respiratory distress* is an increased work of breathing (respiratory effort). *Respiratory failure* is a condition in which there is not enough oxygen in the blood and/or ventilation to meet the demands of body tissues. Respiratory failure is evident when the patient becomes tired and can no longer maintain good oxygenation and ventilation. *Respiratory arrest* occurs when a patient stops breathing.

Respiratory distress is associated with several signs that you will be able to spot (see the following *You Should Know* box). These signs reflect an increased work of breathing (respiratory effort). The child works harder than usual to breathe in order to make up for the low level of oxygen in his blood.

You Should Know

Signs of Respiratory Distress

- Fear, irritability, anxiousness, restlessness
- Noisy breathing (stridor, grunting, gurgling, wheezing)
- A breathing rate that is faster than normal for the patient's age
- An increased depth of breathing
- Nasal flaring
- A mild increase in heart rate
- Retractions
- Seesaw respirations (abdominal breathing)
- The use of neck muscles to breathe
- Changes in skin color

Remember This

Give oxygen to *every* infant and child who is experiencing a respiratory problem. There is no medical reason to avoid giving oxygen to an infant or child. Attempts to deliver oxygen should not delay transport.

You will see signs of respiratory failure as the child tires and can no longer maintain good oxygenation and ventilation (see the following *You Should Know* box). A child in respiratory failure looks very sick. The child becomes limp, peripheral pulses become weak, her color worsens, and her heart rate slows down. The breathing rate slows to below 20 breaths/min in an infant and 10 breaths/min in a child. A slow heart rate in a child with respiratory failure is a red flag. Cardiopulmonary arrest will occur soon if the child's oxygenation and ventilation are not corrected quickly.

You Should Know

Signs of Respiratory Failure

- Sleepiness or agitation
- Combativeness
- Limpness (the patient may be unable to sit up without help)
- A breathing rate that is initially fast with periods of slowing and then eventual slowing
- An altered mental status
- A shallow chest rise
- Nasal flaring
- Retractions
- Head bobbing
- Pale, mottled, or bluish skin
- Weak peripheral pulses

Remember This

When providing care for any patient with a respiratory problem, reassess the patient's condition at least every 5 minutes.

You can assist a child with respiratory distress by doing the following:
- Help the child into a position of comfort.
- Reposition his airway for better airflow if necessary.
- Give oxygen.

A child with respiratory distress will usually be most comfortable in a sitting position. Do not place a child in a sitting position if trauma is suspected. The patient with a respiratory condition such as asthma may need assistance using his metered-dose inhaler. Do not agitate a child with respiratory distress. For example, do not excite the child by taking a blood pressure. If the child shows signs of respiratory failure or respiratory arrest, prepare for immediate transport to the closest appropriate facility. Keep on-scene time to a minimum. Request an early response of ALS personnel to the scene, or consider an ALS intercept while en route to the receiving facility. Do not delay transport for ALS arrival.

Assist the child's breathing with a bag-mask device as needed. Deliver each breath over 1 second. Watch for the rise and fall of the patient's chest with each breath. Stop ventilation when you see gentle chest rise. Allow the patient to exhale between breaths. Breathe at a rate of 12 to 20 breaths/min (1 breath every 3 to 5 seconds). If the child does not tolerate a mask, consider using blow-by oxygen (see the following *You Should Know* box). Although not an ideal method of oxygen delivery, blow-by oxygen is better than no oxygen. Be sure to have suction within arm's reach.

You Should Know

Blow-by oxygen refers to blowing oxygen over the face of an infant or child so that the patient breathes oxygen-enriched air. To give blow-by oxygen, connect oxygen tubing to an oxygen source set to at least 5 L/min. Cup your hand around the tubing. Hold the tube close to the patient's nose and mouth. Alternately, insert the oxygen tubing into a paper cup and direct the tubing at the patient's nose and mouth. You can also ask the child's caregiver to hold an oxygen mask near the patient's nose and mouth.

Check the child's pulse every 1 to 2 minutes to see if chest compressions need to be started. Reassess as often as indicated. Record all patient care information, including the patient's medical history and all emergency care given, on a PCR.

Cardiopulmonary Failure

Objective 6

When a person stops breathing, a respiratory arrest occurs. When a person's heart stops, a cardiac arrest occurs. When the heart and lungs stop working, a cardiopulmonary arrest results. When respiratory failure occurs together with shock, **cardiopulmonary failure** results. Cardiopulmonary failure is a combination of inadequate oxygenation, inadequate ventilation, and poor perfusion (Figure 44-10).

In adults, cardiopulmonary failure and arrest are often the result of underlying heart disease. In children, cardiopulmonary failure and arrest are usually the result of an uncorrected respiratory problem. Some illnesses and injuries are associated with a high risk of cardiopulmonary failure:

- Massive traumatic injuries
- Burns
- Severe dehydration
- Severe asthma, reactive airway disease
- Drowning
- An upper airway obstruction
- Prolonged seizure
- Coma

The signs and symptoms of cardiopulmonary failure are shown in the following *You Should Know* box.

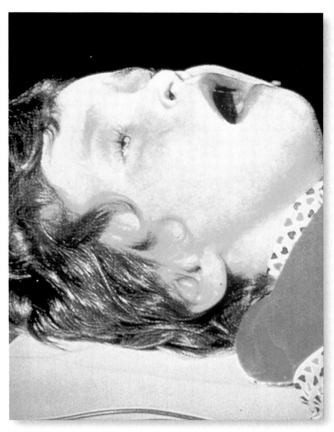

FIGURE 44-10 ▲ Inadequate oxygenation, inadequate ventilation, and poor perfusion can all result in cardiopulmonary failure.

You Should Know

Assessment Findings and Symptoms of Cardiopulmonary Failure

- Mental status changes
- A weak respiratory effort
- Slow, shallow breathing
- Pale, mottled, or bluish skin
- A slow pulse rate
- Weak central pulses and absent peripheral pulses
- Cool extremities
- A delayed capillary refill

Cardiopulmonary failure will progress to cardiopulmonary arrest unless it is recognized and treated promptly. If your patient is showing signs of cardiopulmonary failure, make sure his airway is open. If trauma is suspected, take spinal precautions as necessary. Assist the child's breathing with a bag-mask device. Perform chest compressions if necessary.

Common Problems in Infants and Children ◄ **783**

Altered Mental Status

Objective 7

Altered mental status (also called an *altered level of consciousness,* or *ALOC*) means a change in a patient's level of awareness of her surroundings. For example, a person may be awake and know her name, but she may be unable to answer questions about where she is or what happened to her. In order for you to determine if there has been a change in the patient's behavior, you must find out what the patient's normal behavior is. The patient's caregiver is usually the best person to provide this information. In fact, the child's caregiver is often the person who calls 9-1-1 because he has noticed that the child "isn't acting right." A pediatric patient with an altered mental status may appear agitated, combative, sleepy, difficult to awaken, or unresponsive.

There are many causes of altered mental status. The most common causes in a pediatric patient are a low level of oxygen in the blood, head trauma, seizures, infection, low blood sugar, and drug or alcohol ingestion.

You Should Know

Causes of Altered Mental Status (AEIOU-TIPPS)

- Alcohol, abuse
- Epilepsy (seizures)
- Insulin (diabetic emergency)
- Overdose, (lack of) oxygen (hypoxia)
- Uremia (kidney failure)
- Trauma (head injury), temperature (fever, heat- or cold-related emergency)
- Infection
- Psychiatric conditions
- Poisoning (including drugs and alcohol)
- Shock, stroke

Any patient with an altered mental status is in danger of an airway obstruction. The patient may lose the ability to keep his own airway open because the soft tissues of the airway and the base of the tongue relax. The tongue falls into the back of the throat, blocking the airway. The patient may also have depressed gag and cough reflexes. A blocked airway can result in low blood oxygen levels, respiratory failure, or respiratory arrest. A pulse oximeter should be routinely used and continuously monitored for any infant or child who has an altered mental status. Many causes of an altered mental status may be associated with vomiting. Be prepared to clear the patient's airway with suctioning. Anticipate the need to place the patient in the recovery position (if no trauma is suspected).

If the equipment is available, check the child's blood glucose level. If the child's glucose level is low, notify medical direction. Give oral glucose if appropriate and if ordered by medical direction. Remember that your patient must be awake, with an intact gag reflex. Remember to comfort, calm, and reassure the patient. Reassess as often as indicated. Record all patient care information, including the patient's medical history and all emergency care given, on a PCR.

Shock

Objective 8

Common causes of shock in infants and children include diarrhea and dehydration, trauma, vomiting, blood loss, infection, and abdominal injuries. Less common causes of shock include allergic reactions, poisoning, and cardiac disorders. Shock rarely results from a primary cardiac problem in infants and children. Signs and symptoms of shock are shown in the following *You Should Know* box.

You Should Know

Assessment Findings and Symptoms of Shock in Infants and Children

- Rapid respiratory rate
- Pale, cool, clammy skin
- Weak or absent peripheral pulses
- Delayed capillary refill
- Decreased urine output (determined by asking the caregiver about diaper wetting and looking at the child's diaper)
- Mental status changes
- Absence of tears, even when crying

Remember that infants and children in shock can maintain a normal blood pressure for some time. By the time their blood pressure drops, they are close to death.

Emergency care for an infant or child in shock includes making sure the patient's airway is open and giving oxygen. Request an early response of ALS personnel to the scene, or consider an ALS intercept while en route to the receiving facility. Do not delay transport for ALS arrival. If the patient's breathing is adequate, give oxygen at 15 L/min by nonrebreather mask. If breathing is inadequate, provide positive-pressure ventilation with 100% oxygen. Assess the adequacy of the ventilations delivered. Because of a child's small blood volume, you must quickly control any bleeding, if present. If the child is experiencing anaphylaxis, contact medical direction and request an order to administer epinephrine, or assist the patient with his own autoinjector.

Keep the patient warm and transport rapidly to the closest appropriate facility. Reassess every 5 minutes. Record all patient care information, including the patient's medical history and all emergency care given, on a PCR.

Fever

Objective 9

Fever is a common reason for infant or child calls. Elevated body temperature may be caused by:

- Infection or inflammation
- Heat exposure
- Certain poisonings, such as aspirin
- Severe dehydration
- Uncontrolled seizures

Seizures are common in children. Seizures from fever are most common in children under the age of 5. It is the rapid rise of the child's temperature in a short period—not how high the temperature is—that causes the seizure.

Meningitis is an inflammation of the meninges, the membranes covering the brain and spinal cord. It may be caused by a virus (most common cause), fungus, or bacteria. In children more than 2 years of age, common signs and symptoms include a high fever, headache, and stiff neck. These findings may develop over several hours (less common) or 1 to 2 days (more common). Fever, headache, and neck stiffness may not be present in newborns and young infants (less than 2 to 3 months). Signs and symptoms in newborns and young infants may include poor feeding, decreased activity, and irritability. A bulging fontanel or high-pitched cry may also be present. One form of meningitis (meningococcal meningitis) is potentially life-threatening when the organism that causes it enters the bloodstream. A fever and reddish-purple rash are present in more than half the patients who develop this form of meningitis (Figure 44-11).

Emergency care for an infant or child with a fever includes the following steps:

- Remember to use appropriate PPE. Position the child so that you can maintain an open airway.

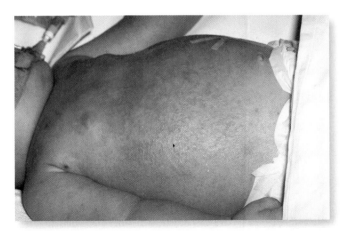

FIGURE 44-11 ▲ A life-threatening form of meningitis is associated with a fever and reddish-purple rash.

- Remove excess clothing.
- Be alert for seizures. Treat for shock if indicated.
- If instructed to begin cooling measures by medical direction, sponge the child with lukewarm water. Do not use cold or ice water or alcohol to cool the child. Ice or cold water baths cause shivering, which is the body's way of generating heat. Alcohol is not used because it can be absorbed through the skin, causing poisoning. Alcohol can also cause very rapid cooling.
- Transport the child for physician evaluation. Reassess as often as indicated. Record all patient care information, including the patient's medical history and all emergency care given, on a PCR.

Seizures

Objective 10

A seizure is a temporary change in behavior or consciousness caused by abnormal electrical activity in one or more groups of brain cells. **Status epilepticus** is recurring seizures without an intervening period of consciousness. Status epilepticus is a medical emergency that can cause brain damage or death if it is not treated.

Many conditions can cause seizures, but sometimes the cause is unknown. It is not necessary for you to determine the cause of a seizure in order to manage a patient who is having one.

You Should Know

Known Causes of Seizures

- A low blood oxygen level
- Low blood sugar
- Brain tumor
- Poisoning
- Head injury
- Previous brain damage
- Seizure disorder
- Fever
- Infection
- An abnormal heart rhythm
- Inherited factors

Seizures generally last about 30 to 45 seconds but can continue for several minutes. During the seizure, the child may have an altered mental status, changes in behavior, uncontrolled muscle movements, and a loss of bowel or bladder control. Depending on its severity, injuries can occur during a seizure. Injuries may include biting of the tongue or cheek, injury to the head, bruises, and broken bones.

When you arrive on the scene, perform a scene size-up before starting emergency medical care. If the scene is safe, approach the child and perform a primary survey. Complete a physical exam as needed. Important assessment findings that can help explain the cause of the seizure include a purplish skin rash, signs of a head injury, or hot skin. The child's arms and/or legs may show signs of trauma from muscle movements during the seizure.

It is most likely that once you have arrived, the seizure will be over. Obtaining a good history is very important when treating these patients. Examples of questions to ask the child's caregiver are listed in the following *Making a Difference* box.

Making a Difference

Questions to Ask About a Seizure

- Is this the child's first seizure?
- If the child has a history of seizures, is he taking a seizure medication? Was this the child's normal seizure pattern? If not, how did it differ?
- What did the caregiver do for the child during the seizure?
- Could the child have ingested any medications, household products, or any potentially toxic item?
- How long did the seizure last?
- Does the child have a fever?
- Does the child have a history of diabetes (possible low blood sugar)?

If the patient is actively seizing when you arrive, look to see if she has bitten her tongue or hit her head during the seizure. If you witness the seizure, you will need to be able to describe what it looked like when transferring patient care. Important information includes how long the seizure lasted and if the seizure involved full body jerking or movement of only an arm or a leg. Note if the child lost bladder or bowel control. If the seizure has stopped, look for clues to the cause. Check for medical jewelry. Look for evidence of burns or suspicious substances that might indicate poisoning or a toxic exposure. Are there signs of recent trauma? If the equipment is available, check the child's blood glucose level. If the child's glucose level is low, notify medical direction.

Comfort, calm, and reassure the patient while he is in your care. Protect the patient's privacy. Ask bystanders (except the caregiver) to leave the area. During the seizure, protect the child from harm by moving hard or sharp objects out of the way. Never attempt to restrain a child having a seizure. Do not put anything in the patient's mouth. Make sure that suction is available because the child may vomit during or after the seizure.

As soon as the seizure is over, make sure the child's airway is clear. Gently suction the child's mouth if secretions are present. Place the child in the recovery position if there is no possibility of spinal trauma. Loosen tight clothing. Give oxygen by nonrebreather mask. Use blow-by oxygen if necessary. If the child's skin appears blue, assist her breathing with a bag-mask device. If the child's skin is hot and she is bundled in blankets, remove the blankets.

The period after a seizure is called the **postictal phase.** During this recovery period, the child often appears limp, has shallow breathing, and has an altered mental status. This altered mental status may appear as confusion, sleepiness, combativeness, memory loss, unresponsiveness, or difficulty talking. The postictal phase may last minutes to hours.

In most cases, the child should be transported to the hospital without using flashing lights and siren. Flashing lights can cause seizures or agitation in susceptible patients. However, if the patient's condition is critical (such as status epilepticus), use lights and siren as needed. Reassess as often as indicated. Record all patient care information, including the patient's medical history and all emergency care given, on a PCR.

Poisonings

Objective 11

Exposure to toxins can happen by eating and drinking, inhaling, absorption through the skin, injection into the body by needle, or bites and stings. Many calls involving a pediatric poisoning become very emotional. You will need to calm the situation, find out what the exposure was, and contact your local poison control center (PCC) at 1-800-222-1222 (the national PCC number). Ask questions using "who, what, where, when, why, and how" to find out what the child was exposed to (see Chapter 28). Keep in mind that trying to find an antidote for a specific poison is not necessary.

Emergency care for an infant or child toxic exposure includes the following steps:

- Use appropriate protection, or have trained rescuers remove the patient from the poisonous environment. Call for additional resources if needed.
- Follow proper decontamination procedures, if necessary, and prepare the ambulance to receive the patient. Methods used for decontamination will depend on the toxin and type of exposure. Call a poison center for advice, as needed, about decontamination procedures and patient care.

- Establish and maintain an open airway. If a child is found unresponsive or trauma is suspected, remember to consider the possibility of spinal injury and take appropriate precautions as needed. Use gloves to remove pills, tablets, or fragments from the patient's mouth, as needed, without injuring yourself. Be alert for vomiting, and have suction within arm's reach.

- Give oxygen. If the child's breathing is adequate, apply oxygen by nonrebreather mask. If the patient's breathing is inadequate, provide positive-pressure ventilation with 100% oxygen. If the child will not tolerate a mask, give blow-by oxygen.

- If the patient has ingested a poison (and is awake), consult medical direction about giving activated charcoal. If the patient is unresponsive or seizing, consult medical direction about checking the child's blood sugar.

- If possible, bring all containers, bottles, labels, and other evidence of suspected poisons to the receiving facility. If the child vomits, save the vomitus in a container (such as a portable suction unit) and transport it to the receiving facility for analysis.

- Anticipate complications, including seizures, vomiting, shock, agitation, and an irregular heart rhythm. Reassess as often as indicated. Record all patient care information, including the patient's medical history and all emergency care given, on a PCR.

Making a Difference

Keep in mind that your line of questioning should not take an accusatory tone. Often, "Why?" questions are misinterpreted as accusations toward the child's caregiver, when most poisonings are accidental. The parents or caregivers are already feeling quite guilty, and any untoward comments made by you or other healthcare professionals at the scene will likely cause further grief for the person responsible for the safety of the child.

Drowning

Objective 12

When you are called to the scene of a possible drowning, first study the scene and determine if approaching the patient is safe. Evaluate the mechanism of injury, and determine (if possible) the length of submersion, cleanliness of the water, and temperature of the water. If needed, call for additional help *before* contact with the patient. Perform a primary survey, and determine

the presence of life-threatening conditions. Stabilize the patient's spine as needed.

Signs and symptoms of drowning will vary depending on the type and length of submersion. Possible signs and symptoms are shown in the next *You Should Know* box. Assess baseline vital signs. Perform a physical examination, carefully assessing the patient for other injuries. Determine the events leading to the present situation. Absence of adult supervision is a factor in most submersion incidents involving infants and children. Questions to ask the caregiver include:

- How long was the child submerged?
- What was the water temperature?
- Where did the incident occur (for example, lake, pool, bathtub, toilet, bucket)?
- Was the child breathing when removed from the water?
- Was there a pulse?
- Did the child experience any loss of consciousness?
- Was the incident witnessed? (This information is useful in determining possible head or spinal injury.)
- Does the child have any significant medical problems?
- Are there any signs of abuse or neglect?

You Should Know

Assessment Findings and Symptoms of Drowning

- Altered mental status, seizures, unresponsiveness
- Coughing, vomiting, choking, or airway obstruction
- Absent or inadequate breathing
- Difficulty breathing
- Fast, slow, or absent pulse
- Cool, clammy, and pale or cyanotic skin
- Vomiting
- Possible abdominal distention

Emergency care for a drowning victim includes ensuring the safety of all rescue personnel. Remove the patient from the water as quickly and safely as possible. Keep on-scene time to a minimum. Request an early response of ALS personnel to the scene, or consider an ALS intercept while en route to the receiving facility. Do not delay transport for ALS arrival. Protect the patient from environmental temperature extremes. Suction the patient's airway as needed. Give oxygen. If breathing is adequate, administer oxygen at 10 to 15 L/min by nonrebreather mask. If breathing is inadequate, provide positive-pressure ventilation with 100% oxygen. Assess the adequacy of the ventilations delivered. Remove wet clothing and dry the patient to prevent heat loss. If trauma is not suspected, place the patient in the recovery position to assist gravity in draining secretions from the patient's airway.

If the patient is unresponsive, is not breathing, and has no pulse or has a pulse rate of less than 60 beats/min with signs of shock, begin CPR once the patient has been removed from the water. If the child has no pulse, attach an automated external defibrillator (AED). Make sure the patient has been dried off before you operate the AED. To avoid electrical injury, take extra precautions to ensure that no one around the patient is in contact with the patient and water or metal during defibrillation.

All drowning victims should be transported to the hospital. Reassess as often as indicated. Record all patient care information, including the patient's medical history and all emergency care given, on a PCR.

Sudden Infant Death Syndrome

Objective 13

The National Institute of Child Health and Human Development defines **sudden infant death syndrome (SIDS)** as "the sudden and unexpected death of an infant that remains unexplained after a thorough case investigation, including performance of a complete autopsy, examination of the death scene, and review of the clinical history."

About 90% of all SIDS deaths occur during the first 6 months of life. Most deaths occur between the ages of 2 and 4 months. SIDS occurs in apparently healthy infants. Boys are affected more often than girls. Most SIDS deaths occur at home, usually during the night after a period of sleep. The baby is most often discovered in the early morning.

The cause of SIDS is not clearly understood. Research is ongoing. The number of SIDS deaths has decreased significantly since 1992 when caregivers were first told that infants should sleep on their backs and sides rather than on their stomachs. SIDS can b diagnosed only by autopsy.

Although not present in all cases, common SIL physical exam findings include an unresponsive bal who is not breathing and has no pulse. The skin ofte.. appears blue or mottled. You may see frothy sputum or vomitus around the mouth and nose. The underside of the baby's body may look dark and bruised because of pooled blood (dependent lividity). General stiffening of the body (rigor mortis) may be present.

The National Institute of Health defines an **apparent life-threatening event (ALTE)** as a sudden event,

frightening to the observer, in which the infant exhibits a combination of symptoms, including apnea, change in color (pallor, redness, cyanosis, plethora), change in muscle tone (floppiness, rigidity), choking, gagging, or coughing.

Unless signs of obvious death are present, you should begin resuscitation according to your local protocols. Rigor mortis is an obvious sign of death. Dependent lividity is considered an obvious sign of death only when there are extensive areas of reddish-purple discoloration of the skin on the underside of the body of an unresponsive, breathless, and pulseless patient. In some EMS systems, both lividity and rigor mortis must be present to be considered signs of obvious death. Check with your instructor about your local protocols regarding obvious death.

Whether or not resuscitation is performed, you must find out about the events leading up to the call for help. Ask questions as tactfully as possible. Start by asking the caregiver the baby's name, and use that name when referring to the baby. Carefully document what you see at the scene and the caregiver's responses to your questions.

Provide emotional support for the baby's caregiver. The caregiver will usually be very distressed. You may observe crying, screaming, yelling, a stony silence, or physical outbursts. The caregiver's feelings of guilt are often enormous.

If the infant is obviously dead, you will need to tell the caregiver. While speaking slowly and quietly, begin by saying, "This is hard to tell you, but…" Explain that the baby is dead. Use the words "dead" or "death." Do not use phrases such as "passed on" or "no longer with us." Explain that there was nothing the caregiver could have done to prevent the baby's death. Before leaving the scene, make sure a friend, relative, member of the clergy, or grief support personnel are available to provide grief support for the family. Remain with the family until law enforcement personnel assume responsibility for the body and grief support personnel are on the scene.

After the call, make sure to assess your own emotional needs. It may be helpful for you and other personnel involved in the call to discuss the feelings that normally follow the death of an infant or child.

On the Scene   Wrap-Up

You apply an oxygen mask to your small patient while calmly reassuring her that it will help her. You quickly assess her, contact medical direction, and then begin assisting her with her prescribed metered-dose inhaler. Within a few minutes of starting the drug, her breathing is improving, but her wheezing is still significant. You secure the patient in the ambulance and reassess her every 5 minutes during the 30-mile trip to the hospital. ∎

► Children are not small adults. Children have unique physical, mental, emotional, and developmental characteristics that you must consider when assessing and caring for them.

► Before responding to any call involving an infant or child, it is essential to know where pediatric equipment is located in your emergency bags. It is not appropriate to search for age-appropriate equipment for the first time at an emergency scene.

► While en route to a call involving an infant or child, think about age-appropriate vital signs and anticipated developmental stage based on the dispatch information given. If you have this information stored on a note card or in a pocket guide, locate it en route to the call and have it readily accessible (such as attached to your clipboard).

► Communicating with scared, concerned parents and family is an important aspect of your responsibilities at the scene of an ill infant or child. Be professional and compassionate, and remember to include them while providing care to their loved one.

► Your assessment of an infant or child should begin "across the room." When forming a general impression of an infant or child, look at his appearance, breathing, and circulation. Quickly determine if the child appears sick or not sick.

► Once your general impression is complete, perform a hands-on ABCDE assessment to determine if life-threatening conditions are present. In a responsive infant or child, use a toes-to-head or trunk-to-head approach. This approach should help reduce the infant's or child's anxiety.

► If a child is unable to speak, cry, cough, or make any other sound, her airway is completely obstructed. If the child has noisy breathing, such as snoring or gurgling, she has a partial airway obstruction. You will need to intervene if the child has a complete airway obstruction.

► In children, pulse regularity normally changes with respirations (increases with inspiration, decreases with expiration).

► Use the carotid artery to assess the pulse in an unresponsive child older than 1 year of age. Feel for a brachial pulse in an unresponsive infant. Feel for a pulse for about 10 seconds. If there is no pulse, or if a pulse is present but the rate is less than 60 beats/min with signs of shock, you must begin chest compressions.

► In infants and children, it is important to compare the pulse of the central blood vessels (such as the femoral artery) with those found in peripheral areas of the body (such as the feet). They should feel the same. If they do not, a circulatory problem is present.

► Assess capillary refill in children 6 years of age or younger. Delayed capillary refill may occur because of shock or hypothermia, among other causes.

► Assess blood pressure in children older than 3 years of age. In children 1 to 10 years of age, the following formula may be used to determine the lower limit of a normal systolic blood pressure: 70 + (2 × child's age in years) = systolic blood pressure. The lower limit of normal systolic blood pressure for a child 10 or more years of age is 90 mm Hg. The diastolic blood pressure should be about two-thirds the systolic pressure.

► The most common medical emergencies in children are respiratory emergencies. Upper airway problems usually occur suddenly. Lower airway problems usually take longer to develop. Respiratory distress is an increased work of breathing (respiratory effort). Respiratory failure is a condition in which there is not enough oxygen in the blood and/or ventilation to meet the demands of body tissues. Respiratory failure becomes evident when the patient becomes tired and can no longer maintain good oxygenation and ventilation. Respiratory arrest occurs when a patient stops breathing.

► Cardiopulmonary arrest results when the heart and lungs stop working. When respiratory failure occurs together with shock, cardiopulmonary failure results. Cardiopulmonary failure will progress to cardiopulmonary arrest unless it is recognized and treated promptly.

► The most common causes of an altered mental status in a pediatric patient are a low level of oxygen in the blood, head trauma, seizures, infection, low blood sugar, and drug or alcohol ingestion. Any patient with an altered mental status is in danger of an airway obstruction. Be prepared to clear the patient's airway with suctioning.

► Shock rarely results from a primary cardiac problem in infants and children. Common causes of shock in infants and children include diarrhea and dehydration, trauma, vomiting, blood loss, infection, and abdominal injuries.

► Seizures from fever are most common in children younger than the age of 5. It is the rapid rise of the child's temperature in a short period—not how high the temperature is—that causes the seizure.

► Meningitis is an inflammation of the meninges, the membranes covering the brain and spinal cord. It may be caused by a virus (most common cause), fungus, or bacteria. One form of meningitis is potentially life-threatening when the organism that causes it enters the bloodstream. A fever and reddish-purple rash are present in more than half the patients who develop this form of meningitis.

- A seizure is a temporary change in behavior or consciousness caused by abnormal electrical activity in one or more groups of brain cells. Status epilepticus is recurring seizures without an intervening period of consciousness. Status epilepticus is a medical emergency that can cause brain damage or death if it is not treated.

- Many calls involving a pediatric poisoning become very emotional. You will need to calm the situation, find out what the exposure was, and contact your local poison control center.

- Absence of adult supervision is a factor in most submersion incidents involving infants and children. Signs and symptoms of drowning will vary depending on the type and length of submersion. All drowning victims should be transported to the hospital.

- Sudden infant death syndrome is the sudden and unexpected death of an infant that remains unexplained after a thorough case investigation, including performance of a complete autopsy, examination of the death scene, and review of the clinical history. The cause of SIDS is not clearly understood.

- An apparent life-threatening event is a sudden event, frightening to the observer, in which the infant exhibits a combination of symptoms, including apnea, change in color (such as pallor, redness, or cyanosis), change in muscle tone (such as floppiness or rigidity), choking, gagging, or coughing.

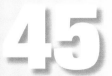
Older Adults

By the end of this chapter, you should be able to:

Knowledge Objectives ▶

1. Describe assessment of the older adult.
2. Discuss techniques that should be used to enhance communication with an older adult.
3. Describe cardiovascular system changes that occur in older adults.
4. Describe respiratory system changes that occur in older adults.
5. Describe nervous system changes that occur in older adults.
6. Differentiate between delirium and dementia.
7. Describe gastrointestinal system changes that occur in older adults.
8. Describe genitourinary system changes that occur in older adults.
9. Describe metabolic and endocrine disorders that occur in older adults.
10. Describe musculoskeletal system changes that occur in older adults.
11. Describe toxicological emergencies in older adults.
12. Describe the sensory changes that occur in older adults.

Attitude Objectives ▶

There are no attitude objectives identified for this lesson.

Skill Objectives ▶

13. Demonstrate the ability to take a relevant history from an older adult.
14. Demonstrate the ability to perform a physical assessment on an older adult.
15. Demonstrate completing a prehospital care report for an older adult.

On the Scene

It is a beautiful spring day, and you are enjoying a great round of golf at a local course when you notice the foursome ahead of you start waving and hollering for assistance. As you run forward to render help, you observe an 80-year-old man seated on the passenger side of a golf cart. This man, the patient, is a member of the foursome and tells you that he is not feeling well. You quickly confirm that one of his friends has already called 9-1-1 and then turn to the patient to begin providing emergency care. ■

THINK ABOUT IT

As you read this chapter, think about the following questions:

- What changes occur with the aging process that may change the way you interview or interact with this patient?
- How does your knowledge of the aging process alter the care you provide to an older adult?

Introduction

The term *elderly* refers to persons 65 years of age and older. The number of adults age 65 years and older grew from 3.1 million in 1900 to 35 million in 2000. It is projected that this age group will increase to almost 71.5 million by 2030. Elderly people are rapidly becoming the largest group of patients who are encountered in the prehospital setting.

Because of the advances in medical technology and treatment, patients are living longer with diseases that were once terminal or required prolonged hospitalization. This has resulted in prehospital professionals dealing with patients who have increased medical needs. Many older adults have at least one chronic medical condition. Some have multiple medical conditions, such as high blood pressure, heart disease, and arthritis. Many of them are on multiple medications. Some may be technology-dependent. Technology-dependent patients have special healthcare needs. These patients depend on medical devices for their survival. Although some older adults have multiple medical conditions, do not assume that every older adult will have age-related health problems. Many elderly patients are healthy and active even into their later years (Figure 45-1).

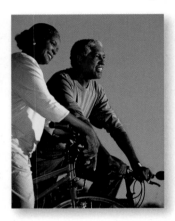

FIGURE 45-1 ▲ Many older people remain healthy and active.

FIGURE 45-2 ▶ Note the position and location of the patient to help determine the cause of the fall.

Assessment of the Older Adult

Objectives 1, 2

The physiologic, cognitive, and psychosocial characteristics of an older adult were discussed in Chapter 8 and should be reviewed if needed. On arrival at the scene, evaluate the scene for safety threats to yourself, your crew, the patient, and others. Survey the patient's environment for clues to the cause of the emergency. Note any hazards or potential hazards. Make a note of the position and location in which the patient is found (Figure 45-2). Determine if you need additional resources before approaching the patient.

Making a Difference

As many as 20% of older adults who seek emergency care are malnourished. The physical signs of malnutrition are not always easy to spot. While you are in a patient's home, take a moment to look around you. Does the patient have adequate food in the house? Is he able to prepare food for himself? Also look for hazards in the home that can contribute to falls, such as extension cords, loose rugs, slick or wet floors, inadequate lighting, a lack of stair or bath rails, and uneven flooring. Be sure to let appropriate personnel within your organization and/or at the receiving facility know your findings.

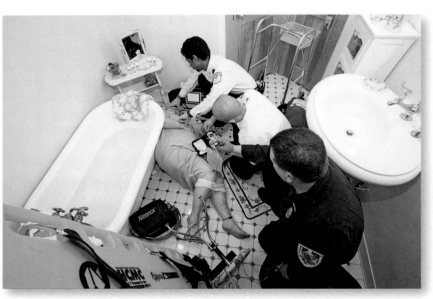

Assessment of an older adult should be approached in the same systematic manner as all other patients. Begin by forming a general impression of the patient from across the room.

- *Appearance.* Is the patient awake and alert? Is she aware of your presence? Does she appear agitated or irritable? Does she appear confused or combative? Does the patient appear well groomed or does she have unkempt hair or soiled clothing? Poor personal grooming can be a sign of an inability to care for oneself, caregiver neglect, and/or depression. If the patient appears unresponsive, proceed immediately to the hands-on assessment.

- *(Work of) breathing.* What is the patient's position? Is he sitting up, lying down, or leaning forward? Does his breathing seem effortless, or is it obvious that he is having breathing difficulty? If the patient appears to be struggling to breathe, has noisy breathing, moves his chest abnormally, or has a rate of breathing that is faster or slower than normal, proceed immediately to the hands-on assessment.

- *Circulation.* Look at the patient's skin color. Is it pink, pale, mottled, flushed, or blue? Do you see any bleeding? If the patient's skin looks pale, mottled, flushed, gray, or blue, proceed immediately to the hands-on assessment.

Next, perform a hands-on assessment to locate and treat any life threats. Assess the patient's airway and level of responsiveness. Assessment of a patient's airway and level of responsiveness occur at the same time. Is the patient awake and alert? If the patient is not alert, try to find out from a family member or caregiver what the patient's normal mental status is. Before deciding that a patient is confused, take a moment to determine if the questions that you routinely ask are appropriate. For example, it is easy for older adults who are no longer working to lose track of time. This is particularly common if the patient is living in an assisted living facility or nursing home. When assessing mental status, an older adult may not know the specific date or even the day of the week, but should be able to tell you if it is morning, noon, or night.

If you suspect trauma to the head, neck, or back or if the patient is unresponsive with an unknown nature of illness, take spinal precautions. Remember that extra padding on a backboard may be necessary to accommodate the anatomic changes that occur in older adults.

Is the patient's airway open? If the patient is unresponsive, it may be difficult to assess and manage the airway due to neck arthritis. If dentures are present and fit well, they should not be removed if bag-mask ventilation is needed because the dentures will help form a good face-to-mask seal. However, ill-fitting dentures increase the risk of an airway obstruction and should be removed.

Difficulty breathing is one of the most common complaints for which an older adult seeks emergency care. When evaluating breathing, keep in mind that the underlying cause of breathing difficulty in an older adult may not be limited to a respiratory system problem. In some patients, difficulty breathing may be the only symptom of a heart attack. As with all patients, quickly determine if breathing is adequate or inadequate. Assess the patient's respiratory rate and work of breathing. Look for equal rise and fall of the chest. Listen to lung sounds. If the patient's breathing is inadequate or absent, begin bag-mask ventilation immediately.

Remember This

Older adults may not show severe symptoms, even if they are very ill.

Assess the patient's pulse and skin and look for signs of obvious bleeding. Note the rate, regularity (rhythm), and quality of the pulse. Remember that an irregular pulse due to heart rhythm problems is common in older adults. Peripheral and central pulses should be assessed simultaneously to determine a comparison of volume and strength.

If the patient's condition appears stable, proceed with a secondary survey, obtaining vital signs and the patient's medical history. When taking vital signs and moving the patient, handle the patient gently as his skin is fragile and can easily tear.

While communicating with the patient, face the patient and speak slowly, clearly, and respectfully at the patient's eye level. Make sure that lighting is adequate to enable the patient to see your face and lips when speaking to her. Locate the patient's hearing aid or eyeglasses if needed. Speak to the patient first rather than to family or others. After asking a question, give the patient ample time to respond unless her condition appears urgent. Your verbal and nonverbal communication should reflect concern and empathy. When a patient has multiple complaints, pay attention to those that indicate a new or changed symptom. The patient's caregiver, family, and friends should be used as needed to obtain answers to the questions you seek.

An older adult may not tell you about important symptoms because she is afraid of being hospitalized. She may be afraid that once she is at the hospital, she will never come home or she may not be able to make decisions about her care. Try to reassure the patient that she will receive the best of care from the hospital. It is extremely important to acknowledge these fears, as they are often justified concerns. You have a greater chance of successfully transporting your patient for appropriate care if you simply listen with empathy to her concerns and carefully explain what you will be doing and what the patient can anticipate at the hospital. Often, encouraging a loved one to meet you at the hospital will help diffuse fears of loss of control.

Comfort, calm, and reassure the patient while he is in your care. Reassess often because an older adult's condition may deteriorate quickly.

Making a Difference

Older adults are sometimes mislabeled as "confused" or "senile" when they do not answer a question but the patient's reason for not answering is impaired hearing or a healthcare professional who simply does not allow the patient sufficient time to respond to the question.

Common Health Problems in Older Adults

Cardiovascular System

Objective 3

Coronary artery disease is the leading cause of death and disability in persons aged 65 years and older. The frequency of sudden cardiac death as the initial sign of coronary artery disease increases with age. Cardiovascular changes that occur in older adults are shown in the following *You Should Know* box.

You Should Know

Cardiovascular System Changes in Older Adults
- Thickening of the blood vessels
- Decreased blood vessel elasticity
- Increased peripheral vascular resistance
- Reduced blood flow to organs
- Hardening and thickening of heart valves
- Degeneration of the conduction system
- Increased blood pressure
- Decreased stroke volume
- Decreased cardiac output
- Abnormal heart rhythms

An older adult who is experiencing an acute coronary syndrome may not show the same assessment findings and symptoms as a younger person. His signs and symptoms are often vague and can be masked by other diseases. Examples of atypical signs and symptoms are shown in the following *You Should Know* box. Signs and symptoms of acute coronary syndromes in women are also atypical and often include shortness of breath and upper abdominal discomfort. Assess the patient's pulse, respirations, blood pressure, and oxygen saturation.

You Should Know

Atypical Assessment Findings and Symptoms of Acute Coronary Syndromes
- Unexplained new onset or worsened difficulty breathing with exertion
- Unexplained nausea, vomiting
- Sweating
- Unexplained tiredness
- Change in mental status
- Weakness
- Fainting
- Abdominal discomfort
- Numbness or tingling in one or both upper extremities

Allow the patient to assume a position of comfort. Do not allow the patient to perform activities that require exertion, such as walking to the stretcher. Give 100% oxygen, preferably by nonrebreather mask. If the patient's breathing is inadequate, give positive-pressure ventilation with 100% oxygen. If ordered by medical direction (and there are no contraindications), aspirin should be given as soon as possible after the patient's onset of chest discomfort. If the patient has prescribed nitroglycerin, contact medical direction, and if instructed to do so, assist the patient with its use. Reassess the patient's vital signs after *each dose* of nitroglycerin. Continue providing supportive care until patient care is transferred to ALS personnel or medical personnel at the receiving facility.

Heart failure is a common condition in older adults. When the left ventricle fails as a pump, blood backs up into the lungs (pulmonary edema). The patient may be anxious and restless and experience mental status changes secondary to hypoxia. The patient is often short of breath with exertion and may experience orthopnea and paroxysmal nocturnal dyspnea. He may have a cough that produces frothy sputum that is sometimes blood-tinged. Lung sounds typically reveal crackles and wheezes. Accessory muscles are often used to improve breathing. The patient often complains of fatigue and recent weight gain. His pulse is usually rapid and may be irregular.

When the right ventricle fails, blood returning to the heart backs up and causes congestion in the organs and tissues of the body. Swelling of the feet and ankles and distention of the jugular veins are usually present.

The patient typically complains of weakness, recent weight gain, nausea, and may complain of abdominal discomfort.

Place the patient in a sitting position, and administer 100% oxygen. If the patient cannot tolerate a nonrebreather mask but her breathing is adequate, try using a nasal cannula. Patients with heart failure will often tell you that they feel like they are smothering when a nonrebreather mask is put on their face. If the patient's breathing is inadequate, you will need to assist her breathing with a bag-mask device. Provide calm reassurance to help reduce the patient's anxiety. Reassess as often as indicated until patient care is transferred. Record all patient care information on a prehospital care report.

Respiratory System

Objective 4

Respiratory system changes that occur in older adults are shown in the following *You Should Know* box. Asthma and chronic obstructive pulmonary disease (COPD) are common in older adults. In fact, the death rate from asthma has increased most significantly in those aged 65 or older. It has been speculated that one possible explanation for this is the patient's decreased awareness of bronchoconstriction and delays in seeking medical attention.

You Should Know

Respiratory System Changes in Older Adults

- Diminished elasticity of the diaphragm
- Decreased strength in chest wall and accessory muscles
- Decreased cough reflex, ineffective coughing
- Decreased number of alveoli that participate in gas exchange
- Reduction in oxygen and carbon dioxide exchange
- Decreased activity of cilia in the lungs, which increases susceptibility to infection
- Inability to increase rate of respiratory effort

The patient with asthma typically presents with tightness in the chest, dyspnea, wheezing, retractions, and coughing. Cyanosis and an absence of wheezing may be present in severe attacks. The patient with COPD generally presents with coughing and shortness of breath on exertion that is often accompanied by wheezing.

More than 50% of all pneumonia cases occur in individuals 65 years of age and older. Possible risk factors include institutionalization, chronic disease processes, immune system compromise, COPD, cancer, inhaled toxins, and aspiration. Typical symptoms of pneumonia include gradual onset, cough productive of sputum,

shortness of breath with or without fever, fatigue, loss of appetite, headache, nausea and vomiting, musculoskeletal pain, weight loss, confusion, and tightness in the chest. Your assessment findings may reveal changes in the patient's circulation; cyanosis and pallor; dry skin; fever; poor skin turgor; pale, dry mucous membranes; furrowed tongue; tachycardia; diminished breath sounds with wheezing, crackles, or rhonchi; and hypotension.

A pulmonary embolism is the sudden blockage of a branch of the pulmonary artery by a venous clot. Experts say that the incidence of a pulmonary embolism triples between the ages of 65 and 90. The patient is often anxious and complains of a sudden onset of dyspnea. She may complain of shoulder, back, or chest pain. Assessment findings may include fever, leg pain with redness and unilateral pedal edema, fatigue, or cardiac arrest. Your assessment findings may reveal changes in the patient's circulation, tachycardia, diminished breath sounds with wheezing or crackles, hypotension, and pulse oximetry readings of 70% or lower.

Allow the patient with a respiratory complaint to assume a position of comfort unless hypotension is present. If the patient is alert but showing signs of breathing difficulty, give oxygen by nonrebreather mask at 15 L/min. Provide positive-pressure ventilation with 100% oxygen as necessary. Continuously monitor the patient's oxygen saturation. Reassess the patient frequently. Transport promptly to the closest appropriate medical facility. Record all patient care information on a PCR.

Nervous System

Objectives 5, 6

Nervous system changes that occur in older adults are shown in the following *You Should Know* box. The incidence of strokes and transient ischemic attacks

You Should Know

Nervous System Changes in Older Adults

- Partial or complete wasting away (atrophy) of brain tissue
- Difficulty with recent memory
- Difficulty retrieving information
- Decreased balance and coordination
- Forgetfulness
- Decreased reaction time
- Deterioration of the nervous system function in controlling the rate and depth of breathing, heart rate, blood pressure, hunger and thirst, temperature, and sensory perception (including audio, visual, olfactory, touch, and pain)
- Peripheral nervous system disorders (neuropathy)

increases with advancing age. It has been estimated that 75% of stroke patients are more than 65 years of age. Some of the more common complications after a stroke include depression, pressure sores, urine incontinence, difficulty swallowing, and venous clots in the legs that can lead to pulmonary emboli.

A patient who has experienced a stroke on the right side of the brain may experience problems such as irritability, confusion, sluggishness, difficulty retaining information, distortions of time, and unawareness of the left side of the body. A patient who has experienced a stroke on the left side of the brain may experience problems such as difficulty starting tasks, compulsive behavior, slow processing of information, repetition of words, and difficulty expressing himself verbally or in writing. Some patients who have experienced a stroke require the use of a cane, walker, or wheelchair for mobility.

Delirium (also known as *acute brain syndrome*) is a sudden change (onset of minutes, hours, days) in mental status that is generally caused by a reversible condition such as hypoglycemia, drug overdose, or trauma. Other possible causes of delirium are shown in the following *You Should Know* box. Delirium is very common in older adults and is characterized by a decreased attention span, disordered stream of thought, and disturbances in perception (such as visual hallucinations or illusions). The patient may have moments of clarity during the day with increasing confusion at night. The term **sundowning** is used to describe an increase in confusion that often occurs in older adults, particularly at night. Anxiety, irritability, fear, anger, and indifference are common. The delirious patient's speech may be incoherent, rambling, hesitant, slow, or rapid. Episodes of delirium can last from hours to weeks.

You Should Know
Causes of Delirium

- Hypoxia
- Hypoglycemia or hyperglycemia
- Drug overdose
- Trauma
- Intoxication or withdrawal from alcohol
- Withdrawal from sedatives
- Urinary tract infection
- Intestinal obstruction
- Dehydration
- Depression
- Malnutrition or vitamin deficiency
- Heat or cold exposure

Dementia refers to a more gradual change in baseline mental status that causes a progressive and sometimes irreversible loss of intellectual functions, psychomotor skills, and social skills. The gradual change in mental status typically occurs over months to years and involves deterioration in mental processes, such as thinking, reasoning, learning, problem solving, memory, language, and speech. Changes in personality and behavior are also common. Causes of potentially reversible dementia include alcoholism, organic poisons, trauma, depression, infections, eye and ear problems, and drug overdose. Huntington's chorea (a hereditary disease that leads to a progressive loss of motor coordination, spasmodic jerking of the limbs, bizarre behavior, and mental deterioration) and Parkinson's disease (a brain disorder characterized by tremors) also are possible causes of dementia. **Alzheimer's disease** is an example of an irreversible dementia. Dementia generally begins after the age of 60 years, but some forms of Alzheimer's disease may begin as early as age 30.

Occasional lapses in memory are normal and must be differentiated from those that are possible symptoms of dementia. A few examples from the Alzheimer's Association will help explain this point. For example, occasionally forgetting the day or date is normal. Getting lost in your own neighborhood or being unable to find your way home may be a symptom of dementia. Occasionally forgetting where you put your car keys or glasses is normal. Putting the iron in the freezer or your wristwatch in the sugar bowl may be a symptom of dementia.

It has been estimated that more than 60% of all dementias are of the Alzheimer's type. The progression of Alzheimer's disease has been divided into three stages that reflect early (mild), middle (moderate), or late (severe) symptoms. In the very early stage of the disease, the patient gets lost in familiar surroundings, is easily angered, has difficulty making decisions, and forgets names, events, and phone numbers. In the early stage of the disease, she becomes disoriented to date, has difficulty managing her finances (such as forgetting to pay bills), forgets messages, and misplaces items. She gets lost while driving, makes poor decisions, has difficulty maintaining good hygiene, complains of neglect by others, and is restless and impatient. In the middle stage of the disease the Alzheimer's patient has difficulty recognizing family or friends, makes up stories to compensate for memory loss, and is disoriented to date and place. She is restless, anxious, and depressed and develops suspicious and paranoid behavior. She has problems with dressing and grooming and often loses control of her bowels and bladder. In the late stage (which can last from 1 to 3 years), the patient must be dressed, fed, bathed, and turned. Her verbal responses are nearly unintelligible, consisting mainly of grunts and agitation to communicate. The patient is no longer in control of her bowels and bladder and becomes susceptible to infection.

Assessment of the patient with an altered mental status can be challenging. Because the patient is generally a poor historian, you will need to obtain the patient's history from sources such as family, friends, neighbors, and the patient's environment. Attempt to find out when the patient's symptoms started. Ask specifically what is different about the patient today compared to yesterday or 2 or 3 days ago. Also, ask about similar episodes, a history of psychiatric illnesses, and medical conditions. Look for medical jewelry that may provide additional clues about the patient's medical history. While on the scene, look at the patient's environment. If medications are present, look at the date the prescription was last refilled and note the number of pills remaining in each bottle. This information will help determine if the patient has been taking his medications as prescribed. As with all patients, obtain vital signs and perform a physical exam, looking for signs of a treatable cause of the patient's altered mental status. Assess the patient's oxygen saturation using a pulse oximeter, and assess the patient's blood glucose level. Administer oxygen, and treat hypoglycemia with oral glucose if the patient can swallow and if ordered by medical direction. When preparing the patient for transport, consider the use of restraints if the patient is combative (and if consistent with your local protocols), recognizing that in some situations the application of restraints may increase the patient's agitation. Reassess as often as indicated until patient care is transferred. Record all patient care information, including the patient's medical history, emergency care given, and the patient's response to your care, on a PCR. If restraints are used, document the following information:

- The reason for the restraints
- The number of personnel used to restrain the patient
- The type of restraint used
- The time the restraints were placed on the patient
- The status of the patient's airway, breathing, circulation (ABCs), and distal pulses before and after the restraints were applied
- Reassessment of the patient's ABCs and distal pulses

Remember This

Before labeling any patient with a sudden deterioration in mental status as confused or disoriented, make sure that you have searched for and ruled out possible treatable causes such as hypoxia, hypoglycemia, infection, and dehydration (among many other possibilities).

Gastrointestinal System

Objective 7

The gastrointestinal (GI) system undergoes many changes with age, which are summarized in the following *You Should Know* box. Dry mouth is a common complaint in older adults. Saliva plays an important role in speech, swallowing, chewing, and taste perception. Reduced amounts of saliva in the mouths of older adults can affect these functions. The most common cause of dry mouth is prescription medications that have this adverse effect. Dry mouth is also associated with dehydration.

You Should Know

Gastrointestinal System Changes in Older Adults
- Tooth decay
- Missing teeth
- Periodontal disease
- Decreased saliva production
- Delayed emptying of the stomach
- Decreased hydrochloric acid in the stomach
- Changes in absorption of nutrients
- Slowing peristalsis causing constipation
- Weakened rectal sphincter resulting in fecal incontinence
- Liver shrinkage
- Decreased blood flow to the liver
- Decreased metabolism in the liver
- Decreased pancreatic secretions

Dysphagia (difficulty swallowing) is a frequent complaint of older adults. The patient may describe this problem as "food getting stuck" shortly after swallowing. Some patients drool or leak fluid or food from the mouth. Coughing before, during, or after swallowing fluids or food is common. The patient may choke while drinking or eating.

Upper GI bleeding may be caused by gastritis, peptic ulcer disease, tumors, esophagitis (inflammation of the esophagus), and esophageal varices (enlarged and twisted veins in the esophagus). Assessment findings and symptoms include hematemesis (vomiting blood), epigastric pain, epigastric tenderness, and nausea. Lower GI bleeding can be caused by tumors, hemorrhoids, and colitis (inflammation of the colon). Assessment findings and symptoms include rectal bleeding, increased frequency of stools, and cramping pain. The color of blood in the stool depends on the source of the bleeding and the amount of time the blood has spent in the GI tract.

Ulcer disease in older adults may result from increased stomach acidity, bacteria, and/or psychological stress caused by hospitalization or nursing home placement. The patient typically complains of upper abdominal pain, vomiting, and a loss of appetite. Hematemesis (vomiting blood) and melena (black, tarry stool) may also occur.

Constipation is a common complaint among older adults. Laxative use in older adults is common, even among those who are not constipated. The patient who is constipated may have abdominal distention and cramping. **Fecal impaction** is the condition in which hardened feces become trapped in the rectum and cannot be expelled. Signs and symptoms of a fecal impaction include abdominal cramping, rectal pain, abdominal distention, loss of appetite, and oozing of a thin or liquid discharge of feces from the rectum without any signs of passing solid stool.

Diarrhea occurs frequently in older adults and can cause dehydration and electrolyte imbalances. An intestinal infection, excessive laxative use, and antibiotic administration are causes of diarrhea. Infectious diarrhea sometimes occurs in nursing home settings because of ingestion of poorly cooked foods of animal origin.

The involuntary leakage of stool is called **fecal incontinence.** Causes of fecal incontinence include fecal impaction, poor access to toileting facilities, damage to the spinal cord, and loss of rectal sphincter tone. Fecal incontinence can occur in patients who have dementia because of difficulty in communicating their needs to caregivers, immobility, or failing to sense or recognize normal cues pertaining to stool elimination. Additional assessment findings in an older adult with a GI complaint may reveal changes in the patient's circulation; pale or yellow, thin skin; frail musculoskeletal system; peripheral, sacral, and periorbital edema; hypertension (or hypotension if the patient is dehydrated); fever; tachycardia; and dyspnea.

Allow the patient with a GI complaint to assume a position of comfort unless hypotension is present. Provide supportive care. If recommended by local policy, obtain blood pressures with the patient lying, sitting, and standing, noting any decrease in BP of 10 mmHg or more as the patient moves to an upright position. Obtain pulses with the patient lying, sitting, and standing, noting any increase in pulse rate of 10 beats/min or more as the patient moves to an upright position. Transport promptly to the closest appropriate medical facility.

Genitourinary System

Objective 8

Genitourinary system changes that occur in older adults are shown in the following *You Should Know* box. Enlargement of the prostate gland is common in men older than 50 years of age. The gland slowly increases in size and gradually leads to problems with urination such as dribbling, urinary frequency and hesitancy, increased urination at night, and involuntary bladder contractions. Urinary tract infections and urinary retention are common complications of prostate gland enlargement. Prostate cancer is the second leading cause of death in men in the United States, and the frequency with which

You Should Know

Genitourinary System Changes in Older Adults
- Reduced kidney function
- Reduced blood flow to the kidneys
- Reduced sphincter muscle control
- Decreased bladder capacity
- Decline in sensation to urinate
- Increase in urinating at night
- Prostate enlargement in males

it occurs increases with age. Annual screening tests for prostate cancer are recommended for men older than 50 years of age.

Urinary incontinence is the involuntary leakage of urine. Although the most common cause of urinary incontinence is an interference with sphincter control, contributing factors include drugs (such as diuretics and sedatives), infections of and injury to the urinary system, and obesity. The patient who is incontinent of urine may be embarrassed, depressed, and socially isolated.

Urinary tract infections (UTIs) are common in older adults, and urinary incontinence is sometimes the only sign of a UTI. Older adults are susceptible to UTIs because of incomplete emptying of the bladder and the use of indwelling urinary catheters. Signs and symptoms of a urinary tract infection in older adults are often vague and missed because they can be attributed to other conditions, such as altered mental status, nausea, vomiting, and abdominal pain.

Provide supportive care, and reassess the patient as often as indicated. Transport to the closest appropriate medical facility. Record all patient care information, including the patient's medical history, emergency care given, and the patient's response to your care, on a PCR.

Metabolic and Endocrine Problems

Objective 9

Endocrine system changes that occur in older adults are shown in the following *You Should Know* box. Older adults have less subcutaneous tissue, inefficient blood vessel constriction, diminished shivering and sweating, diminished perception of temperature, and diminished thirst perception. These factors increase

You Should Know

Endocrine System Changes in Older Adults
- Impaired glucose regulation
- Fluid and electrolyte imbalances
- Reduced thyroid hormone production

an older adult's likelihood of experiencing a heat- or cold-related emergency. Some older adults are at increased risk of heat- and cold-related emergencies because of financial circumstances. For example, despite extreme weather conditions, an older adult may not use a heater or an air conditioner to save money on utilities.

Reduced thyroid hormone production can result in signs and symptoms that progress slowly and are often attributed to other conditions, such as dry skin, decreased skin elasticity, weakness, constipation, arthritis, walking disturbances, and slowed mental responses.

Type 2 diabetes mellitus is the most common form of diabetes in older adults. Inadequate insulin production results in hyperglycemia. The breakdown of protein and fat to provide energy produces waste products, including acids (ketoacidosis). **Hyperosmolar hyperglycemic state (HHS)** is a complication of type 2 diabetes that results in a very high glucose concentration in the blood (usually greater than 600 mg/dL). HHS was previously called *hyperosmolar hyperglycemic nonketotic coma*, but the terminology was changed because coma is found in fewer than 10% of patients with HHS. Although HHS can occur in younger patients, including children, it is more common in older adults. HHS is usually precipitated by an illness that leads to a reduced fluid intake, such as an infection or the flu. Signs and symptoms often worsen over a period of days or weeks and can include weakness, increased thirst, nausea, dizziness, altered mental status, seizures, and, ultimately, coma. Additional signs that are usually present and consistent with dehydration include warm, flushed skin; tachycardia (an early indicator of dehydration); decreased skin elasticity; dry mouth; sunken eyes; and hypotension (a later sign of severe dehydration).

Administer oxygen and provide supportive care. Check and document the patient's blood glucose level. Reassess the patient as often as indicated. Transport to the closest appropriate medical facility. Record all patient care information, including the patient's medical history, emergency care given, and the patient's response to your care, on a PCR.

Musculoskeletal System

Objective 10

Musculoskeletal system changes that occur in older adults are shown in the next *You Should Know* box. **Osteoarthritis (OA)** is the major cause of knee, hip, and back pain in older adults. The knee is the joint most commonly affected by OA. Assessment findings include swelling, crepitus, deformity (enlargement), tenderness, pain, and decreased joint motion.

Osteoporosis, a bone disease that decreases bone mass, can result in a loss of height because of compression fractures of the vertebrae and kyphosis (Figure 45-3).

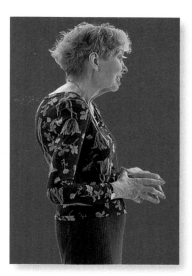

FIGURE 45-3 ▲ Kyphosis is an abnormal curvature of the spine, resulting in stooped posture.

Provide supportive care. Padding a backboard may be necessary to allow for changes in the shape of the patient's spine. Use gentle care when moving your patient. Reassess the patient as often as indicated. Transport to the closest appropriate medical facility. Record all patient care information, including the patient's medical history, emergency care given, and the patient's response to your care, on a PCR.

You Should Know

Musculoskeletal System Changes in Older Adults

- Muscle wasting
- Loss of bone mass
- Loss of muscle strength
- Degenerative changes in joints
- Loss of elasticity in ligaments and tendons
- Thinning of cartilage and thickening of synovial fluid

Toxicological Emergencies

Objective 11

Older adults are at risk of toxicity because of factors that alter drug metabolism and excretion, including decreased kidney function, altered gastrointestinal absorption, and decreased blood flow in the liver. Some older adults see several doctors. If they fail to tell each doctor about the drugs another physician has prescribed, they may be prescribed drugs that can cause serious health problems when taken with the other medicines (Figure 45-4). **Polypharmacy** is the use of multiple medications, often prescribed by different doctors, which can cause adverse reactions in the patient. Be respectful but firm

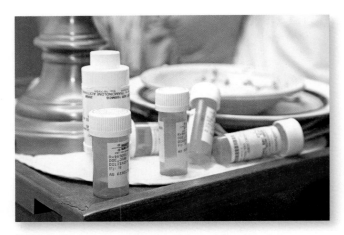

FIGURE 45-4 ▲ The average older adult takes four prescribed and three over-the-counter medications every day.

when questioning the patient about her medical history, including any prescribed medicines and their proper dosages. Check the patient's prescription dates and the number of pills available in the bottle to determine if the patient has been taking her medication as prescribed.

Some older adults are on several medications because they have multiple medical problems. If your elderly patient's chief complaint is unclear or does not seem to fall within the "normal" signs and symptoms of a particular disease, it may be due to his not taking his medication as prescribed. The patient may not take his pills at all, may take them every now and then, or may accidentally overdose from taking too much medication. A patient who is not taking his medication as prescribed may be doing so because he simply cannot afford it. Some prescribed medications are expensive. Many older adults are on fixed incomes and may have to choose between taking their medicine or paying for food and utilities. Other reasons that an older adult may not take medications as prescribed include a lack of motor ability to open the bottle cap, altered mental status, and impaired vision.

Some of the medicines that older adults take can hide the signs and symptoms of an illness. For example, some patients take heart or blood pressure medicines that keep the heart rate low. If they have a blood loss, the drug will prevent the heart rate from increasing to compensate for the shock. When you assess them, you may think that they are stable because the heart rate remains normal despite shock.

Sensory Changes in Older Adults

Objective 12

Visual impairment increases with age. The pupil's ability to dilate decreases with age, and the thickness of the lens increases, reducing the amount of light that reaches the retina. These changes limit the ability to see clearly in dimly lighted areas and at night. **Cataracts**, which cloud the lens of the eye, are the most common disorder of the eye in older adults. According to the National Eye Institute, by age 80, more than half of all Americans either have a cataract or have had cataract surgery.

The ability to focus on near objects decreases with age. For example, the average 16-year-old can clearly see objects as close as 4 inches, but the average 44-year-old cannot clearly see objects closer than about 12 inches, and the average 60-year-old cannot clearly see objects closer than about 40 inches. With age the lens yellows, affecting color vision. Dark colors (particularly blue) appear faded, and the contrast between different colors is less noticeable. Some medications, such as digoxin, can also cause changes in color vision. The lens of the eye becomes cloudy with age. This causes light scatter and increases glare, making night driving difficult.

Glaucoma is a disease associated with a buildup of internal eye pressure that can damage the optic nerve, which sends visual information to the brain. If untreated, glaucoma will eventually cause blindness. Glaucoma is the second leading cause of blindness in the United States. It has been called the "silent thief of sight" because most types of glaucoma produce no symptoms, and irreversible damage to the optic nerve can occur before the disease is recognized. Testing for increased pressure within the eye is easy to perform and should be done on all adults older than 40 years of age. As vision worsens, the patient with glaucoma compensates by using a magnifying lens, large-print books and/or talking books, and large-faced clocks, watches, and telephones.

Macular degeneration is the leading cause of vision loss and legal blindness in Americans aged 65 and older. The macula is the central part of the retina and is responsible for sharp vision, such as that needed to read or drive. The cause of macular degeneration is unknown. Signs of vision loss include shadowy areas in central vision, unusually fuzzy vision, objects that increase or decrease in size, and straight lines that appear bent. As vision worsens, the patient with macular degeneration compensates by using a magnifying lens and high-intensity lighting.

Hearing loss because of aging is called **presbycusis**, which means older hearing. Presbycusis is progressive, occurring gradually over a period of years. It becomes increasingly difficult to tell the difference between the sounds of the consonants *f, g, s,* and *t* because the patient cannot hear high-pitched sounds well. The patient often has difficulty hearing when background noise is present but can hear adequately in a quiet environment. An amplification device such as a hearing aid is often helpful.

Touch sensitivity decreases and the pain threshold increases with age. A decreased ability to differentiate hot from cold or sharp from dull can increase the risk of injury. For example, the inability to distinguish bath water that is too hot or a heating pad that has been left in one place too long can result in burns before the patient is aware of any discomfort.

If your older adult patient is complaining of pain or discomfort, ask carefully worded questions about the discomfort he is having. Because pain sensation can be lessened or absent in older adults, the patient can easily misjudge how serious his condition is. Older adults may live with chronic pain and underreport the discomfort associated with their current medical problem. Acute pain is pain of sudden onset. Chronic pain is pain that is of long duration. Asking an older adult to rate his discomfort on a scale from 0 to 10 may not give a true picture of the pain he is experiencing. Look for visual cues that your patient is in pain. For example, grimacing, wincing, or stiff muscles may be indicators that the patient is experiencing pain. Use the memory aid OPQRST to help identify the type and location of the patient's complaint.

On the Scene Wrap-Up

As you assist your patient to the ground near the cart path, he informs you that he has "a rather hard time hearing" and that he takes "a bunch of heart medications." You immediately recognize the need to stand in front of the patient so that he may see your face, and you remember to speak in a normal tone so that he may understand each question.

You ask the patient if he is having pain or discomfort in his chest, and he responds by stating, "No, but my chest feels heavy." You also understand that older adults may have an altered perception of pain and that the report of heaviness may be the only clue that the patient may be experiencing a heart problem.

You quickly relay the information you have obtained to the fire department personnel who have arrived on the scene. Using a nonrebreather mask, an EMT quickly administers oxygen to the patient. Within minutes the patient reports feeling much better. The patient is secured onto the stretcher, loaded into an ambulance, and transported for additional care. ■

Sum It Up

▶ The term elderly refers to persons 65 years of age and older. Elderly people are rapidly becoming the largest group of patients that are encountered in the prehospital setting.

▶ Assessment of an older adult should be approached in the same systematic manner as all other patients. Keep in mind that an older adult may not show severe symptoms even if very ill.

▶ While communicating with the patient, face the patient and speak slowly, clearly, and respectfully at the patient's eye level. Make sure that lighting is adequate to enable the patient to see your face and lips when speaking to her. Locate the patient's hearing aid or eyeglasses if needed. Speak to the patient first rather than to family or others.

▶ Coronary artery disease is the leading cause of death and disability in persons aged 65 years and older. The frequency of sudden cardiac death as the initial sign of coronary artery disease increases with age. An older adult who is experiencing an acute coronary syndrome may not show the same signs and symptoms as a younger person. His signs and symptoms are often vague and can be masked by other diseases.

▶ Heart failure is a common condition in older adults. When the left ventricle fails as a pump, blood backs up into the lungs (pulmonary edema). When the right ventricle fails, blood returning to the heart backs up and causes congestion in the organs and tissues of the body.

▶ Asthma and chronic obstructive pulmonary disease are common in older adults. In fact, the death rate from asthma has increased most significantly in those aged 65 or over. More than 50% of all pneumonia cases occur in individuals 65 years of age and older. A pulmonary embolism is the sudden blockage of a branch of the pulmonary artery by a venous clot. Experts say that the incidence of a pulmonary embolism triples between the ages of 65 and 90.

▶ The incidence of strokes and transient ischemic attacks increases with advancing age. It has been estimated that 75% of stroke patients are more than 65 years of age and that 40% of stroke survivors have significant dysfunction.

▶ Delirium (also known as acute brain syndrome) is a sudden change (onset of minutes, hours, days) in mental status that is generally caused by a reversible condition, such as hypoglycemia, drug overdose, or trauma.

▶ Dementia refers to a more gradual change in baseline mental status that causes a progressive and sometimes irreversible loss of intellectual functions, psychomotor skills, and social skills. Causes of potentially reversible dementia include alcoholism, organic poisons, trauma, depression, infections, eye and ear problems, and drug overdose. Alzheimer's disease is an example of an irreversible dementia. It has been estimated that more than 60% of all dementias are of the Alzheimer's type. The progression of symptoms of Alzheimer's disease and the time that it first appears vary by individual.

- Before labeling any patient with a sudden deterioration in mental status as confused or disoriented, make sure that you have searched for and ruled out possible treatable causes, such as hypoxia, hypoglycemia, infection, and dehydration (among many other possibilities).

- Dysphagia (difficulty swallowing) is a frequent complaint of older adults. The patient may describe this problem as "food getting stuck" shortly after swallowing.

- Constipation is a common complaint among older adults. Laxative use in older adults is common, even among those who are not constipated. Fecal impaction is the condition in which hardened feces become trapped in the rectum and cannot be expelled.

- The involuntary leakage of stool is called fecal incontinence. Urinary incontinence is the involuntary leakage of urine.

- Enlargement of the prostate gland is common in men over 50 years of age. The gland slowly increases in size and gradually leads to problems with urination.

- Older adults are susceptible to urinary tract infections because of incomplete emptying of the bladder and the use of indwelling urinary catheters.

- Osteoarthritis is the major cause of knee, hip, and back pain in older adults. Osteoporosis can result in a loss of height because of compression fractures of the vertebrae and kyphosis (an abnormal curvature of the spine resulting in stooped posture).

- Older adults are at risk of toxicity because of factors that alter drug metabolism and excretion, including decreased kidney function, altered gastrointestinal absorption, and decreased blood flow in the liver.

- Polypharmacy is the use of multiple medications, often prescribed by different doctors, which can cause adverse reactions in the patient. Be respectful but firm when questioning the patient about his medical history, including any prescribed medicines and their proper dosages.

- The formation of cataracts, clouding of the lens of the eye, is the most common disorder of the eye in older adults.

- Glaucoma is a disease associated with a buildup of internal eye pressure that can damage the optic nerve, which sends visual information to the brain. If untreated, glaucoma will eventually cause blindness. Glaucoma is the second leading cause of blindness in the United States.

- Macular degeneration is the leading cause of vision loss and legal blindness in Americans aged 65 and older. The macula is the central part of the retina and is responsible for sharp vision, such as that needed to read or drive.

- Hearing loss because of aging is called presbycusis, which means older hearing.

- If your older adult patient is complaining of pain or discomfort, ask carefully worded questions about the discomfort she is having. Acute pain is pain of sudden onset. Chronic pain is pain that is of long duration. Asking an older adult to rate her discomfort on a scale from 0 to 10 may not give a true picture of the pain she is experiencing.

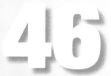

CHAPTER
46

Patients with Special Challenges

By the end of this chapter, you should be able to:

Knowledge Objectives ▶
1. Define child maltreatment, and differentiate among the four primary types of child abuse.
2. Describe possible signs and symptoms and emergency care for child abuse.
3. Define elder abuse, and differentiate among the primary categories of elder abuse.
4. Describe the assessment findings, symptoms, and emergency care for elder abuse.
5. Discuss common illnesses among the homeless.
6. Discuss possible challenges associated with the assessment and provision of emergency care to the homeless patient.
7. Discuss possible challenges associated with the assessment and provision of emergency care to the bariatric patient.
8. Differentiate between home care and home healthcare.
9. Discuss medical devices commonly used by patients with special healthcare needs.
10. Discuss the specific assessment and emergency care considerations for patients with special healthcare needs.
11. Differentiate between palliative care and hospice care.

Attitude Objective ▶
12. Understand the provider's own emotional response to caring for victims of possible abuse or terminal illness.

Skill Objectives ▶

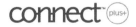

13. Demonstrate the assessment and emergency care of a patient with signs of abuse or neglect.
14. Demonstrate the assessment and emergency care of a bariatric patient.
15. Demonstrate the assessment and emergency care of a homeless patient.
16. Demonstrate the assessment and emergency care of a patient with special healthcare needs.
17. Demonstrate the assessment and emergency care of a hospice patient.
18. Practice completing a prehospital care report for victims of suspected abuse or neglect.
19. Practice completing a prehospital care report for a bariatric patient.
20. Practice completing a prehospital care report for a homeless patient.
21. Practice completing a prehospital care report for a patient with special healthcare needs.
22. Practice completing a prehospital care report for a hospice patient.

It is a cold winter night, and overnight temperatures are expected to drop into the teens. You have been dispatched to the local homeless shelter for a man with chest pain. The shelter is full to capacity, and the patient has been denied a bed for the night. You arrive to find a 60-year-old man seated on a chair in the lobby of the shelter. Although you cannot recall his name, you recognize him as a patient you have transported many times in the past 6 months for various illnesses and injuries. He is complaining of chest pain that is located in the center of his chest and radiates to his left arm. ■

THINK ABOUT IT

As you read this chapter, think about the following questions:

- Which signs of respiratory distress have you observed in this patient?
- Will this patient's circumstances alter the care that you provide?
- What treatment should you consider for this patient?

Introduction

In this chapter we discuss patients with special challenges such as child abuse or neglect, elder abuse, morbid obesity, homelessness, special healthcare needs, or terminal illness. Providing care for patients in these situations is stressful for many healthcare professionals. After the call, assess your own emotional needs. A discussion with other personnel involved in the call may be helpful.

Child Abuse and Neglect

Objectives 1, 2

Child maltreatment is an act or failure to act by a parent, caregiver, or other person as defined by state law that results in physical abuse, neglect, medical neglect, sexual abuse, and/or emotional abuse. It is also defined as an act or failure to act that presents an impending risk of serious harm to a child (Figure 46-1). State laws define the specific acts that make up the various forms of abuse. These laws vary from state to state.

There are four common types of abuse: physical abuse, sexual abuse, emotional abuse, and neglect. **Physical abuse** refers to physical acts that cause or could cause physical injury to a child. Examples of physical abuse include hitting, kicking, shaking, burning, or other acts of harm. Physical signs that may indicate abuse are listed in the following *You Should Know* box. Consider the possibility of physical abuse when the child has unexplained burns, bites, bruises, broken bones, or black eyes; has fading bruises or other marks noticeable after an absence from school; seems frightened of the caregiver and protests or cries when it is

time to go home; shrinks at the approach of adults; or reports an injury caused by a parent or another adult caregiver. You should also consider the possibility of physical abuse when the parent or other adult caregiver offers a conflicting or unconvincing explanation or no explanation for the child's injury.

You Should Know

Physical Signs That May Indicate Abuse

- Multiple bruises in various stages of healing
- Human bite marks
- Inflicted burns—"stockinglike" burns with no associated splash marks; usually present on the buttocks, genitalia, or extremities
- Circular burns from a cigarette or cigar
- Rope burns on the wrists
- Burns in the shape of a household utensil or appliance, such as a spoon or iron
- Fractures
- Head, face, and oral injuries
- Abdominal injuries
- An injury inconsistent with the history or developmental level of the child

It is important to recognize that some medical conditions or cultural practices may look like signs of abuse but are not. For example, **impetigo** is a contagious bacterial skin infection that can look like a burn (Figure 46-2). Chickenpox may resemble cigarette burns. **Mongolian spots** are bluish areas usually seen in non-Caucasian infants and young children that may be mistaken for bruises (Figure 46-3). Some cultures, such as

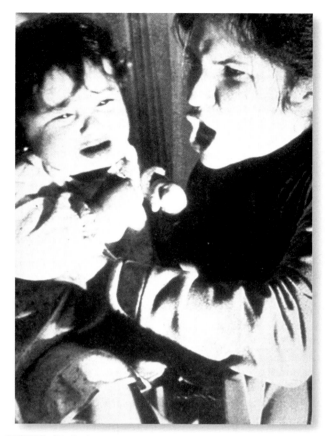

FIGURE 46-1 ▲ Never shake or jiggle a baby.

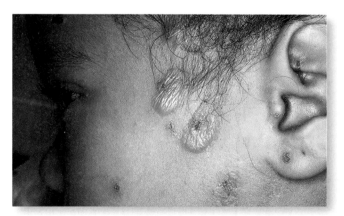

FIGURE 46-2 ▲ Impetigo, a bacterial skin infection, can be mistaken for burns.

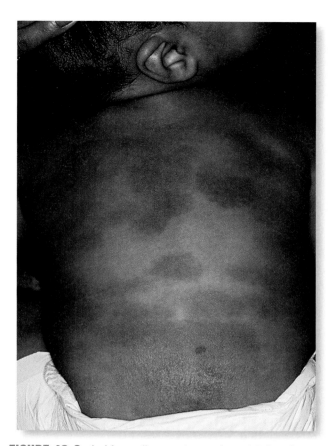

FIGURE 46-3 ▲ Mongolian spots can be mistaken for bruises.

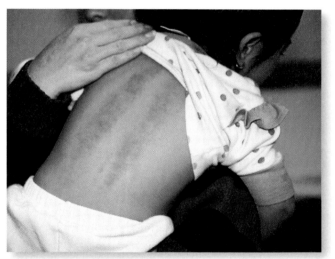

FIGURE 46-4 ▲ Some cultures practice coining, a healing remedy.

those of Southeast Asia, practice **coining.** Coining is a healing remedy in which a coin is heated in hot oil and then rubbed along the patient's spine to heal an illness, such as congestion in the lungs (Figure 46-4). Coining is not considered child abuse.

Sexual abuse is inappropriate adolescent or adult sexual behavior with a child. It includes fondling, rape, and exposing a child to other sexual activities. **Emotional abuse** refers to behaviors that harm a child's

self-worth or emotional well-being. Examples include name calling, shaming, rejection, withholding love, and threatening. **Neglect** is the failure to provide for a child's basic physical, emotional, or educational needs or to protect a child from harm or potential harm

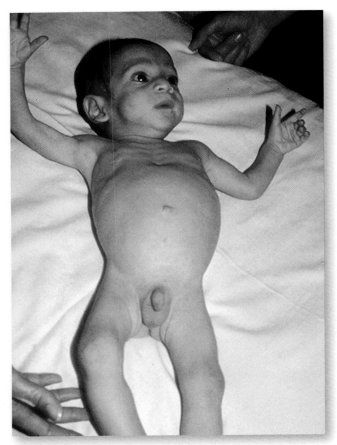

FIGURE 46-5 ▲ Neglect is the failure to provide for a child's basic needs. Neglect can be medical, physical, educational, or emotional.

(Figure 46-5). Neglect can be medical, physical, educational, or emotional. **Medical neglect** is a type of maltreatment characterized by failure of the caregiver to provide for the appropriate healthcare of the child despite being financially able to do so. Signs of neglect that you may see in the child's environment are shown in the following *You Should Know* box.

You Should Know

Signs of Neglect

- Untreated chronic illness (such as a diabetic or asthmatic child with no medication)
- Untreated soft tissue injuries
- A home that is bug- or rodent-infested
- A lack of adult supervision
- A lack of food or basic necessities
- A child who appears to be malnourished
- Stool or urine present on items in the home
- An unsafe living environment
- The presence of alcohol or drug paraphernalia

As a healthcare professional, you must be aware of these conditions and be able to recognize them. Physical abuse and neglect are the two forms of child maltreatment that you are most likely to detect. Do not confront or accuse any caregiver of abuse. Accusation and confrontation delay transportation and may endanger you or your crew. Keep in mind that the caregiver with the child at the scene may not be the abuser.

Reporting known or suspected child abuse is required by law in most states. Individuals who are typically required to report abuse have frequent contact with children. Some states require all citizens to report suspected abuse or neglect regardless of their profession. It is your responsibility to know what the requirements are in your area.

Carefully document your physical exam findings as well as your observations of the child's environment. Document the caregiver's comments exactly as stated, and enclose them in quotation marks. Make sure that your documentation reflects the facts and not your opinion of what may or may not have occurred. Do not comment on what you think. Be objective, and do not document emotions or suspicions. Document only what you see, hear, or witness using your five senses. Report your findings to appropriate personnel when transferring patient care.

Elder Abuse

Objectives 3, 4

Elder abuse is any physical, sexual, or emotional abuse or neglect committed against an older adult. Because definitions of elder abuse vary from state to state, collection of data regarding the frequency with which elder abuse occurs is lacking. It has been estimated that about two-thirds of the individuals who commit elder abuse are family members, usually the victim's adult child or spouse. In many cases, the abuser is financially dependent on the older adult's resources. The National Center on Elder Abuse has identified three basic categories of elder abuse:

- *Domestic elder abuse* refers to maltreatment of an older adult that occurs in the elder's home (or in the home of a caregiver) by an individual who has a special relationship with the elder (such as a spouse, sibling, child, friend, or caregiver).
- *Institutional elder abuse* occurs in residential facilities for older persons, such as nursing homes, foster homes, group homes, or board and care facilities. The abuser is generally an individual who has a legal or contractual obligation to provide care and protection to an older adult, such as a paid caregiver or healthcare professional.

- *Self-neglect* or *self-abuse* is the conscious and voluntary behavior of a mentally competent older adult that threatens her own health or safety as a matter of personal choice. For example, the older adult may refuse or fail to provide herself with adequate food, water, clothing, shelter, personal hygiene, medication (when indicated), and safety precautions.

Types of elder abuse are similar to those encountered with children and include physical, sexual, and emotional abuse and neglect. In addition to hitting, slapping, and other forms of physical abuse previously mentioned in regard to children, physical abuse of an older adult also includes inappropriate use of drugs and physical restraints, force-feeding, and physical punishment of any kind. Signs and symptoms of sexual abuse in older adults can include bruises around the breasts or genital area; unexplained vaginal or anal bleeding; torn, stained, or bloody underclothing; and an older adult's report of being sexually assaulted or raped. Emotional abuse of an older adult includes insulting, threatening, intimidating, and harassing the older adult; treating the older adult like an infant; isolating the older adult from family, friends, or regular activities; and giving the older adult the "silent treatment." Neglect of an older adult may include failure of a person who has a responsibility to care for an elder to provide necessities, such as food, water, clothing, shelter, personal hygiene, medicine, comfort, or personal safety, or to pay for necessary home care services. Examples of older adult neglect are listed in the following *You Should Know* box.

You Should Know

Examples of Older Adult Neglect

- Dehydration
- Malnutrition
- Untreated bedsores
- Poor personal hygiene
- Unattended or untreated health problems
- Hazardous or unsafe living conditions or arrangements (improper wiring, no indoor plumbing, no heat, no running water)
- Unsanitary and unclean living conditions (dirt, fleas, lice on person, soiled bedding, no functioning toilet, fecal or urine smell, inappropriate and/or inadequate clothing)
- Older adult's report of being mistreated

Provide emergency care for the patient as needed. Do not confront or accuse any caregiver of elder abuse. Reporting known or suspected elder abuse is required by law in most states. It is your responsibility to know the requirements in your area. Carefully document your physical exam findings as well as your observations of the patient's environment. Document the patient's comments exactly as stated, and enclose them in quotation marks. Make sure that your documentation reflects the facts and not your opinion of what may or may not have occurred. Report your findings to appropriate personnel when transferring patient care.

Homelessness

Objectives 5, 6

According to the National Coalition for the Homeless, there are two main reasons for the rise in homelessness over the past 20–25 years: a growing shortage of affordable rental housing and an increase in poverty. Homelessness and poverty often go hand in hand because poor individuals are often unable to pay for housing, food, childcare, healthcare, and education. Other factors that contribute to homelessness are listed in the following *You Should Know* box.

You Should Know

Factors That Contribute to Homelessness

- Decreasing work opportunities
- Stagnant or falling incomes
- Less secure jobs that offer fewer benefits
- Lack of affordable healthcare
- Domestic violence
- Mental illness
- Racial discrimination
- Addiction disorders, such as drugs and alcohol

It has been estimated that 40% of homeless men are veterans, about a third of the homeless have mental illnesses, and half have a current or past drug or alcohol addiction. Trauma resulting from violence and conditions caused by exposure to the elements and infections of all types are common among the homeless. Some studies suggest that families with children make up 36% of the homeless population.

EMS is often the primary route that the homeless use to access healthcare. Homeless people typically do not have health insurance or money to pay for healthcare services, and most do not have transportation. Many of the homeless have had identification documents lost or stolen that would otherwise enable them to prove their poverty status and qualify for free or reduced-fee services. Without regular access to healthcare, even relatively minor problems can quickly become urgent medical emergencies. Examples of common illnesses among homeless people are listed in the following *You Should Know* box.

You Should Know

Common Illnesses Among the Homeless

- Upper respiratory tract infections
- Trauma (lacerations, wounds, sprains, contusions, fractures, burns)
- Female genitourinary problems
- Hypertension
- Skin and ear disorders
- Gastrointestinal diseases
- Peripheral vascular disease
- Musculoskeletal problems
- Dental problems
- Vision problems

Tuberculosis is common in some homeless populations. A homeless individual may be infested with lice or have draining sores. With these possibilities in mind, be certain to wear appropriate personal protective equipment, as you must, when providing care to any patient.

When you are called to provide care for a homeless person, recognize that the patient will most likely be distrustful. Runaway teenagers and homeless women with children may worry that you will report them to child protective services. Drug abusers may worry that you will report them to the police. The patient's shoes and clothing are likely to be dirty. He may reek of an odor that is a mix of sweat, urine, and stool. Some patients will be embarrassed about their poor hygiene.

Every patient, regardless of the circumstances, deserves to be treated with respect. Unless the patient is one that you are frequently called to treat and have come to know, it is more likely that you will be unaware of the circumstances that resulted in the patient's homelessness and current situation. Talk with your patient and listen without making a moral judgment. Document your assessment findings and the care provided objectively.

The U.S. Department of Health and Human Services, U.S. Department of Housing and Urban Development (HUD), U.S. Public Health Service, and many other agencies fund programs to help the homeless. These programs are managed by local organizations that provide a range of services, including shelter, food, counseling, and job skills programs. You should become familiar with homeless assistance agencies in your area. Consider visiting a homeless shelter or soup kitchen to learn more about the homeless population and the challenges they face every day.

Bariatric Patients

Objective 7

Bariatrics is the branch of medicine that deals with the causes, prevention, and treatment of obesity and weight-related health problems. The bariatric patient is at increased risk for diabetes, hypertension, heart disease, and stroke.

Proper positioning and handling of the bariatric patient are important. If the patient is conscious and hypotension is not present, allow her to assume a position of comfort, which is usually sitting upright. This position generally offers the patient the best opportunity for adequate ventilation.

Before moving a bariatric patient, know in advance the manufacturer's weight limitations on such EMS equipment as backboards, stair chairs, and stretchers. Some EMS systems have specialized units for transporting bariatric patients. Bariatric stretchers are typically moved into the transport vehicle on a ramp by using a pulley or winch system. Request additional resources if this equipment is unavailable and the patient is large. Lifting a heavy or large patient not only puts your back at risk but also has a greater possibility of dropping the patient. Sometimes, if the patient is very large and bariatric EMS equipment is unavailable, unconventional methods of moving the patient have been necessary, such as the use of forklifts or flatbed trucks.

Patients with Special Healthcare Needs

Objectives 8, 9, 10

Patients with special needs may also be referred to as *technology-assisted patients*. These are patients who are experiencing a chronic or terminal illness, are being cared for at home, and are dependent on high-technology equipment.

Home care is professional assistance that a patient receives in his home. It does not require a doctor's prescription and does not include skilled nursing services. For example, some patients need assistance preparing meals, bathing, dressing, doing light housekeeping, washing laundry, changing bed linens, shopping for groceries, running errands, or moving around their home. These services are offered by homemaker services and are generally provided by nonmedical personal care.

Home healthcare is medical care provided in the home that is deemed medically necessary by a physician (requires a physician's prescription). Home healthcare is provided by home healthcare agencies, which are regulated by state and federal laws. Healthcare workers who provide home healthcare include registered nurses, licensed practical nurses, physical therapists, respiratory therapists, home care aides, occupational therapists, and social workers.

Tracheostomy Tubes

A **tracheostomy** is the creation of a surgical opening into the trachea through the neck, with insertion of a tube to aid passage of air or removal of secretions. The surgical opening created is called a *stoma*. A tracheostomy may be temporary or permanent. A temporary tracheostomy is sewn closed when no longer needed. In a permanent tracheostomy, a tube is inserted to keep the stoma open. Tracheostomy tubes come in a variety of types and sizes. They may be metal or plastic, cuffed or uncuffed. The tube selected depends on the patient's condition and physician preference. Complications that you may encounter include the following:

- Obstruction of the tube by dried secretions, excessive secretions, or airway swelling
- Dislodgment from coughing or patient movement, accidental removal, or inability to reinsert after a routine change
- Bleeding
- Air leak
- Infection

Emergency care includes maintaining an open airway. Request an early response of ALS personnel to the scene, or consider an ALS intercept while en route to the receiving facility. If the tracheostomy tube has become dislodged and the caregiver is unable to replace it, ventilate the patient as needed with a bag-mask device. Seal the bag-mask device over the patient's mouth and nose, and cover the stoma with a gloved hand. If unsuccessful, cover the stoma with a small mask and attempt to ventilate through the stoma. At the same time, cover the patient's mouth and nose with a gloved hand. If external bleeding is present, apply gentle direct pressure to the bleeding site, being careful not to block the airway or apply pressure to the carotid arteries. Allow the patient to maintain a position of comfort. Reassess as often as indicated. Record all patient care information, including the patient's medical history and all emergency care given, on a PCR.

Home Mechanical Ventilators

Mechanical ventilators are used to assist breathing in patients who are unable to breathe adequately on their own. Ventilator equipment is usually managed by a supplier that provides 24-hour emergency service. The home ventilator has an internal backup battery in case of power failure. Ventilator malfunction is usually the result of mechanical failure, power outage, or low oxygen supply.

If the ventilator is malfunctioning and the caregiver cannot quickly determine the cause of the problem, disconnect the patient from the ventilator and provide positive-pressure ventilation with a bag-mask device. Request an early response of ALS personnel to the scene, or consider an ALS intercept while en route to the receiving facility. If the patient has a tracheostomy tube in place, the bag-mask device can be connected directly to the tracheostomy tube. Reassess as often as indicated en route. Record all patient care information, including the patient's medical history and all emergency care given, on a PCR.

Apnea Monitors

Some patients are on home apnea monitors. The patient wears a strap around her chest that is equipped with sensors. The strap is connected to a monitor that has an alarm. The sensors monitor the patient's chest movement and heart rate. If the patient does not breathe for a preset number of seconds or if the patient's heart rate drops below or rises above a predetermined level, an alarm on the monitor sounds. Although apnea monitors are used for patients of all ages, they are probably most often used for premature infants on their discharge home from the hospital.

If you are called to the scene where the alarm on an apnea monitor sounded, chances are the patient will have resumed adequate breathing by the time you arrive. Quickly assess the patient. Ensure that his airway is open, and assess the adequacy of his breathing. If breathing is inadequate, provide positive-pressure ventilation with a bag-mask device. Begin chest compressions, if indicated. Reassess as often as indicated en route to the hospital. Record all patient care information, including the patient's medical history and all emergency care given, on a PCR.

Central Lines

A **central line** is an intravenous line placed near the heart for long-term use. Central lines may be used to give medications and nutritional solutions directly into the venous circulation.

A **peripherally inserted central catheter** is also called a *PICC line*. A PICC line is smaller than those routinely used for central lines. Complications include a cracked line, infection, clotting, and bleeding.

If you are called for a patient who has a problem with a central line or PICC line, request an early response of ALS personnel to the scene, or consider an ALS intercept while en route to the receiving facility. Establish and maintain an open airway. Give the patient oxygen if needed. If the site is bleeding, apply direct pressure to the site with a sterile dressing. Reassess as often as indicated. Record all patient care information, including the patient's medical history and all emergency care given, on a PCR.

Gastrostomy Tubes and Gastric Feeding

A **gastrostomy tube** is a special catheter placed directly into the stomach for feeding. It is most often used when passage of a tube through a patient's mouth, pharynx, or esophagus is contraindicated or impossible or when the tube must be maintained for a long period. A typical gastrostomy tube sticks out about 12–15 inches from the skin. It is sewn in place. A skin-level "feeding button" may be used in patients who require long-term gastrostomy feedings. The button is small and sticks out only slightly from the abdomen. The button has a one-way valve that accepts a feeding tube. It allows the patient greater mobility and comfort and is easier to care for than a gastrostomy tube.

Emergency care for a patient with a gastrostomy tube includes making sure the airway remains open. Request an early response of ALS personnel to the scene, or consider an ALS intercept while en route to the receiving facility. Be prepared to suction if necessary. Be alert for changes in mental status. If the patient is a diabetic, she will become hypoglycemic quickly if she cannot be fed. Give oxygen as needed. Check the site for bleeding, and control bleeding if present. Transport the patient in a sitting (Fowler's) position or lying on the right side, with the head elevated. Reassess as often as indicated. Record all patient care information, including the patient's medical history and all emergency care given, on a PCR.

Shunts

Hydrocephalus (commonly known as "water on the brain") is a condition in which there is an excess of cerebrospinal fluid (CSF) within the brain. A **ventricular shunt** is a drainage system used to remove the excess CSF. A catheter is surgically implanted in a chamber in the brain. The catheter is connected to a reservoir that collects the fluid. The reservoir can usually be felt through the skin behind the ear. A one-way valve prevents fluid from flowing back into the chamber. The reservoir is connected to a drainage catheter that empties into the abdominal cavity. The major complications associated with shunts include infection and equipment failure caused by obstruction, kinking, plugging, displacement, or separation of the tubing. If the shunt becomes blocked, excess CSF will collect in the brain and pressure within the skull will increase. This will produce such signs and symptoms as changes in men-

tal status, headache, irritability, vomiting, seizures, and respiratory depression.

Request an early response of ALS personnel to the scene, or consider an ALS intercept while en route to the receiving facility. Establish and maintain an open airway. Be prepared to suction if necessary. Give oxygen. If the patient's breathing is adequate, apply oxygen by nonrebreather mask at 15 L/min if not already done. If the patient's breathing is inadequate, provide bag-mask ventilation with 100% oxygen. Reassess as often as indicated. Record all patient care information, including the patient's medical history and all emergency care given, on a PCR.

Hospice Care

Objective 11

Palliative care (also called comfort care) is care provided to relieve symptoms of disease, such as pain, nausea, and vomiting, rather than to cure the disease. Palliative care is usually provided for patients with a terminal illness and their families.

The Centers for Disease Control and Prevention define **hospice care** as a program of palliative and supportive care services providing physical, psychological, social, and spiritual care for dying persons, their families, and other loved ones. Most hospice care is provided in the patient's home. Hospice care is provided by a team consisting of a registered nurse, social worker, physician medical director, chaplains, counselors, and support specialists as needed, such as a pharmacist and pediatrician. For a patient to be eligible for hospice care, the patient's physician usually certifies that the patient is terminal (has less than 6 months to live). The patient must no longer be seeking a cure for his disease. Hospice services include grief counseling, which is available to the patient and his family, usually for up to 13 months after the patient's death.

A hospice patient, in consultation with her family and the hospice team, decides the treatment she wants to receive. Many hospice patients have do not resuscitate (DNR) orders that reflect their wishes about what they want done in the event of a cardiopulmonary arrest.

If you are called to a scene where the patient has a terminal illness, you are expected to assess the patient as you would in any other situation. Determine the existence of a valid DNR as a part of your patient assessment. If the patient is breathless and pulseless and his DNR is valid and specifies withholding CPR in the event of a cardiac and/or respiratory arrest, you should honor the patient's request by withholding CPR. You may need to begin resuscitation efforts while you determine the status of the patient's DNR. Contact medical control if you are uncertain about what to do. Begin treatment of the patient, including CPR, if the DNR has been revoked. Avoid confrontation with family. If the family demands care in contrast to that specified in a valid DNR, provide basic care while contacting medical control and providing information pertinent to the situation.

On the Scene Wrap-Up

You put on appropriate personal protective equipment and perform an assessment as you would on any other patient. You find that the patient may have chest pain secondary to a cardiac event. You do not allow the patient's prior history or the fact that he is homeless deter you from offering him the very best of care. You apply a nonrebreather mask and begin gathering the patient's medical history while your partner obtains the patient's vital signs. You then prepare the patient for transport, providing additional care en route to the hospital. ∎

Sum It Up

▶ Child maltreatment is an act or failure to act by a parent, caregiver, or other person as defined by state law that results in physical abuse, neglect, medical neglect, sexual abuse, and/or emotional abuse. It is also defined as an act or failure to act that presents an impending risk of serious harm to a child.

▶ There are four common types of abuse: physical abuse, sexual abuse, emotional abuse, and neglect. Physical abuse refers to physical acts that cause or could cause physical injury to a child. Sexual abuse is inappropriate adolescent or adult sexual behavior with a child. Emotional abuse refers to behaviors that harm a child's self-worth or emotional well-being. Neglect is the failure to provide for a child's basic physical, emotional, or educational needs or to protect a child from harm or potential harm. Medical neglect is a type of maltreatment caused by failure of the caregiver to provide for the appropriate healthcare of the child although financially able to do so.

▶ When providing care for an infant or a child who is ill or injured due to neglect or abuse, show a professional and caring attitude for the patient. Report known or suspected child abuse as required by law in your state. Carefully document your physical exam findings as well as your observations of the child's environment. Document the caregiver's comments exactly as stated, and enclose them in quota-

tion marks. Your documentation must reflect the facts and not your opinion of what may or may not have occurred. Report your findings to appropriate personnel when transferring patient care.

▶ Elder abuse is any physical, sexual, or emotional abuse or neglect committed against an older adult. Domestic elder abuse refers to maltreatment of an older adult that occurs in the elder's home (or in the home of a caregiver) by an individual who has a special relationship with the elder (such as a spouse, sibling, child, friend, or caregiver). Institutional elder abuse occurs in residential facilities for older persons, such as nursing homes, foster homes, group homes, or board and care facilities. Self-neglect or self-abuse is the conscious and voluntary behavior of a mentally competent older adult that threatens his own health or safety as a matter of personal choice. Types of elder abuse are similar to those encountered with children and include physical, sexual, and emotional abuse and neglect.

▶ EMS is often the primary route that the homeless use to access healthcare. Homeless people typically do not have health insurance or money to pay for healthcare services, and most do not have transportation. Talk with your patient and listen without making a moral judgment. Document your assessment findings and the care provided objectively.

▶ Bariatrics is the branch of medicine that deals with the causes, prevention, and treatment of obesity and weight-related health problems. Before moving a bariatric patient, know in advance the manufacturer's weight limitations on such EMS equipment as backboards, stair chairs, and stretchers.

▶ Patients with special needs may also be referred to as technology-assisted patients. These are patients who are experiencing a chronic or terminal illness, are being cared for at home, and are dependent on high-technology equipment.

▶ Home care is professional assistance that a patient receives in her home. It does not require a doctor's prescription and does not include skilled nursing services. Home healthcare is medical care provided in the home that is deemed medically necessary by a physician (requires a physician's prescription). Home healthcare is provided by home healthcare agencies, which are regulated by state and federal laws.

▶ A central line is an intravenous line placed near the heart for long-term use. Central lines may be used to give medications and nutritional solutions directly into the venous circulation. A peripherally inserted central catheter is also called a PICC line. A PICC line is smaller than those routinely used for central lines.

- A gastrostomy tube is a special catheter placed directly into the stomach for feeding. It is most often used when passage of a tube through a patient's mouth, pharynx, or esophagus is contraindicated or impossible or when the tube must be maintained for a long period.
- Hydrocephalus is a condition in which there is an excess of cerebrospinal fluid within the brain. A ventricular shunt is a drainage system used to remove the excess CSF.

- Palliative care (also called comfort care) is care provided to relieve symptoms of disease, such as pain, nausea, and vomiting, rather than to cure the disease. Palliative care is usually provided for patients with a terminal illness and their families.
- Hospice care is a program of palliative and supportive care services providing physical, psychological, social, and spiritual care for dying persons, their families, and other loved ones. Most hospice care is provided in the patient's home.

Module 10

EMS Operations

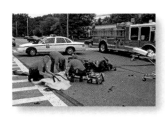

▶ CHAPTER 47

Principles of Emergency Response and Transportation 815

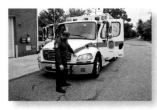

▶ CHAPTER 48

Incident Management 833

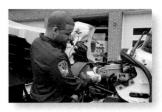

▶ CHAPTER 49

Multiple-Casualty Incidents 838

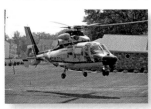

▶ CHAPTER 50

Air Medical Transport 844

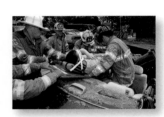

► CHAPTER **51**

Vehicle Extrication   849

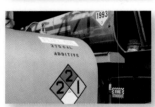

► CHAPTER **52**

Hazardous Materials Awareness   858

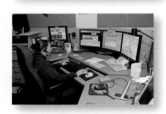

► CHAPTER **53**

Terrorism and Disaster Response   866

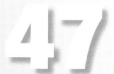

Principles of Emergency Response and Transportation

By the end of this chapter, you should be able to:

Knowledge Objectives ▶

1. Discuss the medical and nonmedical equipment needed to respond to a call.
2. Differentiate among the various methods of moving a patient to the unit on the basis of injury or illness.
3. Discuss the measures necessary to ensure safe operation of an emergency vehicle.
4. State what information is essential in order to respond to a call.
5. Describe the general provisions of state laws relating to the operation of the ambulance and privileges in any or all of the following categories: speed, warning lights, sirens, right-of-way, parking, and turning.
6. Discuss "due regard for the safety of others" while operating an emergency vehicle.
7. List contributing factors to unsafe driving conditions.
8. Give examples of possible driver distractions.
9. Describe the considerations that should be given to a request for escorts, following of an escort vehicle, and intersections.
10. Determine if the scene is safe to enter.
11. Describe the important factors to consider when placing an emergency vehicle at the emergency scene.
12. Discuss communication with dispatch and the receiving facility during the transport phase of an emergency response.
13. Discuss the verbal report provided and the importance of an accurate prehospital care report when transferring patient care.
14. Summarize the importance of preparing the unit for the next response.
15. Distinguish among the terms cleaning, low-level disinfection, intermediate-level disinfection, high-level disinfection, and sterilization.
16. Describe how to clean or disinfect items following patient care.

Attitude Objectives ▶

17. Explain the rationale for appropriate report of patient information.
18. Explain the rationale for having the unit prepared to respond.

Skill Objectives ▶

No skill objectives are identified for this lesson.

You are looking forward to your first day as an EMT. You have arrived early for your shift. You have combed your hair, pressed your uniform, verified that all your certification cards are current, and studied your local protocols to make sure you are up to date with appropriate treatments. Your partner for the day is a 15-year veteran who is known for her extensive knowledge of prehospital care. She introduces you to members of the off-going shift and then asks you to sit while she explains how she likes to have things done on "her shift." At exactly 0800, you ask if you should begin checking the equipment for the day. Your partner explains that the crews have an "arrangement" at this station. No one checks the equipment unless the off-going crew reports that they did not have time to replace something used on a late call. As the off-going crew did not mentioned anything, she says, "The equipment is fine." For the next hour your partner talks to you about her years of experience as an EMT. You are amazed at the amount of information that she has stored inside her head.

You hear your first alarm, dispatching your unit to a possible cardiac arrest at a local shopping mall. You and your partner respond quickly and efficiently to the proper address. While en route, you review the list of equipment that may be needed at the scene and wonder where it might be located. Your unit is the first to arrive. Your partner states that she will get the stretcher as you get the rest of the equipment. It takes you several minutes to find the needed equipment, as you have never looked inside this vehicle before. In fact, you are unable to find an automated external defibrillator (AED) or an airway kit. You decide to assist your partner with the stretcher and hope that the next unit will have additional equipment. You find the patient lying on the ground next to his vehicle in the mall parking lot. The patient is in cardiac arrest. Your partner begins positive-pressure ventilation with a bag-mask device while you start chest compressions. ■

THINK ABOUT IT

As you read this chapter, think about the following questions:

- Could a lack of proper equipment have an unfavorable effect on the care your patient receives?
- If you could turn back the clock, what would you have done differently when you arrived on the job today?

Introduction

An EMT must be familiar with emergency vehicle operations, the medical and nonmedical equipment used in patient care, and the phases of an emergency response. To minimize the risk of exposure to and transmission of infectious diseases, an EMT must understand the primary methods of decontamination. Although an overview of emergency vehicle operations is presented in this chapter, you should consider completing a standardized emergency vehicle operator's course.

Your patient needs and deserves your best effort at all times, including daily vehicle checks and the cleaning and restocking of your apparatus. Be diligent in all duties, and represent your profession with pride and integrity. Remember your life, your partner's life, and the lives of your patients will literally be in your hands.

Principles of Emergency Response

Preparation Phase
Personnel and Basic Supplies

Objective 1

Preparation for an EMS call requires ensuring that appropriately trained personnel are available to respond. Minimum staffing requirements for an ambulance include at least one EMT in the patient compartment. Two EMTs are preferred. In some states, two licensed personnel are required.

In some states, ambulances are licensed. In others, ambulances are certified, and some states do not have such a designation. To be licensed or certified as ambulances, emergency transport vehicles are required to carry specific types and quantities of medical equipment. You must check with your local and state regulatory agencies for the specific equipment requirements. Supplies in addition to those in the next *You Should Know* box may be needed to address the specific needs of your agency or the type of calls that are most common in your area.

In addition to basic medical supplies, nonmedical supplies that must be carried include personal safety equipment as required by local, state, and federal standards, as well as preplanned routes or comprehensive street maps. A ground ambulance must also be equipped to provide, and be capable of providing, voice communication between:

- The ambulance attendant and the dispatch center
- The ambulance attendant and the ground ambulance service's assigned medical direction authority
- The ambulance attendant in the patient compartment and the ground ambulance service's assigned medical direction authority

Remember This

Avoid the temptation to overstock your emergency vehicle. If you believe that there is a need for additional supplies, contact the appropriate individual or committee to change the normal quantity.

Patient Transfer Equipment

Objective 2

In most instances, your agency will have already determined the type of patient transfer equipment that will be available for you to use on each call. You must learn the proper method(s) of using this equipment. The proper use of this equipment and the appropriate techniques for lifting will help ensure your patient's safety and will also reduce your risk of injury during a lifting procedure.

Generally, each patient transport vehicle will have the following basic patient transfer equipment: a wheeled stretcher, a collapsible stretcher, and a long

You Should Know

Ground Ambulance: Basic Medical Equipment and Supplies

- Suction equipment (portable and a fixed apparatus)
- Oxygen cylinders (fixed and portable), each with a variable flow regulator
- Oxygen administration equipment, including tubing, nasal cannula (adult and pediatric), and nonrebreather mask (adult and pediatric)
- Hand-operated, disposable, self-expanding bag-mask devices (adult and pediatric)
- Adult, child, and infant oral airways
- Nasal airways
- Cervical stabilization devices
- Upper- and lower-extremity splints
- Traction splint
- Full-length spine boards
- Supplies to secure a patient to a spine board
- Cervical-thoracic spinal stabilization device for extrication
- Sterile burn sheets
- Triangular bandages
- Multitrauma dressings, 10×30 inches or larger
- Abdominal bandages, 5×7 inches or larger
- Nonsterile 4×4-inch gauze sponges
- Nonsterile soft roller bandages, 4 inches or larger
- Nonsterile elastic roller bandages, 4 inches or larger
- Sterile occlusive dressings, 3×8 inches or larger
- Adhesive tape rolls, 2 or 3 inches in width
- Sterile obstetrical kit containing towels, 4×4-inch dressings, scissors, bulb suction, and clamps or tape for the umbilical cord
- Blood pressure cuffs (child size, adult size, and large adult size)
- Specific emergency medications as determined by protocols
- Automated external defibrillator (AED)
- Stethoscope
- Heavy-duty scissors capable of cutting clothing, belts, or boots
- Blankets, sheets
- Infection control materials, including protective gloves, gowns, masks, shoe coverings, filtration masks, protective eyewear, and nonlatex gloves

backboard or Stokes basket. Some EMS agencies will also have a bariatric stretcher available for use.

Wheeled stretchers are used more often than any other patient transfer device. A collapsible stretcher is designed to be folded. It is generally used when a standard stretcher is too large to be used on scene. Care should be taken to ensure that your patient is properly secured to the stretcher before moving. This requires two straps applied over the patient's shoulders, one strap at the chest, one at the hips, and one at the legs. Kinds of collapsible stretchers include the stair chair and the roll-up stretcher. When using a collapsible stretcher, remember to plan the move before lifting the patient. Someone must be "in charge" to ensure a coordinated and safe move to the stretcher. In most instances, you will need additional personnel to ensure a safe lift. Never try to move these types of stretchers without a clear path to the main stretcher. A stair chair will force your patient into a sitting position. This may cause additional pain or even injury if the chair is used improperly. If the patient has experienced trauma or has the potential for any spinal injury, consider the use of a long backboard or the Stokes-style stretcher.

If needed, request additional resources and personnel before moving a patient. Then secure your patient to the device. Explain your plan to the patient before the first move. An unsuspecting patient who is frightened by suddenly being lifted into the air will reach out for support and grab the closest object, which may be you!

In some instances, you will need to use alternative devices to move a patient during the extrication phase of a rescue. Only trained personnel using proper safety and personal protective equipment should attempt these specialty rescues. If you are part of this kind of rescue, take precautions to securely strap your patient onto the rescue board or into the basket. This style of rescue may place your patient at an extreme angle during the extrication. You must prevent movement or slipping in all planes of travel.

Stop and Think!

Think before you lift. Is there a better path? Have you removed any obstacles that may trip you and cause you to drop the patient? Have all personnel on the scene heard the plan, and do they understand their part in the move?

Daily Inspections

Objective 3

The importance of careful completion of the preparation phase cannot be overemphasized. Preparing your vehicle for daily operation is important.

Your first preparations for duty start before you arrive at the workplace. The knowledge and skills that you acquired during your initial training must be constantly refreshed and practiced. Careful review of your knowledge base and practice with infrequently used equipment will prepare you to give the most efficient and skilled patient care possible.

Planning for duty includes getting a reasonable amount of rest before your shift. You will be required to move your patients to the stretcher and lift them into the transport vehicle. Staying in shape and exercising will protect your back and ensure the safety of your patients during a lift.

Vehicle Inspection

One of your primary responsibilities will be to check the safe condition of your vehicle and determine whether it is ready for operation. Your vehicle inspection begins with a careful consideration of the types of calls that you will respond to and the type of vehicle needed for these responses. The normal operation of an emergency vehicle has the potential to cause wear and damage to the vehicle. You may be held legally responsible if your apparatus is unable to respond or breaks down during an emergency response and the determination is made that the mechanical failure was preventable. At the very least, you may incur legal responsibility if the failure leads to an accident or injury. Or worse, your patient's life may be endangered.

Exterior Begin your vehicle inspection with a conversation with the crew that used the apparatus during the previous shift. They should be able to inform you about any needs or deficits in the apparatus. Next, visually inspect your vehicle for any obvious damage or deficits (Figure 47-1). Note any breakage

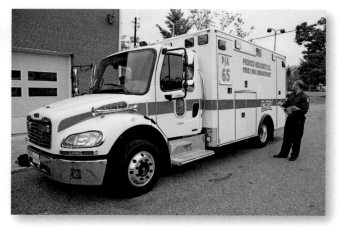

FIGURE 47-1 ▲ Inspect the exterior of the emergency vehicle for any obvious damage. Note any breakage or damage on the appropriate check-off sheet.

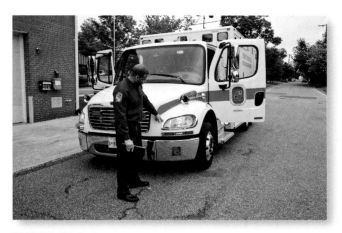

FIGURE 47-2 ▲ Vehicle inspection must include the activation of all lighting devices.

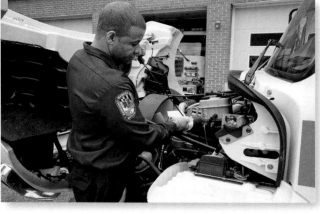

FIGURE 47-3 ▲ Check the vehicle's engine compartment. Inspect the condition of the radiator, hoses and belts and the levels of all fluids.

or damage on the appropriate check-off sheet. Decide if the vehicle needs immediate repair or is safe for operation.

All glass should be inspected and free of breakage, and the windshield wipers should function properly. Tires should have no visible damage to the rims or sidewalls. The tread depth should be no less than the state's accepted minimum; the nationally recognized minimum is about ⅛-inch. Tire pressure should be appropriate to manufacturer's guidelines. In addition, all tire lugs should be inspected to ensure that they are tight and none is missing.

All doors and compartments should open and close with ease. The latching mechanisms should be intact and in working order. External mirrors should be intact and in the proper position for vehicle operation. All external lights should function properly and have no damage to the external housing. This inspection must include the activation of all lighting devices (Figure 47-2).

When inspecting the engine, make sure the motor is off. You should wear gloves to protect your hands from any damage or contamination. Start with a visual inspection of the entire engine compartment, and look for any obviously loose or damaged components. All hoses should be intact and not have any visible cracks or abrasions.

Inspect the radiator for leaks or damage, and verify that the fluid reservoir is at the appropriate level. If fluid must be added, contact the maintenance division or consult your local policies to determine the proper type and amount of fluid to add. All belts should be inspected for cracks or unusual wear. The appropriate personnel should immediately replace any damaged belt. Inspect the battery and cables to confirm that they are intact and that the cables are tightly connected to the battery. Pay particular attention to any visible

corrosion as this may interfere with the proper connection of the cables to the battery.

Check all fluid levels as detailed by the operator's guide (Figure 47-3). Oil levels should match the manufacturer's specifications and generally oil must be clear or tan in color. Black engine oil is an indication of the need for an oil change or may be indicative of a potential failure. Transmission fluid levels are generally checked after the vehicle has been warmed up. The vehicle operator's guide should be consulted for the proper method of inspection. Windshield washer fluid should be checked as a standard part of all vehicle inspections. This fluid may be of critical importance during winter driving conditions.

Patient Area Begin inspection of the patient compartment by looking at the general cleanliness of the area. Next, confirm that all safety equipment and seat belts are in good repair and function properly. All patient care equipment must be checked to ensure that there are appropriate stock levels and that each item functions as required (Figure 47-4). This includes cardiac monitors, suction devices, sharps containers, and your response bag or box. The inspection of any battery-powered device must include verification of proper battery levels and the availability of additional batteries for extended responses. The equipment must then be properly stowed and secured in preparation for a response.

Continued inspection of the patient area should confirm the proper functioning of the heating, cooling, and exhaust system. All oxygen storage devices should be checked to confirm that they contain appropriate levels of oxygen and that the regulators function properly.

In general, most transport vehicles have communications equipment available in the patient area. This

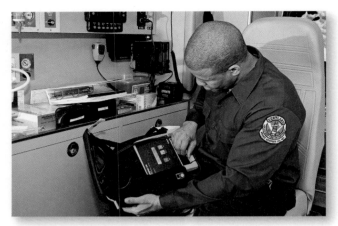

FIGURE 47-4 ▲ Check all patient care equipment to ensure that there are appropriate stock levels and that each item functions as required.

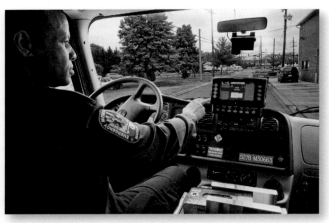

FIGURE 47-5 ▲ In the operator's area, inspect all warning and fluid gauges on the instrument panel to confirm that they are functioning and indicating safe operational levels.

equipment must also be checked to confirm that it functions as required.

Operator Area The operator's area requires not only inspection but also the adjustment of some equipment to your specifications. The first piece of equipment to be checked is the operator's seat. It should be placed at a safe and comfortable distance from the steering wheel and operator's floor pedals. Most new apparatus will allow the operator to change the angle and distance of the steering wheel in relation to the operator's console. Many of the inspections required in the operator's area require that the vehicle to be started and kept running. This check of equipment while the vehicle is running must be performed outside of any structure or in an area where appropriate exhaust-handling systems are in place. Failure to follow this guideline can lead to the potential exposure to carbon monoxide.

First, inspect all warning and fluid gauges on the instrument panel to confirm that all are functioning and indicating safe operational levels (Figure 47-5). Activate the turn signals and then verify that they function properly. Note any deficiencies for immediate follow-up and repair before using the vehicle on a call. Although it is important to verify the proper functioning of the horn and siren, in many instances this is prohibited by the placement of the station and the apparatus. Remember to warn all personnel in the area before activating the horn or sirens. Inappropriate use of the horn or siren during vehicle inspection has the potential to cause hearing damage in any nearby personnel who are not wearing the proper protective devices. Always wear hearing protection before and during this testing.

Adjust all mirrors as needed. Adjust safety belts and restraint devices as needed. Confirm that all interior lights function appropriately. Parking brakes should be checked for proper operation. Communica-

tions equipment also needs to be checked. Follow local protocol for the safe and proper method of verifying the operation of this equipment.

Remember This

Safe operation of an emergency vehicle affects the safety of the crew, the patient, and the general public. You should not leave the station with a vehicle that is not safe for the road.

Dispatch Phase

Objective 4

In the dispatch phase of an EMS response, the patient or a witness reports the emergency by calling 9-1-1 or another emergency number. The call to 9-1-1 goes to a central communications system that is available 24 hours a day. This system links police, fire, and EMS resources. An emergency medical dispatcher (EMD) receives the call and gathers information from the caller (Figure 47-6). The dispatcher then activates (dispatches) an appropriate EMS response based on the information received. The EMD will attempt to gather important information from the caller, including:

- The nature of the call
- The name, location, and callback number of the caller
- The location of the patient
- The number of patients and the severity of their illnesses or injuries
- Other special problems that can be identified by the caller

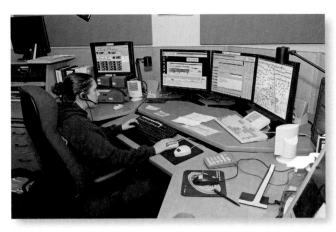

FIGURE 47-6 ▲ An emergency medical dispatcher receives an emergency call, gathers information from the caller, and activates an appropriate EMS response based on the information received.

The EMD is also responsible for coordinating logistics. An EMD is knowledgeable about the geography of the area, the EMS's capabilities, and the activities of other public service agencies. In most EMS systems, the EMD is trained to relay instructions to the caller for life-saving procedures that can be performed, if necessary, while waiting for trained medical personnel to arrive. A good EMD can make a big difference on a call. He or she can shave minutes off your response time by getting precise information about the location of your patient, can keep you safe by asking about hazards on the scene, and can send you appropriate resources in a timely manner.

En Route, or Response, Phase

As you respond to the reported emergency, begin to anticipate the knowledge, equipment, and skills you may need to provide appropriate patient care. Notify the dispatcher that you are responding to the call. Write down the essential information from the dispatcher, including the nature and location of the call.

Determine the responsibilities of the crew members before arriving on the scene. For example, while you and your partner are en route to the scene, decide who will assess the patient and who will document the call. In most agencies, these responsibilities are determined at the start of a shift instead of on the way to a call.

Most states and many companies encourage or even require all emergency vehicle operators to attend and successfully complete an approved driver-training course. The characteristics of good emergency vehicle operators include the following:

- Being physically and mentally fit
- Being able to perform under stress
- Having a positive attitude about their skills
- Being tolerant of other drivers

Safe driving is important in the emergency medical care of the ill or injured patient. Your safe arrival (and that of your crew) at the scene will be one of the most important things that happens during your response. Your late arrival at the scene because of an accident while en route will delay the lifesaving care that your patient needs. Bluntly stated, you may be the best EMT in the world, but you cannot render care if you don't get there!

As you begin your response to the reported emergency, use preplanned routes and street maps. Select the best route on the basis of weather, traffic patterns, and road conditions. You may need to consider many different factors. For instance, you may need to use a different route depending on the time of day, day of the week, detours, road closings, bridges, railroad crossings, tunnels, schools, heavy traffic areas, weather, or local construction. Plan an alternate route if unforeseen conditions are encountered. Consider the need for additional resources if the call is a large incident with multiple patients. Other factors to consider may include checking the wind direction as you approach the scene to confirm that you are upwind from a possible hazardous materials exposure.

Safety guidelines, such as the use of seat belts, should be exercised during each response. The list of actions shown in the following *Remember This* box may be used as a guide for your safe response to an incident or emergency.

Remember This

Response Action List

- Verify the location and type of call.
- Select the most appropriate route.
- Observe weather and road conditions, and modify response if needed.
- Apply safety restraint devices.
- Notify the dispatch agency of your response.
- Modify your emergency response on the basis of your knowledge of the characteristics of your response vehicle. Factors such as length, width, and weight will alter the way your vehicle handles.
- Understand appropriate use of lights and siren.
- Obtain additional information from dispatch.
- Drive with due regard for the safety of others.
- Maintain a safe following distance.
- Approach the scene from uphill and upwind as needed.

Emergency Response

Objectives 5, 6

The general definition of an **emergency response** is the operation of an emergency vehicle while responding to a medical emergency. Laws pertaining to the proper methods of responding to an emergency vary from state to state. These laws also govern the use of emergency signaling devices, such as lights and sirens. In general, most states require that emergency vehicle operators obey all traffic regulations unless a specific exemption has been made and documented in statute. Most states allow these exemptions unless their use endangers life or property. In addition, these exemptions are typically granted only when a true emergency exists. The definition of a "true emergency" can be rather vague. A possible definition of a **true emergency** is a situation in which there is a high possibility of death or serious injury and the rapid response of an emergency vehicle may lessen the risk of death or injury.

When driving in emergency mode, the operator of an emergency vehicle must drive with due regard for the safety of others on the roadway. *Due regard* means that, in similar circumstances, a reasonable and responsible person would act in a way that is safe and considerate of others. The reasonableness of your emergency response will be judged on the basis of some of the following guidelines:

- Your patient care will be compromised if you are in a motor vehicle crash.
- Emergency vehicles should never operate at a speed greater than is warranted by the nature of the call or the condition of the patient being transported. This speed must also not be greater than traffic, road, and weather conditions allow.
- All emergency vehicle warning systems should be used as intended by the manufacturer and must be in operation during an emergency response.
- All emergency vehicle warning systems must be functioning in the prescribed manner before entering any intersection.

The following guidelines are intended to give an overview of motor vehicle laws and are not intended to supersede any local authority. Contact your local or state regulatory agency for the specifics of an emergency response in your area.

Speed and Speed Limits

The posted speed limit on any road or highway is determined by many factors, such as the type of road surface and the normal driving conditions. Most states allow for the increase of your emergency response speed to a maximum of 10 miles an hour over the posted speed limit. This increase is also based on weather and road conditions. Most emergency response training courses discourage any increase in your response speed over the posted limit. In general, an increase in speed also increases the risk to the responding crews and the general public on the roadways. Remember: Speed does not save lives—good patient care does.

Warning Lights and Sirens

Emergency signaling devices such as warning lights and sirens are intended to alert other drivers that an emergency response vehicle is approaching and to request that they yield the right-of-way to that response vehicle. Transportation engineers and emergency response experts calculate that the use of emergency lights and sirens will decrease your overall response time only by seconds. This overall reduction in your response time comes with the added risk of accident and injury.

There are several factors that must be taken into consideration during your emergency response. Do the drivers around your vehicle know that there is an emergency vehicle approaching them? Do they have enough time to make a choice about what to do? Do they have time and space to respond or carry out their choice in an appropriate manner? It is impossible to determine if the drivers around you will notice your approach and react appropriately. You must be prepared for them to make the worst possible decision about how to respond to your approach.

Right-of-Way

Your use of lights and sirens does not automatically grant you the right-of-way. Your use of lights and siren is a *request*, not a *demand*, for the right-of-way. The standard rules of the road apply, even if you are in the emergency response mode. Other drivers may not see

You Should Know

- Headlights are the most visible warning devices on an emergency vehicle because they are mounted at the eye level of other drivers. Use caution during any response that uses lights and siren because of the "excitement factor."
- Most drivers will yield the right-of-way if they notice your approach with lights and siren. However, in many instances they will not know that you are there and may overcorrect their vehicle when they see you. This may potentially put your vehicle in jeopardy. You must be extremely alert when driving in emergency response mode. You must be prepared for these situations.

or hear your vehicle's warning devices because of conversation in their vehicles or the use of air conditioning or stereo equipment, among other reasons. Before taking the right-of-way, make sure other drivers see your emergency vehicle.

General Considerations

In general, most jurisdictions allow emergency response vehicle drivers to alter standard rules in many of the following situations:

- *Parking or standing.* You may be allowed to park or have the vehicle remain stationary even in posted no-parking areas.

- *Red lights, stop signs, intersections.* You must stop at all red lights, stop signs, and intersections even if you are responding to an emergency. However, once you have checked that the intersection is clear and no traffic is preparing to enter the intersection, you may proceed through the red light at a slow rate of speed.

- *Speed limit.* Maintain your speed at the speed limit or below as weather conditions permit. In general, the vehicle may travel up to 10 miles per hour over the posted speed limit if conditions and traffic allow. Because some state laws specify "reasonable speed," be sure to check your state laws pertaining to this topic.

- *Directions of flow and specified turns.* You may use all lanes of travel and even turn against no-turn signs to reach the emergency scene. However, you are responsible for any collision and injury, regardless of your response mode.

- *Emergency or disaster routes.* You may be allowed to use any emergency route or access, but do so with extreme caution.

- *School buses. Do not* proceed past a school bus that has stopped to load or unload unless it has specifically yielded to your lights and siren. Approach the school bus that is stopped to pick up passengers with extreme caution. You should make eye contact with the driver to verify that it is safe to proceed before passing this vehicle.

Contributing Factors to Unsafe Driving Conditions

Objectives 7, 8

Some of the factors that contribute to unsafe driving conditions include heavy traffic, traffic jams, wind, rain, snow and ice, dust, fog, animals, debris, running or standing water, night driving, and fatigue. Examples of possible driver distractions are listed in the following *You Should Know* box.

You Should Know

Possible Driver Distractions

- Mobile computer
- Global positioning systems
- Mobile radio
- Visual and audible devices
- Vehicle stereo
- Wireless devices
- Eating or drinking

Wind has the potential to influence the handling characteristics of your emergency response vehicle. Most emergency response vehicles have a higher center of gravity than other vehicles. A strong crosswind can cause your vehicle to sway or even overturn. As you encounter other vehicles or changes in terrain, the winds may be blocked or even funneled into stronger gusts. Be prepared for these changes, and reduce your speed appropriately. Use extreme caution in high winds, especially around curves or corners and on wet or icy roads.

Rain can reduce tire traction and block your vision during an emergency response. Always verify that the emergency vehicle's windshield wipers are functioning and that there are no cracks or dry spots in the blades. Tire tread depth and design can be a factor when water is on the roadway. Hydroplaning is possible any time there is rain or standing water on the roadway. Reduce speed, and be prepared for hydroplaning or tire pull caused by rain.

Snow and ice can be extremely hazardous and tend to reduce tire traction even in small amounts. Be aware of local weather conditions. Be prepared for ice to form, particularly on bridges or shaded portions of the roadway. Tire tread design and depth are factors that must be considered before your response. Add traction devices or change to traction-type tires when you have advance knowledge of the possibility of adverse weather. The best advice is to *slow down.* Snow and ice can be especially hazardous during braking, turning, and accelerating. Each of these maneuvers may cause sliding. In addition, blowing snow can rapidly reduce visibility. You must reduce speed to avoid collisions during this type of weather. Snow and ice may also build up rapidly on the windshield. You will need good wiper blades and the proper windshield washer fluid to remove it.

Dust and dust storms are a significant hazard in some areas and can reduce driving visibility to zero in just seconds. You must be aware of the potential for these storms. Never knowingly enter a dust storm. If you are already on the roadway when one occurs, reduce your speed and safely exit the roadway as far as you reasonably can. Next, turn off your headlights and emergency lights, and remove your foot from the brake pedal. Traffic on the roadway may mistakenly believe that your taillights are from a moving vehicle on the roadway and may strike you.

Some areas of the country experience fog at almost any time of year. Visibility may be reduced significantly, and your driving will be impaired. Always reduce your speed to match road conditions. Turn on any fog lights with which your vehicle is equipped. Generally, the low-beam setting on your headlights will be more beneficial than the high beams. The increased amount of light produced by the high beams tends to be reflected back by the fog, further reducing visibility. If your vehicle has an Opticom or a strobe that activates traffic signal lights, consider turning it off. Driving for any extended period with this system functioning has the potential to "mesmerize" you or to draw your attention to the reflection and away from the road.

Response to some rural areas can bring you into conflict with everything from livestock to large wild animals. Hitting an elk, moose, or cow even at low speeds can be deadly. Slow down any time there is the possibility of this type of collision.

Be alert to the possibility of debris in the roadway, and reduce your speed to limit the need for extreme maneuvers to dodge this material. Any extreme maneuver such as braking or steering around an object has the potential to cause harm to the personnel and patient in the transport vehicle. It may also contribute to losing control of the vehicle.

Standing water has the potential to either cause hydroplaning or even stall a vehicle, depending on the depth of the water, and should be approached cautiously and at a safe speed. Running water *must not* be entered in any circumstance. Moving water can sweep your vehicle downstream, placing all aboard in jeopardy. In addition, most states that have the possibility of flash flooding have laws that prohibit anyone from entering running water.

Nighttime can cause unsafe driving conditions because of decreased visibility. In addition, the number of sleep-deprived or otherwise impaired drivers increases dramatically at night. Use your headlights to your best advantage. Use your high beams if oncoming traffic will allow. Avoid the tendency to "overdrive" your headlights. Keep your eyes moving between an outside and an inside focal point. This will help to reduce eyestrain. As you approach an oncoming vehicle, scan the right shoulder instead of the centerline. This will help to keep your night vision intact.

Fatigue is another factor that must be considered. Fatigue will impair your judgment, vision, and driving skills. It may even impair your patient care skills. When the opportunity for rest arises, take a nap. Know your limits. Do not drive impaired.

Escorts and Multiple-Vehicle Responses

Objective 9

Escorts and multiple-vehicle responses are extremely dangerous. They should be used only when emergency responders are unfamiliar with the location of the patient or receiving facility or when multiple units from the same location are being called to a multiple-casualty incident. Provide a safe following distance (generally a minimum of 500 feet). Stop and then use the standard right-of-way guidelines to proceed through any intersection. Check your agency's policy regarding the use of siren and/or lights in these situations. Some agencies do not want them used because they may confuse other drivers. Other agencies specify that a different siren time and/or tone must be used to help other motorists distinguish multiple emergency vehicles.

Multiple-vehicle responses pose an even greater-than-normal hazard at intersections. For example, a motorist may see the first emergency vehicle pass and begin to proceed, assuming it was the only emergency vehicle. An accident may occur with the motorist and the second emergency vehicle. Each vehicle must "clear" the intersection by using the guidelines in the following section.

Intersection Crashes

Objective 9

Intersection crashes are the most common collision involving emergency vehicles.

Intersection crashes can occur in the following ways:
- The motorist arrives at an intersection as the light changes and does not stop.
- Multiple emergency vehicles are following closely, and a waiting motorist does not expect more than one vehicle.
- Vision is obstructed by vehicles waiting at an intersection, blocking the view of a pedestrian.

All intersections should be approached and cleared by using the following guidelines:
- Your siren should be in "wail" mode at least 300 feet before the intersection. Change your siren to the "yelp" mode 150 feet before the intersection (Figure 47-7).
- Begin deceleration, and make sure that your vehicle can be at a complete stop at the crosswalk line. Give two short blasts on the vehicle's air horn. Look to your left first, then straight ahead, then to the right, and then again to your left before entering the intersection.
- Verify that all left lanes are stopped and will remain stopped as you proceed into the intersection. The best method to verify that the driver of a stopped vehicle is aware of your

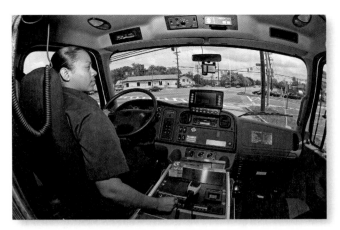

FIGURE 47-7 ▲ When approaching an intersection, your siren should be in "wail" mode at least 300 feet before the intersection. Change your siren to the "yelp" mode 150 feet before the intersection.

presence in the intersection is to make eye contact with each driver.

- Proceed carefully through the intersection at no more than 10 miles per hour. Use extreme caution when crossing the path of a vacant lane to your left or right. Drivers in these lanes may be unaware of your presence in the intersection.
- Right turns from a left lane at an intersection where all traffic has stopped can be very hazardous. Verify that all drivers are stopped and are aware of your need to make a right turn in front of them. Proceed with extreme caution.

You must also be aware of the potential for other emergency vehicles responding through the same intersection at the same time as your vehicle does so. Confirm that they have completely stopped before proceeding with your response.

You Should Know

Contributing Factors to Unsafe Driving Conditions
- Escorts
- Road surface
- Excessive speed
- Reckless driving
- Weather conditions
- Multiple-vehicle response
- Inadequate dispatch information and unfamiliarity with the location
- Failure to heed traffic warning signals
- Disregarding of traffic rules and regulations
- Failure to anticipate the actions of other motorists
- Failure to obey traffic signals or posted speed limits

Arrival Phase and Scene Size-Up
Objective 10

Although your approach to an emergency at a residence may not be influenced by topography and weather, your response to a motor vehicle crash may require your consideration of these factors. If you receive additional information while en route, consider the need for additional resources, and make the appropriate assignments based on this information.

To ensure the safety of all personnel responding to a scene, you will need to be cautious and look for dangers while approaching the scene. You should also be aware of the presence of or the need for other emergency vehicles. Positioning of your emergency vehicle requires careful consideration of the following potential dangers:

- **Hazardous materials.** Indications of hazardous materials dangers may include spills, fumes, and noxious gases. Be alert for the presence of hazardous materials when responding to tractor-trailer accidents, train derailments, industrial incidents, and certain farm incidents.
- **Fires.** Approach the scene of a fire with caution. Avoid driving into a wet area, as the liquid may be flammable. Never drive over hoses unless specifically ordered to do so by fire suppression personnel. Be cautious of smoke clouds as they may be toxic. Coordinate your response and the positioning of your vehicle with the firefighters on scene.
- **Downed power lines.** Power lines that are down or hanging are extremely dangerous. Only trained personnel should try to remove them. Do not touch or try to move any downed power line. Remember that any water or other object that is in contact with a power line may be energized. Set up a **safe zone** (an area safe from exposure or the threat of exposure), also called the *cold zone* or *support zone,* and allow entry to properly trained personnel only. Stay in the safe zone until cleared by trained personnel.
- **Heavy traffic flow.** Transport vehicles should be parked away from the flow of traffic to ensure the protection of the crew, the patient, and the vehicle itself. Unfortunately, many motorists are very interested in observing the scene of an emergency and may not pay close attention to their driving. This can and will place all emergency responders at risk of an additional accident. In addition, if your vehicle is struck or damaged, your ability to transport the patient may be compromised.
- **Large crowds.** Use extreme caution when approaching a scene where a crowd has gathered. Crowds can become hostile to EMS personnel or may "rush" your vehicle, placing themselves in danger.

- *Violent or terrorist acts.* The potential exists for an emergency call to be a violent situation or even a terrorist event. Allow law enforcement personnel to deal with violent or hostile persons. Position your vehicle out of range of gunfire or other violence. Do not approach the scene without clearance from law enforcement personnel.

vehicle, is an important consideration for vehicle placement. If the sides of the vehicle are along the flow of traffic, it will be dangerous for crew members to get to the equipment needed for patient care. Park where access to all compartments is out of dangerous traffic flow. Be conscious of obstacles such as guardrails, trees, additional emergency vehicles, and other hazards that may restrict access to parts of the vehicle if you park too close to them.

In general, the transport vehicle should not be used for scene protection. The primary function of this vehicle is for patient transport. Most jurisdictions have standard operating procedures for such situations and use other emergency vehicles, such as fire apparatus, to protect the scene. Fire apparatus is typically parked downward from the scene and in such a way that a traveling vehicle would be more likely to strike the apparatus and not crew members (see Chapter 51) (Figure 47-8). Call for additional resources if necessary. If there are no additional resources available, then you may have to consider the use of your vehicle as a shield for the scene.

Always attempt to park the transport vehicle far enough away from the scene to protect the crew and the patient. In the case of a vehicle wreck, park at least 100 feet beyond the wreckage. This will generally protect the transport vehicle from broken glass and debris from the wreckage and allow access for fire suppression equipment. In addition, you must be aware of any fuel leaking from wrecked vehicles and park uphill or upwind. Park at least 2,000 feet from a hazardous substance. In situations involving a trench rescue, emergency vehicles are parked 300 feet from the excavation site to minimize vibration. Working apparatuses at these scenes are positioned at least 100 feet from the excavation site.

Vehicle Placement

Objective 11

The tendency to park your vehicle in the first available clear area and rush to assist with patient care may place you and your apparatus at risk. This can lead to more problems and delays because access to your vehicle and equipment may become dangerous or even impossible. There are four things to consider when placing an emergency vehicle at the emergency scene. They include scene safety, traffic volume and flow, egress from the scene, and distance from the patient(s) or scene.

Scene Safety

Personal safety, as well as the safety of the crew when accessing the vehicle and the equipment carried in the

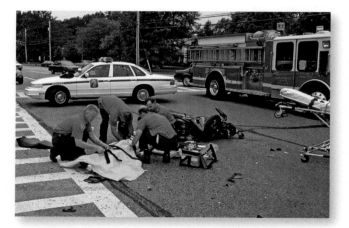

FIGURE 47-8 ▲ At this accident scene, the police and fire vehicles are positioned correctly to block traffic, creating a safe area for the EMTs and their patient.

Avoid placing the transport vehicle where it will block the access of other emergency personnel and vehicles. Use extreme care if you must park on a hill or any other unstable or uneven surface. Be sure to set the vehicle's parking brake. In addition, position the front wheels so that if the vehicle starts to roll, the wheels will hit the curb.

Remember This

When parking, consider access to the patient and the effects of traffic flow, the roadway, known hazards, the public, and other agencies.

Traffic Volume and Flow

The transport vehicle should be positioned so that it does not block traffic. In general, placing the transport vehicle in the path of traffic will limit access to the compartments and needed equipment.

Egress from the Scene

Position the emergency vehicle in preparation for an easy and rapid departure. In general, you should always position the transport vehicle pointed in the direction of the appropriate medical facility. Attempt to avoid having to back into traffic or steer around obstacles once the patient has been loaded.

In most situations, you should not use the driveway of a private residence if you are responding to an emergency in a residential area. It may be better to park in the street, especially if the house is near the street or if the driveway is steep or narrow. Parking on the street will prevent your having to back into or out of a driveway. This can be difficult and dangerous on residential streets because of the presence of children, pets, and obstacles such as bushes and parked cars.

Distance from the Patient or Scene

Your need for equipment to care for your patient and the necessity for ease of departure may require that you position your vehicle closer than you believe is safe. Use common sense and extreme caution in these instances.

On-Scene Care

When you arrive on the scene, notify the EMD of your arrival. Before initiating patient care, put on appropriate PPE. Make certain that your actions at the scene are efficient and organized, keeping in mind the goals of safe and efficient patient care and transport. Determine the mechanism of injury or nature of the patient's illness. Ask for additional resources before making patient contact, and initiate the Incident Command System if needed (see Chapter 48).

When it is safe to do so, gain access to the patient. Perform a primary survey, and provide essential emergency care.

Transferring the Patient to the Ambulance

If patient transport is needed, prepare the patient. Make sure that dressings and splints, if used, are secure. When you are ready, ask for assistance with lifting and moving the patient to the ambulance, using the techniques discussed in Chapter 2. The lifting and moving method and the device used will depend on the patient's illness or injury. They will also be determined by the safety of the scene, such as an emergency move at an unsafe scene versus a move of a stable medical patient. Secure the patient to the stretcher, and lock the stretcher in place (Figure 47-9). Before leaving the scene, the driver should ensure that all outside compartment doors are closed and secure.

Transport Phase

Objective 12

During transport, remember that your safety must be your priority. Wearing a seat belt is one way to ensure your safety. Although some people may consider it cumbersome to wear a seat belt during transport, your risk of injury increases if you are not restrained. Notify the dispatcher when you are leaving the scene. Let the dispatcher know your destination. For example:

Medic 51:	"Medic 51 (five, one) to Dispatch."
Dispatch Center:	"Dispatch. Medic 51 (five, one), go ahead."
Medic 51:	"Dispatch, Medic 51 (five, one) is transporting one patient to Anytown Medical Center, emergent."

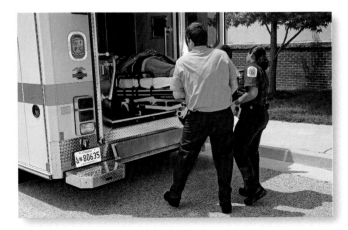

FIGURE 47-9 ▲ Secure the patient to the stretcher, and lock the stretcher in place.

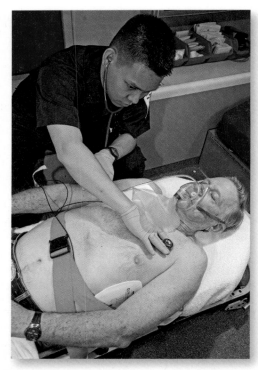

FIGURE 47-10 ▲ Care begun on the scene should be continued throughout patient transport.

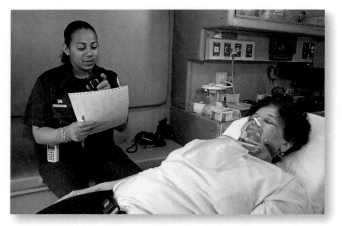

FIGURE 47-11 ▲ When possible, contact the receiving facility while you are en route. Use a standardized medical reporting format to provide patient information.

| Dispatch Center: | "Received, Medic 51 (five, one). Transporting one patient to Anytown Medical Center, emergent. Time: 1532 (fifteen, three, two)." |
| Medic 51: | "Dispatch, Medic 51 (five, one), received, clear." |

Follow your local protocol regarding the communication of additional patient information.

Care begun on the scene should be continued throughout patient transport (Figure 47-10). The frequency of reassessing the patient during transport will be based on the patient's condition. The patient's condition may improve, remain the same, or worsen during transport. A good rule to follow is that an unstable patient should be reassessed at least every 5 minutes. A stable patient should be reassessed at least every 15 minutes. Reassure the patient throughout the transport.

Complete your prehospital care report. Contact the receiving facility, if possible, and use a standardized medical reporting format (Figure 47-11).

In most EMS systems, the information that is relayed to the receiving facility includes:
- Your unit's name and level of service (basic life support or advanced life support)
- The estimated time of arrival
- The patient's age and gender
- The patient's chief complaint

- A brief, pertinent history of the present illness
- Major past illnesses
- The patient's mental status and baseline vital signs
- Pertinent physical exam findings
- The emergency medical care given (and by whom)
- The patient's response to emergency medical care

The following is a sample radio report simulating communication with a receiving facility:

Medic 51:	"Anytown Medical Center, Medic 51 (five, one)"
Anytown Medical Center:	"Anytown Medical Center. Go ahead, Medic 51 (five, one)."
Medic 51:	"Anytown Medical Center, EMT Burgan on Medic 51 (five, one). We are en route to your facility. Expected arrival time: 4 minutes. The patient is a 67-year-old man found unresponsive by his wife on the bedroom floor. On arrival, the patient was unresponsive, not breathing, and had no pulse. The patient's wife states he was last seen about 5 minutes before her call to 9-1-1. CPR was performed and the AED applied. One shock delivered while on scene. After resuming CPR, rhythm analysis by the AED indicated no shock advised. Strong carotid pulse present. Patient now responds to verbal stimuli. Vital signs follow: respirations 14; pulse 98, strong and regular; blood pressure

104/62. Exam reveals clear breath sounds bilaterally. There is a healed surgical scar in the center of the patient's chest. The patient's wife says the patient had a three-vessel coronary bypass 7 months ago. She has provided a typed list of medications. The patient is on oxygen by nonrebreather mask at 15 liters per minute. Any questions or orders?"

Anytown Medical Center:	"Medic 51 (five, one), Anytown Medical Center report received [*your report may be repeated to ensure accuracy*]. No orders or questions. Contact us if there is any change in patient condition before arrival. Anytown Medical Center clear."
Medic 51:	"Medic 51 (five, one) clear."

Making a Difference

Place yourself in this situation. You have just been involved in an MVC. The local emergency responders have just finished cutting you out of your mangled vehicle. You are strapped onto a hard piece of plastic and placed on a stretcher. You cannot see where you are going, and you feel every bump and corner that the emergency transport vehicle hits or travels around. The EMT in the back of the ambulance is busy writing on a clipboard or talking on a radio and doesn't seem to have time for your questions.

Would you feel comforted during this trip? Is this the type of care that you would like to have rendered to you or a family member?

At some point in our careers, we make a statement that sounds something like this, "I got into this business to help people and make a difference." Now is your chance to prove that you meant what you said. On each call, you have an opportunity to make a difference in someone's life. Yes, you need to complete your report. Yes, you will need to talk to the receiving facility. These tasks pale in importance compared with the need to give comfort and care to your patient. In some instances, this may be as simple as listening to your patient's fears. You are charged with the responsibility to use your knowledge and skills to help people in their time of need. Treat the patient as needed, assess the patient's vital signs, and do all the things you were trained to do; just don't forget to listen.

Transfer to Definitive Care

Objective 13

Notify the dispatcher as soon as you arrive at the receiving facility.

Medic 51:	"Dispatch, Medic 51 (five, one). Arrival at Anytown Medical Center."
Dispatch Center:	"Received, Medic 51 (five, one). Arrival at Anytown Medical Center at 1535 (fifteen, three, five)."

Once at the hospital, you must give a verbal report to the hospital staff. As the healthcare professional that provided patient care, you become the only link the hospital staff has to the patient's history and what happened at the scene. Information about how you found the patient, how the scene looked, and the care given to her by family members or bystanders before you arrived will be available to the hospital staff only through your report.

You should give a verbal report to the appropriate hospital staff member at the patient's bedside. Introduce the patient by name (if known).

Summarize the information already provided by radio or telephone to the receiving facility, including:

- The patient's chief complaint
- Pertinent patient history that was not previously given
- Emergency medical care given en route and the patient's response to the treatment given
- Vital signs taken en route

Provide any additional information collected en route but not transmitted by telephone or radio. Be sure to let hospital staff know if there was any delay in reaching the patient or if there were any unusual circumstances at the scene. Make sure the hospital staff member who listens to your report signs your PCR when you transfer patient care.

Leave a copy of your completed PCR with the hospital staff person. Your report will be included in the patient's hospital medical record. Remember that good documentation accurately and completely tells a story about what happened while the patient was in your care. This includes the patient's condition on arrival at the scene, your assessment findings, the emergency care performed, and the patient's response to the care given. Your documentation should contain facts that are supported by what you see, hear, feel, and smell. It should not contain jargon, slang, bias, opinions, or impressions. Subjective information that can be documented includes what the patient says that pertains to his current illness or complaint.

En Route to the Station

Notify the dispatcher when you are en route to your station and again when you arrive.

Medic 51:	"Dispatch, Medic 51 (five, one). En route to the station."
Dispatch Center:	"Received, Medic 51 (five, one). En route at 1551 (fifteen, five, one)."
Medic 51:	"Dispatch, Medic 51 (five, one). Arrival at the station."
Dispatch Center:	"Received, Medic 51 (five, one). Arrival at your station at 1602 (sixteen, zero, two)."

Most transport vehicles carry enough supplies to run multiple calls. Your vehicle should be cleaned and readied for the next call. In most instances, most of the cleaning will take place at the receiving facility. Your transport vehicle should carry enough cleaning supplies to perform a simple decontamination. Most EMS systems have a limited number of vehicles available at any one given time. Your rapid preparation for the next call can be very beneficial to the entire EMS system. It will be your responsibility to clean and disinfect the ambulance and equipment as needed. You will need to restock any disposable equipment that you may have used and return equipment to its storage area. It is very important that you understand your company's policies and arrangements made with receiving hospitals regarding restocking of supplies.

After the Run

Objectives 14, 15

Refuel your vehicle as needed, and remember to file all written reports. Mentally and physically prepare yourself for the next call. Have lunch or dinner, stay hydrated, and try to relax for a few moments. Inspect the vehicle, checking tires, lights, and anything unusual noticed during the run. Replace empty oxygen cylinders. Replace discharged batteries, or reconnect them to vehicle chargers. Replace supplies used during the run. Change soiled uniforms.

Complete cleaning and disinfecting the vehicle and/or equipment. **Decontamination** is the use of physical or chemical means to remove, inactivate, or destroy bloodborne pathogens on a surface or item to the point at which it is no longer capable of transmitting infectious particles and the surface or item is considered safe for handling, use, or disposal. Primary methods of decontamination include low-level disinfection, intermediate-level disinfection, high-level disinfection, and sterilization. **Low-level disinfection** destroys most bacteria, some viruses and fungi, but not tuberculosis bacteria or bacterial spores. It is used for routine cleaning of surfaces, such as floors, countertops, and ambulance seats, when no body fluids are visible. Use a household bleach and water solution or a hospital disinfectant registered with the Environmental Protection Agency (EPA).

Intermediate-level disinfection destroys tuberculosis bacteria, vegetative bacteria, and most viruses and fungi, but not bacterial spores. It is used for surfaces that contact intact skin and have been visibly contaminated with body fluids, such as blood pressure cuffs, stethoscopes, backboards, and splints. Use a household bleach and water solution or an EPA-registered hospital disinfectant that claims it is tuberculocidal.

High-level disinfection destroys all microorganisms except large numbers of bacterial spores. It is used for reusable equipment that has been in contact with mucous membranes, such as laryngoscope blades. Either use hot water pasteurization by placing articles in water 176–212°F (80–100°C) for 30 minutes or immerse them in an EPA-registered chemical sterilizing agent for 10 to 45 minutes according to manufacturer's instructions. Items requiring high-level disinfection should first be cleaned with soap and water to remove debris.

Sterilization destroys all microorganisms, including highly resistant bacterial spores. It is used for instruments that penetrate the skin or contact normally sterile areas of the body during invasive procedures. Methods used include autoclave (steam under pressure) and immersion in an EPA-registered chemical sterilizing agent for 6 to 10 hours. Sterilization is usually performed at the hospital. Items requiring sterilization should first be cleaned with soap and water to remove debris.

Remember This

Medical equipment should never be disinfected in areas such as the kitchen, bathrooms, or living areas of the station or receiving facility.

Infection Control Procedures

Objective 16

Remove any contaminated clothing. If blood or other potentially infectious material contaminates your clothing, remove it as soon as possible. Bag the clothing for decontamination, and place it in an appropriately designated area or container. Thoroughly wash your hands, contaminated skin areas, and areas of skin that were not covered by clothing or PPE. Remember that your hands should be washed after every patient encounter. Also, remember to wash your hands after cleaning and disinfecting procedures are completed. Wear protective gloves, such as cleaning gloves, when cleaning potentially infectious materials. If splashing is likely, wear face and eye protection.

Contaminated sharps must be discarded immediately in an acceptable sharps container. If leakage is possible, or if the outside of the container has become contaminated, the sharps container must be placed in a secondary container that is closable, labeled or color-coded, and leak resistant. If the sharps container is one-half to three-quarters full, close and lock the lid. Follow agency procedures for disposal of the container.

Decontaminate the vehicle and large equipment. Clean up blood and body fluid spills with disposable towels. Dispose the towels in a biohazard-labeled bag. Decontaminate surfaces with soap and water. Wipe or spray with a disinfectant solution as needed, and allow disinfected areas to air dry. Place disposable PPE worn during decontamination procedures in a properly labeled, sealed waste container. Restock the vehicle. Make note of any items needing repair or replacement.

Protective gloves and other appropriate PPE must be worn when handling contaminated laundry. Laundry contaminated with blood or other potentially infectious materials should be handled as little as possible. It must be placed in appropriately marked bags at the location where it was used. Contaminated laundry should be washed according to the uniform or linen manufacturer's recommendations. Contaminated items should always be laundered separately from other laundry to prevent cross-contamination.

Notify dispatch when your tasks are complete and you are ready for another call.

Medic 51: "Dispatch, Medic 51 (five, one). In service and available for traffic."

Dispatch Center: "Received, Medic 51 (five, one). Available for traffic at 1615 (sixteen, one, five)."

You Should Know

When to Notify Dispatch

- Receiving the call
- Responding to the call
- Arriving at the scene
- Leaving the scene for the receiving facility
- Arriving at the receiving facility
- Leaving the hospital for the station
- Arriving at the station

On the Scene   Wrap-Up

Fortunately, your partner knows where the airway kit and the AED are located on your unit. She quickly grabs the needed equipment. The call runs smoothly. After performing CPR, and shocking when prompted by the AED, you hear the patient begin moaning. You can feel a strong pulse. Using proper body mechanics, you and your partner move the patient from the ground to the stretcher and then into the back of the ambulance. En route to the hospital, you make promises to yourself that you will *always* know where the appropriate equipment is located on an emergency vehicle and that you will perform a complete check of the vehicle and equipment at the start of each shift. ∎

Sum It Up

▶ Preparations for an emergency call include having the appropriate personnel and equipment and an emergency response vehicle that is ready for use. Minimum staffing requirements for an ambulance include at least one EMT in the patient compartment. Two EMTs are preferred. In some states, two licensed personnel are required. Emergency transport vehicles are required to carry specific types and quantities of medical equipment to be certified as ambulances. In addition to basic medical supplies, nonmedical supplies that must be carried include personal safety equipment as required by local, state, and federal standards as well as preplanned routes or comprehensive street maps. Daily inspections of the emergency response vehicle and its equipment are necessary to ensure it is in proper working order.

▶ In the dispatch phase of an EMS response, the patient or a witness reports the emergency by calling 9-1-1 or another emergency number. EMD receives the call and gathers information from the caller. The dispatcher then activates (dispatches) an appropriate EMS response based on the information received.

▶ En route to the reported emergency, begin to anticipate the knowledge, equipment, and skills you may need to provide appropriate patient care. Notify the dispatcher that you are responding to the call. Determine the responsibilities of the crew members before arriving on the scene.

▶ Laws pertaining to the proper methods of responding to an emergency vary from state to state. In general, most states require that emergency vehicle operators obey all traffic regulations unless a specific exemption has been made and documented in statute. Most states allow for such exemptions as long as they do not endanger life or property. In addition, these exemptions are typically granted only when a true emergency exists. A true emergency is a situation in which there is a high possibility of death or serious injury and the rapid response of an emergency vehicle may lessen the risk of death or injury.

► When driving in emergency mode, the operator of an emergency vehicle must drive with due regard for the safety of others on the roadway. Due regard means that, in similar circumstances, a reasonable and responsible person would act in a way that is safe and considerate of others. Emergency vehicles should never operate at a speed greater than is warranted by the nature of the call or the condition of the patient being transported. This speed must also not be greater than traffic, road, and weather conditions allow. All emergency vehicle warning systems should be used as intended by the manufacturer and must be in operation during an emergency response. All emergency vehicle warning systems must be functioning in the prescribed manner before entering any intersection.

► Escorts and multiple-vehicle responses are extremely dangerous. They should be used only if emergency responders are unfamiliar with the location of the patient or receiving facility. Provide a safe following distance (generally a minimum of 500 feet). Stop and then proceed through any intersection as directed by the standard right-of-way guidelines.

► While approaching the scene, be cautious, and look for dangers. Position the emergency vehicle with careful consideration of potential dangers such as fire, hazardous materials, downed power lines, crowds, heavy traffic flow, and potential violence. When you arrive on the scene, notify the EMD of your arrival. Before initiating patient care, put on appropriate PPE. Determine the mechanism of injury or nature of the patient's illness. Ask for additional resources before making patient contact, and institute the Incident Command System if needed. When it is safe to do so, gain access to the patient. Perform an initial assessment, and provide essential emergency care.

► If patient transport is needed, prepare the patient. Ask for assistance with lifting and moving the patient to the ambulance. Secure the patient to the stretcher, and lock the stretcher in place. Ensure that outside compartment doors are closed and secure.

► During transport, remember that your safety must be your priority. Wearing a seat belt is one way to ensure your safety. Notify the dispatcher when you are leaving the scene. Perform ongoing patient assessments during transport. Complete your PCR, and contact the receiving facility, if possible, using a standardized medical reporting format.

► Notify the dispatcher as soon as you arrive at the receiving facility. Give a verbal report to the hospital staff. Notify the dispatcher when you are en route to your station and again when you arrive. Clean and disinfect the vehicle and equipment as needed in preparation for the next call. Replace supplies used during the run. Notify the dispatcher when your tasks are complete and you are ready for another call.

Incident Management

By the end of this chapter, you should be able to:

Knowledge Objective ▶   **1.** Describe basic concepts of incident management.

Attitude Objectives ▶   No attitude objectives are identified for this lesson.

Skill Objectives ▶   No skill objectives are identified for this lesson.

On the Scene

The National Weather Service's national Weather Center has issued information on the possibility of a tornado in your county. The local television station is reporting the sighting of a tornado approximately 1 mile from your station, and winds are measured and sustained at approximately 100 miles per hour. You can hear the debris hitting and bouncing off your station, and the roar of the storm as it passes by. The noise has abated a little, and the debris seems to have gotten smaller when the first alarm comes into your station. You are being asked to respond to the report of a possible building collapse with trapped victims at the local high school. You notify your dispatch center that you are responding, and a dispatcher alerts you to the activation of the local "command system" with instructions on the location of staging. ◾

THINK ABOUT IT

As you read this chapter, think about the following questions:

- What is the Incident Command System, and what role do you play as the first responding EMS unit?
- How does your understanding of "ICS-100" alter your response to this call?
- What is *staging,* and how does it help the management of this scene?

All field EMS professionals must know how to establish and work within the National Incident Management System (NIMS). Homeland Security Presidential Directive 5 requires the adoption of NIMS by all state, territorial, local, and tribal jurisdictions. Volunteer fire departments are governed by the section of the directive entitled, "Tribal and Local Jurisdictions." Requirements for entry-level personnel include certification in Incident Command System (ICS)-100: Introduction to ICS, or equivalent, and the Federal Emergency Management Agency (FEMA) IS-700 course called NIMS: An Introduction.

All federal, state, territorial, local, tribal, private sector, and nongovernmental personnel at the entry level, first-line supervisor level, middle management level, and command and general staff level of emergency management operations must complete ICS-100 level training. The United State Fire Administration (USFA), through its National Fire Programs Office, has the ICS-100 course available on the web. The course can be accessed at the following website: www.usfa .fema.gov/training/nfa/independent/.

The web-based awareness level course, IS-700 NIMS: An Introduction, explains NIMS components, concepts, and principles. Although it is designed to be taken online as an interactive web course, course materials may be downloaded and used in a group or classroom setting. To obtain the IS-700 course materials or take the course online, go to http://training.fema .gov/. In this chapter, a brief overview of the Incident Command System is provided. This information is not meant to replace the course completion requirements already specified.

Incident Command System

Objective 1

In 2003, President George W. Bush directed the secretary of Homeland Security to develop and administer a National Incident Management System. The purpose of NIMS is to provide a consistent nationwide template that allows all governmental, private sector, and nongovernmental agencies to work together during domestic incidents. Examples of domestic incidents include acts of terrorism, wildland and urban fires, floods, hazardous materials spills, nuclear accidents, aircraft accidents, earthquakes, tornadoes, hurricanes, typhoons, and war-related disasters. Domestic incidents are often multiple-casualty incidents. A *multiple-casualty incident* is any event that places a great demand on resources—equipment, personnel, or both.

NIMS Components

NIMS is made up of several components that work together as a system. These components include the following:

- Command and management
- Preparedness
- Resource management
- Communications and information management
- Supporting technologies
- Ongoing management and maintenance

Command and Management

NIMS standard incident management structures are based on three primary organizational systems:

1. The Incident Command System
2. Multiagency coordination systems
3. Public information systems

NIMS requires that responses to all domestic incidents use a common management structure. The **Incident Command System (ICS)**—also called the *Incident Management System* (IMS)—is an important part of this comprehensive system. The ICS is a standardized system developed to assist with the control, direction, and coordination of emergency response resources. The ICS is a proved incident management system that is based on organizational best practices. It can be used at an incident of any type and size, from an everyday call to a large and complex incident.

An **incident commander (IC)** is the person who is responsible for managing all operations at the incident site. There is only one IC per incident.

The incident commander has three priorities:

1. **Life safety.** Ensuring the safety of the lives and the physical well-being of emergency personnel and the public
2. **Incident stability.** Minimizing the effect the incident may have on the surrounding area while using resources efficiently
3. **Property conservation.** Minimizing damage to property

Persons on the scene who are familiar with the ICS will also be familiar with the following risk-benefit model:

- We will risk our lives a lot within a calculated plan for lives that are savable.
- We will risk our lives a little within a calculated plan for property that is savable.
- We will not risk our lives at all for lives or property that are already lost.

Remember This

Several ICS features make the system well suited to managing incidents, including the following:

- Common terminology
- Organizational resources
- Manageable span of control
- Organizational facilities
- Use of position titles
- Reliance on an incident action plan
- Integrated communications
- Accountability

Using common terminology within the ICS, including standard titles for facilities and positions within the organization, is essential to ensuring efficient, clear communications. This means communicating without the use of agency-specific codes or jargon. Resources, including all personnel, facilities, and major equipment and supply items used to support incident management activities, are assigned common terms to help avoid confusion. For example, only the incident commander is called "commander"—and there is only one incident commander per incident. The incident commander is found at the incident command post. Command staff are called "officers." Only the heads of sections are called "chiefs."

Incident facilities are established depending on the type and complexity of the incident (Figure 48-1). Typical incident facilities include the following:

- The incident command post
- One or more staging areas
- A base
- One or more camps (when needed)
- A helibase
- One or more helispots

Maintaining an effective span of control throughout an ICS organization is critical. Typically, an effective span of control may vary from three to seven, and a ratio of one supervisor to five reporting elements is recommended. The ICS organizational structure can expand or contract in a modular fashion as needed for each incident. For instance, depending on the size of the incident, the IC may assign others the authority to perform certain activities (Figure 48-2). Scene operations may be broken down into groups. For example, the treatment group is assigned patient treatment, while an extrication group is responsible for extrication. Within the ICS, incident action plans (IAPs) are used to communicate the overall incident objectives. IAPs are developed for operational periods that are usually 12 hours long.

Integrated communications are essential to ensure the transfer of information throughout the ICS organization. Integrated communications include hardware systems, planning for the use of all available communications frequencies and resources, and the procedures and processes for transferring information internally and externally.

To ensure effective accountability, ICS requires an orderly chain of command, check-in for all responders regardless of agency affiliation, and assignment of each individual involved in incident operations to only one supervisor.

Multiagency coordination systems are a combination of facilities, equipment, personnel, procedures, and communications integrated into a common framework for coordinating and supporting incident management. These systems define the operating characteristics, management components, and organizational structure of supporting entities.

Public information systems include the processes, procedures, and systems for communicating timely and accurate information to the public during emergency situations.

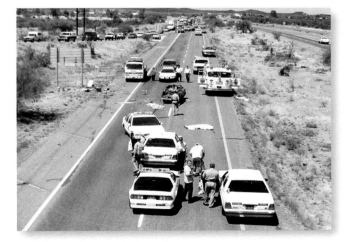

FIGURE 48-1 ▲ When the condition of one or more patients is critical, air medical transport is often used.

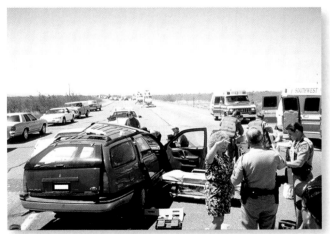

FIGURE 48-2 ▲ A typical ICS structure for a common emergency such as an MVC with two patients entrapped.

Unified and Area Command

NIMS recommends variations in incident management in some situations. Two common variations involve the use of unified command and area command.

Unified command is used when there is more than one responding agency with responsibility for the incident and/or incidents cross political jurisdictions. Under a unified command, agencies with responsibility for the incident work together to analyze available information and establish a common set of objectives and strategies for a single incident action plan. A hazardous materials spill in which more than one agency has responsibility for the response or an explosion that simultaneously involves a fire and crime scene are examples in which unified command may be used. Unified command does not change any of the other features of ICS.

An *area command* is an organization that is established to oversee the management of multiple incidents that are each being managed by an ICS organization and/or to oversee the management of large incidents that cross jurisdictional boundaries. An area command is organized similarly to an ICS structure, but because operations are conducted on-scene, there is no operations section in an area command. A public health emergency that is not site specific (such as an outbreak of a flulike virus throughout a state) is an example of when an area command may be used.

Preparedness

Effective incident management begins with many preparedness activities that are conducted well in advance of any potential incident. Preparedness involves a combination of the following:

- Planning, training, and exercises
- Personnel qualification and certification standards
- Equipment acquisition and certification standards
- Publication management processes and activities
- Mutual aid agreements and emergency management assistance compacts

You Should Know

Mutual aid agreements and emergency management assistance compacts (EMACs) enable one jurisdiction to provide resources or other support to another jurisdiction during an incident.

Resource Management

NIMS defines standardized mechanisms and establishes requirements for describing, inventorying, mobilizing, dispatching, tracking, and recovering resources over the life cycle of an incident.

Communications and Information Management

NIMS identifies the requirements for a standardized framework for communications, information management, and information sharing at all levels of incident management. Incident management organizations must make sure that effective communication processes, procedures, and systems exist across all agencies and jurisdictions. Information management systems help ensure that information flows efficiently. Effective information management enhances incident management and response by helping to ensure that decision making is better informed.

Supporting Technologies

Voice and data communication systems, information management systems, such as record keeping and resource tracking, and data display systems provide supporting capabilities essential to implementing and refining NIMS.

Ongoing Management and Maintenance

The NIMS integration center provides strategic direction, oversight, and continual refinement of both the system and its components.

Remember This

At the beginning of an incident, the IC is typically the most senior EMS professional who arrives at the scene. As more resources arrive, command is transferred to another person on the basis of who has the primary authority for overall control of the incident. When command is transferred, the outgoing IC must give the incoming IC a full report and notify all staff of the change in command.

If you arrive on the scene of a multiple-casualty incident (MCI) where the ICS has been established, report to the command post. Find out who the IC is. Identify yourself and your level of training. Follow the directions given by the IC about your assignment. In most instances, you will be assigned to the staging area. In EMS, *staging* means to wait. The staging area is a location identified by a member of the incident command structure (such as a staging officer) that is located away from the incident scene. Emergency vehicles arriving at the scene stage (or wait) in this area until they are called into action by the incident commander. Do not "self-assign." This only creates confusion and may hinder the responses of others working to resolve the incident.

On the Scene   Wrap-Up

Your knowledge of the Incident Command System allows you to understand the need for the coordination of efforts from any agency that responds to this call. You are the first EMS unit to arrive, and you have been placed in charge of the staging area. You are now the point of contact for all responding EMS units, and your partner assists you with parking the units in a fashion that allows them to rapidly report from staging to the scene when directed. ∎

Sum It Up

▶ The National Incident Management System was created to provide a consistent nationwide template that allows all governmental, private sector, and nongovernmental agencies to work together during domestic incidents.

▶ The Incident Command System is an important part of NIMS. The ICS is a standardized system developed to assist with the control, direction, and coordination of emergency response resources. The ICS can be used at an incident of any type and size.

▶ An incident commander is the person who is responsible for managing all operations at the incident site. Depending on the size of the incident, the incident commander may assign others the authority to perform certain activities. Scene operations may be broken down into groups, such as treatment and extrication.

▶ If you arrive on the scene of an MCI where the ICS has been established, report to the command post. Find out who the IC is. Identify yourself and your level of training. Follow the directions given by the IC about your assignment.

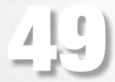
Multiple-Casualty Incidents

By the end of this chapter, you should be able to:

Knowledge Objectives ▶
1. Describe the criteria for a multiple-casualty situation.
2. Evaluate the role of the EMT in a multiple-casualty situation.
3. Summarize the components of basic triage.

Attitude Objectives ▶
No attitude objectives are identified for this lesson.

Skill Objective ▶
4. Given a scenario of a multiple-casualty incident, perform triage.

On the Scene

You drive with caution through the thick, milky fog to the vehicle collision, thankful you are on the ambulance with a seasoned veteran tonight. As you approach the scene, you can see that this is no ordinary car crash. A car has collided with a train. The car lies crushed in the ditch about 10 feet off the road. Bystanders are pointing you to several patients who are scattered in the area.

You and your partner quickly size up the situation. There were six teens in the car—four were ejected and two remain trapped in the mangled wreckage. You open the airway of a young girl. She is not breathing, so you reopen her airway and look, listen, and feel again; there is still no breathing. You know what you have to do, but it's not easy—you tag her black and move on. The others are breathing, but three are unconscious and the remaining two have signs of shock. Your partner radios for more ambulances and equipment, and you begin the overwhelming task of trying to provide some care for your seriously injured patients. ■

THINK ABOUT IT

As you read this chapter, think about the following questions:

- How will you categorize the remaining patients?
- How should incoming units protect the scene from another collision while you move your patients across the road to the ambulance?
- Who will remove the trapped patients?
- What types of additional resources are needed to safely treat all the patients?

Introduction

You may respond to situations involving multiple patients. To do the greatest good for the greatest number of patients, you must be able to effectively triage patients in multiple-casualty situations.

Multiple-Casualty Incidents

Objectives 1, 2

A **multiple-casualty incident (MCI),** also called a *mass-casualty incident* or *multiple-casualty situation (MCS),* is any event that places a great demand on resources—equipment, personnel, or both. An MCI could be four patients for some communities and a much larger number for others. There is no set number of patients that defines an MCI.

In most EMS situations, emergency care is provided first to the most seriously injured patient(s). In an MCI, the goal is to do the most good for the most people. Priority is given to the most salvageable patients with the most urgent problems. *Triage* is a French word that means "to sort." **Triage** is sorting multiple victims into priorities for emergency medical care or transportation to definitive care. By quickly sorting the injured patients and identifying the needs of those patients, you are better able to grasp what resources will be needed to care for them.

START Triage System

Objective 3

Many EMS systems use the **START triage system.** START is an acronym for *simple triage and rapid treatment.* START was developed by the Newport Beach (California) Fire and Marine Department in cooperation with staff at Hoag Hospital in Newport Beach. When you are using the START system, your initial patient assessment and treatment should take less than 30 seconds for each patient.

Four areas are evaluated during your initial START assessment:

1. The ability to walk (ambulation)
2. Respirations
3. Perfusion
4. Mental status

On the basis of your assessment findings, you then place the patient into one of four START categories:

- Immediate—Red—Priority-1 (P-1)
- Delayed—Yellow—Priority-2 (P-2)
- Hold—Green—Priority-3 (P-3); (ambulatory patients; "walking wounded")
- Deceased—Black—Priority-0 (P-0)

Color-coded triage tags that correspond with these categories are placed on the patients and used to identify the level of injury sustained (Figure 49-1).

Identify a triage officer who will remain on the scene for the duration of the event. Request additional resources (personnel and equipment), as needed. Perform triage of all patients, and then assign personnel and equipment to the highest-priority patients.

To triage patients using START, follow these steps (see also Figure 49-2):

- First identify patients who are able to walk. Patients who are able to walk are called the *walking wounded.* Clear them from the area so that you can triage the more seriously injured patients. For example, instruct patients who can walk to go to a predetermined evaluation and treatment area. These patients should be tagged as "green" or "minor" (Figure 49-3).

- Next, determine the patients who are injured but have adequate respirations, perfusion, and mental status. For example, you might ask, "If you can hear me, please raise an arm or leg so we can help you!" These patients should be tagged as "yellow" or "delayed."

- Proceed to the remaining patients. These patients will be tagged as "red" (immediate) or "black" (dead or dying), depending on your assessment. Start with the patient closest to you.

- Assess the patient's respirations. If the patient is not breathing, open his airway. If he is still not breathing, triage the patient as dead (black tag).

- If opening the patient's airway results in breathing, check her respiratory rate. If she is breathing more than 30 times per minute, triage the patient as immediate (red tag).

- If the patient is breathing less than 30 times per minute, check perfusion. To assess perfusion, check the patient's radial pulse.

- If a radial pulse is absent, triage the patient as immediate.

- If a radial pulse is present, check the patient's mental status. If the patient cannot follow simple commands (he is unresponsive or has an altered mental status), triage the patient as immediate. If the patient can follow simple commands, triage the patient as delayed (yellow tag).

- If the patient is triaged as immediate, repositioning the airway and controlling severe bleeding are the only initial treatment efforts that are performed before moving on to the next patient.

- Continue triaging patients until all patients have been assigned a category.

However, do not triage the patients once and think you are done. Triage is an ongoing process. In most

TRIAGE TAG
DO **NOT** REMOVE

PATIENT INFORMATION

☐ MALE ☐ FEMALE   AGE   WEIGHT   **PATIENT NUMBER**

NAME

ADDRESS

CITY   ST   PHONE

TRIAGE STATUS

EVALUATION	TIME	RED	YELLOW	GREEN	BLACK
INITIAL		IMMEDIATE	DELAYED	MINOR	DECEASED
SECONDARY		IMMEDIATE	DELAYED	MINOR	DECEASED
		IMMEDIATE	DELAYED	MINOR	DECEASED
HOSPITAL		IMMEDIATE	DELAYED	MINOR	DECEASED

CHIEF COMPLAINT

Head Injury C-Spine
Blunt Trauma
Penetrating Injury
Burn Fracture
Laceration Amputation

Medical _____
Cardiac Respiratory
Diabetic OB/GYN
Haz-Mat Exposure

COMMENTS

TRANSPORTATION AGENCY/UNIT   DESTINATION   TIME ARRIVED

TREATMENT   HOSPITAL

OTHER   OTHER

OTHER   OTHER

OTHER   OTHER

TRANSPORT RECORD

☐ MALE ☐ FEMALE   AGE   **PATIENT NUMBER**

NAME

CHIEF COMPLAINT

DESTINATION   HOSP NOTIFIED

	TRIAGE STATUS	
RED	YELLOW	GREEN

TRANSPORTATION AGENCY/UNIT   TIME OUT

TRIAGE TAG   DO **NOT** REMOVE

VITAL SIGNS

TIME	RESP	PULSE	MENTAL STATUS	B/P
			A V P U	
			A V P U	
			A V P U	

MEDICAL HISTORY

MEDICATIONS/MEDICAL PROBLEMS

ALLERGIES

TIME	TREATMENT RECORD	INITIALS
	☐ BVM ☐ ET	
	☐ Oxygen by at L/min	
	☐ Bleeding Control ☐ Tourniquet @ _____	
	☐ Spinal Immobilization ☐ Extremity Splint	
	☐ IV Started at Gauge	
	☐ PASG Inflated at _____	
	☐ Gross Decon. ☐ Final Decon.	

TRIAGE TAG

FIGURE 49-1 ▲ An example of a triage tag.

MCIs, reassessing the patient is done in the treatment area and again when she is moved to the transportation area. The patient's triage category is updated as needed. Examples of patient priorities are listed in the following *You Should Know* box.

You Should Know

Examples of Patient Priorities

Immediate

- Airway and breathing difficulties
- Uncontrolled or severe bleeding
- Decreased mental status
- Patients with severe medical problems
- Shock
- Severe burns

Delayed

- Burns without airway problems
- Major or multiple bone or joint injuries
- Back injuries with or without spinal cord damage

Hold

- Minor painful, swollen, deformed extremities
- Minor soft tissue injuries

Deceased

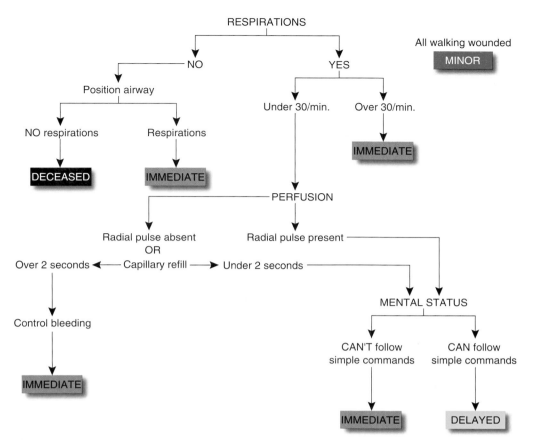

RESPIRATIONS

NO → Position airway
- NO respirations → DECEASED
- Respirations → IMMEDIATE

YES
- Under 30/min.
- Over 30/min. → IMMEDIATE

All walking wounded → MINOR

PERFUSION
- Radial pulse absent OR Capillary refill Over 2 seconds → Control bleeding → IMMEDIATE
- Radial pulse present / Capillary refill Under 2 seconds → MENTAL STATUS
  - CAN'T follow simple commands → IMMEDIATE
  - CAN follow simple commands → DELAYED

FIGURE 49-2 ▲ The START triage algorithm.

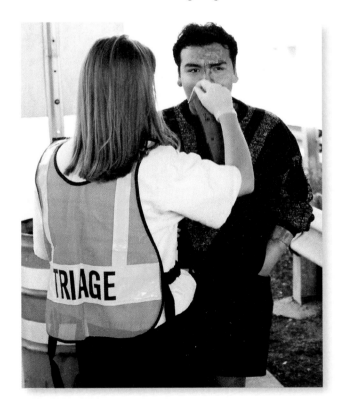

FIGURE 49-3 ▲ A "walking wounded" patient receiving a green tag during the initial triage phase.

Remember This

Triaging patients during an MCI goes against your instincts to help everyone you encounter. Practice using the START triage system so it will be easy to use if you are ever faced with an MCI.

JumpSTART Triage System

Objective 3

The START system works very well for adults. However, Dr. Lou Romig, a well-known pediatric emergency and EMS physician, identified some weaknesses in the START system when applied to children. As a result, in 1995 she developed a modified START system for use with children. This system is called *JumpSTART triage* (Figure 49-4).

In the JumpSTART system:

- All children who are able to walk are triaged in the minor (green) category.
- Begin assessing children who are not able to walk as you come to them. First, assess the

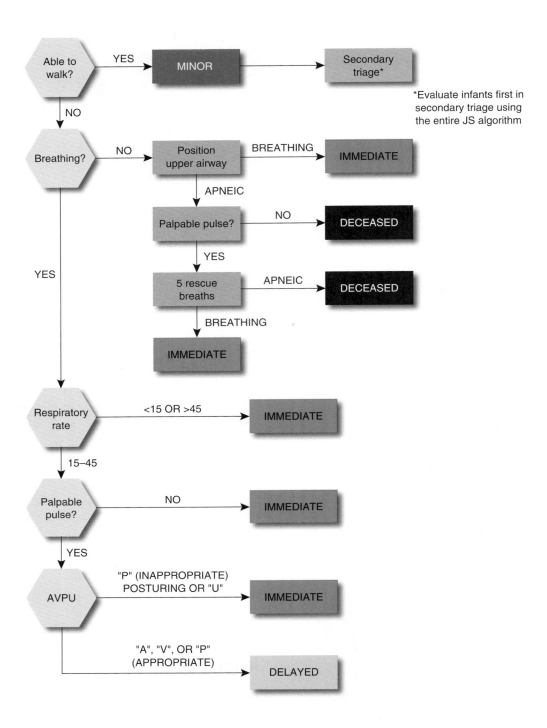

FIGURE 49-4 ▲ The JumpSTART triage algorithm for pediatric patients.

child's breathing. If she is breathing, assess her respiratory rate.

- If the child is not breathing or has very irregular breathing, open his airway by using the jaw thrust without head tilt. If the child begins breathing, triage him as immediate (red) and move on to the next patient.

- If the child does not begin breathing, check for a pulse. If there is no pulse, triage the patient as dead (black) and move on.

- If the child does have a pulse, give 15 seconds of mouth-to-mask breathing (about five breaths).

- If the child begins breathing, triage her as immediate (red) and move on. If she does not begin breathing, triage the patient as dead (black) and move on.

- If a child is breathing on his own when you find him, quickly check his respiratory rate. If the child is breathing faster than 45 times per minute or less than 15 times per minute, or if his breathing is irregular, triage him as immediate.

- If the child is breathing 15–45 times per minute, assess perfusion. If a pulse is present, assess mental status. If no pulse is present in the least injured limb, triage the child as immediate and move on.

- Assess mental status by using the AVPU scale. If the child is alert, responds to a verbal stimulus, or responds appropriately to pain, triage the child as delayed (yellow) and move on.

- If the child responds inappropriately to pain or is unresponsive, triage her as immediate (red) and move on.

- As with adults, children will need to be reassessed in the treatment and transportation areas.

After a multiple-casualty incident, assess your own emotional needs. Discussion with other personnel involved in the call may be helpful.

Making a Difference

A rule of triage is to do the greatest good for the greatest number. To make sure you are ready in the event of an MCI, a MCI drill should be a part of the regular training for you and your agency.

The fire captain on the first engine that arrives positions his truck to block the road behind the ambulance and assumes command of the scene. He tells the rescue squad to extricate the trapped patients. He establishes a staging area for incoming ambulances. He also asks the police to direct traffic and place flares to alert oncoming cars. As each ambulance arrives, you assign each crew a patient. Within 30 minutes, the last teen is en route to the local hospital. In the debriefing later, you discuss how the weather prevented the use of helicopter transport. Overall, everyone felt that all crews performed well and hoped that they will never again be faced with such a scene. ■

Sum It Up

▶ A multiple-casualty incident may also be called a mass-casualty incident or multiple-casualty situation. An MCI is any event that places a great demand on resources—equipment, personnel, or both.

▶ The START triage system is used by many systems in dealing with MCIs. START stands for *simple triage and rapid treatment.* On the basis of your assessment findings, you categorize each patient according to one of four categories. Color-coded triage tags that correspond with these categories are placed on the patients and used to identify the level of injury sustained.

▶ The JumpSTART triage system was developed for use with children. It specifies how the four color-coded tags are applied to pediatric patients.

CHAPTER

50 Air Medical Transport

By the end of this chapter, you should be able to:

Knowledge Objectives ▶

1. Give examples of situations in which air medical transport may be indicated.
2. Discuss the general requirements for a helicopter landing zone.
3. Discuss general safety guidelines for use around helicopters.

Attitude Objectives ▶

No attitude objectives are identified for this lesson.

Skill Objectives ▶

No skill objectives are identified for this lesson.

On the Scene

You are on the scene of a car versus motorcycle crash on a rural road in your jurisdiction. The motorcyclist was not wearing a helmet when he hit a vehicle that pulled out in front of him. Bystanders estimate his speed was about 60 mph. The patient is unconscious with bilateral femur fractures and a closed head injury. The closest hospital is 40 miles away, and the closest trauma center is 60 miles away. ■

THINK ABOUT IT

As you read this chapter, think about the following questions:

- What are the indications for the use of air medical transport?
- What must you consider when landing a helicopter?
- What is the proper method to activate an air medical transport service in your area?

Introduction

An EMT must be familiar with the appropriate use of air transport services. In this chapter we discuss considerations for the use of air medical transport, guidelines for establishing a landing zone, and safety around a helicopter.

Air Medical Transport Considerations

Objectives 1, 2, 3

When air medical transport is necessary, the scene is often complex. In most cases, air transportation is used because the condition of one or more patients is critical (Figure 50-1). In these types of scenes, emotions run high, and safety considerations can be overlooked. Remember that the goal in any EMS operation is to ensure the safety of every person at the scene.

It is important to identify the need for air transport as early as possible.

The mechanisms of injury that may require helicopter transport include:
- A vehicle rollover with unrestrained passengers
- An incident in which a vehicle strikes a pedestrian at a speed greater than 10 mph
- Falls from a height greater than 15 feet
- An incident in which a motorcyclist is thrown from the motorcycle at a speed of more than 20 mph
- Multiple victims

Examples of other conditions that may require helicopter transport include:
- Acute myocardial infarction or a stroke in evolution (in progress) requiring time-sensitive emergency care

- Known high-risk pregnancy with a serious injury

Time and distance must also be considered before transporting by helicopter. For example, what is the projected total time of the air response (air ambulance estimated time of arrival + air ambulance transport time to hospital + loading/unloading time)?

Helicopter transport should be considered in the following circumstances:
- The transport time to a trauma center is more than 45 minutes by ground ambulance and total air transport time is less than 45 minutes.
- The transport time to a local hospital by ground ambulance is more than the transport time to a trauma center by helicopter.
- The patient is entrapped, and extrication will take longer than 15 minutes.
- Using a local ground ambulance leaves the local community without ground ambulance coverage.
- The patient needs rapid transport to a specialty center (for example, a burn center, stroke center, or pediatric center).

Additional considerations regarding air transport should include the following:
- What level of care will the patient receive during the flight? Is the level of care the ground ambulance will provide to the patient the same as that to be provided by air transport?
- Is the patient combative?
- Is the patient contaminated? (A patient who requires decontamination before emergency care can be provided should be transported by ground ambulance.)
- Does the patient's weight exceed the air transport service's requirements for safe transport?

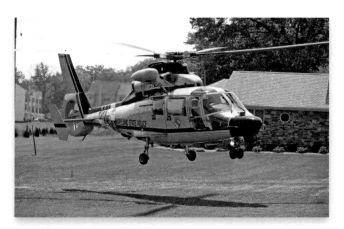
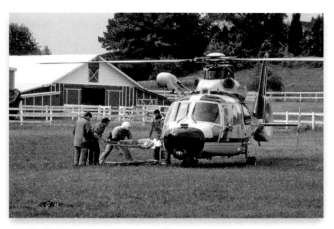

FIGURE 50-1 ▲ When the condition of one or more patients is critical, air medical transportation is often used.

Air Medical Transport Considerations ◄ **845**

Remember This

Local standards and protocols for the use of air transport vary widely, even within a given region, and the guidelines and criteria for the use of air transport are not always black and white. For example, it is not always possible to make absolute statements regarding the use of air transport such as a patient with problem *X* is always flown, whereas a patient with problem *Y* is never flown. The decision to transport a patient by air often requires consideration of individual factors. Many situations require a judgment call by the lead provider on the scene. It is essential that you become familiar with local guidelines regarding the use of air transport.

You will need to notify the appropriate agency for help in securing a **landing zone (LZ).** In most cases, the local fire department will be the agency contacted. However, in some cases, police departments assume this role. When more than one agency is on the scene, each agency should have the ability to communicate on a common radio channel. All healthcare professionals that provide care need to be aware of the loca-

tion of the LZ and the helicopter's estimated time of arrival (ETA).

If your unit is designated to land the helicopter, you will need to locate a secure LZ (Figure 50-2). This means that you must locate an area that is easily controlled for traffic and pedestrians. Check with your local helicopter service for LZ requirements. A good rule to follow is to allow *at least* 100 feet by 100 feet for any helicopter. The area should be relatively level and free of overhead obstacles such as wires, trees, and light poles. Walk the area, look for holes, and remove all garbage and debris. The ground should be clear of rocks and grooves and must be firm enough to support the aircraft. Mark the corners of the landing area with light sticks or cones. Alternatively, you can use emergency vehicles with headlights directed toward the landing area (but not at the approaching aircraft). If the landing area is dirt, lightly moisten the area with water if possible. Under no circumstances should anyone be allowed to enter the LZ after it has been secured.

Constant communication must be maintained throughout the helicopter operation. If you are the ground contact, you may be responsible for relaying

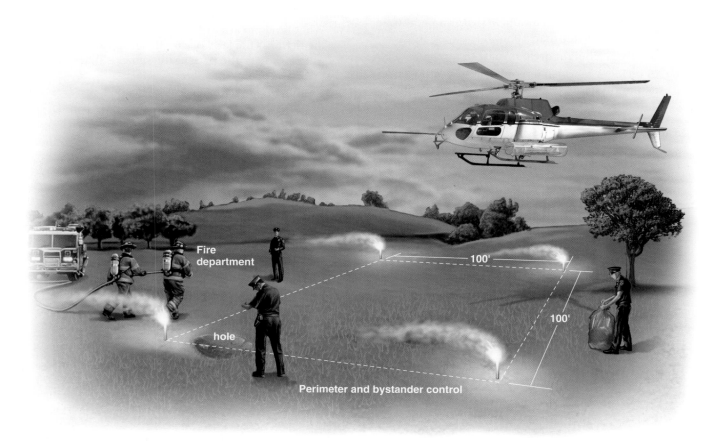

FIGURE 50-2 ▲ A helicopter landing zone requires at least 100 by 100 feet.

important information to the responding flight crew about the patient's condition. All aspects of the LZ, including such hazards as light poles, trees, and power lines, must be relayed to the pilot. The pilot should also be told the approximate ground wind conditions.

As the helicopter approaches, it is important to maintain eye contact with the helicopter and pay attention to any visible hazards on the ground at the same time. At any moment it may be necessary to abort the landing. Your assessment of ground conditions could be the key factor in this decision. As the helicopter is landing (or taking off), lower the face shield on your helmet or turn your head momentarily to avoid getting debris in your eyes from the rotor wash.

Once the helicopter is on the ground, it is very important to pay attention to traffic. The arrival of a helicopter often draws a large crowd with many bystanders. Pay particular attention to bicycles and motorized vehicles because they can approach the scene quickly and without warning. As the patient is moved toward the helicopter, the flight crew will be focused on loading the patient and may not see all the hazards on the ground. Your constant attention to the scene is critical to the safety of the flight crew and all persons on the scene. The rear of a helicopter can be especially dangerous. The tail rotor is often low and invisible when turning. Use extreme caution, and follow the instructions of the crew when you are close to the aircraft. Important safety tips to keep in mind around helicopters are shown in the following *Remember This* box.

Remember This

Safety is critical around a helicopter. Remember to wear appropriate personal protective equipment (such as a helmet, turnout coat, eye shield, etc.). Also, remember to *never* approach a helicopter from the rear.

After the patient is loaded into the helicopter, the pilot will radio you when she is ready for liftoff. A brief response from you that the scene is still clear will assure the pilot that you have been vigilant about surveying the scene for hazards. As the helicopter leaves the scene, advise your coworkers to keep the LZ intact for several minutes. This step is done in case the helicopter must return for an emergency landing.

Make sure your dispatcher is aware of all times associated with helicopter operations. For example, you should notify the EMD when the helicopter has arrived on the scene. You should also notify the dispatcher when the helicopter has left the scene, and you should report its destination. In your PCR, make sure to docu-

ment the time patient care was transferred to the flight crew, the patient's condition at the time care was transferred, and the patient's destination.

Stop and Think!

Working Safely Around Helicopters

- Never move toward a helicopter until signaled by the flight crew.
- Always approach the helicopter from the front so that the pilot can see you.
- Wear ear and eye protection when approaching the helicopter.
- Never raise your arms or equipment above your head.
- Remove loose items, such as hats, that can be blown around or sucked into the rotors or engines.
- If the aircraft is parked on a slope, always approach and exit from the downhill side.
- When moving from one side of the helicopter to the other, always cross in front of the helicopter.
- Do not open or pull on any part of the aircraft.
- Do not allow vehicles or nonaircraft personnel within 60 feet of the aircraft.

On the Scene   Wrap-Up

Recognizing that your patient was thrown from his motorcycle at a speed of more than 20 mph, you know that he will need definitive treatment from a trauma center and the distance to such a facility is too great to be traveled quickly by ground ambulance. Your local guidelines allow you to activate a helicopter based on these criteria. You contact your dispatch and recommend contacting the air medical service to "launch" a helicopter. While you attend to the patient, your partner locates a large clear area and begins to set up a landing zone. She clears the landing zone of any loose objects and debris that may be a hazard. It seems like just a few moments before you hear the sounds of an approaching helicopter. The helicopter pilot talks with you directly by means of your handheld radio and tells you she will be landing shortly after looking at the landing area. In just a few more minutes, the flight crew is at your side. One listens to your report as the other moves to the patient to begin assessment. You assist them in preparing the patient for the flight and then help load the patient into the aircraft. ■

▶ Air medical transport may be necessary when the condition of one or more patients is critical.

▶ Local standards and protocols for the use of air transport vary widely, even within a given region. It is essential that you become familiar with local guidelines regarding the use of air transport.

▶ If your unit is designated to land the helicopter, you will need to locate a secure landing zone. You must locate an area that is easily controlled for traffic and pedestrians. You should allow at least 100 feet by 100 feet to land any helicopter. The area should be free of such overhead obstacles as wires, trees, and light poles. It should also be free of debris and should be relatively level. The ground should be clear of rocks and grooves and must be firm enough to support the aircraft.

▶ Safety is critical around a helicopter. Remember to wear appropriate personal protective equipment (such as a helmet, turnout coat, eye shield, etc.). Also, remember to *never* approach a helicopter from the rear.

Vehicle Extrication

By the end of this chapter, you should be able to:

Knowledge Objectives ▶

1. Describe the purpose of extrication.
2. Discuss the role of the EMT in extrication.
3. Identify what equipment for personal safety is required for the EMT.
4. Define the fundamental components of extrication.
5. Evaluate various methods of gaining access to the patient.
6. State the steps that should be taken to protect the patient during extrication.
7. Distinguish between simple and complex access.

Attitude Objectives ▶

No attitude objectives are identified for this lesson.

Skill Objectives ▶

No skill objectives are identified for this lesson.

On the Scene

While driving back to the station, your unit is dispatched to a motor vehicle crash at the intersection of Central Avenue and Main Street. While en route, the mobile data computer in the unit advises that this will be a two-vehicle crash with injuries. Upon arrival, you find a four-door sedan that has been struck in the passenger side by a full-size pickup truck. There is a patient in the front seat on the passenger side of the four-door sedan who cannot get out of the vehicle. The vehicle's other occupants are standing outside. ∎

THINK ABOUT IT

As you read this chapter, think about the following questions:

- How will you gain access to the interior of the vehicle to treat the patient?
- What types of protection are required for both the patient and yourself while performing extrication?
- How will you determine the route by which to remove the patient from the vehicle?
- What can you determine about the patient's condition from observing the interior and exterior of the vehicle?

Objective 1

Each year thousands of people are involved in motor vehicle collisions on U.S. roadways. Vehicle crashes can range in severity from a minor auto accident involving only damage to the bumpers of the vehicles to a motor vehicle crash involving heavy entrapment of the patient.

Extrication is the use of specialized equipment for the safe removal of a trapped and injured patient. Situations in which a patient cannot get out of the vehicle by himself or should not because of his injuries will require extrication. This chapter prepares you for dealing with patients entrapped in vehicles after a vehicle collision has occurred.

You Should Know

Although the focus of this chapter is patient entrapment in a vehicle, other forms of entrapment occur that require special rescue teams, equipment, and training. Examples of these situations include confined space rescue, trench rescue, high-angle rescue, water rescue, search rescue, wilderness rescue, and tactical rescue, to name a few.

Role of the EMT on an Extrication Scene

Objective 2

As an EMT on an extrication scene, you may be called to perform a variety of tasks to assist in the extrication process. Your main duties will involve ensuring patient safety and delivering patient care by providing cervical spine stabilization, treating any injuries sustained by the patient(s), and assisting paramedics on the scene with any special needs. Patient care precedes extrication unless delayed movement would endanger the life of the patient or rescuers. Patient care should include attention to life-threatening emergencies. All patients should be packaged and moved carefully to minimize the danger of further injury or aggravation of existing injuries.

In some areas, the EMTs are also the rescue providers. If this is the case, you must be trained in the use of extrication tools and proper extrication techniques. A chain of command should be established to ensure patient care priorities. Give necessary care to the patient before extrication, and ensure that the patient is removed in a way that minimizes further injury.

Equipment

Objective 3

Remember that your personal safety is your priority on every call. Protective clothing that is appropriate for the situation must be worn during extrication. This includes protective boots, pants, a coat, eye protection, a helmet, and gloves. Respiratory protection may also be needed if there is a possibility of inhaling particulates from the extrication process. Particulates can come from many sources, such as a deployed airbag or the windshield being cut by a reciprocating saw, just to name a few. Several standards regulate the use of PPE and should be followed when selecting the type of clothing to wear. Hearing protection may also be necessary depending on the amount of noise on the scene. If there is any possibility of a fire, structural firefighting gear should be worn. Fire-resistant jumpsuits are also available and can be worn if your agency permits. A helmet, gloves, boots, and eye protection should be used in conjunction with the jumpsuit. Bloodborne pathogens are another concern and should be addressed with appropriate PPE that is rated against bloodborne pathogens. Structural firefighting gear is rated against bloodborne pathogens, but additional protection may be required, including medical gloves and respiratory protection for airborne pathogens. Always wear the PPE that will give you the most protection from the hazards present at the extrication scene (Figure 51-1).

Stages of Extrication

Objective 4

The stages of extrication include preparation, en route scene size-up, hazards, operations, access, emergency medical care, disentanglement, removal and transfer, and termination.

Preparation

Preparing for the possibility of extrication is the first step in providing good patient care. It begins by doing exactly what you're doing right now: learning. Many textbooks have been written on vehicle extrication that provide valuable information about extrication techniques and procedures for removing patients from motor vehicles. Additionally, several hands-on classes are available that allow practicing learned techniques in a controlled setting before performing them on an extrication scene.

Once you are working in the field and adequately trained, preparation also includes inspecting any

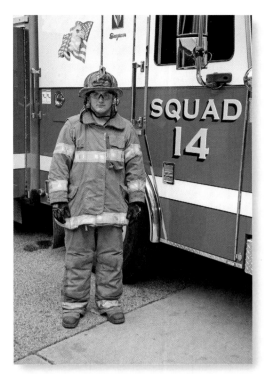
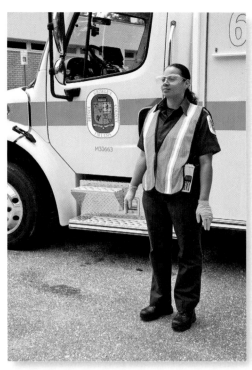

FIGURE 51-1 ▲ Protective clothing that is appropriate for the situation must be worn during extrication.

extrication equipment at the beginning of your shift to ensure it is in good condition; has the proper amount of fuel, if applicable; and is working properly. Postcall reviews from previous calls are also a great way of learning the extrication techniques that proved useful during the call and those that did not. Remember: Continuous training is the key for preparing to handle MVCs that require extrication.

En Route and Scene Size-Up

The scene size-up is an important step in the extrication process because it determines the direction the call is going to take. If done properly, the scene size-up will reveal any hazards present and provide information that will help you determine the need for additional resources. It should also give a good indication of the number of persons injured, the types of injury, and which patient or patients require medical attention first.

Scene size-up begins as you respond to the crash scene. En route to the scene, the dispatcher should advise you of any pertinent information regarding conditions on the scene. Once on the scene, park in a **fend-off position.** The fend-off position involves parking your unit in advance of the scene and in such a way that allows traveling vehicles to strike your unit and not crew members (Figure 51-2). This provides protection to crew members while they are working on the scene.

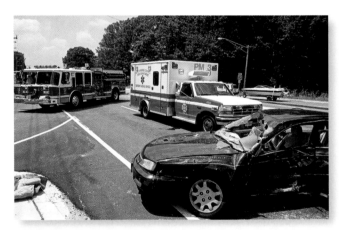

FIGURE 51-2 ▲ Once on the scene, park in a fend-off position. The fend-off position involves parking your unit downward from the scene and in such a way that allows traveling vehicles to strike your unit and not crew members.

Hazard Control and Safety Considerations

Before exiting your unit, make sure that it is safe to do so. Check for passing traffic and any hazards that would prevent you from exiting the vehicle. Either your partner or you will need to establish command, with the most experienced person being the incident commander. A 360-degree assessment (looking at the scene from all angles) should be made around the entire scene to look for any hazards around and underneath the vehicles. Be alert for any of the following:

- Traffic at the scene
- Leaking fuels or fluids
- Hazardous materials
- Broken glass
- Exposed or downed electrical wires
- Fire or possibility of fire
- Explosive materials
- Trapped or ejected patients
- Unstable vehicle or structure
- Environmental conditions (heavy rain, heavy snowfall, flash floods)

Alternative fuels and renewable fuels, such as hydrogen and ethanol, pose special challenges for emergency response personnel. For example, both hydrogen and ethanol can burn with an invisible or almost invisible flame. If you know or suspect that a scene involves alternative or renewable fuels, contact your dispatch center so that this important information can be relayed to responding fire department crews. Do not approach unless you are trained and equipped with appropriate PPE for the situation or the scene has been deemed safe by the proper authorities. If extrication is required, call for the additional resources that will be necessary.

Operations

When vehicles collide, they can wind up in a wide array of configurations that may place the vehicles in unstable positions. **Stabilization** is the process of rendering a vehicle motionless in the position in which it is found. The purpose of stabilization is to eliminate potential movement of a vehicle (or structure) that may cause further harm to entrapped patients or rescuers.

Equipment for stabilization may include a come-along (hand winch), cribbing and wedges, airbags, step chocks, hydraulic rams, jacks, and/or chains. Cribbing is usually used to provide a platform for the vehicle to rest on for stabilization. Cribbing consists of 4×4-inch wooden posts that can range from 18 to 36 inches long depending upon your needs. Step chocks are another form of cribbing. They provide a stairlike platform for the vehicle's frame to rest on. The bottom stair of the step chock is 24 inches long. As the stairs move up, the length of each stair shortens. This allows the step chock to be used for multiple vehicles of different heights.

If the vehicle is in an upright position, stabilization of the vehicle is straightforward. Begin by taking four step chocks and placing two behind the front tires and two in front of the rear tires. Make sure that the frame will rest on the step that is closest to the height of the frame. This will allow the vehicle to come down the least amount possible (Figure 51-3). If step chocks are not available, use 4×4-inch cribbing as a substitute. Next, use a pair of pliers, and remove the valve stems from all four tires. As the vehicle begins to lower, the frame will rest on the step chocks, isolating the frame from the vehicle's springs and tires. Stabilizing the vehicle is the first step in providing spinal stabilization for the patient. If the vehicle is motionless, then the patient will be motionless as well, which protects the patient's spine. With the step chocks in place and the tires deflated, the vehicle is now stable, and the extrication process can begin.

Other tools are available for special situations, including car-on-car situations, vehicles on their sides or roofs, and larger vehicles. These tools include jacks, ratchet straps, and struts, among others. The

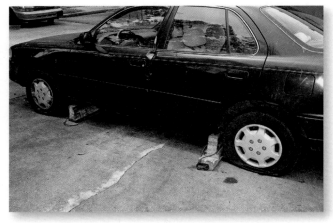

FIGURE 51-3 ▲ If a vehicle is in an upright position, stabilize it by taking four step chocks and placing two behind the front tires and two in front of the rear tires. Make sure that the frame will rest on the step that is closest to the height of the frame.

use of this equipment is covered in advanced extrication courses.

Gaining Access

Objectives 5, 6

Gaining access to the patient inside an entangled vehicle should be accomplished as soon as safely possible after arriving on the scene. Check for deployed and undeployed airbags, and make sure that the ignition key is turned to the off position. To gain access, use the path of least resistance. Try opening each door, roll down windows, or have the patient unlock doors. In many cases, the easiest way to gain access to the interior of a vehicle is through the unaffected side of the vehicle. When collision damage extends to the interior of a vehicle, the main hazards are the airbags inside the vehicle. The 5-10-20 rule is the standard rule regarding strike zones from undeployed airbags. This means that you should be at least 5 inches away from the side airbags, 10 inches away from the driver's airbag, and 20 inches from the passenger's airbag. Placing yourself in the center of the backseat of the vehicle will put you outside all strike zones from undeployed airbags.

Remember This

The route used to reach the patient is not necessarily the route through which the patient will be removed.

If the vehicle is not upright or there is heavy damage to the vehicle, you may need to enter through the vehicle's glass. There are two types of glass commonly found in vehicles today. Laminated glass is found in the front windshield of most vehicles. It is composed of two panes of glass with a laminated sheet between them. The laminated sheet allows the glass to remain intact should it be struck by an object. It is best removed by working around the edges of the glass. Start by taking an ax and working around the edges of the glass, using the ax like a can opener. Continue around the edge until you come back to the starting point. The glass can now be removed from the vehicle (Figure 51-4). The other type of glass is tempered, which breaks into small pieces but does not shatter and leave jagged, sharp edges, as most glass does. It is found in side windows and the rear window. A spring-loaded window punch is the best tool for this type of glass. Simply place the tip of the punch against a corner of the window and push in. The glass will break into very small pieces but should remain relatively intact until you remove it by hand (Figure 51-5).

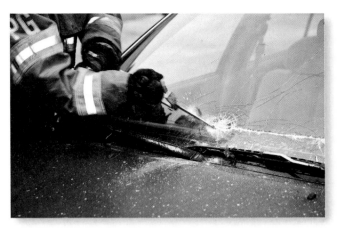

FIGURE 51-4 ▲ The front windshield of most vehicles is made of laminated glass. Remove it by taking an ax or similar tool and working around the edges of the glass. Continue around the edge until you come back to the starting point; then remove the glass.

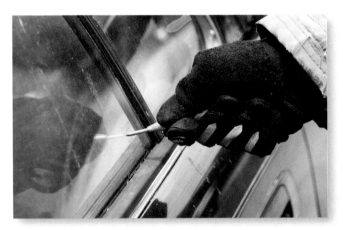

FIGURE 51-5 ▲ A window punch can be used to remove tempered glass from side windows and the rear window.

You Should Know

When using a window punch, use contact paper or duct tape to help keep the glass together during the breakage and removal. Without this, there is occasionally a problem with the glass shattering and going in different directions, and possibly falling on the patient.

After you have gained access to the interior of the vehicle, the next step should be to provide protection for the patient. A heavy tarp or other type of cover specially designed for rescue purposes should be used to protect the patient, and respiratory protection should be used if there is a concern about particulates entering the patient's respiratory tract (Figure 51-6). It is important to remember that the patient does not understand

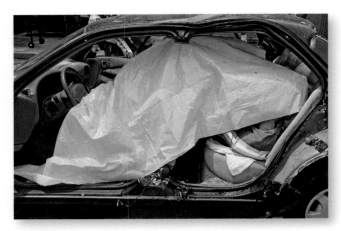

FIGURE 51-6 ▲ A heavy tarp or other type of cover specially designed for rescue purposes should be used to protect the patient during extrication.

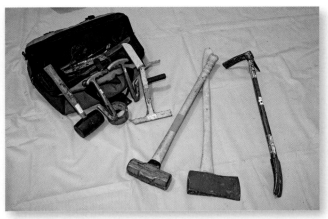

(a)

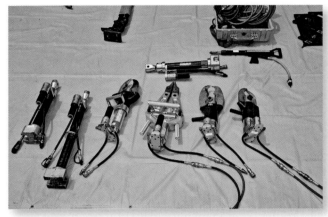

(b)

FIGURE 51-7 ▲ **(a)** Simple extrication is the use of hand tools in order to gain access to and extricate the patient from the vehicle. **(b)** Complex extrication involves the use of powered hydraulic rescue tools, such as cutters, spreaders, and rams.

the extrication process and can become frightened by the sounds and procedures occurring around him. It is often desirable for a rescuer working in the interior of the vehicle to provide psychological support from underneath the tarp during the extrication. This will also give the inside rescuer the opportunity to assess the patient continuously throughout the extrication process.

Extrication Process

Objective 7

Extrication can be divided into two categories: simple and complex. **Simple extrication** is the use of hand tools in order to gain access and extricate the patient from the vehicle. Simple hand tools include hammers, hacksaws, battery-operated saws, center punch, and pry bars (Figure 51-7a). **Complex extrication** involves the use of powered hydraulic rescue tools, such as cutters, spreaders, and rams (Figure 51-7b). The patient's level of entrapment will determine whether the extrication will fall into a simple or complex category.

Degrees of Entrapment

Four levels of entrapment are possible during an MVC:
1. *No entrapment* is the first level. This means no one is entrapped in the vehicle, and occupants were able to get out of the vehicle on their own.
2. *Light entrapment* means that a door or some other object will need to be opened or moved to get the patient out (Figure 51-8a).
3. *Moderate entrapment* is more involved, requiring removal of doors or the roof (Figure 51-8b). A patient in a moderate entrapment situation is confined by the wreckage, but a rescuer can access the entire patient.

4. *Heavy entrapment* is the highest level of entrapment and involves any situation that is above and beyond moderate entrapment. A person who is heavily entrapped in a vehicle is actually pinned by some part of the vehicle that must be moved away from the patient before the patient can be removed from the vehicle (Figure 51-8c).

Light entrapment situations fall into the category of simple extrication. In most cases, only hand tools are needed to gain access to the patient. Moderate entrapment falls into the complex category. It usually involves hydraulic, gas, or electric tools to remove the doors from the vehicle. The same tools can remove the roof and any additional pieces of the vehicle that need to be removed in order to gain patient access and provide egress. Heavy entrapment requires rescuers to actually move a structural component of the vehicle to free the patient for removal from the vehicle.

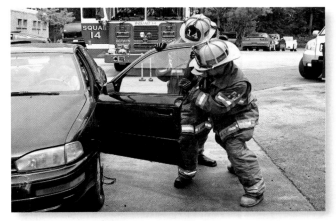

(a)

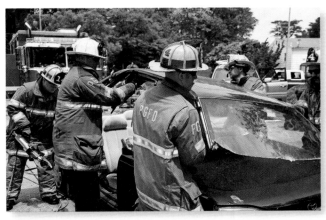

(b)

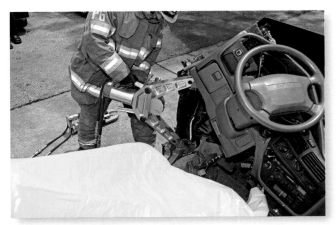

(c)

FIGURE 51-8 ▲ **(a)** Light entrapment requires opening or moving a door or some other object to get the patient out. **(b)** Moderate entrapment requires removal of doors or the roof. **(c)** A person who is heavily entrapped in a vehicle requires that some part of the vehicle must be moved away from the patient before the patient can be moved from the vehicle.

Disentanglement

Disentanglement is the moving or removing of material that is trapping a victim. As disentanglement progresses, the patient can be prepared for removal. You should remove the patient from the vehicle in the manner that provides the greatest amount of spinal protection for the patient. Manual cervical spinal stabilization should be performed upon patient contact. Then a cervical collar should be applied for additional protection. The rest of the patient's spine should also be stabilized. This is best accomplished with the use of a short spine immobilizer. One example of a short spine immobilizer is the Kendrick Extrication Device (KED). The KED allows the patient's spine to be stabilized from her head to her lower lumbar vertebrae (Figure 51-9). If the patient is a child, use a device of appropriate size, such as a Pedi-Immobilizer, that allows for whole-body stabilization (Figure 51-10). Dress and

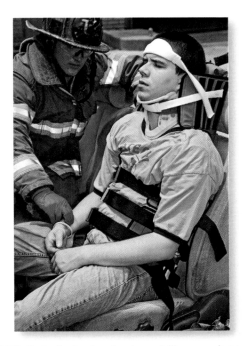

FIGURE 51-9 ▲ A short spine immobilizer, such as the KED, allows the patient's spine to be immobilized from head to lower lumbar vertebrae.

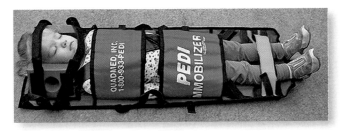

FIGURE 51-10 ▲ A device such as a Pedi-Immobilizer allows for whole-body stabilization.

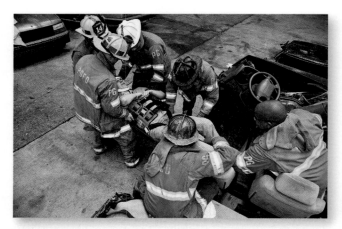

FIGURE 51-11 ▲ In most , but not all, cases, an immobilized patient who is being removed from the vehicle through a doorway should be taken out onto a backboard. Each extrication procedure will ultimately be dictated by what is safest for the patient and the rescuers.

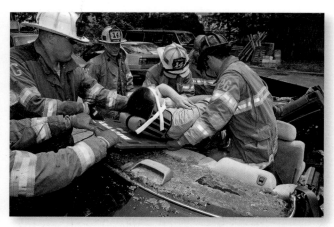

FIGURE 51-12 ▲ Removing a patient over the trunk of a vehicle.

bandage open wounds, and splint or stabilize fractures as time and conditions permit.

In most cases, if an immobilized patient is being removed from the vehicle through a doorway, then he should be taken out onto a backboard (Figure 51-11). Several rescuers will be needed to remove a patient from a vehicle. Always call for additional help if needed, and use proper body mechanics to prevent injury while moving any patient.

Another method of removal from a vehicle is to place a backboard behind the patient while she is still in her seat. This method requires that the roof be totally removed from the vehicle. First, recline the seat into a position that will allow you to place the backboard behind the victim, positioning the backboard between the patient and the seat. Several rescuers will be needed to accomplish this. One rescuer should be at the patient's head and will be in control of patient movement. When the head rescuer calls for the patient to be moved, every rescuer involved in the process moves at once and brings the patient farther up the backboard until the patient is completely on. With the patient on the backboard, the head should be stabilized last by using materials designed for this purpose (such as soft foam blocks and tape). The straps on the backboard should be joined together. The patient is now ready to be taken away from the vehicle. The rescuers can lift the patient on either side and take the backboard out over the trunk of the vehicle (Figure 51-12). Continue to protect the patient from hazards.

Removal, Transfer, and Termination

The patient is now ready for transport to the hospital. Several factors should be considered when determin-

ing whether to go by ground transportation or air, such as time of day, traffic, and weather.

Remember This

The extrication of patients requires special consideration. For instance, if a patient is pinned by the dash, compression syndrome can result. The patient can severely decompensate once the dash is removed (blood can rush into the pinned extremity, which can result in severe circulatory problems from toxins, as well as significant hypotension). If the patient is trapped, try to find out how long the patient has been trapped. If the patient has been trapped for an hour or more, you should suspect crush syndrome. Contact dispatch and request ALS personnel to the scene. In these situations, it will be important for ALS personnel to begin patient treatment before extrication.

Additional Scene Hazards

With the extrication process over and the patient removed, the next step is to secure any hazards created on the scene. These include any pieces of the vehicle that were removed, fuel leaks, or even vehicles still in the roadway that need to be removed. Address the removed pieces of the vehicle by placing them back into the vehicle that was cut. Fuel leaks should be handled by placing an absorbent material on the spill and then collecting the material for disposal. Any additional vehicles on the scene that can be removed from the roadway should be placed outside the traffic area.

Making a Difference

After every extrication, a postcall review should be performed to determine which actions proved to be beneficial and which did not. This is not a blame session. It is a tool to facilitate learning for the next extrication you perform. Each experience will help you become a better EMT.

On the Scene   Wrap-Up

Any extrication is a complex event that requires great skill and a working knowledge of vehicle design and extrication operations. On the basis of the patient's condition, you decide that this patient needs to be extricated from the vehicle. You perform a 360-degree rotation around the vehicle to check for any hazards; none is found. Wearing your PPE, you approach the vehicle. Stabilization of the vehicle is accomplished by using cribbing. You then enter the vehicle through the back door on the driver's side. As you enter the vehicle, you notice that there is a significant amount of intrusion of the passenger side of the vehicle. This gives you an indication of the types and severity of the patient's injuries. The extrication team removes the roof of the vehicle, lifts the patient onto a long backboard, and takes the patient out of the vehicle over the trunk. The patient is placed into the back of your ambulance for transport, and you accompany the patient to the hospital. ■

Sum It Up

► You may be called to assist with extrication. Your main duties will involve ensuring patient safety and delivering patient care by providing cervical spine stabilization, treating any injuries sustained by the patient(s), and assisting paramedics on the scene with any special needs.

► Extrication is the use of specialized equipment for the safe removal of a trapped and injured patient. The EMT on the extrication scene has an important role both as a care provider for the patient and a support member for the extrication team. Base the extrication on the patient's condition to ensure that the techniques used will provide the fastest access and best egress for the patient from the vehicle.

► Protective clothing that is appropriate for the situation must be worn during extrication. This includes protective boots, pants, a coat, eye protection, a helmet, and gloves. Respiratory protection may also be needed.

► Scene size-up is an important step in the extrication process. A proper scene size-up will reveal any hazards present and also give a good indication of the number of persons injured, the types of injury, and which patient or patients require medical attention first.

► Once on the scene, fire apparatus should be parked in the fend-off position, which involves parking your unit in advance of the scene and in such a way that allows traveling vehicles to strike your unit and not crew members.

► Alternative fuels and renewable fuels, such as hydrogen and ethanol, pose special challenges for emergency response personnel. If you know or suspect that a scene involves alternative or renewable fuels, contact your dispatch center so that this important information can be relayed to responding fire department crews. Do not approach unless you are trained and equipped with appropriate PPE for the situation or the scene has been deemed safe by the proper authorities.

► Stabilization is the process of rendering a vehicle motionless in the position in which it is found. The purpose of stabilization is to eliminate potential movement of a vehicle (or structure) that may cause further harm to entrapped patients or rescuers.

► Simple extrication is the use of hand tools in order to gain access and extricate the patient from the vehicle. Complex extrication involves the use of powered hydraulic rescue tools, such as cutters, spreaders, and rams. The patient's level of entrapment will determine whether the extrication will fall into a simple or complex category.

► Four levels of entrapment are possible during a motor vehicle crash. The first level is no entrapment. Light entrapment means that a door or some other object will need to be opened or moved to get the patient out. Moderate entrapment is more involved, requiring removal of doors or the roof. Heavy entrapment is the highest level of entrapment and involves any situation that is above and beyond moderate entrapment.

► Disentanglement is the moving or removing of material that is trapping a victim.

► Continue your education beyond the information contained in this chapter in order to provide the best care for your patient and maintain and improve your skills as you gain more experience in EMS.

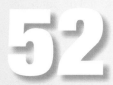
Hazardous Materials Awareness

Note: This material is not intended to replace the need for a hazardous materials, first responder course.

By the end of this chapter, you should be able to:

Knowledge Objectives ▶

1. Define hazardous materials, and explain the EMT's role during a call involving them.
2. Describe what the EMT should do if there is reason to believe that there is a hazard at the scene.
3. Briefly describe the various types of chemical protective clothing.
4. State the role the EMT should perform until appropriately trained personnel arrive at the scene of a hazardous materials situation.
5. Discuss methods used to identify hazardous materials.
6. Discuss the establishment of safety zones at a scene involving hazardous materials.

Attitude Objectives ▶

No attitude objectives are identified for this lesson.

Skill Objectives ▶

No skill objectives are identified for this lesson.

On the Scene

You have been dispatched to a medical emergency at a local manufacturing facility that produces silicone wafers for the computer industry. Dispatch reports that several employees are complaining of a burning sensation in their eyes and throat. You will be the first EMS unit on scene. Your dispatcher has informed you that you are to meet the security guard at the front gate for an escort into the scene. Upon arrival at the main gate, the guard greets you with a map and asks you to follow him to a specific building in a large industrial plant. As you approach the building, you notice a diamond-shaped placard to the right of the door that the guard leads you to. ■

THINK ABOUT IT

As you read this chapter, think about the following questions:

- What indication do you have that this scene may be a hazardous materials incident?
- Do you have the proper personal protective equipment to handle this call?
- What additional resources may be needed to gain access to the patients?

You may respond to situations involving hazardous materials. To prevent further illness or injury, you must be able to recognize when a hazardous materials situation exists.

Hazardous Materials

Objective 1

The National Fire Protection Association (NFPA) defines a *hazardous material* as "a substance (solid, liquid, or gas) that, when released, is capable of creating harm to people, the environment, and property." Hazardous materials may be found in incidents involving vehicle crashes, railroads, pipelines, storage containers and buildings, chemical plants, and acts of terrorism. Hazardous materials can also be found in the home.

The Role of the EMT

Objective 2

Management of a hazardous materials incident requires preplanning, specialized emergency care by trained personnel, identifying the substance or material, treatment protocols specific for the material involved, and emergency department care by personnel trained to handle this type of medical emergency.

During the early stages of a hazardous materials event, local EMS providers will be on their own for the initial phase of the response until specialty teams arrive. You must ensure the safety of yourself and your crew, the patient, and bystanders. To do this effectively, standard operating procedures and protocols must be used. In some cases, you will be able to recognize a hazardous material from the information given by the dispatcher. Alternatively, you may be the one who activates the hazardous materials team because you discovered the incident.

Scene Safety and Reporting

Objective 2

The first phase of dealing with a hazardous materials incident is recognizing that one exists and recognizing the limitations of yourself and your crew. Remember that hazardous materials may pose a threat to the community. As always, your personal safety is your priority in any emergency scene. Dealing with hazardous materials requires extensive training and proper equipment. Without the proper equipment, any intervention could put you and your crew at risk. Access to any patient must not occur without the proper protective equip-

ment. Standard personal protective equipment may not be sufficient or appropriate for this type of response.

Protective Equipment

Objective 3

Many chemicals can cause harm to unprotected skin. Corrosives and strong oxidizers can cause contact dermatitis or chemical burns. Many pesticides and poisons can seep into the skin, resulting in toxic effects. Liquefied or cryogenic gases can cause thermal injuries, such as frostbite. Some liquefied gases may present more than one hazard. For example, chlorine stored as a liquefied gas is corrosive, especially to the eyes and moist skin. It is also a thermal hazard because of the frostbite potential as it rapidly evaporates.

Chemical protective clothing (**CPC**) is designed to protect the skin from exposure to chemicals by either physical or chemical means. Examples of CPC classes include gas-tight encapsulating suits, liquid splash–protective suits, permeable protective suits, nonhazardous chemical–protective clothing, and other protective apparel, such as chemically resistant hoods, gloves, and boots. A variety of materials are used to make the fabric from which CPC is manufactured. Each material provides protection against specific chemicals or mixtures of chemicals but may afford little or no protection against certain others. No material provides satisfactory protection from all chemicals. Protective clothing material needs to be compatible with the chemical substances involved and its use consistent with manufacturers' instructions. When used alone, CPC provides no fire or heat protection.

CPC is commonly categorized as either *limited use* or *heavy use*. Heavy-use CPC is designed to be more highly resistant to abrasions and punctures. Limited-use CPC is generally of lighter-weight construction. It is designed to be used once and then disposed of.

The Environmental Protection Agency has defined four levels of PPE. Level A protection is a vapor-protective suit that is encapsulated. This type of suit provides the highest available level of respiratory, skin, and eye protection from solid, liquid, and gaseous chemicals. Level A PPE includes a pressure-demand, full-face mask; self-contained breathing apparatus (SCBA); inner chemical-resistant gloves; and chemical-resistant safety boots (Figure 52-1). Optional equipment includes a cooling system, outer gloves, hard hat, and two-way radio communication system. Level A protection is intended for situations in which a chemical or chemicals have been identified and pose high levels of hazards to the respiratory system, skin, and eyes. Level A protection is typically used by members of the HazMat (hazardous material) team for entry into the contaminated area (hot zone).

Level B protection is a liquid splash–protective suit. It includes a pressure-demand, full-face mask; SCBA;

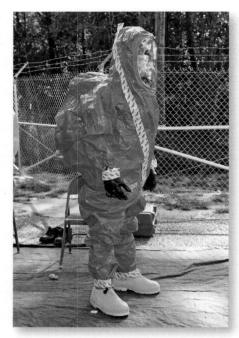

FIGURE 52-1 ▲ Level A protective equipment.

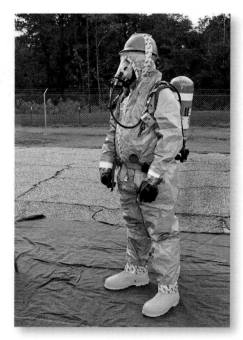

FIGURE 52-2 ▲ Level B protective equipment.

inner chemical-resistant gloves; chemical-resistant safety boots; and a hard hat (Figure 52-2). Level B PPE offers the same level of respiratory protection as level A but less skin protection. It offers no protection against chemical vapors or gases. Level B protection is worn when the chemical or chemicals have been identified but do not require a high level of skin protection. For example, level B protection is used when evaluation of the scene identifies that hazards of the chemical involved are associated with liquid but not vapor contact.

Level C PPE is a support-function protective garment. It includes a full-face mask, chemical-resistant gloves and safety boots, and a canister-equipped respirator that filters chemicals from the air (Figure 52-3). It does not include an SCBA. Level C protective equipment provides the same level of skin protection as level B but a lower level of respiratory protection. It provides liquid splash protection but no protection against chemical vapors or gases. Level C protection is used when the type of airborne substance is known, and contact with the chemical or chemicals will not affect the skin. Level C protective equipment is not acceptable for use in a chemical emergency response.

Level D PPE includes a work uniform, such as firefighter turnout clothing (Figure 52-4). It provides no respiratory protection and minimal skin protection. This level of protective equipment is used when the atmosphere of the involved area contains no known chemical hazards. Level D protective equipment is not acceptable for use in a chemical emergency response. (See Table 52-1 for an overview of the levels of protective equipment.)

No single combination of protective equipment and clothing can protect you from all hazards. Combining PPE ensembles with other types of protective clothing may be appropriate as additional measures for preventing exposure. For example, although CPC alone provides no fire or heat protection, aluminized radiant heat protection worn over CPC will provide limited protection in potential flash fire situations.

A specific PPE ensemble may protect well against some hazards but poorly, or not at all, against others. In many instances, PPE will not provide continuous protection from a particular hazard. In such cases, exposure times should be reduced as necessary and closely monitored. Technical data provided by the PPE manufacturer must be used when determining the most appropriate PPE for the hazards present.

Scene Size-Up

Objective 4

To maximize safety, approach and park uphill and upwind of a hazardous materials scene. In this position, you are less likely to become exposed if the hazardous material becomes airborne or a large spill occurs. Examples of incidents that may involve hazardous materials include vehicle crashes (commercial vehicles, pest

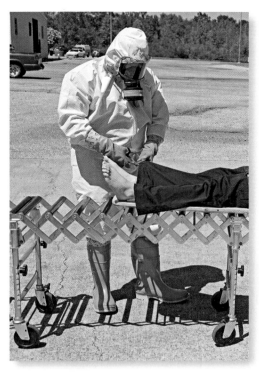

FIGURE 52-3 ▲ Level C protective equipment.

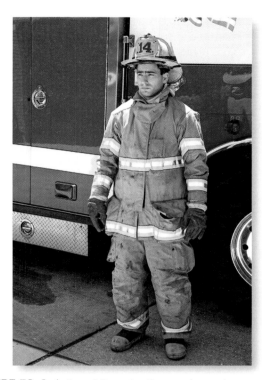

FIGURE 52-4 ▲ Level D protective equipment.

TABLE 52-1	Levels of Personal Protective Equipment	
Level	**When Used**	**Notes**
A	Intended for situations in which the chemical or chemicals have been identified and pose high levels of hazards to the respiratory system, skin, and eyes	• Vapor-protective suit that is encapsulated • Highest available level of respiratory, skin, and eye protection from solid, liquid, and gaseous chemicals
B	Worn when the chemical or chemicals have been identified and a high level of skin protection is not required	• Liquid splash–protective suit • Same level of respiratory protection as level A but less skin protection • No protection against chemical vapors or gases • Usually worn by decontamination team
C	Used when the type of airborne substance is known and contact with the chemical or chemicals will not affect the skin	• Support-function protective garment • Same level of skin protection as level B but a lower level of respiratory protection • Liquid splash protection but no protection against chemical vapors or gases • Not acceptable for use in a chemical emergency response
D	Used when the atmosphere of the involved area contains no known chemical hazards	• No respiratory protection and minimal skin protection • Should not be worn in the hot zone • Not acceptable for use in a chemical emergency response

control vehicles, tankers, cars with alternative fuels, or tractor-trailers), transportation (railroads or pipelines), storage (tanks or storage vessels, warehouses, or hardware or agricultural stores), manufacturing operations (such as chemical plants), and acts of terrorism.

On arrival at the scene, obtain scene control and establish a perimeter. If the call was not initially reported as a hazardous materials incident and you are the first on the scene and suspect hazardous materials involvement, an emergency medical dispatcher (EMD) should be notified so that appropriate measures can be taken. Give dispatch the exact location of the incident or perimeter.

If hazardous substances or conditions are suspected, the scene must be secured by qualified personnel wearing appropriate equipment. If you are not qualified and do not have the appropriate equipment, you may need to wait for additional help to arrive before you can attempt entry into the scene. Stage (wait for instructions) a minimum of 2,000 feet from a suspected hazardous materials incident.

If you have been trained to do so (and are properly equipped), identify and establish safety zones. Initiate the National Incident Management System (NIMS) plan (see Chapter 48). Designate the incident commander, and announce the location of the command post. The command post location may be determined by standard operating procedures or other resources. Generally, the command post should not be less than 300 feet away from the scene. In most cases, apparatus should point away from the scene. If possible, attempt to identify the material by sighting placards or identification numbers through binoculars while remaining at a safe distance from the area.

Remember This

Scene size-up is a continuous process. It allows the incident commander to periodically review strategy and tactics in order to effectively position more resources where necessary.

Identifying Hazardous Substances

Objective 5

The substance involved in an incident can be identified by using a number of resources:

- U.S. Department of Transportation (DOT) *Emergency Response Guidebook*
- United Nations (UN) classification numbers
- NFPA 704 placard system
- UN/DOT placards
- Shipping papers
- Material safety data sheets

Department of Transportation Regulations

Objective 5

The DOT regulates all aspects of transporting hazardous materials in the United States. These regulations include the design of the container, the type of container used, and the means by which hazardous materials are transported. If dangerous materials are being transported, the DOT requires that a placard be displayed on shipping containers and transport vessels (railroad cars, trucks, and ships). The color of the placard tells the class of the hazardous material. The presence of a four-digit number allows more specific identification. This four-digit number is keyed to the DOT's *Emergency Response Guidebook*. This book is a quick reference guide for hazardous materials incidents. Chemicals are listed in the book alphabetically and by their four-digit DOT number. Each chemical is given a reference number that corresponds to a set of instructions and precautions, listed in the back of the book, for dealing with that class of chemical (Figure 52-5).

Remember This

EMTs should attend a 24-hour hazardous materials, first responder course. If you have not received specific hazardous materials training, use the following rule of thumb. Assume that any material that has a colored placard or four-digit number on it is dangerous to your health and safety and that you must set up a safe zone until trained personnel properly identify the material.

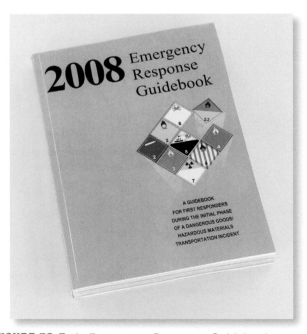

FIGURE 52-5 ▲ *Emergency Response Guidebook.*

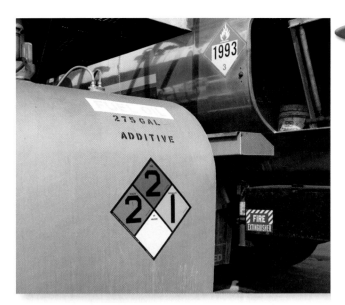

FIGURE 52-6 ▲ The NFPA hazard classification system uses diamond-shaped placards divided into quadrants.

National Fire Protection Association's Standard 704

Objective 5

The NFPA's Standard 704 designates a hazardous material's classification. The NFPA hazard classification system uses diamond-shaped placards divided into quadrants (Figure 52-6). Different background colors and numbers ranging from 0 to 4 (4 representing an extremely high hazard) are used to indicate the dangers presented by the hazardous material:

- Blue quadrant: Health hazard
- Red quadrant: Flammability hazard
- Yellow quadrant: Reactivity hazard
- White quadrant: Specific hazard (such as radioactivity, water reactivity, or biological hazard)

Material Safety Data Sheets

Objective 5

Material safety data sheets (MSDSs) provide detailed information about the material. This information includes the name and physical properties of the substance, fire and explosion hazard information, and first aid treatment. The Occupational Safety and Health Administration (OSHA) requires MSDSs to be kept on-site anywhere chemicals are used. MSDSs may be used to identify materials or products if they can be obtained safely.

Establishing Safety Zones

Objective 6

Hazardous materials scenes are divided into zones according to safety. If you have been trained to do so (and are properly equipped), identify and establish safety zones (Figure 52-7). The **hot zone** is the area of the incident that contains the hazardous material (contaminant). The hot zone is also known as the *exclusion zone*. This is a dangerous area. The size of the hot zone depends on many factors, including the characteristics of the chemical, the amount released (or spilled or escaped), local weather conditions, the local terrain, and other chemicals in the area. Areas around the contaminant that may be exposed to gases, vapors, mist, dust, or runoff are also part of the hot zone. Only personnel with high-level PPE enter this area. The hot zone is considered contaminated and dangerous until cleared by trained personnel.

The **warm zone** (also called the *contamination reduction zone*) is a controlled area for entry into the hot zone. The warm zone is where most operations will take place as a support area for the hot zone. It also serves as the decontamination area after exiting the hot zone. All personnel in the warm zone must wear appropriate protective equipment. If you have not been trained and do not have the appropriate protective gear, you *must* stay out of the hot and warm zones.

The safe zone (also called the *cold zone* or *support zone*) is an area safe from exposure or the threat of exposure. The cold zone serves as the staging area for personnel and equipment. If there is no risk to you, remove patients to a safe zone. You should not move from this zone or allow anyone else access to the scene

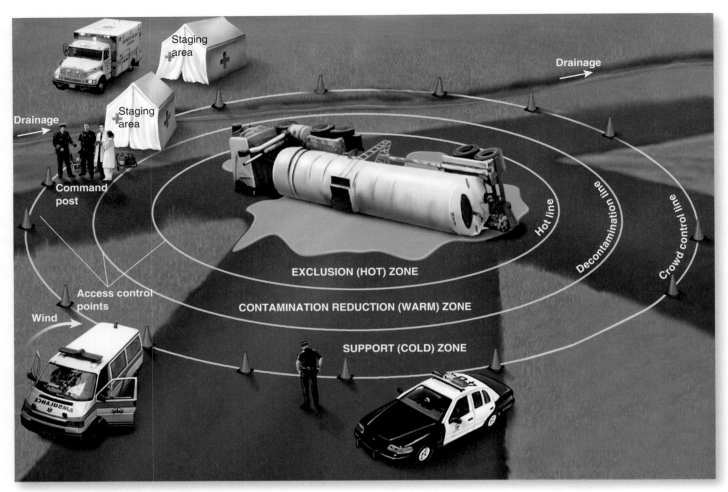

FIGURE 52-7 ▲ Safety zones.

from this zone unless the person has specialized training and PPE. The incident command post is located in the cold zone.

Approaching the Patient

Determine if the scene has been secured to allow for your safe approach to the patient. Do not approach unless you are trained and equipped with appropriate PPE for the situation or the scene has been deemed safe by the proper authorities. Much of the information you will need to properly treat the patient may be gathered initially from a distance with the use of binoculars or spotting scopes.

Remember to stay uphill and upwind as you approach any patient. Patient care must be performed only by trained personnel wearing the appropriate level of PPE, or the patient must have already been decontaminated.

Patients who are unable to walk must be removed from the hot zone by trained personnel. This is usually done by fire department and/or hazardous materials personnel. Even if you have been trained and are properly equipped, emergency care in the hot zone must be limited to spinal stabilization, gross airway management (such as opening the airway, suctioning), and hemorrhage control. Emergency care in the hot zone is limited because of the risk of patient or rescuer exposure to hazardous substances or conditions.

Address life-threatening problems, and carry out gross decontamination before giving emergency care. Gross decontamination means removing all suspected contaminated clothing. Brush off any obvious contaminants. Remove the patient's jewelry and watch, if present. Cover wounds with a waterproof dressing after decontamination. If spinal stabilization appears necessary, begin it as soon as feasible. Perform a primary survey at the same time as decontamination. Request ALS personnel if you suspect hazardous material contamination. Complete a more detailed assessment as conditions allow.

When treating patients, consider the chemical-specific information received from your PCC and other information resources. In multiple-patient situations, begin proper triage procedures according to your local emergency response plan. Triage is discussed in Chapter 49.

Decontamination

At every incident involving hazardous materials, there is a possibility that personnel, their equipment, and members of the public will become contaminated. The contaminant poses a threat to the persons contaminated, as well as to other personnel who may subsequently be exposed to contaminated personnel and equipment. Decontamination (decon) is done to reduce and prevent the spread of contamination from persons and equipment used at a hazardous materials incident by physical and/or chemical processes. The process should be directed toward confinement of the contaminant to maintain the safety and health of response personnel, the public, and the environment. Decon should be performed only by trained personnel wearing the appropriate level of PPE. Decon is usually performed in the warm zone. Decon procedures should be continued until it is determined or judged they are no longer necessary.

On the Scene **Wrap-Up**

The diamond-shaped placard at the door of the building adds to your concern that this is a hazardous materials incident. You ask the guard who has escorted you to the door if he has any additional information about the patients. He says that the on-site hazardous materials team has made contact with the patients and determined that they have been exposed to a chemical in the building. The HazMat team wants you to wait outside the building until it has properly "deconned" the patients. You contact your dispatch to inform that this is a hazardous materials incident and that you will be staging outside the building. ■

Sum It Up

▶ As defined by the NFPA, a hazardous material is any substance that causes or may cause adverse effects on the health or safety of employees, the general public, or the environment.

▶ A hazardous substance can be identified by using a number of resources:
- U.S. DOT *Emergency Response Guidebook*
- UN classification numbers
- NFPA 704 placard system
- UN/DOT placards
- Shipping papers
- MSDSs

▶ The first phase of dealing with a hazardous materials incident is recognizing that one exists. As always, your personal safety is your priority in any emergency scene. If there is no risk to you (and you are properly trained and equipped to do so), remove patients to a safe zone. The safe zone (also called the cold zone) is an area safe from exposure or the threat of exposure. The warm zone is a controlled area for entry into the hot zone. It also serves as the decontamination area after exiting the hot zone. All personnel in the warm zone must wear appropriate protective equipment. The hot zone is the danger zone.

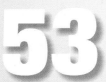

CHAPTER 53

Terrorism and Disaster Response

By the end of this chapter, you should be able to:

Knowledge Objectives ▶
1. Define weapons of mass destruction.
2. Discuss the five main types of weapons of mass destruction.
3. Define biological weapons, give examples, and explain how they are spread.
4. Discuss the types of radiation that may be given off by nuclear weapons.
5. Define chemical agents, give examples of their use as weapons, and their effects on the human body.
6. Discuss your primary responsibilities at a suspected terrorist incident.
7. Discuss incident factors that may suggest possible terrorist activity or weapons of mass destruction.

Attitude Objectives ▶
No attitude objectives are identified for this lesson.

Skill Objectives ▶
No skill objectives are identified for this lesson.

On the Scene

Your community has been chosen as the location for a large sporting event, and your crew has been busy with all of the medical calls associated with the huge number of fans in town for the event. You have just reached your quarters after the last medical call when you hear your station tones alerting you to another incoming call. Your dispatch center is asking for a response to the sporting event where a large number of sick fans have overwhelmed the resources of the aid station on-site. Your partner makes a "loop" around the station as you begin your response. As you respond to the call, the dispatch center adds two additional units to the response as the number of patients is rapidly increasing. You are able to make contact with the aid station on-site via radio, and the EMS crew reports that it has at least 50 patients with the same symptoms. These signs and symptoms include runny nose, watery eyes, excessive drooling, and diarrhea. ▪

THINK ABOUT IT

As you read this chapter, think about the following questions:

- What indication do you have that this scene may be a weapons of mass destruction event or terrorist incident?
- Do you have the proper personal protective equipment to handle this call?
- What additional resources may be needed to treat the patients and handle this event?

Objectives 1, 2

Our world has changed dramatically in just a few short years. Events involving weapons of mass destruction or hazardous materials once would have been unthinkable outside the movie theater but now must be considered possible in the real world. **Weapons of mass destruction (WMD)** are materials used by terrorists that have the potential to cause great harm over a large area.

Terrorists use fear to bring about political change. They want to cause panic and disrupt normal activities. Their goal is to injure (incapacitate), not necessarily kill, large numbers of people. By injuring as many people as possible, terrorists cause mass confusion and panic. This could affect an already overloaded EMS system, bringing it to a standstill. Additionally, healthcare professionals and emergency responders are prime targets. Incapacitating them ensures other victims do not recover. Military experts agree that incapacitating a person creates the need for a minimum of two healthcare professionals to begin any type of care.

There are five main categories of WMD. B-NICE is a simple way to remember these categories:

> Biological
> Nuclear/radiological
> Incendiary
> Chemical
> Explosive

Any material that has a harmful effect on the body can be used as a weapon of mass destruction or as a weapon of mass confusion. The sad reality is that there is an amazing amount of "terrorist" information about such materials available on the Internet. Fortunately, it is hard to "weaponize" most of these materials. For instance, some biological agents must come into contact with the victim's lung tissue to have a harmful effect and thus must be dispersed into the air. Other types of materials, such as nerve agents, need only to come in contact with the victim's skin to have a harmful effect.

Remember This

We must prepare for the unthinkable at all levels of training.

Types of Weapons of Mass Destruction

Biological Weapons

Objective 3

Biological weapons involve the use of bacteria, viruses, rickettsias, or toxins to cause disease or death (Figure 53-1). Diseases can be spread by:

- Inhalation of substances dispersed by spray devices (aerosols)
- Ingestion of contaminated food or water supplies
- Absorption through direct skin contact with the substance

Bacteria are germs that can cause disease in humans, plants, or animals. Bacteria can live outside the human body and do not depend on other organisms to live and grow. Examples of diseases caused by bacteria that may be used as biological weapons include anthrax and tularemia (rabbit fever).

A **virus** is a type of infectious agent that depends on other organisms to live and grow. Viruses that could serve as biological weapons include the smallpox virus and those that cause viral hemorrhagic fevers, such as the Ebola virus. Infection with a hemorrhagic virus causes bleeding from many body tissues. The person may die from shock or from lack of oxygen caused by severe bleeding.

Rickettsias are very small bacteria that require a living host to survive. Rickettsias are transmitted by bloodsucking parasites such as fleas, lice, and ticks. An example of a disease caused by rickettsia is Q fever.

Toxins are substances produced by an animal, a plant, or microorganism. Toxins are not the same as chemical agents. Toxins are natural substances and are generally more deadly than chemical agents, which are man-made. Toxins that could serve as biological weapons include ricin (made from the waste left over from processing castor beans), botulism (found in improperly canned food and in contaminated water supplies, such as rivers and lakes), and enterotoxin B.

Indicators of possible biological weapon use are shown in the following *You Should Know* box.

You Should Know

Indicators of Possible Biological Weapon Use
- Dead or dying animals, fish, or birds
- Unusual casualties
- Unusual widespread illness not typical for that region

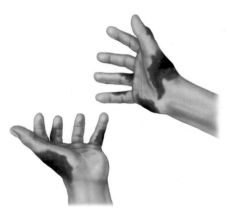

Bacteria: anthrax, tularemia (rabbit fever)

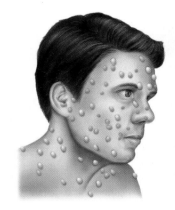

Viruses: smallpox, Ebola virus

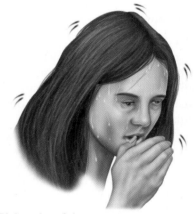

Rickettsias: Q fever

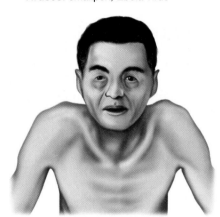

Toxins: ricin, botulism, enterotoxin B

FIGURE 53-1 ▲ Biological weapons use bacteria, viruses, rickettsias, or toxins to cause disease or death.

Creating a biological weapon is not complicated. It can be done by using materials purchased at a local hardware store and techniques learned in a high school chemistry course. Large quantities of biological weapons can often be produced in a few days to a few weeks.

You Should Know

The Centers for Disease Control and Prevention (CDC) categorize biological weapons according to their risk to national security. *Category A* diseases and agents are most likely to be used in an attack and include germs that are rarely seen in the United States. Category A diseases and agents include organisms that pose a risk to national security because they:

- Can be easily spread from person to person
- Result in high death rates and have the potential for major public health impact
- Might cause public panic

- Require special action for public health preparedness

Examples of category A diseases and agents include anthrax, botulism, plague, smallpox, tularemia, and viral hemorrhagic fevers.

Category B diseases and agents are the second-highest priority to the CDC because they are fairly easy to spread but cause moderate amounts of disease and low death rates. These weapons require specific public health action, such as improved diagnostic and detection systems. These agents include Q fever, brucellosis, glanders, ricin, enterotoxin B, viral encephalitis, food safety threats, water safety threats, and typhus fever.

Category C diseases and agents include germs that could be engineered for mass distribution in the future because they are fairly easy to obtain, produce, and spread. They can produce high rates of disease and death. Examples of category C diseases and agents include Nipah virus and hantavirus.

Nuclear Weapons

Objective 4

Nuclear weapons may be used in the form of ballistic missiles or bombs. Nuclear power plants, nuclear medicine machines in hospitals, research facilities, industrial construction sites, and vehicles used to transport nuclear waste may be possible targets for terrorist groups.

Nuclear radiation gives off three main types of radiation: alpha, beta, and gamma (Figure 53-2). It is the charge that makes radiation an immediate problem and disruptive to cell function and structure.

Alpha particles are large, heavy, and charged and cannot penetrate very far into matter. Because clothing or a sheet of paper is of sufficient thickness to stop them, external exposure to alpha particles usually has no effect on people. This is because the outermost dead layer of skin (epidermis) stops the particles from entering a person's body. However, if a person eats, drinks, or breathes in material that is contaminated with alpha-emitting particles, the alpha radiation can cause significant damage inside the body with exposure of live tissues.

Beta particles are much smaller, travel more quickly, have less charge, and can penetrate more deeply than alpha particles. Beta particles can be stopped by layers of clothing or thin metal or plastic, such as several sheets of aluminum foil or Plexiglas. Generally, skin burns (called *beta burns*) can occur if the skin is exposed to large amounts of beta radiation. Internal damage can occur if a person eats, drinks, or breathes in material that is contaminated with beta-emitting particles.

Gamma rays are waves of very high energy, similar to light. These waves of energy penetrate very deeply and can easily go right through a person. To reduce exposure from gamma rays, thick material such as lead must be used. Because gamma rays can penetrate tissues and organs, nausea, vomiting, high fever, hair loss, and skin burns may result if a person is exposed to a large amount of gamma radiation in a short period.

According to the CDC, a dirty bomb is a mix of explosives, such as dynamite, with radioactive powder or pellets. A dirty bomb is also known as a *radiological weapon*. When the dynamite or other explosives are set off, the blast carries radioactive material into the surrounding area. The impact of a dirty bomb depends on factors such as the size of the explosive, the amount and type of radioactive material used, and weather conditions. Any terrorist explosion or WMD incident has the potential of being a dirty bomb.

Remember This

You cannot see, smell, feel, or taste radiation. The longer you are exposed to it, the worse the effect.

Incendiary Weapons

Incendiary materials are substances that burn with a hot flame for a specific period. An incendiary system consists of the materials needed to start a fire, such as the initiator (the source that provides the first fire, such as a match), a delay mechanism (if needed), an igniter or fuse, and incendiary material or filler.

Most terrorist attacks involve the use of explosives, improvised explosive devices, and incendiary materials. Incendiaries are mainly used to set fire to wooden structures and other burnable targets. Firebombs are examples of incendiaries. They may range from a Molotov cocktail (bottle, gasoline, rag, and match) to much larger and sophisticated bombs. Firebombs may contain napalm or other flammable fluid. They are usually ignited with a fuse. Some incendiaries are used to melt, cut, or weld metal.

Chemical Weapons

Objective 5

Chemical agents are poisonous substances that injure or kill people when inhaled, ingested, or absorbed through the skin or eyes. There are five broad categories of chemical weapons: nerve agents, blister agents, blood agents, choking agents, and irritants (Table 53-1). Indicators of possible chemical weapon use are shown in the next *You Should Know* box. The general symptoms of exposure will vary by individual and depend on many factors such as:

- The substance involved
- The concentration of the substance
- The duration of exposure

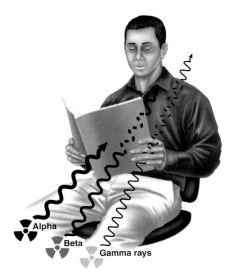

FIGURE 53-2 ▲ Nuclear radiation gives off three main types of radiation: alpha, beta, and gamma.

Alpha

Beta

Gamma rays

TABLE 53-1 Chemical Agents

Chemical Agent	Effects	Examples
Nerve agents	Interrupt nerve signals, causing a loss of consciousness within seconds and death within minutes of exposure	Tabun, sarin, soman, VX
Blister agents	Produce effects like those of a corrosive chemical, such as lye or a strong acid; result in severe burns to the eyes, skin, and tissues of the respiratory tract	Distilled mustard, forms of nitrogen mustard
Blood agents	Cause rapid respiratory arrest and death by blocking the absorption of oxygen to the cells and organs through the bloodstream	Cyanide, arsine, hydrogen chloride
Choking (pulmonary) agents	Inhaled chlorine mixes with the moisture in the lungs and becomes hydrochloric acid, which causes fluid to build up in the lungs (pulmonary edema), interferes with the body's ability to exchange oxygen, and results in asphyxiation that resembles drowning	Chlorine
Irritants	Result in immediate tearing of the eyes, coughing, difficulty breathing, nausea, and vomiting	Mace, pepper spray, tear gas

- The number of exposures
- The route of entry (inhalation, ingestion, injection, or absorption)

Other factors that influence how an individual is affected include the person's age, gender, general health, allergies, smoking habits, alcohol consumption, and medications.

You Should Know

Indicators of Possible Chemical Weapon Use
- Dead or dying animals, fish, or birds
- Lack of insects
- Unexplained casualties
- Multiple victims
- Serious illnesses
- Unusual liquid, spray, vapor, or droplets
- Unexplained odors
- Low clouds or fog unrelated to the weather
- Suspicious devices or packages, including metal debris, abandoned spray devices, unexplained weapons

Stop and Think!

Some chemical agents have a distinctive smell. Remember: If you can smell the chemical agent, you are too close.

Irritants are often used for personal protection and by police in riot control. Examples include Mace, pepper spray, and tear gas. These substances cause burning and intense pain to exposed skin areas. Exposure results in immediate tearing of the eyes, coughing, difficulty breathing, nausea, and vomiting.

Medical attention is needed for any of the following:
- Unconsciousness
- Confusion
- Lightheadedness
- Anxiety
- Dizziness
- Changes in skin color
- Shortness of breath
- Burning of the upper airway
- Coughing or painful breathing
- Drooling
- Chest tightness
- Loss of coordination
- Seizures
- Nausea, vomiting
- Abdominal cramping
- Diarrhea
- Loss of bowel or bladder control
- Dim, blurred, or double vision
- Tingling or numbness of the extremities

All these signs and symptoms can be indicative of some type of chemical exposure. They should be considered as the first warning signs that the call may be a WMD event. The reality of these types of situations is that responders may have already treated a large number of patients before recognizing that this is a WMD situation. Treating a large number of patients with the same signs and symptoms at the same scene should trigger the thought of a WMD event. Can you imagine the difficulty with recognizing the problem when the patients have been transported to multiple hospitals over a period of several days? You must be conscientious in recognizing and reporting these types of scenes.

A growing number of EMS operational systems are or will be carrying autoinjected medications called DuoDote kits. In the event of a mass exposure to a nerve agent, these kits are designed for self-treatment and treatment of other members of the initial emergency response team. ALS personnel may also administer the kits to the general public, when authorized by medical direction.

Remember This

Keep in mind that a hazardous materials incident is accidental. A terrorist attack is deliberate.

Explosives

Most terrorist attacks involve the use of explosives. Explosives are associated with a very rapid release of gas and heat. Examples of explosives include:

- Grenades
- Rockets
- Missiles
- Mines
- Pipe bombs
- Vehicle bombs
- Package or letter bombs
- Bombs carried in devices, such as a knapsack

Weapons of Mass Destruction Incident Response

Objective 6

A scene involving a WMD is a crime scene.

At a possible WMD incident, your primary responsibilities will be to:
- Isolate the scene.
- Preserve evidence and deny entry.
- Ask for additional help (see the following *Remember This* box), and coordinate efforts with other responding fire, EMS, and law enforcement personnel.
- Recognize signs of a potential WMD incident, and alert the proper authorities.
- Recognize the potential of a secondary explosion or attack on emergency responders.
- Make sure you, as well as additional responders, are safe.

Remember This

Depending on the type of WMD incident, additional resources that may be needed include:

- Law enforcement personnel
- Fire, hazardous materials, and other special rescue teams
- Gas, electric, water companies
- Hospitals
- Environmental Protection Agency (EPA)
- CDC
- State health department
- Military
- Public transportation
- Disaster services (Red Cross, Salvation Army)

To work effectively, you must use standard operating procedures (SOPs) and protocols according to your local emergency response plan (LERP). Try to assess the potential for an exposure by using the guidelines in the following sections.

Remember This

Because a terrorist event is a crime scene, it is important that you disturb the scene as little as possible.

Prearrival Response

From the dispatch information you are given, listen for specific clues that may indicate a possible terrorist incident, such as:

- Type of incident
- Incident location
- Number of reported casualties

Prearrival information may be your only opportunity to recognize a WMD incident before you become part of the situation. Your knowledge of the terrain, local events, and local weather may be very important in recognizing a possible WMD event. For instance, knowing that a large open-air event is going on in your response area should trigger the thought of the potential for a mass-casualty incident in the event of an exposure.

Arrival Response

Objective 7

As you approach the scene, consider the safest approach, such as uphill, upwind, or even upstream. Be aware of the terrain and try to avoid bottlenecks or traps. Do not become a victim yourself by rushing in haphazardly.

Be alert for indicators of possible terrorist activity or WMD. Be prepared for a possible rush of contaminated patients. Use the dispatch information provided, your senses, and any other information available. As you approach, you may smell odors indicating a gas leak, chemical spill, or fire.

Look for:
- An unusually large number of people with burns or blast injuries
- Large numbers of people running from the scene or on the ground
- Danger of fire, explosion, electrical hazards, or structural collapse
- Weapons, explosive devices
- Signs of corrosion
- Evidence of use of chemical agents

Listen for:
- Screaming
- Explosion
- Breaking glass
- Hissing sounds indicating pressure releases
- Information from victims or bystanders

Stop and Think!

Remember that responders to the scene may be the target! This means *you*. Terrorists may use a secondary explosive device (equipped with a timer or trigger mechanism) designed to detonate after responders have arrived at a location. The intention is clear: to injure or kill responders.

The location of an incident may also be a clue to the type of problem. For example, targeted locations may include an abortion clinic, religious function, or political event. Approach any large or special event with caution. Examples of high-risk targets include:

- Landmarks: The White House, Hoover Dam, the Statue of Liberty
- Transportation sites: Highways, railways, airports, bridges, tunnels
- Energy sources: Nuclear power plants, oil or gas pipelines
- Financial institutions: The Federal Reserve, a stock exchange
- Government or public safety buildings: Military, EMS, police, fire

- High-attendance sites: Amusement parks, concerts, sporting events, graduations
- Communications centers

The anniversary of an event can be significant. For instance, the 1995 bombing of the Alfred P. Murrah Federal Building in Oklahoma City, Oklahoma, took place on the second anniversary of the 1993 standoff between Branch Davidians and the Federal Bureau of Investigation (FBI) near Waco, Texas. Unfortunately, the significance of a date may not be realized until after the incident has occurred.

Other factors to consider at a possible WMD incident include:

- Time of day
- Temperature
- Wind intensity and direction
- Humidity
- Cloud cover
- Precipitation

These factors can be very important. For example, time of day can be an indicator of the increased possibility of the use of a biological agent. In most cases, wind speed is slower at night, and biological agents will not disperse or thin out as rapidly.

On arrival at the scene, obtain scene control and establish a perimeter. Give dispatch the exact location of the incident or perimeter. Alert responders to potential hazards or danger. Always err on the side of caution.

A WMD is a hazardous material. The presence of hazardous materials is not always easy to detect. In a WMD incident, the presence of identifying placards may not be accurate because the placards may have been deliberately altered by terrorists. If hazardous substances or conditions are suspected, the scene must be secured by qualified personnel wearing appropriate equipment. If you are not qualified and do not have the appropriate equipment, you may need to wait for additional help to arrive before you can attempt entry into the scene. Try to quickly identify the type of incident (e.g., biological, nuclear, chemical). Relay the information to dispatch as soon as possible. Knowing the type of incident is important so that you can take appropriate precautions when providing emergency care.

Approaching the Patient

Access to any patient must not occur without the proper personal protective equipment. Standard personal protective equipment may not be sufficient or appropriate for this type of response.

In most respects, a contaminated patient is like any other patient except that emergency responders must protect themselves and others from dangers resulting from secondary contamination.

The goals for emergency responders at a scene involving a WMD include:

- Terminating the patient's exposure to the contaminant
- Maintaining rescuer safety
- Removing the patient from danger
- Providing emergency patient care

Determine if the scene has been secured to allow for your safe approach to the patient. In many instances, there will be no clear signals that this is a potential WMD event. Approach with caution.

Assuming that you are properly trained and equipped to provide emergency care in the hot zone, limit care to spinal stabilization, gross airway management (such as opening the airway and suctioning), and hemorrhage control. Remember that the patient will be further exposed to any airborne contaminants when you open his airway. Address life-threatening problems and gross decontamination before giving emergency care. If spinal stabilization appears necessary, begin it as soon as feasible.

Stop and Think!

Do not go into the hot zone unless you are properly trained and equipped.

Begin your primary survey at the same time as decontamination. Look for clues that suggest the presence of some type of exposure. Is the patient having a seizure? This may alert you to the presence of some type of nerve agent. Assess the patient's level of responsiveness by shouting a question to her from a distance away. If the patient responds to your voice or is moving, you can safely make some assumptions about the amount of blood flow to her brain. Look at the patient closely. Is she breathing? Can you see the rise and fall of her chest? Is her breathing regular, or is she gasping for breath? As you get closer to the patient, look at her body and limb position. Do you see any obvious signs of trauma, such as limbs in an abnormal position? This may be a sign that there has been some force applied to the patient's body. Is her clothing intact or has it been torn or shredded? Is there evidence of any foreign material on her clothing or skin? This may be indicative of some type of explosive device. Request ALS personnel if you suspect WMD contamination.

Complete a more detailed assessment as conditions allow. When treating patients, consider the chemical-specific information received from your poison control center (PCC) and other information resources. In multiple-patient situations, begin proper triage procedures according to your local emergency response plan.

Stop and Think!

Rushing into a possible WMD event only increases confusion and the potential for harm to yourself and other emergency responders. Stay alert, and remain suspicious of unusual events or circumstances.

Key Safety Points

- *Always consider the possibility of multiple hazards.* Only those emergency personnel wearing appropriate protective gear and actively involved in performing emergency operations should work inside the contaminated area.
- *Identify the materials involved in the incident* **only** *from a safe distance.* Do not approach anyone coming from a contaminated area. The person may be the perpetrator or may be contaminated.

On the Scene   Wrap-Up

You and your partner immediately recognize the possibility of a terrorist or WMD event and ask your dispatch center to announce and declare an MCI event. You also ask for a wind speed and direction report so that you may respond from uphill and upwind. Upon your safe arrival at the entrance of the sporting event, you have your partner stop so that you may perform a scene size-up. The fire department arrives at the same time, and the captain assumes incident command. ■

Sum It Up

▶ Weapons of mass destruction are materials used by terrorists that have the potential to cause great harm over a large area.

▶ There are five main categories of WMD. B-NICE is a simple way to remember these categories:
- Biological
- Nuclear/radiological
- Incendiary
- Chemical
- Explosive

▶ Biological weapons involve the use of bacteria, viruses, rickettsias, or toxins to cause disease or death. Diseases can be spread by inhalation of substances dispersed by spray devices (aerosols), ingestion of contaminated food or water supplies, or absorption through direct skin contact with the substance.

- The Centers for Disease Control and Prevention categorize biological weapons according to their risk to national security.

- Nuclear radiation gives off three main types of radiation: alpha, beta, and gamma. It is the charge that makes radiation an immediate problem and disruptive to cell function and structure. Alpha particles are large, heavy, and charged and cannot penetrate very far into matter. Because clothing or a sheet of paper is of sufficient thickness to stop them, external exposure to alpha particles usually has no effect on people. Beta particles are much smaller, travel more quickly, have less charge, and can penetrate more deeply than alpha particles. Beta particles can be stopped by layers of clothing or thin metal or plastic, such as several sheets of aluminum foil or Plexiglas.

- Gamma rays are waves of very high energy, similar to light. These waves of energy penetrate very deeply and can easily go right through a person. To reduce exposure from gamma rays, thick material such as lead must be used.

- According to the CDC, a dirty bomb is a mix of explosives, such as dynamite, with radioactive powder or pellets. A dirty bomb is also known as a radiological weapon. When the dynamite or other explosives are set off, the blast carries radioactive material into the surrounding area.

- Incendiary materials are substances that burn with a hot flame for a specific period.

- Chemical agents are poisonous substances that injure or kill people when inhaled, ingested, or absorbed through the skin or eyes. There are five broad categories of chemical weapons: nerve agents, blister agents, blood agents, choking agents, and irritants.

- Most terrorist attacks involve the use of explosives. Explosives are associated with a very rapid release of gas and heat.

- At a possible WMD incident, your primary responsibilities will be to isolate the scene; preserve evidence and deny entry; ask for additional help, and coordinate efforts with other responding fire, EMS, and law enforcement personnel; recognize signs of a potential WMD incident and alert the proper authorities; recognize the potential of a secondary explosion or attack on emergency responders; and make sure you, as well as additional responders, are safe.

- If hazardous substances or conditions are suspected, the scene must be secured by qualified personnel wearing appropriate equipment. If you are not qualified and do not have the appropriate equipment, you may need to wait for additional help to arrive before you can attempt entry into the scene.

- Access to any patient must not occur without the proper personal protective equipment. Standard personal protective equipment may not be sufficient or appropriate for this type of response.

Go to http://mhhe.com/aehlertemtb2e for Aehlert's updated instructions for cardiopulmonary resuscitation based on the 2010 guidelines on CPR from the American Heart Association.

▶ SKILL DRILL **A-1**
One-Rescuer Adult Cardiopulmonary Resuscitation 876

▶ SKILL DRILL **A-2**
Two-Rescuer Adult Cardiopulmonary Resuscitation 879

▶ SKILL DRILL **A-3**
One-Rescuer Child Cardiopulmonary Resuscitation 882

▶ SKILL DRILL **A-4**
One-Rescuer Infant Cardiopulmonary Resuscitation 885

▶ SKILL DRILL **A-5**
Adult Automated External Defibrillator Sequence 887

▶ SKILL DRILL **A-6**
Clearing a Foreign Body Airway Obstruction in a Conscious Adult 888

▶ SKILL DRILL **A-7**
Clearing a Foreign Body Airway Obstruction in an Unconscious Adult 890

▶ SKILL DRILL **A-8**
Clearing a Foreign Body Airway Obstruction in a Conscious Child 891

▶ SKILL DRILL **A-9**
Clearing a Foreign Body Airway Obstruction in an Unconscious Child 892

▶ SKILL DRILL **A-10**
Clearing a Foreign Body Airway Obstruction in a Conscious Infant 893

▶ SKILL DRILL **A-11**
Clearing a Foreign Body Airway Obstruction in an Unconscious Infant 894

One-Rescuer Adult Cardiopulmonary Resuscitation

STEP 1 ▶
- Make sure the scene is safe for providing emergency care. If the scene is safe, quickly check the patient's level of responsiveness. Gently squeeze the patient's shoulders, and shout, "Are you all right?"
- If the patient does not respond, shout for help. If you are alone and there is no response to your shout for help, contact your dispatcher and request additional resources, including an AED (if you do not have an AED with you).

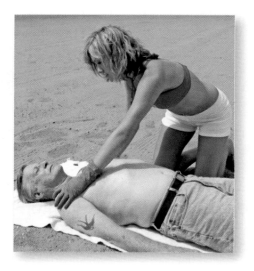

STEP 2 ▶
- If the patient is unresponsive and you do not suspect trauma, open his airway by using the head tilt–chin lift maneuver.
  - If trauma is suspected, open the airway by using the jaw thrust without head tilt maneuver.
  - If trauma is suspected but you are unable to maintain an open the airway by using the jaw thrust maneuver, open the airway by using the head tilt–chin lift maneuver.
- Suction any blood, vomit, or other fluid that may be present from the patient's airway.

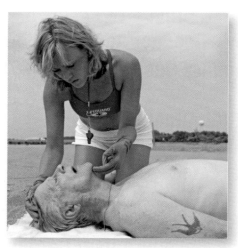

STEP 3 ▶ Place your face near the patient, and look, listen, and feel for adequate breathing. Check for at least 5 seconds but not for more than 10 seconds.

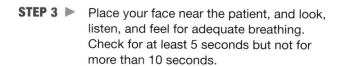

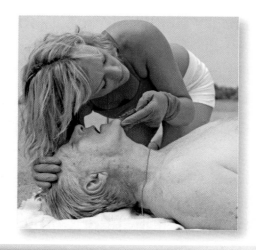

STEP 4 ▶ If the patient's breathing is not adequate, begin rescue breathing by using a pocket mask, mouth-to- barrier device, or BM device. Give 2 breaths (each breath over 1 second), with just enough pressure to make the chest rise with each breath.
—If the first rescue breath does not result in chest rise, reposition the patient's head and try again to ventilate.
—If there is still no chest rise, move on to the next step.

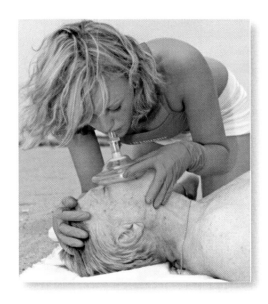

STEP 5 ▶ • Assess the carotid pulse on the side of the patient's neck nearest you. Feel for a pulse for 5 to 10 seconds.
• If you definitely feel a pulse, give 1 breath every 5 to 6 seconds. Reassess the patient's pulse every 2 minutes.
• If you do not definitely feel a pulse within 10 seconds, or if you are uncertain, begin chest compressions.

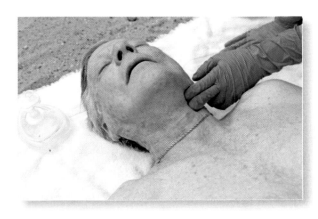

STEP 6 ▶ • If there is no pulse, begin cycles of 30 compressions and 2 breaths. Kneel beside the patient's chest.
• Place the heel of one hand in the center of the patient's chest, between the nipples. Place your other hand on top of the first hand. Interlock the fingers of both hands to keep your fingers off the patient's ribs.

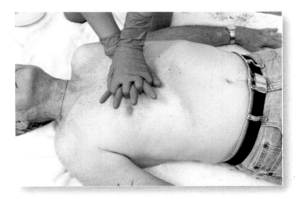

Continued

One-Rescuer Adult Cardiopulmonary Resuscitation *Continued*

STEP 7 ▶
- Position yourself directly above the patient's chest so that your shoulders are directly over your hands.
- With your arms straight and your elbows locked, press down about 1½–2 inches on the patient's breastbone with the heels of your hands. Compress at a rate of 100 per minute.
- Release pressure (let up) after each compression to allow the patient's chest to recoil.

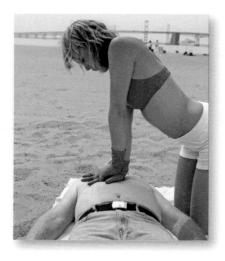

STEP 8 ▶ After 30 compressions, open the patient's airway and deliver 2 breaths.

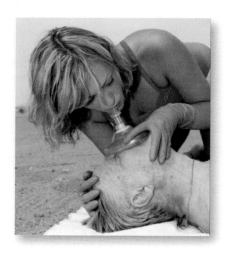

Two-Rescuer Adult Cardiopulmonary Resuscitation

STEP 1 ▶
- Make sure the scene is safe for providing emergency care. If the scene is safe, quickly check the patient's level of responsiveness. Gently squeeze the patient's shoulders, and shout, "Are you all right?"
- If the patient does not respond, one rescuer should call for help.

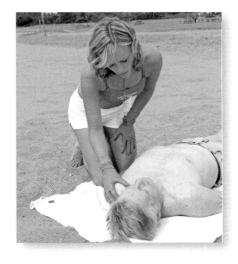

STEP 2 ▶
- If the patient is unresponsive and you do not suspect trauma, open his airway by using the head tilt–chin lift maneuver.
  — If trauma is suspected, open the airway by using the jaw thrust without head tilt maneuver.
  — If trauma is suspected but you are unable to maintain an open the airway by using the jaw thrust maneuver, open the airway by using the head tilt–chin lift maneuver.
- Suction any blood, vomit, or other fluid that may be present from the patient's airway.

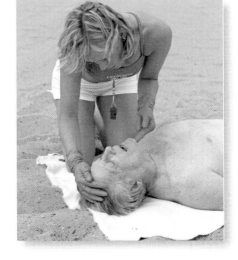

STEP 3 ▶ Place your face near the patient, and look, listen, and feel for adequate breathing. Check for at least 5 seconds but not for more than 10 seconds.

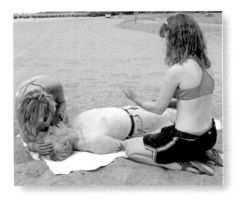

Continued

Two-Rescuer Adult Cardiopulmonary Resuscitation *Continued*

STEP 4 ▶ If the patient's breathing is not adequate, the first rescuer should begin rescue breathing by using a pocket mask, mouth-to-barrier device, or BM device. Give 2 breaths (each breath over 1 second), with just enough pressure to make the chest rise with each breath.

—If the first rescue breath does not result in chest rise, reposition the patient's head and try again to ventilate.

—If there is still no chest rise, move on to the next step.

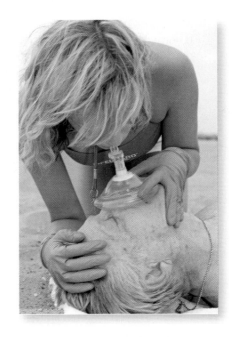

STEP 5 ▶ • The first rescuer should assess the carotid pulse on the side of the patient's neck nearest the rescuer. Feel for a pulse for 5 to 10 seconds.

• If you definitely feel a pulse, give 1 breath every 5 to 6 seconds. Reassess the patient's pulse every 2 minutes. If you do not definitely feel a pulse within 10 seconds, or if you are uncertain, begin chest compressions.

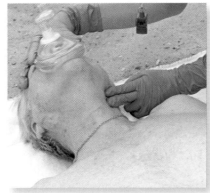

STEP 6 ▶ • If there is no pulse, begin cycles of 30 compressions and 2 breaths.

• The second rescuer should kneel beside the patient's chest and then place the heel of one hand in the center of the patient's chest, between the nipples.

• The rescuer should then place her other hand on top of the first, interlocking the fingers of both hands to keep her fingers off the patient's ribs.

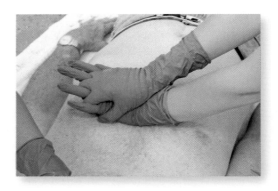

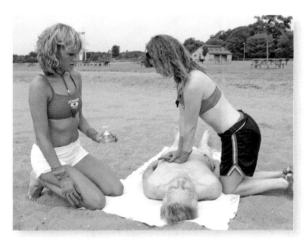

STEP 7 ▲ Position yourself directly above the patient's chest so that your shoulders are directly over your hands.

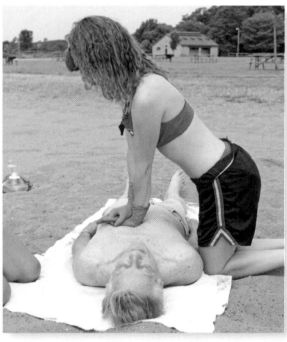

STEP 8 ▲ • With your arms straight and your elbows locked, press down about 1½–2 inches on the patient's breastbone with the heels of your hands. Compress at a rate of 100 per minute.
• Release pressure (let up) after each compression to allow the patient's chest to recoil.

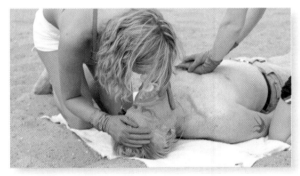

STEP 9 ▲ After 30 compressions, the first rescuer should open the patient's airway and deliver 2 breaths.

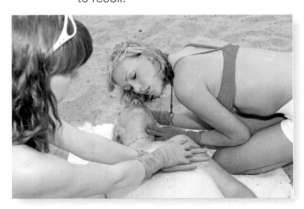

STEP 10 ▲ Because performing chest compressions is tiring, rescuers should switch roles about every 2 minutes or 5 cycles of CPR. The "switch" should ideally take place in 5 seconds or less.

Skill Drill   A-3

One-Rescuer Child Cardiopulmonary Resuscitation

STEP 1 ▶
- Make sure the scene is safe for providing emergency care. If the scene is safe, quickly check the patient's level of responsiveness. Gently squeeze the patient's shoulders, and shout, "Are you all right?"
- If the patient does not respond, you are alone, and you saw the child collapse, phone for help and get an AED, and then begin CPR.
- If the child does not respond, you are alone, and you did not witness the child's collapse, begin CPR. After about 2 minutes of CPR, phone for help and get an AED.

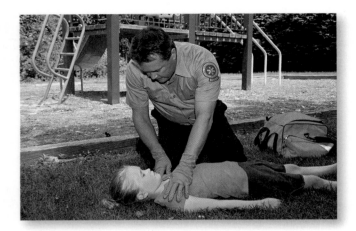

STEP 2 ▶
- If the patient is unresponsive and you do not suspect trauma, open the airway by using the head tilt–chin lift maneuver. Push down on the child's forehead with one hand. Place the fingers of your other hand on the bony part of the chin. Gently lift the chin.
  - If trauma is suspected, open the airway by using the jaw thrust without head tilt maneuver.
  - If trauma is suspected but you are unable to maintain an open the airway by using the jaw thrust maneuver, open the airway by using the head tilt–chin lift maneuver.
- Look for an actual or a potential airway obstruction, such as a foreign body, blood, vomit, teeth, or the patient's tongue. Suction the airway if necessary.

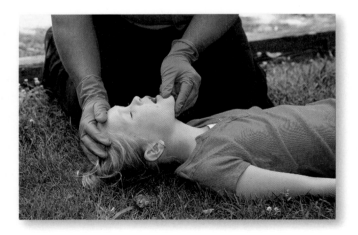

STEP 3 ▶ Hold the airway open, and look, listen, and feel for breathing for at least 5 seconds but not for more than 10 seconds.

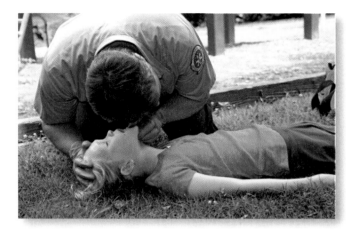

STEP 4 ▶ If the patient's breathing is not adequate, begin rescue breathing by using a pocket mask, mouth-to-barrier device, or BM device. Give 2 breaths (each breath over 1 second), with just enough pressure to make the chest gently rise with each breath.
  —If the first rescue breath does not result in chest rise, reposition the patient's head and try again to ventilate.
  —If there is still no chest rise, move on to the next step.

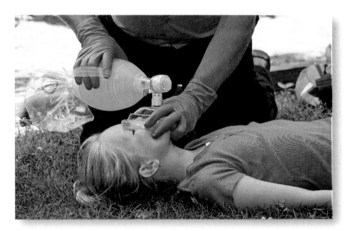

STEP 5 ▶ Assess the carotid pulse on the side of the patient's neck nearest you. Feel for a pulse for at least 5 seconds but not for more than 10 seconds.

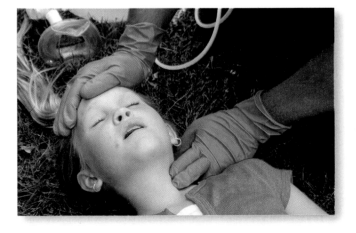

Continued

One-Rescuer Child Cardiopulmonary Resuscitation *Continued*

STEP 6 ▶

- If you definitely feel a pulse, give 1 breath every 3 to 5 seconds. Reassess the patient's pulse every 2 minutes. If you do not definitely feel a pulse within 10 seconds, if you are uncertain, or if a pulse is present but the heart rate is less than 60 beats/min with signs of poor perfusion (pale, cool, mottled skin), begin chest compressions.
- Begin cycles of 30 compressions and 2 breaths. Kneel beside the patient's chest. Place the heel of one hand in the center of the patient's chest, between the nipples. Use one or two hands as needed to compress the child's chest one-third to one-half the depth of the chest. Give compressions at a rate of about 100 per minute.
- Release pressure (let up) after each compression to allow the patient's chest to recoil.
- After 30 compressions, open the airway and deliver 2 breaths.

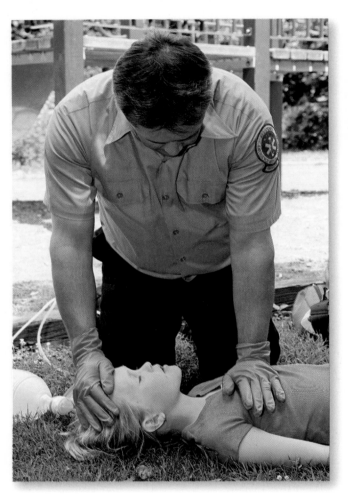

One-Rescuer Infant Cardiopulmonary Resuscitation

STEP 1 ▶
- Make sure the scene is safe for providing emergency care. If the scene is safe, quickly check the infant's level of responsiveness (if the infant is not obviously awake) by gently tapping the infant's feet.
- If the patient does not respond, you are alone, and you saw the infant collapse, phone for help and then begin CPR.
- If the infant does not respond, you are alone, and you did not witness the infant's collapse, begin CPR. After about 2 minutes of CPR, phone for help, then resume CPR.

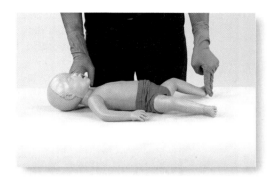

STEP 2 ▶
- If the infant is unresponsive and you do not suspect trauma, open her airway by using the head tilt–chin lift maneuver.
  - If trauma is suspected, open the airway by using the jaw thrust without head tilt maneuver.
  - If trauma is suspected but you are unable to maintain an open the airway by using the jaw thrust maneuver, open the airway by using the head tilt–chin lift maneuver.
- Suction any blood, vomit, or other fluid that may be present from the infant's airway.

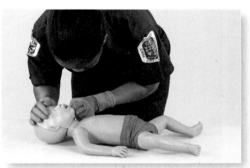

STEP 3 ▶ Hold the airway open, and look, listen, and feel for breathing for at least 5 second but not for more than 10 seconds.

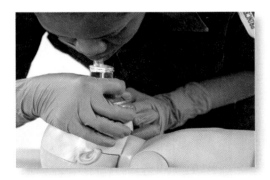

STEP 4 ▶ If the patient's breathing is not adequate, begin rescue breathing by using a pocket mask, mouth-to-barrier device, or BM device. Give 2 breaths (each breath over 1 second), with just enough pressure to make the chest gently rise with each breath.
  - If the first rescue breath does not result in chest rise, reposition the patient's head and try again to ventilate.
  - If there is still no chest rise, move on to the next step.

Continued

One-Rescuer Infant Cardiopulmonary Resuscitation *Continued*

STEP 5 ▶
- Assess the brachial pulse on the inside of the upper arm. Feel for a pulse for at least 5 seconds but not for more than 10 seconds.
- If you definitely feel a pulse, give 1 breath every 3 to 5 seconds. Reassess the patient's pulse every 2 minutes. If you do not definitely feel a pulse within 10 seconds, if you are uncertain, or if a pulse is present but the heart rate is less than 60 beats/min with signs of poor perfusion (pale, cool, mottled skin), begin chest compressions.

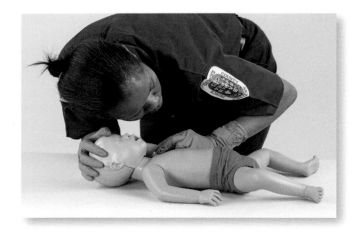

STEP 6 ▶
- Begin cycles of 30 compressions and 2 breaths. Imagine a line between the nipples. Place the flat part of your middle and ring fingers about one finger's width below this imaginary line. Use your other hand to hold the infant's head in a position that keeps the airway open.
- Give compressions at a rate of about 100 per minute. Depress the breastbone one-third to one-half the depth of the chest.
- Release pressure (let up) after each compression to allow the infant's chest to recoil.

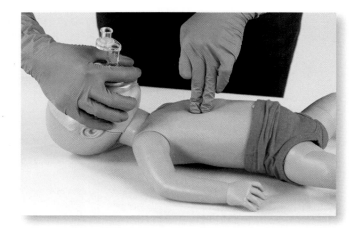

STEP 7 ▶ After 30 compressions, open the airway and deliver 2 breaths.

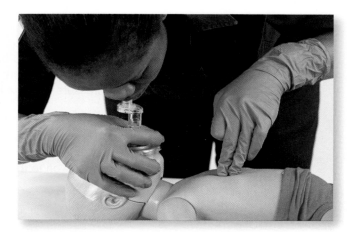

Adult Automated External Defibrillator Sequence

STEP 1 ▶
- If you arrive on the scene and see an adult collapse (you witness a cardiac arrest), assess the patient's airway, breathing, and circulation, and then quickly apply an AED. Perform CPR until the AED is ready. Your medical director may recommend that if you arrive at the scene of an adult cardiac arrest, did not witness the patient's collapse, and your response time is more than 4 to 5 minutes, provide 5 cycles of CPR (about 2 minutes) and then analyze the patient's rhythm with an AED.
- Be sure the patient is lying face up on a firm, flat surface. Place the AED near the rescuer who will be operating it. Turn on the power of the AED. If more than one rescuer is present, one rescuer should continue CPR while the other readies the AED for use. One rescuer should apply the AED pads to the patient's chest.

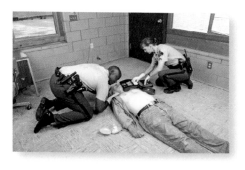

STEP 2 ▶ Analyze the patient's heart rhythm. Do not touch the patient while the AED is analyzing the rhythm. If the AED advises that a shock is indicated, check the patient from head to toe to make sure no one is touching the patient (including you) before pressing the shock control. Shout, "Stand clear!"

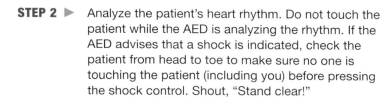
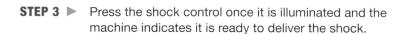

STEP 3 ▶ Press the shock control once it is illuminated and the machine indicates it is ready to deliver the shock.

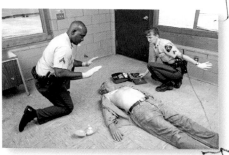

STEP 4 ▶ After delivery of the shock, quickly resume CPR, beginning with chest compressions. After about 2 minutes of CPR, reanalyze the rhythm.

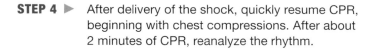
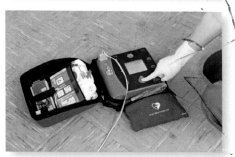
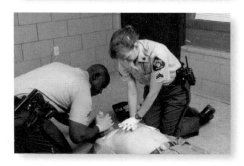

Clearing a Foreign Body Airway Obstruction in a Conscious Adult

STEP 1 ▶
- Find out if the patient can speak or cough. Ask, "Are you choking?"
- If the patient can cough or speak, encourage him to cough out the obstruction. Watch him closely to make sure the object is expelled.

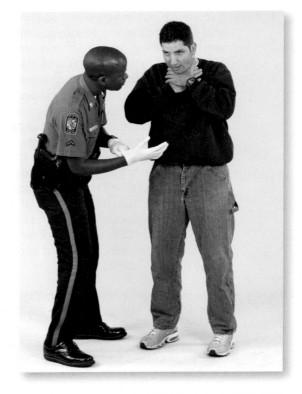

STEP 2 ▶
- If the patient cannot cough or speak, perform abdominal thrusts (the Heimlich maneuver).
- Stand behind the patient and wrap your arms around his waist.
- Make a fist with one hand. Place your fist, thumb side in, just above the patient's navel.

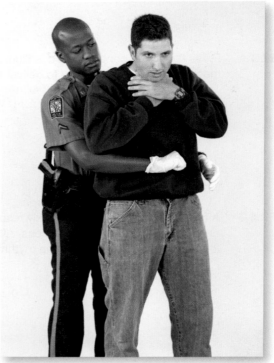

STEP 3 ▶
- Grab your fist tightly with your other hand. Pull your fist quickly inward and upward.
- Continue performing abdominal thrusts until the foreign body is expelled or the patient becomes unresponsive. Perform each abdominal thrust with the intent of relieving the obstruction. If abdominal thrusts are not effective, consider the use of chest thrusts to relieve the obstruction.

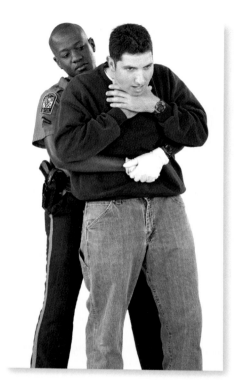

STEP 4 ▶ If your patient is obese or in the later stages of pregnancy, perform chest thrusts instead of abdominal thrusts:
- —Place your arms around the patient's chest, directly under the armpits. Press your hands backward, giving quick thrusts into the middle of the breastbone.
- —Do not place your hands on the patient's ribs or on the bottom of the breastbone (xiphoid process). The xiphoid process can easily be broken off the breastbone and can cut underlying organs, such as the liver.

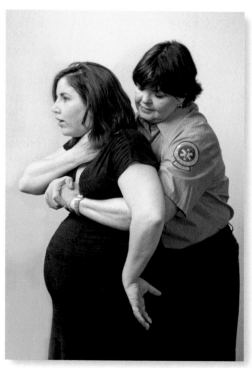

Skill Drill A-7

Clearing a Foreign Body Airway Obstruction in an Unconscious Adult

STEP 1 ▶
- Make sure the scene is safe for providing emergency care. If the scene is safe, quickly check the patient's level of responsiveness. Gently squeeze the patient's shoulders, and shout, "Are you all right?" If the patient does not respond, shout for help.
- If the patient is unresponsive and you do not suspect trauma, open his airway by using the head tilt–chin lift maneuver. If trauma is suspected, open the airway by using the jaw thrust without head tilt maneuver. If trauma is suspected but you are unable to maintain an open airway by using the jaw thrust maneuver, open the airway by using the head tilt–chin lift maneuver.
- Check the nose and mouth for secretions, vomit, a foreign body, or other obstructions. Suction fluids from the airway as needed. If you *see* a solid object in the patient's upper airway, remove it. Do not blindly sweep the mouth in search of a foreign object.

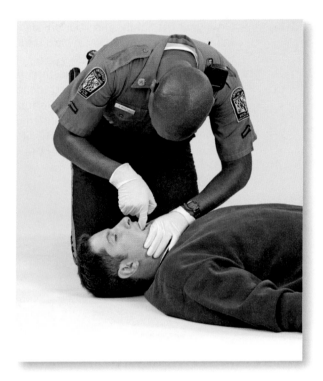

STEP 2 ▶
- Place your face near the patient, and look, listen, and feel for adequate breathing. Check for at least 5 seconds but not for more than 10 seconds.
- If the patient's breathing is not adequate, begin rescue breathing by using a pocket mask, mouth- to-barrier device, or BM device. Give 2 breaths (each breath over 1 second), with just enough pressure to make the chest rise with each breath.
  - If the first rescue breath does not result in chest rise, reposition the patient's head and try again to ventilate.
  - If there is still no chest rise, begin CPR. Check the patient's mouth for the foreign body each time you open the airway to give rescue breaths. If you *see* a solid object in the patient's upper airway, remove it. If no foreign body is seen, continue CPR.

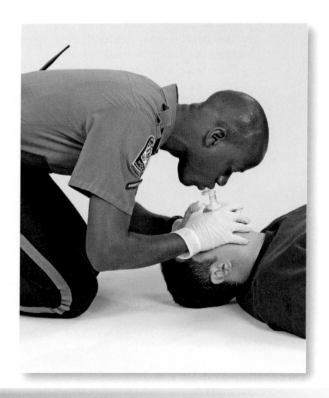

Clearing a Foreign Body Airway Obstruction in a Conscious Child

STEP 1 ▶
- Find out if the child can speak or cough. Ask, "Are you choking?"
- If the patient can cough or speak, encourage her to cough out the obstruction. Watch her closely to make sure the object is expelled.

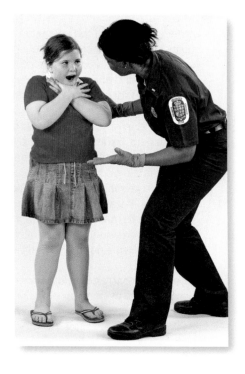

STEP 2 ▶ If the child cannot cough or speak, perform abdominal thrusts (the Heimlich maneuver).
- Stand behind the child and wrap your arms around her waist.
- Make a fist with one hand. Place your fist, thumb side in, just above the patient's navel. Grab your fist tightly with your other hand. Pull your fist quickly inward and upward.
- Continue performing abdominal thrusts until the object is expelled or the child becomes unresponsive.

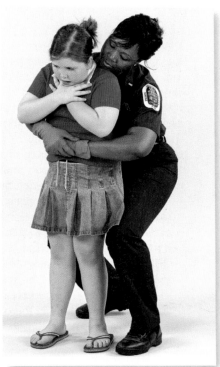

Clearing a Foreign Body Airway Obstruction in an Unconscious Child

STEP 1 ▶
- Make sure the scene is safe for providing emergency care. If the scene is safe, quickly assess the child's level of responsiveness. Gently squeeze the patient's shoulders, and shout, "Are you all right?" If the patient does not respond, shout for help.
- If the child is unresponsive and you do not suspect trauma, open her airway by using the head tilt–chin lift maneuver. If trauma is suspected, open the airway by using the jaw thrust without head tilt maneuver. If trauma is suspected but you are unable to maintain an open the airway by using the jaw thrust maneuver, open the airway by using the head tilt–chin lift maneuver.
- Check the nose and mouth for secretions, vomit, a foreign body, or other obstructions. Suction fluids from the airway as needed. If you *see* a solid object in the patient's upper airway, remove it. Do not blindly sweep the mouth in search of a foreign object.

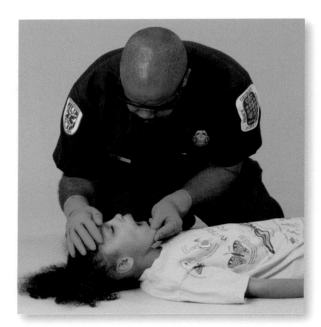

STEP 2 ▶
- Place your face near the patient, and look, listen, and feel for adequate breathing. Check for at least 5 seconds but not for more than 10 seconds.
- If the patient's breathing is not adequate, begin rescue breathing by using a pocket mask, mouth-to-barrier device, or BM device. Give 2 breaths (each breath over 1 second), with just enough pressure to make the chest rise with each breath.
  —If the first rescue breath does not result in chest rise, reposition the patient's head and try again to ventilate.
  —If there is still no chest rise, begin CPR. Check the patient's mouth for the foreign body each time you open the airway to give rescue breaths. If you *see* a solid object in the patient's upper airway, remove it. If no foreign body is seen, continue CPR.

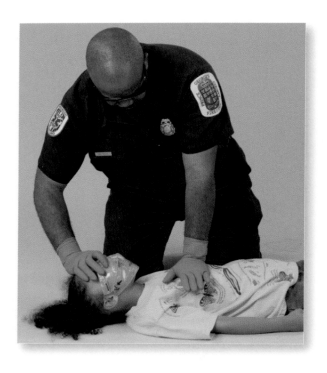

Clearing a Foreign Body Airway Obstruction in a Conscious Infant

STEP 1 ▶ While supporting the infant's head, place the infant facedown over your forearm. You may find it helpful to rest your forearm on your thigh to support the weight of the infant. Keep the infant's head slightly lower than the rest of the body.

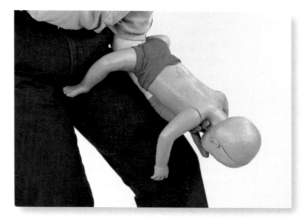

STEP 2 ▶ Using the heel of one hand, forcefully deliver up to 5 back slaps between the infant's shoulder blades.

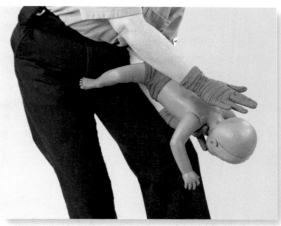

STEP 3 ▶ • If the foreign body is not expelled, deliver chest thrusts. Place your free hand on the infant's back. Turn the infant over onto his back while supporting the back of the head with the palm of your hand. Imagine a line between the infant's nipples. Place the flat part of one finger about one finger width below this imaginary line. Place a second finger next to the first on the infant's sternum. Deliver up to 5 downward chest thrusts at a rate of about 1 per second.
- Check the infant's mouth. If you *see* the foreign body, remove it.
- Continue alternating up to 5 back slaps and up to 5 chest thrusts and attempting to visualize the object until the object is expelled or the infant becomes unconscious.

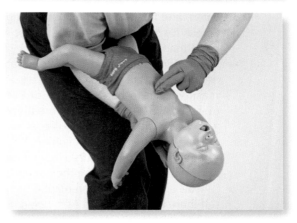

Clearing a Foreign Body Airway Obstruction in an Unconscious Infant

STEP 1 ▶

- Make sure the scene is safe for providing emergency care. If the scene is safe, quickly assess the infant's level of responsiveness. After confirming that the infant is unresponsive, place the infant on her back on a flat surface or on your forearm. Support the infant's head.
- If the infant is unresponsive and you do not suspect trauma, open her airway by using the head tilt–chin lift maneuver. If trauma is suspected, open the airway by using the jaw thrust without head tilt maneuver. If trauma is suspected but you are unable to maintain an open the airway by using the jaw thrust maneuver, open the airway by using the head tilt–chin lift maneuver.
- Check the nose and mouth for secretions, vomit, a foreign body, or other obstructions. Suction fluids from the airway as needed. If you *see* a solid object in the infant's upper airway, remove it. Do not blindly sweep the mouth in search of a foreign object.

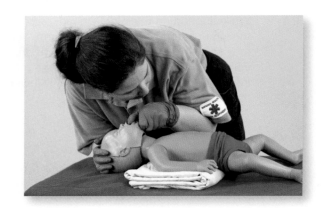

STEP 2 ▶

- Place your face near the infant, and look, listen, and feel for adequate breathing. Check for at least 5 seconds but not for more than 10 seconds.
- If the infant's breathing is not adequate, begin rescue breathing by using a pocket mask, mouth-to-barrier device, or BM device. Give 2 breaths (each breath over 1 second), with just enough pressure to make the chest rise with each breath.
  —If the first rescue breath does not result in chest rise, reposition the patient's head and try again to ventilate.
  —If there is still no chest rise, begin CPR. Check the infant's mouth for the foreign body each time you open the airway to give rescue breaths. If you *see* a solid object in the infant's upper airway, remove it. If no foreign body is seen, continue CPR.

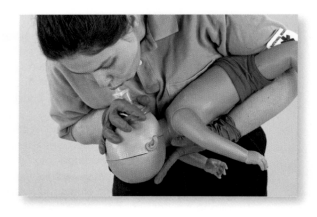

B

Rural and Frontier EMS

Introduction

Emergency Response in Rural and Frontier Areas

EMS is an important part of rural and frontier healthcare. Rural and frontier areas have been defined as the wilderness of woods, hills, mountains, plains, islands, and desert outside urban and suburban centers. In most areas of the United States, when people place a 9-1-1 call for a medical emergency, they expect an immediate dispatch of an ambulance and/or fire equipment. In many areas of the United States, including many rural areas, EMS consistently meets this expectation. However, this expectation is not being met in some rural and frontier areas for a variety of reasons.

You Should Know

In 2004, the National Rural Health Association (NRHA), the National Organization of State Offices of Rural Health (NOSORH), and the National Association of State EMS Directors (NASEMSD) released the final draft of the *Rural/Frontier EMS Agenda for the Future.* This document offers recommendations to support and improve emergency services in rural and frontier communities by focusing on restructuring, reimbursement, and recruitment issues.

The Challenges of Rural and Frontier EMS

Healthcare Resources

The number of hospital and medical practice closures in rural and frontier areas has increased. This increase has resulted in shrinking healthcare resources in these communities. Because of the heavy demands of rural healthcare (such as long hours and no backup), it is hard for many rural areas to recruit and retain doctors, nurses, and other healthcare personnel. Doctors and nurses who choose to work in rural and frontier areas often have limited contact with EMS personnel. They are often unfamiliar with the different levels of EMS professionals and their capabilities.

As the residents of rural and frontier areas age, their need for medical care increases. Residents must often travel great distances to see specialists. As their local healthcare resources disappear, residents of these areas call upon EMS professionals for assistance. Requests for help may include an unofficial assessment, advice, or emergency care.

Some rural and frontier communities are using EMS professionals in doctor's offices, healthcare clinics, hospice, and home health settings. In some settings, EMS professionals are used between EMS calls to supplement the hospital staff. In others, they are used for regular shift coverage. Using EMS professionals in this way helps fill the gap in the community's healthcare resources.

Response Times

In urban areas, fire departments and ambulance services try hard to arrive at the patient's side within 4 to 8 minutes of the patient's call for help. This goal is unrealistic in rural and frontier areas. Rural and frontier EMS professionals cover large, sparsely populated areas and have minimal resources to respond to the scene. Response times in rural and frontier settings may be long because of the following:

- A delay in volunteers' response from home or work
- A failure to respond
- The physical distance that must be covered
- The type of transportation that must be used (land, air, water)

- The type and condition of the roadway, airway, or waterway
- Bad weather, difficult access, unmarked roads, and houses not visible from the street (addresses unmarked and fewer landmarks to help guide response vehicles)

Limited access to communications may delay the detection and reporting of a need for emergency care. Traveling on land to remote locations with unpredictable road conditions (including unmarked roads) can delay the arrival of EMS professionals on the scene.

EMS Workforce

Many rural and frontier EMS professionals often work a full-time job outside their EMS roles. They frequently volunteer their time to provide emergency medical care and transportation to members of their community. When receiving a request to respond to an EMS call, a volunteer often leaves a full-time job to respond in her private vehicle. In areas where an emergency response vehicle is available, the volunteer must travel to the station, pick up the emergency vehicle, and then respond to the emergency. When an EMS call is over, the volunteer returns home, returns to her regular job, or goes back to the station to return the emergency vehicle. Rural and frontier EMS professionals have the following attributes:

- Often know their patient
- Often know about the patient's condition
- Understand the environment in which the patient lives and works
- Know what the patient needs

Making a Difference 〜〜〜〜〜

EMS professionals in rural and frontier areas have a different attitude about their job. It may be because whereas most of us talk about the possibility of providing EMS care for friends and family, these folks literally do. EMS for them is less a job and more a way of giving back to their community. Rural and frontier EMS professionals are often more open to education and technology than some of their urban counterparts. It may be because they are looking at a way to care not only for people but also for people they know—their children's schoolmates, families they see at social gatherings, their colleagues, and so on.

Rural and frontier EMS systems rely heavily on volunteers. However, the increasing expectations of rural and frontier residents about the level and type of prehospital care may result in a demand for services that cannot easily be provided by volunteers. In rural and frontier settings, the level of emergency medical responder and emergency medical technician prehospital care is more likely to be available than advanced-level care. This situation is partly the result of the costs, time, and travel needed to obtain advanced-level training. States have been pressured to use EMTs as the national minimum level of care for personnel who provide patient care on ambulances. Some EMS leaders are concerned that increased training, testing, and certification requirements will jeopardize the interest and availability of their volunteers. At the same time, the number of interested EMS volunteers may be decreasing because of the following factors:

- The increase in two-wage-earner households
- Limited EMS pay or a lack of pay
- Increased exposure to the risks of providing EMS care
- The belief that there is increased personal liability when providing EMS care
- A lack of EMS leadership in the community
- Limited funding or a lack of funding for training, equipment, and supplies
- An increased number of nursing home and routine transfer calls instead of emergency calls

Individuals who do become advanced EMTs and paramedics often do not remain in the rural or frontier area after their training is finished. Low call volumes in some areas make it difficult for some advanced care professionals to keep up their skills. Continuing education opportunities may be limited, and training resources (including qualified instructors) are often scarce.

As in the urban setting, EMS professionals in rural and frontier communities should seek out opportunities for continuing education. Some colleges are recognizing the unique needs of busy professionals and are providing Internet refresher and continuing education courses for rural and long-distance students so that they do not have to leave their communities to obtain education.

Illness and Injury

Many rural and frontier residents are employed in some of the most hazardous occupations in our country—logging, mining, farming, fishing, and hunting. Work-related deaths occur more frequently among these groups of workers than among workers as a whole.

A number of factors may contribute to the severity of injuries and the greater number of injury-related deaths seen in rural and frontier areas:

- There may be long delays between the time of the injury and its discovery by a passerby.
- It may take a considerable amount of time to get a patient from the scene of an accident to a hospital because of distances between the scene, the ambulance service, and the hospital.
- Prehospital care in many rural areas may be performed by volunteers who are unable to provide advanced airway management or fluid resuscitation.
- Emergency departments in small rural hospitals may be staffed by physicians who do not have the knowledge or skills needed to manage critical trauma patients.
- There may be relatively few trauma cases at the rural hospital, making it difficult for physicians and nurses to maintain their skills.
- Rural hospitals may not have 24-hour physician coverage. In addition, laboratory and x-ray services may not be available 24 hours a day.
- In situations involving multiple victims, delays may occur in the initial stabilization of patients because there are too few emergency responders, physicians, or nurses available.
- Injuries from all-terrain vehicles, snowmobile collisions, and other recreational activities are common in rural settings.
- Injuries may occur as a result of farming activities. Adults and children may be injured while operating heavy machinery, operating dangerous tools, caring for large livestock, or handling dangerous pesticides or other chemicals (Figure B-1). Responses to situations that involve large livestock can be unsafe to rescuers. Farm rescues may include such hazards as poisonous gases or low-oxygen atmospheres found in silos; confined-space situations; and unique extrication situations involving farm machinery.
- Industries located in rural and frontier areas may pose potential hazards (Figure B-2).
- Rural emergencies may also include wilderness-related medical situations. These situations include envenomation from poisonous snakes; heat-, cold-, and water-related emergencies; and poisoning from plants.

Factors that may contribute to higher rates of motor vehicle–related injury and death in rural and frontier areas include:

- Poor road conditions
- The absence of safety features (guardrails, appropriately placed shoulder reflectors)

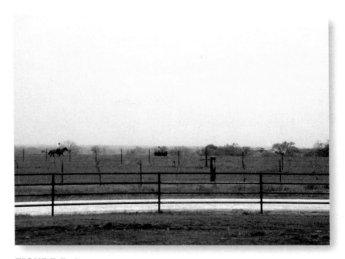

FIGURE B-1 ▲ Adults and children may be injured as a result of farm activities. In this picture, a horse and all-terrain vehicle are being used to herd cattle.

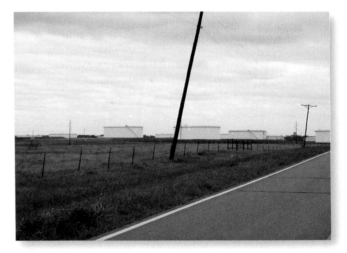

FIGURE B-2 ▲ Industries located in rural and frontier areas may pose potential hazards.

- A greater likelihood of high-speed travel (65 mph or more)
- A greater use of utility vehicles and pickup trucks
- A lack of effective safety measures (seat belts)
- Greater distances between emergency facilities

A motor vehicle crash occurring along an infrequently traveled rural road may not be detected for hours. When the crash is detected, access to the EMS system may be further delayed because phones or other forms of communication or service may not be readily available. The patient may sustain injuries that require the use of specialized services such as a trauma center. Trauma centers are usually not immediately available in rural and frontier areas. It is often necessary to contact an air medical service for

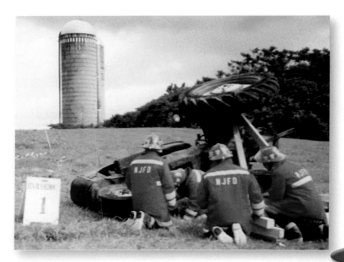

FIGURE B-3 ▲ Farmedic Provider course in North Java, New York. The student team is stabilizing an overturned tractor to rescue the patient who is pinned under the tractor cowling.

patient transport. The air transport team may be located some distance away from the accident site, which delays transporting the patient from the crash site to the hospital.

Making a Difference

In a rural or frontier EMS system, long distances, minimal resources, and road conditions that are less than optimal usually allow a significant length of time for interaction between you and the patient. This prolonged patient contact time will give you an opportunity to talk with your patient, reassess his condition, perform additional skills, and provide frequent reassurance.

If a cardiac arrest occurs, cardiopulmonary resuscitation (CPR) must be started as quickly as possible. Some rural and frontier communities have improved emergency cardiac care in their areas by providing citizen CPR programs. In addition, they have trained basic life support personnel to use automated external defibrillators (AEDs). AEDs are particularly well suited to the needs of rural and frontier areas because they are

easy to use. They are also more affordable now than ever before. Many states have grants and financial assistance programs available. These programs enable agencies to purchase AEDs for use in their community.

Making a Difference

If you will be working in a rural or frontier area, find out from your instructor how you can become a CPR instructor. Teaching CPR regularly and placing AEDs in public areas could save the life of a cardiac arrest patient in your community.

You Should Know

The Unique Training Needs of Rural and Frontier EMS Professionals

In some areas, organizations are working to develop and deliver training programs that meet the unique needs of rural and frontier EMS professionals. Examples of innovative programs include the following:

- The Southern Coastal Agromedicine Center (SCAC), in collaboration with the North Carolina Forestry Association, has developed a Timber Medic program to improve logging-injury outcomes.
- Cornell University offers a First on the Scene program that teaches farm family members, farm employees, and the general community how to make important decisions at the scene of a farm emergency. The program is intended for all farm groups, such as farm managers, employees, spouses, and 4-H and Future Farmers of America groups. Some of the available topics include tractor overturns, machinery entanglements, grain bin emergencies, and silo emergencies.
- The National Farmedic Training Program, owned and operated by McNeil & Company, provides rural fire and rescue responders with a systematic approach to farm rescue procedures that addresses the safety of both patients and responders (Figure B-3). This program has trained more than 28,000 students since it began in 1981. For more information, visit this website: www.farmedic.com.

Glossary

A

Abandonment Termination of patient care without making sure that care will continue at the same level or higher.

Abdomen The part of the body trunk below the ribs and above the pelvis.

Abdominal cavity The body cavity located below the diaphragm and above the pelvis. It contains the stomach, intestines, liver, gallbladder, pancreas, and spleen.

Abnormal behavior A way of acting or conducting that is not consistent with society's norms and expectations, interferes with the individual's well-being and ability to function, and may be harmful to the individual or others.

Abortion Termination of pregnancy before the fetus is able to live on its own outside the uterus.

Abrasion Damage to the outermost layer of skin (epidermis) by shearing forces (such as rubbing or scraping).

Abruptio placentae Condition that occurs when a normally implanted placenta separates prematurely from the wall of the uterus (endometrium) during the last trimester of pregnancy; also called *placental abruption*.

Absence seizures A type of generalized seizures in which the patient experiences a brief loss of consciousness (for 5 to 10 seconds) without a loss of muscle tone; also called *petit mal seizures.*

Absorption The process of moving nutrients, water, and electrolytes into the circulatory system so they can be used by body cells.

Accessory muscles for breathing The internal intercostal muscles; muscles between the ribs, above the collarbones, and in the abdomen used for breathing during periods of respiratory distress.

Accessory organs of digestion The teeth and tongue, salivary glands, liver, gallbladder, and pancreas.

Acetabulum A socket of the hip bone.

Acidosis A buildup of acid in the blood and tissues.

Acrocyanosis Blueness of the hands and feet.

Activated charcoal Medication used to bind many toxic substances in the GI tract, preventing them from being absorbed and then carrying them out of the GI tract

Active rewarming The act of adding heat directly to the surface of the patient's body.

Acute abdomen Phrase that means a sudden onset of abdominal pain.

Acute coronary syndromes (ACSs) Conditions caused by temporary or permanent blockage of a coronary artery as a result of coronary artery disease.

Acute myocardial infarction (acute MI) Death of heart tissue that occurs when a coronary artery becomes severely narrowed or is completely blocked, usually by a blood clot (thrombus); also called a *heart attack.*

Acute renal failure (ARF) A sudden deterioration of kidney function that is potentially reversible; also called *acute kidney injury (AKI).*

Addiction A psychological and/or physical dependence on a substance that has gone beyond voluntary control.

Administrative agency A governmental body responsible for implementing and enforcing particular laws.

Administrative law Rules and regulations made by the executive branch of the government.

Adolescence Stage of human development from 13 to 18 years.

Adrenal glands Endocrine glands located on top of each kidney that release epinephrine in response to stress.

Advance directive A legal document that details a person's healthcare wishes if the person becomes unable to make decisions.

Advanced emergency medical technician (AEMT) EMTs with additional training in skills such as assessing patient, administering IV fluids and medications, and performing advanced airway procedures.

Adverse effects Undesired effects of a drug.

Advocate A person who supports others and acts in their best interests.

AEIOU-TIPPS A memory aid for common causes of altered mental status: **a**lcohol, abuse; **e**pilepsy (seizures); **i**nsulin (diabetic emergency); **o**verdose, (lack of) oxygen (hypoxia); **u**remia (kidney failure); **t**rauma (head injury), temperature (fever, heat-, or cold-related emergency); **i**nfection; **p**sychiatric conditions; **p**oisoning (including drugs and alcohol); and **s**hock, stroke.

Aerobic metabolism Cell metabolism that occurs in the presence of oxygen.

Agonal breathing Slow and shallow breathing that is sometimes seen just before the onset of respiratory failure.

Air embolism The presence of air bubbles in the circulatory system.

Airborne diseases Infections that are spread by droplets produced by coughing or sneezing.

Airway adjuncts Devices used to help keep a patient's airway open.

Alcohol withdrawal syndrome A series of signs and symptoms that occur 6 to 48 hours after a chronic alcoholic reduces intake or stops consuming alcohol.

Allergen An antigen that causes signs and symptoms of an allergic reaction.

Allergic asthma Asthma that is triggered by an allergic reaction.

Allergic reaction An exaggerated response by the body's immune system to a substance.

Altered mental status A change in a patient's level of awareness; also called an *altered level of consciousness* (ALOC).

Alveolar ducts Ducts that end in several alveolar sacs.

Alveoli Grapelike sacs at the end of bronchioles where oxygen and carbon dioxide are exchanged between the air and blood.

Alzheimer's disease A type of irreversible dementia.

Amniotic sac The sac of fluid that surrounds the fetus inside the uterus; also called *bag of waters.*

Amputation The separation of a body part from the rest of the body.

Anabolism One type of cell metabolism where a cell uses energy to make larger molecules from smaller ones.

Anaerobic metabolism Cell metabolism that does not require the presence of oxygen.

Anal canal The end of the large intestine, 1 to 2 inches long, that remains closed except during defecation.

Anaphylactic shock Shock caused by a severe allergic reaction.

Anaphylaxis A severe allergic reaction; a life-threatening emergency.

Anatomic dead space The volume of air contained in the trachea and mainstem bronchi where gas exchange does not occur.

Anatomic splint Use of the body as a splint; also called a *self-splint.*

Anatomical position A position in which a person stands with arms to the sides and with the palms turned forward, feet close together, the head pointed forward, and the eyes open.

Anatomy The study of the structure of an organism (such as the human body).

Anesthesia Without sensation; a loss of feeling.

Aneurysm An abnormal bulging of a blood vessel.

Angina pectoris A symptom of coronary artery disease that occurs when the heart's need for oxygen exceeds its supply; literally, "choking in the chest."

Angioplasty A procedure in which a balloon-tipped catheter is inserted into a partially blocked coronary artery; when the balloon is inflated, plaque is pressed against the walls of the artery, improving blood flow to the heart muscle.

Anisocoria Unequal pupil size that is normal in 2 to 4% of the population.

Ankle drag Emergency move in which the rescuer grabs the patient's ankles or pant cuffs and drags the patient to safety.

Anterior The front portion of the body or body part.

Antibody A substance produced by white blood cells to defend the body against bacteria, viruses, or other antigens.

Antidote A substance that neutralizes a poison.

Antigen Any substance that is foreign to an individual and causes antibody production.

Anxiety A state of worry and agitation that is usually triggered by a real or imagined situation.

Anxiety disorder Condition that involves excessive anxiety ranging from uneasiness to terror.

Aorta One of the two major blood vessels of the abdomen; the largest artery in the body.

Aortic valve A semilunar valve located at the junction of the left ventricle and aorta.

Apgar score Method used to assess five specific signs in newborns at 1 and 5 minutes after birth: **a**ppearance (color), **p**ulse (heart rate), **g**rimace (irritability), **a**ctivity (muscle tone), and **r**espirations.

Apparent life-threatening event (ALTE) An episode in which an infant was about to die but was found early enough for successful resuscitation; also called *near-miss SIDS* or *near-SIDS.*

Appeal When an attorney requests that a higher court hear a case in order to reverse the decision of a lower court.

Appendicitis Inflammation of the appendix; generally requires surgical removal.

Appendicular skeleton The upper and lower extremities (arms and legs), the shoulder girdle, and the pelvic girdle.

Arachnoid Literally, "resembling a spider's web"; middle meningeal layer with delicate fibers resembling a spider's web; it contains few blood vessels.

Arteries Blood vessels that carry blood away from the heart to the rest of the body.

Arterioles The smallest branches of arteries leading to the capillaries.

Arteriosclerosis Hardening *(-sclerosis)* of the walls of the arteries *(arterio-).*

Arteriovenous (AV) fistula A fistula created by a surgeon in which a large artery and vein are joined under the patient's skin, usually at the wrist or near the elbow; used for hemodialysis.

Arteriovenous graft A graft formed by a surgeon for hemodialysis; most commonly placed in the upper or lower arm.

Arteriovenous shunt An external shunt that consists of two pieces of flexible tubing, each with a tip on the end; created by a surgeon for patients requiring short-term dialysis treatment.

Arthropods Animals that have a segmented body, jointed legs, a digestive tract, and, in most cases, a hard outer shell but no backbone.

Ascending colon The part of the large intestine that passes upward from the cecum to the lower edge of the liver where it turns to become the transverse colon.

Aspiration The entry of secretions or foreign material into the trachea and lungs.

Aspirin A nonnarcotic pain reliever, fever reducer, and anti-inflammatory medication.

Assault Threatening, attempting, or causing a fear of offensive physical contact with a patient or another person.

Asthma A widespread, temporary narrowing of the air passages that transport air from the nose and mouth to the lungs; the condition is associated with bronchospasm, swelling of the mucous membranes in the bronchial walls, and excessive mucus secretion; also known as *reactive airway disease (RAD).*

Asymmetry Unevenness.

Atherosclerosis Narrowing and thickening of the inner lining (endothelium) of the walls of large- and medium-size arteries because of a buildup of plaque.

Atmospheric pressure The force exerted by air on the body surface.

Atria The two upper chambers of the heart, which receive blood from the body and lungs (singular, *atrium*).

Atrioventricular (AV) valves Heart valves that lie between an atrium and a ventricle.

Atropine An antidote that reverses some effects of nerve agent poisoning.

Aura A peculiar sensation that comes before a seizure.

Autoinjector A drug delivery system that is designed to work through clothing; when firm, even pressure is applied to the injector, it propels a spring-driven needle into the patient's skin (usually the thigh) and then injects the drug into the muscle.

Automated external defibrillator (AED) A machine that analyzes a patient's heart rhythm and, if indicated, delivers an electrical shock.

Automatic vehicle locator (AVL) A device that uses the Global Positioning System (GPS) to track a vehicle's location.

Automaticity The ability of specialized electrical (pacemaker) cells in the heart to produce an electrical impulse without being stimulated by another source, such as a nerve.

Automatisms Purposeless, repetitive behavior such as lip smacking, eye blinking, chewing or swallowing movements, fumbling of the hands, or shuffling of the feet.

Autonomic division The division of the peripheral nervous system that has receptors and nerves concerned with the internal environment. It controls the involuntary system of glands and smooth muscle and functions to maintain a steady state in the body.

AVPU scale A memory aid used to identify a patient's mental status. Each letter of the scale refers to a level of awareness: **a**lert, **v**erbal stimuli, **p**ainful stimuli, and **u**nresponsive. A patient who is oriented to person, place, time, and event is said to be "alert and oriented × (times) 4" or "A&O×4."

Avulsion A soft tissue injury in which a flap of skin or tissue is torn loose or pulled completely off.

Axial skeleton The part of the skeleton that includes the skull, spinal column, sternum, and ribs.

Axilla Armpit.

B

Bacteria Germs that can cause disease in humans, plants, or animals.

Bag-mask (BM) device A self-inflating bag used to force air into a patient's lungs.

Bag-mask ventilation The use of a self-inflating bag to force air into a patient's lungs.

Bandage Material used to secure a dressing in place.

Barbiturates Drugs prescribed to relieve anxiety, promote sleep, control seizures, and relax muscles; include pentobarbital (Nembutal), secobarbital (Seconal), amobarbital (Amytal), and phenobarbital (Luminal).

Bariatrics The branch of medicine that deals with the causes, prevention, and treatment of obesity and weight-related health problems.

Barotrauma Diving-related injury caused by pressure that can occur on ascent or descent.

Barrier device A thin film of plastic or silicone that is placed on the patient's face to prevent direct contact with the patient's mouth during positive-pressure ventilation.

Base station A transmitter-receiver at a stationary site such as a hospital, mountaintop, or public safety agency.

Baseline vital signs An initial set of vital sign measurements.

Basket stretcher A patient-transfer device that is usually made of plastic and shaped like a long basket and can accommodate a scoop stretcher or a long backboard. It is used for moving patients over rough terrain and is often used in water rescues or high-angle rescues; also called a *Stokes basket* or *basket litter*.

Battery The unlawful touching of another person without consent.

Battle's sign A bluish discoloration behind the ear that is a sign of a possible skull fracture.

Behavior The way in which a person acts or performs.

Behavioral emergency A situation in which a patient displays abnormal behavior that is unacceptable to the patient, family members, or community.

Benign tumor A noncancerous tumor.

Bilateral Pertaining to both sides.

Binaurals The metal pieces of the stethoscope that connect the earpieces to the plastic or rubber tubing.

Biological weapons The use of bacteria, viruses, rickettsias, or toxins to cause disease or death.

Bipolar disorder A brain disorder that causes alternating episodes of mood elevation (mania) and depression; also known as *manic-depressive illness*.

Blanket drag Emergency move in which the rescuer places the patient on a blanket and drags the blanket.

Blast injuries Injuries that result from pressure waves generated by an explosion.

Blastocyst A cluster of cells that forms a few days after the joining of a sperm and egg. In human development, a blastocyst is preceded by a zygote (fertilized egg) and succeeded by an embryo.

Bleb A small air- or fluid-filled sac in the lung.

Blood glucose meter (glucometer) A device used to measure the amount of glucose in a blood sample.

Blood pressure (BP) The force exerted by the blood on the walls of the arteries.

Bloodborne diseases Infections that are spread by contact with the blood or body fluids of an infected person.

Bloody show Mucus and blood that may come out of the vagina as labor begins.

Blow-by oxygen Method of oxygen delivery in which the device used to deliver the oxygen does not make actual contact with the patient.

Blowout fracture Cracks or breaks in the facial bones that make up the orbit of the eye.

Blunt trauma Any mechanism of injury that occurs without actual penetration of the body.

Body The main part of a skeletal muscle; also, the middle portion of the sternum.

Body cavity A hollow space in the body that contains internal organs.

Body mechanics The coordinated effort of the musculoskeletal and nervous systems to maintain proper balance,

posture, and body alignment during lifting, bending, moving, and other activities of daily living.

Body temperature The balance between the heat produced by the body and the heat lost from the body.

Bones Living, growing tissues that are made up mostly of collagen and calcium.

Bradypnea A slower than normal respiratory rate for the patient's age.

Brainstem The portion of the brain that consists of the midbrain, pons, and medulla oblongata.

Breach of duty Violation of the standard of care that applies in a given situation.

Breath stacking A series of breaths without adequate exhalation.

Breathing The mechanical process of moving air into and out of the lungs; also called *pulmonary ventilation*.

Breech delivery A delivery in which the presenting part of the infant is the buttocks or feet instead of the head.

Bronchioles Small, thin-walled branches of a bronchus.

Bronchodilator A medication that relaxes smooth muscles in the bronchioles, reducing airway resistance.

Bronchus Large passageway for air to and from the alveoli.

Bruise A collection of blood under the skin caused by bleeding capillaries.

Buccal Pertaining to the cheek.

Buddy taping Using an anatomic splint by taping an injured finger or toe to an uninjured finger or toe next to it.

Bursitis Condition that occurs when a bursa becomes swollen and inflamed, resulting in pain when the joint is moved.

C

Calcium A mineral that strengthens and hardens the framework of bones.

Capillaries The very thin blood vessels that connect arteries and veins.

Capillary refill Assessment tool used in infants and children; performed by pressing on the patient's skin or nail beds and determining the time for return to initial color; normal capillary refill in infants and children is less than 2 seconds, and delayed (greater than 2 seconds) capillary refill suggests circulatory compromise.

Caplet An oval-shaped tablet that has a film-coated covering.

Capsule A small gelatin container containing a medication dose in powder or granule form.

Cardiac arrest A condition that occurs when the contraction of the heart stops; confirmed by unresponsiveness, absent breathing, and absent pulses.

Cardiac muscle Involuntary muscle found only in the heart.

Cardiac output (CO) The amount of blood the heart pumps each minute.

Cardiac tamponade A condition that occurs when blood enters the pericardial sac because of laceration of a coronary blood vessel, a ruptured coronary artery, laceration of a chamber of the heart, or a significant cardiac contusion. The blood in the pericardial sac compresses the heart, decreasing the amount of blood the heart can pump out with each contraction.

Cardiogenic shock A condition in which the heart fails to function effectively as a pump; as a result, the heart does not pump enough blood to maintain adequate perfusion.

Cardiopulmonary failure Respiratory failure that occurs together with shock.

Cardiopulmonary resuscitation (CPR) The combination of rescue breathing and external chest compressions.

Cardiovascular disease Disease of the heart and blood vessels.

Cardiovascular system The heart, blood vessels, and blood.

Carina The point at which the trachea divides into two primary bronchi, forming an internal ridge.

Carpals Wrist bones.

Cartilage Tissue that provides cushioning between bones and allows easy movement of joints.

Cartilaginous joints Joints in which the bones are attached by cartilage; found in the spine and ribs and allow for only a little movement.

Catabolism Type of cell metabolism where cells break down large molecules into small ones, releasing energy.

Cataract Disorder which features the clouding of the lens of the eye; the most common disorder of the eye in older adults.

Cecum A blind pouch or cul-de-sac that forms the first part of the large intestine.

Cell metabolism The sum of chemical reactions that occur within cells, enabling them to maintain a living state.

Cells The basic building blocks of the body.

Centers for Disease Control and Prevention (CDC) A federal agency of the U.S. government that promotes health and quality of life by preventing and controlling disease, injury, and disability.

Central chemoreceptors Sensory receptors located in the medulla oblongata in the brain that are sensitive to changes in the carbon dioxide content of the blood.

Central cyanosis A bluish tint in the color of a newborn's face, chest, or inside the mouth.

Central line An intravenous line placed near the heart for long-term use.

Central nervous system (CNS) The brain and spinal cord.

Central pulse A pulse found close to the trunk of the body.

Cephalic (head) delivery A delivery in which an infant emerges head first from the birth canal.

Cerebellum The second largest part of the human brain. It is responsible for the precise control of muscle movements and the maintenance of posture and equilibrium.

Cerebral contusion A brain injury in which brain tissue is bruised and damaged in a local area.

Cerebral cortex The outer layer of the cerebrum.

Cerebrospinal fluid (CSF) A clear liquid that acts as a shock absorber for the brain and spinal cord and provides a means for the exchange of nutrients and wastes among the blood, brain, and spinal cord.

Cerebrovascular accident (CVA) Stroke; an infarct in the brain.

Cerebrum The largest part of the brain, made up of two hemispheres.

Certification A designation that ensures a person has met predetermined requirements to perform a particular activity.

Cervical spine (c-spine) The seven cervical vertebrae of the neck.

Cervix The narrow opening at the lower end of the uterus that connects the uterus to the vagina.

Chain of survival The ideal series of events that should take place immediately after recognizing an injury or the onset of sudden illness.

CHART An acronym pertaining to a common format used for documentation: **c**hief complaint, **h**istory, **a**ssessment, **R**x (treatment), and **t**ransport.

Chemical agents Poisonous substances that injure or kill people when inhaled, ingested, or absorbed through the skin or eyes.

Chemical name A description of a drug's composition and molecular structure.

Chemical protective clothing (CPC) Materials designed to protect the skin from exposure to chemicals by either physical or chemical means.

Chemoreceptors Sensory receptors that monitor the levels of oxygen and carbon dioxide in the body.

Chest (thorax) The body cavity located below the neck and above the diaphragm. It contains the heart, major blood vessels, and lungs.

Chief complaint The reason EMS has been called; usually recorded in the patient's own words.

Child maltreatment An act or failure to act by a parent, caregiver, or other person as defined by state law that results in physical abuse, neglect, medical neglect, sexual abuse, and/or emotional abuse; it is also defined as an act or failure to act that presents an impending risk of serious harm to a child.

Childbirth The emergence of an infant from the mother's uterus.

Cholecystitis Inflammation of the gallbladder.

Chronic bronchitis Sputum production for 3 months of a year for at least 2 consecutive years.

Chronic renal failure (CRF) Renal failure that develops over months or years and is usually irreversible.

Chyme Partially digested food that is moved through the digestive tract by peristalsis.

Circulatory system Cardiovascular and lymphatic systems.

Circumferential burns Swellings from burns that encircle extremities.

Civil law A branch of law that deals with complaints by individuals or organizations against a defendant for an illegal act or wrongdoing.

Cleaning The process of washing a contaminated object with soap and water.

Clenched fist injury An injury in which the fist of an individual strikes the teeth of another; also called a *fight bite*. The skin on the hand may or may not be broken.

Closed questions Questions that can be answered with one- or two-word responses; also called *direct questions*.

Closed soft tissue injury A soft tissue injury that results when the body is struck by a blunt object; there is no break in the skin, but the tissues and vessels beneath the skin surface are crushed or ruptured.

Closed wound An injury that occurs when the soft tissues under the skin are damaged but the surface of the skin is not broken.

Clothes drag Emergency move in which a rescuer pulls on the patient's clothing in the neck and shoulder area; also called a *clothing pull* or *shirt drag*.

Cluster headaches Attacks of severe pain that are primarily localized to the eye, temple, forehead, or cheek area.

Cognition The mental functions, including memory, learning, awareness, reasoning, and judgment and the ability to think, plan, form, and comprehend speech, process information, and understand and solve problems.

Cognitive impairment A change in a person's mental functioning caused by an injury or disease process.

Coining A healing remedy practiced by some cultures in which a coin is heated in hot oil and then rubbed along the patient's spine to heal an illness, such as congestion in the lungs.

Collagen A protein that provides a soft framework for bones.

Colles' fracture A break in the distal radius that is usually caused by falling on an outstretched hand in an attempt to break a fall.

Colon (large intestine) The portion of the digestive system that extends from the ileum of the small intestine to the anus. It is subdivided into the following sections (listed in the order in which food passes through them): cecum, ascending colon, transverse colon, descending colon, sigmoid colon, rectum, and anal canal.

Comfort care Measures used to ease the symptoms of an illness or injury; also called *palliative care* or *supportive care*.

Comminuted fracture One in which the bone is splintered or crushed, resulting in several breaks in the bone and multiple bone fragments.

Commotio cordis Literally, "disturbed or agitated heart motion"; a sudden cardiac death due to a blunt force injury to the chest (directly over the left ventricle of the heart) without causing any significant structural injury to the heart.

Communicable disease A contagious infection that can be spread from one person to another.

Communication The exchange of thoughts and messages that occurs by sending and receiving information.

Compartment syndrome A compression injury that develops when the pressure within a compartment causes compression and abnormal function of nerves and blood vessels.

Competence A patient's ability to understand the questions you ask and understand the implications of decisions the patient makes concerning care.

Completed suicide Death by a self-inflicted, consciously intended action.

Complex extrication The use of powered hydraulic rescue tools such as cutters, spreaders, and rams to gain access to and extricate the patient from the vehicle.

Complex partial seizure A type of partial seizure in which the patient's consciousness, responsiveness, or memory is impaired; also called a *temporal lobe seizure* or *psychomotor seizure*.

Compliance The ability of a patient's lung tissue to distend (inflate) with ventilation.

Compound fracture A broken bone that penetrates the skin; also called an *open fracture*.

Compression injury of the abdomen An injury by which abdominal contents are squeezed between the vertebral column and the impacting object.

Compulsions Recurring behaviors or rituals performed with the hope of preventing obsessive thoughts or making them go away.

Computer-aided dispatch (CAD) A computer system that aids dispatch personnel in handling and prioritizing emergency calls.

Concussion A traumatic brain injury that results in a temporary loss of function in some or all of the brain.

Condom catheter Urinary catheter used for male patients that consists of a condom or condomlike device with a tube attached to the distal end that is attached to a drainage bag; also called a *Texas catheter*.

Conduction The transfer of heat between objects that are in direct contact.

Congestive heart failure (CHF) A condition in which one or both sides of the heart fail to pump efficiently.

Conjunctiva A paper-thin mucous membrane that covers the sclera (the white of the eye).

Consent Permission.

Continuous ambulatory peritoneal dialysis (CAPD) A type of peritoneal dialysis that does not require a machine and is performed by the patient three to five times per day while carrying out normal daily activities.

Continuous cyclic peritoneal dialysis (CCPD) A type of peritoneal dialysis that requires the use of a machine called a cycler that automates the exchange procedure.

Contraindications Conditions for which a drug should not be used because it may cause harm to the patient or offer no improvement of the patient's condition or illness.

Contralateral Opposite side.

Contributing risk factors Risk factors that can be part of the cause of a person's risk of heart disease.

Convection The transfer of heat by the movement of air current.

Convulsions The jerking movements during the clonic phase of a tonic-clonic seizure.

Coronary artery bypass graft (CABG) A surgical procedure in which a graft is created from a healthy blood vessel from another part of the patient's body to reroute blood flow around a diseased coronary artery; acronym is pronounced "cabbage."

Coronary artery disease (CAD) Disease that slows or stops blood flow through the arteries that supply the heart muscle with blood.

Coronary heart disease (CHD) Disease of the coronary arteries and the complications that result, such as angina pectoris or a heart attack.

Corpus callosum A collection of nerve fibers in the brain that connect the left and right cerebral hemispheres.

Crackles Abnormal breath sound that indicates the presence of fluid in the alveoli or larger airways.

Cradle carry A move in which the rescuer kneels next to the patient, places one hand under the patient's shoulders and the other under the patient's knees, and then stands up, carrying the patient to safety; also called the *one-person arm carry*.

Cranial cavity The body cavity located in the head that contains the brain.

Cranial nerves Twelve pairs of nerves that connect the brain with the neck and structures in the chest and abdomen.

Cranium The portion of the skull that encloses the brain.

Credentialing A local process by which an individual is permitted by a specific entity to practice medical procedures and functions in a specific setting, such as an EMS agency.

Crepitation (crepitus) A crackling sensation heard and felt beneath the skin; caused by bone ends grating against each other or air trapped between layers of tissue.

Cricoid cartilage The most inferior of the cartilages of the larynx.

Cricoid pressure Application of pressure to the cricoid cartilage; this pushes the trachea backward and compresses the esophagus against the cervical vertebrae, decreasing the amount of air entering the stomach during positive-pressure ventilation; also called the *Sellick maneuver*.

Criminal law The area of law in which individuals are prosecuted on behalf of society for violating laws designed to safeguard society.

Croup A respiratory infection that primarily affects children ages 6 months to 3 years; usually caused by a virus that causes swelling around the larynx and trachea.

Crowing A long, high-pitched sound heard on inhalation.

Crowning The stage of birth when the presenting part of the infant is visible at the vaginal opening.

Crush injuries Traumas caused by a compressing force applied to the body; also called *compression injuries*.

Crush syndrome A compression injury that can occur when a large amount of skeletal muscle is compressed for a long period (usually 4–6 hours, although it may be as little as 1 hour) and compromises local blood flow.

Cumulative stress Tension that results from repeated exposure to smaller stressors that build up over time.

Cushing's triad Three findings (increased systolic blood pressure, abnormal breathing pattern, and decreased heart rate) that indicate increasing intracranial pressure in a head-injured patient.

Cyanosis Blue-gray color of the skin or mucous membranes that suggests inadequate oxygenation or poor perfusion.

Cystic fibrosis (CF) An inherited disease that appears in childhood. A defective gene inherited from each parent results in an abnormality in the glands that produce or secrete sweat and mucus.

Cystitis Inflammation of the bladder.

D

DCAP-BTLS Memory aid used for patient assessment: **d**eformities, **c**ontusions, **a**brasions, **p**unctures or penetrations, **b**urns, **t**enderness, **l**acerations, and **s**welling.

Deceleration injury An injury by which an individual's body stops its forward movement on impact but the organs continue to move forward until structural impact, tear, or rupture occurs.

Decode Interpret a message received from a sender.

Decompression sickness A diving-related injury that results from dissolved nitrogen in the blood and tissues; also called *the bends*.

Decontamination The use of physical or chemical means to remove, inactivate, or destroy bloodborne pathogens on a surface or item to the point at which it is no longer capable of transmitting infectious particles and the surface or item is considered safe for handling, use, or disposal.

Defecation The elimination of undigested waste from the body.

Defendant A person being sued or accused in a lawsuit or criminal prosecution.

Defibrillation The delivery of an electrical shock to a patient's heart to end an abnormal heart rhythm.

Defibrillator A machine that delivers electrical shocks to the heart.

Degloving An avulsion injury where the skin and fatty tissue are stripped away from an extremity like a glove.

Delayed drowning A type of drowning that occurs when a victim appears to have survived an immersion or submersion episode but later dies from respiratory failure or an infection; also called *secondary drowning*.

Delirium A sudden change (onset of minutes, hours, days) in mental status that is generally caused by a reversible condition such as hypoglycemia, drug overdose, or trauma; also known as *acute brain syndrome*.

Delirium tremens (DTs) Signs and symptoms associated with alcohol withdrawal that have progressed beyond the usual symptoms of withdrawal and are potentially fatal.

Delivery The actual birth of the baby at the end of the second stage of labor.

Delusions False beliefs that the patient believes are true, despite facts to the contrary.

Dementia A gradual change in baseline mental status that causes a progressive and sometimes irreversible loss of intellectual functions, psychomotor skills, and social skills.

Denial A defense mechanism used to create a buffer against the shock of dying or dealing with an illness or injury.

Dependent lividity The settling of blood in dependent areas of the body (those areas on which the body has been resting).

Depressants Alcohol, barbiturates, narcotics (opiates), and benzodiazepines.

Depression A state of mind characterized by feelings of sadness, worthlessness, and discouragement.

Dermis The thick layer of skin below the epidermis that contains hair follicles, sweat and oil glands, small nerve endings, and blood vessels.

Descending colon The part of the large intestine descending from the left colic (splenic) flexure to the brim of the pelvis.

Designer drugs Variations of federally controlled substances that have high abuse potential (such as narcotics and amphetamines); they are produced by persons ranging from amateurs to highly skilled chemists (called "cookers") and sold on the street.

Deviated septum A bent nasal septum.

Diabetic ketoacidosis (DKA) Severe, uncontrolled hyperglycemia (usually over 300 mg/dL); also called *diabetic coma*.

Dialysis A procedure, normally performed by the kidneys, that removes waste products from the blood; the two types of dialysis are *hemodialysis* and *peritoneal dialysis*.

Diaphragm The dome-shaped muscle below the lungs that is the primary muscle of respiration.

Diastolic blood pressure The pressure in the arteries when the heart is at rest.

Diazepam A medication that is used to control seizures following severe exposure to nerve agents (and similar toxins); trade name, Valium.

Diencephalon The part of the brain between the cerebrum and the brainstem. It contains the thalamus and hypothalamus.

Digestion The chemical process of breaking down food into small parts so absorption can occur.

Dilate Expand.

Diplomacy Art of tact and skill for dealing with people.

Direct ground lift A nonurgent move used to lift and carry a patient with no suspected spine injury from the ground to a bed or stretcher.

Direct pressure Firm pressure applied to a bleeding site with gloved hands or bandages to control bleeding.

Direct questions Questions that can be answered with one- or two-word responses; also called *closed questions*.

Discovery Legal process to enable each side in a lawsuit or criminal prosecution to learn the facts necessary to prepare its case.

Disease An abnormal condition in which the body's steady state is threatened or cannot be maintained.

Disentanglement The moving or removing of materials that are trapping a victim.

Disinfecting Cleaning with such chemical solutions as alcohol or chlorine.

Dislocation Forceful movement of the ends of bones from their normal positions in a joint.

Distal Farther away from the midline, or center area, of the body.

Distention The state of bulging or swelling.

Distributive shock Condition that causes massive dilation of the blood vessels, redistributing the fluid volume within the circulatory system; as a result, there is an inadequate amount of blood to fill the enlarged vessels, and the vital organs are not perfused.

Do not resuscitate (DNR) order Instructions written by a physician that notify medical professionals not to provide medical care to a patient who has experienced a cardiac arrest.

Dose The amount of a drug that should be given to the patient at one time.

DOTS Memory aid used for patient assessment: **d**eformities, **o**pen injuries, **t**enderness, and **s**welling.

Draw sheet A narrow sheet placed crosswise on a bed under the patient; used to assist in moving a patient or in changing soiled bed sheets.

Dressing Absorbent material placed directly over a wound.

Drowning A process that results in harm to the respiratory system from submersion or immersion in a liquid.

Drug profile A description of a drug's characteristics; includes generic and trade names, mechanism of action, indications, dose, route of administration, contraindications, and adverse effects.

Dry drowning Drowning in which the larynx closes to prevent the passage of water into the lungs.

Duodenum The portion of the small intestine that connects the stomach and jejunum.

Duplex system A mode of radio transmission that uses two frequencies to transmit and receive messages, allowing simultaneous two-way communication.

Dura mater Literally, "hard" or "tough mother"; tough, durable, outermost layer of the meninges, the outermost layer of connective tissue around the brain, that adheres to the inner surface of the cranium.

Duty to act A formal contractual or an implied legal obligation to provide care to a patient requesting services.

Dysphagia Difficulty swallowing.

Dyspnea A sensation of shortness of breath or difficulty breathing.

Dysuria Painful or burning urination.

E

Early adulthood Stage of human development from 19 to 40 years.

Early (compensated) shock Stage of shock where the body's defense mechanisms are still attempting to protect the vital organs (the brain, heart, and lungs); also called *shock with a normal blood pressure.*

Ecchymosis Bluish discoloration caused by leakage of blood into the skin or mucous membrane.

Eclampsia A condition of pregnancy characterized by high blood pressure, swelling, protein in the urine, and seizures.

Ectopic pregnancy A condition that occurs when a fertilized egg implants outside the uterus. An ectopic pregnancy that occurs in a fallopian tube is called a *tubal pregnancy.*

Edema Swelling.

Elder abuse Any physical, sexual, or emotional abuse or neglect committed against an older adult.

Elder speak An inappropriate style of speech that some people use when speaking to older adults; it resembles baby talk.

Elective abortion An abortion performed at the request of the mother.

Elixir Clear liquid made with alcohol, water, flavors, or sweeteners.

Emancipated minor A person who is less than the legal age of consent but who is given the rights of adults.

Embolic stroke A stroke that occurs when an embolus breaks up, travels through the circulatory system, and lodges in a vessel within or leading to the brain.

Embolus A clot that travels through the circulatory system.

Embryo In human development, the third to the eighth week of gestation. At the end of the eighth week, the essentials of the organ systems are present.

Emergency An unexpected illness or injury that requires immediate action to avoid risking the life or health of the person being treated.

Emergency medical dispatchers (EMDS) Certified personnel who receive 9-1-1 calls, verify the address and emergency, assign responders, provide prearrival instructions to the caller, communicate with the responders, and record incident times.

Emergency Medical Radio Service (EMRS) A group of frequencies designated by the FCC exclusively for use by EMS providers.

Emergency medical responder (EMR) A person who has the basic knowledge and skills necessary to provide lifesaving emergency care while waiting for the arrival of additional EMS help; formerly called *first responder.*

Emergency Medical Services (EMS) system A network of resources that provides emergency care and transportation to victims of sudden illness or injury.

Emergency medical technician (EMT) A member of the EMS team who responds to emergency calls, provides efficient emergency treatment to ill or injured patients, and transports the patient to a medical facility.

Emergency move A method used to move, lift, or carry a patient when there is an immediate danger to the rescuer or the patient.

Emergency response Operation of an emergency vehicle while responding to a medical emergency.

Emergency transportation The process of moving a patient from the scene of an emergency to an appropriate healthcare facility.

Emotional abuse Behaviors that harm a child's self-worth or emotional well-being. Examples include name calling, shaming, rejection, withholding love, and threatening.

Empathy The act of understanding, being aware of, and being sensitive to the feelings, thoughts, and experiences of another.

Emphysema A respiratory disease that causes destruction of the alveolar walls; damage to the adjacent capillary walls; abnormal, permanent enlargement of the alveoli; and a loss of lung elasticity.

Emulsion Mixture of two liquids, with one distributed throughout the other in small globules.

Encoding The act of placing a message into words or images so that it is understood by the sender and receiver.

Endocrine system A system of ductless glands that secrete chemicals, such as insulin and adrenalin, which regulate and influence body activities and functions.

Endometriosis A condition in which uterine tissue is located outside the uterus, causing pain and bleeding.

End-stage renal disease (ESRD) Condition when kidney failure is permanent.

Enhanced 9-1-1 (E9-1-1) A system that routes an emergency call to the 9-1-1 center closest to the caller and automatically displays the caller's phone number and address.

Enteral Route of administration for drugs that involves passage of the medication through any portion of the digestive tract.

Enteric-coated tablet Tablet that has a special coating so that it breaks down in the intestines instead of the stomach.

Epidermis The outer layer of the skin.

Epidural hematoma A buildup of blood between the dura and the skull that often involves the tearing of an artery, which is usually the middle meningeal artery.

Epiglottis Leaf-shaped cartilage that covers the opening to the larynx during swallowing, preventing food and liquids from entering the airway.

Epiglottitis A bacterial infection of the upper airway that involves inflammation and swelling between the base of the tongue and the epiglottis.

Epilepsy A condition of recurring seizures in which the cause is usually irreversible.

Epinephrine Medication that works by relaxing the bronchial passages of the airway and constricting the blood vessels; administered by autoinjector.

Epiphyseal plate An area of growing tissue near each end of a long bone in children and adolescents; also called *growth plate.*

Epistaxis Nosebleed.

Erect Standing upright.

Erythrocytes Red blood cells; formed elements of blood.

Esophagus A muscular tube about 9 inches long (in adults) that is a passageway for food.

Essential hypertension Hypertension that has no identifiable cause.

Ethics   Principles of right and wrong, good and bad, that affect our actions and lead to consequences.

Etiology   The study of cause; of disease, for example.

Evaporation   A loss of heat by vaporization of moisture on the body surface.

Evisceration   The protrusion of an organ through an open wound.

Excited delirium   Abnormal behavior characterized by elevated temperature, agitation, aggression, and "superhuman" strength, especially during attempts to restrain the patient; also called *agitated delirium.*

Exhalation   The process of breathing out and moving air out of the lungs; also called *expiration.*

Exhaled carbon dioxide detector   A device that measures a person's exhaled carbon dioxide.

Expiration   See *exhalation.*

Exposure   Direct or indirect contact with infected blood, body fluids, tissues, or airborne droplets.

Expressed consent   A type of consent in which a patient gives specific permission verbally, in writing, or nonverbally for care and transport to be provided.

External bleeding   Bleeding that can be seen.

External nares   Nostrils.

Extracellular fluid (ECF)   Body fluids outside the walls of the billions of body cells.

Extrication   To free from entrapment.

F

Fainting (syncope)   See *syncope (fainting).*

Fallopian tubes (oviducts)   In the female, tubes that receive and transport the ovum to the uterus after ovulation.

False labor pains   Pain that women often have about 2 to 4 weeks before delivery; also called *Braxton-Hicks contractions.*

False ribs   Rib pairs 8 through 10. These ribs attach to the cartilage of the seventh ribs.

Fascia   A tough sheet of fibrous tissue that covers the skeletal muscles of the body.

Fasciotomy   A surgical procedure in which a physician cuts the tough sheet of fibrous tissue covering a muscle to relieve pressure.

Febrile seizures   Seizures caused by fever.

Fecal impaction   Hardened feces that become trapped in the rectum and cannot be expelled.

Fecal incontinence   The involuntary leakage of stool.

Federal Communications Commission (FCC)   The U.S. government agency responsible for regulation of interstate and international communications by radio, television, wire, satellite, and cable.

Feedback   Verbal or nonverbal response from a receiver that allows the sender of a message to know that it has been received.

Femur   The thigh bone. It extends from the hip to the knee.

Fend-off position   The parking of an emergency vehicle downward from the scene and in such a way that allows traveling vehicles to strike the emergency vehicle and not crew members.

Fetus   In human development, the eighth week of gestation through the time of birth.

Fibromyalgia (FM)   A disorder characterized by general fatigue and widespread musculoskeletal pain and stiffness that often persists for months at a time.

Fibula   The bone that lies next to the tibia along the outer side of the lower leg.

Field impression   The conclusion an EMT reaches about what is wrong with a patient.

Firefighter's carry   A move involving a series of maneuvers in which the patient is positioned lengthwise across the rescuer's shoulders and carried to safety.

Firefighter's drag   Emergency move in which the patient is placed on his back with wrists crossed and secured. While the rescuer straddles the patient, the patient's arms are lifted over the rescuer's head so that the patient's wrists are behind the rescuer's neck. The rescuer then crawls forward, dragging the patient to safety.

Flail chest   Condition that occurs when two or more adjacent ribs are fractured in two or more places or when the sternum is detached.

Flail segment   The section of the chest wall between the fractured ribs in a patient with flail chest that becomes free-floating because it is no longer in continuity with the thorax.

Flexible stretcher   A patient-transfer device made of canvas or synthetic flexible material with carrying handles. A flexible stretcher is useful when space to access the patient is limited, such as in narrow hallways, stairs, or cramped corners; examples include the Reeves stretcher, SKED, and Navy stretcher.

Floating ribs   Rib pairs 11 and 12. These ribs have no attachment to the sternum.

Flow meter   A valve that controls the liters of oxygen delivered per minute.

Flow-restricted, oxygen-powered ventilation device (FROPVD)   A manually triggered ventilation (MTV) device used to give positive-pressure ventilation with 100% oxygen.

Focused physical examination   An assessment of specific body areas that relate to a patient's illness or injury.

Focused trauma assessment   An exam concentrating on the specific injury site performed on a trauma patient with no significant MOI; also called a *focused physical examination.*

Foley catheter   An indwelling catheter consisting of a flexible tube that is inserted through the urethra and into the bladder to drain urine.

Fontanels   Soft, diamond-shaped spots in the bones of the head of an infant that allow flexibility during delivery and growth of the brain; they will not completely close until about 6 months of age for the rear fontanel and 18 months for the top one.

Foodborne diseases   Infections that are spread by the improper handling of food or by poor personal hygiene.

Foramen magnum   The large opening in the base of the skull through which the spinal cord passes.

Forearm drag   Emergency move in which the rescuer's hands are positioned under the patient's armpits, the patient's forearms are grasped, and the patient is dragged to safety; also called the *bent-arm drag.*

Foreign body airway obstruction (FBAO)   A partial or complete blockage of the conducting airways due to a foreign body, such as a piece of food, bleeding into the airway, or vomitus.

Fowler's position Lying on the back with the upper body elevated at a 45- to 60-degree angle.

Fraction of inspired oxygen (FiO₂) The percentage of oxygen in the air inhaled.

Fracture A break in a bone; if a bone is broken, chipped, cracked, or splintered, it is said to be fractured.

Frank-Starling law of the heart An increase in the volume of blood in the ventricles that causes fibers in the heart muscle to stretch, resulting in a more forceful contraction.

Free radicals Highly reactive molecules that are a byproduct of normal cellular reactions.

Frontal plane The vertical (lengthwise) field that passes through the body from side to side, dividing the body (or any of its parts) into anterior (ventral) and posterior (dorsal) parts.

Full-thickness burn A burn in which the epidermis and dermis are destroyed; the burn may also involve subcutaneous tissue, muscle, and bone; also called a *third-degree burn.*

G

Gallbladder A pear-shaped sac on the undersurface of the liver that stores bile until it is needed by the small intestine.

Gastritis Inflammation of the stomach lining.

Gastroenteritis Inflammation of the lining of the intestinal tract, most often caused by a virus; also called *stomach flu.*

Gastrostomy tube A special catheter placed directly into the stomach for feeding.

Gelcap A small gelatin container containing a liquid medication dose.

Gel Clear or translucent semisolid substance that liquefies when applied to the skin or a mucous membrane.

General impression An across-the-room assessment of a patient that is completed in 60 seconds or less to decide if the patient looks sick or not sick; also called a *first impression.*

Generalized seizure A type of seizure that begins suddenly and involves a period of altered mental status.

Generic name The name given to a drug by the company that first manufactures it; also called the *nonproprietary name.*

Gestational diabetes Diabetes that begins during pregnancy.

Glasgow Coma Scale (GCS) A minineurological examination used to establish a baseline level of responsiveness and note any obvious problem with central nervous system (brain and spinal cord) function.

Glaucoma A disease associated with a buildup of internal eye pressure that can damage the optic nerve, which sends visual information to the brain.

Global Positioning System (GPS) Technology that uses a system of satellites and receiving devices to compute the receiver's geographic position on the earth.

Glottis The space between the vocal cords.

Glucagon A hormone released from alpha cells in the pancreas that stimulates cells in the liver to break down stores of glycogen into glucose to increase the blood glucose level.

Glucometer See *blood glucose meter (glucometer).*

Glucose A sugar that is the basic fuel for body cells.

Glycolysis The cellular process of breaking down glucose into usable energy.

Golden hour The first 60 minutes after the occurrence of major trauma; the period from the time of the injury to the time the patient should receive definitive care in an operating room.

Great vessels The body's major blood vessels: pulmonary arteries and veins, the aorta, and the superior and inferior vena cavae.

Greater trochanter The large, bony prominence on the lateral shaft of the femur to which the buttock muscles are attached.

Greenstick fracture A break in a bone that occurs in a child where the bone breaks on one side but not the other, like bending a green tree branch.

Grief A normal response that helps a person cope with the loss of someone or something that had great meaning.

Growth plate An area of growing tissue near each end of a long bone in children and adolescents.

Gurgling A wet sound that suggests that fluid is collecting in the patient's upper airway.

Gynecology The study of the female reproductive system.

H

Hallucinations False sensory perceptions that are seen, heard, or felt by a person but not by others.

Hallucinogens Drugs that cause hallucinations; include lysergic acid diethylamine (LSD), PCP (angel dust), and mescaline (street names include *buttons, mess,* and *peyote*).

Hand-foot syndrome One of the earliest changes of sickle cell disease and results from the blockage of blood vessels in the hands or feet by sickle cells; it usually starts with painful swelling, affecting one or both hands and/or feet at the same time.

Hard palate The bony floor of the nasal cavity.

Hazardous material A substance (solid, liquid, or gas) that, when released, is capable of creating harm to people, the environment, and property.

Head bobbing An indicator of increased work of breathing in infants. When the baby breathes out, the head falls forward, and the baby's head comes up when the baby breathes in and its chest expands.

Head injury A traumatic insult to the head that may result in injury to soft tissue, bony structures, and/or the brain.

Head tilt–chin lift maneuver Effective method for opening the airway in a patient with no known or suspected trauma to the head or neck.

Health Insurance Portability and Accountability Act (HIPAA) A law passed by Congress in 1996 to ensure the confidentiality of a person's health information.

Healthcare system A network of people, facilities, and equipment designed to provide for the general medical needs of the population.

Heart The primary organ of the cardiovascular system. It lies in the thoracic cavity (mediastinum) behind the sternum and between the lungs.

Heat cramps Painful muscle spasms caused by an excessive loss of water and electrolytes in a warm environment; the mildest form of heat-related emergency.

Heat exhaustion A medical condition caused by excessive heat and dehydration; the most common heat-related illness.

Heat stroke A medical condition in which the body's heat regulating mechanisms fail; the most severe form of heat-related emergency.

Hematemesis Vomiting blood.

Hematology The study of diseases of the blood and blood-forming organs.

Hematoma A localized collection of blood beneath the skin caused by a tear in a blood vessel.

Hematuria Blood in the urine.

Hemodialysis Removal of waste products and excess water and minerals from the blood using an external machine as the filter.

Hemoglobin An iron-containing protein that chemically binds with oxygen.

Hemophilia An inherited bleeding disorder caused by an abnormality of a blood-clotting factor.

Hemoptysis The coughing up of blood.

Hemorrhage An extreme loss of blood from a blood vessel; also called *major bleeding*.

Hemorrhagic shock Shock caused by severe bleeding.

Hemorrhagic stroke A stroke caused by bleeding into the brain.

Hemostasis The process by which the body stops bleeding.

Hemothorax A collection of blood in the pleural cavity that may result from injury to the chest wall, the major blood vessels, or the lung because of penetrating or blunt trauma.

Hepatitis Inflammation of the liver; most commonly caused by a viral infection.

High-efficiency particulate air (HEPA) mask Mask that should be worn if you suspect a patient has tuberculosis.

High-Fowler's position A position in which a patient sits upright at a 90-degree angle.

High-level disinfection A method of decontamination that destroys all microorganisms except large numbers of bacterial spores. It is used for reusable equipment that has been in contact with mucous membranes, such as laryngoscope blades.

History of the present illness (HPI) A chronological record of the reason a patient is seeking medical assistance that includes the patient's chief complaint and the patient's answers to questions about the circumstances that led up to the request for medical help.

Hollow organs Stomach, intestines, gallbladder, and urinary bladder; when they are cut or burst, their contents spill into the abdominal cavity causing pain and soreness.

Home care Professional assistance that a patient receives in the home; it does not require a doctor's prescription and does not include skilled nursing services.

Home healthcare Medical care provided in the home by home healthcare agencies that is deemed medically necessary by a physician (requires a physician's prescription).

Homeostasis The property of an organism allowing it to regulate its internal processes to maintain a constant internal environment; also called *steady state*.

Hospice care A program of palliative and supportive care services providing physical, psychological, social, and spiritual care for dying persons, their families, and other loved ones.

Hot zone An identified safety zone at a hazardous materials incident that contains the hazardous material (contaminant); also known as the *exclusion zone*.

Human crutch move A move in which a rescuer places the patient's arm across the rescuer's shoulders, holds the patient's wrist with one hand, and places the rescuer's other hand around the patient's waist to help her to safety; also called the *rescuer assist* or *walking assist*.

Human immunodeficiency virus (HIV) Virus that causes AIDS.

Humerus The upper arm bone.

Humidifier A bottle filled with sterile water; when the bottle is connected to oxygen, oxygen passes through the water to gather moisture.

Hydrocephalus A condition in which there is an excess of cerebrospinal fluid within the brain.

Hypercarbia An increase in carbon dioxide in the respiratory system.

Hyperglycemia A higher-than-normal blood sugar level.

Hyperosmolar hyperglycemic state (HHS) A complication of type 2 diabetes that results in a very high glucose concentration in the blood (usually greater than 600 mg/dL).

Hypertension A sustained elevation of the systolic or diastolic blood pressure.

Hypertensive emergencies Situations that require rapid lowering of blood pressure to prevent or limit damage to such organs as the heart, brain, and kidneys.

Hyperthermia A high core body temperature.

Hyperthyroidism Oversecretion of thyroid hormones; also called *overactive thyroid*.

Hyperventilation Condition when the minute volume is higher than normal.

Hyphema A buildup of blood in the anterior chamber of the eye.

Hypoglycemia A lower-than-normal blood sugar level. In adults, hypoglycemia is a blood glucose level less than 70 mg/dL.

Hypoperfusion The inadequate flow of blood through an organ or a part of the body; also called *shock*.

Hypothalamus A part of the brain that plays an important role in the control of thirst, hunger, and body temperature; also serves as a link between the nervous and endocrine systems.

Hypothermia A core body temperature of less than 95°F (35°C).

Hypothyroidism Inadequate secretion of thyroid hormones; also called *underactive thyroid*.

Hypoventilation Condition when the minute volume is below normal.

Hypovolemic shock Condition in which there is a loss of blood, plasma, or water from the body, resulting in an inadequate volume of fluid in the circulatory system to maintain adequate perfusion.

Hypoxemia Lack of oxygen in the arterial blood.

Hypoxia A lack of oxygen available to the tissues.

Hypoxic drive Condition when low levels of oxygen in the blood become the breathing stimulus.

I

Ileum The last portion of the small intestine that connects with the cecum, which is the first part of the large intestine.

Immersion Covering of the face and airway by water or other fluid.

Immovable joint Type of joint that is joined by fibrous connective tissue and does not move; also called *fibrous joint*.

Immune system Specialized cells, tissues, and organs that protect the body against disease by distinguishing the body's healthy cells from pathogens and then killing the foreign invaders.

Impaled object An object that remains embedded in an open wound.

Impetigo A contagious bacterial skin infection that can look like a burn.

Implantable cardioverter-defibrillator (ICD) A surgically implanted device placed in a person who has had, or is at high risk of having, heart rhythm problems; the device is programmed to recognize heart rhythms that are too fast or life-threatening and to deliver a shock to reset the rhythm.

Implied consent Consent assumed from a patient requiring emergency care who is mentally, physically, or emotionally unable to provide expressed consent.

Incendiary materials Substances that burn with a hot flame for a specific period.

Incident Command System (ICS) A standardized system developed to assist with the control, direction, and coordination of emergency response resources at an incident of any type and size; also called the *incident management system (IMS)*.

Incident commander (IC) The person who is responsible for managing all operations during domestic incidents.

Incompetence A patient who does not have the ability to understand the questions asked or does not understand the implications of the decisions the patient makes regarding care.

Incomplete abortion An abortion in which part of the products of conception have been passed, but some remain in the uterus.

Incubation period The interval between exposure to a disease-causing agent and the appearance of signs and symptoms.

Index of suspicion Anticipating potential injuries based on the patient's chief complaint, mechanism of injury, and assessment findings. In the case of a medical patient, anticipating potential complications of an illness based on the patient's chief complaint, SAMPLE history, and assessment findings.

Indications The conditions for which a drug has documented usefulness.

Indwelling catheter A urinary catheter that remains in place for a long period of time; the most commonly used is the Foley catheter; also called a *retention catheter*.

Infancy Stage of human development from birth to 12 months.

Infarct Death of tissues due to ischemia.

Infection An illness that results when the body is invaded by germs capable of producing disease.

Inferior In a position lower than another.

Inferior vena cava One of the two major blood vessels of the abdomen.

Inflammation Tissue reaction to disease, injury, irritation, or infection; characterized by pain, heat, redness, swelling, and sometimes loss of function.

Inflammatory response A series of local cellular and vascular responses that are triggered when the body is injured or invaded by an antigen.

Informed consent A type of consent in which the patient understands the risks and benefits of the EMT's care.

Ingestion The process of taking nutrients, water, and electrolytes into the body's digestive system.

Inhalants Household and commercial products that can be abused by intentionally breathing the product's gas or vapors for its mind-altering effects. Inhalant use is called *huffing* or *sniffing*.

Inhalation The process of breathing in and moving air into the lungs; route of administration for drugs that are a gas or fine mist. Also called *inspiration*.

In-line stabilization A technique used to minimize movement of the head and neck.

Insertion Part of the muscle that is the movable attachment to a bone.

Inspiration See *inhalation*.

Insulin A hormone released from beta cells in the pancreas that helps glucose enter the body's cells to be used for energy.

Insulin resistance A condition in which the pancreas releases insulin, but the amount of insulin released is not enough to cause an effect in body cells.

Integrity Honesty, sincerity, and truthfulness.

Integumentary system The body system made up of the skin, hair, nails, sweat glands, and oil (sebaceous) glands.

Interagency Radio Advisory Committee (IRAC) The federal agency responsible for coordinating radio use by agencies of the federal government.

Intercostal muscles Muscles located between the ribs.

Intercostal retractions Indentations of the skin between the ribs.

Intermediate-level disinfection A method of decontamination that destroys tuberculosis bacteria, vegetative bacteria, and most viruses and fungi, but not bacterial spores. It is used for surfaces that contact intact skin and have been visibly contaminated with body fluids, such as blood pressure cuffs, stethoscopes, backboards, and splints.

Intermittent peritoneal dialysis (IPD) A type of peritoneal dialysis that uses the same type of machine as CCPD, but treatments take longer, sometimes lasting up to 24 hours; usually done in the hospital but can be done at home.

Internal bleeding Bleeding that occurs inside body tissues and cavities.

Intestinal obstruction A blockage of the large or small intestine that prevents food and fluid from passing through.

Intracellular fluid (ICF) Body fluids contained within the walls of the billions of body cells.

Intracerebral hematoma A collection of blood within the brain.

Intracerebral hemorrhage Bleeding within the brain caused by a ruptured blood vessel within the brain itself.

Intramuscular (IM) route   Injection of a liquid form of medication directly into a skeletal muscle.

Ipsilateral   Same side.

Irreversible shock   Stage of shock when the body's defense mechanisms have failed; permanent damage occurs to the vital organs because the cells and organs have been without oxygenated blood for too long; also called *terminal shock*.

Ischemia   Decreased blood flow to an organ or tissue.

Ischemic stroke   A stroke caused by a blood clot (thrombus) or embolus.

Islets of Langerhans   Structures located in the pancreas, which is a part of the endocrine system. Alpha cells secrete glucagon, which increases blood glucose concentration; beta cells secrete insulin, which decreases blood glucose concentration.

J

Jaundiced skin   Yellow skin suggestive of liver or gallbladder problems.

Jaw thrust maneuver   A preferred method for opening the airway of an unresponsive patient when trauma to the head or neck is suspected; also called the *jaw thrust without head tilt maneuver* or the *jaw thrust without head extension maneuver*.

Jejunum   The middle portion of the small intestine that connects the duodenum and ileum.

Joint   A place where two bones come together.

Jugular venous distention (JVD)   Distention (or bulging) of the neck veins when the patient is placed in a sitting position at a 45-degree angle.

K

Kehr's sign   Left upper quadrant pain that radiates to the left shoulder; suggests injury or rupture of the spleen or injury to the diaphragm.

Kidneys   Two organs located at the back of the abdominal cavity on each side of the spinal column that produce urine, maintain water balance, aid in the regulation of blood pressure, and regulate levels of many chemicals in the blood.

Kidney failure   A condition in which the kidneys fail to adequately remove wastes, concentrate urine, and conserve electrolytes to meet the demands of the body; also called *renal failure*.

Kidney stones   Hard masses that form in the kidney from crystallization of excreted substances in the urine; also called *renal calculi*.

Kinematics   The science of analyzing the mechanism of injury and predicting injury patterns.

Kinetic energy   The energy of motion.

Kussmaul respirations   A breathing pattern in which the patient breathes deeply and rapidly in an attempt to get rid of excess acid by "blowing off" carbon dioxide.

Kyphosis   Severely stooped posture.

L

Labia   Structures that protect the vagina and urethra but are prone to soft tissue injury.

Labia major   Parts of the labia that are located laterally.

Labia minora   Parts of the labia that are located more medially.

Labor   The process in which the uterus repeatedly contracts to push the fetus and placenta out of the mother's body; it begins with the first uterine muscle contraction and ends with delivery of the placenta.

Laceration   A cut or tear in the skin of any length, shape, and depth.

Lancet   A device used to prick a patient's skin to obtain a blood sample.

Landing zone (LZ)   A designated area to land a helicopter.

Large intestine (colon)   See *colon*.

Laryngeal stoma   Surgical opening in the neck.

Laryngectomy   The surgical removal of the larynx.

Laryngopharynx   The middle portion of the throat that opens into the mouth and serves as a passageway for both food and air.

Laryngospasm   Contraction of the sensitive tissue near the vocal cords.

Larynx   The voice box; the narrowest part of an adult's airway.

Late adulthood   Stage of human development from 61 years and up.

Late (decompensated) shock   Stage of shock when an ill or injured adult patient's systolic blood pressure drops to less than 90 mm Hg.

Lateral   Toward the side of the body.

Lateral recumbent position   Lying on the side. Left side is the left lateral recumbent position; right side is the right lateral recumbent position.

Left lower quadrant (LLQ)   Abdominal quadrant that along with the other three quadrants contains the intestines.

Left upper quadrant (LUQ)   Abdominal quadrant that contains the stomach, spleen, and pancreas.

Leukocytes   White blood cells; formed elements of blood.

Libel   To injure a person's character, name, or reputation by false or malicious writings.

Licensure   Receipt of a written authorization from an official or legal authority.

Ligaments   Tough groups of connective tissue that attach bones to bones and bones to cartilages.

Linear fracture   A fracture in which the break runs parallel to the long axis of the bone.

Liver   The largest internal organ of the body and one that is responsible for many functions, including the production of bile, the storage of minerals and fat-soluble vitamins, and the storage of blood.

Local cold injury   Tissue damage to a specific area of the body that occurs when a body part, such as the nose, ears, cheeks, chin, hands, or feet, is exposed to prolonged or intense cold; also called *frostbite*.

Local effect   An effect of a drug that usually occurs at the site of drug application.

Logroll   A technique used to move a patient from a facedown to a face-up position while maintaining the head and neck in line with the rest of the body.

Long backboard   A device that is 6 to 7 feet long and commonly made of wood, metal, or plastic, with holes spaced along the head and foot ends and the sides of the board for handholds and insertion of straps.

Lotion   A preparation applied to protect the skin or treat a skin disorder.

Low vision A visual impairment that interferes with a person's ability to perform everyday activities.

Lower extremities The pelvis, upper legs, lower legs, and feet.

Lower GI bleeding Bleeding from the small intestine, colon, or rectum.

Low-level disinfection A method of decontamination that destroys most bacteria, and some viruses and fungi, but not tuberculosis bacteria or bacterial spores. It is used for routine cleaning of surfaces, such as floors, countertops, and ambulance seats, when no body fluids are visible.

Lumen The space in the interior of an artery.

Lungs Spongy, air-filled organs that bring air into contact with the blood so that oxygen and carbon dioxide can be exchanged in the alveoli.

Luxation A complete dislocation.

Lymphatic system Lymph, lymph nodes, lymph vessels, tonsils, spleen, and thymus gland.

M

Macular degeneration Eye deterioration that includes shadowy areas in central vision, unusually fuzzy vision, objects that increase or decrease in size, and straight lines that appear bent; the leading cause of vision loss and legal blindness in Americans aged 65 and older.

Malignant tumor A cancerous tumor.

Mammalian diving reflex A reflex triggered by cold water stimulation of the temperature receptors in the skin that causes shunting of blood to the brain and heart from the skin, gastrointestinal tract, and extremities, resulting in slowing of the victim's heart rate in response to the increased volume of blood in the body's core.

Mammary glands (breasts) Glands in the female that function in milk production after delivery of an infant.

Manual defibrillator A machine that requires the rescuer to analyze and interpret the patient's cardiac rhythm before administering an electrical shock to the patient's heart.

Manubrium The uppermost portion of the breastbone. It connects with the clavicle and the first rib.

Mask-to-stoma breathing The delivery of a rescuer's exhaled air to a patient through a pocket mask that makes contact with a stoma.

Massive hemothorax A life-threatening injury that involves blood loss of more than 1,500 mL in the chest cavity.

Material safety data sheets (MSDSs) Papers required by the Occupational Safety and Health Administration to be kept on-site anywhere where chemicals are used. These sheets include the name of the substance, physical properties of the substance, fire and explosion hazard information, and guidelines for emergency first-aid treatment.

Mechanism of action Method by which a drug exerts its effect on body cells and tissues.

Mechanism of injury (MOI) Method by which an injury occurs, as well as the forces involved in producing the injury.

Meconium Thick, sticky material that collects in the intestines of a fetus and forms the first stools of a newborn. It is usually greenish to black in color.

Medial Anatomic directional term meaning toward the middle.

Mediastinal shift Shifting of the heart and major blood vessels from their normal position.

Mediastinum The part of the thoracic cavity between the lungs that contains the heart, major vessels, esophagus, trachea, and nerves.

Medical director A physician who provides medical oversight and is responsible for ensuring that actions taken on behalf of ill or injured people are medically appropriate.

Medical neglect A type of maltreatment characterized by failure of the caregiver to provide for the appropriate healthcare of the patient despite being financially able to do so.

Medical oversight The process by which a physician directs the emergency care provided by EMS personnel to an ill or injured patient; also referred to as *medical control* or *medical direction*.

Medical patient An individual whose condition is caused by an illness.

Medical practice acts State laws that grant authority to provide medical care to patients and determine the scope of practice for healthcare professionals.

Medication-induced headaches Headaches that result from overuse of medications or substances; also called *rebound headaches*.

Medulla oblongata A part of the brainstem that extends from the pons and is continuous with the upper portion of the spinal cord. It is involved in the regulation of heart rate, blood vessel diameter, respiration, coughing, swallowing, and vomiting.

Melatonin A naturally occurring hormone that has a role in regulating daily rhythms, such as sleep.

Melena Black, tarry stool that reflects partially digested blood from the upper GI tract.

Menarche The onset of menstruation; occurs in early adolescence.

Meninges Literally, membranes; three layers of connective tissue coverings that surround the brain and spinal cord.

Meningitis An inflammation of the membranes covering the brain and spinal cord.

Menopause The cessation of menstruation; occurs in middle adulthood.

Menstruation The periodic discharge of blood and tissue from the uterus; also called a *period*.

Message Information to be communicated.

Metabolism The chemical reactions that occur within a living organism that convert food to energy.

Metacarpals The bones that form the support for the palm of the hand.

Metastasis The spread of cancerous cells from their site of origin to sites elsewhere in the body.

Metatarsals The bones that form the part of the foot to which the toes attach.

Metered-dose inhaler (MDI) A drug delivery system used to inhale respiratory medications.

Midaxillary line An imaginary vertical line drawn from the middle of the armpits (axillae) parallel to the midline of the body.

Midbrain A part of the brainstem that acts as a relay for auditory and visual impulses.

Midclavicular line An imaginary vertical line drawn through the middle portion of the collarbone (clavicle) and nipple; parallel to the midline of the body.

Middle adulthood Stage of human development from 41 to 60 years.

Midline An imaginary line down the center of the body that divides the body into right and left sides.

Migraine headache Headache caused by changes in a major pain pathway in the nervous system and imbalances in brain chemicals; may be accompanied by nausea, vomiting, abdominal pain, or sensitivity to light.

Minimum data set The recommended minimum information that should be included in a prehospital care report.

Minor In most states, a child under the age of 18.

Minute volume The amount of air moved in and out of the lungs in 1 minute; the tidal volume multiplied by the respiratory rate.

Mitral (bicuspid) valve An atrioventricular valve located between the left atrium and the left ventricle.

Mobile data computer (MDC) A computer mounted in an emergency vehicle that displays information pertaining to the calls for which EMS personnel are dispatched.

Mobile two-way radio A vehicular-mounted communication device that usually transmits at a lower power than base stations.

Modifiable risk factors Risk factors that can be changed.

Modified chin lift A variation of the conventional head tilt–chin lift maneuver by which one rescuer stabilizes the patient's head and cervical spine in a neutral position to minimize movement and the second rescuer grasps the patient's chin and lower incisors with gloved fingers and then lifts to pull the lower jaw forward.

Modified jaw thrust maneuver A variation of the conventional jaw thrust where the patient's lower jaw is moved forward while the head and cervical spine are stabilized in a neutral position to minimize movement.

Mongolian spots Bluish areas usually seen in non-Caucasian infants and young children that may be mistaken for bruises.

Motor nerves Nerves that carry responses *from* the brain and spinal cord, stimulating a muscle or organ.

Mottling An irregular or patchy skin discoloration that is usually a mixture of blue and white; usually seen in patients in shock, with hypothermia, or in cardiac arrest.

Mouth-to-barrier device ventilation The delivery of a rescuer's exhaled air to a patient through a barrier device that makes contact with the patient's mouth.

Mouth-to-mask ventilation The delivery of a rescuer's exhaled air to a patient through a pocket mask that makes contact with the patient's mouth.

Multiple-casualty incident (MCI) Any event that places a great demand on resources—equipment, personnel, or both; also called a *mass-casualty incident* or *multiple-casualty situation* (MCS).

Multiplex system A mode of radio transmission that permits simultaneous transmission of voice and other data using one frequency.

Multisystem trauma Trauma from significant forces that affect more than one area of the body at the same time; also called *polytrauma*.

Muscle tone The constant tension produced by muscles of the body over long periods.

Myocardial contusion Bruising of the heart.

Myocardial infarction The process of heart muscle dying; also called a *heart attack*.

N

N-95 Mask that should be worn when you suspect that a patient has tuberculosis.

Narcotics Prescribed drugs used to relieve moderate to severe pain, control diarrhea, and suppress cough; include opium, opium derivatives, and man-made compounds that produce opiumlike effects.

Nasal airway A soft, rubbery tube with a hole in it that is placed in a patient's nose to keep the tongue from blocking the upper airway. Also called a *nasopharyngeal airway (NPA)*.

Nasal cannula An oxygen delivery device that consists of plastic tubing with two soft prongs that are inserted into the patient's nostrils and through which oxygen is delivered to the patient.

Nasal flaring Widening of the nostrils; a sign of increased breathing effort.

Nasopharyngeal airway (NPA) See *nasal airway*.

Nasopharynx The portion of the throat located directly behind the nasal cavity. It serves as a passageway for air only.

National EMS Education Standards A document that specifies the competencies, clinical behaviors, and judgments that each level of EMS professional must meet when completing his or her education.

National EMS Scope of Practice A document that defines four levels of EMS professionals and what each level of EMS professional legally can and cannot do.

Nature of the illness (NOI) The medical condition that resulted in the patient's call to 9-1-1.

Navel (umbilicus) Pit in the center of the abdomen where the umbilical cord entered the fetus.

Near syncope See *presyncope*.

Neglect Failure to provide for a patient's basic needs.

Negligence A deviation from the accepted standard of care, resulting in further injury to the patient.

Nerve agents Chemical weapons that interrupt nerve signals, causing a loss of consciousness within seconds and death within minutes of exposure.

Nervous system A collection of specialized cells that conduct information to and from the brain.

Neurogenic shock Type of distributive shock that causes loss of nervous system control.

Neurons Cells of the nervous system.

Nitroglycerin (NTG) A medication that is used to treat chest discomfort that is believed to be cardiac in origin; it causes dilation of the smooth muscle of blood vessel walls.

Noise Anything that obscures, confuses, or interferes with communication.

Nonallergic asthma Asthma that is triggered by factors not related to allergies.

Nonmodifiable risk factors Risk factors that cannot be changed.

Nonrebreather (NRB) mask An oxygen delivery device with a reservoir that is designed to deliver high-concentration oxygen.

Nonurgent move A method used to move, lift, or carry patients with no known or suspected injury to the head, neck, spine, or extremities.

O

Objective findings A medical or trauma condition of the patient that can be seen, heard, smelled, measured, or felt; also called *signs* or *clinical findings.*

Oblique fracture Fracture in which the break is at about a 45-degree angle to the bone.

Obsessions Recurring thoughts, impulses, or images that cause the person anxiety.

Obsessive-compulsive disorder (OCD) A type of anxiety disorder in which recurring thoughts, impulses, or images cause a person anxiety, which causes the individual to perform recurring behaviors or rituals with the hope of preventing obsessive thoughts or making them go away.

Obstetric emergency An emergency related to pregnancy or childbirth.

Obstructive shock Shock that occurs when blood flow to an organ is slowed or stopped by a mechanical or physical obstruction.

Occlusive Airtight.

Occupational Safety and Health Administration (OSHA) A branch of the U.S federal government responsible for safety in the workplace.

Off-line medical direction Medical supervision of EMS personnel through use of policies, protocols, standing orders, education, and quality management review; also called *indirect, retrospective,* or *prospective medical direction.*

Olecranon The elbow.

Onboard oxygen Large oxygen cylinders carried on an ambulance.

On-line medical direction Direct communication with a physician (or a designee) by radio, telephone, or face-to-face communication at the scene, before a skill is performed or care is given.

Open crush injury A crush injury where broken bone ends may stick out through the skin.

Open fracture See *compound fracture.*

Open pneumothorax The entry of air through an open wound in the chest wall into the pleural cavity; also called a *sucking chest wound.*

Open soft tissue injury A soft tissue injury in which a break occurs in the skin.

Open wound An injury in which the skin surface is broken.

Open-ended questions Questions that require a patient to answer with more than a yes or no, such as, "What is troubling you today?"

OPQRST Memory aid used to help identify the type and location of a patient's complaint: **o**nset, **p**rovocation/palliation/position, **q**uality, **r**egion/radiation, **s**everity, and **t**ime.

Oral airway A curved device made of rigid plastic that is inserted into a patient's mouth and used to keep the tongue away from the back of the throat.

Oral glucose The basic fuel for body cells; may be administered to a patient who has an altered mental status and a history of diabetes controlled by medication and is able to swallow.

Organ Body part that has at least two different types of tissue working together to perform a particular function; examples include the brain, stomach, and liver.

Organ system Tissues and organs that work together to provide a common function; examples of organ systems include the respiratory system and the nervous system.

Organic headaches Headaches that are the result of an abnormality in the brain or skull; also called *structural headaches.*

Origin The stationary attachment of a skeletal muscle to a bone.

Oropharyngeal airway (OPA) A curved device made of rigid plastic that is inserted into a patient's mouth and used to keep the tongue away from the back of the throat.

Oropharynx The middle portion of the throat that opens into the mouth and serves as a passageway for both food and air.

Orthopnea Breathlessness when lying flat that is relieved or lessened when the patient sits or stands.

Osteoarthritis (OA) A chronic condition characterized by the breakdown of the joint's cartilage; also called *degenerative arthritis* or *degenerative joint disease.*

Osteoporosis A condition that develops when the rate of old bone removal occurs too quickly or when old bone replacement occurs too slowly, resulting in bones that are brittle and tend to break easily.

Ovarian cyst A fluid-filled sac that develops on or within an ovary.

Ovaries Paired, almond-shaped organs in a woman's body that produce eggs; located on either side of the uterus in the pelvic cavity.

Overdose An intentional or unintentional overmedication or ingestion of a toxic substance.

Overuse syndromes A group of conditions in which a part of the body is injured from repeated motions performed in the course of normal work or daily activities; other terms used to describe overuse syndromes include *cumulative trauma disorder, occupational overuse syndrome, overuse disorder, overuse strain, repetitive motion disorders, repetitive strain injury,* and *repetitive stress injury.*

Ovulation Release of an egg from an ovary.

Oxygen A molecule that is needed for body metabolism; it is considered a drug when administered by an EMR.

Oxygen saturation A relative measure of the percentage of hemoglobin bound to oxygen.

Oxygenation The process of loading oxygen molecules onto hemoglobin molecules in the bloodstream.

P

Pack-strap carry A move in which the rescuer kneels in front of a seated patient with the rescuer's back to the patient. The patient's arms are placed over the rescuer's shoulders and crossed over the rescuer's chest. The rescuer grasps the patient's wrists, leans forward, rises up on his knees, and pulls the patient up onto the rescuer's back.

Palliative care Care provided to relieve symptoms of disease, such as pain, nausea and vomiting, rather than to cure the disease; usually provided for patients with a terminal illness and their families; also called *comfort care.*

Palpitations An abnormal awareness of one's heartbeat.

Pancreas A gland that secretes juices that contain enzymes for protein, carbohydrate, and fat digestion into the small intestine.

Pancreatitis Inflammation of the pancreas; usually caused by gallstones and excessive alcohol use.

Panic attack An intense fear that occurs for no apparent reason.

Paradoxical chest movement Movement of a segment of the chest wall in an opposite direction from the rest of the chest during respiration.

Paramedic Highest level of prehospital professional. Can perform skills of an advanced EMT plus has additional training in pathophysiology, physical exam techniques, assessment of abnormal heart rhythms, and invasive procedures.

Paranoia A mental disorder characterized by excessive suspiciousness or delusions.

Paraplegia A loss of movement and sensation of the lower half of the body from the waist down.

Parasympathetic division The division of the autonomic nervous system that conserves and restores energy. It provides the "rest and digest" response.

Parathyroid glands Glands located behind the thyroid gland that secrete a hormone that maintains the calcium level in the blood.

Parenteral Route of administration for drugs that does not pass through the digestive tract; drugs given this way are injected, inhaled, or infused.

Paresthesias Abnormal sensations, such as tingling, burning, numbness, or a pins-and-needles feeling.

Parietal pleura The outer pleural lining that lines the wall of the thoracic cavity.

Paroxysmal nocturnal dyspnea (PND) A sudden onset of difficulty breathing that occurs at night because of a buildup of fluid in the alveoli or pooling of secretions during sleep.

Partial rebreather mask An oxygen delivery device that has an attached reservoir bag that is filled with oxygen before patient use.

Partial seizure A category of seizures in which nerve cells fire abnormally in one hemisphere of the brain; this category of seizures includes simple partial seizures and complex partial seizures.

Partial-thickness burn A burn that involves the epidermis and dermis; also called a *second-degree burn.*

Passive rewarming Warming of a patient with minimal or no use of heat sources other than the patient's own heat production; methods include placing the patient in a warm environment, applying clothing and blankets, and preventing drafts.

Patella The flat, triangular, movable bone that forms the anterior part of the knee; the kneecap.

Patent Open.

Pathogenesis The mechanism by which a disease develops.

Pathogens Germs capable of producing disease, such as bacteria and viruses.

Pathology The study of disease.

Pathophysiology The study of the physical, chemical, and mechanical processes that are caused by disease or injury.

Patient assessment The process of evaluating a person for signs of illness or injury.

Patient history The part of the patient assessment that provides pertinent facts about the patient's current medical problem and medical history.

Pelvic cavity The body cavity below the abdominal cavity. It contains the urinary bladder, part of the large intestine, and the reproductive organs.

Pelvic girdle The bones that enclose and protect the organs of the pelvic cavity. It provides a point of attachment for the lower extremities and major muscles of the trunk and supports the weight of the upper body.

Pelvic inflammatory disease (PID) An infection of the uterus, fallopian tubes, and other female reproductive organs.

Pelvis The bony ring formed by three separate bones that fuse to become one in an adult.

Penetrating chest injury A break in the skin over the chest wall.

Penetrating trauma Any mechanism of injury that causes a cut or piercing of the skin.

Penis The male external organ that serves as the outlet for sperm and urine.

Peptic ulcer An open sore in the lining of the stomach (gastric ulcer), duodenum (duodenal ulcer), or esophagus (esophageal ulcer).

Perfusion The flow of blood through the body's tissues.

Pericardial cavity The body cavity containing the heart.

Perineum Area between the vaginal opening and anus.

Peripheral artery disease (PAD) Atherosclerosis that affects the arteries that supply the arms, legs, and feet.

Peripheral chemoreceptors Sensory receptors located in the carotid arteries and arch of the aorta that monitor changes in carbon dioxide and oxygen levels.

Peripheral nervous system (PNS) All nervous tissue found outside the brain and spinal cord.

Peripheral pulse Pulse located far from the heart, such as radial, brachial, posterior, tibial, and dorsal pedis pulses.

Peripheral vascular resistance (PVR) The opposition that blood encounters in the blood vessels as it travels away from the heart.

Peripherally inserted central catheter (PICC) An intravenous line often used for patients requiring only short-term IV therapy for the delivery of medications and nutritional solutions directly into the venous circulation.

Peristalsis The involuntary wavelike contraction of smooth muscle that moves material through the digestive tract.

Peritoneal cavity A potential space between two membranes that line the abdominal cavity, separating the abdominal organs from the abdominal wall.

Peritoneal dialysis Removal of waste products and excess water and minerals from the blood using the lining of the abdomen as the filter.

Peritoneum A smooth, transparent membrane that lines the abdominal cavity.

Peritonitis Inflammation of the abdominal lining.

Personal protective equipment (PPE) Eye protection, protective gloves, gowns, and masks.

Personal space The invisible area immediately around each of us that we feel is our own.

Pertinent negative A finding expected to accompany a patient's chief complaint but not found during the patient assessment.

Pertinent positive A finding expected to accompany a patient's chief complaint that is found during the patient assessment.

Pertussis A highly contagious bacterial infection of the respiratory tract; also called *whooping cough*.

Phalanges The bones of the fingers and toes.

Pharmacodynamics The study of the effects of drugs and their mechanisms of action at target sites in the body.

Pharmacology The study of drugs or medications and their effect on living systems.

Pharynx The throat; a funnel-shaped muscular tube that serves as a passageway for food, liquids, and air.

Phobia An irrational and constant fear of a specific activity, object, or situation (other than a social situation).

Physical abuse Acts that cause or could cause physical injury to an individual.

Physical examination A head-to-toe assessment of the patient's entire body.

Physician Orders for Life-Sustaining Treatment (POLST) Program for individuals with advanced chronic, progressive illness or terminal illness that further defines their end-of-life care wishes; POLSTs do not replace advance directives.

Physiology The study of the normal functions of an organism (such as the human body).

Pia mater Literally, "gentle mother"; delicate inner layer of the meninges that clings gently to the brain and spinal cord; it contains many blood vessels that supply the nervous tissue.

Piggyback carry A move in which the rescuer kneels in front of a seated patient with the rescuer's back to the patient. The patient's arms are placed over the rescuer's shoulders and crossed over the rescuer's chest. The rescuer grasps the patient's wrists, leans forward, rises up on her knees, and pulls the patient up onto the rescuer's back. The rescuer's forearms are positioned under the patient's knees and the patient's wrists are grasped while the patient is carried to safety.

Pineal gland A small gland located near the center of the brain that is responsible for producing the hormone melatonin.

Pituitary gland A small gland located just beneath the hypothalamus in the brain that regulates growth and controls other endocrine glands; the "master gland" of the body.

Placenta A specialized organ through which the fetus exchanges nourishment and waste products during pregnancy; also called *afterbirth*.

Placenta previa A condition that occurs when part or all of the placenta implants in the lower part of the uterus, covering the opening of the cervix.

Plaintiff A person or party that files a formal complaint with the court.

Plasma The liquid portion of the blood.

Platelets Thrombocytes, which are essential for the formation of blood clots. They function to stop bleeding and repair ruptured blood vessels.

Pleurae Serous (oily), double-walled membranes that enclose each lung.

Pleural cavities The body cavities containing the lungs; the right lung is located in the right pleural cavity, and the left lung is located in the left pleural cavity.

Pleural space A space between the visceral and parietal pleura, filled with a small amount of oily fluid, that allows the lungs to glide easily against each other.

Pneumatic antishock garment (PASG) A device that can be used as a pressure splint to help control suspected severe bleeding in the abdomen or pelvis that is accompanied by hypotension; also called *military antishock trousers (MAST)*.

Pneumatic splint One that requires air to be pumped in or suctioned out of it.

Pneumonia A respiratory infection that may involve the lower airways and alveoli, part of a lobe, or an entire lobe of the lung.

Pneumothorax A buildup of air between the outer lining of the lung and the chest wall, causing a complete or partial collapse of the lung.

Pocket mask A piece of equipment used for mouth-to-mask ventilation that provides a physical barrier between the rescuer and the patient's nose, mouth, and secretions; also called a *pocket face mask, ventilation face mask,* or *resuscitation mask*.

Poison Any substance taken into the body that interferes with normal body function.

Poison control center (PCC) A medical facility that provides free telephone advice to the public and medical professionals in case of exposure to poisonous substances.

Poisoning Exposure to a substance that is harmful in any dosage.

Polydipsia Increased thirst.

Polyphagia Increased appetite.

Polypharmacy The use of multiple medications, often prescribed by different doctors, which can cause adverse reactions in the patient.

Polyuria Increased urination.

Pons Literally, "bridge"; a part of the brainstem that connects parts of the brain with one another by means of tracts and that influences respiration.

Portable radio A handheld communication device used for radio communication away from the emergency vehicle.

Position of function The natural position of the hand or foot at rest.

Positive-pressure ventilation Forcing air into a patient's lungs.

Posterior The back side of the body or body part.

Postictal phase The period after a seizure; during this recovery period, pediatric patients often appear limp, have shallow breathing, and have an altered mental status.

Postpartum hemorrhage Condition when a new mother hemorrhages greater than 500 mL following delivery.

Postterm pregnancy Pregnancy that lasts longer than 42 weeks; also called *prolonged pregnancy*.

Pott's fracture A fracture of the lower part of the fibula with displacement of the foot.

Powder Drug ground into fine particles.

Power grip (underhand grip) A method of placing one's hands on an object that is designed to take full advantage of the strength of the rescuer's hands and forearms.

Power lift A technique used to lift a heavy object.

Pralidoxime chloride (2-PAM) An antidote that is given in conjunction with atropine in cases of nerve agent poisoning.

Precipitous labor Labor that lasts less than 3 hours from the start of contractions to delivery.

Preeclampsia A condition of high blood pressure and swelling that occurs in some women during the third trimester of pregnancy; also called *pregnancy-induced hypertension* or *toxemia of pregnancy*.

Prehospital care report (PCR)   Documentation of the emergency care provided and the patient's response to it.

Prehypertension   Condition that exists when the systolic blood pressure is between 120 and 139 or the diastolic blood pressure is between 80 and 89 on multiple readings.

Premature infant   An infant born before the 37th week of gestation or weighing less than 5.5 pounds (2.5 kilograms); also called a *preemie.*

Premature rupture of the membranes (PROM)   When the rupture of the amniotic sac occurs before the onset of labor.

Presbycusis   Hearing loss because of aging; it is progressive, occurring gradually over a period of years.

Preschooler   Stage of human development from 3 to 5 years.

Presenting part   The part of an infant that emerges first during delivery.

Pressure bandage   A bandage with which enough pressure is applied over a wound site to control bleeding.

Pressure regulator   A device used to reduce pressure in an oxygen cylinder to a safe range, allowing the release of oxygen from the cylinder in a controlled manner.

Pressure splint   An air splint that acts as a pressure bandage, applying even pressure to the entire arm or leg; also called an *air* or *pneumatic splint.*

Presyncope   Warning symptoms of an impending loss of consciousness; also called *near syncope.*

Preterm labor   Labor before a woman's 37th week of pregnancy; also called *premature labor.*

Primary hypertension   Hypertension that has no identifiable cause.

Primary spontaneous pneumothorax   A spontaneous pneumothorax that occurs in people with no history of lung disease; most commonly occurs in tall, thin men between the ages of 20 and 40.

Primary survey   A rapid assessment of the patient to find and care for immediate life-threatening conditions.

Prolapsed cord   During childbirth, the portion of the umbilical cord that falls down below the presenting part of the fetus and presents through the birth canal before delivery of the head.

Prone   Facedown.

Prospective medical direction   Activities performed by a physician medical director before an emergency call.

Prostate gland   In the male, a gland that secretes fluid that enhances sperm motility and neutralizes the acidity of the vagina during intercourse.

Protected health information (PHI)   Information that relates to a person's physical or mental health, treatment, or payment that identifies the person or gives a reason to believe that the individual can be identified and that is transmitted or maintained in any form.

Protocols   Written instructions to provide emergency care for specific health-related conditions.

Proximal   Closer to the midline or center area of the body.

Proximate cause   Actions or inactions of the healthcare professional that caused the injury or damages.

Pruritus   An itch.

Psychogenic shock   Type of distributive shock due to psychological causes.

Public health   The science and practice of protecting and improving the health of the community as a whole.

Public safety answering point (PSAP)   A facility equipped and staffed to receive and control 9-1-1 access calls.

Pulmonary contusion   Bruising of the lung.

Pulmonary edema   A buildup of fluid in the alveoli, most commonly caused by failure of the left ventricle of the heart.

Pulmonary embolus   A clot that travels through the circulatory system, eventually becoming trapped in the smaller branches of the pulmonary arteries, causing partial or complete blood-flow obstruction.

Pulmonic valve   A semilunar valve located at the junction of the right ventricle and the pulmonary artery.

Pulse   The regular expansion and recoil of an artery caused by the movement of blood from the heart as it contracts.

Pulse oximeter   A machine that measures oxygen saturation.

Pulse oximetry   A method of measuring the amount of oxygen saturated in the blood; commonly referred to as *pulse ox.*

Puncture wound   Piercing of the skin with a pointed object, such as a nail, pencil, ice pick, splinter, piece of glass, bullet, or a knife, resulting in little or no external bleeding (internal bleeding may be severe); also called a *penetration wound.*

Putrefaction   The decomposition of organic matter, such as body tissues.

Pyelonephritis   An infection of the kidney that is often the result of a bacterial bladder infection and a backflow of urine from the bladder into the ureters or kidney.

Q

Quadriplegia   Loss of movement and sensation in both arms, both legs, and the parts of the body below an area of injury to the spinal cord; also called *tetraplegia.*

Quality management   A system of internal and external reviews and audits of all aspects of an EMS system.

R

Raccoon eyes   Bilateral bluish discoloration (ecchymosis) around the eyes that suggests a possible skull fracture.

Radiation   The transfer of heat, as infrared heat rays, from the surface of one object to the surface of another without contact between the two objects.

Radius   The bone on the thumb (lateral) side of the forearm.

Rapid medical assessment   A quick head-to-toe assessment of a medical patient who is unresponsive or has an altered mental status.

Rapid trauma assessment   A quick head-to-toe assessment of a trauma patient with a significant mechanism of injury.

Reactive airway disease (RAD)   See *asthma.*

Reasonable force   The amount of force necessary to keep a patient from injuring you, himself, or others.

Reassessment   The process of reevaluating a patient's condition to assess the effectiveness of the emergency care provided, identify any missed injuries or conditions, observe subtle changes or trends in the patient's condition, and alter emergency care as needed.

Rebound headaches   See *medication-induced headaches.*

Receiver   The person or group for whom a sender's message is intended.

Recovery position   Placement of an unresponsive patient who is breathing and in no need of CPR (and in whom trauma is not suspected) on the patient's side to help keep the airway open.

Rectum The lower part of the large intestine, about 5 inches long, between the sigmoid colon and the anal canal.

Referred pain Pain that is felt in a part of the body that is away from the tissues or organ that causes the pain.

Regression A return to an earlier or former developmental state.

Renal calculi See *kidney stones.*

Renal failure See *kidney failure.*

Repeater A device that receives a transmission from a low-power portable or mobile radio on one frequency and then retransmits it at a higher power on another frequency so that it can be received at a distant location.

Reproductive system Organs that make cells (sperm, eggs) that allow continuation of the human species.

Residual volume The amount of air left in the lungs after maximal expiration.

Respiration The act of breathing air into the lungs (inhalation) and out of the lungs (exhalation); the exchange of gases between a living organism and its environment.

Respiratory arrest An absence of breathing.

Respiratory distress Increased work of breathing (respiratory effort).

Respiratory failure Inadequate blood oxygenation and/or ventilation to meet the demands of body tissues.

Respiratory system System that supplies oxygen from the air we breathe to the body's cells and transports carbon dioxide to the lungs for removal from the body.

Retention catheter See *indwelling catheter.*

Reticular formation A complex network of nerve fibers located throughout the medulla, pons, and midbrain that connect with nerve fibers of other structures, including the hypothalamus, cerebellum, and cerebrum.

Retractions Soft tissues that "sink in" between and around the ribs or above the collarbones.

Retroperitoneal space The area behind the peritoneum. Also called the *retroperitoneum.*

Retroperitoneum See *retroperitoneal space.*

Retrospective medical direction Activities performed by a physician after an emergency call.

Revised trauma score (RTS) A scoring system used to predict the likelihood of serious injury or death following trauma; it is calculated from a combination of results from three categories: respiratory rate, systolic blood pressure, and Glasgow Coma Scale.

Rheumatoid arthritis Type of arthritis in which the lining of the joints is inflamed.

Rhonchi Abnormal breath sounds produced when air flows through passages narrowed by mucus or fluid.

Rickettsias Very small bacteria that require a living host to survive.

Right lower quadrant (RLQ) Abdominal quadrant that contains the appendix.

Right upper quadrant (RUQ) Abdominal quadrant that contains the liver, gall bladder, portions of the stomach, and major blood vessels.

Rigor mortis Stiffening of body muscles that occurs after death.

Risk factors Conditions that may increase a person's chance of developing a disease.

Route of administration The route and form in which a drug should be given to the patient.

Rule of nines A guide used to estimate the affected body surface area of a burn that divides the body into sections in multiples of 9%.

Rule of palms A guide used to estimate the affected body surface area for small or irregularly shaped burns, or burns that are scattered over the patient's body, using the palm of the *patient's* hand to equal 1% of the patient's BSA.

Ruptured uterus Uterus tear that can result from strong labor for a long period or from abdominal trauma.

S

Safe zone An identified safety zone at a hazardous materials incident that is an area safe from the exposure or the threat of exposure and that serves as the staging area for personnel and equipment; also called the *cold zone* or *support zone.*

Sagittal plane The vertical field that passes through the body from front to back, dividing the body (or any of its parts) into right and left sections.

SAMPLE Memory aid used to standardize the approach to history taking: **s**igns and symptoms, **a**llergies, **m**edication, **p**ast medical history, **l**ast oral intake, and **e**vents leading to the injury or illness.

Saturation of peripheral oxygen (SpO₂) The amount of hemoglobin saturated with oxygen.

Scalp The outermost part of the head that contains tissue, hair follicles, sweat glands, oil glands, and a rich supply of blood vessels.

Scene safety An assessment of the entire scene and surroundings to ensure your well-being and that of other rescuers, the patient(s), and bystanders.

Scene size-up The first phase of patient assessment that includes taking standard precautions, evaluating scene safety, determining the mechanism of injury or nature of the patient's illness, determining the total number of patients, and determining the need for additional resources.

Schizophrenia A group of mental disorders characterized by hallucinations, delusions, disordered thinking, and bizarre or disorganized behavior.

School-age Stage of human development from 6 to 12 years.

Scoop (orthopedic) stretcher A patient-transfer device made of metal and consisting of four sections: two sections support the upper body, and two sections support the lower body. In the absence of spinal injury, the scoop stretcher may be used to carry a supine patient up or down stairs or in other confined spaces; also called a *split litter.*

Scope of practice State laws that detail the medical procedures and functions that can be legally performed by a licensed or certified healthcare professional

Scrotum A loose sac of skin that houses the male testes.

Secondary hypertension Hypertension that has an identifiable cause.

Secondary spontaneous pneumothorax A spontaneous pneumothorax that most often occurs as a complication of lung disease.

Secondary survey A full body assessment performed to discover medical conditions and/or injuries that are not immediately life-threatening but may become so if left untreated. In addition to a head-to-toe (or focused) assessment, it includes obtaining vital signs, reassessing changes in the patient's condition, and determining the patient's chief complaint, history of present illness, and significant past medical history.

Seesaw breathing Abnormal breathing in which the abdominal muscles move in a direction opposite the chest wall.

Seizure A temporary change in behavior or consciousness caused by abnormal electrical activity within one or more groups of brain cells.

Semiautomated external defibrillator (SAED) A type of defibrillator that "advises" the rescuer of the steps to take based on its analysis of the patient's heart rhythm by means of a voice or visual message; also called a *shock-advisory defibrillator.*

Semi-Fowler's position A position in which a patient sits up with her head at a 45-degree angle and her legs out straight.

Semilunar valves Heart valves shaped like half-moons.

Seminal vesicles Accessory glands in the male that secrete fluid that nourishes and protects sperm.

Semisynthetic drugs Naturally occurring substances that have been chemically altered, such as antibiotics.

Sensitization The production of antibodies in response to the body's first exposure to an antigen.

Sensory nerves Nerves that send signals *to* the brain about the activities of the different parts of the body relative to their surroundings.

Septic shock Type of distributive shock that occurs because of a massive infection.

Septum A wall between two cavities.

Sexual abuse Inappropriate adolescent or adult sexual behavior with a child; it includes fondling, rape, and exposing a child to other sexual activities.

Sexually transmitted diseases (STDs) Infections that are spread by either blood or sexual contact.

Shaken baby syndrome A group of signs and symptoms that result from violent shaking or shaking and impacting of the head of an infant or small child; also called *abusive head trauma.*

Shock See *hypoperfusion.*

Short backboard A device made of wood, aluminum, or plastic that is 3 to 4 feet long and serves as an intermediate device for stabilizing the spine of a stable patient found in a seated position. It must be used in conjunction with a long backboard for full spinal stabilization; also called a *half board.*

Shoulder drag Emergency move in which the rescuer's hands are positioned under the patient's armpits and the patient is dragged to safety.

Shoulder girdle The bony arch formed by the collarbones (clavicles) and shoulder blades (scapulae).

Sickle cell anemia Condition in patients with sickle cell disease that occurs because the bone marrow is unable to produce new red blood cells fast enough to replace the dying ones, causing a lower-than-normal number of red blood cells in the body.

Sickle cell crisis Condition by which clumps of sickled cells build up in the blood vessels, blocking blood flow to organs and limbs; impaired circulation causes pain, swelling, infection, and organ damage and death.

Sickle cell disease An inherited disorder that affects red blood cells.

Sigmoid colon The lower part of the descending colon between the iliac crest and the rectum, shaped like the letter S.

Signs See *objective findings.*

Simple extrication The use of hand tools in order to gain access and extricate the patient from the vehicle.

Simple partial seizure A type of partial seizure that involves motor or sensory symptoms with no change in mental status; also called a *focal seizure* or *focal motor seizure.*

Simple pneumothorax A condition in which air enters the chest cavity causing a loss of negative pressure (vacuum) and a partial or total collapse of the lung.

Simplex system A mode of radio transmission that uses a single frequency to transmit and receive messages.

Sinus headache Headache triggered by pressure in the sinuses.

Sinuses Spaces or cavities inside some cranial bones.

Skeletal muscles Voluntary muscles. Most skeletal muscles are attached to bones.

Skeletal system The 206 bones of the body along with the cartilages.

Skull The bony skeleton of the head that protects the brain from injury and gives the head its shape.

Slander To injure a person's character, name, or reputation by false and maliciously spoken words.

Small intestine The portion of the digestive system between the stomach and the beginning of the large intestine that consists of three parts: the duodenum, the jejunum, and the ileum. It receives food from the stomach, secretions from the pancreas and liver, and completes the digestion of food that began in the mouth and stomach.

Smooth (involuntary) muscle An involuntary muscle found in many internal organs (except the heart).

Snoring A loud breathing sound that suggests the upper airway is partially blocked by the tongue.

SOAP Method of documentation that includes subjective findings, objective findings, assessment, and plan.

Social phobia An extreme anxiety response in situations in which the individual may be seen by others and caused by the individual's fear of acting in an embarrassing or shameful manner.

Soft palate The fleshy portion of the nasal cavity that extends behind the hard palate. It marks the boundary between the nasopharynx and the rest of the pharynx.

Soft tissues Layers of the skin and the fat and muscle beneath them.

Solid organs Liver, spleen, and kidneys, for example; solid organs bleed when injured.

Solution Liquid preparation of one or more chemical substances, usually dissolved in water.

Somatic division The voluntary division of the peripheral nervous system that has receptors and nerves concerned with the external environment.

Somatostatin A hormone released by delta cells in the pancreas that inhibits the release of insulin and glucagon.

Sphygmomanometer A device used to take a blood pressure.

Spinal cavity The body cavity that extends from the bottom of the skull to the lower back and contains the spinal cord.

Spinal cord Nervous tissue that extends from the base of the skull to down the back and is responsible for relaying electrical signals to and from the brain and peripheral nerves.

Spinal nerves Any of 31 pairs of nerves that branch from the spinal cord.

Spinal precautions Precautions made to stabilize the head, neck, and back in a neutral position to prevent movement that could cause injury to the spinal cord.

Spine (vertebral column) The 32 to 33 vertebrae that enclose the spinal cord and provide rigidity to the body.

Spiral fracture A bone break caused by a twisting motion; usually occurs in the long bones of the body, such as the humerus and femur.

Spirit Volatile substance dissolved in alcohol.

Splenic crisis A condition in which sickled red blood cells become trapped in the spleen, causing a significant fall in the amount of red blood cells and hemoglobin circulating in the bloodstream; this condition is a leading cause of death in children with sickle cell disease.

Splint A device used to limit the movement of an injured arm or leg and reduce bleeding and discomfort.

Spontaneous abortion The loss of a fetus due to natural causes before the 20th week of pregnancy; also called *miscarriage.*

Spontaneous pneumothorax A type of pneumothorax that does not involve trauma to the lung.

Sprain The stretching or tearing of a ligament.

Stabilization The process of rendering a vehicle motionless in the position in which it is found.

Stable angina pectoris Angina pectoris that is relatively constant and predictable in terms of severity, signs and symptoms, precipitating events, and the patient's response to therapy.

Staging Waiting for further instructions at a safe distance at an emergency scene.

Stair chair A commercially made patient-transfer device designed for patients who can assume a sitting position while being carried to an ambulance. The stair chair is useful for moving patients up or down stairs, through narrow corridors and doorways, into small elevators, and in narrow aisles in aircraft or buses.

Standard of care The minimum level of care expected of similarly trained healthcare professionals.

Standard precautions Self-protection against all body fluids and substances; also referred to as *body substance isolation (BSI) precautions* and *universal precautions.*

Standing orders Written orders that allow EMS personnel to perform certain medical procedures before making direct contact with a physician.

START triage system A nationally recognized method of sorting patients by the severity of their illness or injury; START is an acronym for **s**imple **t**riage **a**nd **r**apid **t**reatment.

Status epilepticus Recurring seizures without an intervening period of consciousness.

Statute of limitations The maximum period within which a plaintiff must begin a lawsuit or a prosecutor must bring charges or lose the right to file the suit.

Statutes Laws established by Congress and state legislatures.

Stent A small plastic or metal tube that is inserted into a vessel or duct to help keep it open and maintain fluid flow through it.

Sterilization A method of decontamination that destroys all microorganisms, including highly resistant bacterial spores. It is used for instruments that penetrate the skin or contact normally sterile areas of the body during invasive procedures.

Sterilizing A process that uses boiling water, radiation, gas, chemicals, or superheated steam to destroy all the germs on an object.

Sternum (breastbone) Bone in the middle of the thorax and consisting of three sections: manubrium, body, and xiphoid process.

Stethoscope An instrument used to hear sounds within the body, such as respirations.

Stoma An artificial opening.

Straight catheter Type of urinary catheter used to drain urine when a patient is temporarily unable to urinate or to obtain a urine specimen; it has no balloon to inflate and no drainage bag.

Strain Condition that results from the twisting, pulling, or tearing of a muscle.

Stress A chemical, physical, or emotional factor that causes bodily or mental tension.

Stressor Any event or condition that has the potential to cause bodily or mental tension.

Stridor A harsh, high-pitched sound that suggests the upper airway is partially blocked.

Stroke An interruption of the blood supply in the brain caused by blockage or rupture of an artery; also called a *cerebrovascular accident (CVA)* or *brain attack.*

Stroke volume The amount of blood ejected by the ventricles of the heart with each contraction.

Subarachnoid hemorrhage Bleeding in the brain caused by a ruptured blood vessel in the subarachnoid space in the brain.

Subcostal retractions Indentations of the skin below the rib cage.

Subcutaneous emphysema Air trapped beneath the skin; a crackling sensation under the fingers that suggests laceration of a lung and the leakage of air into the pleural space.

Subcutaneous layer The thick skin layer that lies below the dermis and is loosely attached to the muscles and bones of the musculoskeletal system.

Subcutaneous (SubQ) route Injection of a liquid form of medication underneath the skin into the subcutaneous tissue.

Subdural hematoma A buildup of blood in the space between the dura and the arachnoid layer of the meninges that usually results from tearing of veins located between the dura and the cerebral cortex after an injury to the head.

Subjective findings See *symptoms.*

Sublingual Medication given under the tongue.

Subluxation A partial dislocation.

Submersion An incident in which the victim's entire body, including the airway, is under the water or other fluid.

Substance abuse The deliberate, persistent, and excessive self-administration of a substance in a way that is not medically or socially approved.

Substance misuse The self-administration of a substance for unintended purposes or for appropriate purposes but in improper amounts or doses, or without a prescription for the person receiving the medication.

Sucking chest wound A chest injury in which air moves into the pleural cavity through an open chest wound, creating a sucking or gurgling sound when air escapes from the wound when the patient breathes in.

Suctioning A procedure used to vacuum vomitus, saliva, blood, food particles, and other material from a patient's airway.

Sudden cardiac death SCD) Unexpected death from cardiac causes early after symptom onset (immediately or within 1 hour) or without the onset of symptoms.

Sudden infant death syndrome (SIDS) The sudden and unexpected death of an infant that remains unexplained after a thorough case investigation, including performance of a complete autopsy, examination of the death scene, and review of the clinical history.

Sudden sniffing death syndrome (SSDS) A condition that can occur when a person sniffs highly concentrated amounts of the chemicals in solvents or aerosol sprays.

Suicide attempt Self-destructive behavior for the purpose of ending one's life that, for unanticipated reasons, fails.

Suicide gesture Self-destructive behavior that is unlikely to have any possibility of being fatal.

Sundowning Term used to describe an increase in confusion that often occurs in older adults, particularly at night.

Superficial burn A burn that affects only the epidermis; also called a *first-degree burn.*

Superior Above or in a higher position than another portion of the body.

Supine Face-up.

Suppository Drugs mixed in a firm base, such as cocoa butter, that when placed into a body opening melt at body temperature.

Supraclavicular retractions Indentations of the skin above the collarbones (clavicles).

Surfactant A thin substance that coats each alveolus and prevents the alveoli from collapsing.

Suspension Drug particle mixed with, but not dissolved in, a liquid.

Swathe A piece of soft material used to secure an injured extremity to the body.

Symmetry Evenness.

Sympathetic division The division of the autonomic nervous system that mobilizes energy, particularly in stressful situations; the fight-or-flight response.

Symptoms Conditions described by the patient, such as shortness of breath; also called *subjective findings.*

Syncope (fainting) A brief loss of responsiveness caused by a temporary decrease in blood flow to the brain; sometimes called a *blackout.*

Syndrome A group of signs and symptoms that together are characteristic of a specific disease or disorder.

Synovial joints Joints that allow movement in many directions.

Synthetic drugs Drugs that are made in a laboratory.

Syrup Drug suspended in sugar and water.

Systemic effect An effect of a drug on the whole body rather than just a single area or part of the body.

Systolic blood pressure The pressure in the arteries when the heart is pumping blood.

T

Tablet Powdered drug, molded or compressed into a small form.

Tachypnea A faster than normal respiratory rate for age.

Tarsals The bones of the heel and back part of the foot.

Teamwork The ability to work with others to achieve a common goal.

Tendonitis An inflammation of a tendon or the covering of the tendon; often associated with pain, tenderness, and (possibly) limited movement of the muscle attached to the affected tendon.

Tendons Cords of connective tissue that firmly attach the end of a muscle to a bone.

Tension pneumothorax A life-threatening condition in which air enters the pleural cavity during inspiration and progressively builds up under pressure.

Tension-type headaches The most common type of headaches with mild to moderate pain that feels like a tight band around the head; also called *muscle contraction headaches, ordinary headaches,* or *stress headaches.*

Terminal illness A disease that cannot be cured and is expected to lead to death.

Testes Two male reproductive glands located in the scrotum that produce reproductive cells and secrete testosterone.

Thalamus An area of the brain that functions as a relay station for impulses going to and from the cerebrum.

Therapeutic abortion An abortion performed for medical reasons, often because the pregnancy posed a threat to the mother's health.

Thoracic (chest) cavity The body cavity located below the neck and above the diaphragm. It contains the heart, major blood vessels, and lungs.

Threatened abortion A condition in which a woman is less than 20 weeks pregnant and experiences vaginal spotting or bleeding and possible mild uterine cramping. The cervix remains closed, and the fetus remains in the uterus.

Thrombocytes (platelets) Irregularly shaped blood cells that have a sticky surface.

Thrombotic stroke A stroke caused by a thrombus (blood clot) that forms in and partially or completely blocks a blood vessel of, or leading to, the brain.

Thrombus Blood clot.

Thymus gland A ductless organ that produces lymphocytes, which play a role in the body's immune system.

Thyroid cartilage The Adam's apple; the largest cartilage of the larynx.

Thyroid gland The endocrine gland that lies in the neck, just below the larynx. It regulates the metabolic rate.

Tibia The shinbone; the larger of the two bones of the lower leg.

Tidal volume The amount of air moved into or out of the lungs during a normal breath.

Tincture Alcohol solution prepared from an animal or a vegetable drug or chemical substance.

Tissues A group of similar cells that cluster together to perform a specialized function.

Toddler Stage of human development from 12 to 36 months.

Tolerance The need for progressively larger doses of a drug to achieve the desired effect.

Tonic-clonic seizure A seizure that involves stiffening and jerking of the patient's body; also called a *generalized motor seizure*; formerly called a *grand mal seizure*.

Tort Legal term for an illegal act or wrongdoing.

Tourniquet A tight bandage that surrounds an arm or leg and is used to stop the flow of blood in the extremity.

Toxidromes Signs, symptoms, and characteristics that often occur together in toxic exposures.

Toxin A poisonous substance.

Trachea The windpipe; the tube through which air passes to and from the lungs. It extends down the front of the neck from the larynx and divides in two to form the primary bronchi.

Tracheal deviation Shifting of the trachea from a midline position.

Tracheal stoma A permanent opening at the front of the neck that extends from the skin surface to the trachea, opening the trachea to the atmosphere.

Tracheostomy The creation of a surgical opening into the trachea through the neck, with insertion of a tube to aid passage of air or removal of secretions; the surgical opening created is called a *stoma or tracheal stoma*.

Traction splint A device used to maintain a constant, steady pull (traction) on a closed fracture of the femur.

Trade name A drug's brand name; also called the *proprietary name*.

Transient ischemic attack (TIA) A temporary interruption of the blood supply to the brain; sometimes called a *ministroke*.

Transmitter A device that sends out data on a given radio frequency.

Transverse colon The portion of the large intestine that extends across the abdomen.

Transverse fracture Fracture in which the break is at about a 90-degree angle to the bone.

Transverse plane The crosswise field that divides the body (or any of its parts) into superior (upper) and inferior (lower) sections.

Trauma patient An individual who has experienced an injury from an external force.

Traumatic asphyxia A condition that occurs because of a severe compression injury to the chest, resulting in a backup of blood into the veins, venules, and capillaries of the head, neck, extremities, and upper torso and subsequent capillary rupture.

Traumatic brain injury (TBI) An injury that occurs when an external force to the head causes the brain to move within the skull or the force causes the skull to break and directly injures the brain.

Traumatic incident A situation that causes a healthcare provider to experience unusually strong emotions.

Traumatic incident stress A normal stress response to an abnormal circumstance; can affect all levels of EMS personnel, healthcare providers, and bystanders.

Treatment protocol A list of steps to be followed during provision of emergency care to an ill or injured patient.

Triage Sorting multiple victims into priorities for emergency medical care or transportation to definitive care.

Tricuspid valve An atrioventricular valve located between the right atrium and the right ventricle.

Tripod position Position in which a patient sits up and leans forward, with the weight of the upper body supported by the hands on the thighs or knees; allows a patient to draw in more air and better expand her lungs than by lying on her back or leaning back in a sitting position.

True emergency A situation in which there is a high possibility of death or serious injury and the rapid response of an emergency vehicle may lessen the risk of death or injury.

True ribs Rib pairs 1–7. These ribs are attached anteriorly to the sternum by cartilage.

Tumor A growth of cells that multiply without a purpose.

Turbinates Several shelflike projections that protrude into the nasal cavity that help protect structures of the lower airway from foreign body contamination.

Two-person carry A move in which rescuers place one arm under the patient's thighs and the other across the patient's back. Each rescuer grasps the arms of the other, locking them in position at the elbows, forming a "seat." Both rescuers rise to a standing position and carry the patient to safety; also called the *two-person seat carry*.

Type 1 diabetes mellitus A disease in which little or no insulin is produced by beta cells in the pancreas, resulting in a buildup of glucose in the blood; usually begins during childhood or young adulthood.

Type 2 diabetes mellitus A disease caused by a combination of insulin resistance and relative insulin shortage that usually affects people older than 40 years of age, especially those who are overweight.

U

UHF Ultrahigh frequency radio band (a band is a group of radio frequencies close together).

Ulna The bone on the medial side of the forearm.

Umbilical cord An extension of the placenta through which the fetus receives nourishment while in the uterus.

Umbilicus See *navel*.

Unstable angina pectoris Angina pectoris that is progressively worsening, occurs at rest, or is brought on by minimal physical exertion.

Upper extremities The shoulder girdle, arms, forearms, and hands.

Upper GI bleeding Bleeding from the esophagus, stomach, or duodenum.

Ureters Two tubes that carry urine from the kidneys to the urinary bladder.

Urethra A canal that passes urine from the urinary bladder to the outside of the body.

Urethritis Inflammation or infection limited to the urethra.

Urgent move A method used to move a patient when there is an immediate threat to life.

Urinary bladder A temporary storage site for urine.

Urinary catheter A tube that is inserted into the bladder to empty it of urine.

Urinary incontinence The involuntary leakage of urine.

Urinary tract infection (UTI) An infection that affects any part of the urinary tract.

Urticaria Hives.

Uterus A hollow, muscular organ of the female reproductive system where a fertilized egg implants and develops into a fetus; also called the *womb*.

Uvula The small piece of tissue that looks like a punching bag and that hangs down in the back of the throat.

V

Vagina (birth canal) In the female, a muscular tube that serves as a passageway between the uterus and the outside. It receives the penis during intercourse and serves as a passageway for menstrual flow and the delivery of an infant.

Vasoconstriction Constriction of a blood vessel.

Vasodilation Dilation of a blood vessel.

Veins Blood vessels that return blood to the heart.

Venous return The amount of blood returning to the ventricles.

Ventricles The two lower chambers of the heart; the right ventricle pumps blood to the lungs and the left ventricle pumps blood to the body.

Ventricular fibrillation (VF or VFib) An abnormal heart rhythm in which the heart's electrical impulses are completely disorganized and the heart cannot pump blood effectively.

Ventricular shunt A drainage system used to remove excess cerebrospinal fluid in a patient who has hydrocephalus.

Venules The smallest branches of veins leading to the capillaries.

Vertebral column See *spine*.

VHF A very high frequency radio band (a band is a group of radio frequencies close together).

Virus A type of infectious agent that depends on other organisms to live and grow.

Visceral pleura The inner pleural layer that covers the surface of the lungs.

Vital capacity The amount of air that can be forcefully expelled from the lungs after breathing in as deeply as possible.

Vital organs The organs essential for life, such as the brain, heart, and lungs.

Vital signs Measurements of breathing, pulse, temperature, pupils, and blood pressure.

Voice over Internet Protocol (VoIP) Technology that allows users to make telephone calls by means of a broadband Internet connection instead of using a regular telephone line; also known as *Internet Voice*.

W

Warm zone An identified safety zone at a hazardous materials incident that serves as a controlled area for entry into the hot zone and where most operations take place. It also serves as the decontamination area after exiting the hot zone; also called the *contamination reduction zone*.

Weapons of mass destruction (WMD) Materials that have the potential to cause great harm over a large area.

Wellness A state of health and happiness that involves lifestyle choices in pursuit of an optimal state of health.

Wet drowning The entry of water into the trachea and lungs.

Wheezing A high- or low-pitched whistling sound that is usually heard on exhalation; wheezing suggests that the lower airways are partially blocked with fluid or mucus.

Whooping cough See *pertussis*.

Withdrawal The condition produced when an individual stops using or abusing a drug to which the individual is physically or psychologically addicted.

Wound An injury to the soft tissues of the body.

X

Xiphoid process The inferior portion of the breastbone.

Z

Zygote Fertilized egg.

Credits

Unless otherwise credited all photos © The McGraw-Hill Companies, Inc./Rick Brady, photographer.

Chapter 1

Figure 1-2: © The McGraw-Hill Companies, Inc./Carin Marter, photographer; **1-3:** © Courtesy of Air Evac Services, Phoenix, Arizona.

Chapter 2

Figure 2-1: © Courtesy of Tempe Fire Department, Tempe, Arizona.

Chapter 6

Figure 6-4: © The McGraw-Hill Companies, Inc./Joe DeGrandis, photographer; **6-11, 6-20, 6-24:** © The McGraw-Hill Companies, Inc./Karl Rubin, photographer; **6-31:** © Branislav Vidic.

Chapter 7

Figure 7-2: © Tony Brain/SPL/Photo Researchers, Inc.

Chapter 8

Figure 8-1: Courtesy of Laura Horowitz; **8-3, 8-4:** EMSC Slide Set (CD-ROM). 1996. Courtesy of the Emergency Medical Services for Children Program, administered by the U.S. Department of Health and Human Services' Health Resources and Services Administration, Maternal and Child Health Bureau; **8-6:** Barbara Aehlert; **8-7:** EMSC Slide Set (CD-ROM). 1996. Courtesy of the Emergency Medical Services for Children Program, administered by the U.S. Department of Health and Human Services' Health Resources and Services Administration, Maternal and Child Health Bureau; **8-9:** © Digital Vision/Getty RF; **8-10, 8-11:** EMSC Slide Set (CD-ROM). 1996. Courtesy of the Emergency Medical Services for Children Program, administered by the U.S. Department of Health and Human Services' Health Resources and Services Administration, Maternal and Child Health Bureau; **8-12:** © Brand X Pictures/Superstock RF; **8-13:** Barbara Aehlert.

Chapter 16

Figure 16-1: © Courtesy of City of Tempe Fire Department, Tempe, Arizona; **16-3, 16-4:** Courtesy of City of Mesa Fire Department. Mesa, Arizona; **16-5:** © Courtesy of City of Tempe Fire Department, Tempe, Arizona.

Chapter 20

Figure 20-3: © L.V. Begman/The Bergman Collection; **20-4:** © Biophoto Associates/Photo Researchers, Inc.

Chapter 21

Figure 21-6a,b: © Randy Budd, RRT, CEP, City of Mesa Fire Department.

Chapter 23

Figure 23-4: Photo by Wilfred Chapleau.

Chapter 24

Figure 24-2: © Hank Morgan/Photo Researchers.

Chapter 26

Figure 26-3, 26-4: © The McGraw-Hill Companies, Inc./ Rebecca Gray, photographer/Don Kincaid, dissections.

Chapter 30

Figure 30-1a,b: © The McGraw-Hill Companies /Joe DeGrandis, photographer.

Chapter 31

Figure 31-1: © Meckes/Ottawa/Photo Researchers, Inc.; **31-2:** Courtesy Dr. Thomas F. Sellers/Emory University/CDC.

Chapter 32

Figure 32-3a,b, 32-4: EMSC Slide Set (CD-ROM). 1996. Courtesy of the Emergency Medical Services for Children Program, administered by the U.S. Department of Health and Human Services' Health Resources and Services Administration, Maternal and Child Health Bureau.

Chapter 33

Figure 33-1b, 33-2b: © David Page.

Chapter 34

Figure 34-8: © The McGraw-Hill Companies, Inc./Carin Marter, photographer; **34-11:** © Mediscan; **34-14:** Trauma.org Image; **34-16:** Matthew D. Sztajnkrycer, MD, PhD, from Knoop, et al., Atlas of Emergency Medicine, 2nd edition, McGraw-Hill Company, Inc; **34-17:** © The McGraw-Hill Companies, Inc./Carin Marter, photographer; **34-19:** Courtesy of Alan B. Storrow, MD, from Knoop, et al., Atlas of Emergency Medicine, 2nd edition, McGraw-Hill Company, Inc.; **34-21:** Matthew D. Sztajnkrycer, MD, PhD, from Knoop, et al., Atlas of Emergency Medicine, 2nd edition, McGraw-Hill Company, Inc.; **34-22, 34-23:** Trauma.org Image; **34-25a:** © David Page; **34-27, 34-31, 34-32:** Trauma.org Image; **34-36, 34-38, 34-40, 34-42:** EMSC Slide Set (CD-ROM). 1996. Courtesy of the Emergency Medical Services for Children Program, administered by the U.S. Department of Health and Human Services' Health Resources and Services Administration, Maternal and Child Health Bureau; **34-43:** Trauma.org Image.

Chapter 35

Figure 35-2, 35-10: Courtesy of Stephen Corbett, MD, from Knoop, et al., Atlas of Emergency Medicine, 2nd edition, McGraw-Hill Company, Inc.

Chapter 37

Figure 37-2, 37-3: © The McGraw-Hill Companies, Inc./ Rebecca Gray, photographer/Don Kincaid, dissections; **37-9, 37-11:** Trauma.org Image.

Chapter 38

Figure 38-2: © Branislav Vidic; **38-3, 38-5:** © The McGraw-Hill Companies, Inc./Karl Rubin, photographer; **38-10:** Trauma. org Image; **38-11:** © Photo Researchers, Inc.; **38-12, 38-13:** © The McGraw-Hill Companies, Inc./Karl Rubin, photographer.

Chapter 39

Figure 39-1: Courtesy of John Fildes, MD, from Knoop, et al., Atlas of Emergency Medicine, 2nd edition, McGraw-Hill Company, Inc.; **39-6:** © Administration on Aging.

Chapter 40

Figure 40-5: Courtesy of James O'Malley, MD, from Knoop, et al., Atlas of Emergency Medicine, 2nd edition, McGraw-Hill Company, Inc.; **40-8–40-10:** Courtesy of R. Jason Thurman, MD, from Knoop, et al., Atlas of Emergency Medicine, 2nd edition, McGraw-Hill Company, Inc.; **40-11, 40-12:** Courtesy of Sean P. Bush, MD, from Knoop, et al., Atlas of Emergency Medicine, 2nd edition, McGraw-Hill Company, Inc.; **40-13:** Courtesy of Stephen Holt, MD, from Knoop, et al., Atlas of Emergency Medicine, 2nd edition, McGraw-Hill Company, Inc.; **40-14:** Courtesy of Sean P. Bush, MD, from Knoop, et al., Atlas of Emergency Medicine, 2nd edition, McGraw-Hill Company, Inc.; **40-17:** Courtesy of Alan B. Storrow, MD, from Knoop, et al., Atlas of Emergency Medicine, 2nd edition, McGraw-Hill Company, Inc.; **40-18:** Courtesy of Gerald O'Malley, DO, from Knoop, et al., Atlas of Emergency Medicine, 2nd edition, McGraw-Hill Company, Inc.; **40-19:** Courtesy of Alan B. Storrow, MD, from Knoop, et al., Atlas of Emergency Medicine, 2nd edition, McGraw-Hill Company, Inc.; **40-20, 40-21:** Centers For Disease Control and Prevention; **40-22:** Courtesy of Kevin J. Knoop, MD, from Knoop, et al., Atlas of Emergency Medicine, 2nd edition, McGraw-Hill Company, Inc.; **40-23:** Courtesy of Sean P. Bush, MD, from Knoop, et al., Atlas of Emergency Medicine, 2nd edition, McGraw-Hill Company, Inc.; **40-24:** Courtesy of Stephen Corbett, MD, from Knoop, et al., Atlas of Emergency Medicine, 2nd edition, McGraw-Hill

Company, Inc.; **40-25, 40-26:** Courtesy of Alan B. Storrow, MD, from Knoop, et al., Atlas of Emergency Medicine, 2nd edition, McGraw-Hill Company, Inc.; **40-27:** Courtesy of Daniel L. Savitt, MD, from Knoop, et al., Atlas of Emergency Medicine, 2nd edition, McGraw-Hill Company, Inc.; **40-28:** Courtesy of Matthew D. Sztajnkrycer, MD, PhD.

Chapter 41

Figure 41-2: © AP Wide World Photos.

Chapter 42

Figure 42-5: Courtesy of Stephen Corbett, MD, from Knoop, et al., Atlas of Emergency Medicine, 2nd edition, McGraw-Hill Company, Inc.

Chapter 44

Figure 44-1: EMSC Slide Set (CD-ROM). 1996. Courtesy of the Emergency Medical Services for Children Program, administered by the U.S. Department of Health and Human Services' Health Resources and Services Administration, Maternal and Child Health Bureau; **44-3:** © James Shaffer; **44-4–44-8, 44-10:** EMSC Slide Set (CD-ROM). 1996. Courtesy of the Emergency Medical Services for Children Program, administered by the U.S. Department of Health and Human Services' Health Resources and Services Administration, Maternal and Child Health Bureau; **44-11:** © Mediscan.

Chapter 45

Figure 45-1: © Corbis RF; **45-3:** © Yoav Levy/PhotoTake.

Chapter 46

Figure 46-1: EMSC Slide Set (CD-ROM). 1996. Courtesy of the Emergency Medical Services for Children Program, administered by the U.S. Department of Health and Human Services' Health Resources and Services Administration, Maternal and Child Health Bureau; **46-2:** Courtesy of Anne W. Lucky, MD, from Knoop, et al., Atlas of Emergency Medicine, 2nd edition, McGraw-Hill Company, Inc.; **46-3:** Courtesy of Douglas R. Landry, MD, from Knoop, et al., Atlas of Emergency Medicine, 2nd edition, McGraw-Hill Company, Inc.; **46-4:** Courtesy of Charles J. Schubert, MD, from Knoop, et al., Atlas of Emergency Medicine, 2nd edition, McGraw-Hill Company, Inc.; **46-5:** EMSC Slide Set (CD-ROM). 1996. Courtesy of the Emergency Medical Services for Children Program, administered by the U.S. Department of Health and Human Services' Health Resources and Services Administration, Maternal and Child Health Bureau.

Chapter 48

Figure 48-1: © The McGraw-Hill Companies, Inc./Carin Marter, photographer; **48-2:** © Courtesy of Air Evac Services, Phoenix, Arizona.

Chapter 49

Figure 49-3: © David Page.

Appendix B

Figure B-1, B-2: Barbara Aehlert; **B-3:** © www.farmedic.com, McNeil and Company Farmedic Training Program.

Index

*Page numbers with *f* indicate figures; page numbers with *t* indicate tables.

Abandonment, 91
Abbreviations
  common medical, 130, 131–135*t*
  for common units of measure, 135*t*
Abdomen
  in children, 774, 774*f*
  defined, 140
  in rapid medical assessment,
    374–375
  in secondary assessment, 360–361,
    360*f*
Abdominal and gastrointestinal
    disorders, 457–465
  acute abdomen, 459–460
    hemorrhagic causes of, 460–461
    nonhemorrhagic causes of,
      461–462
  basic anatomy, 457, 457*f*
  causes of, 464–465*t*
  digestive system organs, 458–459,
    458*f*
  emergency care in, 463–464
  patient assessment in, 462–463, 463*f*
  solid and hollow organs, 457–458
Abdominal aortic aneurysm, 460, 464*t*
Abdominal cavity, 142–143, 143*f*, 457,
    457*f*
Abdominal/chest thrusts, 250
Abdominal injuries
  closed, 607
  open, 608
Abdominal organs by quadrant, 607*t*
Abdominal trauma, 606–607, 606*f*,
    607*ft*, 608*t*
  emergency care for, 610
  patient assessment in, 609
Abdominopelvic cavity, 142
Abnormal behavior, 521
Abortion, 751
  elective, 751
  incomplete, 751
  spontaneous, 751
  therapeutic, 751
  threatened, 751
Abrasion, 567, 567*f*
Abruptio placentae, 685, 687, 753, 753*f*
Absence seizures, 380
Absorbed poisons, 518
  emergency care with, 518
  patient assessment with, 518
Absorption, 165, 458
Abuse
  child, 804–806, 805*f*, 806*f*
  elder, 693, 806–807
  emotional, 805
  pregnancy and, 750
  self-, 807
  sexual, 805
  shaken baby syndrome as, 192, 689
  substance, 750–751
Abusive head trauma, 689
Acceptance as stage of grief, 73
Accessory muscles for breathing,
    155, 264
Accessory organs of digestion, 166
*Accidental Death and Disability, The
    Neglected Disease of Modern
    Society*, 4
Accidental disclosure of protected
    health information, 94
Accidental poisonings, 506

Acclimation, 707
Acclimatization, 707
Accommodation, 653
Achilles tendon, 491
Achilles tendonitis, 490
Acidosis, 711, 712
Acquired immunodeficiency
    syndrome (AIDS), 185
Acrocyanosis, 766
Activated charcoal, 213, 214*f*, 220–
    221, 220*f*, 222*f*, 515, 515*f*
Active listening, 296
Active rewarming, 704–705
Acute abdomen, 459–460
  hemorrhagic causes of, 460–461
  nonhemorrhagic causes of, 461–462
Acute brain syndrome, 796
Acute chest syndrome, 535
Acute coronary syndromes (ACSs),
    434, 435*t*
Acute kidney injury (AKI), 471
Acute myocardial infarction, 435–
    437, 436*f*, 437*t*
Acute pulmonary edema, 421–422
Acute renal failure (ARF), 471
Adam, 511
Adam's apple, 152, 244
Addiction, 507
Adenosine triphosphate (ATP),
    176–177, 177*f*
Administered medications, 220–226
  activated charcoal, 220–221, 220*f*,
    222*f*
  aspirin, 221, 223
  oral glucose, 223–224, 223*f*, 225*f*
  oxygen, 224, 224*f*, 226
Administrative agency, 81
Administrative law, 81
Administrative uses of prehospital
    care report, 96
Adolescents, 197–198
  cognitive changes in, 197
  communication with, 302
  implications for healthcare
    professional, 198, 198*f*
  physiologic changes in, 197
  pregnancy in, 197
  psychosocial changes, 198
Adrenal glands, 167, 468
Adults. *See also* Early adults; Middle
    adults; Older adults
  automated external defibrillator
    sequence in, 452*f*, 887
  cardiopulmonary resuscitation in
    one-rescuer, 876–878
    two-rescuer, 879–881
  clearing foreign body airway
    obstruction
    in conscious, 888–889
    in unconscious, 890
Advanced EMTs (AEMTs), 11, 13
Advance directives, 74, 87, 90*f*
Advanced life support (ALS), 11*t*, 74
  assistance in endocrine disorders,
    398–399
  personnel in, 5
Advocate, 22
Aerobic metabolism, 140, 177
African Americans
  drowning in, 710
  pregnancy and delivery in, 749

Africanized honeybees, 723
Afterbirth, 737
After the run, 830–831
Age
  as disease risk factor, 184
  in endocrine disorders, 399
  as factor in burns, 579
  in immunology, 501–502, 502*t*
Age classification
  of children, 770
  of infants, 770
Agents
  chemical, 185
  physical, 185
Agitated delirium, 526
Agitation, 521
Agonal breathing, 246, 267, 408
Airborne diseases, 37
  signs, symptoms, and complications
    of some, 42*t*
Air embolism, 573, 714
  emergency care for, 714
Air medical transport, 844–848, 845*f*,
    846*f*
Air splint, 560, 560*f*, 627
Airway
  assessment of, 246–248
  in children, 771–772, 772*t*, 778–
    780, 778*f*, 779*f*
  clearing, 250–253
  inspecting, 248–249
  keeping open, 253
  nasal, 255–257, 255*f*
  in newborn, 764–765, 765*f*
  obstruction of, 249–250
    foreign-body, 192
    in infants and children, 781
  opening, 246–247, 247*f*
  oral, 253, 255, 255*f*
  in primary survey, 342–343, 343*f*
  reevaluating, 364
  in secondary survey, 364
  signs of adequate, 246
  signs of inadequate, 246
  trauma to, 263
  upper, 243–244
Airway adjuncts, 253
  in children, 780
Airway management, 243–258
  adjuncts, 253
  assessment, 246–248
  clearing, 250–253
    manual maneuvers, 250
    recovery position, 252–253,
      252*f*
    suctioning, 250–252
  head tilt, 247–248, 247*f*
  inspecting, 248–249
  jaw thrust, 248
  keeping open, 253
    nasal, 255–257, 255*f*
    oral, 253, 255, 255*f*
  mechanics of breathing, 245
  obstruction, 249–250
  opening, 246–247, 247*f*
  opening mouth, 247, 247*f*
  respiratory system in, 243–246
    functions of, 243, 244*f*
    lower, 244–245
    older adult anatomy, 245–246
    upper, 243–244

special patient populations, infant
    and child anatomy, 245
Airway patency, disruption of,
    262–263
Alcohol, 509
  drowning and, 710
  effect on respiratory function, 263
  pregnancy and, 738
Alcohol withdrawal syndrome, 509
Alkali burns, 575
Allergens, 185, 495*f*, 497
  routes of entry of, 496*t*
Allergic asthma, 417
Allergies, 262, 495, 497*t*. *See
    also* Asthma
  in ascertaining current health
    status, 307–308
  causes of, 495, 496*t*, 497, 497*t*
  defined, 495
  in immunology, 497–498, 498*t*, 499*t*
  pregnancy and, 739
All-terrain vehicles (ATVs), 316
Alpha particles, 869
Altered level of consciousness
    (ALOC), 347, 377
Altered mental status, 84, 347,
    377–378, 394
  causes of, 349
  common causes of, 377
  emergency care, 377–378
  in infants and children, 784
  in older adults, 796–797
  in shock, 543
Alveolar-capillary gas exchange, 157
Alveolar ducts, 153
Alveolar sacs, 245
Alveoli, 153, 156–157, 245
Alzheimer's disease, 184, 694
  in older adults, 796
Ambulance, transferring patient to,
    827
American College of Emergency
    Physicians (ACEP), 5
  establishment of, 5
American College of Surgeons (ACS)
  Committee on Trauma, 6
    *Optimal Hospital Resources for Care
      of the Injured Patient*, 5
  Committee on Treatment of
    Fractures, 4
American Heart Association, 2005
    Resuscitation Guidelines of,
    711, 788
*American Hospital Formulary Service
    (AHFS) Drug Information*, 208
American Trauma Society, founding
    of, 5
Amniotic fluid, 764
Amniotic fluid embolism, 760
Amniotic sac, 738
Amobarbital (Amytal), 510
Amphetamines, 508, 512
Amputations, 569, 570*f*, 572, 572*f*
Amy's, 510
Anabolic Steroid Act (1990), 207*t*
Anabolism, 176
Anaerobic metabolism, 140, 176
Anal canal, 166, 458
Anaphylactic reaction, 501
Anaphylactic shock, 540
Anaphylaxis, 185, 498

Anaphylaxis kit, 500, 500*f*
Anatomical position, 127
Anatomic dead space, 155
Anatomic splint, 624
Anatomy, 140
Anemia
  defined, 534
  sickle cell, 534
Anesthesia, 565
Aneurysm, 382
  abdominal aortic, 460
Anger as stage of grief, 73
Angina pectoris, 435
  stable, 435
  unstable, 435
Angioplasty, 436
Anglo-Americans, pregnancy and
  delivery in, 749
Anisocoria, 333
Ankle
  bandage for, 587*f*
  injuries to, 640, 641*t*
Ankle drag, 54–55, 55*f*
Antabuse, 509
Anterior, 127
Anterior nosebleed, 531
Anthrax, 868
Antiarrhythmics, 439
Antibody, 185, 497
Anticholinergic toxidrome, 508*t*
Antidotes, 505
  defined, 233
  nerve agent, 233, 236
Antigen, 185, 497
Antioxidants, 178
Anxiety, 522
Anxiety disorder, 522–523
  phobias as type of, 523–524
Aorta, 160, 430, 457
Aortic aneurysm, abdominal, 460
Aortic valves, 428
Apgar, Virginia, 766
Apgar score in newborn, 766, 767*t*
Aphasia
  expressive, 385
  receptive, 385
Apnea monitors, 809
Apparent life-threatening event
  (ALTE), 788
Apparent sexual assault, 483–484
Appeal, 81
Appearance, 20
  in general impression, 342
  in older adults, 793
Appellate court, 81
Appendicitis, 458, 464*t*
Appendicular skeleton, 144, 614,
  614*f*, 615*t*
Appendix, 458
Aqueous humor, 653
Arab Americans, pregnancy and
  delivery in, 749
Arachnoid, 163, 645
Arc eye, 655
Area command, 836
Arrival at receiving facility, 118, 118*f*
Arrival phase and scene size-up,
  825–827, 826*f*
  egress from scene, 827
  on-scene care, 827
  scene safety, 826–827, 826*f*
  traffic volume and flow, 827
  vehicle placement, 826–827
Arrival response in weapons of mass
  destruction (WMD) incident
  response, 871–872
Arsenic, exposure to, 511
Arterial bleeding, 557, 557*f*
Arteries, 159, 160*f*, 181, 430, 431*f*
  major, 160, 161*t*
Arterioles, 160, 160*f*, 181, 432
Arteriosclerosis, 434
Arteriovenous (AV) fistula, 472, 472*f*
Arteriovenous (AV) graft, 472
Arteriovenous (AV) shunts, 181, 472
Artery pulse, 328*t*
Arthritis, 184, 489
Arthropods, 720
Artificial ventilation, 279–291
  adequacy of respiration, 280, 281*t*
  adequate and inadequate, 288
  positive-pressure, 280, 283*t*
  applying cricoid, 280–282, 281*f*,
    282*f*

bag-mask, 285–288, 285*f*, 286*f*, 287*f*
  flow-restricted, oxygen-powered
    device, 288–289, 288*f*
  mouth-to-barrier device, 283,
    283*f*, 285
  mouth-to-mouth, 282–283, 282*f*,
    285*f*
  signs of adequate and inadequate,
    412, 412*t*
  special considerations
    dental appliances, 291
    infants and children, 291
    tracheal stomas, 289, 291
Ascending colon, 166, 458
Asphyxia, traumatic, 599–600, 600*f*
Aspiration, 244
Aspirin, 213, 221, 223, 512
  in emergency care in cardiovascular
    disease, 441, 441*t*
Assault, 91
Assessment, 105
  with epistaxis, 531
  for hemophilia, 536
  of older adult, 792–794, 792*f*
  for patients with psychiatric
    disorders, 526–527, 527*f*
Assisted medications, 226–233
  epinephrine, 226–227, 227*f*,
    228–229*f*
  inhaled bronchodilators, 227,
    229–230, 229*f*, 231–232*f*
  nitroglycerin, 230, 232–233, 233*f*,
    235*f*
Asthma, 264, 417–418, 417*f*, 596. See
  also Allergies
  allergic, 417
  nonallergic, 417
  in older adults, 795
Asymmetrical (uneven) facial
  movements, 351
  in assessing face, 351
Atherosclerosis, 434
Atlas, 145
Atmospheric pressure, 155
Atria, 158, 428
Atrioventricular (AV) node, 428
Atrioventricular (AV) valves, 428
Atropine, 236–238
Auditory hallucinations, 525
Auditory ossicles, 144
Aura, 379
Auscultation, measuring blood
  pressure by, 336*f*
Autistic disorders, 694
Autoimmune disorders, 185
Automated external defibrillator
  (AED), 444, 448–449, 448*f*
  advantages of, 449
  maintenance, 453
  operation of, 450–451
  sequence of, for adults, 452*f*, 887
Automaticity, 428
Automatic Vehicle Locator (AVL), 112
Automatisms, 380
Automobile restraints, while
  pregnant, 687
Autonomic nervous system (ANS),
  164, 647
  effect of stimulation of, 164*t*
AVPU scale, 695
  in assessing level of consciousness,
    650, 688, 694, 730
  in child, 691
  in primary survey, 343
Avulsion, 569, 569*f*
Axial skeleton, 144, 614, 614*f*
Axilla, 127
Axillary temperature, 699

Backboards, 69–70, 634, 729
  long, 69–70, 69*f*, 729
  in removing victim from vehicle, 856
  short, 70, 70*f*
Backslaps, 250
Bacteria, 178, 868, 869*f*
Bag-mask ventilation, 285–288, 285*f*,
  286*f*, 287*f*
Bag of waters, 738
Ball-and-socket joints, 487, 488*f*, 615,
  616
Bandages, 584–587
  ankle, 587*f*
  Coban, 585*f*
  foot, 587*f*

forearm, 587*f*
  knee, 587*f*
  pressure, 585
  triangular, 585, 585*f*
  types of, 584–585, 587*f*
  wrist, 587*f*
Barbiturates, 510
Barbs, 510
Bargaining as stage of grief, 73
Bariatric patients, 808
Barotrauma, 418, 714
  emergency care for, 714
Barrel chest, 245
Baseline vital signs, 327–328
Base station, 111, 112*f*
Basic life support (BLS) care, 11*t*,
  24–35
Basilar head fracture, 648, 649*f*, 650*f*
Basket litter, 68
Basket stretcher, 68, 69*f*
Battery, 91
Battle's sign, 358, 648, 651
Bed, transferring supine patient to
  stretcher
  direct carry, 60, 63–64*f*
  draw sheet transfer, 62, 65*f*
Behavior
  abnormal, 521
  bizarre, 521
  changes in, in psychiatric
    disorders, 521, 522*t*
  defined, 521
  in psychiatric disorders, 521
Behavioral emergency, 521
Bends, 714
Benign tumor, 177
Bent-arm drag, 54
Benzodiazepines, 510, 510*t*
Beta burns, 869
Beta particles, 869
Biceps, 615
Bicuspid valve, 433
Bicycle crashes, 321
Bicycle helmets, 321
Bicycle-related injuries, 689
Bilateral, 127
Binaurals, 335
Biohazard bags or containers, 39
Biological weapons, 867–868, 868*f*
Biologics Control Act (1902), 206*t*
Bipolar disorder, 524–525
Bipolar traction splint, applying,
  638–639, 638–639*f*
Birth canal, 479, 736
Bites. See also Stings
  cat, 724–725, 725*f*
  dog, 724–725, 725*f*
  human, 725–726
  snake, 715, 716*t*, 717–720, 717*f*
  spider, 720–722, 720*f*, 721*f*
Bizarre thinking and behavior, 521
Black eye, 654
Black widow spider, 720, 720*f*
Blanket drag, 53, 54*f*
Blast injuries, 730–731, 731*f*
Blastocyst, 737
Bleb, 422, 596
Bleeding, 556–563
  arterial, 557, 557*f*
  capillary, 557–558
  external, 558–562
  internal, 562–563, 563*f*
  obvious, in primary survey, 346
  pregnancy and, 751–752
  types of, 557–558, 557*f**t*
  vaginal, 754*t*
  venous, 557
Blistering, 576, 577, 577*f*
Blood, 159, 159*f*, 432–433
  clotting, 557
  obstruction of flow of, 264
  vomited, 461
Bloodborne diseases, 37
Blood glucose meter, 400
Blood glucose test, performing, 400,
  401*f*, 402
  with glucometer, 401*f*
Blood pressure, 160, 162, 182–183,
  183*f*, 334–338, 430, 433
  in children, 773, 780
  common errors in measurement, 338
  diastolic, 433
  measuring
    by auscultation, 336*f*

by palpation, 337*f*
  pregnancy and, 738
  pulse oximetry, 338–339, 338*f*
  systolic, 182, 433
Blood pressure cuff as tourniquet,
  562, 562*f*
Blood vessels, 159–162, 160*f*, 161*f*
  function of, 181, 181*f*
  major, 430, 431*f*, 432
  walls of, 180, 180*f*
Bloody show, 736
Blow-by oxygen, 276, 276*f*
Blow-by oxytocin, 783
Blowout fracture, 654–655
Blue bloater, 418
Blues, 510
Blunt trauma, 315, 316*t*
  to abdomen, 690
  to chest, 690
  to head, 648
BM-to-stoma breathing, steps in
  performing, 289, 289*f*, 291
Body armor, 46
  of skeletal muscle, 616, 617*f*
Body cavities, 142–143, 143*f*
Body mechanics and lifting
  techniques, 48–50
  carrying patients and equipment, 50
  carrying procedure on stairs, 52
  guidelines for safe lifting of cots
    and stretchers, 50
  guidelines for safe pushing and
    pulling, 52
  guidelines for safe reaching, 52
  power grip, 49, 49*f*
  safety precautions and preparation,
    48–49, 49*f*
Body planes, 143–144, 143*f*
Body position and directional terms,
  127, 128–129*t*, 128*f*, 130*t*
Body surface area (BSA), 192
  in children, 190
Body temperature, 699–701
  heat loss, 700–701, 700*f*
  heat production, 699–700
  regulation, 699
Bone marrow, 144
Bones, 144, 147*f*, 487
  nasal, 652
Botulism, 868
Brachial arteries, 160, 430
Brachial pulse, 160, 328*t*, 329, 347,
  347*f*, 430
Bradypnea, 408
Brain, 162–163, 163*f*, 645
  of child, 771
  of infant, 771
  repetitive questioning, 659–660, 659*f*
  respiratory centers in, 263
Brain injuries, 659–660, 659*f*
  concussion, 659–660, 659*f*
  emergency care for, 662
Brainstem, 163
Brain Trauma Foundation on head
  injuries, 645
Brand name, 205
Braxton-Hicks contractions, 742
Breach of duty, 92
Breast cancer, 184
Breathing
  agonal, 246, 267, 408
  assessing patient with difficulty,
    407–412
  in children, 772, 772*t*, 780
  in general impression, 342
  mechanics of, 245
  in newborns, 764–765, 765*f*
  in older adults, 793
  possible signs of labored, 331
  in primary survey, 345–346, 346*f*
  reevaluating, 364
  in secondary survey, 364
  seesaw, 411, 772
Breath sounds, 264–265, 264*f*, 265*f*
  abnormal, 409*t*
Breath stacking, 418
Breech delivery, 741
Breech presentation, 757–758
Bronchioles, 153, 245
Bronchodilators, inhaled, 227,
  229–230, 229*f*, 231–232*f*
Bronchus, 153
Brown recluse spiders, 721, 721*f*
Brucellosis, 868

Bruise, 562, 564, 564*f*
  myocardial (cardiac), 601, 601*f*
  pulmonary, 600–601, 600*f*
Buccal drugs, 214
Buddy taping, 631
Bulb syringe in clearing airway, 779
Bureau of Narcotics and Dangerous
  Drugs (BNDD), 205
Burn centers, 15*t*
  burns best treated in, 579
Burns, 567, 576–582
  age as factor in, 579
  alkali, 575
  best treated in burn center, 579
  chemical, 574, 576, 580–581, 655
  circumferential, 579
  depth of, 576
  electrical, 576, 581–582
  extent of, 578, 578*t*
  factors related to severity of, 578–579
  first-degree, 576
  full-thickness, 577, 577*f*
  location of, 578
  nonchemical, 575
  partial-thickness, 576–577, 577*f*
  second-degree, 576
  superficial, 576, 576*f*
  thermal, 576, 579, 580, 685
    emergency care of, 579, 580
  third-degree, 577
Bursa, 490
Bursitis, 490
  hip, 490
  of kneecap, 491
Bush, George W., 7, 834
Buttons, 510
Bystanders
  assistance from, in emergencies, 48
  responses to injury or illness, 304
  safety of, 314

Caffeine, 508, 512
Calcium, 487
Call, 113–119
  arrival at receiving facility, 118, 118*f*
  arrival at scene, 116–117, 116*f*
  en route to, 116
    receiving facility, 117–118
    station, 118–119
Canal, 458
Cancer, 177, 178*f*, 184
  breast, 184
  cervical, 483
  lung, 184, 596
  primary, 177
Capacitance vessels, 181
Capillaries, 160, 181, 432
Capillary bleeding, 557–558
Capillary refill, 332–333, 333*f*, 541
  in primary survey, 347
Carbon dioxide, 157
  exhaled, 338–339
Carbon monoxide (CO), 512,
  515–516
Cardiac arrest, 247, 249, 443–453
  chain of survival, 443–444
  in children, 190
  in infants, 190
  patient assessment and emergency
    care in, 444–451
  in pregnancy, 687–688
  during transport, 453
Cardiac muscle, 151, 151*t*
Cardiac output, 179
  in regulating blood pressure, 183*f*
Cardiac pain, 460
Cardiac (pericardial) tamponade,
  264, 598–599, 599*f*
Cardiogenic shock, 183, 264, 438,
  540, 712
Cardiopulmonary failure in infants
  and children, 783
Cardiopulmonary resuscitation
  (CPR), 4, 6, 48, 74, 439, 443
  guidelines of, 447*t*
  interruption of, 451
  one-rescuer adult, 876–878
  one-rescuer child, 882–885
  one-rescuer infant, 885–886
  stopping, 453
  two-rescuer adult, 879–881
Cardiovascular disorders, 427–453
  aspirin in emergency care in, 441,
    551*t*

cardiac arrest, 443–453
  chain of survival, 443–444
  patient assessment and
    emergency care, 444–451
  during transport, 453
cardiogenic shock, 438
circulatory system, 428
congestive heart failure, 437
disease, 434–443
  acute coronary syndromes, 434,
    435*t*
  angina pectoris, 435
  cardiogenic shock, 438
  congestive heart failure, 437
  emergency care, 440–443, 441*t*,
    442*t*
  hypertensive emergencies, 438
  patient assessment, 439–440
emergency care in, 440–443, 441*t*,
  442*t*
hypertensive emergencies, 438
MONA in treating, 440–441
NTG in emergency care in, 441–
  442, 442*t*
OPQRST in assessing, 439–440
patient assessment in, 439–440
physiology of circulation, 433–434,
  433*f*
postresuscitation care, 451
system, 428–433, 429*f*, 430*f*
Cardiovascular system, 158, 428–433,
  429*f*, 430*f*
  allergic reactions in, 499*t*
  in older adults, 794–795
  in temperature regulation, 699
Careful delivery of service, 22
Carina, 153, 245
Carotid arteries, 160, 329, 347, 347*f*,
  430, 652, 658
Carotid pulse, 160, 328*t*
Carpals, 149
Carpal tunnel, 490
Carpal tunnel syndrome, 490
Carries, 55–58
  cradle, 55, 57*f*
  firefighter's, 55, 56*f*
  pack-strap, 55–56, 57*f*
  two-person, 57–58, 58*f*
Cartilage, 487
  cricoid, 153
Cartilaginous joints, 487, 616
Catabolism, 176
Cataracts in older adults, 800
Cat bites, 724–725, 725*f*
  emergency care for, 725
Category A diseases and agents, 868
Category B diseases and agents, 868
Catheters
  suction, 251–252, 251*f*
  urinary, 470–471
Cecum, 166, 458
Cell-capillary gas exchange, 158
Cell division, 177
Cell function, 176–178, 177*f*
  factor affecting, 178–184
Cell membrane, 141
Cell metabolism, 140, 176–177, 261
Cells, 140, 141*f*
  injury and death, 177–178
  reproduction of, 177, 178*f*
  structure and function of, 142*t*
Cellular respiration, 156, 262
Cellular telephones, 113
Centers for Disease Control and
  Prevention (CDC), 38
Central chemoreceptors, 155
Central cyanosis, 766
Central lines, 809–810
Central nervous system (CNS), 142,
  162–164, 162*f*, 645, 646*f*
  depression, 511
  stimulation, 511
Central pulses, 328*t*, 329, 433
Cephalic (head) delivery, 741
Cerebellum, 163, 645
Cerebral contusion, 660
Cerebral cortex, 163
Cerebral hemorrhages, 382
Cerebral palsy, 186
Cerebrospinal fluid (CSF), 163, 645,
  648
Cerebrovascular accident (CVA),
  178
Cerebrum, 163, 645, 646*f*

Certification, 12
  emergency medical technician
    (EMT), 12
Cervical cancer, 483
Cervical collars, 669, 669*f*, 670*f*
Cervical spine, 145
  protection of
    in children, 777
    in primary survey, 345, 345*f*
Cervical (neck) vertebrae, 145, 614
Cervicitis, 483
Cervix, 479, 736
Chain of survival in cardiac arrest,
  443–444
CHART, 105–106
Chemical agents, 178
  as cause of disease, 185
Chemical burns, 574, 576, 580–581, 655
  emergency care of, 581
Chemical names, 205
Chemical protective clothing (CPC),
  859
Chemical weapons, 869–871, 870*t*
Chemoreceptors, 155
Chest, 146–147, 148*f*, 615
  assessment of, 359–360
    in rapid medical assessment, 374
    in secondary survey, 359–360
  sucking wound to, 571
Chest compressions
  adult, 445–446
  child, 446
  infant, 446, 446*f*
Chest injuries, 245
  penetrating, 570–571, 571*f*
Chest trauma, 591–604
  anatomy of cavity, 591, 592*f*
  categories of injuries, 591–592, 592*t*
  closed injuries, 592–594
    cardiac (pericardial) tamponade,
      598–599, 599*f*
    commotio cordis, 601–602
    flail chest, 594–596, 595*f*
    hemothorax, 598
    myocardial (cardiac) contusion,
      601, 601*f*
    pulmonary contusion, 600–601,
      600*f*
    rib fractures, 592–594, 593*f*
    simple pneumothorax, 596–597,
      596*f*
    tension pneumothorax, 597–598,
      597*f*
    traumatic asphyxia, 599–600, 600*f*
  open injuries, open pneumothorax,
    602–603, 602*f*
Chickenpox (varicella), 42*t*
  immunizations for, 42–43
Chief complaint, 105, 306, 342
  focused medical assessment by, 373*t*
Childbirth, 737
  precipitous, 756
Children. *See also* Preschoolers;
  School-age children; Toddlers
  abuse and neglect of, 804–806,
    805*f*, 806*f*
  age classification of, 770
  anatomical and physiological
    differences in, 771
    abdomen, 774, 774*f*
    airway, 771–772, 772*t*
    breathing, 772, 772*t*
    circulation, 772–774, 773*t*
    extremities in, 774–775, 775*f*
    face, 771
    head, 771, 771*f*
  assessment of
    primary survey, 776–781, 777*f*,
      778*f*, 779*f*
    scene size-up, 775–776, 775*f*
    secondary survey, 781
  BM device in, 291
  breathing difficulties in, 410–411
  cardiopulmonary resuscitation,
    one-rescuer, 882–885
  clearing foreign airway obstruction
    in conscious, 891
  clearing foreign airway obstruction
    in unconscious, 892
  common problems in
    airway obstruction, 781
    altered mental status, 784
    cardiopulmonary failure, 783
    drowning, 787–788

fever, 785
  poisonings, 786–787
  respiratory emergencies, 781–783
  seizures, 785–786
  shock, 784
  sudden infant death syndrome
    (SIDS), 788
  communication with, 301–302, 302*f*
  JumpSTART triage system for,
    841–843, 842*f*
  respiratory anatomy of, 245
  shock in, 543, 543*f*
  susceptibility of, to pedestrian
    injuries, 321
China white, 511
Chinese Americans, pregnancy and
  delivery in, 749
Chin lift, modified, 248
Choking, 244
Cholecystitis, 459, 461–462, 464*t*
Cholinergic toxidrome, 508*t*
Choroid, 653
Chronic bronchitis, 418–420, 419*f*
Chronic obstructive airway disease, 420
Chronic obstructive lung disease, 420
Chronic obstructive pulmonary
  disease (COPD), 261, 420, 596
  in older adults, 795
Chronic renal failure (CRF), 471
Chyme, 166, 458
Ciliary muscles, 653
Cincinnati Prehospital Stroke Scale,
  384–385, 603
Circuit courts, 81
Circulation
  in children, 772–774, 773*t*, 780–781
  in general impression, 342
  in older adults, 793
  physiology of, 162, 433–434, 433*f*
  in primary survey, 346–347
  reevaluating, 364
  in secondary survey, 364
Circulation compromise, 264
Circulatory system, 158–162, 158*f*,
  159*f*, 160*f*, 161*f*, 170*t*, 428
Circumferential burns, 579
Civil law, 81
Clavicles, 149, 614, 615
Cleaning, 43
Clenched-fist injury, 725
Clinical findings, 327
Clonic phase, 379
Closed abdominal injuries, 607
  specific, 608
Closed bone and joint injuries, 618
Closed chest injuries, 591, 592–594
  cardiac (pericardial) tamponade,
    598–599, 599*f*
  commotio cordis, 601–602
  flail chest, 594–596, 595*f*
  hemothorax, 598
  myocardial (cardiac) contusion,
    601, 601*f*
  pulmonary contusion, 600–601, 600*f*
  rib fractures, 592–594, 593*f*
  simple pneumothorax, 596–597, 596*f*
  tension pneumothorax, 597–598,
    597*f*
  traumatic asphyxia, 599–600, 600*f*
Closed fractures, 620
Closed head injury, 648
Closed questions, 305
Closed wounds, 556, 564–566, 564*f*
  emergency care of, 566–567
Clot-busting drugs (fibrinolytics), 436
Clothes drag, 53, 53*f*
Clothesline injuries, 658
Clothing pull, 53
Cluster headaches, 388
Coban bandage, 585*f*
Cocaine, 508, 512
  use in pregnancy, 751
Coccyx, 146, 614
Cognitive impairment, 694
  trauma in, 694–695
Coining, 805
Cold, exposure to, 701–706, 703*t*,
  704*f*, 706*f*
Cold-related emergencies, 699
Cold-related injury, assessment of
  patient with, 702–703
Cold zone, 863
Colic, 469
Colitis, 461

Collagen, 487
Collapsible stretcher, 818
Colles' fracture, 620
Coma, diabetic, 398
Comfort care, 90–91
Comminuted fracture, 620
Commission on Accreditation of
    Ambulance Services, 6
Commonly misused and abused
    substances, 507
    depressants, 509–510, 510t
    designer drugs, 511
    emergency care in, 513
    hallucinogens, 510–511
    patient assessment in, 511–513
    stimulants, 508–509
Commotio cordis, 601–602
Communicable (contagious)
    diseases, 37
    classification of, 37, 37f
Communications
    with adolescents, 302
    with children, 301–302, 302f
    defined, 110
    with hearing-impaired patients,
        303, 303f
    information management and, 836
    integrated, 835
    with medical direction, 117, 117f
    with non-English-speaking patients,
        303
    with older adults, 302–303
    with preschoolers, 302
    process of, 295, 296f
        with patient, strategies to ascertain
            information, 296–297
        patient's response to illness or
            injury, 297–304, 297f
        receiver, 296
        responses of family, friends, or
            bystanders to injury or illness, 304
        sender in, 295–296
    in professional behavior, 21
    with school-age children, 302
    with speech-impaired patients, 304
    with toddlers, 301–302, 302f
    with visually impaired patients,
        303–304
Community health, 16
Community involvement, 25, 25f
Compartment syndrome, 564–566, 565f
Competence, 83–84
    legal, 84
    medical/situational, 84
    mental, 84
Completed suicide, 525
Complex extrication, 854
Complex partial seizures, 380
Compliance, 285
Compound fracture, 560–561, 560f
Comprehensive Drug Abuse
    Prevention and Control Act
    (1970), 207t
Compression fractures, 662
    of spine, 662
Compression injuries, 564, 564f
    of abdomen, 607
Compulsions, 523
Computer-aided dispatch, 114–115,
    115f
Concussion, 659–660, 659f
Condom catheter, 470
Conductance vessels, 181
Conduction, 700–701, 700f
Conduction system, 158, 428
Cones, 653
Confidentiality, 103
Congestive heart failure (CHF), 437
Conjunctiva, 358, 653
Consent, 84–85
    expressed, 84–85
    implied, 85, 87
    informed, 84–85
    special situations, 85
Constipation in older adults, 797
Contamination reduction zone, 863
Continuing education, 12
Continuous ambulatory peritoneal
    dialysis (CAPD), 473
Continuous cyclic peritoneal dialysis
    (CCPD), 473
Contractions, 741
    Braxton-Hicks, 742
    timing, 741

Contralateral, 127–128
Control, recognizing patient's need
    for, 300
Controlled substances, schedule of,
    207t
Contusion, 564, 564f
    myocardial (cardiac), 601, 601f
    pulmonary, 600–601, 600f
Convection, 700, 700f
Convulsions, 379
Cookers, 511
Coping mechanisms, 297
Copperheads, 715
Coral snakes, 717–718
Core temperature, 699
Cornea, 653
Coronal plane, 144
Coronary arteries, 160, 430
Coronary artery bypass graft
    (CABG), 436–437
Coronary artery disease (CAD), 434
    in older adults, 794–795
Coronary heart disease (CHD), 434
Corpus callosum, 163, 645
Cortex, 167
Cots, guidelines for safe lifting of, 50
Cottonmouth snakes, 715
Coughing, protective reflexes
    involved in, 245–246
Court system, 81
Crackles (rales), 265, 409t, 440
Cradle carry, 55, 57f
Cranial bones, 614
Cranial cavity, 142
Cranial nerves, 164, 647
Cranium, 144
*Crash Injury Management for the Law
    Enforcement Officer* (training
    program), 5
Cravat, 585
Credentialing, 12
Crepitation, 351
Crepitus, 351, 593
    in laryngeal area, 658
Cricoid cartilage, 153, 244, 245
Cricoid pressure, applying, 280–282,
    281f, 282f
Crime scenes, 46–47, 94–95
Criminal law, 81
Crossed-finger technique, 247, 247f
Croup, 262, 413–414, 413t, 414f
    comparison of epiglottitis and, 415t
Crowds, 825–826
Crowing, 331
Crowning, 741, 743, 743f, 745
Crush injuries, 564, 564f
Crush syndrome, 566
Crying in infants, 192
Cultural considerations
    in communication, 301
    in pain expression, 339
Cumulative stress, 34
Current health status, 307–308
Cushing's triad, 660
Cyanide exposure, 511
Cyanosis, 262, 331–332, 332f
Cyst, ovarian, 482
Cystic fibrosis, 416–417
Cystitis, 469

Daily inspections, 818
Damages, 92
Dancer's hip, 490
Danger, warning signs of, 47
DCAP-BTLS
    in assessing abdomen, 463
    in physical exam, 350
Death, 74
    fetal, 685
    helping family of patient, 75–76,
        76f
    resulting from pedestrian injuries,
        689
    signs of obvious, 74–75
    stages of grief, 71–76
Decapitation, 74
Deceleration injury, 607
Decode, 296
Decompression sickness, 714–715
    emergency care for, 715
Decontamination, 830–831, 865
Defecation, 165, 458
Defendant, 81
Defense mechanisms, 297

Defibrillation, 444, 446–451, 446ft
Defibrillator, 444, 446
Definitive care, transfer to, 829
Degenerative arthritis, 489
Degenerative joint disease, 489
Degloving, 569
Dehydration, signs of, 398
Delayed drowning, 709
Delirium
    excited, 526
    in older adults, 796
Delirium tremens (DTs), 509
Delivery, 740, 742
    complications of, 757–758, 759f, 760f
    of placenta, 747
    preparing for, 743–744, 744f
    procedure of, 745–748, 745f, 746f,
        747f, 748f
    prolapsed cord, 758, 759f, 760
    signs of imminent, 743, 743f
Dementia in older adults, 796
Denial as stage of grief, 72–73
Dental appliances, 291
Dependent lividity, 75
Depositions, 82
Depressants, 509–510, 510t
Depression, 524
    central nervous system, 511
    as contributing factor to suicide, 526
    respiratory, 510
    as stage of grief, 73
Dermis, 165, 556
Descending colon, 166, 458
Designer drugs, 511
Destructive behavior, 521
Deviated septum, 243–244
Diabetes
    complications of, 396–397
    gestational, 396, 751
    in older adults, 799
    pregestational, 751
    pregnancy and, 751
Diabetic coma, 398
Diabetic emergency, symptoms of, 394
Diabetic ketoacidosis (DKA), 398
Dialysis, 471
    peritoneal, 473
Diaphragm, 155
    in children, 772
    injury to, 608
    position of, and respiration, 606,
        606f
Diarrhea in older adults, 797
Diastolic blood pressure, 162, 335, 433
Diazepam, 239, 239f
Diencephalon, 163
Diet in ascertaining current health
    status, 308
Digestion, 165, 166, 458
Digestive system, 165–166, 166f, 170t
    functions of, 458
    organs of, 458–459, 458f
Digital radio equipment, 111–112, 113f
Dilated pupils, 333
Dilation, 142
Diplomacy, 21–22
Direct carry, 60, 63–64f
Direct contact, 37
Direct force, 618
Direct ground lift, 58, 60, 61f
    three-person, 61f
Directional terms, 128–129t
Direct pressure in controlling external
    bleeding, 559–560, 559f
Direct questions, 305
Dirty bomb, 869
Disability, 347–349
Discovery, 82
Diseases
    airborne, 37
    bloodborne, 37
    causes of, 184–186
    communicable (contagious), 37
    defined, 176
    foodborne, 37
    of the nose, 530–532
        assessment findings and
            symptoms, 531
        emergency care, 531–532
    risk factors of, 184
    sexually transmitted, 37
    transmission of
        methods of, 37
        preventing, 36–37

Disentanglement in vehicle
    extrication, 855–856, 855f
Disinfection, 43
    high-level, 830
    intermediate-level, 830
    low-level, 830
Dislocation, 620–621f
    hip, 634
Disorders
    autoimmune, 185
    immune, 185
    immunodeficiency, 185
Dispatch, 114–116, 114f
Distal, 127
Distal pulses, 635
Distention, 359
Distributing vessels, 181
Distributive shock, 184, 540
District courts, 81
Disulfiram (Antabuse), 509
Diuretics (water pills), 439
Diving emergencies, 714–715
Doctrine of implied consent, 85
Documentation, 25, 95–106, 95f
    characteristics of good, 102–103,
        103f
    confidentiality, 103
    educational and research uses, 97
    elements of prehospital care
        report, 97–98, 101
    error correction, 104, 104f
    falsification of information on
        prehospital care reports,
        103–104
    formats, 104–106
    general guidelines for, 104
    quality management, 97
    uses of prehospital care report,
        96–97
Dog bites, 724–725, 725f
    emergency care for, 725
Domestic elder abuse, 806
Do no harm, 81
Do-Not-Resuscitate (DNR) orders,
    74, 87–91, 810–811
Dorsalis pedis artery, 432
Dorsalis pedis pulse, 160, 328t, 329
DOTS in physical exam, 350
Double-stage regulator, 270
Downers, 510
Down syndrome, 186, 694
Drags, 53–55
    ankle, 54–55, 55f
    bent-arm, 54
    blanket, 53, 54f
    clothes, 53, 53f
    firefighter's, 55, 55f
    forearm, 54, 54f
Draw sheet transfer, 62, 65f
Dressings, 559, 559f, 583–584
    occlusive, 584
    trauma, 583–584, 583f
    types of, 583
Driving conditions, contributing
    factors to unsafe, 823–824
Drowning, 689, 709–713
    assessment of victim, 711–713
    delayed, 709
    dry, 711
    effects of, 710–711
    emergency care of victim, 713
    in infants and children, 787–788
    risk factors, 709–710
    wet, 711
Drug Enforcement Administration
    (DEA), 205
Drug Importation Act (1848), 206t
Drug profile, 210
Drugs, 178
    administration of, oral route of,
        213–214, 214f
    forms of, 208–209, 209t
    legislation on, in United States,
        205, 206–207t
        federal regulatory agencies and
            services, 205
        forms of, 208–209, 209t
        names of, 205, 207–208t
        profile of, 210
        sources of, 205
    sources of information on, 208
    names of, 205, 207–208t
    semisynthetic, 205
    sources of, 205

sources of information on, 209
synthetic, 205
Dry drowning, 711
Duodenal ulcer, 460
Duodenum, 166, 458
DuoDote kits, 236, 236*f*, 871
Duplex system, 113
Dura mater, 163, 645
Durham-Humphrey Amendment (1951), 206*t*
Dust and dust storms, 823–824
Duty to act, 92
Dwarfism, 186
Dying patient. *See also* Death
  helping, 75, 75*f*
  helping family of, 75–76, 76*f*
Dysphagia in older adults, 797
Dyspnea, 413
Dysuria, 469

Early adults, 198–199. *See also* Middle adults; Older adults
  cognitive changes in, 199
  implications for healthcare professional, 199
  physiologic changes in, 198–199
  psychosocial changes in, 199, 199*f*
Early (compensated) shock, 541–542, 541*f*
Ears
  assessment of, 358–359
  injuries to, 575, 575*f*, 654
  in secondary survey, 358–359
Eastern coral snake, 717
Eating disorders in adolescents, 198
Ecchymosis, 358
Eclampsia, 755
Ecstasy, 511, 512
Ectopic pregnancy, 481–482, 482*f*, 752, 752*f*
Edema, 358
  pulmonary, 261, 264
    acute, 421–422
Educational uses of prehospital care report, 97
Egress from scene, 827
800-megahertz frequencies, 111
Elbow, 615
  golfer's, 490
  injuries to, 628, 630, 630*f*
  tennis, 490
Elder abuse, 693, 806–807
  domestic, 806
  institutional, 806
Elder speak, 201
Elective abortion, 751
Electrical burns, 576, 581–582
  emergency care of, 581–582
Electrolytes, 141
Emancipated minor, 85
Embedded objects, 571
Embolic stroke, 382
Embolism, pulmonary, 795
Embolus, 382
Embryo, 737
Emergency, 4
Emergency! (television program), 5
Emergency care, 24
  in abdominal and gastrointestinal disorders, 463–464
  in abdominal or genitourinary injury, 610
  with absorbed poisons, 518
  in acute pulmonary edema, 422
  in altered medical status, 377
  in asthma, 418
  in brain injuries, 662
  in cardiovascular disease, 440–443, 441*t*, 442*t*
  in chemical burns, 581
  in chronic bronchitis, 419
  in closed wounds, 566–567
  in croup, 414
  in cystic fibrosis, 416–417
  in emphysema, 420
  in endocrine disorders, 399–400
    performing blood glucose test, 400, 401*f*, 402
  in epiglottitis, 415
  in epistaxis, 531–532
  in external bleeding, 558–559, 558*t*
  in facial injuries, 656–657

in genitourinary and renal disorders, 475
in gynecologic patients, 480
in headaches, 390
in head injury, 651–652
in heat-related emergencies, 708–709
in hemophilia, 536
in hypothermia, 704–705, 704*f*
in immunology, 501
in ingested poisons, 514–515, 515*f*
in inhaled poisons, 517
in injected poisons, 517
in internal bleeding, 562–563, 563*f*
in local cold injury, 705–706, 706*f*
in neck injuries, 659
in nontraumatic musculoskeletal disorders, 492
in older adults, 694
in orthopedic trauma, 623–624
in pediatric trauma, 691–692
in pertussis, 416
in pneumonia, 420
in psychiatric disorders, 526–527, 527*f*
in pulmonary embolism, 421
in secondary survey, 362
in seizures, 381–382, 381*f*
in shock, 543–544
in sickle cell crisis, 535
in spinal injury, 668–669
in spontaneous pneumothorax, 422
in strokes, 385
in syncope, 388
in thermal burns, 579, 580
in thyroid disorders, 404
in toxicology, 513
in trauma in pregnancy, 688
Emergency Care Attendants (ECAs), 11
Emergency care interventions, reevaluating, 364
Emergency medical dispatchers (EMDs), 114–116
Emergency Medical Radio Service (EMRS), 110
Emergency medical responder (EMR), 11
Emergency Medical Services (EMS), 3
  for Children (EMSC) Program, 5
  common stressors associated with working in, 32*t*
  Education Agenda for the Future: A Systems Approach, 6, 6*t*
  Education Standards, 26
  levels of training in, 11*t*
  origins of, 4–7, 7–9*t*
  research related to, 26
  workforce in rural and frontier EMS, 896
Emergency Medical Services (EMS) system
  dispatch phase of, 820–821, 821*f*
  overview of, 9–17
  phases of typical, 17–19, 17*f*, 18*ft*, 19*f*
Emergency Medical Services (EMS) system communications, 109–119
  call, 113–119
    dispatch, 114–116, 114*f*
  communications system, 110
    centers, 110
    history, 110
    radio frequencies and ranges, 110–113
    regulation, 110
  equipment, 111–113
    cellular telephones, 113
    transmission modes, 113
Emergency Medical Services Systems (EMSS) Act (1973), 5
Emergency medical technicians (EMTs), 3, 3*f*, 11, 13
  certification of, 12
  curriculum for, 82
  in extrication scene, 850
  goals of training of, 4
  with hazardous materials, 859
  in lifting and moving patients, 47
  primary duties as, 22–26, 23*f*, 25*f*
Emergency medications, 218–240
  administered, 220–226
    activated charcoal, 220–221, 220*f*, 222*f*

aspirin, 221, 223
  oral glucose, 223–224, 223*f*, 225*f*
  oxygen, 224, 224*f*, 226
assisted, 226–233
  epinephrine, 226–227, 227*f*, 228–229*f*
  inhaled bronchodilators, 227, 229–230, 229*f*, 231–232*f*
  nitroglycerin, 230, 232–233, 233*f*, 235*f*
special situations
  atropine, 236–238
  diazepam, 239, 239*f*
  nerve agent antidotes, 233, 236
  pralidoxime chloride, 238–239
Emergency moves, 48
  carries, 55–58, 56*f*, 57*f*, 58*f*
  drags, 53–55, 53*f*, 54*f*, 55*f*
Emergency response and transportation, 815–832
  after the run, 830–831
  arrival phase and scene size-up, 825–827, 826*f*
    egress from scene, 827
    on-scene care, 827
    scene safety, 826–827, 826*f*
    traffic volume and flow, 827
    vehicle placement, 826–827
  en route, or response, phase, 821–825
    contributing factors to unsafe driving conditions, 823–824
    emergency response, 822
    escorts and multiple-vehicle responses, 824
    intersection crashes, 824–825, 825*f*
    right-of-way, 822–823
    speed and speed limits, 822
    warning lights and siren, 822
  en route to station, 830
  patient transfer equipment, 817–821, 818*f*, 819*f*, 820*f*, 821*f*
  dispatch phase, 820–821, 821*f*
  preparation phase, 816–817
    personnel and basic supplies, 816–817
  transferring patient to ambulance, 827
  transfer to definitive care, 829
  transport phase, 827–829, 828*f*
Emergency Response Guidebook, 44, 44*f*
Emergency transportation, 12
Emotional abuse, 805
Emotional support, 582–583
Empathy, 20
  listening with, 300, 301*f*
Emphysema, 264, 420
  subcutaneous, 573, 593
EMT-Basic National Standard Curriculum, 6
Encoding, 295
Endocrine disorders, 393–404
  age-related considerations in, 399
  diabetes mellitus, 396
    complications of, 396–397
    types of, 395–396
  emergency care in, 399–400
    performing blood glucose test, 400, 401*f*, 402
  emergency care in thyroid disorders, 404
  gestational diabetes, 396
  glucose, 394–395, 394*f*
  hyperglycemia, 397*t*, 398
  hypoglycemia, 397–398, 397*t*
  in older adults, 798–799
  patient assessment in, 398–399
  thyroid, 403–404, 403*f*
    hyperthyroidism, 404
    hypothyroidism, 403, 403*f*
Endocrine system, 166–167, 167*f*, 170*t*
Endometriosis, 479
Endometrium, 478
End-stage renal disease (ESRD), 471
Energy
  kinetic, 314
  sources of, and mechanism of injury, 315*t*
Enhanced 9-1-1, 10, 113
Enophthalmos, 655
En route, or response, phase, 821–825
  contributing factors to unsafe driving conditions, 823–824

emergency response, 822
escorts and multiple-vehicle responses, 824
intersection crashes, 824–825, 825*f*
right-of-way, 822–823
speed and speed limits, 822
warning lights and siren, 822
En route and scene size-up in vehicle extrication, 851, 851*f*
En route to receiving facility, 117–118
En route to station, 118–119, 830
Enteral route of administration, 213
Enterotoxin B, 868
Entrapment
  degrees of, 854, 855*f*
  heavy, 854, 855*f*
  light, 854, 855*f*
  moderate, 854, 855*f*
  no, 854
  victims in, 46, 46*f*
Environment
  considering, before approaching patient, 314
  as disease risk factor, 184
Environmental emergencies, 698–727
  bites and stings
    dog and cat bites, 724–725, 725*f*
    human bites, 725–726
    hymenoptera stings (bees, wasps, and ants), 723, 723*f*
    marine life stings, 724
    scorpion stings, 722–723, 722*f*
    snakebites, 715, 716*t*, 717–720, 717*f*
    spider bites, 720–722, 720*f*, 721*f*
  body temperature, 699–701
    heat loss, 700–701, 700*f*
    heat production, 699–700
    regulation, 699
  exposure to cold, 701–706
    hypothermia, 701–705, 703*t*, 704*f*
  exposure to heat, 707–709, 709*f*
    predisposing factors, 707
    types of heat-related emergencies, 707–708
  water-related
    diving, 714–715
    drowning, 709–713
Epidermis, 165, 556
Epidural hematoma, 661, 661*f*
Epiglottis, 152, 244
Epiglottitis, 262, 414–415, 414*f*
  comparison of croup and, 415*t*
Epilepsy, 186, 378
Epinephrine, 226–227, 227*f*, 228–229*f*, 501, 502*t*, 700
  autoinjectors for, 226–227, 227*f*, 501
Epistaxis, 655
  causes of, 531, 531*ft*
Equipment, 66–67
  backboards, 69–70
  cleaning, 43
  for stabilization, 852–853
  stair chair, 69, 69*f*
  stretchers
    basket, 68, 69*f*
    flexible, 68–69, 69*f*
    portable, 67, 68*f*
    scoop, 68, 68*f*
    wheeled, 67, 67*f*
  in vehicle extrication, 850, 851*f*
Erect, 130
Error correction, 104, 104*f*
Erythrocytes, 157, 159, 432
Escorts and multiple-vehicle responses, 824
Esophageal ulcer, 460
Esophageal varices, 461
Esophagitis, 460
Esophagus, 153, 166, 458, 461
  injuries to, 659
Essential hypertension, 438
Estrogen, 735
Ethical care. *See* Legal and ethical care
Ethical responsibilities, 83
Ethics, defined, 83
Ethmoid bone, 648
Etiology, 184
Evaporation, 700*f*, 701
Eviscerations, 571, 572*f*
Excited delirium, 526
Exclusion zone, 863
Exercise, 31

Exhalation, 245, 330
Exhaled carbon dioxide, 338–339
  detector for, 338
Exhaustion, 36
Expiration, 155, 156, 261
Exposure, 37
  to cold, 701–706
    hypothermia, 701–705, 703t, 704f
  documenting and managing, 43
  to heat, 707–709, 709f
    predisposing factors, 707
    types of heat-related
      emergencies, 707–708
Expressed consent, 84–85
Expressive aphasia, 385
External bleeding, 558–562
  controlling, 559–562, 559f, 560f,
    561f, 562f
  emergency care of, 558–559, 558t
External male genitalia, injuries to, 609
External nares, 152
External respiration, 262
Extracellular fluid (ECF), 141
Extremities. See also Lower
    extremities; Upper
    extremities
  in children, 774–775, 775f
  in rapid medical assessment, 375
  in secondary assessment, 361
  in secondary survey, 361
Extremity lift, 60, 62f
  two-person, 62f
Extrication, 24
  complex, 854
  rapid, 729
  simple, 854, 854f
Eye pads, 584
Eyes, 653
  assessment of, 358–359
  black, 654
  injuries to, 573–575, 574f, 654–655,
    655f
  layers and compartments of, 653f
  protection of, 39, 39f
  raccoon, 358, 648, 651
  in secondary survey, 358–359

Face
  in children, 771
  in head-to-toe examination, 351
  injuries to
    anatomy and physiology, 652–
      653, 652f, 653f
    emergency care for, 656–657
    mechanism of, 654
    patient assessment, 655–656
  in secondary survey, 351, 355
FACES Pain Rating Scale,
    Wong-Baker, 306, 307f, 339
Facilities, 14, 14f
  en route to receiving, 117–118
Fainting (syncope), 436
Fallopian tubes, 143, 167, 478, 735
Falls, 648
  as cause of injury in infants and
    children, 689
  as cause of spinal cord injury, 645
  factors to consider in, 321
  injuries from, 319t
False hope, not giving, 300
False labor, 742, 742t
False ribs, 147
Falsification of information on
    prehospital care reports,
    103–104
Family
  responses to injury or illness, 304
  stress and, 35–36, 36f
Fascia, 564
Fasciotomy, 565
FAST assessment for strokes, 384
Fatigue, 824
Fecal impaction in older adults, 797
Fecal incontinence in older adults,
    797–798
Federal Communications
    Commission (FCC), 10, 113
  regulation of interstate and
    international communication,
    110
Federal Food, Drug and Cosmetic
    Act (1938) (FDC), 205, 206t
Federal regulatory agencies and
    services, 205, 206–207t
Feedback, 296

Female reproductive system, 167,
    168f, 169, 478–479, 478f, 479f
  organs in, 735–738, 736f, 737f
Femoral arteries, 160, 329, 432
Femoral pulse, 160, 328t, 432
Femur, 615
Femur acetabulum, 149
Fend-off position, 851
Fentanyl (Sublimaze), 511
Fertilization, 735–736
Fetal alcohol syndrome, 750
  conditions associated with, 751
Fetal death, 685
Fetus, 737
Fever in infants and children, 785
Fibromyalgia, 489
Fibrous joints, 487, 616
Fibula, 149, 616
Fight bite, 725
Fight-or-flight response, 33, 33f, 164,
    647
Fight-or-flight response
  protective reflexes involved in,
    245–246
Finger sweeps, 250
Firearms, injuries caused by, 689
Firebombs, 869
Firefighter's carry, 55, 56f
Firefighter's drag, 55, 55f
Fire hazards, 46
Fire-related deaths, 689
Fires, 825
First-degree burn, 576
First impression, 373
First Responder National Standard
    Curriculum (1979), 5, 6
First Responders, 11
First stage of labor, 741, 741f
First trimester, 738
5-10-20 rule in gaining access to
    vehicle, 853
Fixed suction units, 251
Flail chest, 267, 594–596, 595f
Flail segment, 267, 594, 594f
Flexible, whistle-tip catheter, 252
Flexible stretcher, 68–69, 69f
Flow-restricted, oxygen-powered
    ventilation device, 288–289,
    288f
Flushed (red) skin, 332, 332f
Focal motor seizure, 380
Focal seizure, 380
Focused assessment, repeating, 364
Focused physical examination, 349,
    372, 373t, 549, 552
Focused trauma assessment, 552
Fog, 824
Foley catheter, 470
Follicles, 478
Fontanels, 190, 771
Food and Drug Administration
    (FDA), 205
Food and Drug Administration Act
    (1988), 207t
Foodborne diseases, 37
Food safety threats, 868
Foot
  bandage for, 587f
  injuries to, 640, 641t
Foramen magnum, 163, 648
Forearm, 615
  bandage for, 587f
  drag, 54, 54f
  injuries to, 630–631, 630f, 631f
Foreign body, in eye, 574
Foreign body airway obstruction
    (FBAO), 192, 249–250
  clearing
    in conscious adult, 888–889
    in conscious child, 891
    in conscious infant, 893
    in unconscious adult, 890
    in unconscious child, 892
    in unconscious infant, 894
Foreign body obstruction, 262
Fowler's position, 66, 66f, 130
Fraction of inspired oxygen, 151
Fractures, 489, 618–620, 619f, 620f
  closed, 620
  Colles', 620
  comminuted, 620
  compound, 560–561, 560f
  compression, 662
  jaw, 575f, 654
  linear, 620
  oblique, 620
  open, 560–561, 560f, 620

pelvic, 690
  Pott's, 620
  of spinal column, 693
  spiral, 620
Frank-Starling law of the heart, 179
Free radicals, 178
French suction catheter, 252
Friction burn, 567
Friends
  responses to injury or illness, 304
  stress and, 35–36, 36f
Frontal impact, 316–317
Frontal plane, 144
Frostbite, 705
Frostnip, 705
Fuel leaks, 856
Full-thickness burns, 577, 577f

Gagging, 415
  protective reflexes involved in,
    245–246
Gag reflex, 250
Gallbladder, 166, 458, 459
  inflammation of, 459
  pain from, 460
Gallstones, 462
Gamma rays, 869
Gas forms of drugs, 208
Gastric distention, 245, 280
  in ventilating infants and children,
    291
Gastric feeding, 810
Gastric ulcer, 460
Gastritis, 460, 464t
Gastroenteritis, 462, 464t
Gastroesophageal reflux disease
    (GERD), 460
Gastrointestinal bleeding, lower, 461
Gastrointestinal disorders.
    See Abdominal and
    gastrointestinal disorders
Gastrointestinal system
  allergic reactions in, 499t
  in older adults, 797–798
Gastrostomy tubes, 810
Gender as disease risk factor, 184
General approach in secondary
    survey, 349–350
General impression, 373
  in primary survey, 341–342, 341f,
    776–777
Generalized findings, allergic
    reactions in, 499t
Generalized seizures, 378, 379
Generic name, 205
Genitourinary and renal disorders, 467
  emergency care, 475
  patient assessment, 473–475
  renal disorders
    kidney stones, 469
    pyelonephritis, 471
    renal failure, 471–473, 471t,
      473f
    urinary tract infection, 469–471
  urinary system, 468–469
    anatomy and functions, 468–469
Genitourinary system in older adults,
    798
Genitourinary trauma, 609
  emergency care for, 610
  patient assessment in, 609
German measles, 42t
Germs
  killing, 43
  transmission of, 37
Gestational diabetes, 396, 751
Gestures, 296
Give Me 5 for Stroke, 384
Glanders, 868
Glasgow Coma Scale (GCS), 347–348,
    348t, 551, 650, 691, 694, 695, 730
Glass
  laminated, 853
  tempered, 853
Glaucoma in older adults, 800
Gliding joints, 487
Global Positioning System (GPS),
    112
Glottis, 153, 244
Gloves, 39
  removing, 40
Glucagon, 395, 459
Glucometer, 400

performing blood glucose test
    with, 401f
Glucose, 394–395, 394f
  oral, 223–224, 223f, 225f
Glycolysis, 176, 177f
Goiter, 403, 403f
Golden hour, 548
Golfer's elbow, 490
Gonorrhea, 481
Good Samaritan, 4
Goof balls, 510
Gowns, 39
Grand mal seizures, 379
Greater trochanter, 149
Great vessels, 158
Greenstick fracture, 619
Grief
  defined, 71
  stages of, 71–76
Growth plate, 619
  injuries to, 619
Guidelines for Trauma Care Systems, 5
Gunshot wounds, 568, 648, 654
  as cause of spinal cord injury, 645
Gurgling, 250, 265, 691
Gynecologic disorders
  assessment of patient, 479–480
  emergency care of patient, 480
  female reproductive system,
    478–479, 478f, 479f
  nontraumatic conditions
    cervical cancer, 483
    cervicitis, 483
    ectopic pregnancy, 481–482, 482f
    ovarian cysts, 482
    pelvic inflammatory disease,
      480–481
    sexually transmitted diseases
      (STDs), 481
    uterine fibroids, 483
    vaginitis, 482–483
  traumatic emergencies, 483
    apparent sexual assault, 483–484

Hallucinations, 525
  auditory, 525
  tactile, 525
Hallucinogens, 510–511
Hand, injuries to, 630–631, 630f,
    631f
Hand-foot syndrome, 534–535
Hand-off report, 118
Handwashing in infection control,
    38–39, 38f
Hantavirus, 868
Hard palate, 152, 244
Hard suction catheter, 251
Harrison Narcotic Act (1914), 206t
Hazard control and safety
    considerations in vehicle
    extrication, 851–852
Hazardous materials, 825
  awareness of, 858–865
    approaching patient, 864–865
    decontamination, 865
    role of EMT, 859
    scene safety and reporting,
      859–864
  clues suggesting presence of, 313
  defined, 44, 859
  identifying, 862–863
  scenes involving, 44
Head
  in children, 771, 771f
  in head-to-toe examination, 351
  injuries to, 647–652
    closed, 648
      emergency care for, 651–652
      mechanism of, 648
      open, 648
      patient assessment, 650, 651t
      scalp, 648
      skull, 648, 649, 650, 650f
  in rapid medical assessment, 374
  in secondary survey, 351, 355
Headaches, 387–390
  cluster, 388
  emergency care in, 390
  medication-induced, 388
  migraine, 387–388
  muscle contraction, 387
  ordinary, 387
  organic, 388
  patient assessment in, 389–390

possible signs and symptoms of, 389*t*
sinus, 387
stress, 387
types of, 387–389
Head bobbing, 410
Head fracture, basilar, 648, 649*f*, 650*f*
Headlights, 822
Head-on collision, injuries from, 318*t*
Head tilt–chin lift maneuver, 247–248, 247*f*, 262, 343, 343*f*
Head-to-toe examination, 350–351, 358–362
in secondary survey, 350–351
Health and Human Services Department (DHHS), U.S., Division of Trauma and EMS (DTEMS) of, 6
Healthcare resources in rural and frontier EMS, 895
Healthcare system, defined, 9–10
Health information, protected, 93–94
Health Insurance Portability and Accountability Act (HIPAA) (1996), 93–94, 119
Hearing-impaired patients, communication with, 303, 303*f*
Heart, 158, 158*f*, 428, 429*f*, 430*f*
Heart/cardiovascular centers, 15*t*
Heart disease, 184
Heart failure, 264
in older adults, 794–795
Heart rate
causes of slow, 330
children, 772–774, 773*t*
effect on cardiac output, 179
in newborn, 766
possible cause of rapid, 330
Heat cramps, 707
Heat exhaustion, 707
Heat loss, 700–701, 700*f*
Heat production, 699–700
Heat-related emergencies, 699
emergency care of patients with, 708–709
Heat stroke, 708
Heavy entrapment, 854, 855*f*
Helicobacter pylori, 460
Helicopters, working safety around, 847
Helmets
bicycle, 321
removal of, 678, 679–680*f*
Hematemesis, 461, 607
Hematology, 533–537
hemophilia, 536
assessment findings and symptoms, 536
emergency care for, 536
sickle cell disease, 534–535
assessment findings and symptoms, 534
emergency care for, 535
Hematomas, 564, 660–661, 660*f*, 667*f*
epidural, 661, 661*f*
intracerebral, 661, 661*f*
subdural, 660, 661*f*
Hematuria, 469, 607
Hemodialysis, 472–473, 472*f*
Hemoglobin, 157, 432
Hemophilia, 536, 557
assessment findings and symptoms, 536
emergency care for, 536
Hemoptysis, 598
Hemorrhage, 179, 556, 760
intracerebral, 382
subarachnoid, 382
Hemorrhagic causes of acute abdominal pain, 460–461
Hemorrhagic shock, 540
possible assessment findings and symptoms in, 559*t*
Hemorrhagic strokes, 382, 383*f*
Hemorrhoids, 461
Hemothorax, 265, 598
massive, 598
Hepatitis, 462, 464*t*
Hepatitis B virus (HBV), 37, 462
immunizations, 41–42
Hepatitis C, 37, 462
Hepatitis D, 462
Hepatitis E, 462
Heredity as disease risk factor, 184, 185–186, 307

Hering-Breuer reflex, 156
Hernias, 461
Heroin use in pregnancy, 751
High-efficiency particulate air (HEPA) filter, 282–283, 282*f*
High-efficiency particulate air (HEPA) masks, 39, 40*f*
High-Fowler's position, 66, 66*f*, 130
High-level disinfection, 830
High-risk pregnancy, 756–757
High-risk refusals, examples of, 86
High-visibility vests, 826
Highway Safety Act (1966), 4, 5
Hinge joints, 487, 488*f*, 616
Hip
bursitis, 490
dislocation, 634
immobilizing, 634
injuries to, 631, 634, 634*f*
joints, 615
Histamine, 497, 498
History, 105
importance of thorough, 372
patient, 305
chief complaint, 306
current health status, 307–308
past medical, 307
of present illness, 306–307, 307*f*
SAMPLE, 308
techniques of taking, 305
of present illness, 306–307, 307*f*
Hollow organs, 457–458
Home care, 808
Home healthcare, 808–809
Homeland Security Act (2002), 6–7
Homelessness, 807–808
Home mechanical ventilators, 809
Homeostasis, 140–142
defined, 176
Honesty, 302
Hooding, 599
Horizontal cross section, 144
Hospice care, 810–811
Hot zone, 863
Housemaid's knee, 491
Huffing, 516
Human bites, 725–726
emergency care for, 726
Human body, 138–174
cavities, 142–143, 143*f*
circulatory system, 158–162, 158*f*, 159*f*, 160*f*, 161*f*
digestive system, 165–166, 166*f*
endocrine system, 166–167, 167*f*
homeostasis, 140–142
integumentary system, 165, 165*f*
musculoskeletal system, 144–151
skeletal, 144–150, 145*f*, 146*f*, 148*f*, 149*f*
nervous system, 162–164, 162*f*, 163*f*
planes, 143–144, 143*f*
reproductive system, 167
female, 167, 168*f*, 169, 174*f*
male, 167, 168*f*, 172–173*f*
respiratory system, 151–158, 151*f*, 152*f*, 153*f*, 154*f*, 156*f*, 157*f*
structural organization, 140, 141*f*
urinary system, 169, 169*f*
Human crutch move, 58, 58*f*
Human immunodeficiency virus (HIV), 37, 185
Human papillomavirus (HPV), 481
Human resources and education, 10–12
Humerus, 149, 615, 616
injuries to, 628, 628*f*
Humidifiers, 270, 270*f*, 274
Hydrocephalus, 810
Hydrogen Safety for First Responders course, 852
Hygiene, 20
Hymenoptera stings (bees, wasps, and ants), 723, 723*t*
emergency care for, 723
Hyoid bone, 144
Hyperbaric centers, 15*t*
Hypercarbia, 179
Hyperglycemia, 397*t*, 398
Hyperosmolar hyperglycemic state, 799
Hypertension, 186, 438
Hypertensive disorders, 754–755
Hypertensive emergencies, 438
Hyperthermia, 190, 707

Hyperthyroidism, 404
Hyperventilation, 261
Hyphema, 358, 654, 655*f*
Hypoglycemia, 397–398, 397*t*
Hypoperfusion, 183, 540
Hypothalamus, 163, 699
Hypothermia, 190, 701–705, 703*t*, 704*f*
emergency care of patients with, 704–705, 704*f*
Hypothyroidism, 403, 403*f*
Hypoventilation, 261, 263
Hypovolemic shock, 183, 264, 386, 540, 566
Hypoxemia, 261
Hypoxia, 178, 261–262, 650, 712
cause of, 690
indications of, 408
Hypoxic drive, 155

Ice, 823
Ileum, 166, 458, 615
Illness
mechanism of injury and, 314–321, 315*t*, 316*f*, 317*f*, 318*ft*, 319*t*, 320*t*, 321*f*
responses of family, friends, or bystanders to, 304
in rural and frontier EMS, 896–898
in scene size-up, 321, 321*f*
Immersion, 709
Immovable joint, 487
Immune disorders, 185
Immunizations, 41–43
chickenpox (varicella), 42–43
hepatitis B, 41–42
influenza, 42
measles, mumps, and rubella, 42
pertussis, 416
tetanus, 41
tuberculosis, 43
Immunodeficiency disorders, 185
Immunology, 494–503
age-related considerations in, 501–502, 502*t*
allergic reaction, 497–498, 498*t*, 499*t*
causes of allergic reactions, 495, 495*f*, 496*t*, 497*t*, 498
emergency care in, 501
patient assessment in, 498–501
Impaled objects, 567–568, 568*f*, 571
Impetigo, 804
Implantable cardioverter-defibrillator (ICD), 446–447
Implied consent, 85, 87
Incendiary weapons, 869
Incident commander, 834
Incident command system, 834–837
Incident facilities, 835
Incident management, 833–837
command system, 834–837
Incident Management System (IMS), 834
Incident stability, priorities of, 834–835
Incomplete abortion, 751
Incubation period, 184
Index of suspicion, 548
Indirect contact, 37
Indirect force, 618
Indwelling catheter, 470
Infants, 189–192. *See also* Newborn
age classification of, 770
assessment of
primary survey, 776–781, 777*f*, 778*f*, 779*f*
scene size-up, 775–776, 775*f*
secondary survey, 781
BM device in, 291
breathing difficulties in, 410–411
cardiopulmonary resuscitation of, 885–886
one-rescuer, 885–886
clearing foreign body airway obstruction
in conscious, 893
in unconscious, 894
cognitive changes, 191
common problems in
airway obstruction, 781
altered mental status, 784
cardiopulmonary failure, 783
drowning, 787–788
fever, 785
poisonings, 786–787
respiratory emergencies, 781–783

seizures, 785–786
shock, 784
sudden infant death syndrome (SIDS), 788
implications for healthcare professional, 192, 192*f*
physiologic changes, 189–191, 189*f*, 190*f*, 191*t*
premature, 757
psychosocial changes, 192
respiratory anatomy of, 245
shock in, 543, 543*f*
Infarct, 178
Infection, 36–37
as cause of disease, 185
control procedures of, 830–831
Infection control, 37–44
cleaning equipment, 43
disinfecting, 43
documenting and managing exposure, 43
sterilizing, 44
Inferior, 127
Inferior vena cava, 432, 433, 457
Inflammation as cause of disease, 185
Inflammatory response, 497
Inflation, 156
Influenza, immunizations for, 42
Information, strategies to ascertain, 296–297
Informed consent, 84–85
Ingested poisons, 514–515, 515*f*
emergency care with, 514–515, 515*f*
patient assessment, 514
Ingestion, 165, 458
Inhalants, 516
Inhalation, 245
Inhalation route, 215
Inhaled bronchodilators, 227, 229–230, 229*f*, 231–232*f*
Inhaled poisons, 515–517
emergency care with, 517
patient assessment with, 516
Injected poisons, 517
emergency care with, 517
patient assessment with, 517
Injuries
ear, 575, 575*f*
eye, 573–575, 574*f*
mouth, 575, 575*f*
neck, 572–573, 573*f*
prevention of, 16
hazardous materials scenes, 44
motor vehicle crashes and rescue scenes, 45–46
violent scenes, 46–47
responses of family, friends, or bystanders to, 304
in rural and frontier EMS, 896–898
unintentional, 315*t*
Injury Control Act (1990), 5
Injury in America: A Continuing Public Health Problem, 5
Injury Prevention Act (1990), 5
In-line stabilization, 345, 345*f*
Insertion of skeletal muscle, 616, 617*f*
Inspiration, 155–156, 261, 330
Institutional elder abuse, 806
Insulin, 167, 394, 459
Insulin resistance, 396
Integrated communications, 835
Integrity, 20
Integumentary system, 165, 165*f*, 170*t*
Intentional injuries, 315*t*
Interagency Radio Advisory Committee (IRAC), 110
Intercostal muscles, 155, 245
Intercostal retractions, 409
Intermediate-level disinfection, 830
Intermittent peritoneal dialysis (IPD), 473
Internal bleeding, 562–563, 563*f*
emergency care of, 562–563, 563*f*
Internal female genitalia, injury to, 609
Internal respiration, 262
Internet Voice, 113
Intersection crashes, 824–825, 825*f*
Intestinal obstruction, 461, 464*t*
Intestines, injury to, 608
Intimate partner violence, 684
Intracellular fluid (ICF), 141
Intracerebral hematoma, 661, 661*f*
Intracerebral hemorrhage, 382

Intramuscular (IM) route, 215–216, 216*f*
Intrauterine fetal death, 756–757
Ipsilateral, 130
Iris, 653
Irreversible shock, 542
Ischemia, 178, 434
Ischemic strokes, 382
Ischium, 615
Islets of Langerhans, 167

Japanese Americans, pregnancy and delivery in, 749–750
Jaundice, 774
Jaundiced skin, 332, 332*f*
Jaw fracture, 575*f*, 654
Jaw thrust, 248, 262, 343, 343*f*
    without head extension maneuver, 248
    without head tilt maneuver, 248
Jejunum, 166, 458
Joints, 487, 487*f*, 616
    cartilaginous, 616
    fibrous, 616
    hinge, 616
    synovial, 616
Jugular veins, 658
Jugular venous distention (JVD), 359, 597
JumpSTART triage system, 841–843

Kefauver-Harris Drug Amendment (1962), 206*t*
Kehr's sign, 608
Kendrick Extrication Device (KED), 855, 855*f*
Keratin, 556
Keratitis, ultraviolet, 655
Kidneys, 169, 468–469
    failure of, 471
    injury to, 609
Kidney stones, 462, 465*t*
    pain of, 460
Killer bees, 723
Kinematics, 314
Kinetic energy, 314
Knee, 149, 616
    housemaid's, 491
    injuries to, 635, 635*f*
Knee bandage, 587*f*
Kneecap, bursitis of, 491
Knowledge, maintaining, 12
Kübler-Ross, Elizabeth, 72
Kussmaul respirations, 398
Kyphosis, 489

Labia, 479
Labia major, 479
Labia minora, 479
Labor, 736, 740
    complications of, 757
    false, 742, 742*t*
    precipitous, 756
    preterm, 739
    stages of, 740–742, 741*f*
Laceration, 567, 567*f*
Lactic acid, 176–177, 434
Laminated glass, 853
Lancet, 400
Landing zone, 846
Large intestine, 166, 458
Larrey, Dominique-Jean, 4
Laryngeal injuries, 658
Laryngeal stoma, 359
Laryngopharynx, 152, 244
Laryngospasm, 711
Larynx, 151, 244, 657
Late adulthood, 200–201
    cognitive changes, 201
    implications for healthcare professional, 201
    physiologic changes, 200–201, 200*f*
    psychosocial changes, 201
Lateral, 127
Lateral collision, injuries from, 318*t*
Lateral impact, 316
Lateral recumbent position, 130
Late (decompensated) shock, 542, 542*f*
Latex allergy, 495, 496*t*, 497, 497*t*
Latex allergy decal, 500, 500*f*
Law
    administrative, 81

civil, 81
criminal, 81
    sources of, 81
    statutory or legislative, 81
Lawsuit, steps in, 81–82
Lawyer's letter, 81
Layer, 645
Left lower quadrant (LLQ), 143, 457, 457*f*
Left upper quadrant (LUQ), 143, 457, 457*f*
Legal and ethical care
    abandonment, 91
    advanced directives, 87–91
    assault and battery, 91
    confidentiality, Health Insurance Portability and Accountability Act (HIPAA) (1966), 93–94
    consent, 84–85
    documentation, 95–106, 95*f*
        characteristics of good. 102–103, 103*f*
        educational and research uses, 97
        elements of prehospital care report, 97–98, 101
        quality management, 97
        uses of prehospital care report, 96–97
    do-not-resuscitate (DNR) order, 87–91
    importance of, 80–81
    legal system
        sources of law, 81
        steps in lawsuit, 81–82
    negligence, 91–92
        breach of duty, 92
        damages, 92
        duty to act, 92
        proximate cause, 92–93
    refusals, 85–87, 88*f*, 89*f*
    scope of practice
        competence, 83–84
        ethical responsibilities, 83
        legal duties, 82–83
    special situations
        crime scenes, 94–95
        medical identification devices, 94
        organ donation, 95
        reporting requirements, 95
Legal competence, 84
Legal considerations, communications and, 119
Legal duties, 82–83
Legal uses of prehospital care report, 96
Legislation, 10
Legislative law, 81
Leukocytes, 159
Level A personal protective equipment, 859, 860*f*, 861*t*
Level B personal protective equipment, 859–860, 860*f*, 861*f*
Level C personal protective equipment, 860, 861*ft*
Level D personal protective equipment, 860, 861*ft*
Level of responsiveness in primary survey, 343–344, 344*f*
Libel, 93
Licensure, 12
Life safety, priorities of, 834–835
Life span, 189
Life span development
    adolescents, 197–198, 198*f*
    early adulthood, 198–199, 199*f*
    infants, 189–194, 189*f*, 190*f*, 191*t*, 192*f*
    late adulthood, 200–201, 200*f*
    middle adulthood, 199–200
    preschoolers, 194–196, 194*f*, 195*f*
    school-age children, 196–197, 196*f*, 197*f*
    toddlers, 192–194, 193*f*, 194*f*
Lifestyle
    as disease risk factor, 184
    stress and changes of, 35, 35*f*
Life-threatening emergency, 85
Ligaments, 150, 487, 616
Lightening, 739
Light entrapment, 854, 855*f*
Linear fracture, 620
Lip breathing, pursed, 266
Liquid drugs, 209, 209*t*
Listening, active, 296

Liver, 166, 458–459, 608
    damage to, 608
Local cold injury, 701, 705
    emergency care of patients with, 705–706, 706*f*
Local effect, 208
Long backboard, 69–70, 69*f*, 729
    immobilization of supine patient on, 670, 672–673, 672*f*, 673*f*
Love Drug, 511
Lower airway, 244–245
Lower extremities, 149–150, 149*f*, 615
    injuries to, 631–640, 632–633*f*, 634*f*, 635*f*, 636–637*f*, 638–639*f*, 640*f*
Lower gastrointestinal (GI) bleeding, 461
    in older adults, 797
Low-level disinfection, 830
Low vision, 303
Lumbar vertebrae, 145, 614
Lung cancer, 184, 596
Lungs, 154–155, 154*f*, 245
Luxation, 620
Lymphatic system, 158, 428
Lysergic acid diethylamide (LSD), 510
    drowning and, 710

Macular degeneration in older adults, 800
Magic mushrooms, 510
Major bleeding, 179
Male reproductive system, 167, 168*f*
Malignant tumor, 177
Mammalian diving reflex, 711
Mammary glands, 169
Mandible, 144, 614, 654
    injuries to, 655
Mania, 524
Manic-depressive illness, 524
Manual defibrillator, 446
Manually triggered ventilation (MTV) device, 288
Manual stabilization, 345
Manubrium, 147, 149, 615
Marijuana, drowning and, 710
Marine life stings, 724
Mark I kit, 233, 236, 236*f*
Masks, 39, 40*f*
Mask-to-stoma breathing, steps in performing, 289
Mass-casualty incident, 839
Massive hemothorax, 598
Material Safety Data Sheets (MSDSs), 863
Maxilla, 614, 653, 654
MDMA (3,4-methylene-dioxymethamphetamine) ("Ecstasy"), 511
Measles, 42*t*
    immunizations for, 42
Measure, abbreviations for common units of, 135*t*
Mechanism of injury (MOI)
    in abdominal trauma, 606
    defined, 314–315
    for musculoskeletal injuries, 618, 618*f*
    or nature of illness, 314–321
    predictable injuries based on common, 318–319*t*
    sources of energy and, 315*t*
    in trauma, 548–553, 549*f*, 550*f*, 551*t*
Meconium, 742, 764
Meconium staining, 756
Medial, 127
Medial tibial stress syndrome, 490–491
Mediastinal shift, 597
Mediastinum, 154, 591
Medical abbreviations and acronyms, 130, 131–135*t*
Medical and legal considerations with psychiatric disorders, 528
Medical control, 13
Medical direction, 13
    communicating with, 117, 117*f*
    off-line, 13
    on-line, 13, 13*f*
    prospective, 13
    retrospective, 14
Medical director, 13
Medical history, past, 307
Medical identification devices, 94
Medical neglect, 806

Medical Orders for Life-Sustaining Treatment (MOLST), 91
Medical oversight, 13
Medical overview, 371–375
    responsive patient, 372–374
    unresponsive patient, 374–375
Medical patient, 314
    responsive, 372–374, 372*f*
    unresponsive, 374–375
Medical practice acts, 13
Medical/situational competence, 84
Medical terminology, 121–135
    body positions and directional terms, 127, 128–129*t*, 128*f*, 130*t*
    combining forms, 123, 125
    plural terms, 125, 126–127*t*
    prefixes, 122–123*t*
    root words, 122, 125–126*t*
    suffixes, 123, 124–125*t*
Medical uses of prehospital care report, 96
Medications, 739–740
    administered, 220–226
        activated charcoal, 220–221, 220*f*, 222*f*
        aspirin, 221, 223
        oral glucose, 223–224, 223*f*, 225*f*
        oxygen, 224, 224*f*, 226
    administration of, 211–216
        general guidelines, 212–213
        reassessment and documentation, 216
        routes of, 213–216
        six rights of, 213
    in ascertaining current health status, 308
    assisted, 226–233
        epinephrine, 226–227, 227*f*, 228–229*f*
        inhaled bronchodilators, 227, 229–230, 229*f*, 231–232*f*
        nitroglycerin, 230, 232–233, 233*f*, 235*f*
    emergency (*See* Emergency medications)
    headaches induced by, 388
Medulla, 167
Medulla oblongata, 163, 645
Melatonin, 167
Melena, 461
Menarche, 197
Meninges, 163, 645, 660*f*
Meningitis, 163, 785
Meningococcal meningitis, 785
Menstruation, 197, 478, 736
Mental competence, 84
Mental incompetence, 85
Mental status, reassessment of, 351
Mental well-being, stress and, 31–34, 33*ft*, 34*t*, 35*f*, 36, 36*f*
Mescaline, 510
Mess, 510
Message, 295
Metabolic problems in older adults, 798–799
Metabolism, 699–700
    aerobic, 140
    anaerobic, 140, 176
    cell, 140, 176–177, 261
Metacarpals, 149
Metastasis, 177
Metatarsal bones, 150
Metered-dose inhalant (MDI), 215, 227, 229–230, 229*f*, 231–232*f*, 422, 423*t*
Methamphetamines, 508, 512
    in pregnancy, 751
Mexican Americans, pregnancy and delivery in, 749
Mexican brown, 511
Midaxillary line, 129*t*, 130
Midbrain, 163, 645
Midclavicular line, 129*f*, 130
Middle adults, 199–200. *See also* Early adults; Older adults
    cognitive changes, 200
    implications for healthcare professional, 200
    physiologic changes, 199–200
    psychosocial changes, 200
Midface, 652
    injuries to, 655
Midline, 127
Migraine headaches, 387–388

Military antishock trousers (MAST), 560
Ministroke, 382
Minors, 85
    emancipated, 85
Minute volume, 155, 261, 408
Mitral (bicuspid) valve, 428
Mobile Army Surgical Hospital (MASH) units, 4
Mobile data computers (MDCs), 112
Mobile data terminals (MDTs), 112
Mobile two-way radio, 111, 112*f*
Moderate entrapment, 854, 855*f*
Modifiable risk factors, 434
Modified chin lift, 248
Modified jaw thrust maneuver, 248, 248*f*
Moisture, 347
Molotov cocktail, 869
MONA in treating cardiovascular disease, 440–441
Mongolian spots, 804
Morning sickness, 738
Moro reflex, 190
Motorcycle crashes, injuries from, 319*t*
Motor nerves, 647
Motor vehicle crashes (MVCs), 316–317, 317*f*, 318–319*t*, 318*f*, 648
    as cause of trauma in pregnancy, 684
    flail chest in, 594
    impacts in, 317*f*
    rescue scenes and, 45–46
    rib fractures from, 592
    statistics of, 320
Motor vehicle–pedestrian crashes, 320–321
    injuries from, 318–319*t*
Mottling, 332, 332*f*
Mouth, 166, 458
    injuries to, 575, 575*f*, 654, 654*f*
    opening, 247, 247*f*
Mouth-to-barrier device ventilation, 283, 283*f*, 285
Mouth-to-mask ventilation, 282–283, 282*f*, 285*f*
Movement
    nonpurposeful, 351
    purposeful, 351
Multiagency coordination, 835
Multiple-casualty incidents, 95, 95*f*, 834, 838–843
    defined, 839
    JumpSTART triage system, 841–843
    START triage system, 839–841, 840*f*, 841*f*
Multiple-casualty situation (MCS), 839
Multiple gestation, 756
Multiple-patient situations, triage in, 865
Multiple sclerosis (MS), 184
Multiplex system, 113
Multisystem trauma, 728–732, 729*f*, 731*f*
    blast injuries, 730–731, 731*f*
Mumps, 42*t*
    immunizations for, 43
Muscle contraction headaches, 387
Muscles
    cardiac, 151, 151*t*
    intercostal, 155, 245
    respiratory, 263
    skeletal, 150, 150*f*, 151*t*, 616
    smooth, 150–151, 151*t*
Muscle tissue, 140
Muscle tone, 150
Muscular dystrophy, 186, 263
Muscular system, 150–151, 150*f*, 151*t*, 170*t*, 616, 617*f*
Musculoskeletal injuries
    care of specific, upper-extremity, 627–631, 628*f*, 629*f*, 630*f*, 631*f*
    mechanism of, 618, 618*f*
    types of, 618–622, 619*f*
Musculoskeletal system, 144–151, 613
    in older adults, 799, 799*f*
    review of, 487, 487*f*, 488*f*
    skeletal, 144–150, 145*f*, 146*f*, 148*f*, 149*f*, 613–616
Myocardial (cardiac) contusion, 601, 601*f*
Myocardial infarction, 178

Narcotics, 510
    effect on respiratory function, 263
Narcotics and Dangerous Drugs, Bureau of (BNDD), 205
Narrative documentation format, 106
Nasal airway, 255–257, 255*f*
    sizing and inserting, 256–257*f*
Nasal bones, 652
Nasal cannula, 275*f*, 276*t*
Nasal cavity, 244
Nasal flaring, 358, 410
Nasopharyngeal airway (NPA), 255
Nasopharynx, 152, 244
National Academy of Sciences–National Research Council (NAS/NRC), 4
National Association of Emergency Medical Technicians (NAEMT), 5
National Association of State EMS Directors (NASEMSD), 6, 895
National Center on Shaken Baby Syndrome, 689
National Coalition Against Domestic Violence, 750
National Emergency Medical Services (EMS) information system, components of, 98
National EMS Core Content (document), 7, 26
National EMS Education Standards, 6*t* 10, 11, 12, 26, 82
National EMS Information System (NEMSIS), storage of Emergency Medical Services (EMS) data, 97
National EMS Scope of Practice (document), 7, 10, 26, 82
National Fire Protection Association (NFPA)
    hazardous materials defined by, 44
    Standard 704 of, 863, 863*f*
National Highway Traffic Safety Administration (NHTSA), components of Technical Assistance Program Assessment Standards, 6
National Incident Management System (NIMS), 7, 834, 862
National Institute on Drug Abuse (NIDA), 516
National Organization of State Offices of Rural Health (NOSORH), 895
National Registry of Emergency Medical Technicians (NREMT), 12
    founding of, 5
National Research Council (NRC), 5
National Rural Health Association (NRHA), 895
National Safety Council (NSC), 4
National Spinal Cord Injury Statistical Center on head injuries, 645
Native Americans, pregnancy and delivery in, 749
Nature of illness, 321, 321*f*
Navel (umbilicus), 143
Navy stretcher, 68
Near syncope, 386
Neck
    assessment of, 359
    injuries of, 572–573, 573*f*
        anatomy and physiology, 657–658, 657*f*, 658*f*
        emergency care for, 659
        mechanism of, 658
        patient assessment for, 658–659
    in rapid medical assessment, 374
    in secondary survey, 359
    trauma to, 263
Necrosis, 178
Neglect, 805–806, 806*f*
    child, 804–806, 805*f*, 806*f*
    medical, 806
Negligence, 91–92
Neonatal care, 763–768
    caring for newborn, 764
Neoplasm, 177
Nephrons, 469
Nerve agents
    antidotes for, 233, 236

signs and symptoms of exposure to, 236*t*
Nerves
    cranial, 647
    dysfunction of, 263
    motor, 647
    oculomotor, 647
    sensory, 647
    spinal, 647
Nervous control, interruption of, 263
Nervous system, 162–164, 162*f*, 163*f*, 170*t*
    allergic reactions in, 499*t*
    autonomic, 647
    central, 645, 646*f*
    in older adults, 795–797
    peripheral, 647
Nervous tunic, 653
Neurogenic shock, 184, 540
Neurological disorders, 376–390
    altered mental status, 377–378
        common cause of, 377
        emergency care, 377–378
    headaches, 387–390
        emergency care for, 390
        patient assessment in, 389–390
        types of, 387–389
    seizures, 378–382
        emergency care in, 381–382, 381*f*
    stroke, 382–385, 382*f*
        assessment findings and symptoms, 384–385
        emergency care, 385
        risk factors, 384
        types of, 382, 383*f*, 384
    syncope, 385–387
        emergency care for, 387
        patient assessment, 386–387
Neurons, 162
Newborn. *See also* Infants
    airway and breathing in, 764–765, 765*f*
    Apgar score in, 766, 767*t*
    caring for, 764
    heart rate in, 766
    skin color in, 766, 766*f*
Nicotine, 508
Nightmares, 36
Nighttime, 824
9-1-1 network, 10
Nipah virus, 868
Nitroglycerin (NTG), 178, 215, 230, 232–233, 233*f*, 235*f*, 435, 439
    in emergency care in cardiovascular disease, 441–442, 442*t*
N95 masks, 39, 40*f*
No entrapment, 854
Noise, 296
Nonadherent pads, 584
Nonallergic asthma, 417
Nonchemical burn, 575
Non-English-speaking patients, communication with, 303
Nonhemorrhagic causes of acute abdominal pain, 461
Noninvasive blood pressure (NIBP) monitor, 335
Nonmodifiable risk factors, 434
Nonproprietary name, 205
Nonpurposeful movement, 350, 351
Nonreactive pupils, 333–334
Nonrebreather mask, 274, 274*f*, 276*t*
Nontraumatic gynecologic conditions
    cervical cancer, 483
    cervicitis, 483
    ectopic pregnancy, 481–482, 482*f*
    ovarian cysts, 482
    pelvic inflammatory disease (PID), 480–481
    sexually transmitted diseases (STDs), 481
    uterine fibroids, 483
    vaginitis, 482–483
Nontraumatic musculoskeletal disorders, 486–493
    arthritis, 489
    emergency care, 492
    fibromyalgia, 489
    osteoporosis, 489
    overuse syndromes, 489–491
    patient assessment, 491–492
    review of system, 487, 487*f*, 488*f*

Nonurgent moves, 48, 58
    direct ground lift, 58, 60, 61*f*
    extremity lift, 60, 62*f*
    transferring supine patient from bed to stretcher, 60
        direct carry, 60, 63–64*f*
        draw sheet transfer, 62, 65*f*
Nosebleed, 530, 531
    anterior, 531
    posterior, 532
Noses, 244
    diseases of, 530–532
    injuries to, 654
Nuclear weapons, 869, 869*f*
Nutritional imbalances as cause of disease, 186

Objective findings, 184, 327
Oblique fracture, 620
Oblongata, 155
Obsessions, 523
Obsessive-compulsive disorder, 523
Obstetrics, 734–762
    anatomy and physiology, 735–738, 736*f*, 737*f*
    emergency in, 755
Obstructive shock, 183, 540
Occipital bone, 648
Occipital lobes, 163, 645
Occiput posterior presentation, 757
Occlusive (airtight) dressings, 359, 584
Occupational Safety and Health Administration (OSHA), 38
Oculomotor nerve, 647
Off-line medical direction, 13
Older adults, 791–802, 792*f*. *See also* Early adults; Middle adults
    altered mental status in, 796–797
    Alzheimer's disease in, 796
    appearance in, 793
    assessment of, 792–794, 792*f*
    breathing in, 793
    cataracts in, 800
    circulation in, 793
    common health problems in
        cardiovascular system, 794
        gastrointestinal system, 797–798
        genitourinary system, 798
        metabolic and endocrine, 798–799
        musculoskeletal system in, 799, 799*f*
        nervous system, 795–797
        respiratory system, 795
        toxicological emergencies, 799–800
    communication with, 302–303
    constipation in, 797
    delirium in, 796
    dementia in, 796
    diabetes mellitus in, 799
    diarrhea in, 797
    dysphagia in, 797
    fecal impaction in, 797
    fecal incontinence in, 797–798
    genitourinary system in, 798
    glaucoma in, 800
    lower gastrointestinal (GI) bleeding in, 797
    macular degeneration in, 800
    metabolic and endocrine problems in, 798–799
    musculoskeletal system in, 799, 799*f*
    osteoarthritis (OA) in, 799, 799*f*
    osteoporosis in, 799, 799*f*
    polypharmacy in, 799
    presbycusis in, 800
    respiratory anatomy of, 245–246
    sensory changes in, 800–801
    shock in, 543
    sundowning in, 796
    touch sensitivity in, 801
    toxicological emergencies in, 799–800
    trauma in, 692–694
        emergency care in, 694
        mechanism of injury, 692–693
        patient assessment in, 693–694, 693*f*
        special considerations in, 693
    ulcer disease in, 797
    upper gastrointestinal (GI) bleeding in, 797
    urinary incontinence in, 798
    urinary tract infections (UTIs) in, 798

Olecranon, 149
Onboard oxygen, 269, 269ft
One-person arm carry, 55
One-rescuer adult cardiopulmonary resuscitation, 876–878
One-rescuer child cardiopulmonary resuscitation, 882–885
One-rescuer infant cardiopulmonary resuscitation, 885–886
Ongoing management and maintenance, 836
On-line medical direction, 13, 13f
On-scene care, 827
Open abdominal injuries, 608
Open chest injuries, 591–592
   open pneumothorax, 602–603, 602f
Open crush injury, 569, 569f, 570f
Open-ended questions, 305
Open fracture, 560–561, 560f, 620
Open head injury, 648
Open injury, 618
Open pneumothorax, 597, 602–603, 602f
Open wounds, 556, 564, 567–570, 567f
   emergency care of, 570
Operator area, inspection of vehicle, 820
Opioid (narcotics) toxidrome, 508t
Opium, 510
Opium derivatives, 510
OPQRST assessment
   in abdominal and gastrointestinal disorders, 462–463
   in cardiovascular disease, 439–440
   in nontraumatic musculoskeletal disorders, 491
   in pain/discomfort, 372
Optimal Hospital Resources for Care of the Injured Patient, 5
Oral airway, 253, 255, 255f
   sizing and inserting, 254–255f
Oral cavity, 244
Oral diabetes medications, examples of, 396t
Oral glucose, 214, 223–224, 223f, 225f, 402–403, 402t
Oral intake in ascertaining current health status, 308
Oral route of drug administration, 213–214, 214f
Orbits (eye sockets), 652
Ordinary headaches, 387
Organic headaches, 388
Organophosphate insecticides, exposure to, 511
Organs, 140
   donation of, 95
   vital, 140
Organ systems, 140, 170t
Origin of skeletal muscle, 616, 617f
Oropharyngeal airway (OPA), 253
Oropharynx, 152, 244
Orphan Drug Act (1983), 207t
Orthopedic trauma, 613–642
   emergency care in, 623–624
   musculoskeletal injuries
      mechanism of, 618, 618f
      types of, 618–622, 619f
   musculoskeletal system, 613
      muscular, 616, 617f
      skeletal, 613–616
   patient assessment in, 622–623
   splinting, 624–627
Orthopnea, 407
Osteoarthritis, 186
   in older adults, 799, 799f
Osteoporosis, 489, 620
   in older adults, 799, 799f
Ovarian cyst, 482
Ovaries, 143, 167, 478, 735
Overactive thyroid, 404
Overdose, 507
Overuse syndromes, 489–491
Oviducts, 167
Ovulation, 478, 735
Oximeter, 267
Oxygen, 156–157, 224, 224f, 226
   administration of, 215
   importance to nervous system cells, 243

safe use of, 269–270, 274f, 275f, 276ft
supplemental, 269–276, 269ft, 270f, 271f, 273f
Oxygenation, 178, 261–262
   assessment of, 267–268, 267f, 268f
   defined, 261
Oxygen cylinders, 269–270, 269ft
Oxygen delivery system
   devices in
      blow-by-oxygen, 276, 276f
      nasal cannula, 275f, 276t
      nonrebreather mask, 274, 274f, 276t
      partial rebreather mask, 274, 274f, 276t
      Venturi mask, 275f, 276t
   discontinuing, 273f
   setting up, 271–272f
Oxygen flow meter, 270, 270f
Oxygen saturation, 261

Pack-strap carry, 55–56, 57f
Pads
   eye, 584
   nonadherent, 584
Pain
   acute abdominal, 461
   assessment of, 339
   cardiac, 460
   gallbladder, 460
   kidney stone, 460
   OPQRST assessment of, 372
   pancreatic, 460
   rectal, 460
   referred, 459–460, 459f
   uterine, 460
   Wong-Baker FACES Pain Rating Scale in, 306, 307f, 339
Palate
   hard, 152
   soft, 152
Pale, 331, 332f
Palliative care, 91
Palmar grasp reflex, 190
Palpation, measuring blood pressure by, 337f
Palpitation, 436
Pancreas, 166, 458, 459
   injury to, 608
Pancreatic cell function, 395t
Pancreatic pain, 460
Pancreatitis, 461, 465t
Panic, 521
Panic attack, 523
Paradoxical chest movement, 267, 594, 594f
Paramedic National Standard Curriculum, 6
Paramedics, 11, 13
Paranoia, 525
Paraplegia, 664, 664f
Parasympathetic division, 164
Parathyroid glands, 167
Parenteral route, 213
Paresthesias, 565
Parietal lobes, 163, 645
Parietal pleura, 154
Parkinson's disease, 184
Paroxysmal nocturnal dyspnea, 407
Partial rebreather mask, 274, 274f, 276t
Partial seizures, 380
   complex, 380
   simple, 380
Partial-thickness burns, 576–577, 577f
Passive rewarming, 704
Past medical history, 307
Patella, 149, 616
Patent (open) airway, 343
Pathogen, 37
Pathogenesis, 184
Pathology, 176
Pathophysiology, 176–186
   cell function, 176–178, 177f
   causes of disease, 184–186
   disease risk factors, 184
   factors affecting, 178–184
   defined, 176
Patient(s)
   approaching ill or injured, 298–300, 298f, 299t

assessment of, in headaches, 389–390
communication with, 296–297
complaints and possible significant injury of, 320t
gaining access to, 24
hazardous materials in approaching, 864–865
lifting and moving, 47–48
medical, 314
number of, in scene size-up, 322
positioning of, 64, 66
recognizing need for control, 300
response of, to illness or injury, 297–304, 297f
safety of, 314, 314f
terrorism and approaching, 872–873
trauma, 314
treating, with respect, 300, 300f
Patient advocacy, 22
Patient area, inspection of vehicle, 819–820
Patient assessment, 17–18, 24, 327–365, 339–340, 340t
   in abdominal and gastrointestinal disorders, 462–463, 463f
   with absorbed poisons, 518
   in cardiac arrest, 444–451
   in cardiovascular disease, 439–440
   for facial injuries, 655–656
   in genitourinary and renal disorders, 473–475
   in head injuries, 650, 651t
   in immunology, 498–501
   with ingested poisons, 514
   with inhaled poisons, 516
   with injected poisons, 517
   for neck injuries, 658–659
   in nontraumatic musculoskeletal disorders, 491–492
   in orthopedic trauma, 622–623
   overview of, 339–340, 340t
   in pediatric trauma, 691
   primary survey, 340–349
      airway, 342–343, 343f
      breathing, 345–346, 346f
      capillary refill, 347
      cervical spine protection, 345, 345f
      circulation, 346–347
      disability, 347–349, 348
      expose, 349
      general impression, 341–342, 341f
      identifying priority patients, 349
      level of responsiveness (mental status), 343–345, 344f
      moisture, 347
      pulses, 347, 347f
      skin color, 347
      temperature, 347
   reassessment, 362, 363f
   in scene size-up, 311
   secondary survey, 349–365
      abdomen, 360–361
      chest, 359–360
      ears, 358–359
      emergency care during, 362
      extremities, 361
      eyes, 358–359
      general approach, 349–350
      head and face, 351, 358f
      head-to-toe examination in, 350–351
      of mental status, 351
      neck, 359
      pelvis, 361
      performing, 352–357f
      posterior body, 361–362
      vital signs, 350
   in seizures, 380–381
   in syncope, 386–387
   in trauma in older adults, 693–694, 693f
   for trauma in pregnancy, 688
   vital signs, 327–339
      blood pressure, 334–338
      capillary refill, 332–333, 333f
      pulse, 328–330, 328t, 329ft
      pulse oximetry, 338–339, 338f
      pupils, 333–334, 334ft
      respirations, 330–331, 330f, 331f
      skin color, 331–332, 332f
      skin moisture, 333t, 332
      skin temperature, 332, 332f, 333t

Patient history, 305
   chief complaint, 306
   current health status, 307–308
   past medical, 307
   of present illness, 306–307, 307f
   SAMPLE, 308
   techniques of taking, 305
Patient interview, responses to facilitate good, 299t
Patients with psychiatric disorders, assessment and emergency care for, 526–527, 527f
Patients with special challenges, 803–811
Patients with special healthcare needs, 808–810
Patient transfer equipment, 817–821, 818f, 819f, 820f, 821f
PCP (angel dust), 510, 512
Pedal pulse, 160, 432
Pedestrian injuries, deaths resulting from, 689
Pediarix, 416
Pediatric centers, 15t
Pediatrics, 769–790
   age classification of infants and children, 770
Pediatric trauma, 688–692
   emergency care in, 691–692
   mechanism of injury, 688–689
   patient assessment in, 691
   special considerations, 689–690
Pedi-Immobilizer, 855–856, 855f
Peer groups, importance to adolescents, 198
Pelvic bone, 616
Pelvic cavity, 143
Pelvic fractures, 690
Pelvic girdle, 144, 614
Pelvic inflammatory disease (PID), 462, 465t, 480–481
Pelvis, 149, 615
   immobilizing, 634
   injuries to, 631, 634, 634f
   in rapid medical assessment, 374–375
   in secondary assessment, 361
   in secondary survey, 361
Penetrating chest injuries, 570–571, 571f
Penetrating traumas, 315, 316t, 654
   to head, 648
   injuries from, 319t
   in pregnancy, 687
Penis, 167
Pentobarbital (Nembutal), 510
Peptic ulcer disease, 460
Perfusion, 179, 434, 439
   evaluating, 331
Pericardial cavity, 142
Perinatal centers, 15t
Perineum, 169, 479, 737, 747
Peripheral artery disease (PAD), 434
Peripheral chemoreceptors, 155
Peripherally inserted central catheter (PICC line), 809–810
Peripheral nervous system, 164, 647
Peripheral pulses, 162, 328t, 329, 433
   strength of, 541
Peripheral resistance in regulating blood pressure, 183f
Peripheral (surface) temperature, 699
Peripheral vascular resistance (PVR), 179, 182, 182f
Peristalsis, 166, 458
Peritoneal cavity, 457
Peritoneal dialysis, 473
Peritoneum, 457
Peritonitis, 360–361, 457, 459
Persian white, 511
Personal and other rescuer safety, 313–314, 313f
Personal habits in ascertaining current health status, 308
Personal professional development, 26
Personal protective equipment (PPE), 23, 39–40, 39f, 40f
   bleeding and, 558
   guidelines for using, 41t
   levels of, 859–860, 860f, 861ft
   need for, in scene size-up, 312, 312f
Personal space, 298, 298t
Pertinent negative, 103

Pertinent negative finding, 307
Pertinent positive, 103
Pertinent positive finding, 307
Pertussis, 415–416
  vaccine for, 416
Petit mal seizures, 380
Peyote, 510
Phalanges, 149
Pharmacodynamics, defined, 205
Pharmacology, 204–210
  defined, 205
  drug legislation and federal
    regulatory agencies, 205
Pharynx (throat), 151, 244, 458
Phencyclidine (PCP), 508
  drowning and, 710
Phenobarbital (Luminal), 510
Phobias, 523–524, 524t
Photoreceptor cells, 653
Physical abuse, 804
Physical agents as cause of disease, 185
Physical examination, 349
  focused, 349, 549, 552
Physical well-being, 31
Physician Orders for Life-
  Sustaining Treatment
  (POLST), 91, 321
Physician's Desk Reference (PDR), 208
Physiology
  of circulation, 162
  defined, 140
Pia mater, 163, 645
Piggyback carry, 56–57, 57f
Pill esophagitis, 213
Pineal gland, 167
Pink puffer, 420
Pituitary gland, 167
Pit vipers, 715, 717
  assessment findings and symptoms
    of bites, 717
  signs and symptoms of bites, 715
Placard, 44, 44f
Placenta, 737–738, 737f
  delivery of, 747
  problems dealing with, 752–754,
    753f, 754t
Placental abruption, 685, 687, 751,
  753, 753f
Placenta previa, 752–753, 753f
Plague, 868
Plaintiff, 81
Plaque, 434
Plasma, 159, 432, 433
Platelets, 144, 432
Pleurae, 154
Pleural cavities, 142, 591
Pleural space, 154
Plural medical terms, 125, 126–127t
Pneumatic antishock garments
  (PASG), 560–561, 627
Pneumatic splints, 560, 627, 627f
Pneumonia, 264, 420, 596
  as cause of death in sickle cell
    anemia, 535
  in older adults, 795
Pneumothorax, 265, 359
  open, 597, 602–603, 602f
  primary spontaneous, 596
  secondary spontaneous, 596
  simple, 596–597, 596f
  spontaneous, 596
  tension, 597–598, 597f
Pocket face mask, 282, 282f
Poison control center (PCC), 15t,
  506, 873
Poisonings
  accidental, 506
  in infants and children, 786–787
Poisons, 505–506
  absorbed, 518
  defined, 505
  examples of common, 506t
  ingested, 514–515, 515f
  inhaled, 515–517
  injected, 517
Poliomyelitis, 263
Polypharmacy in older adults, 799
Polytrauma, 729
Pons, 163, 645
Popliteal arteries, 160
Portable radio, 111, 112f
Portable stretcher, 67, 68f
Position of function, 625, 625f

Positive-pressure ventilation, 226,
  280, 283t
  applying cricoid pressure, 280–282,
    281f, 282f
  bag-mask, 285–288, 285f, 286f,
    287f
  flow-restricted, oxygen-powered
    device, 288–289, 288f
  mouth-to-barrier device, 283, 283f,
    285
  mouth-to-mask, 282–283, 282f, 285f
Posterior, 127
Posterior body
  in rapid medical assessment, 375
  in secondary assessment, 361–362
  in secondary survey, 361–362
Posterior nosebleed, 532
Posterior tibial pulse, 328t, 329
Postictal phase of tonic-clonic
  seizures, 379, 786
Postpartum complications, 760
  amniotic fluid embolism, 760
  hemorrhage, 760
Postresuscitation care, 451
Postterm pregnancy, 756
Posture, 296
Pott's fracture, 620
Power grip (underhand grip), in body
  mechanics and lifting, 49, 49f
Power lift, two-person, 51f
Power lines, 45–46
  downed, 825
Pralidoxime chloride, 238–239
Prearrival response in weapons of
  mass destruction (WMD)
  incident response, 871
Precapillary sphincter, 181
Precipitous labor and birth, 756
Predelivery considerations, 742–743
Preeclampsia, 754
Preexisting medical conditions,
  578–579
Prefixes, 122–123t
Pregestational diabetes, 751
Pregnancy
  assessing patient, 739–740
  complications of, 750–755, 752f,
    753f
  cultural considerations in, 748–749
  ectopic, 481–482, 482f, 752, 752f
  emergency care of complications,
    755
  high-risk, 756–757
  hypertensive disorders, 754–755
  normal, 738–739, 739f
  placental and uterine problems,
    752–754, 753f, 754t
  postpartum complications, 760
  postterm, 756
  structures of, 737–738, 737f
  trauma in, 684–688
    emergency care for, 688
    mechanism of injury, 684–685,
      685f
    patient assessment for, 688
Pregnancy-induced hypertension, 754
Prehospital care reports, 25, 95
  administrative or dispatch
    information section, 98, 99t,
    100f
  elements of, 97–98, 101
  minimum data for, 98
  patient and scene information,
    100, 100t, 101f
  patient assessment section, 101, 101f
  uses of, 96–97
Prehospital education, levels of, 11, 11t
Prehypertension, 438
Premature infant, 757
Premature rupture of membranes, 757
Preparation, 23
Preparedness, 836
Presbycusis in older adults, 800
Preschoolers, 194–195. See
    also Children
  cognitive changes, 194
  communication with, 302
  implications for healthcare
    professionals, 195, 195f
  physiologic changes, 194, 194f
  psychosocial changes, 194–195
Presenting part, 739
Pressure bandage, 560, 560f, 573, 585

Pressure immobilization technique,
  718
Pressure regulators, 270, 270f
Presyncope, 386
Preterm labor, 739, 757
Primary blast injury, 730
Primary cancer, 177
Primary hypertension, 438
Primary osteoarthritis, 489
Primary sexual development in
  adolescents, 197
Primary spontaneous pneumothorax,
  422, 596
Primary survey, 340–349
  airway in, 342–343, 343f
  breathing difficulty in, 407–409, 408t
  breathing in, 345–346, 346f
  capillary refill in, 347
  cervical spine protection in, 345, 345f
  circulation in, 346–347
  disability in, 347–349, 348
  in emergency care for shock, 543
  expose in, 349
  general impression in, 341–342, 341f
  identifying priority patients, 349
  in infants and children, 776–781,
    777f, 778f, 779f
  level of responsiveness in, 343–345,
    344f
  moisture in, 347
  pulses in, 347, 347f
  repeating, 362, 364
  skin color in, 347
  temperature in, 347
  in toxicology, 511–512
Primary tumor, 177
Priority patients
  factors to consider when
    identifying, 320t
  identifying, 349
Professional behavior, characteristics
  of, 20–22
  appearance, 20
  careful delivery of service, 22
  communication in, 21
  diplomacy, 21–22
  empathy, 20
  hygiene, 20
  integrity, 20
  patient advocacy, 22
  respect, 21
  self-confidence, 21
  self-motivation, 20
  teamwork, 21–22
  time management, 21
Professional help in managing stress,
  36
Progesterone, 735
Prolapsed cord, 758, 759f, 760
Prone position, 130
Property conservation, priorities of,
  834–835
Proprietary name, 205
Prospective medical direction, 13
Prostate gland, 167
Protected health information (PHI),
  83, 93–94
Protective equipment, 859–860
Protocols, 82
Proximal, 127
Proximate cause, 92–93
Pruritus, 498
Psychiatric disorders, 520–529
  assessment and emergency care for
    patients with, 526–527, 527f
  behavioral change in, 521, 522t
  calming patient who has, 527–528
  excited delirium, 526
  medical and legal considerations
    with, 528
  psychological crisis in, 522–526
    anxiety, 522
    bipolar, 524–525
    depression, 524
    obsessive-compulsive, 523
    panic attack, 523
    paranoia, 525
    phobias, 523–524, 524t
    schizophrenia, 525
    suicide, 525–526
Psychogenic shock, 184, 540
Psychological crises, 521
  in psychiatric disorders, 522–526

Psychomotor seizures, 380
Pubis, 615
Public access and communications, 10
Public health, 16
Public information systems, 835
Public Safety Answering Point
  (PSAP), 10, 113
Pulling, guidelines for safe, 52
Pulmonary artery, blockage of, 264
Pulmonary capillaries, 157
Pulmonary contusion, 600–601, 600f
Pulmonary edema, 261, 264
Pulmonary embolism, 261, 421
  in older adults, 795
Pulmonary veins, 262, 432
Pulmonary ventilation, 170, 261,
  262–263
Pulmonic valve, 158, 428
Pulse oximeter, 261
Pulse oximetry, 267–268, 267f, 268f,
  338–339, 338f
Pulse rates, normal, at rest, 329t
Pulses, 162, 328–330, 328t, 329ft, 433
  brachial, 160, 347f, 430
  carotid, 160
  central, 328t, 433
  distal, 635
  dorsalis pedis, 160
  femoral, 160, 432
  pedal, 432
  peripheral, 162, 328t, 433, 541
  in primary survey, 347, 347f
  radial, 160, 430
Puncture wound, 567, 568f
Pupils, 333–334, 334ft, 653
  dilated (very big), 333
  nonreactive, 333–334
  unequal, 333
Pure Food and Drug Act (1906), 206t
Purkinje fibers, 428
Purple cape, 599
Purposeful movement, 350, 351
Pursed lip breathing, 266
Pushing, guidelines for safe, 52
Putrefaction, 75
Pyelonephritis, 469, 471
Pyruvate, 176
Pyruvic acid, 177, 177f

Q fever, 868
Quadriplegia, 665, 665f
Quality management, 16, 16f, 450
  of prehospital care report, 97
Quaternary blast injury, 731
Questions
  closed, 305
  direct, 305
  open-ended, 305
Quick-sugar foods, 402–403
Quinary blast injury, 731

Raccoon eyes, 358, 648, 651
Radial artery, 430
Radial pulse, 160, 328t, 329, 430
Radiation, 700, 700f
  exposure to, 185
Radio
  frequencies and ranges for, 110–113
  guidelines for effective
    communication with, 115
  mobile two-way, 111, 112f
  portable, 111, 112f
Radiological weapon, 869
Radio waves
  in high-band frequency range, 111
  in low-band frequency range, 111
Radius, 149, 615
Rain, 823
Rainbows, 510
Rales, 265
Rapid extrication, 678
Rapid medical assessment, 349, 372,
  374–375
Rapid trauma assessment, 349, 550–552
Rattlesnakes, 715, 716t
Reaching, guidelines for safe, 52
Reactive airway disease (RAD), 417
Reactivity, 333–334
Rear-end collision, 316
  injuries from, 318t
Reassessment, 362, 363f
  components of, 362
  purpose of, 362, 364–365

Receiver in communication process, 296
Receiving facility, arrival at, 118
Receptive aphasia, 385
Recovery position, 64, 64*f*
Recreational sporting activities as cause of spinal cord injury, 645
Rectal pain, 460
Rectal temperature, 699
Rectum, 166, 458
Red blood cells, 140, 144, 432
  sickle cell disease and, 534
Reds, 510
Reeves stretcher, 68
Referred pain, 459–460, 459*f*
Reflex
  gag, 250
  Moro, 190
  rooting, 190
  sucking, 190
Refresher courses, 12
Refusals, 85–87, 88*f*, 89*f*
Regression, 297
Regulation, 10
Regulation of communications, 110
Rehabilitation services, 15–16
Renal calculi, 469
Renal disorders
  kidney stones, 469
  pyelonephritis, 471
  renal failure, 471–473, 472*f*
  urinary tract infection, 469–471
Renal failure, 471–473, 471*t*, 472*t*
Repeater, 111
Reperfusion injury, 566
Reproduction, cell, 177, 178*f*
Reproductive system, 167, 170*t*
  female, 167, 168*f*, 169
  male, 167, 168*f*
Rescue breathing, 288
Rescue 911 (television program), 6
Rescuer assist, 58
Research uses of prehospital care report, 97
Residual volume, 261
Resistance, insulin, 396
Resistance vessels, 181
Resource management, 836
Resources for Optimal Care of the Injured Patient, 6
Respect, 21
  treating patient with, 300, 300*f*
Respiration, 155, 156–158, 259–276, 330–331, 330*f*, 331*t*
  cellular, 262
  defined, 261
  external, 262, 263–264
  internal, 262, 263–264
  Kussmaul, 398
  pathophysiology of, 262–264
  physiology of, 261
Respiratory arrest, 267
Respiratory centers in brain, 263
Respiratory depression, 510
Respiratory disorders, 407–424
  assessing patient with breathing difficulty, 407
    determining patient's level, 411–412
    infant and child assessment considerations, 410–411
    primary survey, 407–409
    scene size-up, 407
    secondary survey, 410
  metered-dose inhalers, 422, 423*t*
  specific
    acute pulmonary edema, 421–422
    asthma, 417–418, 417*f*
    chronic bronchitis, 418–420, 419*f*
    croup, 413–414, 413*t*, 414*f*
    cystic fibrosis, 416–417
    emphysema, 420
    epiglottitis, 414–415, 414*f*
    pertussis, 415–416
    pneumonia, 420
    pulmonary embolism, 421
    spontaneous pneumothorax, 422
Respiratory distress, 266
  determining patient's level of, 411–412
  signs of, 331*f*
Respiratory emergencies in infants and children, 781–783

Respiratory failure, 267, 594–595, 782
Respiratory muscles, dysfunction of, 263
Respiratory rate, possible causes of change in, 408*t*
Respiratory syncytial virus (RSV), as cause of croup, 413
Respiratory system, 151–158, 151*f*, 152*f*, 153*f*, 154*f*, 156*f*, 157*f*, 170*t*, 243–246
  allergic reactions in, 499*t*
  functions of, 243, 244*f*
  lower airway, 244–245
  in older adults, 795
  upper airway, 243–244
Response, 23
Response times in rural and frontier EMS, 895–896
Responsive medical patient, 372–374, 372*f*
Responsiveness
  assessing, in cardiac arrest, 444
  level of, in children, 777
Restraints, 70–71, 71*f*, 316
Resuscitation mask, 282, 282*f*
Retention catheter, 470
Reticular activating system (RAS), 163–164
Reticular formation, 163–164
Retina, 653
Retractions, 266, 408–409
  intercostal, 409
  subcostal, 409
  supraclavicular, 409
Retroperitoneal space, 457, 468
Retroperitoneum, 457
Retrospective medical direction, 14
Returning to service, 25
Revised trauma score, 551*t*, 552, 730
Rewarming
  active, 704–705
  passive, 704
Rheumatoid arthritis (RA), 184, 185, 489
Rhonchi, 265, 409*t*
Rib cage, 591, 592*f*
Rib fractures, 592–594, 593*f*
  as cause of hemothorax, 598
Ribs, 591
  in children, 772
Ricin, 868
Rickettsias, 868, 869*f*
Right lower quadrant (RLQ), 143, 457, 457*f*
Right-of-way, 822–823
Right to practice, 12
Right upper quadrant (RUQ), 143, 457, 457*f*
Rigid splints, 626, 626*f*
Rigor mortis, 79
Risk factors, 434
  modifiable, 434
  nonmodifiable, 434
Road rash, 567
Roads, 653
Roller bandage, 584–585, 585*f*, 586*f*
Roller gauze, 584, 584*f*
Rollover, injuries from, 318*t*
Rollover impact, 316
Romig, Lou, 842*f*
Rooting reflex, 190
Root words, 122, 125–126*t*
Rotational collision, injuries from, 318*t*
Rotational impact, 316
Rubella, 42
  immunizations for, 42
Rule of nines, 578
Rule of palms, 578
Ruptured uterus, 687, 753–754
Rural and frontier EMS, 895–898
  challenges of, 895
    healthcare resources, 895
    illness and injury, 896–898
    response times in, 895–896
    workforce in, 896
  unique training needs of, 898
Rx (treatment), 105

Sacrum, 145, 614
Safety, 23
Safety precautions and preparation in body mechanics and lifting, 48–49, 49*f*

Safety zones, establishing, 863–864, 864*f*
Safe zone, 825, 863
Sager Emergency Fracture Response System (SEFRS), 631
  application of adaptor, 632–633*f*
Sager SX 405 unipolar traction splint, applying, 636–637, 636–637*f*
Sagittal plane, 144
Salivary glands, 166, 458
Salmonella (food poisoning), 37
SAM Splint, 626
Saturation of peripheral oxygen (SPO₂), 268
Scalp, injuries to, 648
Scapula, 149, 614, 616
Scene hazards, 48
Scene safety, 312–314, 313*f*, 826–827, 826*f*
  defined, 312
Scene size-up, 17, 23, 310–324
  in assessing breathing difficulty, 407
  hazardous materials and, 860
  infants and children in, 775–776, 775*f*
  mechanism of injury or nature of illness, 314–321
  multisystem trauma and, 729, 729*f*
  number of patients, 322
  overview of, 311–312, 311*f*
  resources for, 322, 322*t*
  safety, 312–314, 313*f*
    bystander, 314
    patient, 314, 314*f*
    personal and other rescuer, 313–314
  standard precautions review, 312, 312*f*
  in toxicology, 511
Schizophrenia, 525
School-age children, 196–197
  cognitive changes, 196
  communication with, 302
  implications for healthcare professional, 196–197, 197*f*
  physiologic changes, 196
  psychosocial changes, 196, 196*f*
Sclera, 653
Scoop stretcher, 68, 68*f*
Scope of practice, 12
Scorpion stings, 722–723, 822*f*
  emergency care for, 722–723
Scrotum, 167
Seated patient, spinal stabilization of, 673, 674–675*f*
Secobarbital (Seconal), 510
Secondary blast injury, 731, 731*f*
Secondary hypertension, 438
Secondary osteoarthritis, 489
Secondary sexual development in adolescents, 197
Secondary spontaneous pneumothorax, 422, 596
Secondary survey, 340, 349–365
  abdomen, 360–361
  in assessing breathing difficulties, 410–411
  chest, 359–360
  ears, 358–359
  emergency care during, 362
  extremities, 361
  eyes, 358–359
  general approach, 349–350
  head and face, 351, 358*f*
  head-to-toe examination in, 350–351
  in infants and children, 781
  of mental status, 351
  neck, 359
  pelvis, 361
  performing, 352–357*f*
  posterior body, 361–362
  in syncope, 386
  in toxicology, 512–513
  vital signs, 350
Second-degree burn, 576
Second stage of labor, 741
Second trimester, 738
Sedative/hypnotic toxidrome, 508*t*
Seesaw breathing, 411, 772
Seizures, 378–382
  absence, 380
  causes of, 378

emergency care in, 381–382, 381*f*
  generalized, 378
  generalized motor, 379
  grand mal, 379
  in infants and children, 785–786
  partial, 380
  petit mal, 380
  tonic-clonic, 379, 379*f*
  types of, 378–380
Self-abuse, 807
Self-confidence, 21
Self-contained breathing apparatus (SCBA), 44, 45*f*
Self-destructive behavior, 521
Self-motivation, 20
Self-neglect, 807
Self-splint, 624
Sellick maneuver, 153, 281
Semiautomated external defibrillator (SAED), 448
Semi-Fowler position, 66, 66*f*, 130
Semilunar valves, 428
Seminal vesicles, 167
Semisynthetic drugs, 205
Sender in communication process, 295, 296*f*
Sensitization, 497
Sensory changes in older adults, 800–801
Sensory nerves, 647
Separation anxiety, 192
Septic shock, 184, 540
Septum, 243–244
  deviated, 243–244
Service, careful delivery of, 22
Sexual abuse, 805
Sexual assault, apparent, 483–484
Sexual development
  primary, 197
  secondary, 197
Sexually transmitted diseases (STDs), 37, 197, 481
Shaken baby syndrome, 192, 689
Shirley Amendment (1912), 206*t*
Shirt drag, 53
Shivering, 699, 703
Shock, 434, 539–544
  anaphylactic, 540
  cardiogenic, 183, 264, 438, 540, 712
  in children, 543, 543*f*
  defined, 183
  distributive, 184, 540
  early (compensated), 541–542, 541*f*
  emergency care of, 543–544
  hemorrhagic, 540, 559*t*
  hypovolemic, 183, 264, 386, 540, 566
  in infants, 543, 543*f*
  in infants and children, 784
  irreversible, 542
  late (decompensated), 542, 542*f*
  multisystem trauma and, 729
  neurogenic, 184, 540
  obstructive, 183, 540
  in older adults, 543
  psychogenic, 184, 540
  septic, 184
  stages of, 541–542
  types of, 540
Shock advisory defibrillator, 448
Shocks, inappropriate delivery of, 451
Short backboard, 70, 70*f*
Shoulder, injuries to, 628
Shoulder drag, 53, 54*f*
Shoulder girdle, 144, 614, 615
Shoulder injury, immobilizing, 629*f*
Shrooms, 510
Shunts, 810
Sickle cell anemia, 186, 534
Sickle cell crisis, 534
Sickle cell disease, 534–535
  assessment findings and symptoms, 534
  defined, 534
  emergency care for, 535
  red blood cells and, 534
Sickle cell trait, 534
Sigmoid colon, 166, 458
Signs, 184
  baseline vital, 327–328
  defined, 327
Silent myocardial infarction, 399
Simple extrication, 854, 854*f*

Simple partial seizures, 380
Simple pneumothorax, 596–597, 596*f*
Simplex system, 113
Single-stage regulator, 270
Sinoatrial (SA) node, 428
Sinuses, 152
Sinus headaches, 387
SKED, 68
Skeletal muscles, 150, 150*f*, 151*t*, 616
Skeletal system, 144–150, 145*f*, 146*f*,
    148*f*, 149*f*, 170*t*, 613–616
Skills, maintaining, 12
Skin, 576
    functions of, 556
    layers of, 556
    role in temperature regulation,
        699
Skin color, 331–332, 332*f*, 347
    abnormal, 331–332
    in newborn, 766, 766*f*
Skin integumentary system, allergic
    reactions in, 499*t*
Skin moisture, 332, 333*t*
Skin temperature, 332, 332*f*, 333*t*
Skull, 144, 147*f*, 614
    injuries to, 648, 649, 650, 650*f*
Slander, 93
Sling and swathe, 628
Small intestine, 166, 458
Smallpox, 868
Smooth muscle, 150–151, 151*t*
Snakebites, 715, 716*t*, 717–720, 717*f*
    emergency care for, 718–720, 719*f*
Snapping hip syndrome, 490
Sniffing, 516
Snoring, 246, 265
Snow and ice, 823
Snow blindness, 655
SOAP method of documentation, 105
Social phobia, 523
Socket joints, 487
Soft palate, 152, 244
Soft splints, 626, 626*f*
Soft tissues, 556
    injuries to, 563–575
        closed wounds, 564–566, 564*f*
        compartment syndrome, 564–
            566, 565*f*
        crush syndrome, 566
Solid drugs, 209, 209*t*
Solid organs, 457–458
Somatic (voluntary) division, 164
Somatostatin, 395, 459
Sonoran (Arizona) coral snake, 717
Special considerations in trauma in
    older adults, 693
Special reporting requirements, 95
Special situations
    crime scenes, 94–95
    medical identification devices, 94
    organ donation, 95
    reporting requirements, 95
Specialty centers, 14
    types of, 15*t*
Speech-impaired patients,
    communication with, 304
Speed and speed limits, 822
Sphenoid bone, 648
Sphygmomanometer, 328
Spider bites, 720–722, 720*f*, 721*f*
    emergency care for, 722
Spinal cavity, 142
Spinal column, 645
    fractures of, 693
Spinal cord, 164, 645, 647, 647*f*
    of infant and child, 771
    injuries to, 662–664
        mechanism of, 662–664, 663*f*, 664*f*
        statistics on, 645
        trauma to, 263
Spinal cord injury centers, 15*t*
Spinal injury
    emergency care of, 668–669
    signs and symptoms of, 664–666,
        664*f*, 665*f*
Spinal nerves, 164, 647
Spinal precautions, 345
Spinal stabilization, 669
    cervical collars, 669, 669*f*, 670*f*
    immobilization of supine patient
        on long backboard, 670,
        672–673, 672*f*, 673*f*
    three-person logroll, 670, 671–672*f*

of seated patient, 673, 674–675*f*
of standing patient, 673, 676–677*f*
Spine, 144–146, 147*f*
Spine-injured patient, assessing
    potential, 666–668, 667*f*
Spiral fracture, 620
Spleen
    function of, 535
    injury to, 608
Splenic crisis, 535
Splint, 560
Splint, SAM, 626
Splinting, 492, 624–627
    general rules of, 624–625
Splints
    for bone and joint injuries, 641*t*
    in controlling bleeding, 560–561,
        560*f*
    pneumatic, 627, 627*f*
    rigid, 626, 626*f*
    soft, 626, 626*f*
    traction, 626–627, 627*f*
    types of, 625–627
Split litter, 68
Spontaneous abortion, 751
Spontaneously breathing patients,
    ventilating, 287
Spontaneous pneumothorax, 422, 596
    primary, 596
    secondary, 596
Sprain, 621–621*f*
Stabilization, 852
    equipment for, 852–853
Stable angina pectoris, 435
Stab wounds, 568, 648
    in pregnancy, 687
Stair chair, 69, 69*f*
Stairs, carrying procedure on, 52
Standard of care, 22
Standard precautions, 38, 39–40, 39*f*,
    40*f*
Standard precautions review in scene
    size-up, 312, 312*f*
Standing orders, 14, 82
Standing patient, spinal stabilization
    of, 673, 676–677*f*
Standing water, 824
START triage system, 839–841, 840*f*,
    841*f*
Station, en route to, 118–119
Status epilepticus, 380, 785
Statute of limitations, 81
Statutory law, 81
Steady state, 140
Stem, 122
Stent, 436
Sterile gauze pads, 583, 583*f*
Sterilization, 44, 830
Sternum, 127, 147, 149, 615
Stethoscope, 328, 430
    using, 335, 335*f*
Stimulants, 508–509
Stimulation
    central nervous system (CNS),
        511
    effects of, of autonomic nervous
        system, 164*t*
Stingrays, 724
Stings. *See also* Bites
    hymenoptera (bees, wasps, and
        ants), 723, 723*f*
    marine life, 724
    scorpion, 722–723, 722*f*
Stokes basket, 68
Stoma, 809
    laryngeal, 359
Stomach, 458
    injury to, 608
Stomach flu, 462
Stomas, 289
    tracheal, 289, 291
Straight catheter, 470
Strain, 621–622, 622*f*
Stress, 31
    cumulative, 34
    managing, 34–36, 35*f*
    recognizing warning signs of, 34, 34*t*
    signs of, 34*t*
    stressful situations and additional
        factors that may cause, 33*t*
    traumatic incident, 36
Stress headaches, 387
Stressor, defined, 32

Stressors, common, associated with
    working in Emergency Medical
    Services (EMS), 32*t*
Stretcher
    basket, 68, 69*f*
    collapsible, 818
    flexible, 68–69, 69*f*
    guidelines for safe lifting of, 50
    Navy, 68
    portable, 67, 68*f*
    Reeves, 68
    scoop, 68, 68*f*
    transferring supine patient from
        bed to
        direct carry, 60, 63–64*f*
        draw sheet transfer, 62, 65*f*
    wheeled, 67, 67*f*, 818
Stridor, 246, 265, 691
Stroke(s), 184, 263, 382–385, 382*f*, 694
    assessment findings and symptoms,
        384–385
    embolic, 382
    emergency care for, 385
    hemorrhagic, 382, 383*f*
    ischemic, 382
    risk factors for, 384
    risk of, in sickle cell disease, 535
    types of, 382, 383*f*, 384
Stroke alert patient, 385
Stroke centers, 15*t*
Stroke volume, 179
Stumblers, 510
Subarachnoid hemorrhage, 382
Subclavian arteries, 160
Subcostal retractions, 409
Subcutaneous emphysema, 359, 573,
    593
Subcutaneous layer, 165
Subcutaneous (SubQ) route, 215, 216*f*
Subdural hematoma, 660, 661*f*
Subjective findings, 184, 327
Sublingual drugs, 215
Subluxation, 620
Submersion, 709
Substance abuse, 507
    pregnancy and, 750–751
Substance misuse, 507
Sucking chest wound, 571
Sucking reflex, 190
Suction catheters, 251–252, 251*f*
Suctioning, 250–252
Suction units, 250–251, 251*f*
Sudden cardiac death (SCD), 443
Sudden infant death syndrome
    (SIDS), 788
Sudden sniffing death syndrome
    (SSDS), 516
Suffixes, 123, 124–125*t*
Suicide, 525–526
    completed, 525
    risk factors for, 525–526
Suicide attempt, 525
Suicide gesture, 521, 525
Sundowning in older adults, 796
Superficial burns, 576, 576*f*
Superior, 127
Superior vena cava, 432, 433
Supine patient, transferring, from
    bed to stretcher, 60
Supine position, 130
Supplemental oxygen, 269–276,
    269*f*t, 270*f*, 271*f*, 273*f*
Supporting technologies, 836
Supportive care, 91
Support zone, 863
Supraclavicular retractions, 409
Surfactant, 153
Swallowing
    protective reflexes involved in,
        245–246
    structures involved in, 152*f*
Swathe, 626
Sweat glands, 556
Sweating, 699
Symmetry, 351
    in assessing face, 351
Sympathetic division, 164
Sympathomimetic toxidrome, 508*t*
Symptoms, 184, 327
Syncope, 385–387, 436
    causes of, 386
    emergency care for, 387, 388
    patient assessment, 386–387

Syndrome, 184
Synovial joints, 487, 616
Synovial membrane, 487
Synthetic drugs, 205
Synthetic heroin, 511
Syphilis, 37, 481
Systemic effects, 208
Systemic (peripheral) vascular
    resistance (SVR), 182
Systolic blood pressure, 162, 182,
    334–335, 433

Tachycardia, 693
Tachypnea, 408
Tactile hallucinations, 525
Tarsal bones, 149–150, 616
Teamwork, 21–22
Technical Assistance Program (TAP), 5
Teenagers. *See* Adolescents
Teeth, 166, 458
Temperature, 347
    axillary, 699
    rectal, 699
Temperature regulation, 699
Tempered glass, 853
Temporal bone, 648
Temporal lobes, 163, 645
Temporal lobe seizures, 380
Tendonitis, 490
    Achilles, 491
    wrist, 490
Tendons, 150, 487, 616
Tennis elbow, 490
Tension pneumothorax, 264, 359,
    597–598, 597*f*
Tension-type headaches, 387
Terminal bronchioles, 245
Terrorism and disaster response,
    866–874. *See also* Weapons of
    mass destruction (WMD)
Terrorist acts, 826
Tertiary blast injury, 731
Testes, 167
Tetanus, immunizations for, 41
Tetraplegia, 665, 665*f*
Texas catheter, 470
Texas coral snake, 717
Thalamus, 163
Therapeutic abortion, 751
Thermal burns, 576, 685
Third-degree burn, 577
Third stage of labor, 741–742
Third trimester, 738–739, 739*f*
Thoracic (chest) cavity, 142
Thoracic vertebrae, 614
Thorax. *See* Chest
    dysfunction of, 263
    trauma to, 263
Threatened abortion, 751
Three-person direct ground lift, 61*f*
Three-person logroll, 670, 671–672*f*
Thrombocytes (platelets), 159
Thrombotic stroke, 382, 383*f*
Thrombus, 382, 383*f*
Thymus gland, 167
Thyroid, overactive, 404
Thyroid cartilage, 152
Thyroid disorders, 403–404, 403*f*
    hyperthyroidism, 404
    hypothyroidism, 403–404, 403*f*
Thyroid gland, 167, 657
Tibia, 149, 616
Tibial arteries, 160
Tidal volume, 155, 261, 408
Time management, 21
Tissues, 140
    muscle, 140
    soft, 556
        injuries to, 563–575, 564*f*, 565*f*
Toddlers, 192–194. *See also* Children
    cognitive changes, 193
    communication with, 301–302, 302*f*
    implications for healthcare
        professional, 193–194, 194*f*
    physiologic changes, 192–193, 193*f*
    psychosocial changes, 193
Tolerance, 507
Tones out, 114
Tongue, 166, 245, 458
    lacerations of, 654
Tonic-clonic seizures, 379, 379*f*
Tonic phase, 379
    of tonic-clonic seizures, 379

Tonsil sucker, 251
Tonsil tip catheter, 251
Touch, using reassuring, 301
Touch sensitivity in older adults, 801
Tourniquets, 561, 561*f*
 in treating snakebites, 719
Toxemia of pregnancy, 754
Toxic exposure, signs and symptoms of, 506
Toxicological emergencies in older adults, 799–800
Toxicology, 504–519
 absorbed poisons, 518
  emergency care with, 518
  patient assessment with, 518
 commonly misused and abused substances, 507
  depressants, 509–510, 510*t*
  designer drugs, 511
  emergency care in, 513
  hallucinogens, 510–511
  patient assessment in, 511–513
  stimulants, 508–509
 ingested poisons, 514–515, 515*f*
  emergency care with, 514–515, 515*f*
  patient assessment, 514
 inhaled poisons, 515–517
  emergency care with, 517
  patient assessment with, 516
 injected poisons, 517
  emergency care with, 517
  patient assessment with, 517
 poison in, 504–506
Toxidromes, 506, 508*t*
 common, 508*t*
Toxins, 178, 505, 507*f*, 868, 869*f*
 exposure to, 506
Trachea, 151, 153, 244–245, 657–658, 657*f*, 658*f*
 in children, 772
Tracheal deviation, 359, 597
Tracheal shift, 597
Tracheal stomas, 289, 291
Tracheostomy, 289, 809
Tracheostomy tubes, 809
Traction splints, 626–627, 627*f*
 bipolar, 638–639, 638–639*f*
 Sager SX 405 unipolar, 636–637, 636–637*f*
Trade name, 205, 207–208*t*
Traffic, 45
 heavy, 825
 volume and flow of, 827
Transfer to definitive care, 829
Transient ischemic attack (TIA), 382, 434
Transmission modes, 113
Transmitter, 111
Transport, 105
 of priority trauma patient, 552
Transportation, emergency, 12
Transportation, U.S. Department of (DOT)
 National Highway Traffic Safety Administration (NHTSA) of, 4–5
 regulations in transporting hazardous materials, 862, 863*f*
Transport phase, 827–829, 828*f*
Transport/transfer of care, 24–25
Transverse colon, 166, 458
Transverse fracture, 620
Transverse plane, 144
Trauma, 178, 547–553
 to airway, 263
 blunt, 315, 316*t*
 in cognitively impaired patient, 694–695
 mechanism of injury in, 548–553, 549*f*, 550*f*, 551*t*
 multisystem, 728–732, 729*f*, 731*f*
 to neck, 263
 in older adults, 692–694
  emergency care in, 694
  mechanism of injury, 692–693
  patient assessment in, 693–694, 693*f*

 special considerations in, 693
 penetrating, 315, 316*t*, 654
 in pregnancy, 684–688
  emergency care for, 688
  mechanism of injury, 684–685, 685*f*
  patient assessment for, 688
  special considerations, 685, 686*f*, 687–688
 to spinal cord, 263
 to thorax, 263
Trauma assessment, focused, 552
Trauma center, 14, 15*f*
Trauma chin lift, 248
Trauma dressings, 583–584, 583*f*
Trauma jaw thrust, 248
Trauma patient, 314
 transport of priority, 552
Trauma Systems Planning and Development Act (1990), 6
Traumatic asphyxia, 599–600, 600*f*
Traumatic brain injury, 647–648, 694
Traumatic gynecologic emergencies, 483
 apparent sexual assault, 483–484
Traumatic incident stress, 36
Treatment protocols, 14
Triage, 322, 839
 JumpSTART system in, 841–843, 842*f*
 START system in, 839–841, 840*f*, 841*f*
Triangular bandage, 585, 585*f*
Triceps, 615
Tricuspid valve, 158, 428
TriHIBit, 416
Tripod position, 266, 407
True emergency, 822
True ribs, 147
Trumpet airway, 255
Tubal pregnancy, 481
Tuberculosis, 596, 808
 immunizations for, 43
Tularemia, 868
Tumor, 177, 460, 461
 benign, 177
 malignant, 177
Tunica adventitia, 180
Tunica externa, 180
Tunics, 653
Turbinates, 152
Twisting force, 618
2-PAM autoinjector, 238
Two-person carry, 57–58, 58*f*
Two-person extremity lift, 62*f*
Two-person power lift, 51*f*
Two-person seat carry, 57
Two-rescuer adult cardiopulmonary resuscitation, 879–881
Type 1 diabetes mellitus, 395–396
Type 2 diabetes mellitus, 396
Typhus fever, 868

UHF (ultrahigh frequency) bands, 110
Ulcers
 duodenal, 460
 esophageal, 460
 gastric, 460
 in older adults, 797
 in sickle cell disease, 535, 535*f*
Ulna, 149, 615
Ultrahigh frequency, 111
Ultraviolet keratitis, 655
Umbilical cord, 738
Underactive thyroid, 403
Unequal pupils, 333
Unified command, 836
Unintentional injuries, 315*t*
United States Pharmacopeia – National Formulary, 208
Unresponsive medical patient, 374–375
Unstable angina pectoris, 435
Upper airway, 243–244
Upper extremities, 149, 149*f*, 615
 injuries to, 627–631, 628, 628*f*, 629*f*, 630*f*, 631*f*

Upper gastrointestinal bleeding, 460–461
 in older adults, 797
Upper thigh, injuries to, 634–635, 635*f*
Ureters, 169, 469
 penetrating trauma to, 609
Urethra, 169, 469
Urethritis, 469
Urgent moves (rapid extrication), 58, 59–60*f*
Urinary bladder, 169, 469
Urinary bladder injuries, 609
Urinary catheters, 470–471
Urinary incontinence in older adults, 798
Urinary system, 169, 169*f*, 170*t*
Urinary tract infections, 469–471
 in older adults, 798
Urine collection bag, 470
Urticaria, 498
Uterine fibroids, 483
Uterine massage, steps for performing, 748
Uterine pain, 460
Uterine problems, 752–754, 753*f*, 754*t*
Uterine tubes, 478, 735
Uterus, 143, 167, 478, 736
 ruptured, 687, 753–754
Uvula, 152

Vaccines. *See* Immunizations
Vacuum mattresses, 70
Vacuum splint, 627
Vagina, 167, 736–737
Vaginal bleeding, causes of, 754*t*
Vaginitis, 482–483
Value judgments, 83
Varicella, 42*t*
 immunizations for, 42–43
Vascular dementia, 694
Vascular tunic, 653
Vasoconstriction, 182, 182*f*, 699
Vasodilation, 182, 182*f*, 699
Vehicle extrication, 849–857
 additional scene hazards, 856
 equipment, 850, 851*f*
 role of EMT on, 850
 stages of, 850–856
  disentanglement, 855–856, 855*f*
  en route and scene size-up, 851, 851*f*
  gaining access, 853–854, 853*f*
  hazard control and safety considerations, 851–852
  operations, 852–853, 853*f*
  preparation, 850–851
  removal, transfer, and termination, 856
Vehicle inspection, 818–820, 818*f*, 819*f*
Vehicle placement, 826–827
Veins, 160, 160*f*, 181, 432
 major, 162
 pulmonary, 262
Venous bleeding, 557
Venous return, 179
Ventilation, 155–156, 178
 assessment of, 264–267, 264*f*, 265*f*
 positive-pressure, 226
 pulmonary, 261
 signs of adequate, 266
 signs of inadequate, 266
Ventilation face mask, 282, 282*f*
Ventricles, 158, 428
Ventricular fibrillation (VF or VFib), 444
Ventricular shunt, 810
Venturi mask, 275*f*, 276*t*
Venules, 160, 181, 432
Vertebral column, 145, 614
Vests, high-visibility, 826
VHF (very high frequency) bands, 110, 111
Victims, entrapped, 46, 46*f*
Violence
 clues indicating potential for, 313
 intimate partner, 684
Violent acts, 826
Violent scenes, 46–47

Viral croup, 413
Viral encephalitis, 868
Viral hemorrhagic fevers, 868
Viruses, 178, 868, 869*f*
Visceral pleura, 154
Visual hallucinations, 525
Visually impaired patients, communication with, 303–304
Vital capacity, 261
Vital organs, 140
Vital signs, 24, 327–339
 assessment of, 350
 blood pressure, 334–338
 capillary refill, 332–333, 333*f*
 defined, 327
 in hypothermia, 703
 items for taking, 328
 pulse, 328–330, 328*t*, 329*ft*
 pulse oximetry, 338–339, 338*f*
 pupils, 333–334, 334*ft*
 reassessing, 364, 365*f*
 respirations, 330–331, 330*f*, 331*t*
 in secondary survey, 350
 skin color, 331–332, 332*f*
 skin moisture, 332, 333*t*
 skin temperature, 332, 332*f*, 333*t*
Vitreous humor, 653
Vocal cords, 244
Voice over Internet Protocol (VoIP), 113–114
Vomited blood, 461

Waddell's triad, 689
Walking assist, 58
Warm zone, 863
Warning lights and sirens, 822
Water moccasins, 715, 716*t*
Water-related emergencies
 diving, 714–715
 drowning, 709–713
Water safety threats, 868
Weapons of mass destruction (WMD), 867
 incident response, 871
  approaching patient, 872–873
  arrival, 871–872
  prearrival, 871
 types of, 867–871, 868*f*, 869*f*, 870*t*
Welder's flash, 655
Welfare check, 310
Wellness, 31–36
 infection control, 37–44
 mental well-being, 31–36, 31*f*, 32*f*
 physical well-being, 31
 recognizing warning signs of stress, 34, 34*t*
Wet drowning, 711
Wheeled stretchers, 67, 67*f*, 818
Wheezing, 179, 249, 265, 409*t*
 causes of, 265
 in children, 780
White blood cells, 144, 432
Wind, 823
Withdrawal, 507
Wong-Baker FACES Pain Rating Scale, 306, 307*f*, 339
Work environment changes, stress and, 36
Wounds, 556
 closed, 556, 564–566, 564*f*
 gunshot, 568, 648
 open, 556, 564, 567–570, 567*f*
 puncture, 567, 568*f*
 stab, 568, 648
Wrist, injuries to, 630–631, 630*f*, 631*f*
Wrist bandage, 587*f*
Wrist tendonitis, 490

Xiphoid process, 149, 615
XTC, 511

Yankauer catheter, 251
Yellow jackets, 510

Zygomatic arch, 652–653
Zygomatic bones, 652
Zygote, 737

Organic Chemistry
Laboratory I and II
for Chem 36 and 130

Stanford University

Donald L. Pavia
Western Washington University

Gary M. Lampman
Western Washington University

George S. Kriz
Western Washington University

Randall G. Engel
Edmunds Community College

Kenneth Doxsee
University of Oregon

James Hutchison
University of Oregon

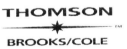

THOMSON

BROOKS/COLE

Australia · Canada · Mexico · Singapore · Spain · United Kingdom · United States

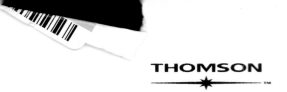

THOMSON
BROOKS/COLE

Organic Chemistry Laboratory I and II
Pavia/Lampman/Kriz/Engel/Doxsee/Hutchison

Executive Editors:
Michele Baird, Maureen Staudt &
Michael Stranz

Project Development Manager:
Linda deStefano

Sr. Marketing Coordinators:
Lindsay Annett and Sara Mercurio

Production/Manufacturing Manager:
Donna M. Brown

Production Editorial Manager:
Dan Plofchan

Pre-Media Services Supervisor:
Becki Walker

Rights and Permissions Specialist:
Kalina Ingham Hintz

Cover Image
Getty Images*

The Adaptable Courseware Program
consists of products and additions to
existing Brooks/Cole products that are
produced from camera-ready copy.
Peer review, class testing, and
accuracy are primarily the responsibility
of the author(s).

Organic Chemistry Laboratory I and II /
Pavia/Lampman/Kriz/Engel/Doxsee/
Hutchison
ISBN: 978-0-495-43053-7
ISBN: 0-495-43053-6

International Divisions List

Asia (Including India):
Thomson Learning
(a division of Thomson Asia Pte Ltd)
5 Shenton Way #01-01
UIC Building
Singapore 068808
Tel: (65) 6410-1200
Fax: (65) 6410-1208

Australia/New Zealand:
Thomson Learning Australia
102 Dodds Street
Southbank, Victoria 3006
Australia

Latin America:
Thomson Learning
Seneca 53
Colonia Polano
11560 Mexico, D.F., Mexico
Tel (525) 281-2906
Fax (525) 281-2656

Canada:
Thomson Nelson
1120 Birchmount Road
Toronto, Ontario
Canada M1K 5G4
Tel (416) 752-9100
Fax (416) 752-8102

UK/Europe/Middle East/Africa:
Thomson Learning
High Holborn House
50-51 Bedford Row
London, WC1R 4LS
United Kingdom
Tel 44 (020) 7067-2500
Fax 44 (020) 7067-2600

Spain (Includes Portugal):
Thomson Paraninfo
Calle Magallanes 25
28015 Madrid
España
Tel 34 (0)91 446-3350
Fax 34 (0)91 445-6218

CONTENTS

Introduction 1

Technique 1: Laboratory Safety 5

Technique 2: The Laboratory Notebook, Calculations, and Laboratory Records 23

Technique 3: Laboratory Glassware: Care and Cleaning 31

Technique 4: How to Find Data for Compounds 40

Technique 5: Masurement of Volume and Weight 49

Technique 6: Heating and Cooling Methods 62

Technique 7: Reaction Methods 74

Technique 8: Filtration 96

Technique 9: Physical Constants of Solids 111

Technique 10: Solubility 122

Technique 11: Crystallization 132

Technique 12: Extractions, Separations, and Drying Agents 152

Technique 13: Physical Constant of Liquids 178

Technique 14: Simple Distillation 189

Technique 15: Fractional Distillation, Azeotropes 200

Technique 19: Column Chromatography 221

Technique 20: Thin-Layer Chromatography 247

Technique 21: High-Performance Liquid Chromatography 260

Technique 22: Gas Chromatography 266

Technique 25: Infrared Spectroscopy 287

Technique 29: Guide to Chemical Literature 324

Appendix A 338

Experiment 8: Microwave Synthesis of 5, 10, 15, 20-Tetraphenylporphyrin 340

Essay: Analgesics 345

Experiment 8 (a): Acetanilide 350

Essay: Aspirin 354

Experiment 8 (b): Acetylsalicylic Acid 357

Essay: Fireflies and Photochemistry 361

Experiment 51: Luminol 365

Experiment 24: 4-Methylcyclohexene 371

Essay: Identification of Drugs 375

Experiment 10: TLC Analysis of Analgesic Drugs 377

Essay: The Chemistry of Vision 383

Experiment 16: Isolation of Chlorophyll and Carotenoid Pigments from Spinach 388

Essay: Esters - Flavors and Fragrances 396

Experiment 12: Isopentyl Acetate (Banana Oil) 400

Experiment 57: A Separation and Purification Scheme 404

Experiment 8: The Diels-Alder Reaction:
      Preparation of 4-Cyclohexene-cis-1,2-dicarboxylic Anhydride .407

Experiment 7: Isolation of Eugenol from Cloves 411

Experiment SYNT 721:
      Synthesis of trans-9-(2-Phenylethenyl) anthracene: A Wittig Reaction 417

Experiment 44: 1,4-Diphenyl-1,3-butadiene 429

Experiment 14: Extraction of Oil of Cloves by Steam Distillation
      and Liquid Carbon Dioxide 437

Experiment 1: Solventless Reactions: The Aldol Reaction 445

WELCOME TO ORGANIC CHEMISTRY!

Organic chemistry can be fun, and we hope to prove it to you. The work in this laboratory course will teach you a lot. The personal satisfaction that comes with performing a sophisticated experiment skillfully and successfully will be great.

To get the most out of the laboratory course, you should strive to do several things. First, you must review all relevant safety material. Second, you need to understand the organization of this laboratory manual and how to use it effectively. The manual is your guide to learning. Third, you must try to understand both the purpose and the principles behind each experiment you do. Finally, you must try to organize your time effectively before each laboratory period.

LABORATORY SAFETY

Before undertaking any laboratory work, it is essential that you familiarize yourself with the appropriate safety procedures and that you understand what precautions you should take. We strongly urge you to read Technique 1, "Laboratory Safety" (pp. 558–575), before starting any laboratory experiments. It is your responsibility to know how to perform the experiments safely and how to understand and evaluate the risks that are associated with laboratory experiments. Knowing what to do and what not to do in the laboratory is of paramount importance, because the laboratory has many potential hazards associated with it.

ORGANIZATION OF THE TEXTBOOK

Consider briefly how this textbook is organized. After this introduction, the textbook is divided into six parts. Part One consists of 17 experiments that introduce you to most of the important basic laboratory techniques in organic chemistry. Part Two contains 2 experiments that introduce you to the modern, computer-based techniques of molecular modeling and computational chemistry. Part Three consists of 35 experiments that may be assigned as part of your laboratory course. Your instructor will choose a set of these experiments.

Part Four is devoted to the identification of organic compounds and contains 1 experiment that provides experience in the analytical aspects of organic chemistry. Interspersed within these first four parts of the textbook are numerous covering essays that provide background information related to the experiments and that place the experiments into a larger, overall context, showing how the experiments and compounds can be applied to areas of everyday concern and interest. Part Five contains 11 project-based experiments that require you to develop important critical thinking skills. Many of these experiments have a result that is not easily predicted in advance. To arrive at an appropriate conclusion, you may have to use many of the thought processes that are important in research. Part Six is composed of a series of detailed instructions and explanations dealing with the techniques of organic chemistry. The techniques are extensively developed and used, and you will become familiar

1

with them in the context of the experiments. The techniques chapters include infrared spectroscopy, nuclear magnetic resonance, ^{13}C nuclear magnetic resonance, and mass spectrometry. Many of the experiments included in Parts One through Five utilize these spectroscopic techniques, and your instructor may choose to add them to other experiments. Within each experiment, you will find the section "Required Reading," which indicates which techniques you should study to do that experiment. Extensive cross-referencing to the techniques chapters in Part Six is included in the experiments. Many experiments also contain a section called "Special Instructions," which lists special safety precautions and specific instructions to you, the student. Finally, most experiments contain a section entitled "Suggested Waste Disposal," which provides instruction on the correct means of disposing of the reagents and materials used during the experiment.

ADVANCE PREPARATION

It is essential to plan carefully for each laboratory period so that you will be able to keep abreast of the material you will learn in your organic chemistry laboratory course. You should not treat these experiments as a novice cook would treat *The Good Housekeeping Cookbook*. You should come to the laboratory with a plan for the use of your time and some understanding of what you are about to do. A really good cook does not follow the recipe line by line with a finger, nor does a good mechanic fix your car with the instruction manual in one hand and a wrench in the other. In addition, it is unlikely that you will learn much if you try to follow the instructions blindly, without understanding them. We can't emphasize strongly enough that you should come to the lab *prepared*.

If there are items or techniques that you do not understand, you should not hesitate to ask questions. You will learn more, however, if you figure things out on your own. Don't rely on others to do your thinking for you.

You should read Technique 2, "The Laboratory Notebook, Calculations, and Laboratory Records" right away. Although your instructor will undoubtedly have a preferred format for keeping records, much of the material here will help you learn to think constructively about laboratory experiments in advance. It would also save time if, as soon as possible, you read the first nine techniques chapters in Part Six. These techniques are basic to all experiments in this textbook. The laboratory class will begin with experiments almost immediately, and a thorough familiarity with this particular material will save you much valuable laboratory time.

BUDGETING TIME

As just mentioned in "Advance Preparation," you should read several techniques chapters of this book even before your first laboratory class meeting. You should also read the assigned experiment carefully before every class meeting. Having read the experiment will allow you to schedule your time wisely. Often you will be doing more than one experiment at a time. Experiments such as the fermentation of sugar or the chiral reduction of ethyl acetoacetate require a few minutes of advance preparation several days ahead of the actual experiment. At other times you will have to catch up on some unfinished details of a previous experiment. For instance, usually it is not possible to determine a yield accurately or a melting point of a product immediately after you first obtain the product. Products must be free of solvent to give an accurate weight or melting point range; they have to be "dried." Usually, this drying is done by leaving the product in an open container on your desk or in your locker. Then, when you have a pause in your schedule during the subsequent experiment, you can determine these missing data using a sample that is dry. Through careful planning you can set aside the time required to perform these miscellaneous experimental details.

PURPOSE

The main purpose of an organic laboratory course is to teach you the techniques necessary for a person dealing with organic chemicals. You will also learn the techniques needed for separating and purifying organic compounds. If the appropriate experiments are included in your course, you may also learn how to identify unknown compounds. The experiments themselves are only the vehicles for learning these techniques. The techniques chapters in Part Six are the heart of this textbook, and you should learn these techniques thoroughly. Your instructor may provide laboratory lectures and demonstrations explaining the techniques, but the burden is on you to master them by familiarizing yourself with the chapters in Part Six.

Besides good laboratory technique and the methods of carrying out basic laboratory procedures, other things you will learn from this laboratory course are

1. How to take data carefully
2. How to record relevant observations
3. How to use your time effectively
4. How to assess the efficiency of your experimental method
5. How to plan for the isolation and purification of the substance you prepare
6. How to work safely
7. How to solve problems and think like a chemist

In choosing experiments, we have tried whenever possible to make them relevant and, more important, interesting. To that end, we have tried to make them a learning experiment of a different kind. Most experiments are prefaced by a background essay to place things in context and to provide you with some new information. We hope to show you that organic chemistry pervades your lives (drugs, foods, plastics, perfumes, and so on). Furthermore, you should leave your course well trained in organic laboratory techniques. We are enthusiastic about our subject and hope you will receive it with the same spirit.

This textbook discusses the important laboratory techniques of organic chemistry and illustrates many important reactions and concepts. In the traditional approach to teaching this subject (called **macroscale**), the quantities of chemicals used were on the order of 5–100 grams. The approach used in this textbook, a **small-scale** approach, differs from the traditional laboratory in that nearly all of the experiments use smaller amounts of chemicals (1–10 grams). However, the glassware and methods used in small-scale experiments are identical to the glassware and methods used in macroscale experiments.

The advantages of the small-scale approach include improved safety in the laboratory, reduced risk of fire and explosion, and reduced exposure to hazardous vapors. This approach decreases the need for hazardous waste disposal, leading to reduced contamination of the environment.

Another approach, a **microscale** approach, differs from the traditional laboratory in that the experiments use very small amounts of chemicals (0.050–1.000 grams). Some microscale glassware is very different from macroscale scale glassware, and there are a few techniques that are unique to the microscale laboratory. Because of the widespread use of microscale methods, some reference to microscale techniques will be made in the techniques chapters. A few experiments in this textbook feature microscale methods. These experiments have been designed to use ordinary glassware; they do not require specialized microscale equipment.

TECHNIQUE 1

Laboratory Safety

In any laboratory course, familiarity with the fundamentals of laboratory safety is critical. Any chemistry laboratory, particularly an organic chemistry laboratory, can be a dangerous place in which to work. Understanding potential hazards will serve you well in minimizing that danger. It is ultimately your responsibility, along with your laboratory instructor's, to make sure that all laboratory work is carried out in a safe manner.

1.1 SAFETY GUIDELINES

It is vital that you take necessary precautions in the organic chemistry laboratory. Your laboratory instructor will advise you of specific rules for the laboratory in which you work. The following list of safety guidelines should be observed in all organic chemistry laboratories.

A. Eye Safety

Always Wear Approved Safety Glasses or Goggles. It is essential to wear eye protection whenever you are in the laboratory. Even if you are not actually carrying out an experiment, a person near you might have an accident that could endanger your eyes. Even dish washing can be hazardous. We know of cases in which a person has been cleaning glassware only to have an undetected piece of reactive material explode, throwing fragments into the person's eyes. To avoid such accidents, wear your safety glasses or goggles at all times.

Learn the Location of Eyewash Facilities. If there are eyewash fountains in your laboratory, determine which one is nearest to you before you start to work. If any chemical enters your eyes, go immediately to the eyewash fountain and flush your eyes and face with large amounts of water. If an eyewash fountain is not available, the laboratory will usually have at least one sink fitted with a piece of flexible hose. When the water is turned on, this hose can be aimed upward, and the water can be directed into the face, working much as an eyewash fountain does. To avoid damaging the eyes, the water flow rate should not be set too high, and the water temperature should be slightly warm.

B. Fires

Use Care with Open Flames in the Laboratory. Because an organic chemistry laboratory course deals with flammable organic solvents, the danger of fire is frequently present. Because of this danger, DO NOT SMOKE IN THE LABORATORY. Furthermore, use extreme caution when you light matches or use any open flame. Always check to see whether your neighbors on either side, across the bench, and behind you are using flammable solvents. If so, either wait or move to a safe location, such as a fume hood, to use your open flame. Many flammable organic substances are the source of dense vapors that can travel for some distance down a bench. These vapors present a fire danger, and you should be careful, because the source of those vapors may be far away from you. Do not use the bench sinks to dispose of flammable solvents. If your bench has a trough running along it, pour only *water* (no flammable solvents!) into it. The troughs and sinks are designed to carry water—not flammable materials—from the condenser hoses and aspirators.

Learn the Location of Fire Extinguishers, Fire Showers, and Fire Blankets. For your own protection in case of a fire, you should immediately determine the location of the nearest fire extinguisher, fire shower, and fire blanket. You should learn how to operate these safety devices, particularly the fire extinguisher. Your instructor can demonstrate this.

If there is a fire, the best advice is to get away from it and let the instructor or laboratory assistant take care of it. DON'T PANIC! Time spent in thought before action is never wasted. If it is a small fire in a container, it can usually be extinguished quickly by placing a wire-gauze screen with a ceramic fiber center or, possibly, a watch glass over the mouth of the container. It is good practice to have a wire screen or watch glass handy whenever you are using a flame. If this method does not extinguish the fire and if help from an experienced person is not readily available, then extinguish the fire yourself with a fire extinguisher.

Should your clothing catch on fire, DO NOT RUN. Walk *purposefully* toward the fire shower station or the nearest fire blanket. Running will fan the flames and intensify them.

C. Organic Solvents: Their Hazards

Avoid Contact with Organic Solvents. It is essential to remember that most organic solvents are flammable and will burn if they are exposed to an open flame or a match. Remember also that on repeated or excessive exposure, some organic solvents may be toxic, carcinogenic (cancer causing), or both. For example, many chlorocarbon solvents, when accumulated in the body, result in liver deterioration similar to cirrhosis caused by excessive use of ethanol. The body does not easily rid itself of chlorocarbons nor does it detoxify them; they build up over time and may cause future illness. Some chlorocarbons are also suspected of being carcinogens. MINIMIZE YOUR EXPOSURE. Long-term exposure to benzene may cause a form of leukemia. Do not sniff benzene and avoid spilling it on yourself. Many other solvents, such as chloroform and ether, are good anesthetics and will put you to sleep if you breathe too much of them. They subsequently cause nausea. Many of these solvents have a synergistic effect with ethanol, meaning that they enhance its effect. Pyridine causes temporary impotence. In other words, organic solvents are just as dangerous as corrosive chemicals, such as sulfuric acid, but manifest their hazardous nature in other, more subtle ways.

If you are pregnant, you may want to consider taking this course at a later time. Some exposure to organic fumes is inevitable, and any possible risk to an unborn baby should be avoided.

Minimize any direct exposure to solvents and treat them with respect. The laboratory room should be well ventilated. Normal cautious handling of solvents should not result in any health problem. If you are trying to evaporate a solution in an open container, you must do the evaporation in the hood. Excess solvents should be discarded in a container specifically intended for waste solvents, rather than down the drain at the laboratory bench.

A sensible precaution is to wear gloves when working with solvents. Gloves made from polyethylene are inexpensive and provide good protection. The disadvantage of polyethylene gloves is that they are slippery. Disposable surgical gloves provide a better grip on glassware and other equipment, but they do not offer as much protection as polyethylene gloves. Nitrile gloves offer better protection (see p. 563).

Do Not Breathe Solvent Vapors. In checking the odor of a substance, be careful not to inhale very much of the material. The technique for smelling flowers is not advisable here; you could inhale dangerous amounts of the compound. Rather, a technique for smelling minute amounts of a substance is used. Pass a stopper or spatula moistened with the substance (if it is a liquid) under your nose. Or hold the substance away from you and waft the vapors toward you with your hand. But *never* hold your nose over the container and inhale deeply!

The hazards associated with organic solvents you are likely to encounter in the organic laboratory are discussed in detail beginning on page 571. If you use proper safety precautions, your exposure to harmful organic vapors will be minimized and should present no health risk.

Safe Transportation of Chemicals. When transporting chemicals from one location to another, particularly from one room to another, it is always best to use some form of **secondary containment.** This means that the bottle or flask is carried inside another, larger container. This outer container serves to contain the contents of the inner vessel in case a leak or breakage should occur. Scientific suppliers offer a variety of chemical-resistant carriers for this purpose.

D. Waste Disposal

Do Not Place Any Liquid or Solid Waste in Sinks; Use Appropriate Waste Containers. Many substances are toxic, flammable, and difficult to degrade; it is neither legal nor advisable to dispose of organic solvents or other liquid or solid reagents by pouring them down the sink.

The correct disposal method for wastes is to put them in appropriately labeled waste containers. These containers should be placed in the hoods in the laboratory. The waste containers will be disposed of safely by qualified persons using approved protocols.

Specific guidelines for disposing of waste will be determined by the people in charge of your particular laboratory and by local regulations. Two alternative systems for handling waste disposal are presented here. For each experiment that you are assigned, you will be instructed to dispose of all wastes according to the system that is in operation in your laboratory.

In one model of waste collection, a separate waste container for each experiment is placed in the laboratory. In some cases, more than one container, each labeled according to the type of waste that is anticipated, is set out. The containers will be labeled with a list that details each substance that is present in the container. In this model, it is common practice to use separate waste containers for aqueous solutions, organic halogenated solvents, and other organic nonhalogenated materials. At the end of the laboratory class period, the waste containers are transported to a central hazardous materials storage location. These wastes may be later consolidated and poured into large drums for shipping. Complete labeling, detailing each chemical contained in the waste, is required at each stage of this waste-handling process, even when the waste is consolidated into drums.

In a second model of waste collection, you will be instructed to dispose of all wastes in one of the following ways:

Nonhazardous solids. Nonhazardous solids such as paper and cork can be placed in an ordinary wastebasket.

Broken glassware. Broken glassware should be put into a container specifically designated for broken glassware.

Organic solids. Solid products that are not turned in or any other organic solids should be disposed of in the container designated for organic solids.

Inorganic solids. Solids such as alumina and silica gel should be put in a container specifically designated for them.

Nonhalogenated organic solvents. Organic solvents such as diethyl ether, hexane, and toluene, or any solvent that does not contain a halogen atom, should be disposed of in the container designated for nonhalogenated organic solvents.

Halogenated solvents. Methylene chloride (dichloromethane), chloroform, and carbon tetrachloride are examples of common halogenated organic solvents. Dispose of all halogenated solvents in the container designated for them.

Strong inorganic acids and bases. Strong acids such as hydrochloric, sulfuric, and nitric acid will be collected in specially marked containers. Strong bases such as sodium hydroxide and potassium hydroxide will also be collected in specially designated containers.

Aqueous solutions. Aqueous solutions will be collected in a specially marked waste container. It is not necessary to separate each type of aqueous solution (unless the solution contains heavy metals); rather, unless otherwise instructed, you may combine all aqueous solutions into the same waste container. Although many types of solutions (aqueous sodium bicarbonate, aqueous sodium chloride, and so on) may seem innocuous and it may seem that their disposal down the sink drain is not likely to cause harm, many communities are becoming increasingly restrictive about what substances they will permit to enter municipal sewage-treatment systems. In light of this trend toward greater caution, it is important to develop good laboratory habits regarding the disposal of *all* chemicals.

Heavy metals. Many heavy metal ions such as mercury and chromium are highly toxic and should be disposed of in specifically designated waste containers.

Whichever method is used, the waste containers must eventually be labeled with a complete list of each substance that is present in the waste. Individual waste containers are collected, and their contents are consolidated and placed into drums for transport to the waste-disposal site. Even these drums must bear labels that detail each of the substances contained in the waste.

In either waste-handling method, certain principles will always apply:

- Aqueous solutions should not be mixed with organic liquids.
- Concentrated acids should be stored in separate containers; certainly they must *never* be allowed to come into contact with organic waste.

■ Organic materials that contain halogen atoms (fluorine, chlorine, bromine, or iodine) should be stored in separate containers from those used to store materials that do not contain halogen atoms.

In each experiment in this textbook, we have suggested a method of collecting and storing wastes. Your instructor may opt to use another method for collecting wastes.

E. Use of Flames

Even though organic solvents are frequently flammable (for example, hexane, diethyl ether, methanol, acetone, and petroleum ether), there are certain laboratory procedures for which a flame must be used. Most often, these procedures involve an aqueous solution. In fact, as a general rule, use a flame to heat only aqueous solutions. Heating methods that do not use a flame are discussed in detail in Technique 6, starting on page 612. Most organic solvents boil below 100°C, and an aluminum block, heating mantle, sand bath, or water bath may be used to heat these solvents safely. Common organic solvents are listed in Technique 10, Table 10.3, page 676. Solvents marked in the table with boldface type will burn. Diethyl ether, pentane, and hexane are especially dangerous, because in combination with the correct amount of air, they may explode.

Some commonsense rules apply to using a flame in the presence of flammable solvents. Again, we stress that you should check to see whether anyone in your vicinity is using flammable solvents before you ignite any open flame. If someone is using a flammable solvent, move to a safer location before you light your flame. Your laboratory should have an area set aside for using a burner to prepare micropipets or other pieces of glassware.

The drainage troughs or sinks should never be used to dispose of flammable organic solvents. They will vaporize if they are low boiling and may encounter a flame farther down the bench on their way to the sink.

F. Inadvertently Mixed Chemicals

To avoid unnecessary hazards of fire and explosion, never pour any reagent back into a stock bottle. There is always the chance that you may accidentally pour back some foreign substance that will react explosively with the chemical in the stock bottle. Of course, by pouring reagents back into the stock bottles, you may introduce impurities that could spoil the experiment for the person using the stock reagent after you. Pouring things back into bottles is not only a dangerous practice but an inconsiderate one. Thus, you should not take more chemicals than you need.

G. Unauthorized Experiments

Never undertake any unauthorized experiments. The risk of an accident is high, particularly if the experiment has not been completely checked to reduce hazards. Never work alone in the laboratory. The laboratory instructor or supervisor must always be present.

H. Food in the Laboratory

Because all chemicals are potentially toxic, avoid accidentally ingesting any toxic substance; therefore, never eat or drink any food while in the laboratory. There is always

9

the possibility that whatever you are eating or drinking may become contaminated with a potentially hazardous material.

I. Clothing

Always wear closed shoes in the laboratory; open-toed shoes or sandals offer inadequate protection against spilled chemicals or broken glass. Do not wear your best clothing in the laboratory because some chemicals can make holes in or permanent stains on your clothing. To protect yourself and your clothing, it is advisable to wear a full-length laboratory apron or coat.

When working with chemicals that are very toxic, wear some type of gloves. Disposable gloves are inexpensive, offer good protection, provide acceptable "feel," and can be bought in many departmental stockrooms and college bookstores. Disposable latex surgical or polyethylene gloves are the least expensive type of glove; they are satisfactory when working with inorganic reagents and solutions. Better protection is afforded by disposable nitrile gloves. This type of glove provides good protection against organic chemicals and solvents. Heavier nitrile gloves are also available.

Finally, hair that is shoulder length or longer should be tied back. This precaution is especially important if you are working with a burner.

J. First Aid: Cuts, Minor Burns, and Acid or Base Burns

If any chemical enters your eyes, immediately irrigate the eyes with copious quantities of water. Tempered (slightly warm) water, if available, is preferable. Be sure that the eyelids are kept open. Continue flushing the eyes in this way for 15 minutes.

In case of a cut, wash the wound well with water unless you are specifically instructed to do otherwise. If necessary, apply pressure to the wound to stop the flow of blood.

Minor burns caused by flames or contact with hot objects may be soothed by immediately immersing the burned area in cold water or cracked ice until you no longer feel a burning sensation. Applying salves to burns is discouraged. Severe burns must be examined and treated by a physician. For chemical acid or base burns, rinse the burned area with copious quantities of water for at least 15 minutes.

If you accidentally ingest a chemical, call the local poison control center for instructions. Do not drink anything until you have been told to do so. It is important that the examining physician be informed of the exact nature of the substance ingested.

1.2 RIGHT-TO-KNOW LAWS

The federal government and most state governments now require that employers provide their employees with complete information about hazards in the workplace. These regulations are often referred to as **Right-to-Know Laws.** At the federal level, the Occupational Safety and Health Administration (OSHA) is charged with enforcing these regulations.

In 1990, the federal government extended the Hazard Communication Act, which established the Right-to-Know Laws, to include a provision that requires the establishment of a Chemical Hygiene Plan at all academic laboratories. Every college and university chemistry department should have a Chemical Hygiene Plan. Having this plan means that all the safety regulations and laboratory safety procedures should be written in a manual. The plan also provides for the training of all employees in laboratory safety. Your laboratory instructor and assistants should have this training.

One of the components of Right-to-Know Laws is that employees and students have access to information about the hazards of any chemicals with which they are working. Your instructor will alert you to dangers to which you need to pay particular attention. However, you may want to seek additional information. Two excellent sources of information are labels on the bottles that come from a chemical manufacturer and **Material Safety Data Sheets** (MSDSs). The MSDSs are also provided by the manufacturer and must be kept available for all chemicals used at educational institutions.

A. Material Safety Data Sheets

Reading an MSDS for a chemical can be a daunting experience, even for an experienced chemist. MSDSs contain a wealth of information, some of which must be decoded to understand. The MSDS for methanol is shown on pages 565–569. Only the information that might be of interest to you is described in the paragraphs that follow.

Section 1. The first part of Section 1 identifies the substance by name, formula, and various numbers and codes. Most organic compounds have more than one name. In this case, the systematic (or International Union of Pure and Applied Chemistry [IUPAC]) name is methanol, and the other names are common names or are from an older system of nomenclature. The Chemical Abstract Service Number (CAS No.) is often used to identify a substance, and it may be used to access extensive information about a substance found in many computer databases or in the library.

Section 3. The Baker SAF-T-DATA System is found on all MSDSs and bottle labels for chemicals supplied by J. T. Baker, Inc. For each category listed, the number indicates the degree of hazard. The lowest number is 0 (very low hazard), and the highest number is 4 (extreme hazard). The Health category refers to damage involved when the substance is inhaled, ingested, or absorbed. Flammability indicates the tendency of a substance to burn. Reactivity refers to how reactive a substance is with air, water, or other substances. The last category, Contact, refers to how hazardous a substance is when it comes in contact with external parts of the body. Note that this rating scale is applicable only to Baker MSDSs and labels; other rating scales with different meanings are also in common use.

Section 4. This section provides helpful information for emergency and first aid procedures.

Section 6. This part of the MSDS deals with procedures for handling spills and disposal. The information could be very helpful, particularly if a large amount of the chemical was spilled. More information about disposal is also given in Section 13.

Section 8. Much valuable information is found in Section 8. To help you understand this material, some of the more important terms used in this section are defined:

Threshold Limit Value (TLV). The American Conference of Governmental Industrial Hygienists (ACGIH) developed the TLV: This is the maximum concentration of a substance in air that a person should be exposed to on a regular basis. It is usually expressed in ppm or mg/m^3. Note that this value assumes that a person is exposed to the substance 40 hours per week, on a long-term basis. This value may not be particularly

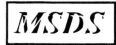 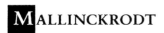 **Material Safety Data Sheet**

24 Hour Emergency Telephone: 908-859-2151
CHEMTREC: 1-800-424-9300

National Response in Canada
CANUTEC: 613-996-6666

From: Mallinckrodt Baker, Inc.
222 Red School Lane
Phillipsburg, NJ 08865

Outside U.S. and Canada
Chemtrec: 202-483-7616

MALLINCKRODT   J.T.Baker

NOTE: CHEMTREC, CANUTEC and National Response Center emergency numbers to be used only in the event of chemical emergencies involving a spill, leak, fire, exposure or accident involving chemicals.

All non-emergency questions should be directed to Customer Service (1-800-582-2537) for assistance.

METHYL ALCOHOL

1. Product Identification

Synonyms: Wood alcohol; methanol; carbinol
CAS No: 67-56-1
Molecular Weight: 32.04
Chemical Formula: CH_3OH
Product Codes: **J.T. Baker:**

5217, 5370, 5794, 5807, 5811, 5842, 5869, 9049, 9063, 9066, 9067, 9069, 9070, 9071, 9073, 9075, 9076, 9077, 9091, 9093, 9096, 9097, 9098, 9263, 9893

Mallinckrodt:

3004, 3006, 3016, 3017, 3018, 3024, 3041, 3701, 4295, 5160, 8814, H080, H488, H603, V079, V571

2. Composition/Information on Ingredients

Ingredient	CAS No.	Percent	Hazardous
Methyl Alcohol	67-56-1	100%	Yes

3. Hazards Identification

Emergency Overview

POISON! DANGER! VAPOR HARMFUL. MAY BE FATAL OR CAUSE BLINDNESS IF SWALLOWED. HARMFUL IF INHALED OR ABSORBED THROUGH SKIN. CANNOT BE MADE NONPOISONOUS. FLAMMABLE LIQUID AND VAPOR. CAUSES IRRITATION TO SKIN, EYES AND RESPIRATORY TRACT. AFFECTS THE LIVER.

J.T. Baker SAF-T-DATA(tm) Ratings
(Provided here for your convenience)

Health:	Flammability:	Reactivity:	Contact:
3 - Severe (Poison)	4 - Extreme (Flammable)	1 - Slight	1 - Slight
Lab Protection Equip:	GOGGLES & SHIELD; LAB COAT & APRON; VENT HOOD; PROPER GLOVES; CLASS B EXTINGUISHER		
Storage Color Code:	Red (Flammable)		

Potential Health Effects

Inhalation:

A slight irritant to the mucous membranes. Toxic effects exerted upon nervous system, particularly the optic nerve. Once absorbed into the body, it is very slowly eliminated. Symptoms of overexposure may include headache, drowsiness, nausea, vomiting, blurred vision, blindness, coma, and death. A person may get better but then worse again up to 30 hours later.

Ingestion:

Toxic. Symptoms parallel inhalation. Can intoxicate and cause blindness. Usual fatal dose: 100-125 milliliters.

Skin Contact:

Methyl alcohol is a defatting agent and may cause skin to become dry and cracked. Skin absorption can occur; symptoms may parallel inhalation exposure.

Eye Contact:

Irritant. Continued exposure may cause eye lesions.

Chronic Exposure:

Marked impairment of vision and enlargement of the liver has been reported. Repeated or prolonged exposure may cause skin irritation.

Aggravation of Pre-existing Conditions:

Persons with pre-existing skin disorders or eye problems or impaired liver or kidney function may be more susceptible to the effects of the substance.

---

4.   First Aid Measures

Inhalation:

Remove to fresh air. If not breathing, give artificial respiration. If breathing is difficult, give oxygen. Call a physician.

Ingestion:

Induce vomiting immediately as directed by medical personnel. Never give anything by mouth to an unconscious person.

Skin Contact:

Remove any contaminated clothing. Wash skin with soap or mild detergent and water for at least 15 minutes. Get medical attention if irritation develops or persists.

Eye Contact:

Immediately flush eyes with plenty of water for at least 15 minutes, lifting lower and upper eyelids occasionally. Get medical attention immediately.

---

5.   Fire Fighting Measures

Fire:

Flash point: 12°C (54°F) CC
Autoignition temperature: 464°C (867°F)
Flammable limits in air % by volume:
lel: 7.3; uel: 36
Flammable.

Explosion:

Above flash point, vapor-air mixtures are explosive within flammable limits noted above. Moderate explosion hazard and dangerous fire hazard when exposed to heat, sparks or flames. Sensitive to static discharge.

Fire Extinguishing Media:

Water spray, dry chemical, alcohol foam, or carbon dioxide.

Special Information:

In the event of a fire, wear full protective clothing and NIOSH-approved self-contained breathing apparatus with full facepiece operated in the pressure demand or other positive pressure mode. Use water spray to blanket fire, cool fire exposed containers, and to flush non-ignited spills or vapors away from fire. Vapors can flow along surfaces to distant ignition source and flash back.

6. Accidental Release Measures

Ventilate area of leak or spill. Remove all sources of ignition. Wear appropriate personal protective equipment as specified in Section 8. Isolate hazard area. Keep unnecessary and unprotected personnel from entering. Contain and recover liquid when possible. Use non-sparking tools and equipment. Collect liquid in an appropriate container or absorb with an inert material (e. g., vermiculite, dry sand, earth), and place in a chemical waste container. Do not use combustible materials, such as saw dust. Do not flush to sewer! J. T. Baker SOLUSORB® solvent adsorbent is recommended for spills of this product.

7. Handling and Storage

Protect against physical damage. Store in a cool, dry well-ventilated location, away from any area where the fire hazard may be acute. Outside or detached storage is preferred. Separate from incompatibles. Containers should be bonded and grounded for transfers to avoid static sparks. Storage and use areas should be No Smoking areas. Use non-sparking type tools and equipment, including explosion proof ventilation. Containers of this material may be hazardous when empty since they retain product residues (vapors, liquid); observe all warnings and precautions listed for the product.

8. Exposure Controls/Personal Protection

Airborne Exposure Limits:

For Methyl Alcohol:
- OSHA Permissible Exposure Limit (PEL):
    200 ppm (TWA)
- ACGIH Threshold Limit Value (TLV):
    200 ppm (TWA), 250 ppm (STEL) skin

Ventilation System:

A system of local and/or general exhaust is recommended to keep employee exposures below the Airborne Exposure Limits. Local exhaust ventilation is generally preferred because it can control the emissions of the contaminant at its source, preventing dispersion of it into the general work area. Please refer to the ACGIH document, "Industrial Ventilation, A Manual of Recommended Practices", most recent edition, for details.

Personal Respirator (NIOSH Approved)

If the exposure limit is exceeded, wear a supplied air, full-facepiece respirator, airlined hood, or full-facepiece self-contained breathing apparatus.

Skin Protection:

Rubber or neoprene gloves and additional protection including impervious boots, apron, or coveralls, as needed in areas of unusual exposure.

Eye Protection:

Use chemical safety goggles. Maintain eye wash fountain and quick-drench facilities in work area.

9. Physical and Chemical Properties

Appearance:	**Boiling Point:**
Clear, colorless liquid.	64.5°C (147°F)
Odor:	**Melting Point:**
Characteristic odor.	-98°C (-144°F)
Solubility:	**Vapor Density (Air=1):**
Miscible in water.	1.1
Specific Gravity:	**Vapor Pressure (mm Hg):**
0.8	97 @ 20°C (68°F)
pH:	**Evaporation Rate (BuAc=1):**
No information found.	5.9
% Volatiles by volume @ 21°C (70°F):	
100	

10. Stability and Reactivity

Stability:

Stable under ordinary conditions of use and storage.

Hazardous Decomposition Products:

May form carbon dioxide, carbon monoxide, and formaldehyde when heated to decomposition.

Hazardous Polymerization:

Will not occur.

Incompatabilities:

Strong oxidizing agents such as nitrates, perchlorates or sulfuric acid. Will attack some forms of plastics, rubber, and coatings. May react with metallic aluminum and generate hydrogen gas.

Conditions to Avoid:

Heat, flames, ignition sources and incompatibles.

11. Toxicological Information

Methyl Alcohol (Methanol) Oral rat LD50: 5628 mg/kg; inhalation rat LC50: 64000 ppm/4H; skin rabbit LD50: 15800 mg/kg; Irritation data-standard Draize test: skin, rabbit: 20mg/24 hr. Moderate; eye, rabbit: 100 mg/24 hr. Moderate; Investigated as a mutagen, reproductive effector.

Cancer Lists			
	---NTP Carcinogen---		
Ingredient	Known	Anticipated	IARC Category
Methyl Alcohol (67-56-1)	No	No	None

12. Ecological Information

Environmental Fate:

When released into the soil, this material is expected to readily biodegrade. When released into the soil, this material is expected to leach into groundwater. When released into the soil, this material is expected to quickly evaporate. When released into the water, this material is expected to have a half-life between 1 and 10 days. When released into water, this material is expected to readily biodegrade. When released into the air, this material is expected to exist in the aerosol phase with a short half-life. When released into the air, this material is expected to be readily degraded by reaction with photochemically produced hydroxyl radicals. When released into air, this material is expected to have a half-life between 10 and 30 days. When released into the air, this material is expected to be readily removed from the atmosphere by wet deposition.

Environmental Toxicity:

This material is expected to be slightly toxic to aquatic life.

13. Disposal Considerations

Whatever cannot be saved for recovery or recycling should be handled as hazardous waste and sent to a RCRA approved incinerator or disposed in a RCRA approved waste facility. Processing, use or contamination of this product may change the waste management options. State and local disposal regulations may differ from federal disposal regulations.

Dispose of container and unused contents in accordance with federal, state and local requirements.

14. Transport Information

Domestic (Land, D.O.T.)

Proper Shipping Name:	METHANOL
Hazard Class:	3
UN/NA:	UN1230 **Packing Group:** II

Information reported for product/size:		350LB	
International (Water, I.M.O.)			
Proper Shipping Name:	METHANOL		
Hazard Class:	3.2, 6.1		
UN/NA:	UN1230	**Packing Group:**	II
Information reported for product/size:		350LB	

15. Regulatory Information

Chemical Inventory Status

						---Canada---		
Ingredient	TSCA	EC	Japan	Australia	Korea	DSL	NDSL	Phil.
Methyl Alcohol (67-56-1)	Yes	Yes	Yes	Yes	Yes	Yes	No	Yes

Federal, State & International Regulations

	---SARA 302---		----------SARA 313----------			-RCRA-	-TSCA-
Ingredient	RQ	TPQ	List	Chemical Catg.	CERCLA	261.33	8(d)
Methyl Alcohol (67-56-1)	No	No	Yes	No	5000	U154	No

Chemical Weapons Convention: No   **TSCA 12(b):** No   **CDTA:** No

SARA 311/312: Acute: Yes   Chronic: Yes   Fire: Yes   Pressure: No   Reactivity: No   (Pure / Liquid)

Australian Hazchem Code: 2PE   **Australian Poison Schedule:** S6

WHMIS: This MSDS has been prepared according to the hazard criteria of the Controlled Products
Regulations (CPR) and the MSDS contains all of the information required by the CPR.

16. Other Information

NFPA Ratings:

Health: 1 Flammability: 3 Reactivity: 0

Label Hazard Warning:

POISON! DANGER! VAPOR HARMFUL. MAY BE FATAL OR CAUSE BLINDNESS IF SWALLOWED.
HARMFUL IF INHALED OR ABSORBED THROUGH SKIN. CANNOT BE MADE NONPOISONOUS.
FLAMMABLE LIQUID AND VAPOR. CAUSES IRRITATION TO SKIN, EYES AND RESPIRATORY TRACT.
AFFECTS THE LIVER.

Label Precautions:

Keep away from heat, sparks and flame.
Keep container closed.
Use only with adequate ventilation.
Wash thoroughly after handling.
Avoid breathing vapor.
Avoid contact with eyes, skin and clothing.

Label First Aid:

If swallowed, induce vomiting immediately as directed by medical personnel. Never give anything by mouth to
an unconscious person. In case of contact, immediately flush eyes or skin with plenty of water for at least 15
minutes while removing contaminated clothing and shoes. Wash clothing before reuse. If inhaled, remove to
fresh air. If not breathing give artificial respiration. If breathing is difficult, give oxygen. In all cases get medical
attention immediately.

Product Use:

Laboratory Reagent.

Revision Information:

New 16 section MSDS format, all sections have been revised.

Disclaimer:

Prepared By: Strategic Services Division
              Phone Number: (314) 539-1600 (U.S.A.)

applicable in the case of a student performing an experiment in a single laboratory period.

Permissible Exposure Limit (PEL). This has the same meaning as TLV; however, PELs were developed by OSHA. Note that for methanol, the TLV and PEL are both 200 ppm.

Section 10. The information contained in Section 10 refers to the stability of the compound and the hazards associated with mixing of chemicals. It is important to consider this information before carrying out an experiment not previously done.

Section 11. More information about the toxicity is given in this section. Another important term must first be defined:

Lethal Dose, 50% Mortality (LD$_{50}$). This is the dose of a substance that will kill 50% of the animals administered a single dose. Different means of administration are used, such as oral, intraperitoneal (injected into the lining of the abdominal cavity), subcutaneous (injected under the skin), and application to the surface of the skin. The LD$_{50}$ is usually expressed in milligrams (mg) of substance per kilogram (kg) of animal weight. The lower the value of LD$_{50}$, the more toxic the substance. It is assumed that the toxicity in humans will be similar.

Unless you have considerably more knowledge about chemical toxicity, the information in Sections 8 and 11 is most useful for comparing the toxicity of one substance with another. For example, the TLV for methanol is 200 ppm, whereas the TLV for benzene is 10 ppm. Clearly, performing an experiment involving benzene would require much more stringent precautions than an experiment involving methanol. One of the LD$_{50}$ values for methanol is 5628 mg/kg. The comparable LD$_{50}$ value of aniline is 250 mg/kg. Clearly, aniline is much more toxic, and because it is easily absorbed through the skin, it presents a significant hazard. It should also be mentioned that both TLV and PEL ratings assume that the worker comes in contact with a substance on a repeated and long-term basis. Thus, even if a chemical has a relatively low TLV or PEL, it does not mean that using it for one experiment will present a danger to you. Furthermore, by performing experiments using small amounts of chemicals and with proper safety precautions, your exposure to organic chemicals in this course will be minimal.

Section 16. Section 16 contains the National Fire Protection Association (NFPA) rating. This is similar to the Baker SAF-T-DATA (discussed in Section 3), except that the number represents the hazards when a fire is present. The order here is Health, Flammability, and Reactivity. Often, this is presented in graphic form on a label (see figure). The small diamonds are often color coded: blue for Health, red for Flammability, and yellow for Reactivity. The bottom diamond (white) is sometimes used to display graphic symbols denoting unusual reactivity, hazards, or special precautions to be taken.

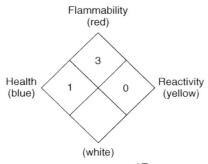

B. Bottle Labels

Reading the label on a bottle can be a very helpful way of learning about the hazards of a chemical. The amount of information varies greatly, depending on which company supplied the chemical.

Apply some common sense when you read MSDSs and bottle labels. Using these chemicals does not mean you will experience the consequences that can potentially result from exposure to each chemical. For example, an MSDS for sodium chloride states, "Exposure to this product may have serious adverse health effects." Despite the apparent severity of this cautionary statement, it would not be reasonable to expect people to stop using sodium chloride in a chemistry experiment or to stop sprinkling a small amount of it (as table salt) on eggs to enhance their flavor. In many cases, the consequences described in MSDSs from exposure to chemicals are somewhat overstated, particularly for students using these chemicals to perform a laboratory experiment.

1.3 COMMON SOLVENTS

Most organic chemistry experiments involve an organic solvent at some step in the procedure. A list of common organic solvents follows, with a discussion of toxicity, possible carcinogenic properties, and precautions that you should use when handling these solvents. A tabulation of the compounds currently suspected of being carcinogens appears at the end of Technique 1.

Acetic Acid. Glacial acetic acid is corrosive enough to cause serious acid burns on the skin. Its vapors can irritate the eyes and nasal passages. Care should be exercised not to breathe the vapors and not to allow them to escape into the laboratory.

Acetone. Relative to other organic solvents, acetone is not very toxic. It is flammable, however. Do not use acetone near open flames.

Benzene. Benzene can damage bone marrow, it causes various blood disorders, and its effects may lead to leukemia. Benzene is considered a serious carcinogenic hazard. It is absorbed rapidly through the skin and also poisons the liver and kidneys. In addition, benzene is flammable. Because of its toxicity and its carcinogenic properties, benzene should not be used in the laboratory; you should use some less dangerous solvent instead. Toluene is considered a safer alternative solvent in procedures that specify benzene.

Carbon Tetrachloride. Carbon tetrachloride can cause serious liver and kidney damage as well as skin irritation and other problems. It is absorbed rapidly through the skin. In high concentrations, it can cause death as a result of respiratory failure. Moreover, carbon tetrachloride is suspected of being a carcinogenic material. Although this solvent has the advantage of being nonflammable (in the past, it was used on occasion as a fire extinguisher), it causes health problems, so it should not be used routinely in the laboratory. If no reasonable substitute exists, however, it must be used in small quantities, as in preparing samples for infrared (IR) and nuclear magnetic resonance (NMR) spectroscopy. In such cases, you must use it in a hood.

Chloroform. Chloroform is similar to carbon tetrachloride in its toxicity. It has been used as an anesthetic. However, chloroform is currently on the list of suspected carcinogens. Because of this, do not use chloroform routinely as a solvent in the laboratory. If it is occasionally necessary to use chloroform as a solvent for special samples, then you must use it in a hood. Methylene chloride is usually found to be a safer substitute in procedures that specify chloroform as a solvent. Deuterochloroform, $CDCl_3$, is a common solvent for NMR spectroscopy. Caution dictates that you should treat it with the same respect as chloroform.

1,2-Dimethoxyethane (Ethylene Glycol Dimethyl Ether or Monoglyme). Because it is miscible with water, 1,2-dimethoxyethane is a useful alternative to solvents such as dioxane and tetrahydrofuran, which may be more hazardous. 1,2-Dimethoxyethane is flammable and should not be handled near an open flame. On long exposure of 1,2-dimethoxyethane to light and oxygen, explosive peroxides may form. 1,2-Dimethoxyethane is a possible reproductive toxin.

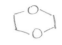

Dioxane. Dioxane has been used widely because it is a convenient, water-miscible solvent. It is now suspected, however, of being carcinogenic. It is also toxic, affecting the central nervous system, liver, kidneys, skin, lungs, and mucous membranes. Dioxane is also flammable and tends to form explosive peroxides when it is exposed to light and air. Because of its carcinogenic properties, it is no longer used in the laboratory unless absolutely necessary. Either 1,2-dimethoxyethane or tetrahydrofuran is a suitable, water-miscible alternative solvent.

Ethanol. Ethanol has well-known properties as an intoxicant. In the laboratory, the principal danger arises from fires, because ethanol is a flammable solvent. When using ethanol, take care to work where there are no open flames.

Ether (diethyl ether). The principal hazard associated with diethyl ether is fire or explosion. Ether is probably the most flammable solvent found in the laboratory. Because ether vapors are much denser than air, they may travel along a laboratory bench for a considerable distance from their source before being ignited. Before using ether, it is very important to be sure that no one is working with matches or any open flame. Ether is not a particularly toxic solvent, although in high enough concentrations it can cause drowsiness and perhaps nausea. It has been used as a general anesthetic. Ether can form highly explosive peroxides when exposed to air. Consequently, you should never distill it to dryness.

Hexane. Hexane may be irritating to the respiratory tract. It can also act as an intoxicant and a depressant of the central nervous system. It can cause skin irritation because it is an excellent solvent for skin oils. The most serious hazard, however, comes from its flammability. The precautions recommended for using diethyl ether in the presence of open flames apply equally to hexane.

Ligroin. See Hexane.

Methanol. Much of the material outlining the hazards of ethanol applies to methanol. Methanol is more toxic than ethanol; ingestion can cause blindness and even death. Because methanol is more volatile, the danger of fires is more acute.

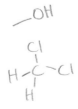

Methylene Chloride (Dichloromethane). Methylene chloride is not flammable. Unlike other members of the class of chlorocarbons, it is not currently considered a serious carcinogenic hazard. Recently, however, it has been the subject of much serious investigation, and there have been proposals to regulate it in industrial situations in which workers have high levels of exposure on a day-to-day basis. Methylene chloride is less toxic than chloroform and carbon tetrachloride. It can cause liver damage when ingested, however, and its vapors may cause drowsiness or nausea.

Pentane. See Hexane.

Petroleum Ether. See Hexane.

Pyridine. Some fire hazard is associated with pyridine. However, the most serious hazard arises from its toxicity. Pyridine may depress the central nervous system; irritate the skin and respiratory tract; damage the liver, kidneys, and gastrointestinal system; and even cause temporary sterility. You should treat pyridine as a highly toxic solvent and handle it only in the fume hood.

Tetrahydrofuran. Tetrahydrofuran may cause irritation of the skin, eyes, and respiratory tract. It should never be distilled to dryness because it tends to form potentially explosive peroxides on exposure to air. Tetrahydrofuran does present a fire hazard.

Toluene. Unlike benzene, toluene is not considered a carcinogen. However, it is at least as toxic as benzene. It can act as an anesthetic and damage the central nervous system. If benzene is present as an impurity in toluene, expect the usual hazards associated with benzene. Toluene is also a flammable solvent, and the usual precautions about working near open flames should be applied.

You should not use certain solvents in the laboratory because of their carcinogenic properties. Benzene, carbon tetrachloride, chloroform, and dioxane are among these solvents. For certain applications, however, notably as solvents for infrared or NMR spectroscopy, there may be no suitable alternative. When it is necessary to use one of these solvents, use safety precautions and refer to the discussions in Techniques 25–28.

Because relatively large amounts of solvents may be used in a large organic laboratory class, your laboratory supervisor must take care to store these substances safely. Only the amount of solvent needed for a particular experiment should be kept in the laboratory. The preferred location for bottles of solvents being used during a class period is in a hood. When the solvents are not being used, they should be stored in a fireproof storage cabinet for solvents. If possible, this cabinet should be ventilated into the fume hood system.

1.4 CARCINOGENIC SUBSTANCES

A **carcinogen** is a substance that causes cancer in living tissue. The usual procedures for determining whether a substance is carcinogenic is to expose laboratory animals to high dosages over a long period. It is not clear whether short-term exposure to these chemicals carries a comparable risk, but it is prudent to use these substances with special precautions.

Many regulatory agencies have compiled lists of carcinogenic substances or substances suspected of being carcinogenic. Because these lists are inconsistent, compiling a definitive list of carcinogenic substances is difficult. The following common substances are included in many of these lists.

Acetamide	4-Methyl-2-oxetanone (β-butyrolactone)
Acrylonitrile	1-Naphthylamine
Asbestos	2-Naphthylamine
Benzene	*N*-Nitroso compounds
Benzidine	2-Oxetanone (β-propiolactone)
Carbon tetrachloride	Phenacetin
Chloroform	Phenylhydrazine and its salts
Chromic oxide	Polychlorinated biphenyl (PCB)

Coumarin	Progesterone
Diazomethane	Styrene oxide
1,2-Dibromoethane	Tannins
Dimethyl sulfate	Testosterone
p-Dioxane	Thioacetamide
Ethylene oxide	Thiourea
Formaldehyde	*o*-Toluidine
Hydrazine and its salts	Trichloroethylene
Lead (II) acetate	Vinyl chloride

REFERENCES

Aldrich Catalog and Handbook of Fine Chemicals. Milwaukee, WI: Aldrich Chemical Co., current edition.

Armour, M. A., *Pollution Prevention and Waste Minimization in Laboratories.* Edited by Peter A. Reinhardt, K. Leigh Leonard, Peter C. Ashbrook. Boca Raton, Florida: Lewis Publishers, 1996.

Fire Protection Guide on Hazardous Materials, 10th ed. Quincy, MA: National Fire Protection Association, 1991.

Flinn Chemical Catalog Reference Manual. Batavia, IL: Flinn Scientific, current edition.

Gosselin, R. E., Smith, R. P., and Hodge, H. C. *Clinical Toxicology of Commercial Products,* 5th ed. Baltimore, MD: Williams & Wilkins, 1984.

Lenga, R. E., ed. *The Sigma-Aldrich Library of Chemical Safety Data.* Milwaukee, WI: Sigma-Aldrich, 1985.

Lewis, R. J. *Carcinogenically Active Chemicals: A Reference Guide.* New York: Van Nostrand Reinhold, 1990.

Lewis, R. J., *Sax's Dangerous Properties of Industrial Materials,* 8th edition, New York: Van Nostrand Reinhold, 1992.

The Merck Index, 13th ed. Rahway, NJ: Merck and Co., 2001.

Prudent Practices in the Laboratory: Handling and Disposal of Chemicals. Washington, DC: Committee on Prudent Practices for Handling, Storage, and Disposal of Chemicals in Laboratories, Board on Chemical Sciences and Technology, Commission on Physical Sciences, Mathematics, and Applications, National Research Council, National Academy Press, 1995.

Renfrew, M. M., ed. *Safety in the Chemical Laboratory.* Easton, PA: Division of Chemical Education, American Chemical Society, 1967–1991.

Safety in Academic Chemistry Laboratories, 4th ed. Washington, DC: Committee on Chemical Safety, American Chemical Society, 1985.

Sax, N. I., and Lewis, R. J. *Dangerous Properties of Industrial Materials,* 7th ed. New York: Van Nostrand Reinhold, 1988.

Sax, N. I., and Lewis, R. J., eds. *Rapid Guide to Hazardous Chemicals in the Work Place,* 2nd ed. New York: Van Nostrand Reinhold, 1990.

Useful Safety-Related Internet Addresses

Interactive Learning Paradigms, Inc.

http://www.ilpi.com/msds/

This is an excellent general site for MSDS sheets. The site lists chemical manufacturers and suppliers. Selecting a company will take you directly to the appropriate place to obtain an MSDS sheet. Many of the sites listed require you to register in order to obtain a MSDS sheet for a particular chemical. Ask your departmental or college safety supervisor to obtain the information for you.

Acros chemicals and Fisher Scientific
https://www1.fishersci.com/

Alfa Aesar
http://www.alfa.com/alf/index.htm

Cornell University, Department of Environmental Health and Safety
http://msds.pdc.cornell.edu/msdssrch.asp
This is an excellent searchable database of more than 325,000 MSDS files. No registration is required.

Eastman Kodak
http://msds.kodak.com/ehswww/external/index.jsp

EMD Chemicals (formerly EM Science) and Merck
http://www.emdchemicals.com/corporate/emd_corporate.asp

J. T. Baker and Mallinckrodt Laboratory Chemicals
http://www.jtbaker.com/asp/Catalog.asp

National Institute for Occupational Safety and Health (NIOSH) has an excellent website that includes databases and information resources, including links:
http://www.cdc.gov/niosh/topics/chemical-safety/default.html

Sigma, Aldrich and Fluka
http://www.sigmaaldrich.com/Area_of_Interest/The_Americas/United_States.html

VWR Scientific Products
http://www.vwrsp.com/search/index.cgi?tmpl=msds

T E C H N I Q U E   2

The Laboratory Notebook, Calculations, and Laboratory Records

In the Introduction to this book, we mentioned the importance of advance preparation for laboratory work. Presented here are some suggestions about what specific information you should try to obtain in your advance studying. Because much of this information must be obtained while preparing your laboratory notebook, the two subjects, advance study and notebook preparation, are developed simultaneously.

An important part of any laboratory experience is learning to maintain very complete records of every experiment undertaken and every item of data obtained. Far too often, careless recording of data and observations has resulted in mistakes, frustration, and lost time due to needless repetition of experiments. If reports are required, you will find that proper collection and recording of data can make your report writing much easier.

Because organic reactions are seldom quantitative, special problems result. Frequently, reagents must be used in large excess to increase the amount of product. Some reagents are expensive, and, therefore, care must be used in measuring the amounts of these substances. Very often, many more reactions take place than you desire. These extra reactions, or **side reactions,** may form products other than the desired product. These are called **side products.** For all these reasons, you must plan your experimental procedure carefully before undertaking the actual experiment.

2.1 THE NOTEBOOK

For recording data and observations during experiments, use a *bound notebook.* The notebook should have consecutively numbered pages. If it does not, number the pages immediately. A spiral-bound notebook or any other notebook from which the pages can be removed easily is not acceptable, because the possibility of losing the pages is great.

All data and observations must be recorded in the notebook. Paper towels, napkins, toilet tissue, or scratch paper tend to become lost or destroyed. It is bad laboratory practice to record information on such random and perishable pieces of paper. All entries must be recorded in *permanent ink.* It can be frustrating to have important information disappear from the notebook because it was recorded in washable ink or pencil and could not survive a flood caused by the student at the next position on the bench. Because you will be using your notebook in the laboratory, the book will probably become soiled or stained by chemicals, filled with scratched-out entries, or even slightly burned. That is expected and is a normal part of laboratory work.

Your instructor may check your notebook at any time, so you should always have it up to date. If your instructor requires reports, you can prepare them quickly from the material recorded in the laboratory notebook.

2.2 NOTEBOOK FORMAT

A. Advance Preparation

Individual instructors vary greatly in the type of notebook format they prefer; such variation stems from differences in philosophies and experience. You must obtain specific directions from your own instructor for preparing a notebook. Certain features, however, are common to most notebook formats. The following discussion indicates what might be included in a typical notebook.

It will be very helpful and you can save much time in the laboratory if for each experiment you know the main reactions, the potential side reactions, the mechanism, and the stoichiometry and you understand fully the procedure and the theory underlying it before you come to the laboratory. Understanding the procedure by which the desired product is to be separated from undesired materials is also very important. If you examine each of these topics before coming to class, you will be prepared to do the experiment efficiently. You will have your equipment and reagents already prepared when they are to be used. Your reference material will be at hand when you need it. Finally, with your time efficiently organized, you will be able to take advantage of long reaction or reflux periods to perform other tasks, such as doing shorter experiments or finishing previous ones.

For experiments in which a compound is synthesized from other reagents, that is, **preparative experiments,** it is essential to know the main reaction. To perform stoichiometric calculations, you should balance the equation for the main reaction. Therefore, before you begin the experiment, your notebook should contain the balanced equation for the pertinent reaction. Using the preparation of isopentyl acetate, or banana oil, as an example, you should write the following:

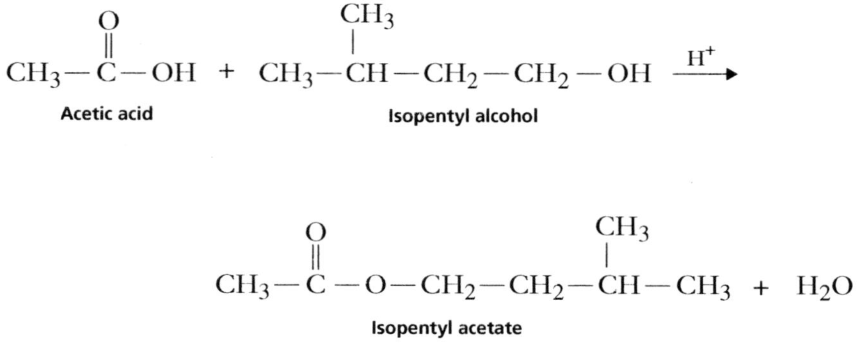

$$CH_3-\overset{\overset{\displaystyle O}{\|}}{C}-OH \; + \; CH_3-\overset{\overset{\displaystyle CH_3}{|}}{CH}-CH_2-CH_2-OH \; \xrightarrow{\; H^+ \;}$$

Acetic acid　　　　　　**Isopentyl alcohol**

$$CH_3-\overset{\overset{\displaystyle O}{\|}}{C}-O-CH_2-CH_2-\overset{\overset{\displaystyle CH_3}{|}}{CH}-CH_3 \; + \; H_2O$$

Isopentyl acetate

Also enter in the notebook the possible side reactions that divert reagents into contaminants (side products), before beginning the experiment. You will have to separate these side products from the major product during purification.

You should list physical constants such as melting points, boiling points, densities, and molecular weights in the notebook when this information is needed to perform an experiment or to do calculations. These data are located in sources such as the *CRC Handbook of Chemistry and Physics, The Merck Index, Lange's Handbook of Chemistry,* or *Aldrich Handbook of Fine Chemicals.* Write physical constants required for an experiment in your notebook before you come to class.

Advance preparation may also include examining some subjects, information not necessarily recorded in the notebook, that should prove useful in understanding the experiment. Included among these subjects are an understanding of the mechanism of the reaction, an examination of other methods by which the same compound might be prepared, and a detailed study of the experimental procedure. Many students find that an outline of the procedure, prepared *before* they come to class, helps them use their time more efficiently once they begin the experiment. Such an outline could very well be prepared on some loose sheet of paper rather than in the notebook itself.

Once the reaction has been completed, the desired product does not magically appear as purified material; it must be isolated from a frequently complex mixture of side products, unreacted starting materials, solvents, and catalysts. You should try to outline a **separation scheme** in your notebook for isolating the product from its contaminants. At each stage, you should try to understand the reason for the particular instruction given in the experimental procedure. This not only will familiarize you with the basic separation and purification techniques used in organic chemistry but also will help you understand when to use these techniques. Such an outline might take the form of a flowchart. For example, see the separation scheme for isopentyl acetate (Figure 2.1). Careful attention to understanding the separation, besides familiarizing you with the procedure by which the desired product is separated from impurities in your particular experiments, may prepare you for original research in which no experimental procedure exists.

In designing a separation scheme, note that the scheme outlines those steps undertaken once the reaction period has been concluded. For this reason, the represented scheme does not include steps such as the addition of the reactants (isopentyl alcohol and acetic acid) and the catalyst (sulfuric acid) or the heating of the reaction mixture.

For experiments in which a compound is isolated from a particular source and is not prepared from other reagents, some information described in this section will not be applicable. Such experiments are called **isolation experiments.** A typical isolation experiment involves isolating a pure compound from a natural source. Examples include isolating caffeine from tea or isolating cinnamaldehyde from cinnamon. Although isolation experiments require somewhat different advance preparation, this advance study may include looking up physical constants for the compound isolated and outlining the isolation procedure. A detailed examination of the separation scheme is very important here because it is the heart of such an experiment.

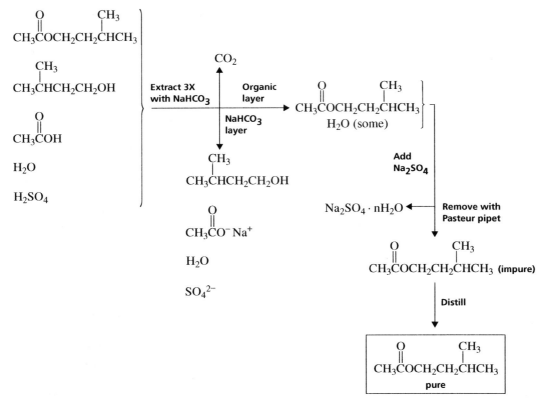

Figure 2.1 Separation scheme for isopentyl acetate.

B. Laboratory Records

When you begin the actual experiment, keep your notebook nearby so you will be able to record those operations you perform. When working in the laboratory, the notebook serves as a place in which to record a rough transcript of your experimental method. Data from actual weighings, volume measurements, and determinations of physical constants are also noted. This section of your notebook should *not* be prepared in advance. The purpose is not to write a recipe but rather to record what you *did* and what you *observed*. These observations will help you write reports without resorting to memory. They will also help you or other workers repeat the experiment in as nearly as possible the same way. The sample notebook pages found in Figures 2.2 and 2.3 illustrate the type of data and observations that should be written in your notebook.

When your product has been prepared and purified, or isolated if it is an isolation experiment, record pertinent data such as the melting point or boiling point of the substance, its density, its index of refraction, and the conditions under which spectra were determined.

C. Calculations

A chemical equation for the overall conversion of the starting materials to products is written on the assumption of simple ideal stoichiometry. Actually, this assumption is sel-

26

dom realized. Side reactions or competing reactions will also occur, giving other products. For some synthetic reactions, an equilibrium state will be reached in which an appreciable amount of starting material is still present and can be recovered. Some of the reactant may also remain if it is present in excess or if the reaction was incomplete. A reaction involving an expensive reagent illustrates another reason for needing to know how far a particular type of reaction converts reactants to products. In such a case, it is preferable to use the most efficient method for this conversion. Thus, information about the efficiency of conversion for various reactions is of interest to the person contemplating the use of these reactions.

The quantitative expression for the efficiency of a reaction is found by calculating the **yield** for the reaction. The **theoretical yield** is the number of grams of the product expected from the reaction on the basis of ideal stoichiometry, with side reactions, reversibility, and losses ignored. To calculate the theoretical yield, it is first necessary to determine the **limiting reagent.** The limiting reagent is the reagent that is not present in excess and on which the overall yield of product depends. The method for determining the limiting reagent in the isopentyl acetate experiment is illustrated in the sample notebook pages shown in Figures 2.2 and 2.3. You should consult your general chemistry textbook for more complicated examples. The theoretical yield is then calculated from the expression

Theoretical yield = (moles of limiting reagent)(ratio)(molecular weight of product)

The ratio here is the stoichiometric ratio of product to limiting reagent. In preparing isopentyl acetate, that ratio is 1:1. One mole of isopentyl alcohol, under ideal circumstances, should yield 1 mole of isopentyl acetate.

The **actual yield** is simply the number of grams of desired product obtained. The **percentage yield** describes the efficiency of the reaction and is determined by

$$\text{Percentage yield} = \frac{\text{Actual yield}}{\text{Theoretical yield}} \times 100$$

Calculation of the theoretical yield and percentage yield can be illustrated using hypothetical data for the isopentyl acetate preparation:

$$\text{Theoretical yield} = (6.94 \times 10^{-2} \text{ mol isopentyl alcohol})\left(\frac{1 \text{ mol isopentyl acetate}}{1 \text{ mol isopentyl alcohol}}\right)$$

$$\times \left(\frac{130.2 \text{ g isopentyl acetate}}{1 \text{ mol isopentyl acetate}}\right) = 9.03 \text{ g isopentyl acetate}$$

$$\text{Actual yield} = 3.81 \text{ g isopentyl acetate}$$

$$\text{Percentage yield} = \frac{3.81 \text{ g}}{9.03 \text{ g}} \times 100 = 42.2\%$$

For experiments that have the principal objective of isolating a substance such as a natural product rather than preparing and purifying some reaction product, the **weight percentage recovery** and not the percentage yield is calculated. This value is determined by

27

THE PREPARATION OF ISOPENTYL ACETATE (BANANA OIL)

Main Reaction

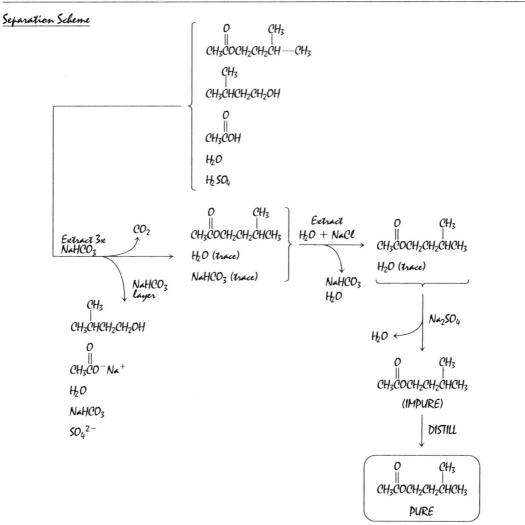

Table of Physical Constants

	MW	BP	Density
Isopentyl alcohol	88.2	132°C	0.813 g/ml
Acetic acid	60.1	118	1.06
Isopentyl acetate	130.2	142	0.876

Separation Scheme

Figure 2.2   A sample notebook, page 1.

Data and Observations

7.5 ml of isopentyl alcohol was added to a pre-weighed 50-ml round-bottomed flask:

Flask + alcohol	139.75 g
Flask	133.63 g
	6.12 g isopentyl alcohol

Glacial acetic acid (10 ml) and 2 ml of concentrated sulfuric acid were also added to the flask, with swirling, along with several boiling stones. A water-cooled condenser was attached to the flask. The reaction was allowed to boil, using a heating mantle, for about one hour. The color of the reaction mixture was brownish-yellow.

After the reaction mixture had cooled to room temperature, the boiling stones were removed, and the reaction mixture was poured into a separatory funnel. About 30 ml of cold water was added to the separatory funnel. The reaction flask was rinsed with 5 ml of cold water, and the water was also added to the separatory funnel. The separatory funnel was shaken, and the lower aqueous layer was removed and discarded. The organic layer was extracted twice with two 10–15-ml portions of 5% aqueous sodium bicarbonate. During the first extraction, much CO_2 was given off, but the amount of gas evolved was markedly diminished during the second extraction. The organic layer was a light yellow in color. After the second extraction, the aqueous layer turned red litmus blue. The bicarbonate layers were discarded, and the organic layer was extracted with a 10–15-ml portion of water. A 2–3 ml portion of saturated sodium chloride solution was added during this extraction. When the aqueous layer had been removed, the upper, organic phase was transferred to a 15-ml Erlenmeyer flask. 2 g of anhydrous magnesium sulfate was added. The flask was stoppered, swirled gently, and allowed to stand for 15 mins.

The product was transferred to a 25-ml round-bottomed flask, and it was distilled by simple distillation. The distillation continued until no liquid could be observed dripping into the collection flask. After the distillation, the ester was transferred to a pre-weighed sample vial.

Sample vial + product	9.92 g
Sample vial	6.11 g
	3.81 g isopentyl acetate

The product was colorless and clear. The observed boiling point obtained during the distillation, was 140°C. An IR spectrum was obtained of the product.

Calculations

Determine limiting reagent:

$$\text{isopentyl alcohol } 6.12 \text{ g} \left(\frac{1 \text{ mol isopentyl alcohol}}{88.2 \text{ g}} \right) = 6.94 \times 10^{-2} \text{ mol}$$

$$\text{acetic acid: } (10 \text{ ml}) \left(\frac{1.06 \text{ g}}{\text{ml}} \right) \left(\frac{1 \text{ mol acetic acid}}{60.1 \text{ g}} \right) = 1.76 \times 10^{-1} \text{ mol}$$

Since they react in a 1:1 ratio, isopentyl alcohol is the limiting reagent. Theoretical yield:

$$(6.94 \times 10^{-2} \text{ mol isopentyl alcohol}) \left(\frac{1 \text{ mol isopentyl acetate}}{1 \text{ mol isopentyl alcohol}} \right) \left(\frac{130.2 \text{ g isopentyl acetate}}{1 \text{ mol isopentyl acetate}} \right)$$

$$= 9.03 \text{ g isopentyl acetate}$$

$$\text{Percentage yield} = \frac{3.81 \text{ g}}{9.03 \text{ g}} \times 100 = 42.2\%$$

Figure 2.3   A sample notebook, page 2.

$$\text{Weight percentage recovery} = \frac{\text{Weight of substance isolated}}{\text{Weight of original material}} \times 100$$

Thus, for instance, if 0.014 g of caffeine was obtained from 2.3 g of tea, the weight percentage recovery of caffeine would be

$$\text{Weight percentage recovery} = \frac{0.014 \text{ g caffeine}}{2.3 \text{ g tea}} \times 100 = 0.61\%$$

2.3 LABORATORY REPORTS

Various formats for reporting the results of the laboratory experiments may be used. You may write the report directly in your notebook in a format similar to the sample notebook pages included in this section. Alternatively, your instructor may require a more formal report that is not written in your notebook. When you do original research, these reports should include a detailed description of all the experimental steps undertaken. Frequently, the style used in scientific periodicals such as *Journal of the American Chemical Society* is applied to writing laboratory reports. Your instructor is likely to have his or her own requirements for laboratory reports and should describe the requirements to you.

2.4 SUBMISSION OF SAMPLES

In all preparative experiments and in some isolation experiments, you will be required to submit to your instructor the sample of the substance you prepared or isolated. How this sample is labeled is very important. Again, learning a correct method of labeling bottles and vials can save time in the laboratory, because fewer mistakes will be made. More important, learning to label properly can decrease the danger inherent in having samples of material that cannot be identified correctly at a later date.

Solid materials should be stored and submitted in containers that permit the substance to be removed easily. For this reason, narrow-mouthed bottles or vials are not used for solid substances. Liquids should be stored in containers that will not let them escape through leakage. Be careful not to store volatile liquids in containers that have plastic caps, unless the cap is lined with an inert material such as Teflon. Otherwise, the vapors from the liquid are likely to contact the plastic and dissolve some of it, thus contaminating the substance being stored.

On the label, print the name of the substance, its melting or boiling point, the actual and percentage yields, and your name. An illustration of a properly prepared label follows:

Isopentyl Acetate
BP 140°C
Yield 3.81 g (42.2%)
Joe Schmedlock

T E C H N I Q U E   3

Laboratory Glassware: Care and Cleaning

Because your glassware is expensive and you are responsible for it, you will want to give it proper care and respect. If you read this section carefully and follow the procedures presented here, you may be able to avoid some unnecessary expense. You may also save time, because cleaning problems and replacing broken glassware are time consuming.

If you are unfamiliar with the equipment found in an organic chemistry laboratory or are uncertain about how such equipment should be treated, this section provides some useful information, such as cleaning glassware and caring for glassware when using corrosive or caustic reagents. At the end of this section are illustrations that show and name most of the equipment you are likely to find in your drawer or locker.

3.1 CLEANING GLASSWARE

Glassware can be cleaned easily if you clean it immediately after use. It is good practice to do your "dish washing" right away. With time, organic tarry materials left in a container begin to attack the surface of the glass. The longer you wait to clean glassware, the more extensively this interaction will have progressed. If you wait, cleaning is more difficult, because water will no longer wet the surface of the glass as effectively. If you cannot wash your glassware immediately after use, soak the dirty pieces of glassware in soapy water. A half-gallon plastic container is convenient for soaking and washing glassware. Using a plastic container also helps prevent the loss of small pieces of equipment.

Various soaps and detergents are available for washing glassware. They should be tried first when washing dirty glassware. Organic solvents can also be used, because the residue remaining in dirty glassware is likely to be soluble. After the solvent has been used, the glass item probably will have to be washed with soap and water to remove the residual solvent. When you use solvents to clean glassware, use caution, because the solvents are hazardous (see Technique 1). Use fairly small amounts of a solvent for cleaning purposes. Usually less than 5 mL (or 1–2 mL for microscale glassware) will be sufficient. Acetone is commonly used, but it is expensive. Your **wash acetone** can be used effectively several times before it is "spent." Once your acetone is spent, dispose of it as your instructor directs. If acetone does not work, other organic solvents such as methylene chloride or toluene can be used.

Caution: Acetone is very flammable. Do not use it around flames.

For troublesome stains and residues that adhere to the glass despite your best efforts, use a mixture of sulfuric acid and nitric acid. Cautiously add about 20 drops of concentrated sulfuric acid and 5 drops of concentrated nitric acid to the flask or vial.

Caution: You must wear safety glasses when you are using a cleaning solution made from sulfuric acid and nitric acid. Do not allow the solution to come into contact with your skin or clothing. It will cause severe burns on your skin and create holes in your clothing. The acids may also react with the residue in the container.

Swirl the acid mixture in the container for a few minutes. If necessary, place the glassware in a warm water bath and heat it cautiously to accelerate the cleaning process. Continue heating the glassware until any sign of a reaction ceases. When the cleaning procedure is completed, decant the mixture into an appropriate waste container.

Caution: Do not pour the acid solution into a waste container that is intended for organic wastes.

Rinse the piece of glassware thoroughly with water and then wash it with soap and water. For most common organic chemistry applications, any stains that survive this treatment are not likely to cause difficulty in subsequent laboratory procedures.

If the glassware is contaminated with stopcock grease, rinse the glassware with a small amount (1–2 mL) of methylene chloride. Discard the rinse solution into an appropriate waste container. Once the grease is removed, wash the glassware with soap or detergent and water.

3.2 DRYING GLASSWARE

The easiest way to dry glassware is to let it stand overnight. Store vials, flasks, and beakers upside down on a piece of paper towel to permit the water to drain from them. Drying ovens can be used to dry glassware if they are available and if they are not being used for other purposes. Rapid drying can be achieved by rinsing the glassware with acetone and air drying it or placing it in an oven. First, thoroughly drain the glassware of water. Then rinse it with one or two *small* portions (1–2 mL) of acetone. Do not use any more acetone than is suggested here. Return the used acetone to an acetone waste container for recycling. After you rinse the glassware with acetone, dry it by placing it in a drying oven for a few minutes or allow it to air dry at room temperature. The acetone can also be removed by aspirator suction. In some laboratories, it may be possible to dry the glassware by blowing a *gentle* stream of dry air into the container. (Your laboratory instructor will indicate if you should do this.) Before drying the glassware with air, make sure that the air line is not filled with oil. Otherwise, the oil will be blown into the container, and you will have to clean it again. It is not necessary to blast the acetone out of the glassware with a wide-open stream of air; a gentle stream of air is just as effective and will not startle other people in the room.

Do not dry your glassware with a paper towel unless the towel is lint free. Most paper will leave lint on the glass that can interfere with subsequent procedures. Sometimes it is not necessary to dry a piece of equipment thoroughly. For example, if you are going to place water or an aqueous solution in a container, it does not need to be completely dry.

3.3 GROUND-GLASS JOINTS

It is likely that the glassware in your organic kit has **standard-taper ground-glass joints.** For example, the Claisen head in Figure 3.1 consists of an inner (male) ground-glass joint at the bottom and two outer (female) joints at the top. Each end is ground to a precise size, which is designated by the symbol ⊺ followed by two numbers. A common joint size in many macroscale organic glassware kits is ⊺ 19/22. The first number indicates the diameter (in millimeters) of the joint at its widest point, and the second number refers to its length (see Figure 3.1). One advantage of standard-taper joints is that the pieces fit together snugly and form a good seal. In addition, standard-taper joints allow all glassware components with the same joint size to be connected, thus permitting the assembly of a wide variety of apparatuses. One disadvantage of glassware with ground-glass joints, however, is that it is expensive.

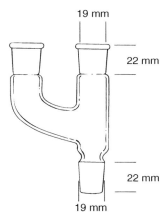

Figure 3.1 Illustration of inner and outer joints, showing dimensions. A Claisen head with ⊺ 19/22 joints.

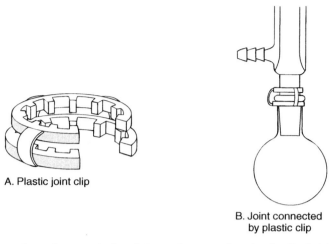

A. Plastic joint clip

B. Joint connected
by plastic clip

Figure 3.2 Connection of ground-glass joints. The use of a plastic clip (A) is also shown (B).

3.4 CONNECTING GROUND-GLASS JOINTS

It is a simple matter to connect pieces of macroscale glassware using standard-taper ground-glass joints. Figure 3.2B illustrates the connection of a condenser to a round-bottom flask. At times, however, it may be difficult to secure the connection so that it does not come apart unexpectedly. Figure 3.2A shows a plastic clip that serves to secure the connection. Methods to secure ground-glass connections with macroscale apparatus, including the use of plastic clips, are covered in Technique 7.

It is important to make sure no solid or liquid is on the joint surfaces. Either of these will decrease the efficiency of the seal, and the joints may leak. With microscale glassware, the presence of solid particles could cause the ground-glass joints to break when the plastic cap is tightened. Also, if the apparatus is to be heated, material caught between the joint surfaces will increase the tendency for the joints to stick. If the joint surfaces are coated with liquid or adhering solid, you should wipe the surfaces with a cloth or a lint-free paper towel before assembling.

3.5 CAPPING FLASKS, CONICAL VIALS, AND OPENINGS

The sidearms in two-necked or three-necked round-bottom flasks can be capped using the Ⅎ19/22 ground-glass stoppers that are part of a normal macroscale organic kit. Figure 3.3 shows such a stopper being used to cap the sidearm of a three-necked flask.

3.6 SEPARATING GROUND-GLASS JOINTS

When ground-glass joints become "frozen" or stuck together, you are faced with the often vexing problem of separating them. The techniques for separating ground-glass

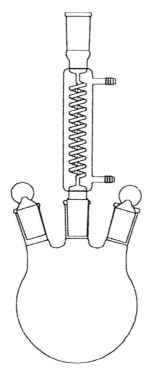

Figure 3.3 Capping a sidearm with a ⊤ 19/22 stopper.

joints, or for removing stoppers that are stuck in the openings of flasks and vials, are the same for both macroscale and microscale glassware.

The most important thing you can do to prevent ground-glass joints from becoming frozen is to disassemble the glassware as soon as possible after a procedure is completed. Even when this precaution is followed, ground-glass joints may become stuck tightly together. The same is true of glass stoppers in bottles or conical vials. Because certain items of microscale glassware may be small and very fragile, it is relatively easy to break a piece of glassware when trying to pull two pieces apart. If the pieces do not separate easily, you must be careful when you try to pull them apart. The best way is to hold the two pieces, with both hands touching, as close as possible to the joint. With a firm grasp, try to loosen the joint with a slight twisting motion (do not twist very hard). If this does not work, try to pull your hands apart without pushing sideways on the glassware.

If it is not possible to pull the pieces apart, the following methods may help. A frozen joint can sometimes be loosened if you tap it *gently* with the wooden handle of a spatula. Then try to pull it apart as already described. If this procedure fails, you may try heating the joint in hot water or a steam bath. If heating fails, the instructor may be able to advise you. As a last resort, you may try heating the joint in a flame. You should not try this unless the apparatus is hopelessly stuck, because heating by flame often causes the joint to expand rapidly and crack or break. If you use a flame, make sure the joint is clean and dry. Heat the outer part of the joint slowly, in the yellow portion of a low flame, until it expands and separates from the inner section. Heat the joint very slowly and carefully, or it may break.

3.7 ETCHING GLASSWARE

Glassware that has been used for reactions involving strong bases such as sodium hydroxide or sodium alkoxides must be cleaned thoroughly *immediately* after use. If these caustic materials are allowed to remain in contact with the glass, they will etch the glass permanently. The etching makes later cleaning more difficult, because dirt particles may become trapped within the microscopic surface irregularities of the etched glass. Furthermore, the glass is weakened, so the lifetime of the glassware is shortened. If caustic materials are allowed to come into contact with ground-glass joints without being removed promptly, the joints will become fused or "frozen." It is extremely difficult to separate fused joints without breaking them.

3.8 ATTACHING RUBBER TUBING TO EQUIPMENT

When you attach rubber tubing to the glass apparatus or when you insert glass tubing into rubber stoppers, first lubricate the rubber tubing or the rubber stopper with either water or glycerin. Without such lubrication, it can be difficult to attach rubber tubing to the sidearms of items of glassware such as condensers and filter flasks. Furthermore, glass tubing may break when it is inserted into rubber stoppers. Water is a good lubricant for most purposes. Do not use water as a lubricant when it might contaminate the reaction. Glycerin is a better lubricant than water and should be used when there is considerable friction between the glass and rubber. If glycerin is the lubricant, be careful not to use too much.

3.9 DESCRIPTION OF EQUIPMENT

Figures 3.4 and 3.5 include examples of glassware and equipment that are commonly used in the organic laboratory. Your glassware and equipment may vary slightly from the pieces shown on pages 589–591.

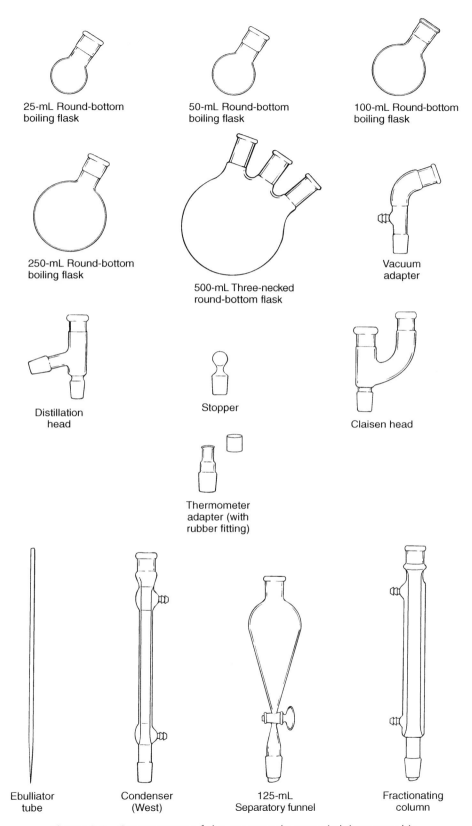

25-mL Round-bottom boiling flask

50-mL Round-bottom boiling flask

100-mL Round-bottom boiling flask

250-mL Round-bottom boiling flask

500-mL Three-necked round-bottom flask

Vacuum adapter

Distillation head

Stopper

Claisen head

Thermometer adapter (with rubber fitting)

Ebulliator tube

Condenser (West)

125-mL Separatory funnel

Fractionating column

Figure 3.4 Components of the macroscale organic laboratory kit.

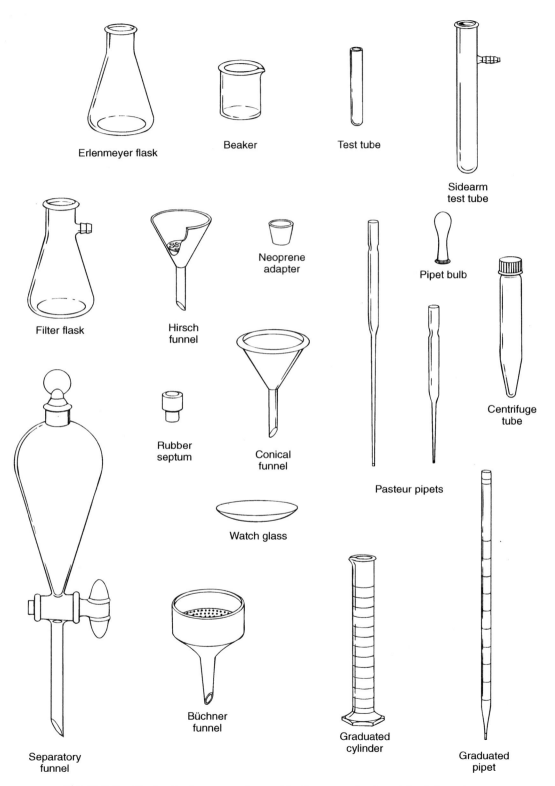

Figure 3.5 Equipment commonly used in the organic chemistry laboratory.

Erlenmeyer flask

Beaker

Test tube

Sidearm test tube

Filter flask

Hirsch funnel

Neoprene adapter

Pipet bulb

Centrifuge tube

Rubber septum

Conical funnel

Pasteur pipets

Watch glass

Separatory funnel

Büchner funnel

Graduated cylinder

Graduated pipet

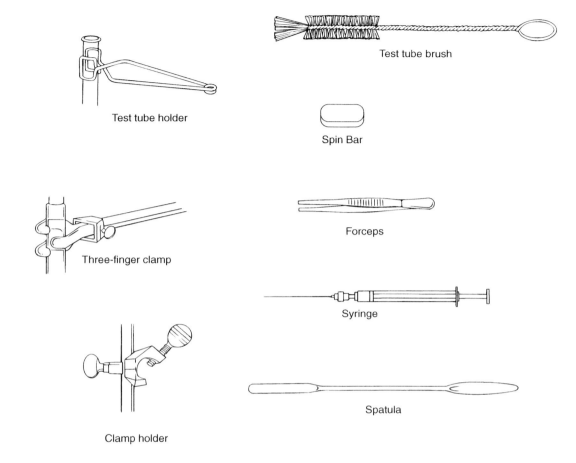

Test tube holder

Test tube brush

Spin Bar

Three-finger clamp

Forceps

Syringe

Clamp holder

Spatula

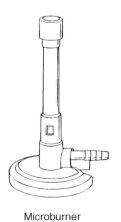

Microburner

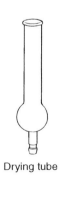

Drying tube

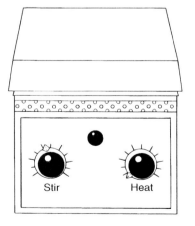

Hot plate / Stirrer

TECHNIQUE 4

How to Find Data for Compounds: Handbooks and Catalogs

The best way to find information quickly on organic compounds is to consult a handbook. We will discuss the use of the *CRC Handbook of Chemistry and Physics, Lange's Handbook of Chemistry, The Merck Index,* and the *Aldrich Handbook of Fine Chemicals.* Complete citations to these handbooks are provided in Technique 29. Depending on the type of handbook consulted, the following information may be found:

Name and common synonyms

Formula

Molecular weight

Boiling point for a liquid or melting point for a solid

Beilstein reference

Solubility data

Density

Refractive index

Flash point

Chemical Abstracts Service (CAS) Registry Number

Toxicity data

Uses and synthesis

4.1 CRC HANDBOOK OF CHEMISTRY AND PHYSICS

This is the handbook that is most often consulted for data on organic compounds. Although a new edition of the handbook is published each year, the changes that are made are often minor. An older copy of the handbook will often suffice for most purposes. In addition to the extensive tables of properties of organic compounds, the *CRC Handbook* includes sections on nomenclature and ring structures, an index of synonyms, and an index of molecular formulas.

The nomenclature used in this book most closely follows the Chemical Abstracts system of naming organic compounds. This system differs, but only slightly, from standard IUPAC nomenclature. Table 4.1 lists some examples of how some commonly encountered compounds are named in this handbook. The first thing you will notice is that this handbook is not like a dictionary. Instead, you must first identify the *parent* name of the compound of interest. The parent names are found in alphabetical order. Once the parent name is identified and found, then you look for the particular substituent or substituents that may be attached to this parent.

For most compounds, it is easy to find what you are looking for as long as you know the parent name. Alcohols are, as expected, named by IUPAC nomenclature. Notice in Table 4.1 that the branched-chain alcohol, isopentyl alcohol, is listed as 1-butanol, 3-methyl.

TABLE 4.1 Examples of Names of Compounds in the *CRC Handbook*

Name of Organic Compound	Location in *CRC Handbook*
1-Chloropentane	Pentane, 1-chloro-
1,4-Dichlorobenzene	Benzene, 1,4-dichloro-
4-Chlorotoluene	Benzene, 1-chloro-4-methyl-
Ethanoic acid	Acetic acid
tert-Butyl acetate (ethanoate)	Acetic acid, 1,1-dimethylethyl ester
Ethyl propanoate	Propanoic acid, ethyl ester
Isopentyl alcohol	1-Butanol, 3-methyl-
Isopentyl acetate (banana oil)	1-Butanol, 3-methyl-, acetate
Salicylic acid	Benzoic acid, 2-hydroxy-
Acetylsalicylic acid (aspirin)	Benzoic acid, 2-acetyloxy-

Esters, amides, and acid halides are usually named as derivatives of the parent carboxylic acid. Thus, in Table 4.1, you find ethyl propanoate listed under the parent carboxylic acid, propanoic acid. If you have trouble finding a particular ester under the parent carboxylic acid, try looking under the alcohol part of the name. For example, isopentyl acetate is not listed under acetic acid, as expected, but instead is found under the alcohol part of the name (see Table 4.1). Fortunately, this handbook has a Synonym Index that nicely locates isopentyl acetate for you in the main part of the handbook.

Once you locate the compound by its name, you will find the following useful information:

CRC number	This is an identification number for the compound. You can use this number to find the molecular structure located elsewhere in the handbook. This is especially useful when the compound has a complicated structure.
Name and synonym	The Chemical Abstracts name and possible synonyms.
Mol. form.	Molecular formula for the compound.
Mol. wt.	Molecular weight.
CAS RN	Chemical Abstracts Service Registry Number. This number is very useful for locating additional information on the compound in the primary chemical literature (see Technique 29, Section 29.11).
mp/°C	Melting point of the compound in degrees Celsius.
bp/°C	Boiling point of the compound in degrees Celsius. A number without a superscript indicates that the recorded boiling point was obtained at 760 mm Hg pressure (atmospheric pressure). A number with a superscript indicates that the boiling point was obtained at reduced pressure. For example, an entry of 234; 122^{16} would indicate that the compound boils at 234°C at 760 mm Hg and 122°C at 16 mm Hg pressure.
Den/g cm^{-3}	Density of a liquid. A superscript indicates the temperature in degrees Celsius at which the density was obtained.

n_D	Refractive index determined at a wavelength of 589 nm, the yellow line in a sodium lamp (D line). A superscript indicates the temperature at which the refractive index was obtained (see Technique 24).
Solubility	

Solubility classification	Solvent abbreviations
1 = insoluble	ace = acetone
2 = slightly soluble	bz = benzene
3 = soluble	chl = chloroform
4 = very soluble	EtOH = ethanol
5 = miscible	eth = ether
6 = decomposes	hx = hexane

Beil. ref.	Beilstein reference. An entry of 4-02-00-00157 would indicate that the compound is found in the 4th supplement in Volume 2, with no subvolume, on page 157 (see Technique 29, Section 29.10 for details on the use of Beilstein).
Merck No.	*Merck Index* number in the 11th edition of the handbook. These numbers change each time a new edition of *The Merck Index* is issued.

Examples of sample handbook entries for isopentyl alcohol (1-butanol, 3-methyl) and isopentyl acetate (1-butanol, 3-methyl, acetate) are shown in Table 4.2.

4.2 LANGE'S HANDBOOK OF CHEMISTRY

This handbook tends not to be as available as the *CRC Handbook,* but it has some interesting differences and advantages. *Lange's Handbook* has synonyms listed at the bottom of each page, along with structures of more complicated molecules. The most noticeable difference is in how compounds are named. For many compounds, the system lists names as they would appear in a dictionary. Table 4.3 lists examples of how some commonly encountered compounds are named in this handbook. Most often, you do not need to identify the *parent* name. Unfortunately, *Lange's Handbook* frequently uses common names that

TABLE 4.2 Properties of Isopentyl Alcohol and Isopentyl Acetate as Listed in the *CRC Handbook*

No.	Name Synonym	Mol. Form. Mol. Wt.	CAS RN mp/°C	Merck No. bp/°C	Beil. Ref. den/g cm^{-3}	Solubility n_D
3627	1-Butanol, 3-methyl	$C_5H_{12}O$	123-51-3	5081	4-01-00-01677	ace 4; eth 4; EtOH 4
	Isopentyl alcohol	88.15	−117.2	131.1	0.8104[20]	1.4053[20]
3631	1-Butanol, 3-methyl, acetate	$C_7H_{14}O_2$	123-92-2	4993	4-02-00-00157	H_2O 2; EtOH 5; eth 5; ace 3
	Isopentyl acetate	130.19	−78.5	142.5	0.876[15]	1.4000[20]

TABLE 4.3   Examples of Names of Compounds in *Lange's Handbook*

Name of Organic Compound	Location in *Lange's Handbook*
1-Chloropentane	1-Chloropentane
1,4-Dichlorobenzene	1,4-Dichlorobenzene
4-Chlorotoluene	4-Chlorotoluene
Ethanoic acid	Acetic acid
tert-Butyl acetate (ethanoate)	*tert*-Butyl acetate
Ethyl propanoate	Ethyl propionate
Isopentyl alcohol	3-Methyl-1-butanol
Isopentyl acetate (banana oil)	Isopentyl acetate
Salicylic acid	2-Hydroxybenzoic acid
Acetylsalicylic acid (aspirin)	Acetylsalicylic acid

are becoming obsolete. For example, propionate is used rather than propanoate. Nevertheless, this handbook often names compounds as a practicing organic chemist would tend to name them. Notice how easy it is to find the entries for isopentyl acetate and acetylsalicylic acid (aspirin) in this handbook.

Once you locate the compound by its name, you will find the following useful information:

Lange's number	This is an identification number for the compound.
Name	See examples in Table 4.3.
Formula	Structures are drawn out. If they are complicated, then the structures are shown at the bottom of the page.
Formula weight	Molecular weight of the compound.
Beilstein reference	An entry of 2, 132 would indicate that the compound is found in Volume 2 of the main work on page 132. An entry of 3^2, 188 would indicate that the compound is found in Volume 3 of the second supplement on page 188 (see Technique 29, Section 29.10 for details on the use of *Beilstein*).
Density	Density is usually expressed in units of g/mL or g/cm^3. A superscript indicates the temperature at which the density was measured. If the density is also subscripted, usually 4°, it indicates that the density was measured at a certain temperature relative to water at its maximum density, 4°C. Most of the time you can simply ignore the subscripts and superscripts.
Refractive index	A superscript indicates the temperature at which the refractive index was determined (see Technique 24).
Melting point	Melting point of the compound in degrees Celsius. When a "d" or "dec" appears with the melting point, it indicates that the compound decomposes at the melting point. When decomposition occurs, you will often observe a change in color of the solid.
Boiling point	Boiling point of the compound in degrees Celsius. A number

without a superscript indicates that the recorded boiling point was obtained at 760 mmHg pressure (atmospheric pressure). A number with a superscript indicates that the boiling point was obtained at reduced pressure. For example, an entry of $102^{11\ mm}$ would indicate that the compound boils at 102°C at 11 mmHg pressure.

Flash point | This number is the temperature in degrees Celsius at which the compound will ignite when heated in air and a spark is introduced into the vapor. There are a number of different methods that are used to measure this value, so this number varies considerably. It gives a crude indication of flammability. You may need this information when heating a substance with a hot plate. Hot plates can be a serious source of trouble because of the sparking action that can occur with switches and thermostats used in hot plates.

Solubility in 100 parts solvent | Parts by weight of a compound that can be dissolved in 100 parts by weight of solvent at room temperature. In some cases, the values given are expressed as the weight in grams that can be dissolved in 100 mL of solvent. This handbook is not consistent in describing solubility. Sometimes gram amounts are provided, but in other cases the description will be more vague, using terms such as *soluble, insoluble,* or *slightly soluble.*

Solvent abbreviations	Solubility characteristics
acet = acetone	i = insoluble
bz = benzene	s = soluble
chl = chloroform	sls = slightly soluble
aq = water	vs = very soluble
alc = ethanol	misc = miscible
eth = ether
HOAc = acetic acid

Examples of sample handbook entries for isopentyl alcohol (3-methyl-1-butanol) and isopentyl acetate are shown in Table 4.4.

4.3 THE MERCK INDEX

The Merck Index is a very useful book because it has additional information not found in the other two handbooks. This handbook, however, tends to emphasize medicinally related compounds, such as drugs and biological compounds, although it also lists many other common organic compounds. It is not revised each year; new editions are published in five- or six-year cycles. It does not contain all of the compounds listed in *Lange's Handbook* or the *CRC Handbook.* However, for the compounds listed, it provides a wealth of useful information. The handbook will provide you with some or all of the following data for each entry.

Merck number, which changes each time a new edition is issued

Name, including synonyms and stereochemical designation

44

Molecular formula and structure

Molecular weight

Percentages of each of the elements in the compound

Uses

Source and synthesis, including references to the primary literature

Optical rotation for chiral molecules

Density, boiling point, and melting point

Solubility characteristics, including crystalline form

Pharmacology information

Toxicity data

One of the problems with looking up a compound in this handbook is trying to decide the name under which the compound will be listed. For example, isopentyl alcohol can also be named as 3-methyl-1-butanol or isoamyl alcohol. In the 12th edition of the handbook, it is listed under the name isopentyl alcohol (#5212) on page 886. Finding isopentyl acetate is even a more challenging task. It is located in the handbook under the name isoamyl acetate (#5125) on page 876. Often, it is easier to look up the name in the name index or to find it in the formula index.

The handbook has some useful appendices that include the CAS registry numbers, a biological activity index, a formula index, and a name index that also includes synonyms. When looking up a compound in one of the indexes, you need to remember that the numbers provided are compound numbers, rather than page numbers. There is also a very useful section on organic name reactions that includes references to the primary literature.

4.4 ALDRICH HANDBOOK OF FINE CHEMICALS

The *Aldrich Handbook* is actually a catalog of chemicals sold by the Aldrich Chemical Company. The company includes in its catalog a large body of useful data on each compound that it sells. Because the catalog is reissued each year at no cost to the user, you should be able to find an old copy when the new one is issued. As you are mainly interested in the data on a particular compound and not the price, an old volume is perfectly fine. Isopentyl alcohol is listed as 3-methyl-1-butanol, and isopentyl acetate is listed as isoamyl acetate in the *Aldrich Handbook*. The following includes some of the properties and information listed for individual compounds.

Aldrich catalog number

Name: Aldrich uses a mixture of common and IUPAC names. It takes a bit of time to master the names. Fortunately, the catalog does a good job of cross-referencing compounds and has a very good molecular formula index.

CAS Registry Number

Structure

Synonym

Formula weight

Boiling point/melting point

TABLE 4.4 Properties of 3-Methyl-1-Butanol and Isopentyl Acetate as Listed in *Lange's Handbook*

No.	Name	Formula	Formula Weight	Beilstein Reference	Density	Refractive Index	Melting Point	Boiling Point	Flash Point	Solubility in 100 Parts Solvent
m155	3-methyl-1-butanol	$(CH_3)_2CHCH_2CH_2OH$	88.15	1, 392	0.8129^{15}_{4}	1.4085^{15}	-117.2	132.0	45	2 aq; misc alc, bz, chl, eth, HOAc
i80	Isopentyl acetate	$CH_3COOCH_2CH_2CH(CH_3)_2$	130.19	2, 132	0.876^{15}_{4}	1.4007^{20}	-78.5	142.0	80	0.25 aq; misc alc, eth

Index of refraction

Density

Beilstein reference

Merck reference

Infrared spectrum reference to the Aldrich Library of FT-IR spectra

NMR spectrum reference to the Aldrich Library of ^{13}C and ^1H FT-NMR spectra

Literature references to the primary literature on the uses of the compound

Toxicity

Safety data and precautions

Flash point

Prices of chemicals

4.5 STRATEGY FOR FINDING INFORMATION: SUMMARY

Most students and professors find *The Merck Index* and *Lange's Handbook* easier and more "intuitive" to use than the *CRC Handbook*. You can go directly to a compound without rearranging the name according to the parent or base name followed by its substituents. Another great source of information is the *Aldrich Handbook*, which contains those compounds that are easily available from a commercial source. Many compounds are found in the *Aldrich Handbook* that you may never find in any of the other handbooks. The Sigma–Aldrich Web site (*http://www.sigmaaldrich.com/*) allows you to search by name, synonym, and catalog number.

PROBLEMS

1. Using *The Merck Index,* find and draw structures for the following compounds:
    a. atropine
    b. quinine
    c. saccharin
    d. benzo[*a*]pyrene (benzpyrene)
    e. itaconic acid
    f. adrenosterone
    g. chrysanthemic acid (chrysanthemumic acid)
    h. cholesterol
    i. vitamin C (ascorbic acid)
2. Find the melting points for the following compounds in the *CRC Handbook, Lange's Handbook,* or the *Aldrich Handbook:*
    a. biphenyl
    b. 4-bromobenzoic acid
    c. 3-nitrophenol
3. Find the boiling point for each compound in the references listed in problem 2:
    a. octanoic acid at reduced pressure
    b. 4-chloroacetophenone at atmosphere and reduced pressure
    c. 2-methyl-2-heptanol
4. Find the index of refraction n_D and density for the liquids listed in problem 3.

5. Using the *Aldrich Handbook,* report the specific rotations for the enantiomers of camphor.

6. Read the section on carbon tetrachloride in *The Merck Index* and list some of the health hazards for this compound.

TECHNIQUE 5

Measurement of Volume and Weight

Performing successful organic chemistry experiments requires the ability to measure solids and liquids accurately. This ability involves both selecting the proper measuring device and using this device correctly.

Liquids to be used for an experiment will usually be found in small containers in a hood. For *macroscale* experiments, a graduated cylinder, a dispensing pump, or a graduated pipet will be used for measuring the volume of a liquid. For **limiting reactants,** it is best to preweigh the container before adding the liquid to the container and then reweigh after adding the liquid. This gives an exact weight and avoids the experimental error involved in using densities to calculate weights when working with smaller amounts of a liquid. For **nonlimiting** liquid reactants, you may calculate the weight of the liquid from the volume you have delivered and the density of the liquid:

$$\text{Weight (g)} = \text{density (g/mL)} \times \text{volume (mL)}$$

For *microscale* experiments, an automatic pipet, dispensing pump, or calibrated Pasteur pipet will be used for measuring the volume of a liquid. It is even more critical that limiting reactants be weighed as described in the preceding paragraph. Measurement of a small volume of a liquid is subject to a large experimental error when converted to a weight using a density of the liquid. Weights of nonlimiting liquid reactants, however, can be calculated using the previous expression.

You will usually transfer the required volume of liquid to a round-bottom flask or an Erlenmeyer flask in macroscale experiments, or to a conical vial or round-bottom flask in microscale experiments. When transferring the liquid to a round-bottom flask, place the flask in a beaker and tare both the flask and the beaker. The beaker keeps the round-bottom flask in a upright position and prevents spills from occurring. The same advice should be followed if a conical vial is being used.

When using a graduated cylinder to measure small volumes of a limiting reagent, it is important to preweigh the cylinder and transfer the required amount of liquid reagent to it using a Pasteur pipet. Reweigh the cylinder to obtain the exact weight of liquid reagent. To *quantitatively* transfer the liquid from the graduated cylinder, pour as much of the liquid as possible into the reaction container. The remaining liquid in the graduated cylinder can be removed by rinsing the cylinder with small amounts of the solvent being used for the reaction. By this procedure, all of the limiting reagent will be transferred from the graduated cylinder to the reaction container.

Using a small amount of solvent to transfer a liquid quantitatively can also be applied in other situations. For example, if your product is dissolved in a solvent and the procedure instructs you to transfer the reaction mixture from a round-bottom flask to a separatory funnel, after pouring most of the liquid into the funnel, a small amount of solvent could be used to transfer the rest of the product quantitatively.

Solids are usually found near the balance. For *macroscale* experiments, it is usually sufficient to weigh solids on a balance that reads at least to the nearest decigram (0.01 g). For *microscale* experiments, solids must be weighed on a balance that reads to the nearest milligram (0.001 g) or tenth of a milligram (0.0001 g). To weigh a solid, place your conical vial or round-bottom flask in a small beaker and take these with you to the balance. Place a smooth piece of paper that has been folded once on the balance pan. The folded paper will enable you to pour the solid into the conical vial or flask without spilling. Use a spatula to aid the transfer of the solid to the paper. Never weigh directly into a conical vial or flask, and never pour, dump, or shake a material from a bottle. While still at the balance, carefully transfer the solid from the paper to your vial or flask. The vial or flask should be in a beaker while you transfer the solid. The beaker traps any material that fails to make it into the container. It also supports the vial or flask so that it does not fall over. It is not necessary to obtain the exact amount specified in the experimental procedure, and trying to be exact requires too much time at the balance. For example, if you obtained 0.140 g of a solid, rather than the 0.136 g specified in a procedure, you could use it, but the actual amount weighed should be recorded in your notebook. Use the actual amount you weighed to calculate the theoretical yield, if this solid is the limiting agent.

Careless dispensing of liquids and solids is a hazard in any laboratory. When reagents are spilled, you may be subjected to an unnecessary health or fire hazard. In addition, you may waste expensive chemicals, destroy balance pans and clothing, and damage the environment. Always clean up any spills immediately.

5.1 GRADUATED CYLINDERS

Graduated cylinders are most often used to measure liquids for macroscale experiments (see Figure 5.1). The most common sizes are 10 mL, 25 mL, 50 mL, and 100 mL, but it is possible that not all of these will be available in your laboratory. Volumes from about 2 mL to 100 mL can be measured with reasonably good accuracy provided that the correct cylinder is used. You should use the *smallest* cylinder available that can hold all of the liquid that is being measured. For example, if a procedure calls for 4.5 mL of a reagent, use a 10-mL graduated cylinder. Using a large cylinder in this case will result in a less accurate measurement. Furthermore, using any cylinder to measure less than 10% of the total capacity of that cylinder will likely result in an inaccurate measurement. Always remember that whenever a graduated cylinder is used to measure the volume of a limiting reagent, you must weigh the liquid to determine the amount used accurately. You should use a grad-

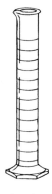

Figure 5.1 Graduated cylinder.

uated pipet, a dispensing pump, or an automatic pipet for accurate transfer of liquids with a volume of less than 2 mL.

If the storage container is reasonably small (< 1.0 L) and has a narrow neck, you may pour most of the liquid into the graduated cylinder and use a Pasteur pipet to adjust to the final line. If the storage container is large (> 1.0 L) or has a wide mouth, two strategies are possible. First, you may use a pipet to transfer the liquid to the graduated cylinder. Alternatively, you may pour some of the liquid into a beaker first and then pour this liquid into a graduated cylinder. Use a Pasteur pipet to adjust to the final line. Remember that you should not take more than you need. Excess material should never be returned to the storage bottle. Unless you can convince someone else to take it, it must be poured into the appropriate waste container. You should be frugal in your estimation of amounts needed.

Note: Never return used reagents to the stock bottle.

5.2 DISPENSING PUMPS

Dispensing pumps are simple to operate, chemically inert, and quite accurate. Because the plunger assembly is made of Teflon, the dispensing pump may be used with most corrosive liquids and organic solvents. Dispensing pumps come in a variety of sizes, ranging from 1 mL to 300 mL. When used correctly, dispensing pumps can be used to deliver accurate volumes ranging from 0.1 mL to the maximum capacity of the pump. The pump is attached to a bottle containing the liquid being dispensed. The liquid is drawn up from this reservoir into the pump assembly through a piece of inert plastic tubing.

Dispensing pumps are somewhat difficult to adjust to the proper volume. Normally, the instructor or assistant will carefully adjust the unit to deliver the proper amount of liquid. As shown in Figure 5.2, the plunger is pulled up as far as it will travel to draw in the liquid from the glass reservoir. To expel the liquid from the spout into a container, you slowly guide the plunger down. With low-viscosity liquids, the weight of the plunger will expel the liquid. With more viscous liquids, however, you may need to push the plunger gently to deliver the liquid into a container. Remove the last drop of liquid on the end of the spout by touching the tip on the interior wall of the container. When the liquid being transferred is a limiting reagent or when you need to know the weight precisely, you should weigh the liquid to determine the amount accurately.

As you pull up the plunger, look to see if the liquid is being drawn up into the pump unit. Some volatile liquids may not be drawn up in the expected manner, and you will observe an air bubble. Air bubbles commonly occur when the pump has not been used for a while. The air bubble can be removed from the pump by dispensing, and discarding, several volumes of liquid to "reprime" the dispensing pump. Also check to see if the spout is filled completely with liquid. An accurate volume will not be dispensed unless the spout is filled with liquid before you lift up the plunger.

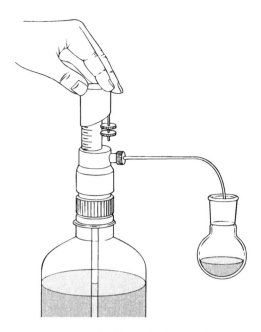

Figure 5.2   Use of a dispensing pump.

5.3 GRADUATED PIPETS

A widely used measuring device is the graduated serological pipet. These *glass* pipets are available commercially in a number of sizes. "Disposable" graduated pipets may be used many times and discarded only when the graduations become too faint to be seen. A good assortment of these pipets consists of the following:

1.00-mL pipets calibrated in 0.01-mL divisions (1 in 1/100 mL)

2.00-mL pipets calibrated in 0.01-mL divisions (2 in 1/100 mL)

5.0-mL pipets calibrated in 0.1-mL divisions (5 in 1/10 mL)

Never draw liquids into the pipets using mouth suction. A pipet pump or a pipet bulb, not a rubber dropper bulb, must be used to fill pipets. Two types of pipet pumps and a pipet bulb are shown in Figure 5.3. A pipet fits snugly into the pipet pump, and the pump can be controlled to deliver precise volumes of liquids. Control of the pipet pump is accomplished by rotating a knob on the pump. Suction created when the knob is turned draws the liquid into the pipet. Liquid is expelled from the pipet by turning the knob in the opposite direction. The pump works satisfactorily with organic, as well as aqueous, liquids.

The style of pipet pump shown in Figure 5.3A is available in four sizes. The top of the pipet must be inserted securely into the pump and held there with one hand to obtain an adequate seal. The other hand is used to load and release the liquid. The pipet pump shown in Figure 5.3B may also be used with graduated pipets. With this style of pipet, the top of the pipet is held securely by a rubber O-ring, and it is easily handled with one hand. You should be certain that the pipet is held securely by the O-ring before using it. Disposable pipets may not fit tightly in the O-ring because they often have smaller diameters than nondisposable pipets.

An alternative, and less expensive, approach is to use a rubber pipet bulb, shown in Figure 5.3C. Use of the pipet bulb is made more convenient by inserting a plastic automatic pipet tip into a rubber pipet bulb.[1] The tapered end of the pipet tip fits snugly into the end of a pipet. Drawing the liquid into the pipet is made easy, and it is also convenient to remove the pipet bulb and place a finger over the pipet opening to control the flow of liquid.

The calibrations printed on graduated pipets are reasonably accurate, but you should practice using the pipets in order to achieve this accuracy. When accurate quantities of liquids are required, the best technique is to weigh the reagent that has been delivered from the pipet.

The following description, along with Figure 5.4, illustrates how to use a graduated

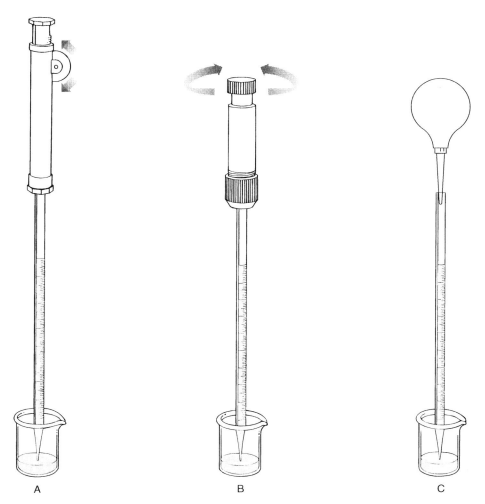

A   B   C

Figure 5.3 Pipet pumps (A, B) and a pipet bulb (C).

---

[1] This technique was described in G. Deckey, "A Versatile and Inexpensive Pipet Bulb," *Journal of Chemical Education, 57* (July 1980): 526.

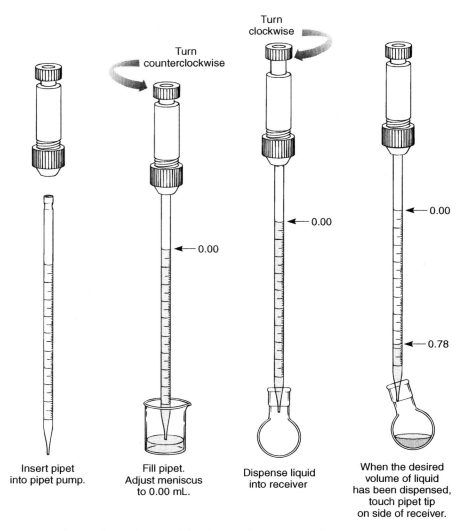

Figure 5.4 Use of a graduated pipet. (The figure shows, as an illustration, the technique required to deliver a volume of 0.78 mL from a 1.00-mL pipet.)

pipet. Insert the end of the pipet firmly into the pipet pump. Rotate the knob of the pipet pump in the correct direction (counterclockwise or up) to fill the pipet. Fill the pipet to a point just above the uppermost mark and then reverse the direction of rotation of the knob to allow the liquid to drain from the pipet until the meniscus is adjusted to the 0.00-mL mark. Move the pipet to the receiving vessel. Rotate the knob of the pipet pump (clockwise or down) to force the liquid from the pipet. Allow the liquid to drain from the pipet until the meniscus arrives at the mark corresponding to the volume that you wish to dispense. Be sure to touch the tip of the pipet to the inside of the container before withdrawing the pipet. Remove the pipet and drain the remaining liquid into a waste receiver. Avoid transferring the entire contents of the pipet when measuring volumes with a pipet. Remember that to achieve the greatest possible accuracy with this method, you should deliver volumes as a *difference* between two marked calibrations.

Pipets may be obtained in a number of styles, but only three types will be described here (Figure 5.5). One type of graduated pipet is calibrated "to deliver" (TD) its total capacity when the last drop is blown out. This style of pipet, shown in Figure 5.5A, is probably the most common type of graduated pipet in use in the laboratory; it is designated by two rings at the top. Of course, it is not necessary to transfer the entire volume to a container. To deliver a more accurate volume, you should transfer an amount less than the total capacity of the pipet using the graduations on the pipet as a guide.

Another type of graduated pipet is shown in Figure 5.5B. This pipet is calibrated to deliver its total capacity when the meniscus is located on the last graduation mark near the bottom of the pipet. For example, the pipet shown in the Figure 5.5B delivers 10.0 mL of liquid when it has been drained to the point where the meniscus is located on the 10.0-mL mark. With this type of pipet, you must not drain the entire pipet or blow it out. In contrast, notice

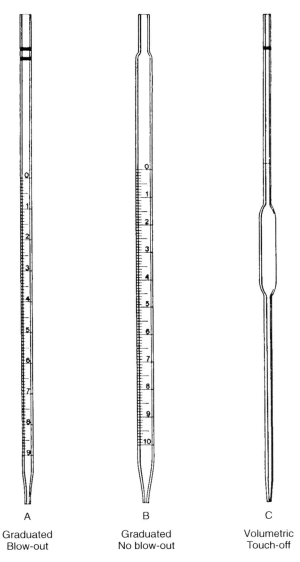

A
Graduated
Blow-out

B
Graduated
No blow-out

C
Volumetric
Touch-off

Figure 5.5 Pipets.

55

that the pipet discussed in Figure 5.5A has its last graduation at 0.90 mL. The last 0.10-mL volume is blown out to give the 1.00-mL volume.

A nongraduated volumetric pipet is shown in Figure 5.5C. It is easily identified by the large bulb in the center of the pipet. This pipet is calibrated so that it will retain its last drop after the tip is touched on the side of the container. It must not be blown out. These pipets often have a single colored band at the top that identifies it as a "touch-off" pipet. The color of the band is keyed to its total volume. This type of pipet is commonly used in analytical chemistry.

5.4 PASTEUR PIPETS

The Pasteur pipet is shown in Figure 5.6A with a 2-mL rubber bulb attached. There are two sizes of Pasteur pipets: a short one (5¾-inch), which is shown in the figure, and a long one (9-inch). It is important that the pipet bulb fit securely. You should not use a medicine dropper bulb because of its small capacity. A Pasteur pipet is an indispensable piece of equipment for the routine transfer of liquids. It is also used for separations (Technique 12). Pasteur pipets may be packed with cotton for use in gravity filtration (Technique 8) or packed with an adsorbent for small-scale column chromatography (Technique 19). Although Pasteur pipets are considered disposable, you should be able to clean them for reuse as long as the tip remains unchipped.

A Pasteur pipet may be supplied by your instructor for dropwise addition of a particular reagent to a reaction mixture. For example, concentrated sulfuric acid is often dispensed in this way. When sulfuric acid is transferred, you should take care to avoid getting the acid into the rubber or latex dropper bulb.

The rubber dropper bulb may be avoided entirely by using one-piece transfer pipets made entirely of polyethylene (Figure 5.6B). These plastic pipets are available in 1- or 2-mL sizes. They come from the manufacturers with approximate calibration marks stamped on them. These pipets can be used with all aqueous solutions and most organic liquids. They cannot be used with a few organic solvents or with concentrated acids.

Pasteur pipets may be calibrated for use in operations in which the volume does not need to be known precisely. Examples include measurement of solvents needed for extraction and for washing a solid obtained following crystallization. A calibrated Pasteur pipet is shown in Figure 5.6C. It is suggested that you calibrate several 5¾-inch pipets using the following procedure. On a balance, weigh 0.5 g (0.5 mL) of water into a small test tube. Select a short Pasteur pipet and attach a rubber bulb. Squeeze the rubber bulb before inserting the tip of the pipet into the water. Try to control how much you depress the bulb so that when the pipet is placed into the water and the bulb is completely released, only the desired amount of liquid is drawn into the pipet. When the water has been drawn up, place a mark with an indelible marking pen at the position of the meniscus. A more durable mark can be made by scoring the pipet with a file. Repeat this procedure with 1.0 g of water, and make a 1-mL mark on the same pipet.

Your instructor may provide you with a calibrated Pasteur pipet and bulb for transferring liquids where an accurate volume is not required. The pipet may be used to transfer a volume of 1.5 mL or less. You may find that the instructor has taped a test tube to the side of the storage bottle. The pipet is stored in the test tube with that particular reagent.

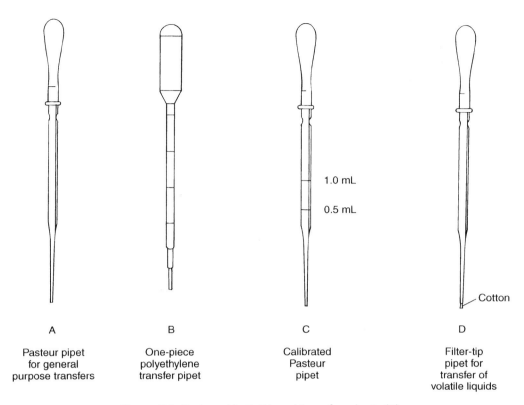

1.0 mL			
0.5 mL			Cotton
A	B	C	D
Pasteur pipet for general purpose transfers	One-piece polyethylene transfer pipet	Calibrated Pasteur pipet	Filter-tip pipet for transfer of volatile liquids

Figure 5.6 Pasteur (A, C, D) and transfer pipets (B).

Note: You should not assume that a certain number of drops equals a 1-mL volume. The common rule that 20 drops equal 1 mL, often used for a buret, does not hold true for a Pasteur pipet!

A Pasteur pipet may be packed with cotton to create a filter-tip pipet as shown in Figure 5.6D. This pipet is prepared by the instructions given in Technique 8, Section 8.6, page 655. Pipets of this type are very useful in transferring volatile solvents during extractions and in filtering small amounts of solid impurities from solutions. A filter-tip pipet is very useful for removing small particles from a solution of a sample prepared for nuclear magnetic resonance (NMR) analysis.

5.5 SYRINGES

Syringes may be used to add a pure liquid or a solution to a reaction mixture. They are especially useful when anhydrous conditions must be maintained. The needle is inserted through a septum, and the liquid is added to the reaction mixture. Caution should be used with some disposable syringes as they often use solvent-soluble rubber gaskets on the plungers. A syringe should be cleaned carefully after each use by drawing acetone or another volatile solvent into it and expelling the solvent with the plunger. Repeat this procedure several times to clean the syringe thoroughly. Remove the plunger and draw air through the barrel with an aspirator to dry the syringe.

Syringes are usually supplied with volume graduations inscribed on the barrel. Large-volume syringes are not accurate enough to be used for measuring liquids in small-scale experiments. A small microliter syringe, such as that used in gas chromatography, delivers a very precise volume.

5.6 AUTOMATIC PIPETS

Automatic pipets are commonly used in microscale organic laboratories and in biochemistry laboratories. Several types of adjustable automatic pipets are shown in Figure 5.7. The automatic pipet is very accurate with aqueous solutions, but it is not as accurate with organic liquids. These pipets are available in different sizes and can deliver accurate volumes ranging from 0.10 mL to 1.0 mL. They are very expensive and must be shared by the entire laboratory. Automatic pipets should never be used with corrosive liquids, such as sulfuric acid or hydrochloric acid. *Always use the pipet with a plastic tip.*

Automatic pipets may vary in design, according to the manufacturer. The following description, however, should apply to most models. The automatic pipet consists of a handle that contains a spring-loaded plunger and a micrometer dial. The dial controls the travel of the

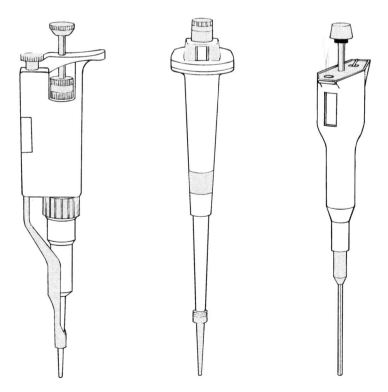

Figure 5.7 The adjustable automatic pipet.

plunger and is the means used to select the amount of liquid that the pipet is intended to dispense. Automatic pipets are designed to deliver liquids within a particular range of volumes. For example, a pipet may be designed to cover the range 10–100 μL (0.010–0.100 mL) or 100–1000 μL (0.100–1.000 mL).

5.7 MEASURING VOLUMES WITH CONICAL VIALS, BEAKERS, AND ERLENMEYER FLASKS

Conical vials, beakers, and Erlenmeyer flasks all have graduations inscribed on them. Beakers and flasks can be used to give only a crude approximation of the volume. They are much less precise than graduated cylinders for measuring volume. In some cases, a conical vial may be used to estimate volumes. For example, the graduations are sufficiently accurate for measuring a solvent needed to wash a solid obtained on a Hirsch funnel after a crystallization. You should use an automatic pipet, dispensing pump, or graduated transfer pipet for accurate measurement of liquids in microscale experiments.

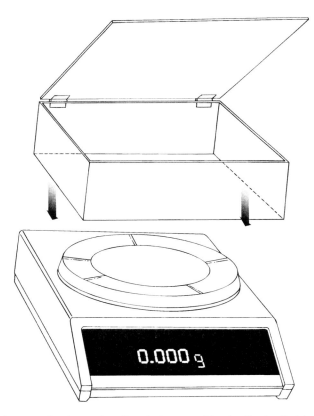

Figure 5.8 A top-loading balance with plastic draft shield.

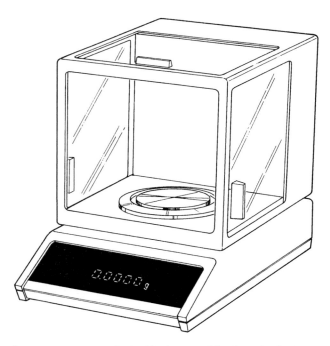

Figure 5.9 An analytical balance with glass draft shield.

5.8 BALANCES

Solids and some liquids will need to be weighed on a balance that reads to at least the nearest milligram (0.001 g) for microscale experiments or at least to the nearest decigram (0.01 g) for macroscale experiments. A top-loading balance (see Figure 5.8) works well if the balance pan is covered with a plastic draft shield. The shield has a flap that opens to allow access to the balance pan. An analytical balance (see Figure 5.9) may also be used. This type of balance will weigh to the nearest tenth of a milligram (0.0001 g) when provided with a glass draft shield.

Modern electronic balances have a tare device that automatically subtracts the weight of a container or a piece of paper from the combined weight to give the weight of the sample. With solids, it is easy to place a piece of paper on the balance pan, press the tare device so that the paper appears to have zero weight, and then add your solid until the balance gives the weight you desire. You can then transfer the weighed solid to a container. You should always use a spatula to transfer a solid and never pour material from a bottle. In addition, solids must be weighed on paper and not directly on the balance pan. Remember to clean any spills.

With liquids, you should weigh the flask to determine the tare weight, transfer the liquid with a graduated cylinder, dispensing pump, or graduated pipet into the flask, and then reweigh it. With liquids, it is usually necessary to weigh only the limiting reagent. The other liquids may be transferred using a graduated cylinder, dispensing pump, or graduated pipet. Their weights can be calculated by knowing the volumes and densities of the liquids.

PROBLEMS

1. What measuring device would you use to measure the volume under each of the conditions described below? In some cases, there may be more than one answer to the question.

    a. 25 mL of a solvent needed for a crystallization

    b. 2.4 mL of a liquid needed for a reaction

    c. 0.64 mL of a liquid needed for a reaction

    d. 5 mL of a solvent needed for an extraction

2. Assume that the liquid used in problem 1b is a limiting reagent for a reaction. What should you do after measuring the volume?

3. Calculate the weight of a 2.5-mL sample of each of the following liquids:

    a. Diethyl ether (ether)

    b. Methylene chloride (dichloromethane)

    c. Acetone

4. A laboratory procedure calls for 5.46 g of acetic anhydride. Calculate the volume of this reagent needed in the reaction.

5. Criticize the following techniques:

    a. A 100-mL graduated cylinder is used to measure accurately a volume of 2.8 mL.

    b. A one-piece polyethylene transfer pipet (Figure 5.6B) is used to transfer precisely 0.75 mL of a liquid that is being used as the limiting reactant.

    c. A calibrated Pasteur pipet (Figure 5.6C) is used to transfer 25 mL of a solvent.

    d. The volume markings on a 100-mL beaker are used to transfer accurately 5 mL of a liquid.

    e. An automatic pipet is used to transfer 10 mL of a liquid.

    f. A graduated cylinder is used to transfer 0.126 mL of a liquid.

    g. For a small-scale reaction, the weight of a liquid limiting reactant is calculated from its density and volume.

T E C H N I Q U E 6

Heating and Cooling Methods

Most organic reaction mixtures need to be heated in order to complete the reaction. In general chemistry, you used a Bunsen burner for heating because nonflammable aqueous solutions were used. In an organic chemistry laboratory, however, the student must heat non-aqueous solutions that may contain *highly flammable* solvents. You *should not heat organic mixtures with a Bunsen burner* unless you are directed to do so by your laboratory instructor. Open flames present a potential fire hazard. Whenever possible you should use one of the alternative heating methods, as described in the following sections.

6.1 HEATING MANTLES

A useful source of heat for most macroscale experiments is the heating mantle, illustrated in Figure 6.1. The heating mantle shown here consists of a ceramic heating shell with electric heating coils embedded within the shell. The temperature of a heating mantle is regulated with the heat controller. Although it is difficult to monitor the actual temperature of

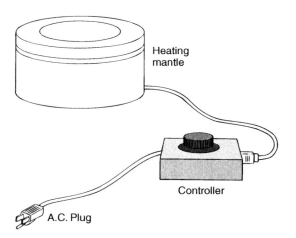

Heating
mantle

Controller

A.C. Plug

Figure 6.1 A heating mantle.

the heating mantle, the controller is calibrated so that it is fairly easy to duplicate approximate heating levels after one has gained some experience with this apparatus. Reactions or distillations requiring relatively high temperatures can be easily performed with a heating mantle. For temperatures in the range of 50–80°C, you should use a water bath (Section 6.3) or a steam bath (Section 6.8).

In the center of the heating mantle shown in Figure 6.1 is a well that can accommodate round-bottom flasks of several different sizes. Some heating mantles, however, are designed to fit only specific sizes of round-bottom flasks. Some heating mantles are also made to be used with a magnetic stirrer so that the reaction mixture can be heated and stirred at the same time. Figure 6.2 shows a reaction mixture being heated with a heating mantle.

Heating mantles are very easy to use and safe to operate. The metal housing is grounded to prevent electrical shock if liquid is spilled into the well; however, flammable liquids may ignite if spilled into the well of a hot heating mantle.

Caution: You should be very careful to avoid spilling liquids into the well of the heating mantle. The surface of the ceramic shell may be very hot and could cause the liquid to ignite.

Raising and lowering the apparatus is a much more rapid method of changing the temperature within the flask than changing the temperature with the controller. For this reason, the entire apparatus should be clamped above the heating mantle so that it can be raised quickly if overheating occurs. Some laboratories may provide a lab jack or blocks of wood that can be placed under the heating mantle. In this case, the heating mantle itself is lowered and the apparatus remains clamped in the same position.

There are two situations in which it is relatively easy to overheat the reaction mixture. The first situation occurs when a larger heating mantle is used to heat a relatively small flask. You should be very careful when doing this. Many laboratories provide heating mantles of different sizes to prevent this from happening. The second situation occurs when the reaction mixture is first brought to a boil. To bring the mixture to a boil as rapidly as possible, the heat controller is often turned up higher than it will need to be set in order to keep the mixture boiling. When the mixture begins boiling very rapidly, turn the controller to a

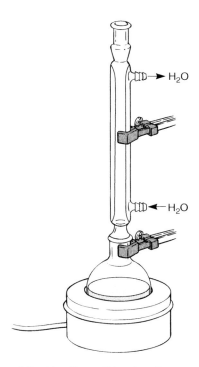

Figure 6.2 Heating with a heating mantle.

lower setting and raise the apparatus until the mixture boils less rapidly. As the temperature of the heating mantle cools down, lower the apparatus until the flask is resting on the bottom of the well.

6.2 HOT PLATES

Hot plates are a very convenient source of heat; however, it is difficult to monitor the actual temperature, and changes in temperature occur somewhat slowly. Care must be taken with flammable solvents to ensure against fires caused by "flashing" when solvent vapors come into contact with the hot-plate surface. Never evaporate large quantities of a solvent by this method; the fire hazard is too great.

Some hot plates *heat constantly* at a given setting. They have no thermostat, and you will have to control the temperature manually, either by removing the container being heated or by adjusting the temperature up or down until a balance point is found. Some hot plates have a thermostat to control the temperature. A good thermostat will maintain a very even temperature. With many hot plates, however, the temperature may vary greatly ($> 10–20°C$), depending upon whether the heater is in its "on" cycle or its "off" cycle. These hot plates will have a cycling (or oscillating) temperature, as shown in Figure 6.3. They too will have to be adjusted continually to maintain even heat.

Some hot plates also have built-in magnetic stirring motors that enable the reaction mixture to be stirred and heated at the same time. Their use is described in Section 6.5.

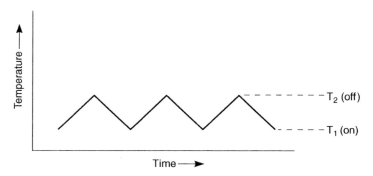

Figure 6.3   Temperature response for a hot plate with a thermostat.

6.3 WATER BATH WITH HOT PLATE/STIRRER

A hot water bath is a very effective heat source when a temperature below 80°C is required. A beaker (250-mL or 400-mL) is partially filled with water and heated on a hot plate. A thermometer is clamped into position in the water bath. You may need to cover the water bath with aluminum foil to prevent evaporation, especially at higher temperatures. The water bath is illustrated in Figure 6.4. A mixture can be stirred with a magnetic stir bar (Technique 7, Section 7.3, p. 630). A hot water bath has some advantage over a heating mantle in that the temperature in the bath is uniform. In addition, it is sometimes easier to establish a lower temperature with a water bath than with other heating devices. Finally, the temperature of the reaction mixture will be closer to the temperature of the water, which allows for more precise control of the reaction conditions.

6.4 OIL BATH WITH HOT PLATE/STIRRER

In some laboratories, oil baths may be available. An oil bath can be used when carrying out a distillation or heating a reaction mixture that needs a temperature above 100°C. An oil bath can be heated most conveniently with a hot plate, and a *heavy-walled* beaker provides a suitable container for the oil.[1] A thermometer is clamped into position in the oil bath. In some laboratories, the oil may be heated electrically by an immersion coil. Because oil baths have a high heat capacity and heat slowly, it is advisable to heat the oil bath partially before the actual time at which it is to be used.

An oil bath with ordinary mineral oil cannot be used above 200–220°C. Above this temperature, the oil bath may "flash," or suddenly burst into flame. A hot oil fire is not ex-

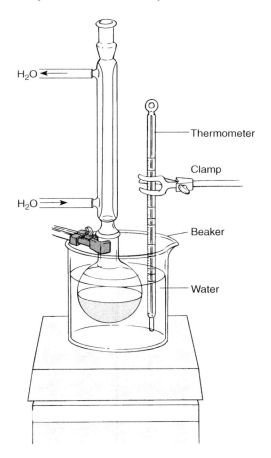

Figure 6.4   A water bath with a hot plate/stirrer.

[1] It is very dangerous to use a thin-walled beaker for an oil bath. Breakage due to heating can occur, spilling hot oil everywhere!

tinguished easily. If the oil starts smoking, it may be near its flash temperature; discontinue heating. Old oil, which is dark, is more likely to flash than new oil. Also, hot oil causes bad burns. Water should be kept away from a hot oil bath, because water in the oil will cause it to splatter. Never use an oil bath when it is obvious that there is water in the oil. If water is present, replace the oil before using the heating bath. An oil bath has only a finite lifetime. New oil is clear and colorless but, after extended use, becomes dark brown and gummy from oxidation.

Besides ordinary mineral oil, a variety of other types of oils can be used in an oil bath. Silicone oil does not begin to decompose at as low a temperature as does mineral oil. When silicone oil is heated high enough to decompose, however, its vapors are far more hazardous than mineral oil vapors. The polyethylene glycols may be used in oil baths. They are water soluble, which makes cleaning up after using an oil bath much easier than with mineral oil. One may select any one of a variety of polymer sizes of polyethylene glycol, depending on the temperature range required. The polymers of large molecular weight are often solid at room temperature. Wax may also be used for higher temperatures, but this material also becomes solid at room temperature. Some workers prefer to use a material that solidifies when not in use because it minimizes both storage and spillage problems.

6.5 ALUMINUM BLOCK WITH HOT PLATE/STIRRER

Although aluminum blocks are most commonly used in microscale organic chemistry laboratories, they can also be used with the smaller round-bottom flasks used in macroscale experiments.[2] The aluminum block shown in Figure 6.5A can be used to hold 25-, 50-, or 100-mL round-bottom flasks, as well as a thermometer. Heating will occur more rapidly if the flask fits all the way into the hole; however, heating is also effective if the flask only partially fits into the hole. The aluminum block with smaller holes, as shown in Figure 6.5B, is designed for microscale glassware. It will hold a conical vial, a Craig tube or small test tubes, and a thermometer.

There are several advantages to heating with an aluminum block. The metal heats very quickly, high temperatures can be obtained, and you can cool the aluminum rapidly by removing it with crucible tongs and immersing it in cold water. Aluminum blocks are also inexpensive or can be fabricated readily in a machine shop.

Figure 6.6 shows a reaction mixture being heated with an aluminum block on a hot plate/stirrer unit. The thermometer in the figure is used to determine the temperature of the aluminum block. *Do not use a mercury thermometer:* use a thermometer containing a liquid other than mercury or use a metal dial thermometer that can be inserted into a smaller-diameter hole drilled into the side of the block.[3] Make sure that the thermometer fits loosely in the hole, or it may break. Secure the thermometer with a clamp.

To avoid the possibility of breaking a glass thermometer, your hot plate may have a hole drilled into the metal plate so that a metal dial thermometer can be inserted into the

---

[2] The use of solid aluminum heating devices was developed by Siegfried Lodwig at Centralia College, Centralia, WA: Lodwig, S. N., *Journal of Chemical Education, 66* (1989): 77.

[3] C. M. Garner, "A Mercury-Free Alternative for Temperature Measurement in Aluminum Blocks," *Journal of Chemical Education, 68* (1991): A244.

unit (Figure 6.7A). These metal thermometers, such as the one shown in Figure 6.7B, can be obtained in a number of temperature ranges. For example, a 0–250°C thermometer with 2-degree divisions can be obtained at a reasonable price. Also shown in Figure 6.7 (inset) is an aluminum block with a small hole drilled into it so that a metal thermometer can be inserted. An alternative to the metal thermometer is a digital electronic temperature-measuring device that can be inserted into the aluminum block or hot plate. It is strongly recommended that mercury thermometers be avoided when measuring the surface temperature of the hot plate or aluminum block. If a mercury thermometer is broken on a hot surface, you will introduce toxic mercury vapors into the laboratory. Nonmercury thermometers filled with high-boiling colored liquids are available as alternatives.

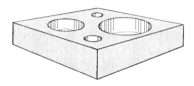

A. Large holes for 25-, 50- or 100-mL round-bottom flasks.

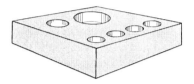

B. Small holes for Craig tube, 3-mL and 5-mL conical vials, and small test tubes.

Figure 6.5 Aluminum heating blocks.

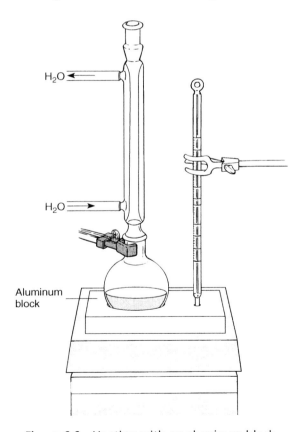

H₂O

H₂O

Aluminum block

Figure 6.6 Heating with an aluminum block.

As already mentioned, aluminum blocks are often used in the microscale organic chemistry laboratory. The use of an aluminum block to heat a microscale reflux apparatus is shown in Figure 6.8. The reaction vessel in the figure is a conical vial, which is used in many microscale experiments. Also shown in Figure 6.8 is a split aluminum collar that may be used when very high temperatures are required. The collar is split to facilitate easy placement around a 5-mL conical vial. The collar helps to distribute heat further up the wall of the vial.

You should first calibrate the aluminum block so that you have an approximate idea where to set the control on the hot plate to achieve a desired temperature. Place the aluminum block on the hot plate and insert a thermometer into the small hole in the block. Select five equally spaced temperature settings, including the lowest and highest settings, on the heating control of the hot plate. Set the dial to the first of these settings and monitor the temperature recorded on the thermometer. When the thermometer reading arrives at a constant value,[4] record this final temperature, along with the dial setting. Repeat this procedure with the remaining four settings. Using these data, prepare a calibration curve for future reference.

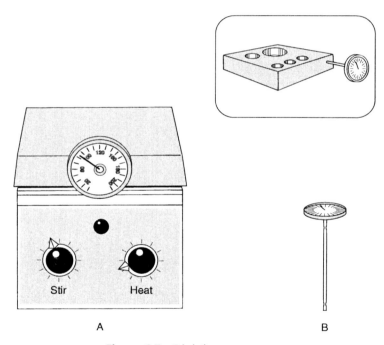

A   B

Figure 6.7 Dial thermometers.

It is a good idea to use the same hot plate each time, as it is very likely that two hot plates of the same type may give different temperatures with identical settings. Record in your notebook the identification number printed on the unit that you are using to ensure that you always use the same hot plate.

For many experiments, you can determine what the approximate setting on the hot

[4]See, however, Section 6.2, page 614.

plate should be from the boiling point of the liquid being heated. Because the temperature inside the flask is lower than the aluminum block temperature, you should add at least 20°C to the boiling point of the liquid and set the aluminum block at this higher temperature. In fact, you may need to raise the temperature even higher than this value in order to bring the liquid to a boil.

Many organic mixtures need to be stirred as well as heated to achieve satisfactory results. To stir a mixture, place a magnetic stir bar (Technique 7, Figure 7.8A, p. 630) in a round-bottom flask containing the reaction mixture as shown in Figure 6.9A. If the mixture is to be heated as well as stirred, attach a water condenser as shown in Figure 6.6. With the combination hot plate/stirrer unit, it is possible to stir and heat a mixture simultaneously. With conical vials, a magnetic spin vane must be used to stir mixtures (Figure 7.8B, p. 630). This is shown in Figure 6.9B. More uniform stirring will be obtained if the flask or vial is placed in the aluminum block so that it is centered on the hot plate. Mixing may also be achieved by boiling the mixture. A boiling stone (Section 7.4, p. 631) must be added when a mixture is boiled without magnetic stirring.

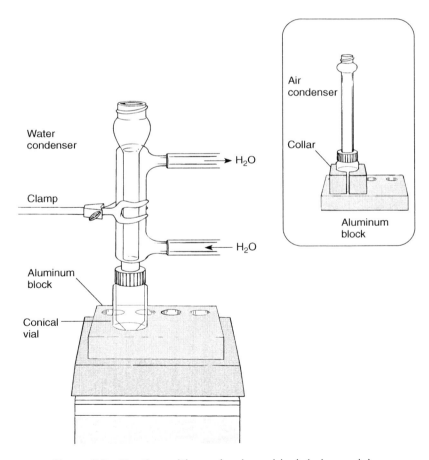

Figure 6.8 Heating with an aluminum block (microscale).

6.6 SAND BATH WITH HOT PLATE/STIRRER

The sand bath is used in some microscale laboratories to heat organic mixtures. It can also be used as a heat source in some macroscale experiments. Sand provides a clean way of distributing heat to a reaction mixture. To prepare a sand bath for microscale use, place about a 1-cm depth of sand in a crystallizing dish and then set the dish on a hot plate/stirrer unit. The apparatus is shown in Figure 6.10. Clamp the thermometer into position in the sand bath. You should calibrate the sand bath in a manner similar to that used with the aluminum block (see previous section). Because sand heats more slowly than an aluminum block, you will need to begin heating the sand bath well before using it.

Do not heat the sand bath much above 200°C, or you may break the dish. If you need to heat at very high temperatures, you should use a heating mantle or an aluminum block rather than a sand bath. With sand baths, it may be necessary to cover the dish with aluminum foil to achieve a temperature near 200°C. Because of the relatively poor heat conductivity of sand, a temperature gradient is established within the sand bath. It is warmer near the bottom of the sand bath and cooler near the top for a given setting on the hot plate. To make use of this gradient, you may find it convenient to bury the flask or vial in the sand to heat a mixture more rapidly. Once the mixture is boiling, you can then slow the rate of heat-

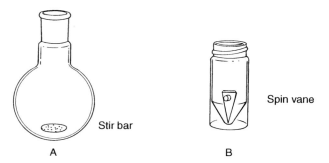

Figure 6.9 Methods of stirring in a round-bottom flask or conical vial.

ing by raising the flask or vial. These adjustments may be made easily and do not require a change in the setting on the hot plate.

6.7 FLAMES

The simplest technique for heating mixtures is to use a Bunsen burner. Because of the high danger of fires, however, the use of the Bunsen burner should be strictly limited to those cases for which the danger of fire is low or for which no reasonable alternative source of heat is available. A flame should generally be used only to heat aqueous solutions or solutions with very high boiling points. You should always check with your instructor about using a burner. If you use a burner at your bench, great care should be taken to ensure that others in the vicinity are not using flammable solvents.

In heating a flask with a Bunsen burner, you will find that using a wire gauze can produce more even heating over a broader area. The wire gauze, when placed under the object being heated, spreads the flame to keep the flask from being heated in one small area only.

Bunsen burners may be used to prepare capillary micropipets for thin-layer chromatography or to prepare other pieces of glassware requiring an open flame. For these purposes, burners should be used in designated areas in the laboratory and not at your laboratory bench.

6.8 STEAM BATHS

The steam cone or steam bath is a good source of heat when temperatures around 100°C are needed. Steam baths are used to heat reaction mixtures and solvents needed for crystallization. A steam cone and a portable steam bath are shown in Figure 6.11. These methods of heating have the disadvantage that water vapor may be introduced, through condensation of steam, into the mixture being heated. A slow flow of steam may minimize this difficulty.

Because water condenses in the steam line when it is not in use, it is necessary to purge the line of water before the steam will begin to flow. This purging should be accomplished before the flask is placed on the steam bath. The steam flow should be started with

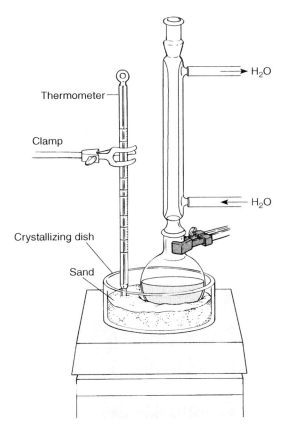

Figure 6.10 Heating with a sand bath.

71

a high rate to purge the line; then the flow should be reduced to the desired rate. When using a portable steam bath, be certain that condensate (water) is drained into a sink. Once the steam bath or cone is heated, a slow steam flow will maintain the temperature of the mixture being heated. There is no advantage to having a Vesuvius on your desk! An excessive steam flow may cause problems with condensation in the flask. This condensation problem can often be avoided by selecting the correct place at which to locate the flask on top of the steam bath.

The top of the steam bath consists of several flat concentric rings. The amount of heat delivered to the flask being heated can be controlled by selecting the correct sizes of these rings. Heating is most efficient when the largest opening that will still support the flask is used. Heating large flasks on a steam bath while using the smallest opening leads to slow heating and wastes laboratory time.

6.9 COLD BATHS

At times, you may need to cool an Erlenmeyer flask or round-bottom flask below room temperature. A cold bath is used for this purpose. The most common cold bath is an **ice bath,** which is a highly convenient source of 0°C temperatures. An ice bath requires water along

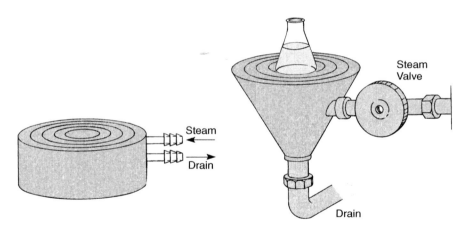

Figure 6.11 A steam bath and a steam cone.

with ice to work well. If an ice bath is made up of only ice, it is not a very efficient cooler because the large pieces of ice do not make good contact with the flask. Enough water should be present with ice so that the flask is surrounded by water but not so much that the temperature is no longer maintained at 0°C. In addition, if too much water is present, the buoyancy of a flask resting in the ice bath may cause it to tip over. There should be enough ice in the bath to allow the flask to rest firmly.

For temperatures somewhat below 0°C, you may add some solid sodium chloride to the ice-water bath. The ionic salt lowers the freezing point of the ice so that temperatures in the range of 0 to −10°C can be reached. The lowest temperatures are reached with ice-water mixtures that contain relatively little water.

A temperature of $-78.5°C$ can be obtained with solid carbon dioxide or dry ice. However, large chunks of dry ice do not provide uniform contact with a flask being cooled. A liquid such as isopropyl alcohol is mixed with small pieces of dry ice to provide an efficient cooling mixture. Acetone and ethanol can be used in place of isopropyl alcohol. Be careful when handling dry ice because it can inflict severe frostbite. Extremely low temperatures can be obtained with liquid nitrogen ($-195.8°C$).

PROBLEMS

1. What would be the preferred heating device(s) in each of the following situations?
   a. Reflux a solvent with a 56°C boiling point
   b. Reflux a solvent with a 110°C boiling point
   c. Distillation of a substance that boils at 220°C
2. Obtain the boiling points for the following compounds by using a handbook (Technique 4). In each case, suggest a heating device(s) that should be used for refluxing the substance.
   a. Butyl benzoate
   b. 1-Pentanol
   c. 1-Chloropropane
3. What type of bath would you use to get a temperature of $-10°C$?
4. Obtain the melting point and boiling point for benzene and ammonia from a handbook (Technique 4) and answer the following questions.
   a. A reaction was conducted in benzene as the solvent. Because the reaction was very exothermic, the mixture was cooled in a salt–ice bath. This was a bad choice. Why?
   b. What bath should be used for a reaction that is conducted in liquid ammonia as the solvent?
5. Criticize the following techniques:
   a. Refluxing a mixture that contains diethyl ether using a Bunsen burner
   b. Refluxing a mixture that contains a large amount of toluene using a hot water bath
   c. Refluxing a mixture using the apparatus shown in Figure 6.6, but with an unclamped thermometer
   d. Using a mercury thermometer that is inserted into an aluminum block on a hot plate
   e. Running a reaction with *tert*-butyl alcohol (2-methyl-2-propanol) that is cooled to 0°C in an ice bath

TECHNIQUE 7

Reaction Methods

The successful completion of an organic reaction requires the chemist to be familiar with a variety of laboratory methods. These methods include operating safely, assembling the apparatus, heating and stirring reaction mixtures, adding liquid reagents, maintaining anhydrous and inert conditions in the reaction, and collecting gaseous products. Several techniques that are used in bringing a reaction to a successful conclusion are discussed here.

7.1 ASSEMBLING THE APPARATUS

Care must be taken when assembling the glass components into the desired apparatus. You should always remember that Newtonian physics applies to chemical apparatus, and unsecured pieces of glassware are certain to respond to gravity.

Assembling an apparatus in the correct manner requires that the individual pieces of glassware be connected to each other securely and the entire apparatus is held in the correct position. This can be accomplished by using **adjustable metal clamps** or a combination of adjustable metal clamps and **plastic joint clips.**

Two types of adjustable metal clamps are shown in Figure 7.1. Although these two types of clamps can usually be interchanged, the extension clamp is more commonly used to hold round-bottom flasks in place, and the three-finger clamp is frequently used to clamp

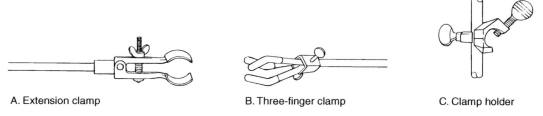

A. Extension clamp   B. Three-finger clamp   C. Clamp holder

Figure 7.1 Adjustable metal clamps.

condensers. Both types of clamps must be attached to a ring stand using a clamp holder, shown in Figure 7.1C.

A. Securing Macroscale Apparatus Assemblies

It is possible to assemble an apparatus using only adjustable metal clamps. An apparatus used to perform a distillation is shown in Figure 7.2. It is held together securely with three metal clamps. Because of the size of the apparatus and its geometry, the various clamps would likely be attached to three different ring stands. This apparatus would be somewhat difficult to assemble, because it is necessary to ensure that the individual pieces stay together while securing and adjusting the clamps required to hold the entire apparatus in place. In addition, one must be very careful not to bump any part of the apparatus or the ring stands after the apparatus is assembled.

A more convenient alternative is to use a combination of metal clamps and plastic joint clips. A plastic joint clip is shown in Figure 7.3A. These clips are very easy to use (they just clip on), will withstand temperatures up to 140°C, and are quite durable. They hold together two pieces of glassware that are connected by ground-glass joints, as shown in Figure 7.3B. These clips come in different sizes to fit ground-glass joints of different sizes and they are color coded for each size.

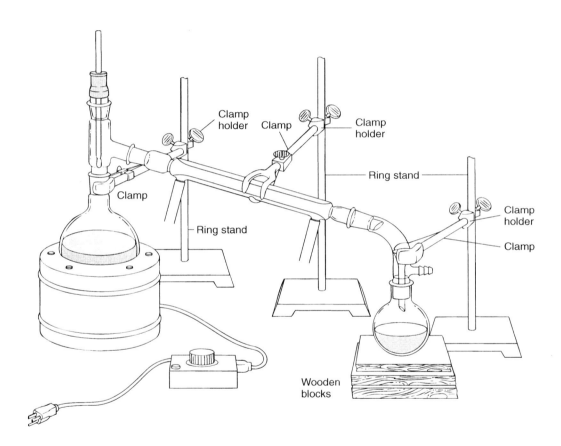

Figure 7.2 Distillation apparatus secured with metal clamps.

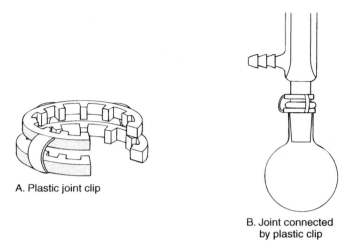

A. Plastic joint clip

B. Joint connected
by plastic clip

Figure 7.3   Plastic joint clip.

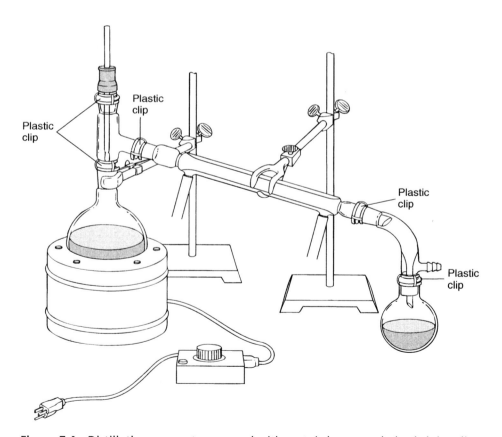

Plastic
clip

Plastic
clip

Plastic
clip

Plastic
clip

Figure 7.4   Distillation apparatus secured with metal clamps and plastic joint clips.

When used in combination with metal clamps, the plastic joint clips make it much easier to assemble most apparatus in a secure manner. There is less chance of dropping the glassware while assembling the apparatus, and once the apparatus is set up, it is more secure. Figure 7.4 shows the same distillation apparatus held in place with both adjustable metal clamps and plastic joint clips.

To assemble this apparatus, first connect all of the individual pieces together using the plastic clips. The entire apparatus is then connected to the ring stands using the adjustable metal clamps. Note that only two ring stands are required and the wooden blocks are not needed.

B. Securing Microscale Apparatus Assemblies

The glassware in most microscale kits is made with standard-taper ground joints. The most common joint size is ⊤ 14/10. Some microscale glassware with ground-glass joints also has threads cast into the outside surface of the outer joints (see top of air condenser in Figure 7.5). The threaded joint allows the use of a plastic screw cap with a hole in the top to fasten two pieces of glassware together securely. The plastic cap is slipped over the inner joint of the upper piece of glassware, followed by a rubber O-ring (see Figure 7.5). The O-ring should be pushed down so that it fits snugly on top of the ground-glass joint. The inner ground-glass joint is then fitted into the outer joint of the bottom piece of glassware. The screw cap is tightened, without excessive force, to attach the entire apparatus firmly together. The O-ring provides an additional seal that makes this joint airtight. With this connecting system, it is unnecessary to use any type of grease to seal the joint. The O-ring *must be used* to obtain a good seal and to lessen the chances of breaking the glassware when you tighten the plastic cap.

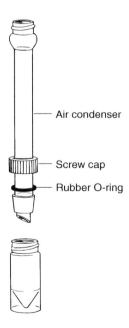

— Air condenser

— Screw cap
— Rubber O-ring

Figure 7.5 A microscale standard-taper joint assembly.

Microscale glassware connected together in this fashion can be assembled very easily. The entire apparatus is held together securely, and usually only one metal clamp is required to hold the apparatus onto a ring stand.

7.2 HEATING UNDER REFLUX

Often we wish to heat a mixture for a long time and to leave it untended. A **reflux apparatus** (see Figure 7.6) allows such heating. The liquid is heated to a boil, and the hot vapors are cooled and condensed as they rise into the water-jacketed condenser. Therefore, very little liquid is lost by evaporation, and the mixture is kept at a constant temperature, the boiling point of the liquid. The liquid mixture is said to be **heating under reflux.**

Condenser.   The **water-jacketed condenser** shown in Figure 7.6 consists of two concentric tubes with the outer cooling tube sealed onto the inner tube. The vapors rise within the inner tube, and water circulates through the outer tube. The circulating water removes heat from the vapors and condenses them. Figure 7.6 also shows a typical microscale apparatus for heating small quantities of material under reflux (Figure 7.6B).

When using a water-jacketed condenser, make sure that the direction of the water flow is such that the condenser will fill with cooling water. The water should enter the bottom of the condenser and leave from the top. The water should flow fast enough to withstand any

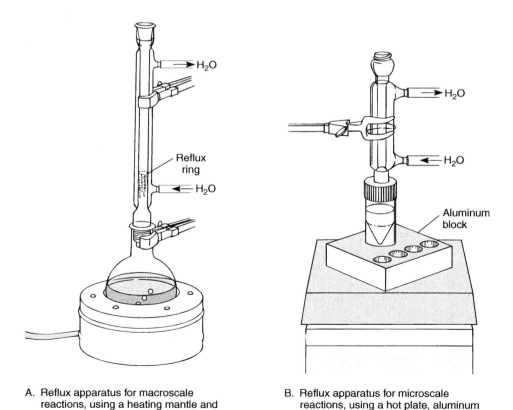

A. Reflux apparatus for macroscale
    reactions, using a heating mantle and
    water-jacketed condenser.

B. Reflux apparatus for microscale
    reactions, using a hot plate, aluminum
    block, and water-jacketed condenser.

Figure 7.6   Heating under reflux.

78

changes in pressure in the water lines, but it should not flow any faster than absolutely necessary. An excessive flow rate greatly increases the chance of a flood, and high water pressure may force the hose from the condenser. Cooling water should be flowing before heating is begun! If the water is to remain flowing overnight, it is advisable to fasten the rubber tubing securely with wire to the condenser. If a flame is used as a source of heat, it is wise to use a wire gauze beneath the flask to provide an even distribution of heat from the flame. In most cases, a heating mantle, water bath, oil bath, aluminum block, sand bath, or steam bath is preferred over a flame.

Stirring. When heating a solution, always use a magnetic stirrer or a boiling stone (see Sections 7.3 and 7.4) to keep the solution from "bumping" (see next section).

Rate of Heating. If the heating rate has been correctly adjusted, the liquid being heated under reflux will travel only partway up the condenser tube before condensing. Below the condensation point, solvent will be seen running back into the flask; above it, the interior of the condenser will appear dry. The boundary between the two zones will be clearly demarcated, and a **reflux ring,** or a ring of liquid, will appear there. The reflux ring can be seen in Figure 7.6A. In heating under reflux, the rate of heating should be adjusted so that the reflux ring is no higher than a third to a half the distance to the top of the condenser. With microscale experiments, the quantities of vapor rising in the condenser frequently are so small that a clear reflux ring cannot be seen. In those cases, the heating rate must be adjusted so that the liquid boils smoothly but not so rapidly that solvent can escape the condenser. With such small volumes, the loss of even a small amount of solvent can affect the reaction. With macroscale reactions, the reflux ring is much easier to see, and one can adjust the heating rate more easily.

Tended Reflux. It is possible to heat small amounts of a solvent under reflux in an Erlenmeyer flask. By heating gently, the evaporated solvent will condense in the relatively cold neck of the flask and return to the solution. This technique (see Figure 7.7) requires constant attention. The flask must be swirled frequently and removed from the heating source for a short period if the boiling becomes too vigorous. When heating is in progress, the reflux ring should not be allowed to rise into the neck of the flask.

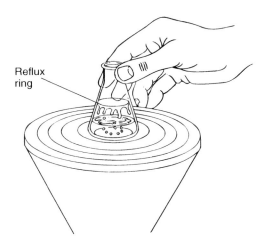

Figure 7.7 Tended reflux of small quantities on a steam cone (this can also be done with a hot plate).

7.3 STIRRING METHODS

When a solution is heated, there is a danger that it may become superheated. When this happens, very large bubbles sometimes erupt violently from the solution; this is called **bumping.** Bumping must be avoided because of the risk that material may be lost from the apparatus, that a fire may start, or that the apparatus may break.

Magnetic stirrers are used to prevent bumping because they produce turbulence in the solution. The turbulence breaks up the large bubbles that form in boiling solutions. An additional purpose for using a magnetic stirrer is to stir the reaction to ensure that all the reagents are thoroughly mixed. A magnetic stirring system consists of a magnet that is rotated by an electric motor. The rate at which this magnet rotates can be adjusted by a potentiometric control. A small magnet, which is coated with a nonreactive material such as Teflon or glass, is placed in the flask. The magnet within the flask rotates in response to the rotating magnetic field caused by the motor-driven magnet. The result is that the inner magnet stirs the solution as it rotates. A very common type of magnetic stirrer includes the stirring system within a hot plate. This type of hot plate/stirrer permits one to heat the reaction and stir it simultaneously. In order for the magnetic stirrer to be effective, the contents of the flask being stirred should be placed as close to the center of the hot plate as possible and not offset.

For macroscale apparatus, magnetic stirring bars of various sizes and shapes are available. For microscale apparatus, a **magnetic spin vane** is often used. It is designed to contain a tiny bar magnet and to have a shape that conforms to the conical bottom of a reaction vial. A small Teflon-coated magnetic stirring bar works well with very small round-bottom boiling flasks. Small stirring bars of this type (often sold as "disposable" stirring bars) can be obtained very cheaply. A variety of magnetic stirring bars is illustrated in Figure 7.8.

There is also a variety of simple techniques that may be used to stir a liquid mixture in a centrifuge tube or conical vial. A thorough mixing of the components of a liquid can be achieved by repeatedly drawing the liquid into a Pasteur pipet and then ejecting the liquid back into the container by pressing sharply on the dropper bulb. Liquids can also be stirred effectively by placing the flattened end of a spatula into the container and twirling it rapidly.

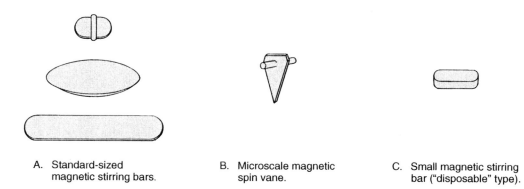

A. Standard-sized magnetic stirring bars.

B. Microscale magnetic spin vane.

C. Small magnetic stirring bar ("disposable" type).

Figure 7.8 Magnetic stirring bars.

7.4 BOILING STONES

A **boiling stone,** also known as a **boiling chip** or **Boileezer,** is a small lump of porous material that produces a steady stream of fine air bubbles when it is heated in a solvent. This stream of bubbles and the turbulence that accompanies it break up the large bubbles of gases in the liquid. In this way, it reduces the tendency of the liquid to become superheated, and it promotes the smooth boiling of the liquid. The boiling stone decreases the chances for bumping.

Two common types of boiling stones are carborundum and marble chips. Carborundum boiling stones are more inert, and the pieces are usually quite small, suitable for most applications. If available, carborundum boiling stones are preferred for most purposes. Marble chips may dissolve in strong acid solutions, and the pieces are larger. The advantage of marble chips is that they are cheaper.

Because boiling stones act to promote the smooth boiling of liquids, you should always make certain that a boiling stone has been placed in a liquid *before* heating is begun. If you wait until the liquid is hot, it may have become superheated. Adding a boiling stone to a superheated liquid will cause all the liquid to try to boil at once. The liquid, as a result, would erupt entirely out of the flask or froth violently.

As soon as boiling ceases in a liquid containing a boiling stone, the liquid is drawn into the pores of the boiling stone. When this happens, the boiling stone no longer can produce a fine stream of bubbles; it is spent. You may have to add a new boiling stone if you have allowed boiling to stop for a long period.

Wooden applicator sticks are used in some applications. They function in the same manner as boiling stones. Occasionally, glass beads are used. Their presence also causes sufficient turbulence in the liquid to prevent bumping.

7.5 ADDITION OF LIQUID REAGENTS

Liquid reagents and solutions are added to a reaction by several means, some of which are shown in Figure 7.9. The most common type of assembly for macroscale experiments is shown in Figure 7.9A. In this apparatus, a separatory funnel is attached to the sidearm of a Claisen head adapter. The separatory funnel must be equipped with a standard-taper, ground-glass joint to be used in this manner. The liquid is stored in the separatory funnel (which is called an **addition funnel** in this application) and is added to the reaction. The rate of addition is controlled by adjusting the stopcock. When it is being used as an addition funnel, the upper opening must be kept open to the atmosphere. If the upper hole is stoppered, a vacuum will develop in the funnel and will prevent the liquid from passing into the reaction vessel. Because the funnel is open to the atmosphere, there is a danger that atmospheric moisture can contaminate the liquid reagent as it is being added. To prevent this outcome, a drying tube (see Section 7.6) may be attached to the upper opening of the addition funnel. The drying tube allows the funnel to maintain atmospheric pressure without allowing the passage of water vapor into the reaction. For reactions that are particularly sensitive to moisture, it is also advisable to attach a second drying tube to the top of the condenser.

Another macroscale assembly, suitable for larger amounts of material, is shown in

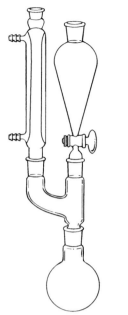

A. Macroscale equipment, using a separatory funnel as an addition funnel.

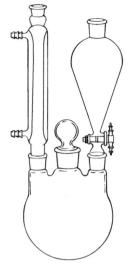

B. Macroscale, for larger amounts.

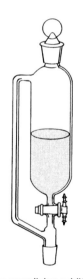

C. A pressure-equalizing addition funnel.

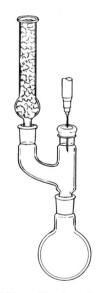

D. Addition with a hypodermic syringe inserted through a rubber septum.

Figure 7.9   Methods for adding liquid reagents to a reaction.

Figure 7.9B. Drying tubes may also be used with this apparatus to prevent contamination from atmospheric moisture.

Figure 7.9C shows an alternative type of addition funnel that is useful for reactions that must be maintained under an atmosphere of inert gas. This is the **pressure-equalizing addition funnel.** With this glassware, the upper opening is stoppered. The sidearm allows the pressure above the liquid in the funnel to be in equilibrium with the pressure in the rest of the apparatus, and it allows the inert gas to flow over the top of the liquid as it is being added.

With either type of macroscale addition funnel, you can control the rate of addition of the liquid by carefully adjusting the stopcock. Even after careful adjustment, changes in pressure can occur, causing the flow rate to change. In some cases, the stopcock can become clogged. It is important, therefore, to monitor the addition rate carefully and to refine the adjustment of the stopcock as needed to maintain the desired rate of addition.

A fourth method, shown in Figure 7.9D, is suitable for use in microscale and some macroscale experiments where the reaction should be kept isolated from the atmosphere. In this approach, the liquid is kept in a hypodermic syringe. The syringe needle is inserted through a rubber septum, and the liquid is added dropwise from the syringe. The septum seals the apparatus from the atmosphere, which makes this technique useful for reactions that are conducted under an atmosphere of inert gas or in which anhydrous conditions must be maintained. The drying tube is used to protect the reaction mixture from atmospheric moisture.

7.6 DRYING TUBES

With certain reactions, atmospheric moisture must be prevented from entering the reaction vessel. A **drying tube** can be used to maintain anhydrous conditions within the apparatus. Two types of drying tubes are shown in Figure 7.10. The typical drying tube is prepared by placing a small, loose plug of glass wool or cotton into the constriction at the end of the tube nearest the ground-glass joint or hose connection. The plug is tamped gently with a glass rod or piece of wire to place it in the correct position. A drying agent, typically calcium sulfate ("Drierite") or calcium chloride (see Technique 12, Section 12.9, p. 713), is poured on top of the plug to the approximate depth shown in Figure 7.10. Another loose plug of glass wool or cotton is placed on top of the drying agent to prevent the solid material from falling out of the drying tube. The drying tube is then attached to the flask or condenser.

Air that enters the apparatus must pass through the drying tube. The drying agent absorbs any moisture from air passing through it so that air entering the reaction vessel has had the water vapor removed from it.

7.7 REACTIONS CONDUCTED UNDER AN INERT ATMOSPHERE

Some reactions are very sensitive to oxygen and water vapor present in air and require an inert atmosphere in order to obtain satisfactory results. The usual reactions in which it is desirable to exclude air often include organometallic reagents, such as organomagnesium or organo-

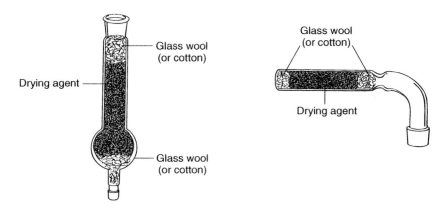

A. Macroscale drying tube.   B. Microscale drying tube.

Figure 7.10 Drying tubes.

lithium reagents, where water vapor and oxygen (air) react with these compounds. The most common inert gases available in a laboratory are nitrogen and argon, which are available in gas cylinders. Nitrogen is probably the gas most often used to carry out reactions under an inert atmosphere, although argon has a distinct advantage because it is denser than air. This allows the argon to push air away from the reaction mixture.

When laboratories are not equipped with individual gas lines to benches or hoods, it is very useful to supply nitrogen or argon to the reaction apparatus using a balloon assembly (shown in Figure 7.11). Your instructor will provide you with the apparatus.

Construct the balloon assembly by cutting off the top of a 3-mL disposable plastic syringe. Attach a small balloon snugly to the top of the syringe, securing it with a small rubber band that has been doubled to hold the balloon securely to the body of the syringe. Attach a needle to the syringe. Fill the balloon with the inert gas through the needle using a piece of rubber tubing attached to the gas source. When the balloon has been inflated to 2–3 inches in diameter, quickly pinch off the neck of the balloon while removing the gas source. Now push the needle into a rubber stopper to keep the balloon inflated. It is possible to keep an assembly like this filled with inert gas for several days without the balloon deflating.

Before you start the reaction, you may need to dry your apparatus thoroughly in an oven. Add all reagents carefully to avoid water. The following instructions are based on the assumption that you are using an apparatus consisting of a round-bottom flask equipped with a condenser. Attach a rubber septum to the top of your condenser. Now flush the air out of the apparatus with the inert gas. It is best not to use the balloon assembly for this purpose, unless you are using argon (see next paragraph). Instead, remove the round-bottom flask from the apparatus and, with the help of your instructor, flush it with the inert gas using a Pasteur pipet to bubble the gas through the solvent and reaction mixture in the flask. In this way, you can remove air from the reaction assembly prior to attaching the balloon assembly. Quickly reattach the flask to the apparatus. Pinch off the neck of the balloon between your fingers, remove the rubber stopper, and insert the needle into the rubber septum. The reaction apparatus is now ready for use.

When argon is employed as an inert gas, you can use the balloon assembly to remove

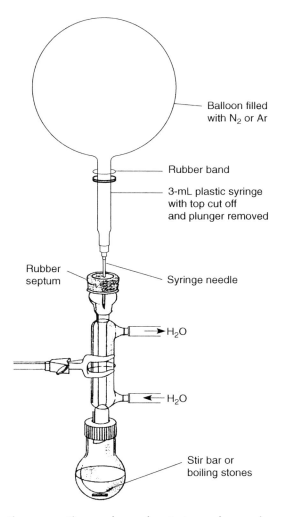

Figure 7.11 Conducting a reaction under an inert atmosphere using a balloon assembly.

air from the reaction apparatus in the following way. Insert the balloon assembly into the rubber septum as previously described. Also insert a second needle (no syringe attached) through the septum. The pressure from the balloon will force argon down the reflux condenser (argon is denser than air) and push the less dense air out through the second syringe needle. When the apparatus has been thoroughly flushed with argon, remove the second needle. Nitrogen does not work as well with this method because it is less dense than air and it will be difficult to remove the air that is in contact with the reaction mixture in the round-bottom flask.

For reactions conducted at room temperature, you can remove the condenser shown in Figure 7.11. Attach the rubber septum directly to the round-bottom flask and insert the needle of an argon-filled balloon assembly through the rubber septum. To flush the air out of the reaction flask, insert a second syringe needle into the rubber septum. Any air present in the flask will be flushed out through this second syringe needle, and the air will be replaced with argon. Now remove the second needle, and you have a reaction mixture free of air.

7.8 CAPTURING NOXIOUS GASES

Many organic reactions involve the production of a noxious gaseous product. The gas may be corrosive, such as hydrogen chloride, hydrogen bromide, or sulfur dioxide, or it may be toxic, such as carbon monoxide. The safest way to avoid exposure to these gases is to conduct the reaction in a ventilated hood where the gases can be safely drawn away by the ventilation system.

In many instances, however, it is quite safe and efficient to conduct the experiment on the laboratory bench, away from the hood. This is particularly true when the gases are soluble in water. Some techniques for capturing noxious gases are presented in this section.

A. External Gas Traps

One approach to capturing gases is to prepare a trap that is separate from the reaction apparatus. The gases are carried from the reaction to the trap by means of tubing. There are several variations on this type of trap. With macroscale reactions, a trap using an inverted funnel placed in a beaker of water is used. A piece of glass tubing, inserted through a thermometer adapter attached to the reaction apparatus, is connected to flexible tubing. The tubing is attached to a conical funnel. The funnel is clamped in place inverted over a beaker of water. The funnel is clamped so that its lip *almost touches* the water surface but is not placed below the surface of the water. With this arrangement, water cannot be sucked back into the reaction if the pressure in the reaction vessel changes suddenly. This type of trap can also be used in microscale applications. An example of the inverted-funnel type of gas trap is shown in Figure 7.12.

One method that works well for macroscale and microscale experiments is to place a thermometer adapter into the opening in the reaction apparatus. A Pasteur pipet is inserted upside down through the adapter, and a piece of flexible tubing is fitted over the narrow tip. It might be helpful to break the Pasteur pipet before using it for this purpose so that only the narrow tip and a short section of the barrel are used. The other end of the flexible tubing is placed through a large plug of moistened glass wool in a test tube. The water in the glass wool absorbs the water-soluble gases. This method is shown in Figure 7.13.

B. Drying-Tube Method

Some macroscale and most microscale experiments have the advantage that the amounts of gases produced are very small. Hence, it is easy to trap them and prevent them from escaping into the laboratory room. You can take advantage of the water solubility of corrosive gases such as hydrogen chloride, hydrogen bromide, and sulfur dioxide. A simple technique is to attach the drying tube (see Figure 7.10) to the top of the reaction flask or condenser. The drying tube is filled with moistened glass wool. The moisture in the glass wool absorbs the gas, preventing its escape. To prepare this type of gas trap, fill the drying tube with glass wool and then add water dropwise to the glass wool until it has been moistened to the desired degree. Moistened cotton can also be used, although cotton will absorb so much water that it is easy to plug the drying tube.

When using glass wool in a drying tube, moisture from the glass wool must not be al-

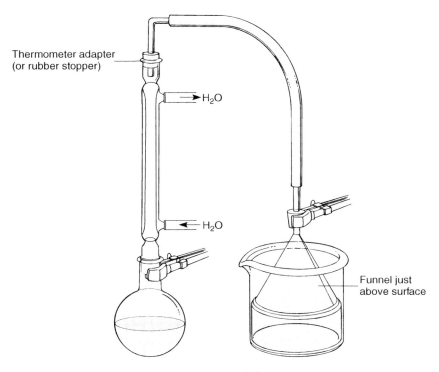

Figure 7.12 An inverted-funnel gas trap.

lowed to drain from the drying tube into the reaction. It is best to use a drying tube that has a constriction between the part where the glass wool is placed and the neck, where the joint is attached (see Figure 7.10B). The constriction acts as a partial barrier preventing the water from leaking into the neck of the drying tube. Make certain not to make the glass wool too moist. When it is necessary to use the drying tube shown in Figure 7.10A as a gas trap and it is essential that water not be allowed to enter the reaction flask, the modification shown in Figure 7.14 should be used. The rubber tubing between the thermometer adapter and the drying tube should be heavy enough to prevent crimping.

C. Removal of Noxious Gases Using an Aspirator

An aspirator can be used to remove noxious gases from the reaction. The simplest approach is to clamp a disposable Pasteur pipet so that its tip is placed well into the condenser atop the reaction flask. An inverted funnel clamped over the apparatus can also be used. The pipet or funnel is attached to an aspirator with flexible tubing. A trap should be placed between the pipet or funnel and the aspirator. As gases are liberated from the reaction, they rise into the condenser. The vacuum draws the gases away from the apparatus. Both types of systems are shown in Figure 7.15. In the special case in which the noxious gases are soluble in water, connecting a water aspirator to the pipet or funnel removes the gases from the reaction and traps them in the flowing water without the need for a separate gas trap.

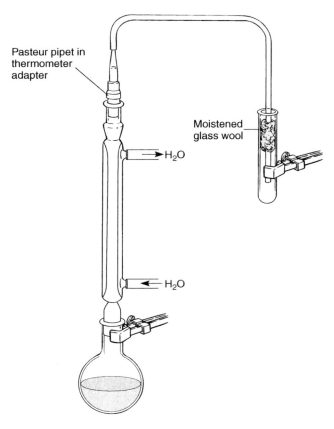

Pasteur pipet in
thermometer
adapter

Moistened
glass wool

H_2O

H_2O

Figure 7.13 An external gas trap.

7.9 COLLECTING GASEOUS PRODUCTS

In Section 7.8, means for removing unwanted gaseous products from the reaction system were examined. Some experiments produce gaseous products that you must collect and analyze. Methods to collect gaseous products are all based on the same principle. The gas is carried through tubing from the reaction to the opening of a flask or a test tube, which has been filled with water and is inverted in a container of water. The gas is allowed to bubble into the inverted collection tube (or flask). As the collection tube fills with gas, the water is displaced into the water container. If the collection tube is graduated, as in a graduated cylinder or a centrifuge tube, you can monitor the quantity of gas produced in the reaction.

If the inverted gas collection tube is constructed from a piece of glass tubing, a rubber septum can be used to close the upper end of the container. This type of collection tube is shown in Figure 7.16. A sample of the gas can be removed using a gas-tight syringe equipped with a needle. The gas that is removed can be analyzed by gas chromatography (see Technique 22).

In Figure 7.16, a piece of glass tubing is attached to the free end of the flexible hose. This piece of glass tubing sometimes makes it easier to fix the open end in the proper position in the opening of the collection tube or flask. The other end of the flexible tubing is at-

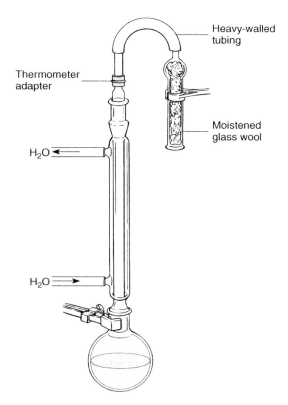

Figure 7.14 A drying tube used to capture evolved gases.

tached to a piece of glass tubing or a Pasteur pipet that has been inserted into a thermometer adapter.

7.10 EVAPORATION OF SOLVENTS

In many experiments, it is necessary to remove excess solvent from a solution. An obvious approach is to allow the container to stand unstoppered in the hood for several hours until the solvent has evaporated. This method is generally not practical, however, and a quicker, more efficient means of evaporating solvents must be used.

Caution: You must always evaporate solvents in the hood.

A. Large-Scale Methods

A large-scale method to remove excess solvent is to evaporate the solvent from an open Erlenmeyer flask (Figure 7.17A and B). Such an evaporation must be conducted in a hood, because many solvent vapors are toxic or flammable. A boiling stone must be used.

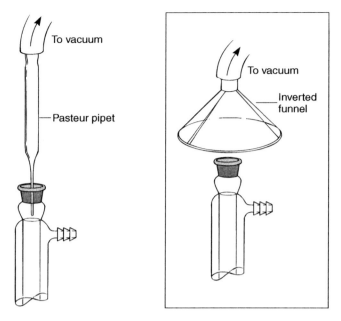

Figure 7.15 Removal of noxious gases under vacuum. (The inset shows an alternative assembly, using an inverted funnel in place of the Pasteur pipet.)

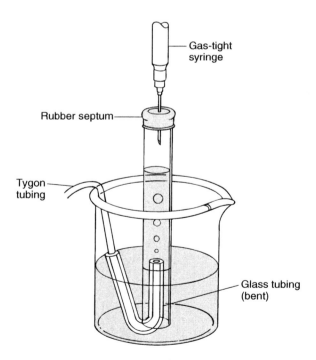

Figure 7.16 A gas collection tube, with rubber septum.

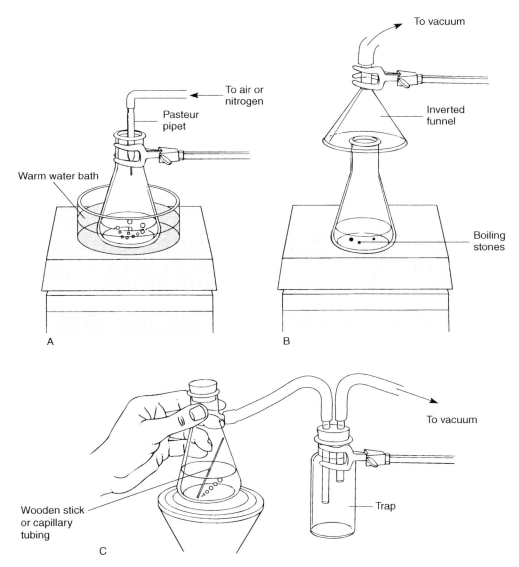

Figure 7.17 Evaporation of solvents (heat source can be varied among those shown).

A gentle stream of air directed toward the surface of the liquid will remove vapors that are in equilibrium with the solution and accelerate the evaporation. A Pasteur pipet connected by a short piece of rubber tubing to the compressed air line will act as a convenient air nozzle (Figure 7.17A). A tube or an inverted funnel connected to an aspirator may also be used (Figure 7.17B). In this case, vapors are removed by suction. It is better to use an Erlenmeyer flask than a beaker for this procedure because deposits of solid will usually build up on the sides of the beaker where the solvent evaporates. The refluxing action in an Erlenmeyer flask does not allow this buildup. If a hot plate is used as the heat source, care must be taken with flammable solvents to ensure against fires caused by "flashing," when solvent vapors come into contact with the hot-plate surface.

It is also possible to remove low-boiling solvents under reduced pressure (Fig-

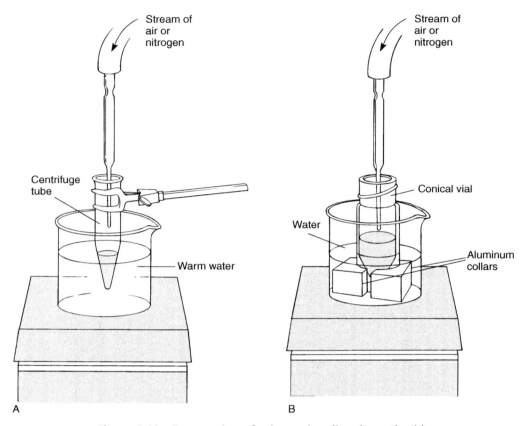

Figure 7.18 Evaporation of solvents (small-scale methods).

ure 7.17C). In this method, the solution is placed in a filter flask, along with a wooden applicator stick or a short length of capillary tubing. The flask is stoppered, and the sidearm is connected to an aspirator (by a trap), as described in Technique 8, Section 8.3, p. 651. Under reduced pressure, the solvent begins to boil. The wooden stick or capillary tubing serves the same function as a boiling stone. By this method, solvent can be evaporated from a solution without using much heat. This technique is often used when heating the solution might decompose thermally sensitive substances. The method has the disadvantage that when low-boiling solvents are used, solvent evaporation cools the flask below the freezing point of water. When this happens, a layer of frost forms on the outside of the flask. Because frost is insulating, it must be removed to keep evaporation proceeding at a reasonable rate. Frost is best removed by one of two methods: either the flask is placed in a bath of warm water (with constant swirling) or it is heated on the steam bath (again with swirling). Either method promotes efficient heat transfer.

Large amounts of a solvent should be removed by distillation (see Technique 14). *Never evaporate ether solutions to dryness,* except on a steam bath or by the reduced-pressure method. The tendency of ether to form explosive peroxides is a serious potential hazard. If peroxides should be present, the large and rapid temperature increase in the flask once the ether evaporates could bring about the detonation of any residual peroxides. The temperature of a steam bath is not high enough to cause such a detonation.

B. Small-Scale Methods

A simple means of evaporating a small amount of solvent is to place a centrifuge tube in a warm water bath. The heat from the water bath will warm the solvent to a temperature at which it can evaporate within a short time. The heat from the water can be adjusted to provide the best rate of evaporation, but the liquid should not be allowed to boil vigorously. The evaporation rate can be increased by allowing a stream of dry air or nitrogen to be directed into the centrifuge tube (Figure 7.18A). The moving gas stream will sweep the vapors from the tube and accelerate the evaporation. As an alternative, a vacuum can be applied above the tube to draw away solvent vapors.

A convenient water bath suitable for microscale methods can be constructed by placing the aluminum collars, which are generally used with aluminum heating blocks, into a 150-mL beaker (Figure 7.18B). In some cases, it may be necessary to round off the sharp edges of the collars with a file in order to allow them to fit properly into the beaker. Held by the aluminum collars, the conical vial will stand securely in the beaker. This assembly can be filled with water and placed on a hot plate for use in the evaporation of small amounts of solvent.

7.11 ROTARY EVAPORATOR

In some organic chemistry laboratories, solvents are evaporated under reduced pressure using a **rotary evaporator.** This is a motor-driven device that is designed for rapid evaporation of solvents, with heating, while minimizing the possibility of bumping. A vacuum is applied to the flask, and the motor spins the flask. The rotation of the flask spreads a thin film of the liquid over the surface of the glass, which accelerates evaporation. The rotation also agitates the solution sufficiently to reduce the problem of bumping. A water bath can be placed under the flask to warm the solution and increase the vapor pressure of the solvent. One can select the speed at which the flask is rotated and the temperature of the water bath to attain the desired evaporation rate. As the solvent evaporates from the rotating flask, the vapors are cooled by the condenser, and the resulting liquid collects in the flask. The product remains behind in the rotating flask. A complete rotary evaporator assembly is shown in Figure 7.19. If the coolant is sufficiently cold, virtually all of the solvent can be recovered and recycled. This is a good example of *Green Chemistry* (see Green Chemistry essay, p. 254).

PROBLEMS

1. What is the best type of stirring device to use for stirring a reaction that takes place in the following type of glassware?
   a. A conical vial
   b. A 10-mL round-bottom flask
   c. A 250-mL round-bottom flask
2. Should you use a drying tube for the following reaction? Explain.

$$CH_3-\overset{\overset{\displaystyle O}{\|}}{C}-OH + CH_3-\underset{\underset{\displaystyle CH_3}{|}}{C}H-CH_2-CH_2-OH \rightleftharpoons CH_3-\overset{\overset{\displaystyle O}{\|}}{C}-O-CH_2-CH_2-\underset{\underset{\displaystyle CH_3}{|}}{C}H-CH_3 + H_2O$$

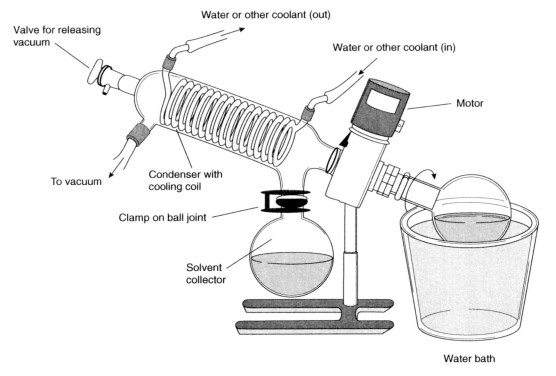

Water or other coolant (out)

Valve for releasing
vacuum

Water or other coolant (in)

Motor

To vacuum

Condenser with
cooling coil

Clamp on ball joint

Solvent
collector

Water bath

Figure 7.19   A rotary evaporator.

3. For which of the following reactions should you use a trap to collect noxious gases?

a. Benzoic acid + SOCl₂ $\xrightarrow{\text{heat}}$ benzoyl chloride + SO₂ + HCl

b. Benzoyl chloride + CH₃—CH₂—OH ⟶ ethyl benzoate + HCl

c. $C_{12}H_{22}O_{11} + H_2O \longrightarrow 4\,CH_3-CH_2-OH + 4\,CO_2$
   (Sucrose)

d. $CH_3-\underset{H}{C}=NH + H_2O \xrightarrow[\text{heat}]{\text{base}} CH_3-\underset{H}{C}=O + NH_3$

4. Criticize the following techniques:
   a. A reflux is conducted with a stopper in the top of the condenser.
   b. Water is passed through the reflux condenser at the rate of 1 gallon per minute.
   c. No water hoses are attached to the condenser during a reflux.
   d. A boiling stone is not added to the round-bottom flask until the mixture is boiling vigorously.
   e. To save money, you decide to save your boiling stones for another experiment.
   f. The reflux ring is located near the top of the condenser in a reflux setup.
   g. A rubber O-ring is omitted when the water condenser is attached to a conical vial.

94

h. A gas trap is assembled with the funnel in Figure 7.12 completely submerged in the water in the beaker.

i. Powdered drying agent is used rather than granular material.

j. A reaction involving hydrogen chloride is conducted on the laboratory bench and not in a hood.

k. An air-sensitive reaction apparatus is set up as shown in Figure 7.6.

l. Air is used to evaporate solvent from an air-sensitive compound.

T E C H N I Q U E   8

Filtration

Filtration is a technique used for two main purposes. The first is to remove solid impurities from a liquid. The second is to collect a desired solid from the solution from which it was precipitated or crystallized. Several different kinds of filtration are commonly used: two general methods include gravity filtration and vacuum (or suction) filtration. Two techniques specific to the microscale laboratory are filtration with a filter-tip pipet and filtration with a Craig tube. The various filtration techniques and their applications are summarized in Table 8.1. These techniques are discussed in more detail in the following sections.

8.1 GRAVITY FILTRATION

The most familiar filtration technique is probably filtration of a solution through a paper filter held in a funnel, allowing gravity to draw the liquid through the paper. Because even a small piece of filter paper will absorb a significant volume of liquid, this technique is useful only when the volume of mixture to be filtered is greater than 10 mL. For many macroscale and microscale procedures, a more suitable technique, which also makes use of gravity, is to use a Pasteur (or disposable) pipet with a cotton or glass wool plug (called a filtering pipet).

A. Filter Cones

This filtration technique is most useful when the solid material being filtered from a mixture is to be collected and used later. The filter cone, because of its smooth sides, can easily be scraped free of collected solids. Because of the many folds, fluted filter paper, described in the next section, cannot be scraped easily. The filter cone is likely to be used in experiments only when a relatively large volume (greater than 10 mL) is being filtered and when a Büchner or Hirsch funnel (Section 8.3) is not appropriate.

The filter cone is prepared as indicated in Figure 8.1. It is then placed into a funnel of an appropriate size. With filtrations using a simple filter cone, solvent may form seals between the filter and the funnel and between the funnel and the lip of the receiving flask. When a seal forms, the filtration stops because the displaced air has no possibility of escaping. To avoid the solvent seal, you can insert a small piece of paper, a paper clip, or some other bent wire between the funnel and the lip of the flask to let the displaced air escape. As an alternative, you can support the funnel by a clamp fixed *above* the flask rather than placed on the neck of the flask. A gravity filtration using a filter cone is shown in Figure 8.2.

TABLE 8.1 Filtration Methods

Method	Application	Section
Gravity filtration		
Filter cones	The volume of liquid to be filtered is about 10 mL or greater, and the solid collected in the filter is saved.	8.1A
Fluted filters	The volume of liquid to be filtered is greater than about 10 mL, and solid impurities are removed from a solution; often used in crystallization procedures.	8.1B
Filtering pipets	Used with volumes less than about 10 mL to remove solid impurities from a liquid.	8.1C
Decantation	Although not a filtration technique, decantation can be used to separate a liquid from large, insoluble particles.	8.1D
Vacuum filtration		
Büchner funnels	Primarily used to collect a desired solid from a liquid when the volume is greater than about 10 mL; used frequently to collect the crystals obtained from crystallization.	8.3
Hirsch funnels	Used in the same way as Büchner funnels, except the volume of liquid is usually smaller (1–10 mL).	8.3
Filtering media	Used to remove finely divided impurities.	8.4
Filter-tip pipets	May be used to remove a small amount of solid impurities from a small volume (1–2 mL) of liquid; also useful for pipetting volatile liquids, especially in extraction procedures.	8.6
Craig tubes	Used to collect a small amount of crystals resulting from crystallizations in which the volume of the solution is less than 2 mL.	8.7
Centrifugation	Although not strictly a filtration technique, centrifugation may be used to remove suspended impurities from a liquid (1–25 mL).	8.8

B. Fluted Filters

This filtration method is also most useful when filtering a relatively large amount of liquid. Because a fluted filter is used when the desired material is expected to remain in solution, this filter is used to remove undesired solid materials, such as dirt particles, decolorizing charcoal, and undissolved impure crystals. A fluted filter is often used to filter a hot solution saturated with a solute during a crystallization procedure.

The technique for folding a fluted filter paper is shown in Figure 8.3. An advantage of a fluted filter is that it increases the speed of filtration in two ways. First, it increases the surface area of the filter paper through which the solvent seeps; second, it allows air to enter the flask along its sides to permit rapid pressure equalization. If pressure builds up in the flask from hot vapors, filtering slows down. This problem is especially pronounced with filter cones. The fluted filter tends to reduce this problem considerably, but it may be a good idea to clamp the funnel above the receiving flask or to use a piece of

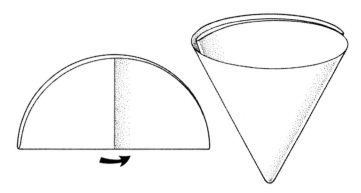

Figure 8.1 Folding a filter cone.

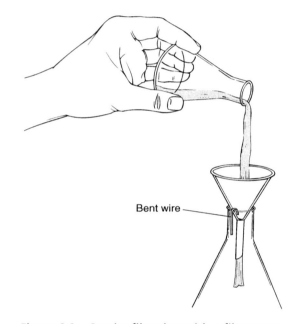

Bent wire ——

Figure 8.2 Gravity filtration with a filter cone.

paper, paper clip, or wire between the funnel and the lip of the flask as an added precaution against solvent seals.

Filtration with a fluted filter is relatively easy to perform when the mixture is at room temperature. However, when it is necessary to filter a hot solution saturated with a dissolved solute, a number of steps must be taken to ensure that the filter does not become clogged by solid material accumulated in the stem of the funnel or in the filter paper. When the hot, saturated solution comes in contact with a relatively cold funnel (or a cold flask, for that matter), the solution is cooled and may become supersaturated. If crystallization then occurs in the filter, either the crystals will fail to pass through the filter paper or they will clog the stem of the funnel.

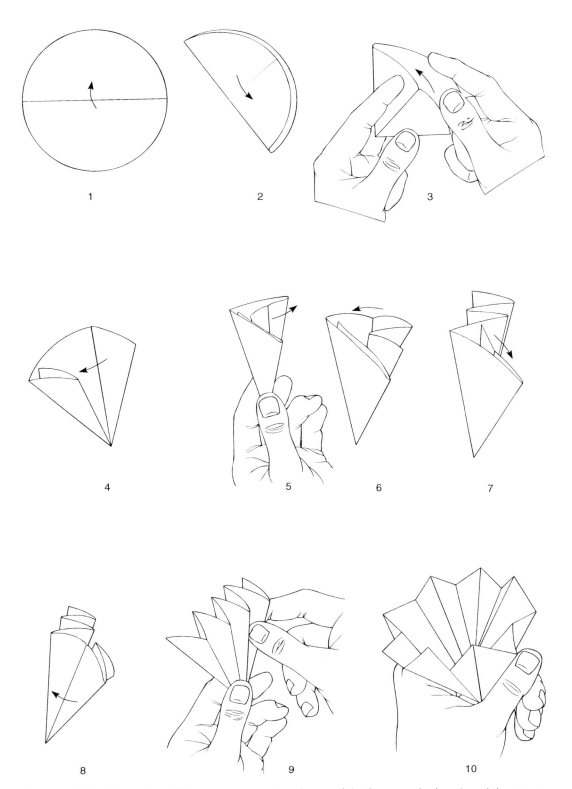

Figure 8.3 Folding a fluted filter paper, or origami at work in the organic chemistry laboratory.

To keep the filter from clogging, use one of the following four methods. The first is to use a short-stemmed or a stemless funnel. With these funnels, it is less likely that the stem of the funnel will become clogged by solid material. The second method is to keep the liquid to be filtered at or near its boiling point at all times. The third way is to preheat the funnel by pouring hot solvent through it before the actual filtration. This keeps the cold glass from causing instantaneous crystallization. And fourth, it is helpful to keep the **filtrate** (filtered solution) in the receiver hot enough to continue boiling *slightly* (by setting it on a hot plate, for example). The refluxing solvent heats the receiving flask and the funnel stem and washes them clean of solids. This boiling of the filtrate also keeps the liquid in the funnel warm.

C. Filtering Pipets

A filtering pipet is a microscale technique most often used to remove solid impurities from a liquid with a volume less than 10 mL. It is important that the mixture being filtered be at or near room temperature because it is difficult to prevent premature crystallization in a hot solution saturated with a solute.

To prepare this filtration device, a small piece of cotton is inserted into the top of a Pasteur (disposable) pipet and pushed down to the beginning of the lower constriction in the pipet, as shown in Figure 8.4. It is important to use enough cotton to collect all the solid being filtered; however, the amount of cotton used should not be so large that the flow rate

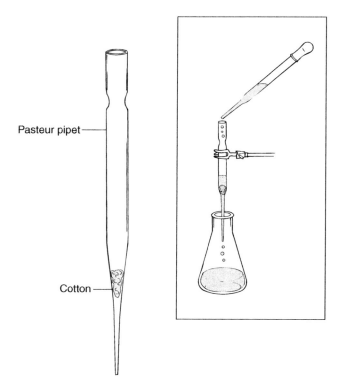

Pasteur pipet

Cotton

Figure 8.4 A filtering pipet.

through the pipet is significantly restricted. For the same reason, the cotton should not be packed too tightly. The cotton plug can be pushed down gently with a long thin object such as a glass stirring rod or a wooden applicator stick. It is advisable to wash the cotton plug by passing about 1 mL of solvent (usually the same solvent that is to be filtered) through the filter.

In some cases, such as when filtering a strongly acidic mixture or when performing a very rapid filtration to remove dirt or impurities of large particle size from a solution, it may be better to use glass wool in place of the cotton. The disadvantage in using glass wool is that the fibers do not pack together as tightly, and small particles will pass through the filter more easily.

To conduct a filtration (with either a cotton or glass wool plug), the filtering pipet is clamped so that the filtrate will drain into an appropriate container. The mixture to be filtered is usually transferred to the filtering pipet with another Pasteur pipet. If a small volume of liquid is being filtered (less than 1 mL or 2 mL), it is advisable to rinse the filter and plug with a small amount of solvent after the last of the filtrate has passed through the filter. The rinse solvent is then combined with the original filtrate. If desired, the rate of filtration can be increased by gently applying pressure to the top of the pipet using a pipet bulb.

Depending on the amount of solid being filtered and the size of the particles (small particles are more difficult to remove by filtration), it may be necessary to put the filtrate through a second filtering pipet. This should be done with a new filtering pipet rather than with the one already used.

D. Decantation

It is not always necessary to use filter paper to separate insoluble particles. If you have large, heavy, insoluble particles, with careful pouring you can decant the solution, leaving behind the solid particles that will settle to the bottom of the flask. The term *decant* means "to carefully pour out the liquid, leaving the insoluble particles behind." For example, boiling stones or sand granules in the bottom of an Erlenmeyer flask filled with a liquid can easily be separated in this way. This procedure is often preferred over filtration and usually results in a smaller loss of material. If there are a large number of particles and they retain a significant amount of the liquid, they can be rinsed with solvent and a second decantation performed. The term *decant* was coined in the wine industry, where it is often necessary to let the wine settle and then carefully pour it out of the original bottle into a clean one, leaving the "must" (insoluble particles) behind.

8.2 FILTER PAPER

Many kinds and grades of filter paper are available. The paper must be correct for a given application. In choosing filter paper, you should be aware of its various properties. **Porosity** is a measure of the size of the particles that can pass through the paper. Highly porous paper does not remove small particles from solution; paper with low porosity removes very small particles. **Retentivity** is a property that is the opposite of porosity. Paper with low retentivity does not remove small particles from the filtrate. The **speed** of filter paper is a measure of the time it takes a liquid to drain through the filter. Fast paper allows the liquid to drain quickly; with slow paper, it takes much longer to complete the filtration. Be-

TABLE 8.2 Some Common Qualitative Filter Paper Types and Approximate Relative Speeds and Retentivities

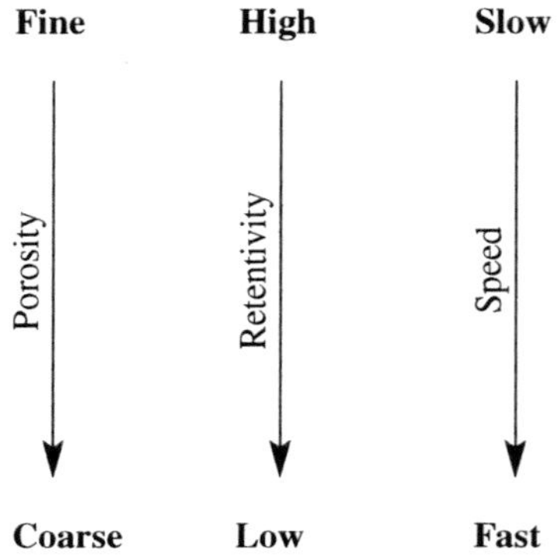

				Type (by number)		
			Speed	E&D	S&S	Whatman
			Very slow	610	576	5
			Slow	613	602	3
			Medium	615	597	2
			Fast	617	595	1
			Very fast	—	604	4

Fine / Porosity ↓ Coarse

High / Retentivity ↓ Low

Slow / Speed ↓ Fast

cause all these properties are related, fast filter paper usually has a low retentivity and high porosity, and slow filter paper usually has high retentivity and low porosity.

Table 8.2 compares some commonly available qualitative filter paper types and ranks them according to porosity, retentivity, and speed. Eaton–Dikeman (E&D), Schleicher and Schuell (S&S), and Whatman are the most common brands of filter paper. The numbers in the table refer to the grades of paper used by each company.

8.3 VACUUM FILTRATION

Vacuum, or suction, filtration is more rapid than gravity filtration and is most often used to collect solid products resulting from precipitation or crystallization. This technique is used primarily when the volume of liquid being filtered is more than 1–2 mL. With smaller volumes, use of the Craig tube (Section 8.7) is the preferred technique. In a vacuum filtration, a receiver flask with a sidearm, a **filter flask,** is used. For macroscale laboratory work, the most useful sizes of filter flasks range from 50 mL to 500 mL, depending on the volume of liquid being filtered. For microscale work, the most useful size is a 50-mL filter flask. The sidearm is connected by *heavy-walled* rubber tubing (see Technique 16, Figure 16.2, p. 767) to a source of vacuum. Thin-walled tubing will collapse under vacuum, due to atmospheric pressure on its outside walls, and will seal the vacuum source from the flask. Because this apparatus is unstable and can tip over easily, it must be clamped, as shown in Figure 8.5.

Caution: It is essential that the filter flask be clamped.

Two types of funnels are useful for vacuum filtration, the Büchner funnel and the Hirsch funnel. The **Büchner funnel** is used for filtering larger amounts of solid from solution in macroscale applications. Büchner funnels are usually made from polypropylene or

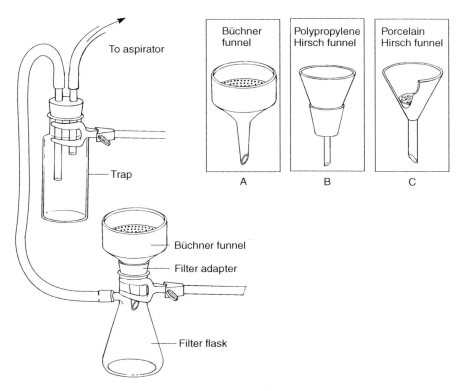

Figure 8.5 Vacuum filtration.

porcelain. A Büchner funnel (see Figures 8.5 and 8.5A) is sealed to the filter flask by a rubber stopper or a filter (neoprene) adapter. The flat bottom of the Büchner funnel is covered with an unfolded piece of circular filter paper. To prevent the escape of solid materials from the funnel, you must be certain that the filter paper fits the funnel exactly. It must cover all the holes in the bottom of the funnel but not extend up the sides. Before beginning the filtration, it is advisable to moisten the paper with a small amount of solvent. The moistened filter paper adheres more strongly to the bottom of the funnel and prevents unfiltered mixture from passing around the edges of the filter paper.

The **Hirsch funnel,** which is shown in Figures 8.5B and C, operates on the same principle as the Büchner funnel, but it is usually smaller, and its sides are sloped rather than vertical. The Hirsch funnel is used primarily in microscale experiments. The polypropylene Hirsch funnel (see Figure 8.5B) is sealed to a 50-mL filter flask by a small section of Gooch tubing or a one-hole rubber stopper. This Hirsch funnel has a built-in adapter that forms a tight seal with some 25-mL filter flasks without the Gooch tubing. A polyethylene fritted disk fits into the bottom of the funnel. To prevent the holes in this disk from becoming clogged with solid material, the funnel should always be used with a circular filter paper that has the same diameter (1.27 cm) as the polyethylene disk. With a polypropylene Hirsch funnel, it is also important to moisten the paper with a small amount of solvent before beginning the filtration.

The porcelain Hirsch funnel is sealed to the filter flask with a rubber stopper or a neoprene adapter. In this Hirsch funnel, the filter paper must also cover all the holes in the bottom but must not extend up the sides.

Because the filter flask is attached to a source of vacuum, a solution poured into a Büchner funnel or Hirsch funnel is literally "sucked" rapidly through the filter paper. For this reason, vacuum filtration is generally not used to separate fine particles such as decolorizing charcoal, because the small particles would likely be pulled through the filter paper. However, this problem can be alleviated, when desired, by the use of specially prepared filter beds (see Section 8.4).

8.4 FILTERING MEDIA

It is occasionally necessary to use specially prepared filter beds to separate fine particles when using vacuum filtration. Often, very fine particles either pass right through a paper filter or clog it so completely that the filtering stops. This is avoided by using a substance called Filter Aid, or Celite. This material is also called **diatomaceous earth** because of its source. It is a finely divided inert material derived from the microscopic shells of dead diatoms (a type of phytoplankton that grows in the sea).

> **Caution:** Diatomaceous earth is a lung irritant. When using Filter Aid, take care not to breathe the dust.

Filter Aid will not clog the fiber pores of filter paper. It is **slurried,** mixed with a solvent to form a rather thin paste, and filtered through a Hirsch or Büchner funnel (with filter paper in place) until a layer of diatoms about 2–3 mm thick is formed on top of the filter paper. The solvent in which the diatoms were slurried is poured from the filter flask, and, if necessary, the filter flask is cleaned before the actual filtration is begun. Finely divided particles can now be suction-filtered through this layer and will be caught in the Filter Aid. This technique is used for removing impurities, not for collecting a product. The filtrate (filtered solution) is the desired material in this procedure. If the material caught in the filter were the desired material, you would have to try to separate the product from all those diatoms! Filtration with Filter Aid is not appropriate when the desired substance is likely to precipitate or crystallize from solution.

In microscale work, it may sometimes be more convenient to use a column prepared with a Pasteur pipet to separate fine particles from a solution. The Pasteur pipet is packed with alumina or silica gel, as shown in Figure 8.6.

8.5 THE ASPIRATOR

The most common source of vacuum (approximately 10–20 mmHg) in the laboratory is the water aspirator, or "water pump," illustrated in Figure 8.7. This device passes water rapidly past a small hole to which a sidearm is attached. The water pulls air in through the

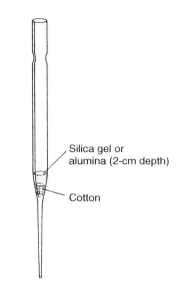

Figure 8.6 A Pasteur pipet with filtering media.

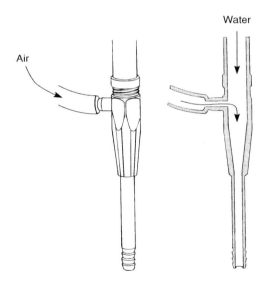

Figure 8.7 An aspirator.

sidearm. This phenomenon, called the Bernoulli effect, causes a reduced pressure along the side of the rapidly moving water stream and creates a partial vacuum in the sidearm.

> **Note:** The aspirator works most effectively when the water is turned on to the fullest extent.

A water aspirator can never lower the pressure beyond the vapor pressure of the water used to create the vacuum. Hence, there is a lower limit to the pressure (on cold days)

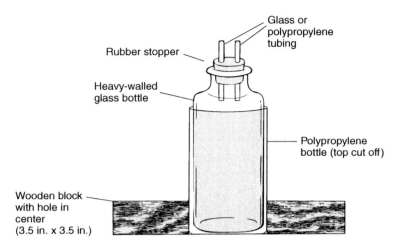

Glass or
polypropylene
tubing

Rubber stopper

Heavy-walled
glass bottle

Polypropylene
bottle (top cut off)

Wooden block
with hole in
center
(3.5 in. x 3.5 in.)

Figure 8.8 A simple aspirator trap and holder.

of 9–10 mmHg. A water aspirator does not provide as high a vacuum in the summer as in the winter, due to this water-temperature effect.

A trap must be used with an aspirator. One type of trap is illustrated in Figure 8.5. Another method for securing this type of trap is shown in Figure 8.8. This simple holder can be constructed from readily available material and can be placed anywhere on the laboratory bench. Although not often needed, a trap can prevent water from contaminating your experiment. If the water pressure in the laboratory drops suddenly, the pressure in the filter flask may suddenly become lower than the pressure in the water aspirator. This would cause water to be drawn from the aspirator stream into the filter flask and contaminate the filtrate or even the material in the filter. The trap stops this reverse flow. A similar flow will occur if the water flow at the aspirator is stopped before the tubing connected to the aspirator side-arm is disconnected.

Note: Always disconnect the tubing before stopping the aspirator.

If a "backup" begins, disconnect the tubing as rapidly as possible before the trap fills with water. Some chemists like to fit a stopcock into the stopper on top of the trap. A three-hole stopper is required for this purpose. With a stopcock in the trap, the system can be vented before the aspirator is shut off. Then water cannot back up into the trap.

Aspirators do not work well if too many people use the water line at the same time because the water pressure is lowered. Also, the sinks at the ends of the lab benches or the lines that carry away the water flow may have a limited capacity for draining the resultant water flow from too many aspirators. Care must be taken to avoid floods.

8.6 FILTER-TIP PIPET

The filter-tip pipet, illustrated in Figure 8.9, has two common uses. The first is to remove a small amount of solid, such as dirt or filter paper fibers, from a small volume of liq-

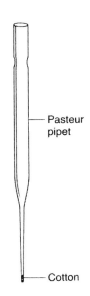

Pasteur pipet

Cotton

Figure 8.9 A filter-tip pipet.

uid (1–2 mL). It can also be helpful when using a Pasteur pipet to transfer a highly volatile liquid, especially during an extraction procedure (see Technique 12, Section 12.5, p. 706).

Preparing a filter-tip pipet is similar to preparing a filtering pipet, except that a much smaller amount of cotton is used. A *very tiny* piece of cotton is loosely shaped into a ball and placed into the large end of a Pasteur pipet. Using a wire with a diameter slightly smaller than the inside diameter of the narrow end of the pipet, push the ball of cotton to the bottom of the pipet. If it becomes difficult to push the cotton, you have probably started with too much cotton; if the cotton slides through the narrow end with little resistance, you probably have not used enough.

To use a filter-tip pipet as a filter, the mixture is drawn up into the Pasteur pipet using a pipet bulb and then expelled. With this procedure, a small amount of solid will be captured by the cotton. However, very fine particles, such as activated charcoal, cannot be removed efficiently with a filter-tip pipet, and this technique is not effective in removing more than a trace amount of solid from a liquid.

Transferring many organic liquids with a Pasteur pipet can be a somewhat difficult procedure for two reasons. First, the liquid may not adhere well to the glass. Second, as you handle the Pasteur pipet, the temperature of the liquid in the pipet increases slightly, and the increased vapor pressure may tend to "squirt" the liquid out the end of the pipet. This problem can be particularly troublesome when separating two liquids during an extraction procedure. The purpose of the cotton plug in this situation is to slow the rate of flow through the end of the pipet so you can control the movement of liquid in the Pasteur pipet more easily.

8.7 CRAIG TUBES

The **Craig tube,** illustrated in Figure 8.10, is used primarily to separate crystals from a solution after a microscale crystallization procedure has been performed (Technique 11,

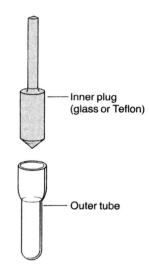

Figure 8.10 A Craig tube (2 mL).

Section 11.4, p. 689). Although it may not be a filtration procedure in the traditional sense, the outcome is similar. The outer part of the Craig tube is similar to a test tube, except that the diameter of the tube becomes wider part of the way up the tube, and the glass is ground at this point so that the inside surface is rough. The inner part (plug) of the Craig tube may be made of Teflon or glass. If this part is glass, the end of the plug is also ground. With either a glass or a Teflon inner plug, there is only a partial seal where the plug and the outer tube come together. Liquid may pass through, but solid will not. This is the place where the solution is separated from the crystals.

After crystallization has been completed in the outer Craig tube, replace the inner plug (if necessary) and connect a thin copper wire or strong thread to the narrow part of the inner plug, as indicated in Figure 8.11A. While holding the Craig tube in an upright position, place a plastic centrifuge tube over the Craig tube so that the bottom of the centrifuge tube rests on top of the inner plug, as shown in Figure 8.11B. The copper wire should extend just below the lip of the centrifuge tube and is now bent upward around the lip of the centrifuge tube. This apparatus is then turned over so that the centrifuge tube is in an upright position. The Craig tube is spun in a centrifuge (be sure it is balanced by placing another tube filled with water on the opposite side of the centrifuge) for several minutes until the **mother liquor** (solution from which the crystals grew) goes to the bottom of the centrifuge tube and the crystals collect on the end of the inner plug (see Figure 8.11C). Depending on the consistency of the crystals and the speed of the centrifuge, the crystals may spin down to the inner plug, or (if you are unlucky) they may remain at the other end of the Craig tube.[1] If the latter situation occurs, it may be helpful to centrifuge the Craig tube longer or, if this

---

[1] Note to the instructor: In some centrifuges, the bottom of the Craig tube may be very close to the center of the centrifuge when the Craig tube assembly is placed into the centrifuge. In this situation, very little centrifugal force will be applied to the crystals, and it likely that the crystals will not spin down. It may then be helpful to use an inner plug with a shorter stem. The stem on a Teflon inner plug can be easily cut off about 0.5 inch with a pair of wire cutters. This will help to spin down the crystals to the inner plug and also the centrifuge can be run at a lower speed, which can help prevent breakage of the Craig tube.

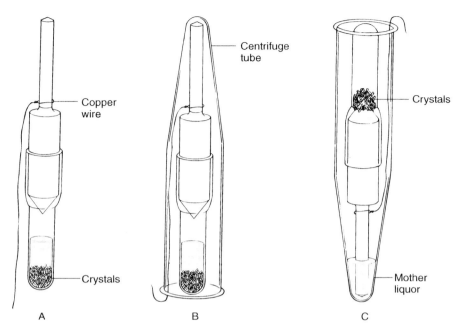

Figure 8.11 Separation with a Craig tube.

problem is anticipated, to stir the crystal-and-solution mixture with a spatula or stirring rod before centrifugation.

Using the copper wire, then pull the Craig tube out of the centrifuge tube. If the crystals collected on the end of the inner plug, it is now a simple procedure to remove the plug and scrape the crystals with a spatula onto a watch glass, a clay plate, or a piece of smooth paper. Otherwise, it will be necessary to scrape the crystals from the inside surface of the outer part of the Craig tube.

8.8 CENTRIFUGATION

Sometimes, centrifugation is more effective in removing solid impurities than conventional filtration techniques. Centrifugation is particularly effective in removing suspended particles, which are so small that the particles would pass through most filtering devices. Centrifugation may also be useful when the mixture must be kept hot to prevent premature crystallization while the solid impurities are removed.

Centrifugation is performed by placing the mixture in one or two centrifuge tubes (be sure to balance the centrifuge) and centrifuging for several minutes. The supernatant liquid is then decanted (poured off) or removed with a Pasteur pipet.

PROBLEM

1. In each of the following situations, what type of filtration device would you use?
   a. Remove powdered decolorizing charcoal from 20 mL of solution
   b. Collect crystals obtained from crystallizing a substance from about 1 mL of solution

c. Remove a very small amount of dirt from 1 mL of liquid
d. Isolate 2.0 g of crystals from about 50 mL of solution after performing a crystallization
e. Remove dissolved colored impurities from about 3 mL of solution
f. Remove solid impurities from 5 mL of liquid at room temperature

T E C H N I Q U E   9

Physical Constants of Solids: The Melting Point

9.1 PHYSICAL PROPERTIES

The physical properties of a compound are those properties that are intrinsic to a given compound when it is pure. A compound may often be identified simply by determining a number of its physical properties. The most commonly recognized physical properties of a compound include its color, melting point, boiling point, density, refractive index, molecular weight, and optical rotation. Modern chemists would include the various types of spectra (infrared, nuclear magnetic resonance, mass, and ultraviolet-visible) among the physical properties of a compound. A compound's spectra do not vary from one pure sample to another. Here, we look at methods of determining the melting point. Boiling point and density of compounds are covered in Technique 13. Refractive index, optical rotation, and spectra are also considered separately.

Many reference books list the physical properties of substances. You should consult Technique 4 for a complete discussion on how to find data for specific compounds. The works most useful for finding lists of values for the nonspectroscopic physical properties include

The Merck Index

The CRC Handbook of Chemistry and Physics

Lange's Handbook of Chemistry

Aldrich Handbook of Fine Chemicals

Complete citations for these references can be found in Technique 29 (p. 984). Although the *CRC Handbook* has very good tables, it adheres strictly to IUPAC nomenclature. For this reason, it may be easier to use one of the other references, particularly *The Merck Index* or the *Aldrich Handbook of Fine Chemicals*, in your first attempt to locate information (see Technique 4).

9.2 THE MELTING POINT

The melting point of a compound is used by the organic chemist not only to identify the compound, but also to establish its purity. A small amount of material is heated *slowly* in a special apparatus equipped with a thermometer or thermocouple, a heating bath or heating coil, and a magnifying eyepiece for observing the sample. Two temperatures are noted. The first is the point at which the first drop of liquid forms among the crystals; the second is the point at which the whole mass of crystals turns to a *clear* liquid. The melting point is recorded by giving this range of melting. You might say, for example, that the melting point of a substance is 51–54°C. That is, the substance melted over a 3-degree range.

The melting point indicates purity in two ways. First, the purer the material, the higher

111

its melting point. Second, the purer the material, the narrower its melting-point range. Adding successive amounts of an impurity to a pure substance generally causes its melting point to decrease in proportion to the amount of impurity. Looking at it another way, adding impurities lowers the freezing point. The freezing point, a colligative property, is simply the melting point (solid → liquid) approached from the opposite direction (liquid → solid).

Figure 9.1 is a graph of the usual melting-point behavior of mixtures of two substances, A and B. The two extremes of the melting range (the low and high temperature) are shown for various mixtures of the two. The upper curves indicate the temperatures at which all the sample has melted. The lower curves indicate the temperature at which melting is observed to begin. With pure compounds, melting is sharp and without any range. This is shown at the left- and right-hand edges of the graph. If you begin with pure A, the melting point decreases as impurity B is added. At some point, a minimum temperature, or **eutectic,** is reached, and the melting point begins to increase to that of substance B. The vertical distance between the lower and upper curves represents the melting range. Notice that for mixtures that contain relatively small amounts of impurity (< 15%) and are not close to the eutectic, the melting range increases as the sample becomes less pure. The range indicated by the lines in Figure 9.1 represents the typical behavior.

We can generalize the behavior shown in Figure 9.1. Pure substances melt with a narrow range of melting. With impure substances, the melting range becomes wider, and the entire melting range is lowered. Be careful to note, however, that at the minimum point of the melting-point–composition curves, the mixture often forms a eutectic, which also melts sharply. Not all binary mixtures form eutectics, and some caution must be exercised in assuming that every binary mixture follows the previously described behavior. Some mixtures may form more than one eutectic; others might not form even one. In spite of these variations, both the melting point and its range are useful indications of purity, and they are easily determined by simple experimental methods.

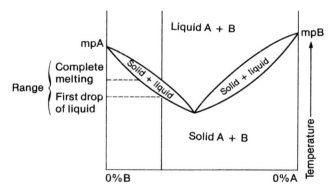

Figure 9.1   A melting-point–composition curve.

9.3 MELTING-POINT THEORY

Figure 9.2 is a phase diagram describing the usual behavior of a two-component mixture (A + B) on melting. The behavior on melting depends on the relative amounts of A and

B in the mixture. If A is a pure substance (no B), then A melts sharply at its melting point t_A. This is represented by point A on the left side of the diagram. When B is a pure substance, it melts at t_B; its melting point is represented by point B on the right side of the diagram. At either point A or point B, the pure solid passes cleanly, with a narrow range, from solid to liquid.

In mixtures of A and B, the behavior is different. Using Figure 9.2, consider a mixture of 80% A and 20% B on a mole-per-mole basis (that is, mole percentage). The melting point of this mixture is given by t_M at point M on the diagram. That is, adding B to A has lowered the melting point of A from t_A to t_M. It has also expanded the melting range. The temperature t_M corresponds to the **upper limit** of the melting range.

Lowering the melting point of A by adding impurity B comes about in the following way. Substance A has the lower melting point in the phase diagram shown, and if heated, it begins to melt first. As A begins to melt, solid B begins to dissolve in the liquid A that is formed. When solid B dissolves in liquid A, the melting point is depressed. To understand this, consider the melting point from the opposite direction. When a liquid at a high temperature cools, it reaches a point at which it solidifies, or "freezes." The temperature at which a liquid freezes is identical to its melting point. Recall that the freezing point of a liquid can be lowered by adding an impurity. Because the freezing point and the melting point are identical, lowering the freezing point corresponds to lowering the melting point. Therefore, as more impurity is added to a solid, its melting point becomes lower. There is, however, a limit to how far the melting point can be depressed. You cannot dissolve an infinite amount of the impurity substance in the liquid. At some point, the liquid will become saturated with the impurity substance. The solubility of B in A has an upper limit. In Figure 9.2, the solubility limit of B in liquid A is reached at point C, the **eutectic point.** The melting point of the mixture cannot be lowered below t_C, the melting temperature of the eutectic.

Now consider what happens when the melting point of a mixture of 80% A and 20% B is approached. As the temperature is increased, A begins to "melt." This is not really a visible phenomenon in the beginning stages; it happens before liquid is visible. It is a softening of the compound to a point at which it can begin to mix with the impurity. As A begins to soften, it dissolves B. As it dissolves B, the melting point is lowered. The lowering continues until all B is dissolved or until the eutectic composition (saturation) is reached.

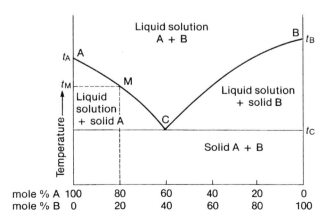

Figure 9.2 A phase diagram for melting in a two-component system.

113

When the maximum possible amount of B has been dissolved, actual melting begins, and one can observe the first appearance of liquid. The initial temperature of melting will be below t_A. The amount below t_A at which melting begins is determined by the amount of B dissolved in A but will never be below t_C. Once all B has been dissolved, the melting point of the mixture begins to rise as more A begins to melt. As more A melts, the semisolid solution is diluted by more A, and its melting point rises. While all this is happening, you can observe *both* solid and liquid in the melting-point capillary. Once all A has begun to melt, the composition of the mixture M becomes uniform and will reach 80% A and 20% B. At this point, the mixture finally melts sharply, giving a clear solution. The maximum melting-point range will be $t_C - t_M$, because t_A is depressed by the impurity B that is present. The lower end of the melting range will always be t_C; however, melting will not always be observed at this temperature. An observable melting at t_C comes about only when a large amount of B is present. Otherwise, the amount of liquid formed at t_C will be too small to observe. Therefore, the melting behavior that is actually observed will have a smaller range, as shown in Figure 9.1.

9.4 MIXTURE MELTING POINTS

The melting point can be used as supporting evidence in identifying a compound in two different ways. Not only may the melting points of the two individual compounds be compared but a special procedure called a **mixture melting point** may also be performed. The mixture melting point requires that an authentic sample of the same compound be available from another source. In this procedure, the two compounds (authentic and suspected) are finely pulverized and mixed together in equal quantities. Then the melting point of the mixture is determined. If there is a melting-point depression or if the range of melting is expanded by a large amount compared to that of the individual substances, you may conclude that one compound has acted as an impurity toward the other and that they are not the same compound. If there is no lowering of the melting point for the mixture (the melting point is identical with those of pure A and pure B), then A and B are almost certainly the same compound.

9.5 PACKING THE MELTING-POINT TUBE

Melting points are usually determined by heating the sample in a piece of thin-walled capillary tubing (1 mm $\times$ 100 mm) that has been sealed at one end. To pack the tube, press the open end gently into a *pulverized* sample of the crystalline material. Crystals will stick in the open end of the tube. The amount of solid pressed into the tube should correspond to a column no more than 1–2 mm high. To transfer the crystals to the closed end of the tube, drop the capillary tube, closed end first, down a ⅔-m length of glass tubing, which is held upright on the desktop. When the capillary tube hits the desktop, the crystals will pack down into the bottom of the tube. This procedure is repeated if necessary. Tapping the capillary on the desktop with fingers is not recommended because it is easy to drive the small tubing into a finger if the tubing should break.

114

Some commercial melting-point instruments have a built-in vibrating device that is designed to pack capillary tubes. With these instruments, the sample is pressed into the open end of the capillary tube, and the tube is placed in the vibrator slot. The action of the vibrator will transfer the sample to the bottom of the tube and pack it tightly.

9.6 DETERMINING THE MELTING POINT— THE THIELE TUBE

There are two principal types of melting-point apparatus available: the Thiele tube and commercially available, electrically heated instruments. The Thiele tube, shown in Figure 9.3, is the simpler device and was once widely used. It is a glass tube designed to contain a heating oil (mineral oil or silicone oil) and a thermometer to which a capillary tube containing the sample is attached. The shape of the Thiele tube allows convection currents to form in the oil when it is heated. These currents maintain a uniform temperature distribution through the oil in the tube. The sidearm of the tube is designed to generate these convection currents and thus transfer the heat from the flame evenly and rapidly throughout the oil. The sample, which is in a capillary tube attached to the thermometer, is held by a rub-

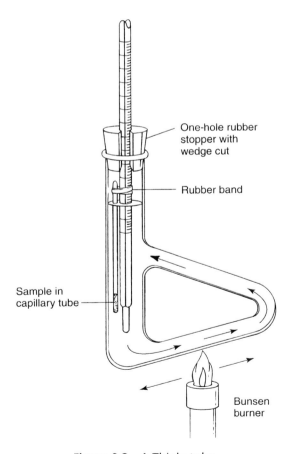

One-hole rubber stopper with wedge cut

Rubber band

Sample in capillary tube

Bunsen burner

Figure 9.3 A Thiele tube.

115

ber band or a thin slice of rubber tubing. It is important that this rubber band be above the level of the oil (allowing for expansion of the oil on heating) so that the oil does not soften the rubber and allow the capillary tubing to fall into the oil. If a cork or a rubber stopper is used to hold the thermometer, a triangular wedge should be sliced in it to allow pressure equalization.

The Thiele tube is usually heated by a microburner. During the heating, the rate of temperature increase should be regulated. Hold the burner by its cool base and, using a low flame, move the burner slowly back and forth along the bottom of the arm of the Thiele tube. If the heating is too fast, remove the burner for a few seconds and then resume heating. The rate of heating should be *slow* near the melting point (about 1°C per minute) to ensure that the temperature increase is not faster than the rate at which heat can be transferred to the sample being observed. At the melting point, it is necessary that the mercury in the thermometer and the sample in the capillary tube be at temperature equilibrium.

9.7 DETERMINING THE MELTING POINT— ELECTRICAL INSTRUMENTS

Three types of electrically heated melting-point instruments are illustrated in Figure 9.4. In each case, the melting-point tube is filled as described in Section 9.5 and placed in a holder located just behind the magnifying eyepiece. The apparatus is operated by moving the switch to the ON position, adjusting the potentiometric control dial for the desired rate of heating, and observing the sample through the magnifying eyepiece. The temperature is read from a thermometer or, in the most modern instruments, from a digital display attached to a thermocouple. Your instructor will demonstrate and explain the type used in your laboratory.

Most electrically heated instruments do not heat or increase the temperature of the sample linearly. Although the rate of increase may be linear in the early stages of heating, it usually decreases and leads to a constant temperature at some upper limit. The upper-limit temperature is determined by the setting of the heating control. Thus, a family of heating curves is usually obtained for various control settings, as shown in Figure 9.5. The four hypothetical curves shown (1–4) might correspond to different control settings. For a compound melting at temperature t_1, the setting corresponding to curve 3 would be ideal. In the beginning of the curve, the temperature is increasing too rapidly to allow determination of an accurate melting point, but after the change in slope, the temperature increase will have slowed to a more usable rate.

If the melting point of the sample is unknown, you can often save time by preparing two samples for melting-point determination. With one sample, you can rapidly determine a crude melting-point value. Then repeat the experiment more carefully using the second sample. For the second determination, you already have an approximate idea of what the melting-point temperature should be, and a proper rate of heating can be chosen.

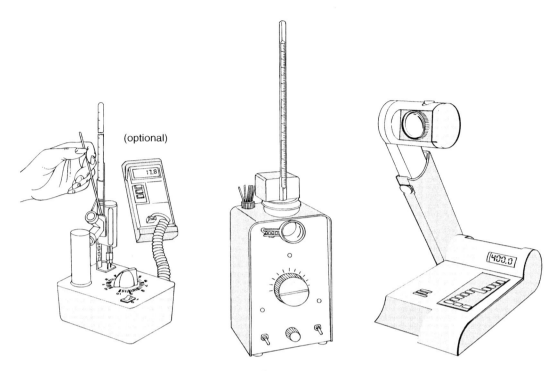

Figure 9.4 Melting-point apparatus.

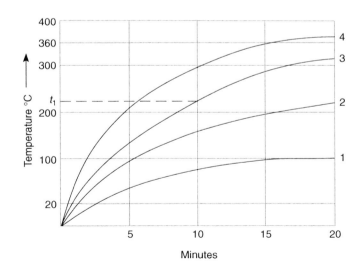

Figure 9.5 Heating-rate curves.

When measuring temperatures above 150°C, thermometer errors can become significant. For an accurate melting point with a high-melting solid, you may wish to apply a **stem correction** to the thermometer as described in Technique 13, Section 13.4. An even better solution is to calibrate the thermometer as described in Section 9.9.

9.8 DECOMPOSITION, DISCOLORATION, SOFTENING, SHRINKAGE, AND SUBLIMATION

Many solid substances undergo some degree of unusual behavior before melting. At times it may be difficult to distinguish these types of behavior from actual melting. You should learn, through experience, how to recognize melting and how to distinguish it from decomposition, discoloration, and particularly, softening and shrinkage.

Some compounds decompose on melting. This decomposition is usually evidenced by discoloration of the sample. Frequently, this decomposition point is a reliable physical property to be used in lieu of an actual melting point. Such decomposition points are indicated in tables of melting points by placing the symbol *d* immediately after the listed temperature. An example of a decomposition point is thiamine hydrochloride, whose melting point would be listed as 248°d, indicating that this substance melts with decomposition at 248°C. When decomposition is a result of reaction with the oxygen in air, it may be avoided by determining the melting point in a sealed, evacuated melting-point tube.

Figure 9.6 shows two simple methods of evacuating a packed tube. Method A uses an ordinary melting-point tube, and method B constructs the melting-point tube from a disposable Pasteur pipet. Before using method B, be sure to determine that the tip of the pipet will fit into the sample holder in your melting-point instrument.

Method A. In method A, a hole is punched through a rubber septum using a large pin or a small nail, and the capillary tube is inserted from the inside, sealed end first. The septum is placed over a piece of glass tubing connected to a vacuum line. After the tube is evacuated, the upper end of the tube may be sealed by heating and pulling it closed.

Method B. In method B, the thin section of a 9-inch Pasteur pipet is used to construct the melting-point tube. Carefully seal the tip of the pipet using a flame. Be sure to hold the tip *upward* as you seal it. This will prevent water vapor from condensing inside the pipet. When the sealed pipet has cooled, the sample may be added through the open end using a microspatula. A small wire may be used to compress the sample into the closed tip. (If your melting-point apparatus has a vibrator, it may be used in place of the wire to simplify the packing.) When the sample is in place, the pipet is connected to the vacuum line with tubing and evacuated. The evacuated sample tube is sealed by heating it with a flame and pulling it closed.

Some substances begin to decompose *below* their melting points. Thermally unstable substances may undergo elimination reactions or anhydride formation reactions during heating. The decomposition products formed represent impurities in the original sample, so the melting point of the substance may be lowered due to their presence.

It is normal for many compounds to soften or shrink immediately before melting. Such behavior represents not decomposition but a change in the crystal structure or a mixing with impurities. Some substances "sweat," or release solvent of crystallization, before melting. These changes do not indicate the beginning of melting. Actual melting begins

118

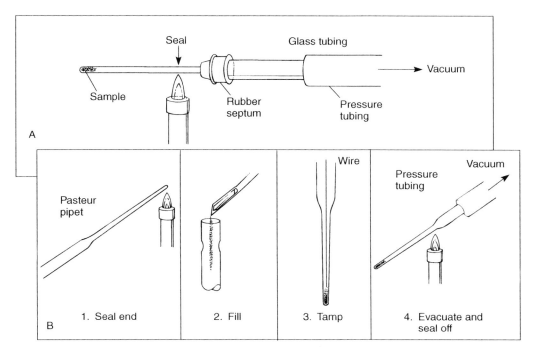

Figure 9.6 Evacuation and sealing of a melting-point capillary.

when the first drop of liquid becomes visible, and the melting range continues until the temperature is reached at which all the solid has been converted to the liquid state. With experience, you soon learn to distinguish between softening, or "sweating," and actual melting. If you wish, the temperature of the onset of softening or sweating may be reported as a part of your melting-point range: 211°C (softens), 223–225°C (melts).

Some solid substances have such a high vapor pressure that they sublime at or below their melting points. In many handbooks, the sublimation temperature is listed along with the melting point. The symbols *sub, subl,* and sometimes *s* are used to designate a substance that sublimes. In such cases, the melting-point determination must be performed in a sealed capillary tube to avoid loss of the sample. The simplest way to accomplish sealing a packed tube is to heat the open end of the tube in a flame and pull it closed with tweezers or forceps. A better way, although more difficult to master, is to heat the center of the tube in a small flame, rotating it about its axis, and keeping the tube straight, until the center collapses. If this is not done quickly, the sample may melt or sublime while you are working. With the smaller chamber, the sample will not be able to migrate to the cool top of the tube that may be above the viewing area. Figure 9.7 illustrates the method.

9.9 THERMOMETER CALIBRATION

When a melting-point or boiling-point determination has been completed, you expect to obtain a result that exactly duplicates the result recorded in a handbook or in the original literature. It is not unusual, however, to find a discrepancy of several degrees from the lit-

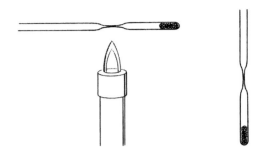

Figure 9.7 Sealing a tube for a substance that sublimes.

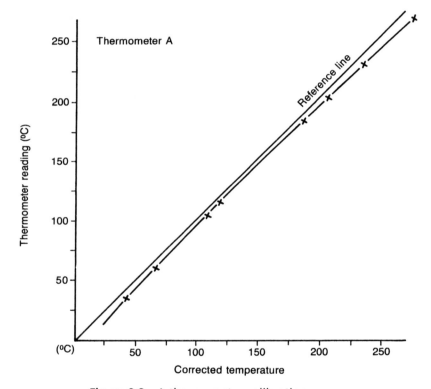

Figure 9.8 A thermometer-calibration curve.

erature value. Such a discrepancy does not necessarily indicate that the experiment was incorrectly performed or that the material is impure; rather, it may indicate that the thermometer used for the determination was slightly in error. Most thermometers do not measure the temperature with perfect accuracy.

To determine accurate values, you must calibrate the thermometer that is used. This calibration is done by determining the melting points of a variety of standard substances with the thermometer. A plot is drawn of the observed temperature vs. the published value of each standard substance. A smooth line is drawn through the points to complete the chart. A correction chart prepared in this way is shown in Figure 9.8. This chart is used to correct

120

TABLE 9.1 Melting-Point Standards

Compound	Melting Point (°C)
Ice (solid–liquid water)	0
Acetanilide	115
Benzamide	128
Urea	132
Succinic acid	189
3,5-Dinitrobenzoic acid	205

any melting point determined with that particular thermometer. Each thermometer requires its own calibration curve. A list of suitable standard substances for calibrating thermometers is provided in Table 9.1. The standard substances, of course, must be pure in order for the corrections to be valid.

PROBLEMS

1. Two substances, A and B, have the same melting point. How can you determine if they are the same without using any form of spectroscopy? Explain in detail.

2. Using Figure 9.5, determine which heating curve would be most appropriate for a substance with a melting point of about 150°C.

3. What steps can you take to determine the melting point of a substance that sublimes before it melts?

4. A compound melting at 134°C was suspected to be either aspirin (mp 135°C) or urea (mp 133°C). Explain how you could determine whether one of these two suspected compounds was identical to the unknown compound without using any form of spectroscopy.

5. An unknown compound gave a melting point of 230°C. When the molten liquid solidified, the melting point was redetermined and found to be 131°C. Give a possible explanation for this discrepancy.

TECHNIQUE 10

Solubility

The solubility of a **solute** (a dissolved substance) in a **solvent** (the dissolving medium) is the most important chemical principle underlying three basic techniques you will study in the organic chemistry laboratory: crystallization, extraction, and chromatography. In this discussion of solubility you will gain an understanding of the structural features of a substance that determine its solubility in various solvents. This understanding will help you to predict solubility behavior and to understand the techniques that are based on this property. Understanding solubility behavior will also help you understand what is going on during a reaction, especially when there is more than one liquid phase present or when a precipitate is formed.

10.1 DEFINITION OF SOLUBILITY

Although we often describe solubility behavior in terms of a substance being **soluble** (dissolved) or **insoluble** (not dissolved) in a solvent, solubility can be described more precisely in terms of the *extent* to which a substance is soluble. Solubility may be expressed in terms of grams of solute per liter (g/L) or milligrams of solute per milliliter (mg/mL) of solvent. Consider the solubilities at room temperature for the following three substances in water:

Cholesterol	0.002 mg/mL
Caffeine	22 mg/mL
Citric acid	620 mg/mL

In a typical test for solubility, 40 mg of solute is added to 1 mL of solvent. Therefore, if you were testing the solubility of these three substances, cholesterol would be insoluble, caffeine would be partially soluble, and citric acid would be soluble. Note that a small amount (0.002 mg) of cholesterol would dissolve. It is very unlikely, however, that you would be able to observe this small amount dissolving, and you would report that cholesterol is insoluble. On the other hand, 22 mg (55%) of the caffeine would dissolve. It is likely that you would be able to observe this, and you would state that caffeine is partially soluble.

When describing the solubility of a liquid solute in a solvent, it is sometimes helpful to use the terms **miscible** and **immiscible.** Two liquids that are miscible will mix homogeneously (one phase) in all proportions. For example, water and ethyl alcohol are miscible. When they are mixed in any proportion, only one layer will be observed. When two liquids are miscible, it is also true that either one of them will be completely soluble in the other one. Two immiscible liquids do not mix homogeneously in all proportions, and under some conditions they will form two layers. Water and diethyl ether are immiscible. When mixed in roughly equal amounts, they will form two layers. However, each liquid is slightly soluble in the other one. Even when two layers are present, a small amount of water will be soluble in the diethyl ether, and a small amount of diethyl ether will be soluble in the water. Furthermore, if only a small amount of either one is added to the other, it may dissolve completely, and only one layer will be observed. For example, if a small amount of water (less than 1.2% at 20°C) is added to diethyl ether, the water will dissolve completely in the diethyl ether, and only one layer will be observed. When more water is added (more than 1.2%), some of the water will not dissolve, and two layers will be present.

Although the terms *solubility* and *miscibility* are related in meaning, it is important to understand that there is one essential difference. There can be different degrees of solubility, such as slightly, partially, very, and so on. Unlike solubility, miscibility does not have any degrees—a pair of liquids is either miscible, or it is not.

10.2 PREDICTING SOLUBILITY BEHAVIOR

A major goal of this section is to explain how to predict whether a substance will be soluble in a given solvent. This is not always easy, even for an experienced chemist. However, guidelines will help you make a good guess about the solubility of a compound in a specific solvent. In discussing these guidelines, it is helpful to separate the types of solutions we will be looking at into two categories: solutions in which both the solvent and the solute are covalent (molecular); and ionic solutions, in which the solute ionizes and dissociates.

A. Solutions in Which the Solvent and Solute Are Molecular

A very useful generalization in predicting solubility is the widely used rule "Like dissolves like." This rule is most commonly applied to polar and nonpolar compounds. According to this rule, a polar solvent will dissolve polar (or ionic) compounds, and a nonpolar solvent will dissolve nonpolar compounds.

The reason for this behavior involves the nature of intermolecular forces of attraction. Although we will not be focusing on the nature of these forces, it is helpful to know what they are called. The force of attraction between polar molecules is called **dipole–dipole interaction;** between nonpolar molecules, forces of attraction are called **van der Waals forces** (also called **London** or **dispersion forces**). In both cases, these attractive forces can occur between molecules of the same compound or different compounds. Consult your lecture textbook for more information on these forces.

To apply the rule "Like dissolves like," you must first determine whether a substance is polar or nonpolar. The polarity of a compound is dependent on both the polarities of the individual bonds and the shape of the molecule. For most organic compounds, evaluating these factors can become quite complicated because of the complexities of the molecules. However, it is possible to make some reasonable predictions just by looking at the types of atoms that a compound possesses. As you read the following guidelines, it is important to understand that although we often describe compounds as being polar or nonpolar, polarity is a matter of degree, ranging from nonpolar to highly polar.

Guidelines for Predicting Polarity and Solubility

1. All hydrocarbons are nonpolar.
   Examples:

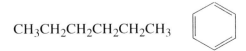

$$CH_3CH_2CH_2CH_2CH_2CH_3$$

123

Hydrocarbons such as benzene are slightly more polar than hexane because of their pi (π) bonds, which allow for greater van der Waals or London attractive forces.

2. Compounds possessing the electronegative elements oxygen or nitrogen are polar. *Examples:*

$$\underset{\text{Acetone}}{CH_3\overset{\overset{\displaystyle O}{\|}}{C}CH_3} \qquad \underset{\text{Ethyl alcohol}}{CH_3CH_2OH} \qquad \underset{\text{Ethyl acetate}}{CH_3\overset{\overset{\displaystyle O}{\|}}{C}OCH_2CH_3}$$

$$\underset{\text{Ethylamine}}{CH_3CH_2NH_2} \qquad \underset{\text{Diethyl ether}}{CH_3CH_2OCH_2CH_3} \qquad \underset{\text{Water}}{H_2O}$$

The polarity of these compounds depends on the presence of polar $C-O$, $C{=}O$, OH, NH, and CN bonds. The compounds that are most polar are capable of forming hydrogen bonds (see guideline 6) and have NH or OH bonds. Although all these compounds are polar, the degree of polarity ranges from slightly polar to highly polar. This is due to the effect on polarity of the shape of the molecule and size of the carbon chain, and whether the compound can form hydrogen bonds.

3. The presence of halogen atoms, even though their electronegativities are relatively high, does not alter the polarity of an organic compound in a significant way. Therefore, these compounds are only slightly polar. The polarities of these compounds are more similar to those of hydrocarbons, which are nonpolar, than to that of water, which is highly polar. *Examples:*

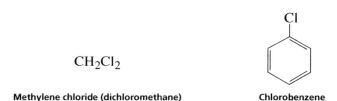

$$CH_2Cl_2$$

Methylene chloride (dichloromethane)   **Chlorobenzene**

4. When comparing organic compounds within the same family, note that adding carbon atoms to the chain decreases the polarity. For example, methyl alcohol (CH_3OH) is more polar than propyl alcohol ($CH_3CH_2CH_2OH$). The reason is that hydrocarbons are nonpolar, and increasing the length of a carbon chain makes the compound more hydrocarbon-like.

5. Compounds that contain four or fewer carbons and also contain oxygen or nitrogen are often soluble in water. Almost any functional group containing these elements will lead to water solubility for low-molecular-weight (up to C_4) compounds. Compounds having five or six carbons and containing one of these elements are often insoluble in water or have borderline solubility.

6. As mentioned earlier, the force of attraction between polar molecules is dipole–dipole interaction. A special case of dipole–dipole interaction is hydrogen bonding. Hydrogen bonding is a possibility when a compound possesses a hydrogen atom bonded to a nitrogen, oxygen, or fluorine atom. The bond is formed by the

attraction between this hydrogen atom and a nitrogen, oxygen, or fluorine atom in another molecule. Hydrogen bonding may occur between two molecules of the same compound or between molecules of different compounds:

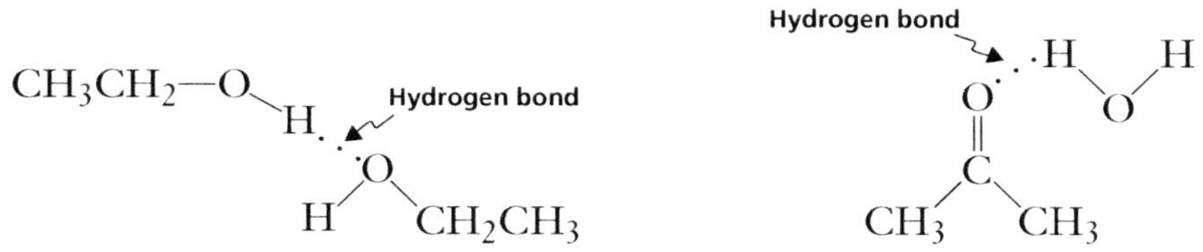

Hydrogen bonding is the strongest type of dipole–dipole interaction. When hydrogen bonding between solute and solvent is possible, solubility is greater than one would expect for compounds of similar polarity that cannot form hydrogen bonds. Hydrogen bonding is very important in organic chemistry, and you should be alert for situations in which hydrogen bonding may occur.

7. Another factor that can affect solubility is the degree of branching of the alkyl chain in a compound. Branching of the alkyl chain in a compound lowers the intermolecular forces between the molecules. This is usually reflected in a greater solubility in water for the branched compound than for the corresponding straight-chain compound. This occurs simply because the molecules of the branched compounds are more easily separated from one another.

8. The solubility rule ("Like dissolves like") may be applied to organic compounds that belong to the same family. For example, 1-octanol (an alcohol) is soluble in the solvent ethyl alcohol. Most compounds within the same family have similar polarity. However, this generalization may not apply if there is a substantial difference in size between the two compounds. For example, cholesterol, an alcohol with a molecular weight (MW) of 386.64, is only slightly soluble in methanol (MW 32.04). The large hydrocarbon component of cholesterol negates the fact that they belong to the same family.

9. The stability of the crystal lattice also affects solubility. Other things being equal, the higher the melting point (the more stable the crystal) is, the less soluble the compound. For instance, *p*-nitrobenzoic acid (mp 242°C) is, by a factor of 10, less soluble in a fixed amount of ethanol than the *ortho* (mp 147°C) and *meta* (mp 141°C) isomers.

You can check your understanding of some of these guidelines by studying the list given in Table 10.1, which is given in order of increasing polarity. The structures of these compounds were given on pages 671–672.

This list can be used to make some predictions about solubility, based on the rule "Like dissolves like." Substances that are close to one another on this list will have similar polarities. Thus, you would expect hexane to be soluble in methylene chloride but not in water. Acetone should be soluble in ethyl alcohol. On the other hand, you might predict that ethyl alcohol would be insoluble in hexane. However, ethyl alcohol is soluble in hexane, because ethyl alcohol is somewhat less polar than methyl alcohol or water. This last example demonstrates that you must be careful in using the guidelines on polarity for predicting solubilities. Ultimately, solubility tests must be done to confirm predictions until you gain more experience.

125

The trend in polarities shown in Table 10.1 can be expanded by including more organic families. The list in Table 10.2 gives an approximate order for the decreasing polarity of organic functional groups. It may appear that there are some discrepancies between the information provided in these two tables. The reason is that Table 10.1 provides information about specific compounds, whereas the trend shown in Table 10.2 is for major organic families and is approximate.

B. Solutions in Which the Solute Ionizes and Dissociates

Many ionic compounds are highly soluble in water because of the strong attraction be-

TABLE 10.1   Compounds in Increasing Order of Polarity

	Increasing Polarity
Aliphatic hydrocarbons	
Hexane (nonpolar)	
Aromatic hydrocarbons (π bonds)	
Benzene (nonpolar)	
Halocarbons	
Methylene chloride (slightly polar)	
Compounds with polar bonds	
Diethyl ether (slightly polar)	
Ethyl acetate (intermediate polarity)	
Acetone (intermediate polarity)	
Compounds with polar bonds and hydrogen bonding	
Ethyl alcohol (intermediate polarity)	
Methyl alcohol (intermediate polarity)	
Water (highly polar)	

TABLE 10.2   Solvents in Decreasing Order of Polarity

Decreasing Polarity (Approximate)

H_2O	Water
RCOOH	Organic acids (acetic acid)
$RCONH_2$	Amides (*N,N*-dimethylformamide)
ROH	Alcohols (methanol, ethanol)
RNH_2	Amines (triethylamine, pyridine)
RCOR	Aldehydes, ketones (acetone)
RCOOR	Esters (ethyl acetate)
RX	Halides ($CH_2Cl_2 > CHCl_3 > CCl_4$)
ROR	Ethers (diethyl ether)
ArH	Aromatics (benzene, toluene)
RH	Alkanes (hexane, petroleum ether)

tween ions and the highly polar water molecules. This also applies to organic compounds that can exist as ions. For example, sodium acetate consists of Na^+ and CH_3COO^- ions, which are highly soluble in water. Although there are some exceptions, you may assume that all organic compounds that are in the ionic form will be water soluble.

The most common way by which organic compounds become ions is in acid–base reactions. For example, carboxylic acids can be converted to water-soluble salts when they react with dilute aqueous NaOH:

$$CH_3CH_2CH_2CH_2CH_2CH_2\overset{\displaystyle O}{\overset{\|}{C}}OH + NaOH \text{ (aq)} \longrightarrow$$

Water-insoluble carboxylic acid

$$CH_3CH_2CH_2CH_2CH_2CH_2\overset{\displaystyle O}{\overset{\|}{C}}O^-\ Na^+ + H_2O$$

Water-soluble salt

The water-soluble salt can then be converted back to the original carboxylic acid (which is insoluble in water) by adding another acid (usually aqueous HCl) to the solution of the salt. The carboxylic acid precipitates out of solution.

Amines, which are organic bases, can also be converted to water-soluble salts when they react with dilute aqueous HCl:

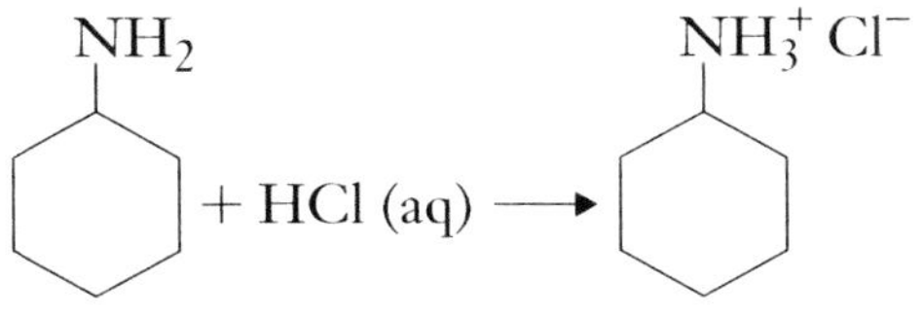

Water-insoluble amine   **Water-soluble salt**

This salt can be converted back to the original amine by adding a base (usually aqueous NaOH) to the solution of the salt.

10.3 ORGANIC SOLVENTS

Organic solvents must be handled safely. Always remember that organic solvents are all at least mildly toxic and that many are flammable. You should become thoroughly familiar with laboratory safety (see Technique 1, pp. 558–575).

The most common organic solvents are listed in Table 10.3 along with their boiling points. Solvents marked in boldface type will burn. Ether, pentane, and hexane are especially dangerous; if they are combined with the correct amount of air, they will explode.

The terms **petroleum ether** and **ligroin** are often confusing. Petroleum ether is a mixture of hydrocarbons with isomers of formulas C_5H_{12} and C_6H_{14} predominating. Petroleum ether is not an ether at all because there are no oxygen-bearing compounds in the mixture. In organic chemistry, an ether is usually a compound containing an oxygen atom to which two alkyl groups are attached. Figure 10.1 shows some of the hydrocarbons that appear commonly in petroleum ether. It also shows the structure of ether (diethyl ether). Use special care when instructions call for either **ether** or **petroleum ether;** the two must not become accidentally confused. Confusion is particularly easy when one is selecting a container of solvent from the supply shelf.

Ligroin, or high-boiling petroleum ether, is like petroleum ether in composition except that compared with petroleum ether, ligroin generally includes higher-boiling alkane isomers. Depending on the supplier, ligroin may have different boiling ranges. Whereas some brands of ligroin have boiling points ranging from about 60°C to about 90°C, other brands have boiling points ranging from about 60°C to about 75°C. The boiling-point ranges of petroleum ether and ligroin are often included on the labels of the containers.

PROBLEMS

1. For each of the following pairs of solutes and solvent, predict whether the solute would be soluble or insoluble. After making your predictions, you can check your answers by looking up the compounds in *The Merck Index* or the *CRC Handbook of Chemistry and Physics*. Generally, *The Merck*

TABLE 10.3 Common Organic Solvents

Solvent	Bp (°C)	Solvent	Bp (°C)
Hydrocarbons		Ethers	
Pentane	36	**Ether** (diethyl)	35
Hexane	69	**Dioxane**[a]	101
Benzene[a]	80	**1,2-Dimethoxyethane**	83
Toluene	111	Others	
Hydrocarbon mixtures		Acetic acid	118
Petroleum ether	30–60	Acetic anhydride	140
Ligroin	60–90	**Pyridine**	115
Chlorocarbons		**Acetone**	56
Methylene chloride	40	**Ethyl acetate**	77
Chloroform[a]	61	Dimethylformamide	153
Carbon tetrachloride[a]	77	Dimethylsulfoxide	189
Alcohols			
Methanol	65		
Ethanol	78		
Isopropyl alcohol	82		

Note: **Boldface type** indicates flammability.

[a] Suspect carcinogen (see p. 573).

Index is the easier reference book to use. If the substance has a solubility greater than 40 mg/mL, you may conclude that it is soluble.

   a. Malic acid in water

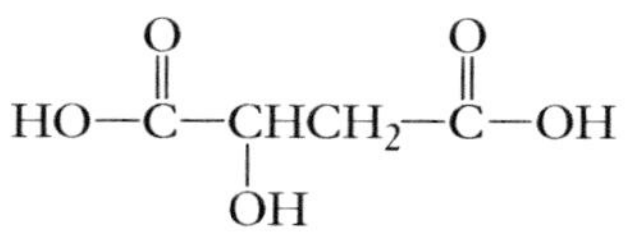

Malic acid

128

b. Naphthalene in water

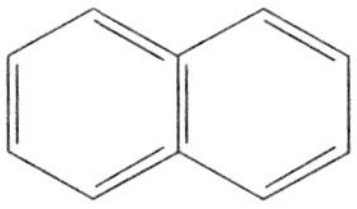

Naphthalene

c. Amphetamine in ethyl alcohol

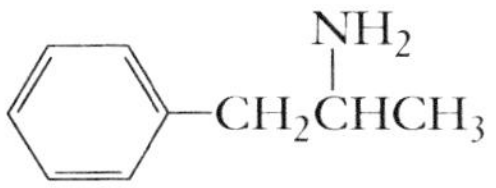

Amphetamine

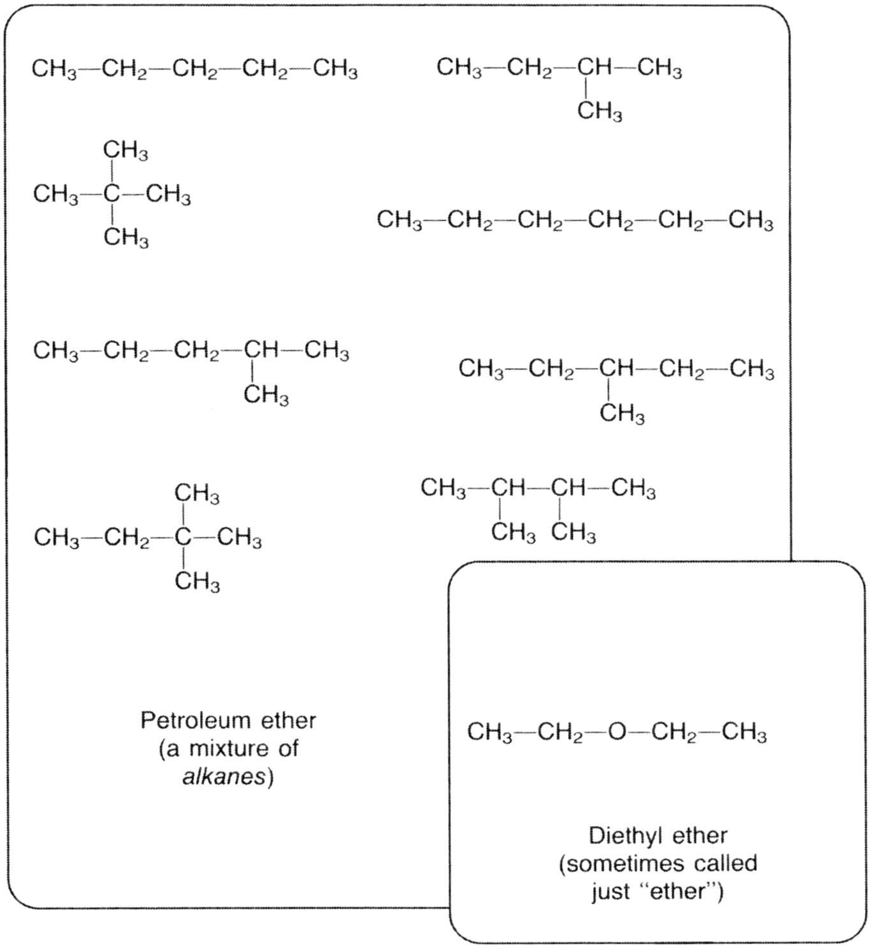

$CH_3-CH_2-CH_2-CH_2-CH_3$

$CH_3-CH_2-\underset{\underset{CH_3}{|}}{CH}-CH_3$

$CH_3-\underset{\underset{CH_3}{|}}{\overset{\overset{CH_3}{|}}{C}}-CH_3$

$CH_3-CH_2-CH_2-CH_2-CH_2-CH_3$

$CH_3-CH_2-CH_2-\underset{\underset{CH_3}{|}}{CH}-CH_3$

$CH_3-CH_2-\underset{\underset{CH_3}{|}}{CH}-CH_2-CH_3$

$CH_3-CH_2-\underset{\underset{CH_3}{|}}{\overset{\overset{CH_3}{|}}{C}}-CH_3$

$CH_3-\underset{\underset{CH_3}{|}}{CH}-\underset{\underset{CH_3}{|}}{CH}-CH_3$

Petroleum ether
(a mixture of
alkanes)

$CH_3-CH_2-O-CH_2-CH_3$

Diethyl ether
(sometimes called
just "ether")

Figure 10.1 A comparison between "ether" (diethyl ether) and "petroleum ether."

d. Aspirin in water

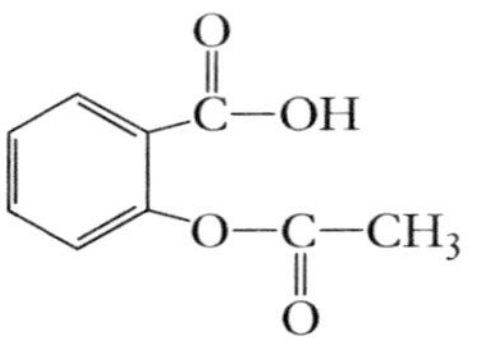

Aspirin

e. Succinic acid in hexane (*Note:* the polarity of hexane is similar to that of petroleum ether.)

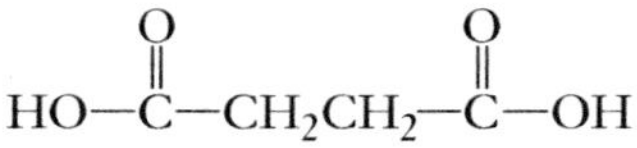

Succinic acid

f. Ibuprofen in diethyl ether

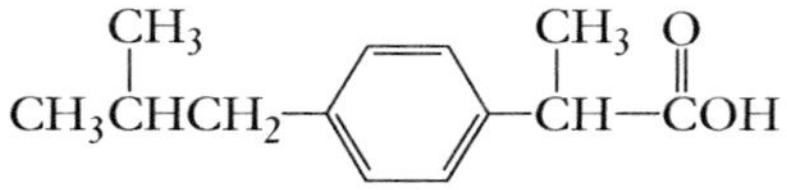

Ibuprofen

g. 1-Decanol (*n*-decyl alcohol) in water

$$CH_3(CH_2)_8CH_2OH$$

1-Decanol

2. Predict whether the following pairs of liquids would be miscible or immiscible:
   a. Water and methyl alcohol
   b. Hexane and benzene
   c. Methylene chloride and benzene
   d. Water and toluene

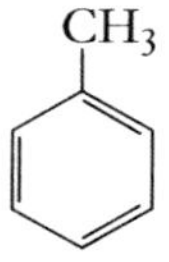

Toluene

   e. Ethyl alcohol and isopropyl alcohol

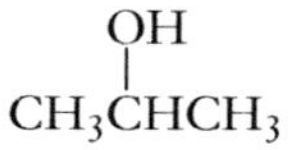

Isopropyl alcohol

3. Would you expect ibuprofen (see problem 1f) to be soluble or insoluble in 1.0 *M* NaOH? Explain.
4. Thymol is very slightly soluble in water and very soluble in 1.0 *M* NaOH. Explain.

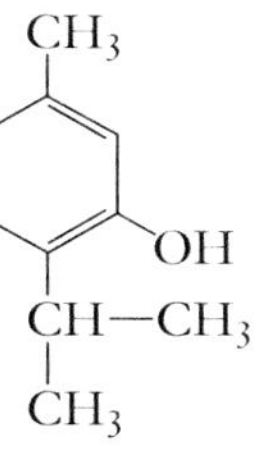

Thymol

5. Although cannabinol and methyl alcohol are both alcohols, cannabinol is very slightly soluble in methyl alcohol at room temperature. Explain.

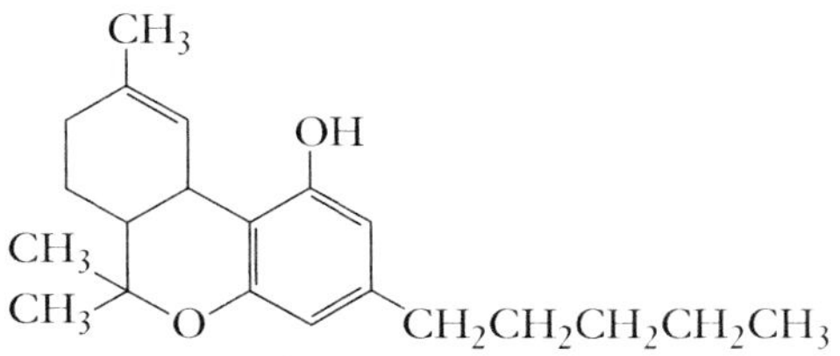

Cannabinol

6. What is the difference between the compounds in each of the following pairs?
   a. Ether and petroleum ether
   b. Ether and diethyl ether
   c. Ligroin and petroleum ether

TECHNIQUE 11

Crystallization: Purification of Solids

In most organic chemistry experiments, the desired product is first isolated in an impure form. If this product is a solid, the most common method of purification is crystallization. The general technique involves dissolving the material to be crystallized in a *hot* solvent (or solvent mixture) and cooling the solution slowly. The dissolved material has a decreased solubility at lower temperatures and will separate from the solution as it is cooled. This phenomenon is called either **crystallization,** if the crystal growth is relatively slow and selective, or **precipitation,** if the process is rapid and nonselective. Crystallization is an equilibrium process and produces very pure material. A small seed crystal is formed initially, and it then grows layer by layer in a reversible manner. In a sense, the crystal "selects" the correct molecules from the solution. In precipitation, the crystal lattice is formed so rapidly that impurities are trapped within the lattice. Therefore, any attempt at purification with too rapid a process should be avoided. Because the impurities are usually present in much smaller amounts than the compound being crystallized, most of the impurities will remain in the solvent even when it is cooled. The purified substance can then be separated from the solvent and from the impurities by filtration.

The method of crystallization described here is called **macroscale crystallization.** This technique, which is carried out with an Erlenmeyer flask to dissolve the material and a Büchner funnel to filter the crystals, is normally used when the weight of solid to be crystallized is more than 0.1 g. Another method, which is performed with a Craig tube, is used with smaller amounts of solid. Referred to as **microscale crystallization,** this technique is discussed briefly in Section 11.4.

When the macroscale crystallization procedure described in Section 11.3 is used with a Hirsch funnel, the procedure is sometimes referred to as a **semi-microscale crystallization.** This procedure is commonly used in microscale work when the amount of solid is greater than 0.1 g or in macroscale work when the amount of solid is less than about 0.5 g.

Part A. Theory

11.1 SOLUBILITY

The first problem in performing a crystallization is selecting a solvent in which the material to be crystallized shows the desired solubility behavior. In an ideal case, the material should be sparingly soluble at room temperature and yet quite soluble at the boiling point of the solvent selected. The solubility curve should be steep, as can be seen in line A of Figure 11.1. A curve with a low slope (line B) would not cause significant crystallization when the temperature of the solution was lowered. A solvent in which the material is very soluble at all temperatures (line C) also would not be a suitable crystallization solvent. The basic problem in performing a crystallization is to select a solvent (or mixed solvent) that provides a steep solubility-vs.-temperature curve for the material to

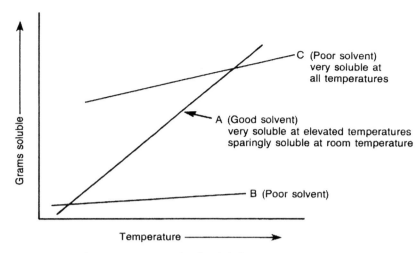

Figure 11.1 Graph of solubility vs. temperature.

be crystallized. A solvent that allows the behavior shown in line A is an ideal crystallization solvent. It should also be mentioned that solubility curves are not always linear, as they are depicted in Figure 11.1. This figure represents an idealized form of solubility behavior. The solubility curve for sulfanilamide in 95% ethyl alcohol, shown in Figure 11.2, is typical of many organic compounds and shows what solubility behavior might look like for a real substance.

The solubility of organic compounds is a function of the polarities of both the solvent and the **solute** (dissolved material). A general rule is "Like dissolves like." If the solute is very polar, a very polar solvent is needed to dissolve it; if the solute is nonpolar, a nonpolar solvent is needed. Applications of this rule are discussed extensively in Technique 10, Section 10.2, page 670 and in Section 11.5, page 689.

11.2 THEORY OF CRYSTALLIZATION

A successful crystallization depends on a large difference between the solubility of a material in a hot solvent and its solubility in the same solvent when it is cold. When the impurities in a substance are equally soluble in both the hot and the cold solvent, an effective purification is not easily achieved through crystallization. A material can be purified by crystallization when both the desired substance and the impurity have similar solubilities, but only when the impurity represents a small fraction of the total solid. The desired substance will crystallize on cooling, but the impurities will not.

For example, consider a case in which the solubilities of substance A and its impurity B are both 1 g/100 mL of solvent at 20°C and 10 g/100 mL of solvent at 100°C. In the impure sample of A, the composition is 9 g of A and 2 g of B. In the calculations for this example, it is assumed that the solubilities of both A and B are unaffected by the presence of the other substance. To make the calculations easier to understand, 100 mL of solvent are used in each crystallization. Normally, the minimum amount of solvent required to dissolve the solid would be used.

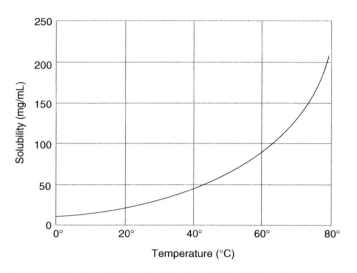

Figure 11.2 Solubility of sulfanilamide in 95% ethyl alcohol.

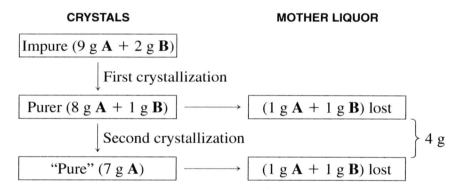

Figure 11.3 Purification of a mixture by crystallization.

At 20°C, this total amount of material will not dissolve in 100 mL of solvent. However, if the solvent is heated to 100°C, all 11 g dissolve. The solvent has the capacity to dissolve 10 g of A *and* 10 g of B at this temperature. If the solution is cooled to 20°C, only 1 g of each solute can remain dissolved, so 8 g of A and 1 g of B crystallize, leaving 2 g of material in the solution. This crystallization is shown in Figure 11.3. The solution that remains after a crystallization is called the **mother liquor.** If the process is now repeated by treating the crystals with 100 mL of fresh solvent, 7 g of A will crystallize again, leaving 1 g of A and 1 g of B in the mother liquor. As a result of these operations, 7 g of pure A are obtained, but with the loss of 4 g of material (2 g of A plus 2 g of B). Again, this second crystallization step is illustrated in Figure 11.3. The final result illustrates an important aspect of crystallization—it is wasteful. Nothing can be done to prevent this waste; some A must be lost along with the impurity B for the method to be successful. Of course, if the impurity B were *more* soluble than A in the solvent, the losses would be reduced. Losses could also be reduced if the impurity were present in *much smaller* amounts than the desired material.

Note that in the preceding case, the method operated successfully because A was present in substantially larger quantity than its impurity B. If there had been a 50-50 mixture of A and B initially, no separation would have been achieved. In general, a crystallization is successful only if there is a *small* amount of impurity. As the amount of impurity increases, the loss of material must also increase. Two substances with nearly equal solubility behavior, present in equal amounts, cannot be separated. If the solubility behavior of two components present in equal amounts is different, however, a separation or purification is frequently possible.

In the preceding example, two crystallization procedures were performed. Normally, this is not necessary; however, when it is, the second crystallization is more appropriately called **recrystallization.** As illustrated in this example, a second crystallization results in purer crystals, but the yield is lower.

In some experiments, you will be instructed to cool the crystallizing mixture in an ice-water bath before collecting the crystals by filtration. Cooling the mixture increases the yield by decreasing the solubility of the substance; however, even at this reduced temperature, some of the product will be soluble in the solvent. It is not possible to recover all your product in a crystallization procedure even when the mixture is cooled in an ice-water bath. A good example of this is illustrated by the solubility curve for sulfanilamide shown in Figure 11.2. The solubility of sulfanilamide at 0°C is still significant, 14 mg/mL.

Part B. Macroscale Crystallization

11.3 MACROSCALE CRYSTALLIZATION

The crystallization technique described in this section is used when the weight of solid to be crystallized is more than 0.1 g. There are four main steps in a macroscale crystallization:

1. Dissolving the solid
2. Removing insoluble impurities (when necessary)
3. Crystallizing
4. Collecting and drying

These steps are illustrated in Figure 11.4. An Erlenmeyer flask of an appropriate size must be chosen. It should be pointed out that a microscale crystallization with a Craig tube involves the same four steps, although the apparatus and procedures are somewhat different (see Section 11.4).

A. Dissolving the Solid

To minimize losses of material to the mother liquor, it is desirable to *saturate* the boiling solvent with solute. This solution, when cooled, will return the maximum possible amount of solute as crystals. To achieve this high return, the solvent is brought to its boiling point, and the solute is dissolved in the *minimum amount* (!) *of boiling solvent.* For this procedure, it is advisable to maintain a container of boiling solvent (on a hot plate). From this container, a small portion (about 1–2 mL) of the solvent is added to the Erlenmeyer

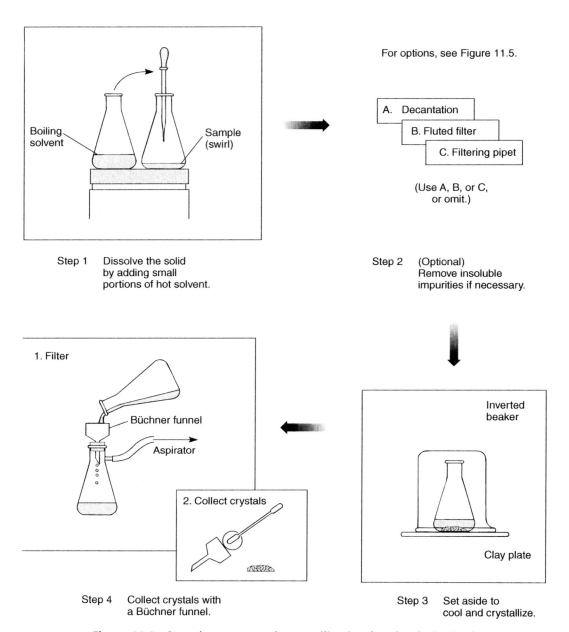

For options, see Figure 11.5.

A. Decantation

B. Fluted filter

C. Filtering pipet

(Use A, B, or C, or omit.)

Boiling solvent

Sample (swirl)

Step 1   Dissolve the solid by adding small portions of hot solvent.

Step 2   (Optional) Remove insoluble impurities if necessary.

1. Filter

Büchner funnel

Aspirator

2. Collect crystals

Inverted beaker

Clay plate

Step 4   Collect crystals with a Büchner funnel.

Step 3   Set aside to cool and crystallize.

Figure 11.4   Steps in a macroscale crystallization (no decolorization).

flask containing the solid to be crystallized, and this mixture is heated while swirling occasionally until it resumes boiling.

Caution: Do not heat the flask containing the solid until after you have added the first portion of solvent.

If the solid does not dissolve in the first portion of boiling solvent, then another small portion of boiling solvent is added to the flask. The mixture is swirled and heated again until it resumes boiling. If the solid dissolves, no more solvent is added. But if the solid has not dissolved, another portion of boiling solvent is added, as before, and the process is repeated until the solid dissolves. It is important to stress that the portions of solvent added each time are small, so only the *minimum* amount of solvent necessary for dissolving the solid is added. It is also important to emphasize that the procedure requires the addition of solvent to solid. You must never add portions of solid to a fixed quantity of boiling solvent. By this latter method, it may be impossible to determine when saturation has been achieved. This entire procedure should be performed fairly rapidly, or you may lose solvent through evaporation nearly as quickly as you are adding it, and this procedure will then take a very long time. This is most likely to happen when using highly volatile solvents such as methyl alcohol or ethyl alcohol. The time from the first addition of solvent until the solid dissolves completely should not be longer than 15–20 minutes.

Comments on This Procedure for Dissolving the Solid

1. One of the most common mistakes is to add too much solvent. This can happen most easily if the solvent is not hot enough or if the mixture is not stirred sufficiently. If too much solvent is added, the percentage recovery will be reduced; it is even possible that no crystals will form when the solution is cooled. If too much solvent is added, you must evaporate the excess by heating the mixture. A nitrogen or air stream directed into the container will accelerate the evaporation process (see Technique 7, Section 7.10, p. 639).

2. It is very important not to heat the solid until you have added some solvent. Otherwise, the solid may melt and possibly form an oil or decompose, and it may not crystallize easily (see p. 691).

3. It is also important to use an Erlenmeyer flask rather than a beaker for performing the crystallization. A beaker should not be used because the large opening allows the solvent to evaporate too rapidly and allows dust particles to get in too easily.

4. In some experiments, a specified amount of solvent for a given weight of solid will be recommended. In these cases, you should use the amount specified rather than the minimum amount of solvent necessary to dissolve the solid. The amount of solvent recommended has been selected to provide the optimum conditions for good crystal formation.

5. Occasionally, you may encounter an impure solid that contains small particles of insoluble impurities, pieces of dust, or paper fibers that will not dissolve in the hot crystallizing solvent. A common error is to add too much of the hot solvent in an attempt to dissolve these small particles, not realizing that they are insoluble. In such cases, you must be careful not to add too much solvent.

6. It is sometimes necessary to decolorize the solution by adding activated charcoal or by passing the solution through a column containing alumina or silica gel (see Section 11.7 and Technique 19, Section 19.15, p. 814). A decolorization step should be performed only if the mixture is *highly* colored and it is clear that the color is due to impurities and not to the actual color of the substance being crys-

tallized. If decolorization is necessary, it should be accomplished before the following filtration step.

B. Removing Insoluble Impurities

It is necessary to use one of the following three methods only if insoluble material remains in the hot solution or if decolorizing charcoal has been used.

Caution: Indiscriminate use of the procedure can lead to needless loss of your product.

Decantation is the easiest method of removing solid impurities and should be considered first. If filtration is required, a filtering pipet is used when the volume of liquid to be filtered is less than 10 mL (see Technique 8, Section 8.1C, p. 649), and you should use gravity filtration through a fluted filter when the volume is 10 mL or greater (see Technique 8, Section 8.1B, p. 646). These three methods are illustrated in Figure 11.5, and each is discussed below.

Decantation.   If the solid particles are relatively large in size or they easily settle to the bottom of the flask, it may be possible to separate the hot solution from the impurities by carefully pouring off the liquid, leaving the solid behind. This is accomplished most easily by holding a glass stirring rod along the top of the flask and tilting the flask so that the liquid pours out along one end of the glass rod into another container. A technique similar in principle to decantation, which may be easier to perform with smaller amounts of liquid, is to use a **preheated Pasteur pipet** to remove the hot solution. With this method, it may be helpful to place the tip of the pipet against the bottom of the flask when removing the last portion of solution. The small space between the tip of the pipet and the inside surface of the flask prevents solid material from being drawn into the pipet. An easy way to preheat the pipet is to draw up a small portion of hot *solvent* (not the *solution* being transferred) into the pipet and expel the liquid. Repeat this process several times.

Fluted Filter.   This method is the most effective way to remove solid impurities when the volume of liquid is greater than 10 mL or when decolorizing charcoal has been used (see Technique 8, Section 8.1B, p. 646 and Section 11.7). You should first add a small amount of extra solvent to the hot mixture. This action helps prevent crystal formation in the filter paper or the stem of the funnel during the filtration. The funnel is then fitted with a fluted filter and installed at the top of the Erlenmeyer flask to be used for the actual filtration. It is advisable to place a small piece of wire between the funnel and the mouth of the flask to relieve any increase in pressure caused by hot filtrate.

The Erlenmeyer flask containing the funnel and fluted paper is placed on top of a hot plate (low setting). The liquid to be filtered is brought to its boiling point and poured through the filter in portions. (If the volume of the mixture is less than 10 mL, it may be more convenient to transfer the mixture to the filter with a preheated Pasteur pipet.) It is necessary to keep the solutions in both flasks at their boiling temperatures to prevent premature crystallization. The refluxing action of the filtrate keeps the funnel warm and reduces the chance that the filter will clog with crystals that may have formed during the filtration.

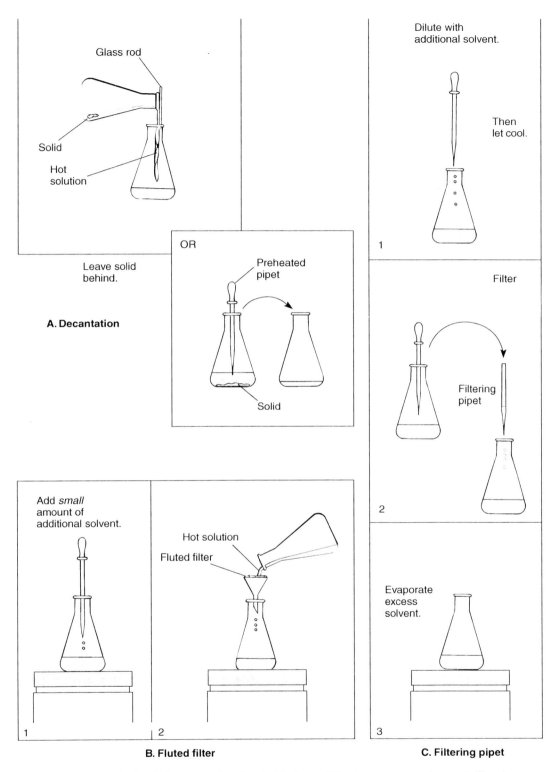

Figure 11.5 Methods for removing insoluble impurities in a macroscale crystallization.

With low-boiling solvents, be aware that some solvent may be lost through evaporation. Consequently, extra solvent must be added to make up for this loss. If crystals begin to form in the filter during filtration, a minimum amount of boiling solvent is added to redissolve the crystals and to allow the solution to pass through the funnel. If the volume of liquid being filtered is less than 10 mL, a small amount of hot solvent should be used to rinse the filter after all the filtrate has been collected. The rinse solvent is then combined with the original filtrate.

After the filtration, it may be necessary to remove extra solvent by evaporation until the solution is once again saturated at the boiling point of the solvent (see Technique 7, Section 7.10, p. 639).

Filtering Pipet. If the volume of solution after dissolving the solid in hot solvent is less than 10 mL, gravity filtration with a filtering pipet may be used to remove solid impurities. However, using a filtering pipet to filter a hot solution saturated with solute can be difficult without premature crystallization. The best way to prevent this from occurring is to add enough solvent to dissolve the desired product at room temperature (be sure not to add too much solvent) and perform the filtration at room temperature, as described in Technique 8, Section 8.1C, p. 649. After filtration, the excess solvent is evaporated by boiling until the solution is saturated at the boiling point of the mixture (see Technique 7, Section 7.10, p. 639). If powdered decolorizing charcoal was used, it will probably be necessary to perform two filtrations with a filtering pipet to remove all of the charcoal, or a fluted filter can be used.

C. Crystallizing

An Erlenmeyer flask, not a beaker, should be used for crystallization. The large open top of a beaker makes it an excellent dust catcher. The narrow opening of the Erlenmeyer flask reduces contamination by dust and allows the flask to be stoppered if it is to be set aside for a long period. Mixtures set aside for long periods must be stoppered after cooling to room temperature to prevent evaporation of solvent. If all the solvent evaporates, no purification is achieved, and the crystals originally formed become coated with the dried contents of the mother liquor. Even if the time required for crystallization to occur is relatively short, it is advisable to cover the top of the Erlenmeyer flask with a small watch glass or inverted beaker to prevent evaporation of solvent while the solution is cooling to room temperature.

The chances of obtaining pure crystals are improved if the solution cools to room temperature slowly. When the volume of solution is 10 mL or less, the solution is likely to cool more rapidly than is desired. This can be prevented by placing the flask on a surface that is a poor heat conductor and covering the flask with a beaker to provide a layer of insulating air. Appropriate surfaces include a clay plate or several pieces of filter paper on top of the laboratory bench. It may also be helpful to use a clay plate that has been warmed slightly on a hot plate or in an oven.

After crystallization has occurred, it is sometimes desirable to cool the flask in an ice-water bath. Because the solute is less soluble at lower temperatures, this will increase the yield of crystals.

If a cooled solution does not crystallize, it will be necessary to induce crystallization. Several techniques are described in Section 11.8A.

D. Collecting and Drying

After the flask has been cooled, the crystals are collected by vacuum filtration through a Büchner (or Hirsch) funnel (see Technique 8, Section 8.3, p. 651, and Figure 8.5). The crystals should be washed with a small amount of *cold* solvent to remove any mother liquor adhering to their surface. Hot or warm solvent will dissolve some of the crystals. The crystals should then be left for a short time (usually 5–10 minutes) in the funnel, where air, as it passes, will dry them free of most of the solvent. It is often wise to cover the Büchner funnel with an oversized filter paper or towel during this air drying. This precaution prevents accumulation of dust in the crystals. When the crystals are nearly dry, they should be gently scraped off the filter paper (so paper fibers are not removed with the crystals) onto a watch glass or clay plate for further drying (see Section 11.9).

The four steps in a macroscale crystallization are summarized in Table 11.1.

TABLE 11.1   Steps in a Macroscale Crystallization

A. Dissolving the Solid

1. Find a solvent with a steep solubility-vs.-temperature characteristic (done by trial and error using small amounts of material or by consulting a handbook).
2. Heat the desired solvent to its builing point.
3. Dissolve the solid in a **minimum** of boiling solvent in a flask.
4. If necessary, add decolorizing charcoal or decolorize the solution on a silica gel or alumina column.

B. Removing Insoluble Impurities

1. Decant or remove the solution with a Pasteur pipet.
2. Alternatively, filter the hot solution through a fluted filter, a filtering pipet, or a filter-tip pipet to remove insoluble impurities or charcoal.

> **Note:** If no decolorizing charcoal has been added or if there are no undissolved particles, Part B should be omitted.

C. Crystallizing

1. Allow the solution to cool.
2. If crystals appear, cool the mixture in an ice-water bath (if desired) and go to Part D. If crystals do not appear, go to the next step.
3. Inducing crystallization
    a. Scratch the flask with a glass rod.
    b. Seed the solution with original solid, if available.
    c. Cool the solution in an ice-water bath.
    d. Evaporate excess solvent and allow the solution to cool again.

D. Collecting and Drying

1. Collect crystals by vacuum filtration using a Büchner funnel.
2. Rinse crystals with a small portion of **cold** solvent.
3. Continue suction until crystals are nearly dry.
4. Drying (three options)
    a. Air-dry the crystals.
    b. Place the crystals in a drying oven.
    c. Dry the crystals under a vacuum.

Part C. Microscale Crystallization

11.4 MICROSCALE CRYSTALLIZATION

In many microscale experiments, the amount of solid to be crystallized is small enough (generally less than 0.1 g) that a **Craig tube** (see Technique 8, Figure 8.10, p. 657) is the preferred method for crystallization. The main advantage of the Craig tube is that it minimizes the number of transfers of solid material, thus resulting in a greater yield of crystals. Also, the separation of the crystals from the mother liquor with the Craig tube is very efficient, and little time is required for drying the crystals. The steps involved are, in principle, the same as those performed when a crystallization is accomplished with an Erlenmeyer flask and a Büchner funnel.

The solid is transferred to the Craig tube, and small portions of hot solvent are added to the tube while the mixture is stirred with a spatula and heated. If there are any insoluble impurities present, they can be removed with a filter-tip pipet. The inner plug is then inserted into the Craig tube and the hot solution is cooled slowly to room temperature. When the crystals have formed, the Craig tube is placed into a centrifuge tube, and the crystals are separated from the mother liquor by centrifugation (see Technique 8, Section 8.7, p. 656). The crystals are then scraped off the end of the inner plug or from inside the Craig tube onto a watch glass or piece of paper. Minimal drying will be necessary (see Section 11.9).

Part D. Additional Experimental Considerations: Macroscale and Microscale

11.5 SELECTING A SOLVENT

A solvent that dissolves little of the material to be crystallized when it is cold but a great deal of the material when it is hot is a good solvent for crystallization. Quite often, correct crystallization solvents are indicated in the experimental procedures that you will be following. When a solvent is not specified in a procedure, you can determine a good crystallization solvent by consulting a handbook or making an educated guess based on polarities, both discussed in this section. A third approach, involving experimentation, is discussed in Section 11.6.

With compounds that are well known, the correct crystallization solvent has already been determined through the experiments of earlier researchers. In such cases, the chemical literature can be consulted to determine which solvent should be used. Sources such as *The Merck Index* or the *CRC Handbook of Chemistry and Physics* may provide this information.

For example, consider naphthalene, which is found in *The Merck Index*. It states under the entry for naphthalene: "Monoclinic prismatic plates from ether." This statement means that naphthalene can be crystallized from ether. It also gives the type of crystal structure. Unfortunately, the crystal structure may be given without reference to the solvent. Another way to determine the best solvent is by looking at solubility-vs.-temperature data. When this is given, a good solvent is one in which the solubility of the compound increases significantly as the temperature increases. Sometimes, the solubility data will be given for only cold solvent and boiling solvent. This should provide enough information to determine whether this would be a good solvent for crystallization.

In most cases, however, the handbooks will state only whether a compound is soluble or not in a given solvent, usually at room temperature. Determining a good solvent for crystallization from this information can be somewhat difficult. The solvent in which the compound is soluble may or may not be an appropriate solvent for crystallization. Sometimes, the compound may be too soluble in the solvent at all temperatures, and you would recover very little of your product if this solvent were used for crystallization. It is possible that an appropriate solvent would be the one in which the compound is nearly insoluble at room temperature because the solubility-vs.-temperature curve is very steep. Although the solubility information may give you some ideas about what solvents to try, you will most likely need to determine a good crystallizing solvent by experimentation as described in Section 11.6.

When using *The Merck Index* or *Handbook of Chemistry and Physics,* you should be aware that alcohol is frequently listed as a solvent. This generally refers to 95% or 100% ethyl alcohol. Because 100% (absolute) ethyl alcohol is more expensive than 95% ethyl alcohol, the cheaper grade is usually used in the chemistry laboratory. Another solvent frequently listed is benzene. Benzene is a known carcinogen, so it is rarely used in student laboratories. Toluene is a suitable substitute; the solubility behavior of a substance in benzene and toluene is so similar that you may assume any statement made about benzene also applies to toluene.

Another way to identify a solvent for crystallization is to consider the polarities of the compound and the solvents. Generally, you would look for a solvent that has a polarity somewhat similar to that of the compound to be crystallized. Consider the compound sulfanilamide, shown in the figure. There are several polar bonds in sulfanilamide, the NH and

Sulfanilamide

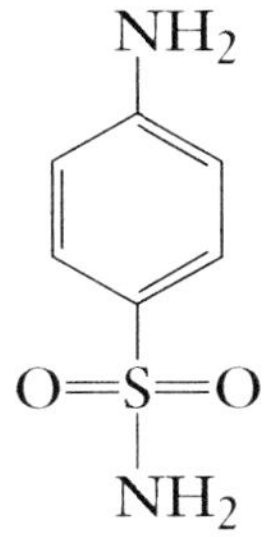

the SO bonds. In addition, the NH_2 groups and the oxygen atoms in sulfanilamide can form hydrogen bonds. Although the benzene ring portion of sulfanilamide is nonpolar, sulfanilamide has an intermediate polarity because of the polar groups. A common organic solvent of intermediate polarity is 95% ethyl alcohol. Therefore, it is likely that sulfanilamide would be soluble in 95% ethyl alcohol because they have similar polarities. (Note that the other 5% in 95% ethyl alcohol is usually a substance such as water or isopropyl alcohol, which does not alter the overall polarity of the solvent.) Although this kind of analysis is a good first step in determining an appropriate solvent for crystallization, without more information it is not enough to predict the shape of the solubility curve for the temperature-vs.-solubility data (see Figure 11.1, p. 680). Therefore, knowing that sulfanilamide is soluble in 95% ethyl alcohol does not necessarily mean that this is a good solvent for crystallizing sulfanilamide. You would still need to test the solvent to see if it is appropriate. The solubility curve for sulfanilamide (see Figure 11.2, page 681) indicates that 95% ethyl alcohol is a good solvent for crystallizing this substance.

When choosing a crystallization solvent, do not select one whose boiling point is higher than the melting point of the substance (solute) to be crystallized. If the boiling point of the solvent is too high, the substance may come out of solution as a liquid rather than a crystalline solid. In such a case, the solid may **oil out.** Oiling out occurs when on cooling the solution to induce crystallization, the solute begins to come out of solution at a temperature above its melting point. The solute will then come out of solution as a liquid. Furthermore, as cooling continues, the substance may still not crystallize; rather, it will become a supercooled liquid. Oils may eventually solidify if the temperature is lowered, but often they will not actually crystallize. Instead, the solidified oil will be an amorphous solid or a hardened mass. In this case, purification of the substance will not have occurred as it does when the solid is crystalline. It can be very difficult to deal with oils when trying to obtain a pure substance. You must try to redissolve them and hope that the substance will crystallize with slow, careful cooling. During the cooling period, it may be helpful to scratch the glass container where the oil is present with a glass stirring rod that has not been fire polished. Seeding the oil as it cools with a small sample of the original solid is another technique that is sometimes helpful in working with difficult oils. Other methods of inducing crystallization are discussed in Section 11.8.

One additional criterion for selecting the correct crystallization solvent is the **volatility** of that solvent. Volatile solvents have low boiling points or evaporate easily. A solvent with a low boiling point may be removed from the crystals through evaporation without much difficulty. It will be difficult to remove a solvent with a high boiling point from the crystals without heating them under vacuum.

Table 11.2 lists common crystallization solvents. The solvents used most commonly are listed in the table first.

11.6 TESTING SOLVENTS FOR CRYSTALLIZATION

When the appropriate solvent is not known, select a solvent for crystallization by experimenting with various solvents and a very small amount of the material to be crystallized. Experiments are conducted on a small test tube scale before the entire quantity of material is committed to a particular solvent. Such trial-and-error methods are common when trying to purify a solid material that has not been previously studied.

Procedure

1. Place about 0.05 g of the sample in a test tube.
2. Add about 0.5 mL of solvent at room temperature and stir the mixture by rapidly twirling a microspatula between your fingers. If all (or almost all) of the solid dissolves at room temperature, then your solid is *probably* too soluble in this solvent and little compound would be recovered if this solvent were used. Select another solvent.
3. If none (or very little) of the solid dissolves at room temperature, heat the tube carefully and stir with a spatula. (A hot water bath is perhaps better than an alu-

TABLE 11.2 Common Solvents for Crystallization

	Boils (°C)	Freezes (°C)	Soluble in H₂O	Flammability
Water	100	0	+	−
Methanol	65	*	+	+
95% Ethanol	78	*	+	+
Ligroin	60–90	*	−	+
Toluene	111	*	−	+
Chloroform**	61	*	−	−
Acetic acid	118	17	+	+
Dioxane**	101	11	+	+
Acetone	56	*	+	+
Diethyl ether	35	*	Slightly	+ +
Petroleum ether	30–60	*	−	+ +
Methylene chloride	41	*	−	−
Carbon tetrachloride**	77	*	−	−

*Lower than 0°C (ice temperature).

**Suspected carcinogen.

minum block because you can more easily control the temperature of the hot water bath. The temperature of the hot water bath should be slightly higher than the boiling point of the solvent.) Add more solvent dropwise, while continuing to heat and stir. Continue adding solvent until the solid dissolves, but do not add more than about 1.5 mL (total) of solvent. If all the solid dissolves, go to step 4. If all the solid has not dissolved by the time you have added 1.5 mL of solvent, this is probably not a good solvent. However, if most of the solid has dissolved at this point, you might try adding a little more solvent. Remember to heat and stir at all times during this step.

4. If the solid dissolves in about 1.5 mL or less of boiling solvent, then remove the test tube from the heat source, stopper the tube, and allow it to cool to room temperature. Then place it in an ice-water bath. If a lot of crystals come out, this is most likely a good solvent. If crystals do not come out, scratch the sides of the tube with a glass stirring rod to induce crystallization. If crystals still do not form, this is probably not a good solvent.

Comments about This Procedure

1. Selecting a good solvent is something of an art. There is no perfect procedure that can be used in all cases. You must think about what you are doing and use some common sense in deciding whether to use a particular solvent.
2. Do not heat the mixture above the melting point of your solid. This can occur most easily when the boiling point of the solvent is higher than the melting point of the solid. Normally, do not select a solvent that has a higher boiling point than the melt-

ing point of the substance. If you do, make certain that you do not heat the mixture beyond the melting point of your solid.

11.7 DECOLORIZATION

Small amounts of highly colored impurities may make the original crystallization solution appear colored; this color can often be removed by **decolorization,** either by using activated charcoal (often called Norit) or by passing the solution through a column packed with alumina or silica gel. A decolorizing step should be performed only if the color is due to impurities, not to the color of the desired product, and if the color is significant. Small amounts of colored impurities will remain in solution during crystallization, making the decolorizing step unnecessary. The use of activated charcoal is described separately for macroscale and microscale crystallizations, and then the column technique, which can be used with both crystallization techniques, is described.

A. Macroscale—Powdered Charcoal

As soon as the solute is dissolved in the minimum amount of boiling solvent, the solution is allowed to cool slightly, and a small amount of Norit (powdered charcoal) is added to the mixture. The Norit adsorbs the impurities. When performing a crystallization in which the filtration is performed with a fluted filter, you should add powdered Norit because it has a larger surface area and can remove impurities more effectively. A reasonable amount of Norit is what could be held on the end of a microspatula, or about 0.01–0.02 g. If too much Norit is used, it will adsorb product as well as impurities. A small amount of Norit should be used, and its use should be repeated if necessary. (It is difficult to determine if the initial amount added is sufficient until after the solution is filtered, because the suspended particles of charcoal will obscure the color of the liquid.) Caution should be exercised so that the solution does not froth or erupt when the finely divided charcoal is added. The mixture is boiled with the Norit for several minutes and then filtered by gravity, using a fluted filter (see Section 11.3 and Technique 8, Section 8.1B, p. 646), and the crystallization is carried forward as described in Section 11.3.

The Norit preferentially adsorbs the colored impurities and removes them from the solution. The technique seems to be most effective with hydroxylic solvents. In using Norit, be careful not to breathe the dust. Normally, small quantities are used so that little risk of lung irritation exists.

B. Microscale—Pelletized Norit

If the crystallization is being performed in a Craig tube, it is advisable to use pelletized Norit. Although this is not as effective in removing impurities as powdered Norit, it is easier to remove, and the amount of pelletized Norit required is more easily determined because you can see the solution as it is being decolorized. Again, the Norit is added to the hot solution (the solution should not be boiling) after the solid has dissolved. This should be performed in a test tube rather than in a Craig tube. About 0.02 g is added, and the mixture is boiled for a minute or so to see if more Norit is required. More Norit is added, if necessary, and the liquid is boiled again. It is important not to add too much pelletized Norit because the Norit will also adsorb some of the desired material, and it is possible that not all the color can be removed no matter how much is added. The decolorized solution is then removed with a preheated filter-tip pipet (see Technique 8, Section 8.6, p. 655) to filter the mixture and transferred to a Craig tube for crystallization as described in Section 11.4.

C. Decolorization on a Column

The other method for decolorizing a solution is to pass the solution through a column containing alumina or silica gel. The adsorbent removes the colored impurities while allowing the desired material to pass through (see Technique 8, Figure 8.6, p. 654, and Technique 19, Section 19.15, p. 814). If this technique is used, it will be necessary to dilute the solution with additional solvent to prevent crystallization from occurring during the process. The excess solvent must be evaporated after the solution is passed through the column (Technique 7, Section 7.10, p. 639) and the crystallization procedure is continued as described in Sections 11.3 or 11.4.

11.8 INDUCING CRYSTALLIZATION

If a cooled solution does not crystallize, several techniques may be used to induce crystallization. Although identical in principle, the actual procedures vary slightly when performing macroscale and microscale crystallizations.

A. Macroscale

In the first technique, you should try scratching the inside surface of the flask vigorously with a glass rod that *has not been* fire polished. The motion of the rod should be vertical (in and out of the solution) and should be vigorous enough to produce an audible scratching. Such scratching often induces crystallization, although the effect is not well understood. The high-frequency vibrations may have something to do with initiating crystallization; or perhaps—a more likely possibility—small amounts of solution dry by evaporation on the side of the flask, and the dried solute is pushed into the solution. These small amounts of material provide "seed crystals," or nuclei, on which crystallization may begin.

A second technique that can be used to induce crystallization is to cool the solution in an ice bath. This method decreases the solubility of the solute.

A third technique is useful when small amounts of the original material to be crystallized are saved. The saved material can be used to "seed" the cooled solution. A small crystal dropped into the cooled flask often will start the crystallization—this is called **seeding.**

If all these measures fail to induce crystallization, it is likely that too much solvent was added. The excess solvent must then be evaporated (Technique 7, Section 7.10, p. 639) and the solution allowed to cool.

B. Microscale

The strategy is basically the same as described for macroscale crystallizations. Scratching vigorously with a glass rod *should be avoided,* however, because the Craig tube is fragile and expensive. Scratching *gently* is allowed.

Another measure is to dip a spatula or glass stirring rod into the solution and allow the solvent to evaporate so that a small amount of solid will form on the surface of the spatula or glass rod. When placed back into the solution, the solid will seed the solution. A small amount of the original material, if some was saved, may also be used to seed the solution.

A third technique is to cool the Craig tube in an ice-water bath. This method may also be combined with either of the previous suggestions.

If none of these measures is successful, it is possible that too much solvent is present, and it may be necessary to evaporate some of the solvent (Technique 7, Section 7.10, p. 639) and allow the solution to cool again.

11.9 DRYING CRYSTALS

The most common method of drying crystals involves allowing them to dry in air. Several different methods are illustrated in Figure 11.6, below. In all three methods, the crystals must be covered to prevent accumulation of dust particles. Note that in each method, the spout on the beaker provides an opening so that solvent vapor can escape from the system. The advantage of this method is that heat is not required, thus reducing the danger of decomposition or melting; however, exposure to atmospheric moisture may cause the hydration of strongly hygroscopic materials. A **hygroscopic** substance is a substance that absorbs moisture from the air.

Another method of drying crystals is to place the crystals on a watch glass, a clay plate, or a piece of absorbent paper in an oven. Although this method is simple, some possible difficulties deserve mention. Crystals that sublime readily should not be dried in an oven because they might vaporize and disappear. Care should be taken that the temperature of the oven does not exceed the melting point of the crystals. Remember that the melting point of crystals is lowered by the presence of solvent; allow for this melting-point depression when selecting a suitable oven temperature. Some materials decompose on exposure to heat, and they should not be dried in an oven. Finally, when many different samples are being dried in the same oven, crystals might be lost due to confusion or reac-

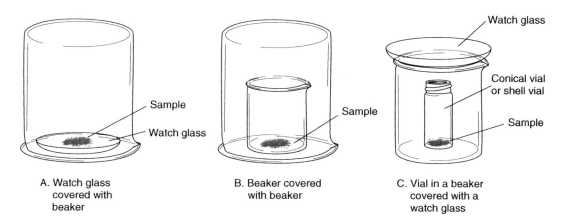

A. Watch glass covered with beaker

B. Beaker covered with beaker

C. Vial in a beaker covered with a watch glass

Figure 11.6 Methods for drying crystals in air.

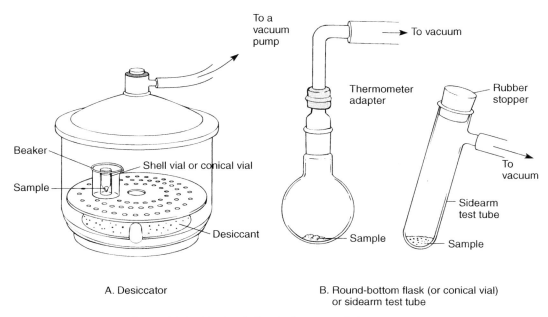

Figure 11.7 Methods for drying crystals in a vacuum.

tion with another person's sample. It is important to label the crystals when they are placed in the oven.

A third method, which requires neither heat nor exposure to atmospheric moisture, is drying *in vacuo*. Two procedures are illustrated in Figure 11.7.

Procedure A. In this method, a desiccator is used. The sample is placed under vacuum in the presence of a drying agent. Two potential problems must be noted. The first deals with samples that sublime readily. Under vacuum, the likelihood of sublimation is increased. The second problem deals with the vacuum desiccator itself. Because the surface area of glass that is under vacuum is large, there is some danger that the desiccator could implode. A vacuum desiccator should never be used unless it has been placed within a protective metal container (cage). If a cage is not available, the desiccator can be wrapped with electrical or duct tape. If you use an aspirator as a source of vacuum, you should use a water trap (see Figure 8.5, p. 652).

Procedure B. This method can be accomplished with a round-bottom flask and a thermometer adapter equipped with a short piece of glass tubing, as illustrated in Figure 11.7B. In microscale work, the apparatus with the round-bottom flask can be modified by replacing the round-bottom flask with a conical vial. The glass tubing is connected by vacuum tubing to either an aspirator or a vacuum pump. A convenient alternative, using a sidearm test tube, is also shown in Figure 11.7B. With either apparatus, install a water trap when an aspirator is used.

11.10 MIXED SOLVENTS

Often, the desired solubility characteristics for a particular compound are not found in a single solvent. In these cases, a mixed solvent may be used. You simply select a first

149

TABLE 11.3   Common Solvent Pairs for
Crystallization

Methanol–water	Ether–acetone
Ethanol–water	Ether–petroleum ether
Acetic acid–water	Toluene–ligroin
Acetone–water	Methylene chloride–methanol
Ether–methanol	Dioxane[a]–water

[a] Suspected carcinogen.

solvent in which the solute is soluble and a second solvent, miscible with the first, in which the solute is relatively insoluble. The compound is dissolved in a minimum amount of the boiling solvent in which it is soluble. Following this, the second hot solvent is added to the boiling mixture, dropwise, until the mixture barely becomes cloudy. The cloudiness indicates precipitation. At this point, more of the first solvent should be added. Just enough is added to clear the cloudy mixture. At that point, the solution is saturated, and as it cools, crystals should separate. Common solvent mixtures are listed in Table 11.3.

It is important not to add an excess of the second solvent or to cool the solution too rapidly. Either of these actions may cause the solute to oil out, or separate as a viscous liquid. If this happens, reheat the solution and add more of the first solvent.

PROBLEMS

1. Listed below are solubility-vs.-temperature data for an organic substance A dissolved in water.

Temperature (°C)	Solubility of A in 100 mL of Water (g)
0	1.5
20	3.0
40	6.5
60	11.0
80	17.0

    a. Graph the solubility of A vs. temperature. Use the data given in the table. Connect the data points with a smooth curve.

    b. Suppose 0.1 g of A and 1.0 mL of water were mixed and heated to 80°C. Would all the substance A dissolve?

    c. The solution prepared in (b) is cooled. At what temperature will crystals of A appear?

    d. Suppose the cooling described in (c) were continued to 0°C. How many grams of A would come out of solution? Explain how you obtained your answer.

2. What would likely happen if a hot saturated solution were filtered by vacuum filtration using a Büchner funnel? (*Hint:* The mixture will cool as it comes in contact with the Büchner funnel.)

3. A compound you have prepared is reported in the literature to have a pale yellow color. When the substance is dissolved in hot solvent to purify it by crystallization, the resulting solution is yellow. Should you use decolorizing charcoal before allowing the hot solution to cool? Explain your answer.

4. While performing a crystallization, you obtain a light tan solution after dissolving your crude product in hot solvent. A decolorizing step is determined to be unnecessary, and there are no solid impurities present. Should you perform a filtration to remove impurities before allowing the solution to cool? Why or why not?

5. a. Draw a graph of a cooling curve (temperature vs. time) for a solution of a solid substance that shows no supercooling effects. Assume that the solvent does not freeze.

    b. Repeat the instructions in (a) for a solution for a solid substance that shows some supercooling behavior but eventually yields crystals if the solution is cooled sufficiently.

6. A solid substance A is soluble in water to the extent of 10 mg/mL of water at 25°C and 100 mg/mL of water at 100°C. You have a sample that contains 100 mg of A and an impurity B.

    a. Assuming that 2 mg of B are present along with 100 mg of A, describe how you can purify A if B is completely insoluble in water. Your description should include the volume of solvent required.

    b. Assuming that 2 mg of the impurity B are present along with 100 mg of A, describe how you can purify A if B has the same solubility behavior as A. Will one crystallization produce pure A? (Assume that the solubilities of both A and B are unaffected by the presence of the other substance.)

    c. Assume that 25 mg of the impurity B are present along with 100 mg of A. Describe how you can purify A if B has the same solubility behavior as A. Each time, use the minimum amount of water to just dissolve the solid. Will one crystallization produce absolutely pure A? How many crystallizations would be needed to produce pure A? How much A will have been recovered when the crystallizations have been completed?

7. An organic chemistry student dissolved 0.30 g of a crude product in 10.5 mL (the minimum amount required) of ethanol at 25°C. He cooled the solution in an ice-water bath for 15 minutes and obtained beautiful crystals. He filtered the crystals on a Hirsch funnel and rinsed them with about 2.0 mL of ice-cold ethanol. After drying, the weight of the crystals was found to be 0.015 g. Why was the recovery so low?

TECHNIQUE 12

Extractions, Separations, and Drying Agents

Part A. Theory

12.1 EXTRACTION

Transferring a solute from one solvent into another is called **extraction,** or more precisely, liquid–liquid extraction. The solute is extracted from one solvent into the other because the solute is more soluble in the second solvent than in the first. The two solvents must not be **miscible** (mix freely), and they must form two separate **phases or layers,** in order for this procedure to work. Extraction is used in many ways in organic chemistry. Many **natural products** (organic chemicals that exist in nature) are present in animal and plant tissues having high water content. Extracting these tissues with a water-immiscible solvent is useful for isolating the natural products. Often, diethyl ether (commonly referred to as "ether") is used for this purpose. Sometimes, alternative water-immiscible solvents such as hexane, petroleum ether, ligroin, and methylene chloride are used. For instance, caffeine, a natural product, can be extracted from an aqueous tea solution by shaking the solution successively with several portions of methylene chloride.

A generalized extraction process, using a specialized piece of glassware called a **separatory funnel,** is illustrated in Figure 12.1. The first solvent contains a mixture of black-and-white molecules (Figure 12.1A). A second solvent that is not miscible with the first is added. After the separatory funnel is capped and shaken, the layers separate. In this example, the second solvent (shaded) is less dense than the first, so it becomes the top layer (Figure 12.1B). Because of differences in physical properties, the white molecules are more soluble in the second solvent, whereas the black molecules are more soluble in the first solvent. Most of the white molecules are in the upper layer, but there are some black molecules there, too. Likewise, most of the black molecules are in the lower layer. However, there are still a few white molecules in this lower phase. The lower phase may be separated from the upper phase by opening the stopcock at the bottom of the separatory funnel and allowing the lower layer to drain into a beaker (Figure 12.1C). In this example, notice that it was not possible to effect a complete separation of the two types of molecules with a single extraction. This is a common occurrence in organic chemistry.

Many substances are soluble in both water and organic solvents. Water can be used to extract, or "wash," water-soluble impurities from an organic reaction mixture. To carry out a "washing" operation, you add water and an immiscible organic solvent to the reaction mixture contained in a separatory funnel. After stoppering the funnel and shaking it, you allow the organic layer and the aqueous (water) layer to separate. A water wash removes highly polar and water-soluble materials, such as sulfuric acid, hydrochloric acid, and sodium hy-

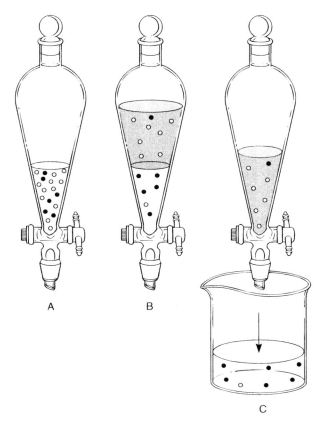

A. Solvent 1 contains a mixture of molecules (black and white).

B. After shaking with solvent 2 (shaded), most of the white molecules have been extracted into the new solvent. The white molecules are more soluble in the second solvent, whereas the black molecules are more soluble in the original solvent.

C. With removal of the lower phase, the black and white molecules have been partially separated.

Figure 12.1 The extraction process.

droxide, from the organic layer. The washing operation helps to purify the desired organic compound present in the original reaction mixture.

12.2 DISTRIBUTION COEFFICIENT

When a solution (solute A in solvent 1) is shaken with a second solvent (solvent 2) with which it is not miscible, the solute distributes itself between the two liquid phases. When the two phases have separated again into two distinct solvent layers, an equilibrium will have been achieved such that the ratio of the concentrations of the solute in each layer defines a constant. The constant, called the **distribution coefficient** (or partition coefficient) K, is defined by

$$K = \frac{C_2}{C_1}$$

where C_1 and C_2 are the concentrations at equilibrium, in grams per liter or milligrams per milliliter of solute A in solvent 1 and in solvent 2, respectively. This relationship is a ratio of two concentrations and is independent of the actual amounts of the two solvents mixed. The distribution coefficient has a constant value for each solute considered and depends on the nature of the solvents used in each case.

Not all the solute will be transferred to solvent 2 in a single extraction unless K is very large. Usually, it takes several extractions to remove all the solute from solvent 1. In extracting a solute from a solution, it is always better to use several small portions of the second solvent than to make a single extraction with a large portion. Suppose, as an illustration, a particular extraction proceeds with a distribution coefficient of 10. The system consists of 5.0 g of organic compound dissolved in 100 mL of water (solvent 1). In this illustration, the effectiveness of three 50-mL extractions with ether (solvent 2) is compared with one 150-mL extraction with ether. In the first 50-mL extraction, the amount extracted into the ether layer is given by the following calculation. The amount of compound remaining in the aqueous phase is given by x.

$$K = 10 = \frac{C_2}{C_1} = \frac{\left(\dfrac{5.0 - x}{50} \dfrac{g}{mL \ ether}\right)}{\left(\dfrac{x}{100 \ mL \ H_2O} \ g\right)}; \qquad 10 = \frac{(5.0 - x)(100)}{50x}$$

$$500x = 500 - 100x$$
$$600x = 500$$
$$x = 0.83 \text{ g remaining in the aqueous phase}$$
$$5.0 - x = 4.17 \text{ g in the ether layer}$$

As a check on the calculation, it is possible to substitute the value 0.83 g for x in the original equation and demonstrate that the concentration in the ether layer divided by the concentration in the water layer equals the distribution coefficient.

$$\frac{\left(\dfrac{5.0 - x}{50} \dfrac{g}{mL \ ether}\right)}{\left(\dfrac{x}{100 \ mL \ H_2O} \ g\right)} = \frac{\dfrac{4.17}{50}}{\dfrac{0.83}{100}} = \frac{0.083 \ g/mL}{0.0083 \ g/mL} = 10 = K$$

The second extraction with another 50-mL portion of fresh ether is performed on the aqueous phase, which now contains 0.83 g of the solute. The amount of solute extracted is given by the calculation shown in Figure 12.2. Also shown in the figure is a calculation for a third extraction with another 50-mL portion of ether. This third extraction will transfer 0.12 g of solute into the ether layer, leaving 0.02 g of solute remaining in the water layer. A total of 4.98 g of solute will be extracted into the combined ether layers, and 0.02 g will remain in the aqueous phase.

Figure 12.3 shows the result of a *single* extraction with 150 mL of ether. As shown there, 4.69 g of solute were extracted into the ether layer, leaving 0.31 g of compound in

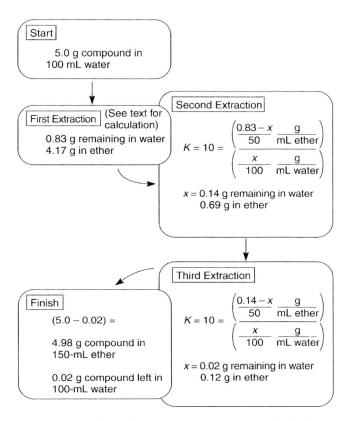

Figure 12.2 The result of extraction of 5.0 g of compound in 100 mL of water by three successive 50-mL portions of ether. Compare this result with that of Figure 12.3.

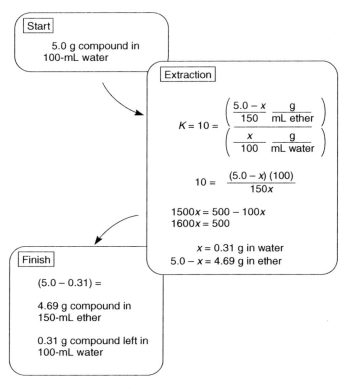

Figure 12.3 The result of extraction of 5.0 g of compound in 100 mL of water with one 150-mL portion of ether. Compare this result with that of Figure 12.2.

the aqueous phase. Three successive 50-mL ether extractions (Figure 12.2) succeeded in removing 0.29 g more solute from the aqueous phase than using one 150-mL portion of ether (Figure 12.3). This differential represents 5.8% of the total material.

> **Note:** Several extractions with smaller amounts of solvent are more effective than one extraction with a larger amount of solvent.

12.3 CHOOSING AN EXTRACTION METHOD AND A SOLVENT

Three types of apparatus are used for extractions: conical vials, centrifuge tubes, and separatory funnels (Figure 12.4). Conical vials may be used with volumes of less than 4 mL; volumes of up to 10 mL may be handled in centrifuge tubes. A centrifuge tube equipped with a screw cap is particularly useful for extractions. Conical vials and centrifuge tubes are most often used in microscale experiments, although a centrifuge tube may also be used in some macroscale applications. The separatory funnel is used with larger volumes of liquid in macroscale experiments. The separatory funnel is discussed in Part B and the conical vial and centrifuge tube are discussed in Part C.

TABLE 12.1 Densities of Common Extraction Solvents

Solvent	Density (g/mL)
Ligroin	0.67–0.69
Diethyl ether	0.71
Toluene	0.87
Water	1.00
Methylene chloride	1.330

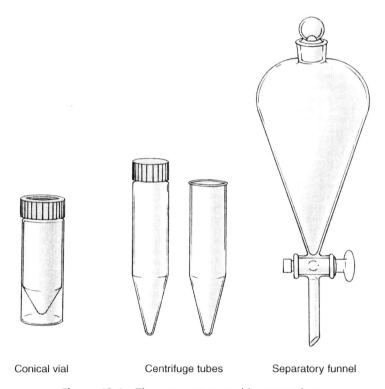

Conical vial   Centrifuge tubes   Separatory funnel

Figure 12.4 The apparatus used in extraction.

Most extractions consist of an aqueous phase and an organic phase. To extract a substance from an aqueous phase, you must use an organic solvent that is not miscible with water. Table 12.1 lists a number of the common organic solvents that are not miscible with water and are used for extractions.

Solvents that have a density less than that of water (1.00 g/mL) will separate as the top layer when shaken with water. Solvents that have a density greater than that of water will separate into the lower layer. For instance, diethyl ether ($d = 0.71$ g/mL) when shaken with water will form the upper layer, whereas methylene chloride ($d = 1.33$ g/mL) will form the lower layer. When an extraction is performed, slightly different methods are used to separate the lower layer (whether or not it is the aqueous layer or the organic layer) than to separate the upper layer.

Part B. Macroscale Extraction

12.4 THE SEPARATORY FUNNEL

A separatory funnel is illustrated in Figure 12.5. It is the piece of equipment used for carrying out extractions with medium to large quantities of material. To fill the separatory funnel, support it in an iron ring attached to a ring stand. Since it is easy to break a separa-

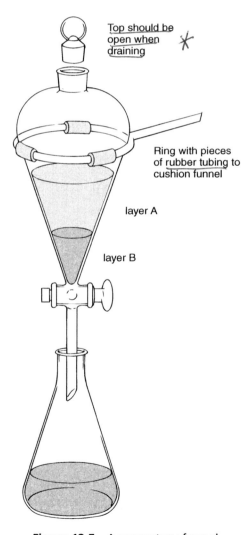

Figure 12.5 A separatory funnel.

tory funnel by "clanking" it against the metal ring, pieces of rubber tubing are often attached to the ring to cushion the funnel, as shown in Figure 12.5. These are short pieces of tubing cut to a length of about 3 cm and slit open along their length. When slipped over the inside of the ring, they cushion the funnel in its resting place.

When beginning an extraction, first close the stopcock. (Don't forget!) Using a powder funnel (wide bore) placed in the top of the separatory funnel, fill the funnel with both the solution to be extracted and the extraction solvent. Swirl the funnel gently by holding it by its upper neck and then stopper it. Pick up the separatory funnel with two hands and hold it as shown in Figure 12.6. Hold the stopper in place firmly because the two immiscible liquids will build pressure when they mix, and this pressure may force the stopper out of the separatory funnel. To release this pressure, vent the funnel by holding it upside down (hold the stopper securely) and slowly open the stopcock. Usually, the rush of vapors out of the opening can be heard. Continue shaking and venting until the "whoosh" is no longer audible. Now continue shaking the mixture gently for about 1 minute. This can be done by inverting the funnel in a rocking motion repeatedly or, if the formation of an emulsion is not a problem (see Section 12.10, p. 716), by shaking the funnel more vigorously for less time.

Note: There is an art to shaking and venting a separatory funnel correctly, and it usually seems awkward to the beginner. The technique is best learned by observing a person, such as your instructor, who is thoroughly familiar with the separatory funnel's use.

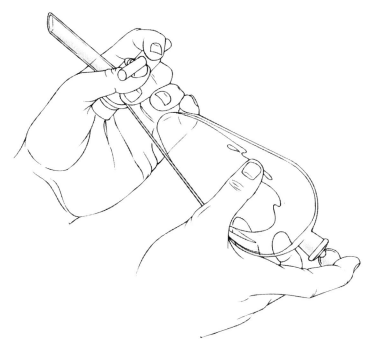

Figure 12.6 The correct way of shaking and venting a separatory funnel.

When you have finished mixing the liquids, place the separatory funnel in the iron ring and remove the top stopper immediately. The two immiscible solvents separate into two layers after a short time, and they can be separated from one another by draining most of the lower layer through the stopcock.[1] Allow a few minutes to pass so that any of the lower phase adhering to the inner glass surfaces of the separatory funnel can drain down. Open the stopcock again and allow the remainder of the lower layer to drain until the interface between the upper and lower phases just begins to enter the bore of the stopcock. At this moment, close the stopcock and remove the remaining upper layer by pouring it from the top opening of the separatory funnel.

> **Note:** To minimize contamination of the two layers, the lower layer should always be drained from the bottom of the separatory funnel and the upper layer poured out from the top of the funnel.

When methylene chloride is used as the extracting solvent with an aqueous phase, it will settle to the bottom and be removed through the stopcock. The aqueous layer remains in the funnel. A second extraction of the remaining aqueous layer with fresh methylene chloride may be needed.

With a diethyl ether (ether) extraction of an aqueous phase, the organic layer will form on top. Remove the lower aqueous layer through the stopcock and pour the upper ether layer from the top of the separatory funnel. Pour the aqueous phase back into the separatory funnel and extract it a second time with fresh ether. The combined organic phases must be dried using a suitable drying agent (Section 12.9) before the solvent is removed.

The usual macroscale procedure requires the use of a 125-mL or 250-mL separatory funnel. For microscale procedures, a 60-mL or 125-mL separatory funnel is recommended. Because of surface tension, water has a difficult time draining from the bore of smaller funnels.

Part C. Microscale Extraction

12.5 THE CONICAL VIAL—SEPARATING THE LOWER LAYER

Before using a conical vial for an extraction, make sure that the capped conical vial does not leak when shaken. To do this, place some water in the conical vial, place the Teflon liner in the cap, and screw the cap securely onto the conical vial. Shake the vial vigorously and check for leaks. Conical vials that are used for extractions must not be chipped on the edge of the vial or they will not seal adequately. If there is a leak, try tightening the cap or

---

[1] A common error is to try to drain the separatory funnel without removing the top stopper. Under this circumstance, the funnel will not drain because a partial vacuum is created in the space above the liquid.

replacing the Teflon liner with another one. Sometimes it helps to use the silicone rubber side of the liner to seal the conical vial. Some laboratories are supplied with Teflon stoppers that fit into the 5-mL conical vials. You may find that this stopper eliminates leakage.

When shaking the conical vial, do it gently at first in a rocking motion. When it is clear that an emulsion will not form (see Section 12.10, p. 716), you can shake it more vigorously.

In some cases, adequate mixing can be achieved by spinning your microspatula for at least 10 minutes in the conical vial. Another technique of mixing involves drawing the mixture up into a Pasteur pipet and squirting it rapidly back into the vial. Repeat this process for at least 5 minutes to obtain an adequate extraction.

The 5-mL conical vial is the most useful piece of equipment for carrying out extractions on a microscale level. In this section, we consider the method for removing the lower layer. A concrete example would be the extraction of a desired product from an aqueous layer using methylene chloride ($d = 1.33$ g/mL) as the extraction solvent. Methods for removal of the upper layer are discussed in the next section.

Note: Always place a conical vial in a small beaker to prevent the vial from falling over.

Removing the Lower Layer.　Suppose that we extract an aqueous solution with methylene chloride. This solvent is denser than water and will settle to the bottom of the conical vial. Use the following procedure, which is illustrated in Figure 12.7, to remove the lower layer.

1. Place the aqueous phase containing the dissolved product into a 5-mL conical vial (Figure 12.7A).
2. Add about 1 mL of methylene chloride, cap the vial, and shake the mixture gently at first in a rocking motion and then more vigorously when it is clear that an emulsion will not form. Vent or unscrew the cap slightly to release the pressure in the vial. Allow the phases to separate completely so that you can detect two distinct layers in the vial. The organic phase will be the lower layer in the vial (Figure 12.7B). If necessary, tap the vial with your finger or stir the mixture gently if some of the organic phase is suspended in the aqueous layer.
3. Prepare a Pasteur filter-tip pipet (Technique 8, Section 8.6, p. 655) using a 5¾-inch pipet. Attach a 2-mL rubber bulb to the pipet, depress the bulb, and insert the pipet into the vial so that the tip touches the bottom (Figure 12.7C). The filter-tip pipet gives you better control in removing the lower layer. In some cases, however, you may be able to use a Pasteur pipet (no filter tip), but considerably more care must be taken to avoid losing liquid from the pipet during the transfer operation. With experience, you should be able to judge how much to squeeze the bulb to draw in the desired volume of liquid.
4. Slowly draw the lower layer (methylene chloride) into the pipet in such a way that you exclude the aqueous layer and any emulsion (Section 12.10) that might be at the interface between the layers (Figure 12.7D). Be sure to keep the tip of the pipet squarely in the V at the bottom of the vial.

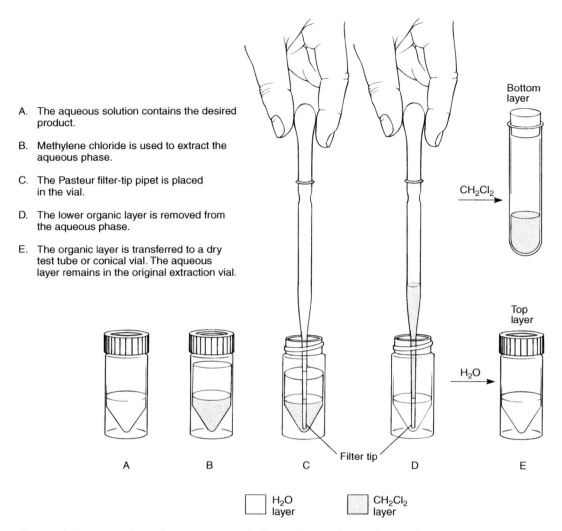

A. The aqueous solution contains the desired product.

B. Methylene chloride is used to extract the aqueous phase.

C. The Pasteur filter-tip pipet is placed in the vial.

D. The lower organic layer is removed from the aqueous phase.

E. The organic layer is transferred to a dry test tube or conical vial. The aqueous layer remains in the original extraction vial.

Bottom layer

CH_2Cl_2 →

Top layer

H_2O →

Filter tip

A   B   C   D   E

☐ H_2O layer   ▨ CH_2Cl_2 layer

Figure 12.7   Extraction of an aqueous solution using a solvent denser than water: methylene chloride.

5. Transfer the withdrawn organic phase into a *dry* test tube or another *dry* conical vial if one is available. It is best to have the test tube or vial located next to the extraction vial. Hold the vials in the same hand between your index finger and thumb, as shown in Figure 12.8. This avoids messy and disastrous transfers. The aqueous layer (upper layer) is left in the original conical vial (Figure 12.7E).

In performing an actual extraction in the laboratory, you would extract the aqueous phase with a second 1-mL portion of fresh methylene chloride to achieve a more complete extraction. Steps 2–5 would be repeated, and the organic layers from both extractions would be combined. In some cases, you may need to extract a third time with yet another 1-mL portion of methylene chloride. Again, the methylene chloride would be combined with the other extracts. The overall process would use three 1-mL portions of methylene chloride to transfer the product from the

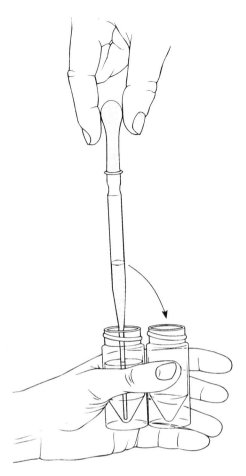

Figure 12.8 Method for holding vials while transferring liquids.

water layer into methylene chloride. Sometimes you will see the statement "extract the aqueous phase with three 1-mL portions of methylene chloride" in an experimental procedure. This statement describes in a shorter fashion the process described previously. Finally, the methylene chloride extracts will contain some water and must be dried with a drying agent as indicated in Section 12.9.

> **Note:** If an organic solvent has been extracted with water, it should be dried with a drying agent (see Section 12.9) before proceeding.

In this example, we extracted water with the heavy solvent methylene chloride and removed it as the lower layer. If you were extracting a light solvent (for instance, diethyl ether) with water and you wished to keep the water layer, the water would be the lower layer and would be removed using the same procedure. You would not dry the water layer, however.

12.6 THE CONICAL VIAL—SEPARATING THE UPPER LAYER

In this section, we consider the method used when you wish to remove the upper layer. A concrete example would be the extraction of a desired product from an aqueous layer using diethyl ether ($d = 0.71$ g/mL) as the extraction solvent. Methods for removing the lower layer were discussed previously.

> **Note:** Always place a conical vial in a small beaker to prevent the vial from falling over.

Removing the Upper Layer.   Suppose we extract an aqueous solution with diethyl ether (ether). This solvent is less dense than water and will rise to the top of the conical vial. Use the following procedure, which is illustrated in Figure 12.9, to remove the upper layer.

1. Place the aqueous phase containing the dissolved product in a 5-mL conical vial (Figure 12.9A).
2. Add about 1 mL of ether, cap the vial, and shake the mixture vigorously. Vent or unscrew the cap slightly to release the pressure in the vial. Allow the phases to separate completely so that you can detect two distinct layers in the vial. The ether phase will be the upper layer in the vial (Figure 12.9B).
3. Prepare a Pasteur filter-tip pipet (Technique 8, Section 8.6, p. 655) using a 5¾-inch pipet. Attach a 2-mL rubber bulb to the pipet, depress the bulb, and insert the pipet into the vial so that the tip touches the bottom. The filter-tip pipet gives you better control in removing the lower layer. In some cases, however, you may be able to use a Pasteur pipet (no filter tip), but considerably more care must be taken to avoid losing liquid from the pipet during the transfer operation. With experience, you should be able to judge how much to squeeze the bulb to draw in the desired volume of liquid. Slowly draw the lower *aqueous* layer into the pipet. Be sure to keep the tip of the pipet squarely in the V at the bottom of the vial (Figure 12.9C).
4. Transfer the withdrawn aqueous phase into a test tube or another conical vial for temporary storage. It is best to have the test tube or vial located next to the extraction vial. This avoids messy and disastrous transfers. Hold the vials in the same hand between your index finger and thumb, as shown in Figure 12.8. The ether layer is left behind in the conical vial (Figure 12.9D).
5. The ether phase remaining in the original conical vial should be transferred with a Pasteur pipet into a test tube for storage and the aqueous phase returned to the original conical vial (Figure 12.9E).

In performing an actual extraction, you would extract the aqueous phase with another 1-mL portion of fresh ether to achieve a more complete extraction. Steps 2–5 would be repeated, and the organic layers from both extractions would be combined in the test tube. In some cases, you may need to extract the aqueous layer a third time with yet another 1-mL portion of ether. Again, the ether would be combined with the other two layers. This over-

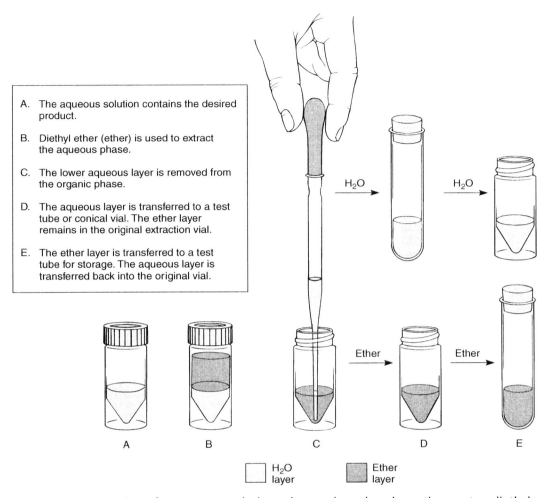

A. The aqueous solution contains the desired product.

B. Diethyl ether (ether) is used to extract the aqueous phase.

C. The lower aqueous layer is removed from the organic phase.

D. The aqueous layer is transferred to a test tube or conical vial. The ether layer remains in the original extraction vial.

E. The ether layer is transferred to a test tube for storage. The aqueous layer is transferred back into the original vial.

H_2O layer

Ether layer

Figure 12.9 Extraction of an aqueous solution using a solvent less dense than water: diethyl ether.

all process uses three 1-mL portions of ether to transfer the product from the water layer into ether. The ether extracts contain some water and must be dried with a drying agent as indicated in Section 12.9.

12.7 THE SCREW-CAP CENTRIFUGE TUBE

If you require an extraction that uses a larger volume than a conical vial can accommodate (about 4 mL), a centrifuge tube can often be used. A centrifuge tube can also be used instead of a separatory funnel for some macroscale applications in which the total volume of liquid is less than about 12 mL. A commonly available size of centrifuge tube has a volume of about 15 mL and is supplied with a screw cap. In performing an extraction with a screw-cap centrifuge tube, use the same procedures outlined for the conical vial (Sections 12.5 and 12.6). As is the case for a conical vial, the tapered bottom of the centrifuge tube makes it easy to withdraw the lower layer with a Pasteur pipet.

> **Note:** A centrifuge tube has a great advantage over other methods of extraction. If an emulsion (Section 12.10) forms, you can use a centrifuge to aid in the separation of the layers.

You should check the capped centrifuge tube for leaks by filling it with water and shaking it vigorously. If it leaks, try replacing the cap with a different one. A **vortex mixer,** if available, provides an alternative to shaking the tube. In fact, a vortex mixer works well with a variety of containers, including small flasks, test tubes, conical vials, and centrifuge tubes. You start the mixing action on a vortex mixer by holding the test tube or other container on one of the neoprene pads. The unit mixes the sample by high-frequency vibration.

Part D. Additional Experimental Considerations: Macroscale and Microscale

12.8 HOW DO YOU DETERMINE WHICH ONE IS THE ORGANIC LAYER?

A common problem encountered during an extraction is trying to determine which of the two layers is the organic layer and which is the aqueous (water) layer. The most common situation occurs when the aqueous layer is on the bottom in the presence of an upper organic layer consisting of ether, ligroin, petroleum ether, or hexane (see densities in Table 12.1). However, the aqueous layer will be on the top when you use methylene chloride as a solvent (again, see Table 12.1). Although a laboratory procedure may frequently identify the expected relative positions of the organic and aqueous layers, sometimes their actual positions are reversed. Surprises usually occur in situations in which the aqueous layer contains a high concentration of sulfuric acid or a dissolved ionic compound, such as sodium chloride. Dissolved substances greatly increase the density of the aqueous layer, which may lead to the aqueous layer being found on the bottom even when coexisting with a relatively dense organic layer such as methylene chloride.

> **Note:** Always keep both layers until you have actually isolated the desired compound or until you are certain where your desired substance is located.

To determine if a particular layer is the aqueous one, add a few drops of water to the layer. Observe closely as you add the water to see where it goes. If the layer is water, then the drops of added water will dissolve in the aqueous layer and increase its volume. If the added water forms droplets or a new layer, however, you can assume that the suspected aqueous layer is actually organic. You can use a similar procedure to identify a suspected organic layer. This time, try adding more of the solvent, such as methylene chloride. The organic layer should increase in size, without separation of a new layer, if the tested layer is actually organic.

When performing an extraction procedure on the microscale level, you can use the following approach to identify the layers. When both layers are present, it is always a good idea to think carefully about the volumes of materials that you have added to the conical vial. You can use the graduations on the vial to help determine the volumes of the layers in the vial. If, for example, you have 1 mL of methylene chloride in a vial and you add 2 mL of water, you should expect the water to be on top because it is less dense than methylene chloride. As you add the water, *watch to see where it goes.* By noting the relative volumes of the two layers, you should be able to tell which is the aqueous layer and which is the organic layer. This approach can also be used when performing an extraction procedure using a centrifuge tube. Of course, you can always test to see which layer is the aqueous layer by adding one or two drops of water, as described previously.

12.9 DRYING AGENTS

After an organic solvent has been shaken with an aqueous solution, it will be "wet"; that is, it will have dissolved some water even though its solubility with water is not great. The amount of water dissolved varies from solvent to solvent; diethyl ether represents a solvent in which a fairly large amount of water dissolves. To remove water from the organic layer, use a **drying agent**. A drying agent is an *anhydrous* inorganic salt that acquires waters of hydration when exposed to moist air or a wet solution:

$$\underset{\substack{\text{Anhydrous} \\ \text{drying agent}}}{\overset{\text{Insoluble}}{\text{Na}_2\text{SO}_4(s)}} + \text{Wet Solution }(n\text{H}_2\text{O}) \rightarrow \underset{\substack{\text{Hydrated} \\ \text{drying agent}}}{\overset{\text{Insoluble}}{\text{Na}_2\text{SO}_4 \cdot n\text{H}_2\text{O (s)}}} + \text{Dry Solution}$$

The insoluble drying agent is placed directly into the solution, where it acquires water molecules and becomes hydrated. If enough drying agent is used, all of the water can be removed from a wet solution, making it "dry," or free of water.

The following anhydrous salts are commonly used: sodium sulfate, magnesium sulfate, calcium chloride, calcium sulfate (Drierite), and potassium carbonate. These salts vary in their properties and applications. For instance, not all will absorb the same amount of water for a given weight, nor will they dry the solution to the same extent. **Capacity** refers to the amount of water a drying agent absorbs per unit weight. Sodium and magnesium sulfates absorb a large amount of water (high capacity), but magnesium sulfate dries a solution more completely. **Completeness** refers to a compound's effectiveness in removing all the water from a solution by the time equilibrium has been reached. Magnesium ion, a strong Lewis acid, sometimes causes rearrangements of compounds such as epoxides. Calcium chloride is a good drying agent but cannot be used with many compounds containing oxygen or nitrogen because it forms complexes. Calcium chloride absorbs methanol and ethanol in addition to water, so it is useful for removing these materials when they are present as impurities. Potassium carbonate is a base and is used for drying solutions of basic substances, such as amines. Calcium sulfate dries a solution completely but has a low capacity.

Anhydrous sodium sulfate is the most widely used drying agent. The granular variety is recommended because it is easier to remove the dried solution from it than from the powdered variety. Sodium sulfate is mild and effective. It will remove water from most common solvents, with the possible exception of diethyl ether, in which case a prior drying with saturated salt solution may be advised (see p. 715). Sodium sulfate must be used at room temperature to be effective; it cannot be used with boiling solutions. Table 12.2 compares the various common drying agents.

Macroscale. An Erlenmeyer flask is the most convenient container for drying a large volume of an organic layer. Before attempting to dry an organic layer, check closely to see that there are no visible signs of water. If you see droplets of water in the organic layer or clinging to the sides of the flask, transfer the organic layer to a *dry* flask before adding any drying agent. If a puddle (water layer) is present, separate the layers, using a separatory funnel if necessary, and place the organic layer in a clean, dry flask. To dry a large amount of solution, you should add enough granular anhydrous sodium sulfate to give a 1–3-mm layer on the bottom of the flask, depending on the volume of the solution. Stop-

TABLE 12.2 Common Drying Agents

	Acidity	Hydrated	Capacity[a]	Complete-ness[b]	Rate[c]	Use
Magnesium sulfate	Neutral	$MgSO_4 \cdot 7H_2O$	High	Medium	Rapid	General
Sodium sulfate	Neutral	$Na_2SO_4 \cdot 7H_2O$ $Na_2SO_4 \cdot 10H_2O$	High	Low	Medium	General
Calcium chloride	Neutral	$CaCl_2 \cdot 2H_2O$ $CaCl_2 \cdot 6H_2O$	Low	High	Rapid	Hydro-carbons Halides
Calcium sulfate (Drierite)	Neutral	$CaSO_4 \cdot \frac{1}{2}H_2O$ $CaSO_4 \cdot 2H_2O$	Low	High	Rapid	General
Potassium carbonate	Basic	$K_2CO_3 \cdot 1\frac{1}{2}H_2O$ $K_2CO_3 \cdot 2H_2O$	Medium	Medium	Medium	Amines, esters, bases, ketones
Potassium hydroxide	Basic	—	—	—	Rapid	Amines only
Molecular sieves (3 or 4 Å)	Neutral	—	High	Extremely high	—	General

[a]Amount of water removed per given weight of drying agent.

[b]Refers to amount of H_2O still in solution at equilibrium with drying agent.

[c]Refers to rate of action (drying).

168

TABLE 12.3 Common Signs That Indicate a Solution Is Dry

1. There are no visible water droplets on the side of flask or suspended in solution.
2. There is not a separate layer of liquid or a "puddle."
3. The solution is clear, not cloudy. Cloudiness indicates water is present. ✕
4. The drying agent (or a portion of it) flows freely on the bottom of the container when stirred or swirled and does not "clump" together as a solid mass.

per the flask and dry the solution for at least 15 minutes, occasionally swirling the flask. The mixture is dry if it appears clear and shows the common signs of a dry solution given in Table 12.3.

If the solution remains cloudy after treatment with the first batch of drying agent, add more drying agent and repeat the drying procedure. If the drying agent clumps badly, with no drying agent that will flow freely when the flask is swirled, you should transfer (decant) the solution to a clean, dry flask and add a fresh portion of drying agent. When the solution is dry, the drying agent should be removed by using decantation (pouring carefully to leave the drying agent behind). With granular sodium sulfate, decantation is quite easy to perform because of the size of the drying agent particles. If a powdered drying agent, such as magnesium sulfate, is used, it may be necessary to use gravity filtration (Technique 8, Section 8.1B, p. 646) to remove the drying agent. The solvent is removed by distillation (Technique 14, Section 14.3, p. 738) or evaporation (Technique 7, Section 7.10, p. 639).

Microscale. Before attempting to dry an organic layer, check closely to see that there are no visible signs of water. If you see droplets of water in the organic layer or water droplets clinging to the sides of the conical vial or test tube, transfer the organic layer with a *dry* Pasteur pipet to a *dry* container before adding any drying agent. Now add one spatulaful of granular anhydrous sodium sulfate (or other drying agent) from the V-grooved end of a microspatula into a solution contained in a conical vial or test tube. If all the drying agent "clumps," add another spatulaful of sodium sulfate. Dry the solution for at least 15 minutes. Stir the mixture occasionally with a spatula during that period. The mixture is dry if there are no visible signs of water and the drying agent flows freely in the container when stirred with a microspatula. The solution should not be cloudy. Add more drying agent if necessary. You should not add more drying agent if a "puddle" (water layer) forms or if drops of water are visible. Instead, you should transfer the organic layer to a dry container before adding fresh drying agent. When dry, use a *dry* Pasteur pipet or a *dry* filter-tip pipet (Technique 8, Section 8.6, p. 655) to remove the solution from the drying agent and transfer the solution to a *dry* conical vial. Rinse the drying agent with a small amount of fresh solvent and transfer this solvent to the vial containing the solution. Remove the solvent by evaporation using heat and a stream of air or nitrogen (Technique 7, Section 7.10, p. 639).

An alternative method of drying an organic phase is to pass it through a filtering pipet (Technique 8, Section 8.1C, p. 649) that has been packed with a small amount (ca. 2 cm) of drying agent. Again, the solvent is removed by evaporation.

Saturated Salt Solution. At room temperature, diethyl ether (ether) dissolves 1.5% by weight of water, and water dissolves 7.5% of ether. Ether, however, dissolves a much smaller amount of water from a saturated aqueous sodium chloride solution. Hence, the bulk of water in ether, or ether in water, can be removed by shaking it with a saturated aqueous sodium chloride solution. A solution of high ionic strength is usually not compatible with an organic solvent and forces separation of it from the aqueous layer. The water migrates into the concentrated salt solution. The ether phase (organic layer) will be on top, and the saturated sodium chloride solution will be on the bottom ($d = 1.2$ g/mL). After removing the organic phase from the aqueous sodium chloride, dry the organic layer completely with sodium sulfate or with one of the other drying agents listed in Table 12.2.

12.10 EMULSIONS

An **emulsion** is a colloidal suspension of one liquid in another. Minute droplets of an organic solvent are often held in suspension in an aqueous solution when the two are mixed or shaken vigorously; these droplets form an emulsion. This is especially true if any gummy or viscous material was present in the solution. Emulsions are often encountered in performing extractions. Emulsions may require a long time to separate into two layers and are a nuisance to the organic chemist.

Fortunately, several techniques may be used to break a difficult emulsion once it has formed.

1. Often an emulsion will break up if it is allowed to stand for some time. Patience is important here. Gently stirring with a stirring rod or spatula may also be useful.
2. If one of the solvents is water, adding a saturated aqueous sodium chloride solution will help destroy the emulsion. The water in the organic layer migrates into the concentrated salt solution.
3. If the total volume is less than 13 mL, the mixture may be transferred to a centrifuge tube. The emulsion will often break during centrifugation. Remember to place another tube filled with water on the opposite side of the centrifuge to balance it. Both tubes should weigh the same.
4. Adding a very small amount of a water-soluble detergent may also help. This method has been used in the past for combating oil spills. The detergent helps to solubilize the tightly bound oil droplets.
5. Gravity filtration (see Technique 8, Section 8.1, p. 645) may help to destroy an emulsion by removing gummy polymeric substances. With large volumes, you might try filtering the mixture through a fluted filter (Technique 8, Section 8.1B, p. 646) or a piece of cotton. With small-scale reactions, a filtering pipet may work (Technique 8, Section 8.1C, p. 649). In many cases, once the gum is removed, the emulsion breaks up rapidly.
6. If you are using a separatory funnel, you might try to use a gentle swirling action in the funnel to help break an emulsion. Gently stirring with a stirring rod may also be useful.

When you know through prior experience that a mixture may form a difficult emulsion, you should avoid shaking the mixture vigorously. When using conical vials for extractions, it may be better to use a magnetic spin vane for mixing and not shake the mixture at all. When using separatory funnels, extractions should be performed with gentle swirling instead of shaking or with several gentle inversions of the separatory funnel. Do not shake

170

the separatory funnel vigorously in these cases. It is important to use a longer extraction period if the more gentle techniques described in this paragraph are being employed. Otherwise, you will not transfer all the material from the first phase to the second one.

12.11 PURIFICATION AND SEPARATION METHODS

In nearly all synthetic experiments undertaken in the organic laboratory, a series of operations involving extractions is used after the actual reaction has been concluded. These extractions form an important part of the purification. Using them, you separate the desired product from unreacted starting materials or from undesired side products in the reaction mixture. These extractions may be grouped into three categories, depending on the nature of the impurities they are designed to remove.

The first category involves extracting or "washing" an organic mixture with water. Water washes are designed to remove highly polar materials, such as inorganic salts, strong acids or bases, and low-molecular-weight, polar substances including alcohols, carboxylic acids, and amines. Many organic compounds containing fewer than five carbons are water soluble. Water extractions are also used immediately following extractions of a mixture with either acid or base to ensure that all traces of acid or base have been removed.

The second category concerns extraction of an organic mixture with a dilute acid, usually 1–2 M hydrochloric acid. Acid extractions are intended to remove basic impurities, especially such basic impurities as organic amines. The bases are converted to their corresponding cationic salts by the acid used in the extraction. If an amine is one of the reactants or if pyridine or another amine is a solvent, such an extraction might be used to remove any excess amine present at the end of a reaction.

$$RNH_2 + HCl \longrightarrow RNH_3^+Cl^-$$
(water-soluble ammonium salt)

Cationic ammonium salts are usually soluble in the aqueous solution, and they are thus extracted from the organic material. A water extraction may be used immediately following the acid extraction to ensure that all traces of the acid have been removed from the organic material.

The third category is extraction of an organic mixture with a dilute base, usually 1 M sodium bicarbonate, although extractions with dilute sodium hydroxide can also be used. Such basic extractions are intended to convert acidic impurities, such as organic acids, to their corresponding anionic salts. For example, in the preparation of an ester, a sodium bicarbonate extraction might be used to remove any excess carboxylic acid that is present.

$$RCOOH + NaHCO_3 \longrightarrow RCOO^-Na^+ + H_2O + CO_2$$
$(pK_a \sim 5)$ **(water-soluble carboxylate salt)**

Anionic carboxylate salts, being highly polar, are soluble in the aqueous phase. As a result, these acid impurities are extracted from the organic material into the basic solution. A water extraction may be used after the basic extraction to ensure that all the base has been removed from the organic material.

Occasionally, phenols may be present in a reaction mixture as impurities, and removing them by extraction may be desired. Because phenols, although they are acidic, are about 10^5 times less acidic than carboxylic acids, basic extractions may be used to separate phenols from carboxylic acids by a careful selection of the base. If sodium bicarbonate is used as a base, carboxylic acids are extracted into the aqueous base, but phenols are not. Phenols are not sufficiently acidic to be deprotonated by the weak base bicarbonate. Extraction with sodium hydroxide, on the other hand, extracts both carboxylic acids and phenols into the aqueous basic solution, because hydroxide ion is a sufficiently strong base to deprotonate phenols.

weak base:
sel. deprot.
stronger acid

$$R-\bigcirc-OH + NaOH \longrightarrow R-\bigcirc-O^-Na^+ + H_2O$$

(pK$_a$ ~10)   (water-soluble salt)

Mixtures of acidic, basic, and neutral compounds are easily separated by extraction techniques. One such example is shown in Figure 12.10.

Organic acids or bases that have been extracted can be regenerated by neutralizing the extraction reagent. This would be done if the organic acid or base were a product of a reaction rather than an impurity. For example, if a carboxylic acid has been extracted with the aqueous base, the compound can be regenerated by acidifying the extract with 6 M HCl until the solution becomes *just* acidic, as indicated by litmus or pH paper. When the solution becomes acidic, the carboxylic acid will separate from the aqueous solution. If the acid is a solid at room temperature, it will precipitate and can be purified by filtration and crystallization. If the acid is a liquid, it will form a separate layer. In this case, it would usually be necessary to extract the mixture with ether or methylene chloride. After removing the organic layer and drying it, the solvent can be evaporated to yield the carboxylic acid.

In the example shown in Figure 12.10, you also need to perform a drying step at (3) before isolating the neutral compound. When the solvent is ether, you should first extract the ether solution with saturated aqueous sodium chloride to remove much of the water. The ether layer is then dried over a drying agent such as anhydrous sodium sulfate. If the solvent were methylene chloride, it would not be necessary to do the step with saturated sodium chloride.

When performing acid–base extractions, it is common practice to extract a mixture several times with the appropriate reagent. For example, if you were extracting a carboxylic acid from a mixture, you might extract the mixture three times with 2-mL portions of 1 M NaOH. In most published experiments, the procedure will specify the volume and concentration of extracting reagent and the number of times to do the extractions. If this information is not given, you must devise your own procedure. Using a carboxylic acid as an example, if you know the identity of the acid and the approximate amount present, you can actually calculate how much sodium hydroxide is needed. Because the carboxylic acid (assuming it is monoprotic) will react with sodium hydroxide in a 1:1 ratio, you would need the same number of moles of sodium hydroxide as there are moles of acid. To ensure that

172

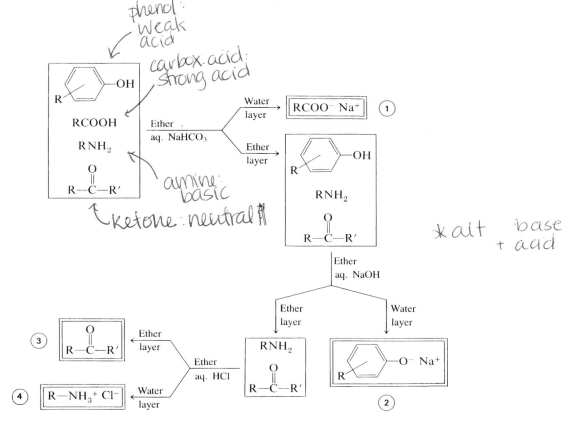

Handwritten annotations:
phenol: weak acid
carbox. acid: strong acid
amine: basic
ketone: neutral
*alt + base + acid

Figure 12.10 Separating a four-component mixture by extraction.

all the carboxylic acid is extracted, you should use about a *twofold* excess of the base. From this, you could calculate the number of milliliters of base needed. This should be divided into two or three equal portions, one portion for each extraction. In a similar fashion, you could calculate the amount of 5% sodium bicarbonate required to extract an acid or the amount of 1 *M* HCl required to extract a base. If the amount of organic acid or base is not known, then the situation is more difficult. A guideline that sometimes works is to do two or three extractions so that the total volume of the extracting reagent is approximately equal to the volume of the organic layer. To test this procedure, neutralize the aqueous layer from the last extraction. If a precipitate or cloudiness results, perform another extraction and test again. When no precipitate forms, you know that all the organic acid or base has been removed.

For some applications of acid–base extraction, an additional step, called **backwashing** or **back extraction,** is added to the scheme shown in Figure 12.10. Consider the first step, in which the carboxylic acid is extracted by sodium bicarbonate. This aqueous layer may contain some unwanted neutral organic material from the original mixture. To remove this contamination, backwash the aqueous layer with an organic solvent such as ether or methylene chloride. After shaking the mixture and allowing the layers to separate, remove and discard the organic layer. This technique may also be used when an amine is extracted with hydrochloric acid. The resulting aqueous layer is backwashed with an organic solvent to remove unwanted neutral material.

Part E. Continuous Extraction Methods

12.12 CONTINUOUS SOLID–LIQUID EXTRACTION

The technique of liquid–liquid extraction was described in Sections 12.1–12.8. In this section, solid–liquid extraction is described. Solid–liquid extraction is often used to extract a solid natural product from a natural source, such as a plant. A solvent is chosen that selectively dissolves the desired compound but that leaves behind the undesired insoluble solid. A continuous solid–liquid extraction apparatus, called a Soxhlet extractor, is commonly used in a research laboratory.

As shown in Figure 12.11, the solid to be extracted is placed in a thimble made from filter paper, and the thimble is inserted into the central chamber. A low-boiling solvent, such as diethyl ether, is placed in the round-bottom distilling flask and is heated to reflux. The vapor rises through the left sidearm into the condenser where it liquefies. The condensate (liquid) drips into the thimble containing the solid. The hot solvent begins to fill the thimble and extracts the desired compound from the solid. Once the thimble is filled with sol-

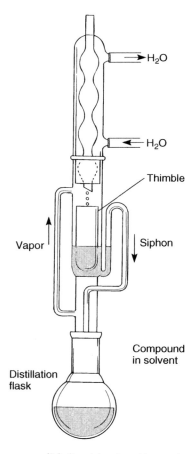

Figure 12.11 Continuous solid–liquid extraction using a Soxhlet extractor.

vent, the sidearm on the right acts as a siphon, and the solvent, which now contains the dissolved compound, drains back into the distillation flask. The vaporization–condensation–extraction–siphoning process is repeated hundreds of times, and the desired product is concentrated in the distillation flask. The product is concentrated in the flask because the product has a boiling point higher than that of the solvent or because it is a solid.

12.13 CONTINUOUS LIQUID–LIQUID EXTRACTION

When a product is very soluble in water, it is often difficult to extract using the techniques described in Sections 12.4–12.7 because of an unfavorable distribution coefficient. In this case, you need to extract the aqueous solution numerous times with fresh batches of an immiscible organic solvent to remove the desired product from water. A less labor-intensive technique involves the use of a continuous liquid–liquid extraction apparatus. One type of extractor, used with solvents that are less dense than water, is shown in Figure 12.12. Diethyl ether is usually the solvent of choice.

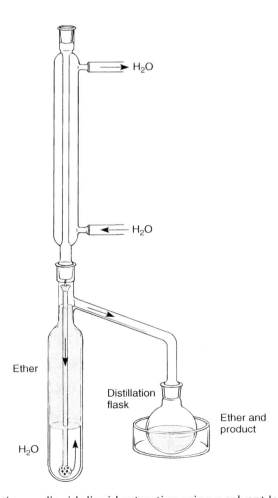

Figure 12.12 Continuous liquid–liquid extraction using a solvent less dense than water.

175

The aqueous phase is placed in the extractor, which is then filled with diethyl ether up to the sidearm. The round-bottom distillation flask is partially filled with ether. The ether is heated to reflux in the round-bottom flask, and the vapor is liquefied in the water-cooled condenser. The ether drips into the central tube, passes through the porous sintered glass tip, and flows through the aqueous layer. The solvent extracts the desired compound from the aqueous phase, and the ether is recycled back into the round-bottom flask. The product is concentrated in the flask. The extraction is rather inefficient and must be placed in operation for at least 24 hours to remove the compound from the aqueous phase.

PROBLEMS

1. Suppose solute A has a distribution coefficient of 1.0 between water and diethyl ether. Demonstrate that if 100 mL of a solution of 5.0 g of A in water were extracted with two 25-mL portions of ether, a smaller amount of A would remain in the water than if the solution were extracted with one 50-mL portion of ether.

2. Write an equation to show how you could recover the parent compounds from their respective salts (1, 2, and 4) shown in Figure 12.10.

3. Aqueous hydrochloric acid was used *after* the sodium bicarbonate and sodium hydroxide extractions in the separation scheme shown in Figure 12.10. Is it possible to use this reagent earlier in the separation scheme to achieve the same overall result? If so, explain where you would perform this extraction.

4. Using aqueous hydrochloric acid, sodium bicarbonate, or sodium hydroxide solutions, devise a separation scheme using the style shown in Figure 12.10 to separate the following two-component mixtures. All the substances are soluble in ether. Also indicate how you would recover each of the compounds from its respective salts.

   a. Give two different methods for separating this mixture.

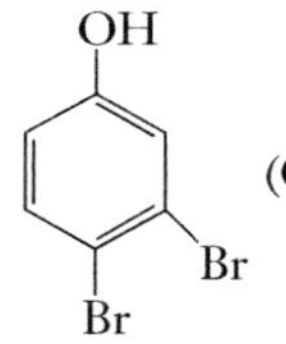

$(CH_3CH_2CH_2CH_2)_3N$

   b. Give two different methods for separating this mixture.

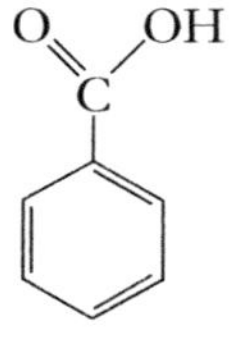

$CH_3CH_2CH_2CH_2CH_2CH_2OH$

   c. Give one method for separating this mixture.

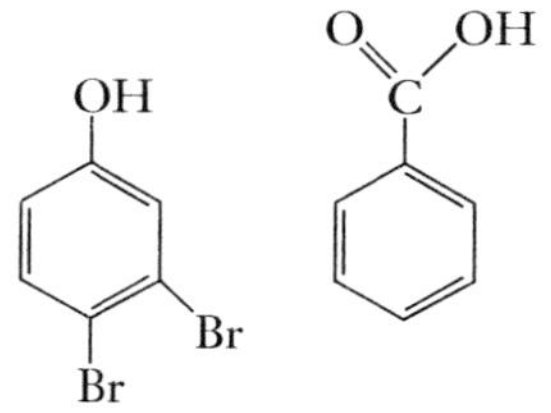

5. Solvents other than those in Table 12.1 may be used for extractions. Determine the relative positions of the organic layer and the aqueous layer in a conical vial or separatory funnel after shaking each of the following solvents with an aqueous phase. Find the densities for each of these solvents in a handbook (see Technique 4, p. 592).

 a. 1,1,1-Trichloroethane

 b. Hexane

6. A student prepares ethyl benzoate by the reaction of benzoic acid with ethanol using a sulfuric acid catalyst. The following compounds are found in the crude reaction mixture: ethyl benzoate (major component), benzoic acid, ethanol, and sulfuric acid. Using a handbook, obtain the solubility properties in water for each of these compounds (see Technique 4, p. 592). Indicate how you would remove benzoic acid, ethanol, and sulfuric acid from ethyl benzoate. At some point in the purification, you should also use an aqueous sodium bicarbonate solution.

7. Calculate the weight of water that could be removed from a wet organic phase using 50.0 mg of magnesium sulfate. Assume that it gives the hydrate listed in Table 12.2.

8. Explain exactly what you would do when performing the following laboratory instructions:

 a. "Wash the organic layer with 5.0 mL of 1 M aqueous sodium bicarbonate."

 b. "Extract the aqueous layer three times with 2-mL portions of methylene chloride."

9. Just prior to drying an organic layer with a drying agent, you notice water droplets in the organic layer. What should you do next?

10. What should you do if there is some question about which layer is the organic one during an extraction procedure?

11. Saturated aqueous sodium chloride (d = 1.2 g/mL) is added to the following mixtures in order to dry the organic layer. Which layer is likely to be on the bottom in each case?

 a. Sodium chloride layer or a layer containing a high-density organic compound dissolved in methylene chloride (d = 1.4 g/mL)

 b. Sodium chloride layer or a layer containing a low-density organic compound dissolved in methylene chloride (d = 1.1 g/mL)

TECHNIQUE 13

Physical Constants of Liquids: The Boiling Point and Density

Part A. Boiling Points and Thermometer Correction

13.1 THE BOILING POINT

As a liquid is heated, the vapor pressure of the liquid increases to the point at which it just equals the applied pressure (usually atmospheric pressure). At this point, the liquid is observed to boil. The normal boiling point is measured at 760 mmHg (760 torr) or 1 atm. At a lower applied pressure, the vapor pressure needed for boiling is also lowered, and the liquid boils at a lower temperature. The relation between applied pressure and tempera-

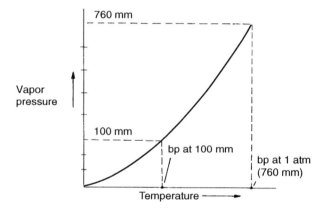

Figure 13.1 The vapor pressure–temperature curve for a typical liquid.

ture of boiling for a liquid is determined by its vapor pressure–temperature behavior. Figure 13.1 is an idealization of the typical vapor pressure–temperature behavior of a liquid.

Because the boiling point is sensitive to pressure, it is important to record the barometric pressure when determining a boiling point if the determination is being conducted at an elevation significantly above or below sea level. Normal atmospheric variations may affect the boiling point, but they are usually of minor importance. However, if a boiling point is being monitored during the course of a vacuum distillation (Technique 16) that is being performed with an aspirator or a vacuum pump, the variation from the atmospheric value will be especially marked. In these cases, it is quite important to know the pressure as accurately as possible.

As a rule of thumb, the boiling point of many liquids drops about 0.5°C for a 10-mm decrease in pressure when in the vicinity of 760 mmHg. At lower pressures, a 10°C drop in boiling point is observed for each halving of the pressure. For example, if the observed boiling point of a liquid is 150°C at 10 mm pressure, then the boiling point would be about 140°C at 5 mmHg.

A more accurate estimate of the change in boiling point with a change of pressure can be made by using a nomograph. In Figure 13.2, a nomograph is given, and a method is described for using it to obtain boiling points at various pressures when the boiling point is known at some other pressure.

13.2 DETERMINING THE BOILING POINT—MACROSCALE METHODS

Two experimental methods of determining boiling points are easily available. When you have large quantities of material, you can simply record the boiling point (or boiling range) as viewed on a thermometer while you perform a simple distillation (see Technique 14).

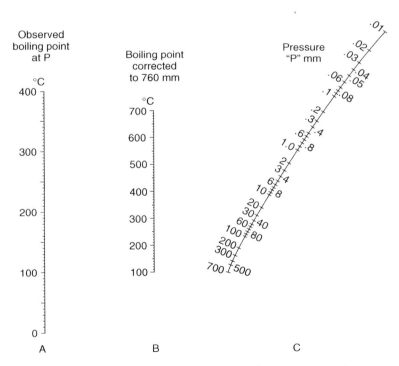

Figure 13.2 Pressure–temperature alignment nomograph. How to use the nomograph: Assume a reported boiling point of 100°C (column A) at 1 mm. To determine the boiling point at 18 mm, connect 100°C (column A) to 1 mm (column C) with a transparent plastic rule and observe where this line intersects column B (about 280°C). This value would correspond to the normal boiling point. Next, connect 280°C (column B) with 18 mm (column C) and observe where this intersects column A (151°C). The approximate boiling point will be 151°C at 18 mm. (Reprinted courtesy of EMD Chemicals, Inc.)

179

Alternatively, you may find it convenient to use a direct method, shown in Figure 13.3. With this method, the bulb of the thermometer can be immersed in vapor from the boiling liquid for a period long enough to allow it to equilibrate and give a good temperature reading. A 13-mm × 100-mm test tube works well in this procedure. Use 0.3–0.5 mL of liquid and a small, inert carborundum (black) boiling stone. This method works best with a partial immersion (76 mm) mercury thermometer (see Section 13.4, p. 729). It is not necessary to perform a stem correction with this type of thermometer.

Place the bulb of the thermometer as close as possible to the boiling liquid without actually touching it. The best heating device is a hot plate with either an aluminum block or a sand bath.[1]

While you are heating the liquid, it is helpful to record the temperature at 1-minute intervals. This makes it easier to keep track of changes in the temperature and to know when you have reached the boiling point. The liquid must boil vigorously, such that you see a reflux ring above the bulb of the thermometer and drops of liquid condensing on the sides of the test tube. Note that with some liquids, the reflux ring will be very faint, and you must looked closely to see it. The boiling point is reached when the temperature reading on the thermometer has remained constant at its highest observed value for 2–3 minutes. It is usually best to turn the heat control on the hot plate to a relatively high setting initially, especially if you are starting with a cold hot plate and aluminum block or sand bath. If the temperature begins to level off at a relatively low temperature (less than about 100°C) or if the

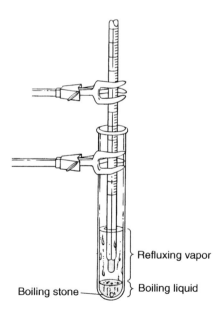

Figure 13.3 Macroscale method of determining the boiling point.

---

[1] Note to the instructor: The aluminum block should have a hole drilled in it that goes *all the way through* the block and is just slightly larger than the outside diameter of the test tube. A sand bath can be conveniently prepared by adding 40 mL of sand to a 150-mL beaker or by using a heating mantle partially filled with sand. For additional comments about these heating methods, see the Instructor's Manual, Experiment 6, "Infrared Spectroscopy and Boiling-Point Determination."

reflux ring reaches the immersion ring on the thermometer, you should turn down the heat-control setting immediately.

Two problems can occur when you perform this boiling-point procedure. The first is much more common and occurs when the temperature appears to be leveling off at a temperature below the boiling point of the liquid. This is more likely to happen with a relatively high-boiling liquid (boiling points greater than about 150°C) or when the sample is not heated sufficiently. The best way to prevent this problem is to heat the sample more strongly. With high-boiling liquids, it may be helpful to wait for the temperature to remain constant for 3–4 minutes to make sure that you have reached the actual boiling point.

The second problem, which is rare, occurs when the liquid evaporates completely, and the temperature inside the dry test tube may rise higher than the actual boiling point of the liquid. This is more likely to happen with low-boiling liquids (boiling point less than 100°C) or if the temperature on the hot plate is set too high for too long. To check for this possibility, observe the amount of liquid remaining in the test tube as soon as you have finished with procedure. If there is no liquid remaining, it is possible that the highest temperature you observed is greater than the boiling point of the liquid. In this case, you should repeat the boiling-point determination, heating the sample less strongly or using more sample.

Depending on the skill of the person performing this technique, boiling points may be slightly inaccurate. When experimental boiling points are inaccurate, it is more common for them to be lower than the literature value, and inaccuracies are more likely to occur for higher-boiling liquids. With higher-boiling liquids, the difference may be as much as 5°C. Carefully following the previous instructions will make it more likely that your experimental value will be close to the literature value.

13.3 DETERMINING THE BOILING POINT— MICROSCALE METHODS

With smaller amounts of material, you can carry out a microscale or semi-microscale determination of the boiling point by using the apparatus shown in Figure 13.4.

Semi-microscale Method.   To carry out the semi-microscale determination, attach a piece of 5-mm glass tubing (sealed at one end) to a thermometer with a rubber band or a thin slice of rubber tubing. The liquid whose boiling point is being determined is introduced with a Pasteur pipet into this piece of tubing, and a short piece of melting-point capillary (sealed at one end) is dropped in with the open end down. The whole unit is then placed in a Thiele tube. The rubber band should be placed above the level of the oil in the Thiele tube; otherwise the band may soften in the hot oil. When positioning the band, keep in mind that the oil will expand when heated. Next, the Thiele tube is heated in the same fashion as described in Technique 9, Section 9.6, p. 663, for determining a melting point. Heating is continued until a rapid and continuous stream of bubbles emerges from the inverted capillary. At this point, you should stop heating. Soon, the stream of bubbles slows down and stops. When the bubbles stop, the liquid enters the capillary tube. The moment at which the liquid enters the capillary tube corresponds to the boiling point of the liquid, and the temperature is recorded.

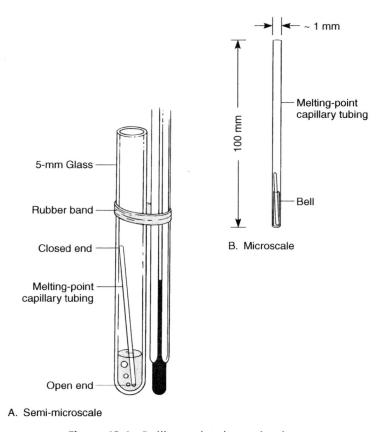

A. Semi-microscale

B. Microscale

Figure 13.4 Boiling-point determinations.

Microscale Method. In microscale experiments, there often is too little product available to use the semi-microscale method just described. However, the method can be scaled down in the following manner. The liquid is placed in a 1-mm melting-point capillary tube to a depth of about 4–6 mm. Use a syringe or a Pasteur pipet that has had its tip drawn thinner to transfer the liquid into the capillary tube. It may be necessary to use a centrifuge to transfer the liquid to the bottom of the tube. Next, prepare an appropriately-sized inverted capillary, or **bell.**

The easiest way to prepare a bell is to use a commercial micropipet, such as a 10-μL Drummond "microcap." These are available in vials of 50 or 100 microcaps and are very inexpensive. To prepare the bell, cut the microcap in half with a file or scorer and then seal one end by inserting it a small distance into a flame, turning it on its axis until the opening closes.

If microcaps are not available, a piece of 1-mm open-end capillary tubing (same size as a melting-point capillary) can be rotated along its axis in a flame while being held horizontally. Use your index fingers and thumbs to rotate the tube; do not change the distance between your two hands while rotating. When the tubing is soft, remove it from the flame and pull it to a thinner diameter. When pulling, keep the tube straight by *moving both your hands and your elbows outward* by about 4 inches. Hold the pulled tube in place a few moments until it cools. Using the edge of a file or your fingernail, break out the thin center section. Seal one end of the thin section in the flame; then break it to a length that is about one and one-half times the height of your sample liquid (6–9 mm). Be sure the break is done squarely. Invert the bell (open end down), and place it in the capillary tube containing the sample liquid. Push the bell to the bottom with a fine copper wire if it adheres to the side of the capillary tube. A centrifuge may be used if you prefer. Figure 13.5 shows the construction method for the bell and the final assembly.

Place the microscale assembly in a standard melting-point apparatus (or a Thiele tube if an electrical apparatus is not available) to determine the boiling point. Heating is continued until a rapid and continuous stream of bubbles emerges from the inverted capillary. At this point, stop heating. Soon, the stream of bubbles slows down and stops. When the bubbles stop, the liquid enters the capillary tube. The moment at which the liquid enters the capillary tube corresponds to the boiling point of the liquid, and the temperature is recorded.

Explanation of the Method. During the initial heating, the air trapped in the inverted bell expands and leaves the tube, giving rise to a stream of bubbles. When the liquid begins boiling, most of the air has been expelled; the bubbles of gas are due to the boiling action of the liquid. Once the heating is stopped, most of the vapor pressure left in the bell comes from the vapor of the heated liquid that seals its open end. There is always vapor in equilibrium with a heated liquid. If the temperature of the liquid is above its boiling point, the pressure of the trapped vapor will either exceed or equal the atmospheric pressure. As the liquid cools, its vapor pressure decreases. When the vapor pressure drops just below atmospheric pressure (just below the boiling point), the liquid is forced into the capillary tube.

Difficulties. Three problems are common to this method. The first arises when the liquid is heated so strongly that it evaporates or boils away. The second arises when the liquid is not heated above its boiling point before heating is discontinued. If the heating is stopped at any point below the actual boiling point of the sample, the liquid enters the bell *immediately,* giving an apparent boiling point that is too low. Be sure you observe a continuous stream of bubbles, too fast for individual bubbles to be distinguished, before lowering the temperature. Also be sure the bubbling action decreases slowly before the liquid enters the bell. If your melting-point apparatus has fine enough control and fast response, you can actually begin heating again and force the liquid out of the bell before it becomes completely filled with the liquid. This allows a second determination to be performed on the same sample. The third problem is that the bell may be so light that the bubbling action of the liquid causes the bell to move up the capillary tube. This problem can sometimes be solved by using a longer (heavier) bell or by sealing the bell so that a larger section of solid glass is formed at the sealed end of the bell.

When measuring temperatures above 150°C, thermometer errors can become significant. For an accurate boiling point with a high-boiling liquid, you may wish to apply a *stem correction* to the thermometer, as described in Section 13.4, or to calibrate the thermometer, as described in Technique 9, Section 9.9, p. 667.

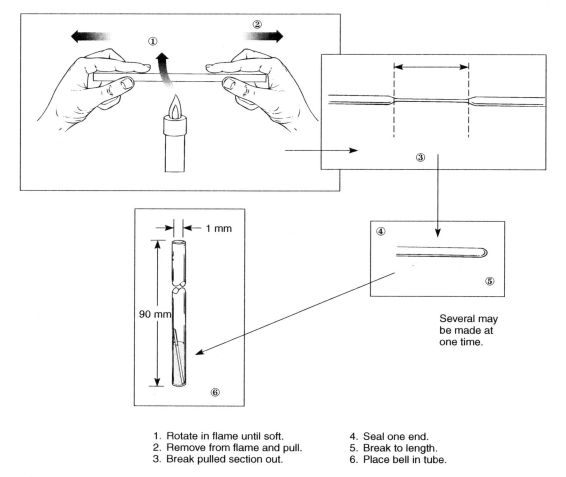

1. Rotate in flame until soft.
2. Remove from flame and pull.
3. Break pulled section out.
4. Seal one end.
5. Break to length.
6. Place bell in tube.

Figure 13.5 Construction of a microcapillary bell for microscale boiling-point determination.

13.4 THERMOMETERS AND STEM CORRECTIONS

Three types of thermometers are available: bulb immersion, partial immersion (stem immersion), and total immersion. Bulb immersion thermometers are calibrated by the manufacturer to give correct temperature readings when only the bulb (not the rest of the thermometer) is placed in the medium to be measured. Partial immersion thermometers are calibrated to give correct temperature readings when they are immersed to a specified depth in the medium to be measured. Partial immersion thermometers are easily recognized because the manufacturer always scores a mark, or immersion ring, completely around the stem at the specified depth of immersion. The immersion ring is normally found below any of the temperature calibrations. Total immersion thermometers are calibrated when the entire thermometer is immersed in the medium to be measured. The three types of thermometer are often marked on the back (opposite side from the calibrations) by the words *bulb, immersion,* or *total,* but this may vary from one manufacturer to another.

Boiling-point determination and distillation are two techniques in which an accurate temperature reading may be obtained most easily with a partial immersion thermometer. A common immersion length for this type of thermometer is 76 mm. This length works well for these two techniques because the hot vapors are likely to surround the bottom of the thermometer up to a point fairly close to the immersion line. If a total immersion thermometer is used in these applications, a stem correction, which is described later, must be used to obtain an accurate temperature reading.

The liquid used in thermometers may be either mercury or a colored organic liquid such as an alcohol. Because mercury is highly poisonous and is difficult to clean up completely when a thermometer is broken, many laboratories now use nonmercury thermometers. When a highly accurate temperature reading is required, such as in a boiling-point determination or in some distillations, mercury thermometers may have an advantage over nonmercury thermometers for two reasons. Mercury has a lower coefficient of expansion than the liquids used in nonmercury thermometers. Therefore, a partial immersion mercury thermometer will give a more accurate reading when the thermometer is not immersed in the hot vapors exactly to the immersion line. In other words, the mercury thermometer is more forgiving. Furthermore, because mercury is a better conductor of heat, a mercury thermometer will respond more quickly to changes in the temperature of the hot vapors. If the temperature is read before the thermometer reading has stabilized, which is more likely to occur with a nonmercury thermometer, the temperature reading will be inaccurate.

Manufacturers design total immersion thermometers to read correctly only when they are immersed totally in the medium to be measured. The entire mercury thread must be covered. Because this situation is rare, a **stem correction** should be added to the observed temperature. This correction, which is positive, can be fairly large when high temperatures are being measured. Keep in mind, however, that if your thermometer has been calibrated for its desired use (such as described in Technique 9, Section 9.9 for a melting-point apparatus), a stem correction should not be necessary for any temperature within the calibration limits. You are most likely to want a stem correction when you are performing a distillation. If you determine a melting point or boiling point using an uncalibrated, total immersion thermometer, you will also want to use a stem correction.

When you wish to make a stem correction for a total immersion thermometer, the following formula may be used. It is based on the fact that the portion of the mercury thread in the stem is cooler than the portion immersed in the vapor or the heated area around the thermometer. The mercury will not have expanded in the cool stem to the same extent as in the warmed section of the thermometer. The equation used is

$$(0.000154)(T - t_1)(T - t_2) = \text{correction to be added to } T \text{ observed}$$

1. The factor 0.000154 is a constant, the coefficient of expansion for the mercury in the thermometer.
2. The term $T - t_1$ corresponds to the length of the mercury thread not immersed in the heated area. Use the temperature scale on the thermometer itself for this measurement rather than an actual length unit. T is the observed temperature, and t_1 is

the *approximate* place where the heated part of the stem ends and the cooler part begins.

3. The term $T - t_2$ corresponds to the difference between the temperature of the mercury in the vapor T and the temperature of the mercury in the air outside the heated area (room temperature). The term T is the observed temperature, and t_2 is measured by hanging another thermometer so the bulb is close to the stem of the main thermometer.

Figure 13.6 shows how to apply this method for a distillation. By the formula just given, it can be shown that high temperatures are more likely to require a stem correction and that low temperatures need not be corrected. The following sample calculations illustrate this point.

Example 1	**Example 2**
$T = 200°C$	$T = 100°C$
$t_1 = 0°C$	$t_1 = 0°C$
$t_2 = 35°C$	$t_2 = 35°C$
$(0.000154)(200)(165) = 5.1°$ stem correction	$(0.000154)(100)(165) = 1.0°$ stem correction
$200°C + 5°C = 205°C$ corrected temperature	$100°C + 1°C = 101°C$ corrected temperature

Part B.   Density

13.5 DENSITY

Density is defined as mass per unit volume and is generally expressed in units of grams per milliliter (g/mL) for a liquid and grams per cubic centimeter (g/cm^3) for a solid.

$$\text{Density} = \frac{\text{mass}}{\text{volume}} \quad \text{or} \quad D = \frac{M}{V}$$

In organic chemistry, density is most commonly used in converting the weight of liquid to a corresponding volume, or vice versa. It is often easier to measure a volume of a liquid than to weigh it. As a physical property, density is also useful for identifying liquids in much the same way that boiling points are used.

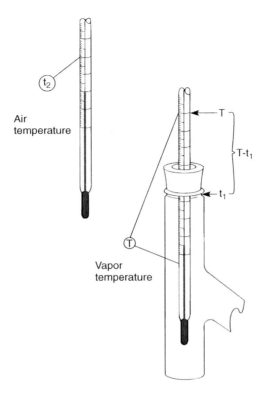

Figure 13.6 Measurement of a thermometer stem correction during distillation.

Although precise methods that allow the measurements of the densities of liquids at the microscale level have been developed, they are often difficult to perform. An approximate method for measuring densities can be found in using a 100-μL (0.100-mL) automatic pipet (Technique 5, Section 5.6, p. 609). Clean, dry, and preweigh one or more conical vials (including their caps and liners) and record their weights. Handle these vials with a tissue to avoid getting your fingerprints on them. Adjust the automatic pipet to deliver 100 μL and fit it with a clean, new tip. Use the pipet to deliver 100 μL of the unknown liquid to each of your tared vials. Cap them so that the liquid does not evaporate. Reweigh the vials and use the weight of the 100 μL of liquid delivered to calculate a density for each case. It is recommended that from three to five determinations be performed, that the calculations be performed to three significant figures, and that all the calculations be averaged to obtain the final result. This determination of the density will be accurate to within two significant figures. Table 13.1 compares some literature values with those that could be obtained by this method.

PROBLEMS

1. Using the pressure–temperature alignment chart in Figure 13.2, answer the following questions.
    a. What is the normal boiling point (at 760 mmHg) for a compound that boils at 150°C at 10 mmHg pressure?

TABLE 13.1 Densities Determined by the
Automatic Pipet Method (g/mL)

Substance	BP	Literature	100 μL
Water	100	1.000	1.01
Hexane	69	0.660	0.66
Acetone	56	0.788	0.77
Dichloromethane	40	1.330	1.27
Diethyl ether	35	0.713	0.67

   b. At what temperature would the compound in (a) boil if the pressure were 40 mmHg?

   c. A compound was distilled at atmospheric pressure and had a boiling point of 285°C. What would be the approximate boiling range for this compound at 15 mmHg?

2. Calculate the corrected boiling point for nitrobenzene by using the method given in Section 13.4. The boiling point was determined using an apparatus similar to that shown in Figure 13.3. Assume that a total immersion thermometer was used. The observed boiling point was 205°C. The reflux ring in the test tube just reached up to the 0°C mark on the thermometer. A second thermometer suspended alongside the test tube, at a slightly higher level than the one inside, gave a reading of 35°C.

3. Suppose that you had calibrated the thermometer in your melting-point apparatus against a series of melting-point standards. After reading the temperature and converting it using the calibration chart, should you also apply a stem correction? Explain.

4. The density of a liquid was determined by the automatic pipet method. A 100-μL automatic pipet was used. The liquid had a mass of 0.082 g. What was the density in grams per milliliter of the liquid?

5. During the microscale boiling-point determination of an unknown liquid, heating was discontinued at 154°C and the liquid immediately began to enter the inverted bell. Heating was begun again at once, and the liquid was forced out of the bell. Heating was again discontinued at 165°C, at which time a very rapid stream of bubbles emerged from the bell. On cooling, the rate of bubbling gradually diminished until the liquid reached a temperature of 161°C and entered and filled the bell. Explain this sequence of events. What was the boiling point of the liquid?

TECHNIQUE 14

Simple Distillation

Distillation is the process of vaporizing a liquid, condensing the vapor, and collecting the condensate in another container. This technique is very useful for separating a liquid mixture when the components have different boiling points or when one of the components will not distill. It is one of the principal methods of purifying a liquid. Four basic distillation methods are available to the chemist: simple distillation, fractional distillation, vacuum distillation (distillation at reduced pressure), and steam distillation. Fractional distillation will be discussed in Technique 15; vacuum distillation, in Technique 16; and steam distillation, in Technique 18.

A typical modern distillation apparatus is shown in Figure 14.1. The liquid to be distilled is placed in the distilling flask and heated, usually by a heating mantle. The heated liquid vaporizes and is forced upward past the thermometer and into the condenser. The vapor is condensed to liquid in the cooling condenser, and the liquid flows downward through the vacuum adapter (no vacuum is used) and into the receiving flask.

14.1 THE EVOLUTION OF DISTILLATION EQUIPMENT

There are probably more types and styles of distillation apparatus than exist for any other technique in chemistry. Over the centuries, chemists have devised just about every conceivable design. The earliest known types of distillation apparatus were the **alembic** and the **retort** (Figure 14.2). They were used by alchemists in the Middle Ages and the Renaissance, and probably even earlier by Arabic chemists. Most other distillation equipment has evolved as variations on these designs.

Figure 14.2 shows several stages in the evolution of distillation equipment as it relates to the organic laboratory. It is not intended to be a complete history; rather, it is representative. Up until recent years, equipment based on the retort design was common in the laboratory. Although the retort itself was still in use early in the last century, it had evolved by that time into the distillation flask and water-cooled condenser combination. This early equipment was connected with drilled corks. By 1958, most introductory laboratories were beginning to use "organic lab kits" that included glassware connected by standard-taper glass joints. The original lab kits contained large ᚏ 24/40 joints. Within a short time, they became smaller with ᚏ 19/22 and even ᚏ 14/20 joints. These later kits are still being used today in many "macroscale" laboratory courses such as yours.

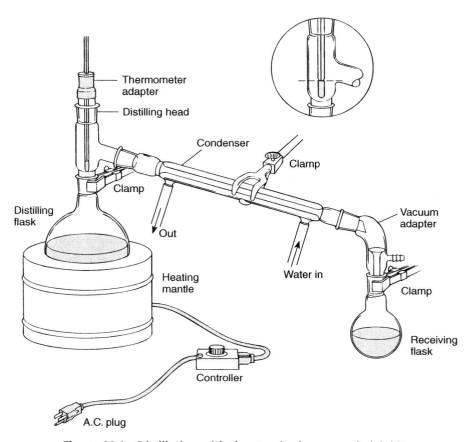

Figure 14.1 Distillation with the standard macroscale lab kit.

In the 1960s, researchers developed even smaller versions of these kits for working at the "microscale" level (in Figure 14.2, see the box labeled "Research use only"), but this glassware is generally too expensive to use in an introductory laboratory. However, in the mid-1980s, several groups developed a different style of microscale distillation equipment based on the alembic design (see the box labeled "Modern microscale organic lab kit"). This new microscale equipment has ᵀ 14/10 standard-taper joints, threaded outer joints with screw-cap connectors, and an internal O-ring for a compression seal. Microscale equipment similar to this is now used in many introductory courses. The advantages of this glassware are that there is less material used (lower cost), lower personal exposure to chemicals, and less waste generated. Because both types of equipment are in use today, after we describe macroscale equipment, we will also show the equivalent microscale distillation apparatus.

14.2 DISTILLATION THEORY

In the traditional distillation of a pure substance, vapor rises from the distillation flask and comes into contact with a thermometer that records its temperature. The vapor then passes through a condenser, which reliquefies the vapor and passes it into the receiving

190

flask. The temperature observed during the distillation of a **pure substance** remains constant throughout the distillation so long as both vapor *and* liquid are present in the system (see Figure 14.3A). When a **liquid mixture** is distilled, often the temperature does not remain constant but increases throughout the distillation. The reason for this is that the composition of the vapor that is distilling varies continuously during the distillation (see Figure 14.3B).

For a liquid mixture, the composition of the vapor in equilibrium with the heated solution is different from the composition of the solution itself. This is shown in Figure 14.4, which is a phase diagram of the typical vapor–liquid relation for a two-component system (A + B).

In this diagram, horizontal lines represent constant temperatures. The upper curve represents vapor composition, and the lower curve represents liquid composition. For any horizontal line (constant temperature), such as that shown at *t,* the intersections of the line

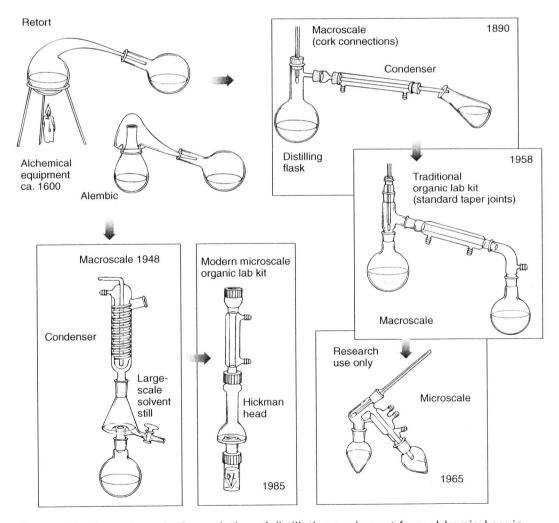

Figure 14.2 Some stages in the evolution of distillation equipment from alchemical equipment (dates represent approximate time of use).

191

with the curves give the compositions of the liquid and the vapor that are in equilibrium with each other at that temperature. In the diagram, at temperature t, the intersection of the curve at x indicates that liquid of composition w will be in equilibrium with vapor of composition z, which corresponds to the intersection at y. Composition is given as a mole percentage of A and B in the mixture. Pure A, which boils at temperature t_A, is represented at the left. Pure B, which boils at temperature t_B, is represented at the right. For either pure A or pure B, the vapor and liquid curves meet at the boiling point. Thus, either pure A or pure B will distill at a constant temperature (t_A or t_B). Both the vapor and the liquid must have the same composition in either of these cases. This is not the case for mixtures of A and B.

A mixture of A and B of composition w will have the following behavior when heated. The temperature of the liquid mixture will increase until the boiling point of the mixture is reached. This corresponds to following line wx from w to x, the boiling point of the mixture t. At temperature t the liquid begins to vaporize, which corresponds to line xy. The vapor has the composition corresponding to z. In other words, the first vapor obtained in distilling a mixture of A and B does not consist of pure A. It is richer in A than the original

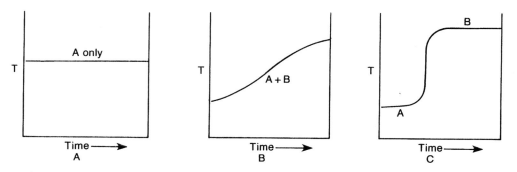

Figure 14.3 Three types of temperature behavior during a simple distillation. (A) A single pure component. (B) Two components of similar boiling points. (C) Two components with widely differing boiling points. Good separations are achieved in A and C.

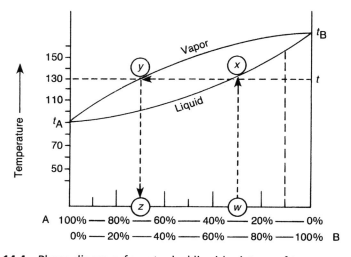

Figure 14.4 Phase diagram for a typical liquid mixture of two components.

mixture but still contains a significant amount of the higher-boiling component B, *even from the very beginning of the distillation.* The result is that it is never possible to separate a mixture completely by a simple distillation. However, in two cases it is possible to get an acceptable separation into relatively pure components. In the first case, if the boiling points of A and B differ by a large amount ($> 100°$) and if the distillation is carried out carefully, it will be possible to get a fair separation of A and B. In the second case, if A contains a fairly small amount of B ($< 10\%$), a reasonable separation of A from B can be achieved. When the boiling-point differences are not large and when highly pure components are desired, it is necessary to perform a **fractional distillation.** Fractional distillation is described in Technique 15, where the behavior during a simple distillation is also considered in detail. Note that only as vapor distills from the mixture of composition *w* (Figure 14.4), is it richer in A than is the solution. Thus, the composition of the material left behind in the distillation becomes richer in B (moves to the right from *w* toward pure B in the graph). A mixture of 90% B (dotted line on the right side in Figure 14.4) has a higher boiling point than at *w*. Hence, the temperature of the liquid in the distillation flask will increase during the distillation, and the composition of the distillate will change (as is shown in Figure 14.3B).

When two components that have a large boiling-point difference are distilled, the temperature remains constant while the first component distills. If the temperature remains constant, a relatively pure substance is being distilled. After the first substance distills, the temperature of the vapors rises, and the second component distills, again at a constant temperature. This is shown in Figure 14.3C. A typical application of this type of distillation might be an instance of a reaction mixture containing the desired component A (bp 140°C) contaminated with a small amount of undesired component B (bp 250°C) and mixed with a solvent such as diethyl ether (bp 36°C). The ether is removed easily at low temperature. Pure A is removed at a higher temperature and collected in a separate receiver. Component B can then be distilled, but it usually is left as a residue and not distilled. This separation is not difficult and represents a case where simple distillation might be used to advantage.

14.3 SIMPLE DISTILLATION—STANDARD APPARATUS

For a simple distillation, the apparatus shown in Figure 14.1 is used. Six pieces of specialized glassware are used:

1. Distilling flask
2. Distillation head
3. Thermometer adapter
4. Water condenser
5. Vacuum adapter
6. Receiving flask

The apparatus is usually heated electrically, using a heating mantle. The distilling flask, condenser, and vacuum adapter should be clamped. Two different methods of clamping this apparatus were shown in Technique 7 (Figure 7.2, p. 625 and Figure 7.4, p. 626). The receiving flask should be supported by removable wooden blocks or a wire gauze on an iron ring attached to a ring stand. The various components are each discussed in the following sections, along with some other important points.

Distilling Flask.   The distilling flask should be a round-bottom flask. This type of flask is designed to withstand the required input of heat and to accommodate the boiling action. It gives a maximized heating surface. The size of the distilling flask should be chosen so that it is never filled more than two-thirds full. When the flask is filled beyond this point, the neck constricts and "chokes" the boiling action, resulting in bumping. The surface area of the boiling liquid should be kept as large as possible. However, too large a distilling flask should also be avoided. With too large a flask, the **holdup** is excessive; the holdup is the amount of material that cannot distill because some vapor must fill the empty flask. When you cool the apparatus at the end, this material drops back into the distilling flask.

Boiling Stones.   A boiling stone (Technique 7, Section 7.4, p. 631) should be used during distillation to prevent bumping. As an alternative, the liquid being distilled may be rapidly stirred using a magnetic stirrer and stir bar (Technique 7, Section 7.3, p. 630). If you forget a boiling stone, cool the mixture before adding it. If you add a boiling stone to a hot superheated liquid, it may "erupt" into vigorous boiling, breaking your apparatus and spilling hot solvent everywhere.

Grease.   In most cases, it is unnecessary to grease standard-taper joints for a simple distillation. The grease makes cleanup more difficult, and it may contaminate your product.

Distillation Head.   The distillation head directs the distilling vapors into the condenser and allows the connection of a thermometer via the thermometer adapter. The thermometer should be positioned in the distillation head so that the thermometer is directly in the stream of vapor that is distilling. This can be accomplished if the entire bulb of the thermometer is positioned *below* the sidearm of the distilling head (see the circular inset in Figure 14.1). The entire bulb must be immersed in the vapor to achieve an accurate temperature reading. When distilling, you should be able to see a reflux ring (Technique 7, Section 7.2, p. 628) positioned well above both the thermometer bulb and the bottom of the sidearm.

Thermometer Adapter.   The thermometer adapter connects to the top of the distillation head (see Figure 14.1). There are two parts to the thermometer adapter: a glass joint with an open rolled edge on the top, and a rubber adapter that fits over the rolled edge and holds the thermometer. The thermometer fits in a hole in the top of the rubber adapter and can be adjusted upward and downward by sliding it in the hole. Adjust the bulb to a point below the sidearm. The distillation temperature can be monitored most accurately by using a partial immersion mercury thermometer (see Technique 13, Section 13.4, p. 729).

Water Condenser.   The joint between the distillation head and the water condenser is the joint most prone to leak in this entire apparatus. Because the distilling liquid is both hot and vaporized when it reaches this joint, it will leak out of any small opening between the two joint surfaces. The odd angle of the joint, neither vertical or horizontal, also makes a good connection more difficult. Be sure this joint is well sealed. If possible, use one of the plastic joint clips described in Technique 7, Figure 7.3, p. 626. Otherwise, adjust your clamps to be sure that the joint surfaces are pressed together and not pulled apart.

The condenser will remain full of cooling water only if the water flows *upward,* not downward. The water input hose should be connected to the lower opening in the jacket, and the exit hose should be attached to the upper opening. Place the other end of the exit hose in a sink. A moderate water flow will perform a good deal of cooling. A high rate of water flow may cause the tubing to pop off the joints and cause a flood. If you hold the exit hose horizontally and point the end into a sink, the flow rate is correct if the water stream continues horizontally for about two inches before bending downward.

If a distillation apparatus is to be left untended for a period of time, it is a good idea to wrap copper wire around the ends of the tubing and twist it tight. This will help to prevent the hoses from popping off of the connectors if there is an unexpected water-pressure change.

Vacuum Adapter. In a simple distillation, the vacuum adapter is not connected to a vacuum but is left open. It is merely an opening to the outside air so that pressure does not build up in the distillation system. If you plug this opening, you will have a **closed system** (no outlet). It is always dangerous to heat a closed system. Enough pressure can build up in the closed system to cause an explosion. The vacuum adapter, in this case, merely directs the distillate into the receiving, or collection, flask.

If the substance you are distilling is water sensitive, you can attach a calcium chloride drying tube to the vacuum connection to protect the freshly distilled liquid from atmospheric water vapor. Air that enters the apparatus will have to pass through the calcium chloride and be dried. Depending on the severity of the problem, drying agents other than calcium chloride may also be used.

The vacuum adapter has a disturbing tendency to obey the laws of Newtonian physics and fall off the slanted condenser onto the desk and break. If plastic joint clips are available, it is a good idea to use them on both ends of this piece. The top clip will secure the vacuum adapter to the condenser, and the bottom clip will secure the receiving flask, preventing it from falling.

Rate of Heating. The rate of heating for the distillation can be adjusted to the proper rate of **takeoff,** the rate at which distillate leaves the condenser, by watching drops of liquid emerge from the bottom of the vacuum adapter. A rate of from one to three drops per second is considered a proper rate of takeoff for most applications. At a greater rate, equilibrium is not established within the distillation apparatus, and the separation may be poor. A slower rate of takeoff is also unsatisfactory because the temperature recorded on the thermometer is not maintained by a constant vapor stream, thus leading to an inaccurate low boiling point.

Receiving Flask. The receiving flask, which is usually a round-bottom flask, collects the distilled liquid. If the liquid you are distilling is extremely volatile and there is danger of losing some of it to evaporation, it is sometimes advisable to cool the receiving flask in an ice-water bath.

Fractions. The material being distilled is called the **distillate.** Frequently, a distillate is collected in contiguous portions, called **fractions.** This is accomplished by replacing the collection flask with a clean one at regular intervals. If a small amount of liquid is collected at the beginning of a distillation and not saved or used further, it is called a **forerun.** Subsequent fractions will have higher boiling ranges, and each fraction should be labeled with its correct boiling range when the fraction is taken. For a simple distillation of a pure material, most of the material will be collected in a single, large **midrun** fraction, with only a small forerun. In some small-scale distillations, the volume of the forerun will be so small that you will not be able to collect it separately from the midrun fraction. The material left behind is called the **residue.** It is usually advised that you discontinue a distillation before the distilling flask becomes empty. Typically, the residue becomes increasingly dark in color during distillation, and it frequently contains thermal decomposition products. In addition, a dry residue may explode on overheating, or the flask may melt or crack when it becomes dry. Don't distill until the distilling flask is completely dry!

14.4 MICROSCALE AND SEMI-MICROSCALE EQUIPMENT

When you wish to distill quantities that are smaller than 4–5 mL, different equipment is required. What you use depends on how small a quantity you wish to distill.

A. Semi-Microscale

One possibility is to use equipment identical in style to that used with conventional macroscale procedures, but to "downsize" it using ᴛ 14/10 joints. The major manufacturers do make distillation heads and vacuum takeoff adapters with ᴛ 14/10 joints. This equipment will allow you to handle quantities of 5–15 mL. An example of such a "semi-microscale" apparatus is given in Figure 14.5. Although the manufacturers make ᴛ 14/10 condensers, the condenser has been left out in this example. This can be done if the material to be distilled is not extremely volatile or is high boiling. It is also possible to omit the condenser if you not have a large amount of material and can cool the receiving flask in an ice-water bath as shown in the figure.

B. Microscale—Student Equipment

Figure 14.6 shows the typical distillation setup for those students who are taking a microscale laboratory course. Instead of a distillation head, condenser, and vacuum takeoff, this equipment uses a single piece of glassware called a **Hickman head.** The Hickman head provides a "short path" for the distilled liquid to travel before it is collected. The liquid is boiled, moves upward through the central stem of the Hickman

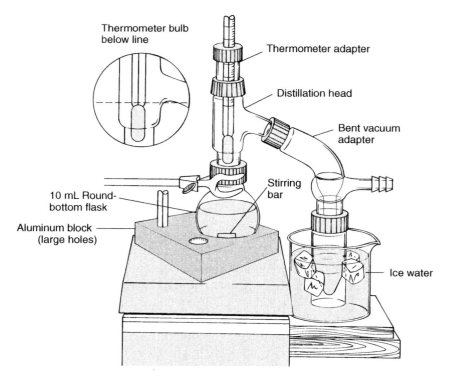

Figure 14.5 Semi-microscale distillation.

196

head, condenses on the walls of the "chimney," and then runs down the sides into the circular well surrounding the stem. With very volatile liquids, a condenser can be placed on top of the Hickman head to improve its efficiency. The apparatus shown uses a 5-mL conical vial as the distilling flask, meaning that this apparatus can distill 1–3 mL of liquid. Unfortunately, the well in most Hickman heads holds only about 0.5–1.0 mL. Thus, the well must be emptied several times using a disposable Pasteur pipet, as shown in Figure 14.7. The figure shows two different styles of Hickman head. The one with the side port makes removal of the distillate easier.

C.   Microscale—Research Equipment

Figure 14.8 shows a very well designed research-style, short-path distillation head. Note how the equipment has been "unitized," eliminating several joints and decreasing the holdup.

PROBLEMS

1. Using Figure 14.4, answer the following questions.
   a. What is the molar composition of the vapor in equilibrium with a boiling liquid that has a composition of 60% A and 40% B?

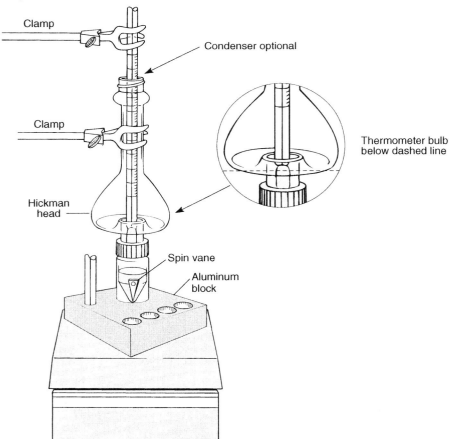

Figure 14.6   Basic microscale distillation.

197

b. A sample of vapor has the composition 50% A and 50% B. What is the composition of the boiling liquid that produced this vapor?

2. Use an apparatus similar to that shown in Figure 14.1 and assume that the round-bottom flask holds 100 mL and the distilling head has an internal volume of 12 mL in the vertical section. At the end of a distillation, vapor would fill this volume, but it could not be forced through the system. No liquid would remain in the distillation flask. Assuming this holdup volume of 112 mL, use the ideal gas law and assume a boiling point of 100°C (760 mmHg) to calculate the number of milliliters of liquid ($d =$ 0.9 g/mL, $MW = 200$) that would recondense into the distillation flask upon cooling.

3. Explain the significance of a horizontal line connecting a point on the lower curve with a point on the upper curve (such as line xy) in Figure 14.4.

4. Using Figure 14.4, determine the boiling point of a liquid having a molar composition of 50% A and 50% B.

5. Where should the thermometer bulb be located in the following setups:

a. A microscale distillation apparatus using a Hickman head

b. A macroscale distillation apparatus using a distilling head, condenser, and vacuum takeoff adapter

6. Under what conditions can a good separation be achieved with a simple distillation?

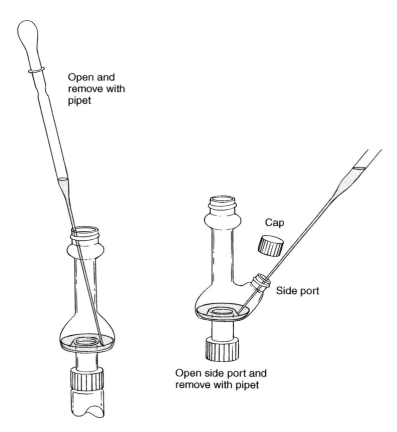

Figure 14.7 Two styles of Hickman head.

198

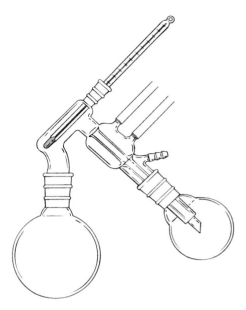

Figure 14.8 A research-style short-path distillation apparatus.

TECHNIQUE 15

Fractional Distillation, Azeotropes

Simple distillation, described in Technique 14, works well for most routine separation and purification procedures for organic liquids. When the boiling-point differences of the components to be separated are not large, however, fractional distillation must be used to achieve a good separation.

A typical fractional distillation apparatus is shown in Figure 15.2 in Section 15.1, where the differences between simple and fractional distillation are discussed in detail. This apparatus differs from that for simple distillation by the insertion of a **fractionating column** between the distilling flask and the distillation head. The fractionating column is filled with a **packing,** a material that causes the liquid to condense and revaporize repeatedly as it passes through the column. With a good fractionating column, better separations are possible, and liquids with small boiling-point differences may be separated by using this technique.

Part A.   Fractional Distillation

15.1 DIFFERENCES BETWEEN SIMPLE AND FRACTIONAL DISTILLATION

When an ideal solution of two liquids, such as benzene (bp 80°C) and toluene (bp 110°C), is distilled by simple distillation, the first vapor produced will be enriched in the lower-boiling component (benzene). However, when that initial vapor is condensed and analyzed, the distillate will not be pure benzene. The boiling point difference of benzene and toluene (30°C) is too small to achieve a complete separation by simple distillation. Following the principles outlined in Technique 14, Section 14.2 (pp. 735–738), and using the vapor-liquid composition curve given in Figure 15.1, you can see what would happen if you started with an equimolar mixture of benzene and toluene.

Following the dashed lines shows that an equimolar mixture (50 mole percent benzene) would begin to boil at about 91°C and, far from being 100% benzene, the distillate would contain about 74 mole percent benzene and 26 mole percent toluene. As the distillation continued, the composition of the undistilled liquid would move in the direction of A' (there would be increased toluene due to removal of more benzene than toluene), and the corresponding vapor would contain a progressively smaller amount of benzene. In effect, the temperature of the distillation would continue to increase throughout the distillation (as in Figure 14.3B, p. 737), and it would be impossible to obtain any fraction that consisted of pure benzene.

Suppose, however, that we are able to collect a small quantity of the first distillate that was 74 mole percent benzene and redistill it. Using Figure 15.1, we can see that this liquid would begin to boil at about 84°C and would give an initial distillate containing 90 mole percent of benzene. If we were experimentally able to continue taking small fractions at the

200

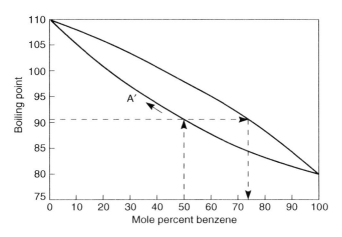

Figure 15.1 The vapor-liquid composition curve for mixtures of benzene and toluene.

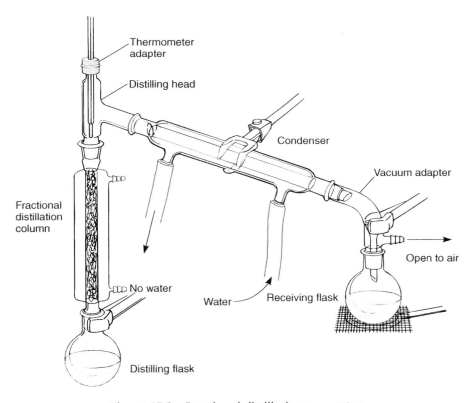

Figure 15.2 Fractional distillation apparatus.

beginning of each distillation and redistill them, we would eventually reach a liquid with a composition of nearly 100 mole percent benzene. However, since we took only a small amount of material at the beginning of each distillation, we would have lost most of the material we started with. To recapture a reasonable amount of benzene, we would have to process each of the fractions left behind in the same way as our early fractions. As each of them was partially distilled, the material advanced would become progressively richer in benzene, and that left behind would become progressively richer in toluene. It would require thousands (maybe millions) of such microdistillations to separate benzene from toluene.

Obviously, the procedure just described would be very tedious; fortunately, it need not be performed in usual laboratory practice. **Fractional distillation** accomplishes the same result. You simply have to use a column inserted between the distillation flask and the distilling head, as shown in Figure 15.2. This **fractionating column** is filled, or **packed,** with a suitable material, such as a stainless steel sponge. This packing allows a mixture of benzene and toluene to be subjected continuously to many vaporization–condensation cycles as the material moves up the column. With each cycle within the column, the composition of the vapor is progressively enriched in the lower-boiling component (benzene). Nearly pure benzene (bp 80°C) finally emerges from the top of the column, condenses, and passes into the receiving head or flask. This process continues until all the benzene is removed. The distillation must be carried out slowly to ensure that numerous vaporization–condensation cycles occur. When nearly all the benzene has been removed, the temperature begins to rise, and a small amount of a second fraction, which contains some benzene and toluene, may be collected. When the temperature reaches 110°C, the boiling point of pure toluene, the vapor is condensed and collected as the third fraction. A plot of boiling point versus volume of condensate (distillate) would resemble Figure 14.3C (p. 737). This separation would be much better than that achieved by simple distillation (Figure 14.3B, p. 737).

15.2 VAPOR–LIQUID COMPOSITION DIAGRAMS

A vapor–liquid composition phase diagram like the one in Figure 15.3 can be used to explain the operation of a fractionating column with an **ideal solution** of two liquids, A and B. An ideal solution is one in which the two liquids are chemically similar, are miscible (mutually soluble) in all proportions, and do not interact. Ideal solutions obey **Raoult's Law.** Raoult's Law is explained in detail in Section 15.3.

The phase diagram relates the compositions of the boiling liquid (lower curve) and its vapor (upper curve) as a function of temperature. Any horizontal line drawn across the diagram (a constant-temperature line) intersects the diagram in two places. These intersections relate the vapor composition to the composition of the boiling liquid that produces that vapor. By convention, composition is expressed either in **mole fraction** or in **mole percentage.** The mole fraction is defined as follows:

$$\text{Mole fraction A} = N_A = \frac{\text{Moles A}}{\text{Moles A} + \text{Moles B}}$$

$$\text{Mole fraction B} = N_B = \frac{\text{Moles B}}{\text{Moles A} + \text{Moles B}}$$

$$N_A + N_B = 1$$

$$\text{Mole percentage A} = N_A \times 100$$

$$\text{Mole percentage B} = N_B \times 100$$

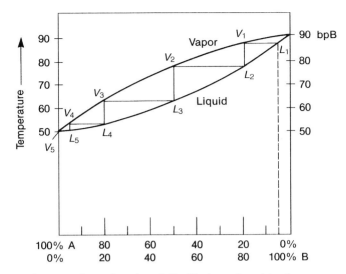

Figure 15.3 Phase diagram for a fractional distillation of an ideal two-component system.

The horizontal and vertical lines shown in Figure 15.3 represent the processes that occur during a fractional distillation. Each of the **horizontal lines** (L_1V_1, L_2V_2, and so on) represents both the **vaporization** step of a given vaporization–condensation cycle and the composition of the vapor in equilibrium with liquid at a given temperature. For example, at 63°C a liquid with a composition of 50% A (L_3 on the diagram) would yield vapor of composition 80% A (V_3 on diagram) at equilibrium. The vapor is richer in the lower-boiling component A than the original liquid was.

Each of the **vertical lines** (V_1L_2, V_2L_3, and so on) represents the **condensation** step of a given vaporization–condensation cycle. The composition does not change as the temperature drops on condensation. The vapor at V_3, for example, condenses to give a liquid (L_4 on the diagram) of composition 80% A with a drop in temperature from 63° to 53°C.

In the example shown in Figure 15.3, pure A boils at 50°C, and pure B boils at 90°C. These two boiling points are represented at the left- and right-hand edges of the diagram, respectively. Now consider a solution that contains only 5% of A but 95% of B. (Remember that these are *mole* percentages.) This solution is heated (following the dashed line) until it is observed to boil at L_1 (87°C). The resulting vapor has composition V_1 (20% A, 80% B). The vapor is richer in A than the original liquid was, but it is by no means pure A. In a simple distillation apparatus, this vapor would be condensed and passed into the receiver in a very impure state. However, with a fractionating column in place, the vapor is condensed in the **column** to give liquid L_2 (20% A, 80% B). Liquid L_2 is immediately revaporized (bp 78°C) to give a vapor of composition V_2 (50% A, 50% B), which is condensed to give liquid L_3. Liquid L_3 is revaporized (bp 63°C) to give vapor of composition V_3 (80% A, 20% B), which is condensed to give liquid L_4. Liquid L_4 is revaporized (bp 53°C) to give vapor of composition V_4 (95% A, 5% B). This process continues to V_5, which condenses to give nearly pure liquid A. The fractionating process follows the stepped lines in the figure downward and to the left.

As this process continues, all of liquid A is removed from the distillation flask or vial, leaving nearly pure B behind. If the temperature is raised, liquid B may be distilled as a

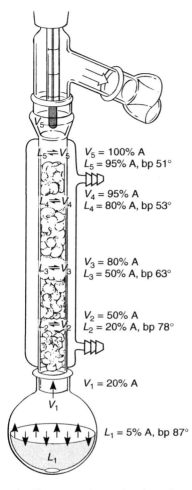

$V_5 = 100\%$ A
$L_5 = 95\%$ A, bp 51°

$V_4 = 95\%$ A
$L_4 = 80\%$ A, bp 53°

$V_3 = 80\%$ A
$L_3 = 50\%$ A, bp 63°

$V_2 = 50\%$ A
$L_2 = 20\%$ A, bp 78°

$V_1 = 20\%$ A

$L_1 = 5\%$ A, bp 87°

Figure 15.4 Vaporization–condensation in a fractionation column.

nearly pure fraction. Fractional distillation will have achieved a separation of A and B, a separation that would have been nearly impossible with simple distillation. Notice that the boiling point of the liquid becomes lower each time it vaporizes. Because the temperature at the bottom of a column is normally higher than the temperature at the top, successive vaporizations occur higher and higher in the column as the composition of the distillate approaches that of pure A. This process is illustrated in Figure 15.4, where the composition of the liquids, their boiling points, and the composition of the vapors present are shown alongside the fractionating column.

15.3 RAOULT'S LAW

Two liquids (A and B) that are miscible and that do not interact form an **ideal solution** and follow Raoult's Law. The law states that the partial vapor pressure of component A in the solution (P_A) equals the vapor pressure of pure A (P_A^0) times its mole fraction (N_A)

(equation 1). A similar expression can be written for component B (equation 2). The mole fractions N_A and N_B were defined in Section 15.2.

$$\text{Partial vapor pressure of A in solution} = P_A = (P_A^0)(N_A) \tag{1}$$

$$\text{Partial vapor pressure of B in solution} = P_B = (P_B^0)(N_B) \tag{2}$$

P_A^0 is the vapor pressure of pure A, independent of B. P_B^0 is the vapor pressure of B, independent of A. In a mixture of A and B, the partial vapor pressures are added to give the total vapor pressure above the solution (equation 3). When the total pressure (sum of the partial pressures) equals the applied pressure, the solution boils.

$$P_{total} = P_A + P_B = P_A^0 N_A + P_B^0 N_B \tag{3}$$

The composition of A and B in the vapor produced is given by equations 4 and 5.

$$N_A \text{ (vapor)} = \frac{P_A}{P_{total}} \tag{4}$$

$$N_B \text{ (vapor)} = \frac{P_B}{P_{total}} \tag{5}$$

Several exercises involving applications of Raoult's Law are illustrated in Table 15.1. Note, particularly in the result from equation 4, that the vapor is richer ($N_A = 0.67$) in the lower-boiling (higher vapor pressure) component A than it was before vaporization ($N_A = 0.50$). This proves mathematically what was described in Section 15.2.

The consequences of Raoult's Law for distillations are shown schematically in Figure 15.5. In Part A the boiling points are identical (vapor pressures the same), and no separation is attained regardless of how the distillation is conducted. In Part B a fractional distillation is required, while in Part C a simple distillation provides an adequate separation.

When a solid B (rather than another liquid) is dissolved in a liquid A, the boiling point is increased. In this extreme case, the vapor pressure of B is negligible, and the vapor will be pure A no matter how much solid B is added. Consider a solution of salt in water.

$$P_{total} = P_{water}^0 N_{water} + P_{salt}^0 N_{salt}$$

$$P_{salt}^0 = 0$$

$$P_{total} = P_{water}^0 N_{water}$$

A solution whose mole fraction of water is 0.7 will not boil at 100°C, because $P_{total} = (760)(0.7) = 532$ mmHg and is less than atmospheric pressure. If the solution is heated to 110°C, it will boil because $P_{total} = (1085)(0.7) = 760$ mmHg. Although the solution must be heated at 110°C to boil it, the vapor is pure water and has a boiling-point temperature of 100°C. (The vapor pressure of water at 110°C can be looked up in a handbook; it is 1085 mmHg.)

TABLE 15.1 Sample Calculations with Raoult's Law

Consider a solution at 100°C where $N_A = 0.5$ and $N_B = 0.5$.

1. What is the partial vapor pressure of A in the solution if the vapor pressure of pure A at 100°C is 1020 mmHg?

   Answer: $P_A = P_A^0 N_A = (1020)(0.5) = 510$ mmHg

2. What is the partial vapor pressure of B in the solution if the vapor pressure of pure B at 100°C is 500 mmHg?

   Answer: $P_B = P_B^0 N_B = (500)(0.5) = 250$ mmHg

3. Would the solution boil at 100°C if the applied pressure were 760 mmHg?

   Answer: Yes. $P_{total} = P_A + P_B = (510 + 250) = 760$ mmHg

4. What is the composition of the vapor at the boiling point?

   Answer: The boiling point is 100°C.

$$N_A \text{ (vapor)} = \frac{P_A}{P_{total}} = 510/760 = 0.67$$

$$N_B \text{ (vapor)} = \frac{P_B}{P_{total}} = 250/760 = 0.33$$

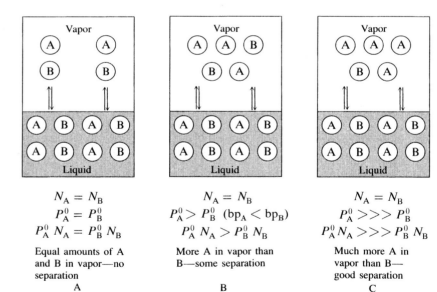

$N_A = N_B$	$N_A = N_B$	$N_A = N_B$
$P_A^0 = P_B^0$	$P_A^0 > P_B^0$ (bp$_A$ < bp$_B$)	$P_A^0 >>> P_B^0$
$P_A^0 N_A = P_B^0 N_B$	$P_A^0 N_A > P_B^0 N_B$	$P_A^0 N_A >>> P_B^0 N_B$
Equal amounts of A and B in vapor—no separation	More A in vapor than B—some separation	Much more A in vapor than B—good separation
A	B	C

Figure 15.5 Consequences of Raoult's Law. (A) Boiling points (vapor pressures) are identical—no separation. (B) Boiling points somewhat less for A than for B—requires fractional distillation. (C) Boiling points much less for A than for B—simple distillation will suffice.

15.4 COLUMN EFFICIENCY

A common measure of the efficiency of a column is given by its number of **theoretical plates.** The number of theoretical plates in a column is related to the number of vaporization–condensation cycles that occur as a liquid mixture travels through it. Using the example mixture in Figure 15.3, if the first distillate (condensed vapor) had the composition at L_2 when starting with liquid of composition L_1, the column would be said to have *one theoretical plate.* This would correspond to a simple distillation, or one vaporization–condensation cycle. A column would have two theoretical plates if the first distillate had the composition at L_3. The two-theoretical-plate column essentially carries out "two simple distillations." According to Figure 15.3, *five theoretical plates* would be required to separate the mixture that started with composition L_1. Notice that this corresponds to the number of "steps" that need to be drawn in the figure to arrive at a composition of 100% A.

Most columns do not allow distillation in discrete steps, as indicated in Figure 15.3. Instead, the process is *continuous,* allowing the vapors to be continuously in contact with liquid of changing composition as they pass through the column. Any material can be used to pack the column as long as it can be wetted by the liquid and does not pack so tightly that vapor cannot pass.

The approximate relationship between the number of theoretical plates needed to separate an ideal two-component mixture and the difference in boiling points is given in Table 15.2. Notice that more theoretical plates are required as the boiling-point differences between the components decrease. For instance, a mixture of A (bp 130°C) and B (bp 166°C) with a boiling-point difference of 36°C would be expected to require a column with a minimum of five theoretical plates.

TABLE 15.2 Theoretical Plates Required to Separate Mixtures, Based on Boiling-Point Differences of Components

Boiling-Point Difference	Number of Theoretical Plates
108	1
72	2
54	3
43	4
36	5
20	10
10	20
7	30
4	50
2	100

15.5 TYPES OF FRACTIONATING COLUMNS AND PACKINGS

Several types of fractionating columns are shown in Figure 15.6. The Vigreux column (A), has indentations that incline downward at angles of 45° and are in pairs on opposites sides of the column. The projections into the column provide increased possibilities for condensation and for the vapor to equilibrate with the liquid. Vigreux columns are popular in cases where only a small number of theoretical plates are required. They are not very efficient (a 20-cm column might have only 2.5 theoretical plates), but they allow for rapid distillation and have a small **holdup** (the amount of liquid retained by the column). A column packed with a stainless steel sponge is a more effective fractionating column than a Vigreux column, but not by a large margin. Glass beads or glass helices can also be used as a packing material, and they have even a slightly greater efficiency. The air condenser or the water condenser can be used as an improvised column if an actual fractionating column is unavailable. If a condenser is packed with glass beads, glass helices, or sections of glass tubing, the packing must be held in place by inserting a small plug of stainless steel sponge into the bottom of the condenser.

The most effective type of column is the **spinning-band column.** In the most elegant form of this device, a tightly fitting, twisted platinum screen or a Teflon rod with helical threads is rotated rapidly inside the bore of the column (Figure 15.7). A spinning-band column that is available for microscale work is shown in Figure 15.8. This spinning-band column has a band about 2–3 cm in length and provides four or five theoretical plates. It can separate 1–2 mL of a mixture with a 30°C boiling-point difference. Larger research models of this spinning-band column can provide as many as 20

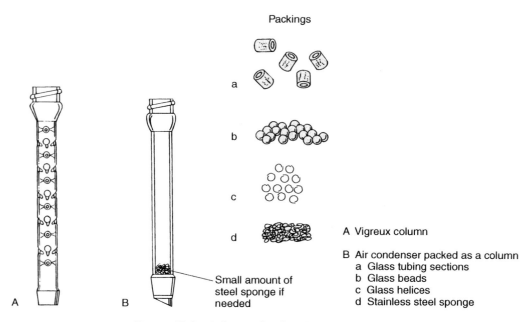

Packings

a

b

c

d

Small amount of steel sponge if needed

A Vigreux column

B Air condenser packed as a column
  a Glass tubing sections
  b Glass beads
  c Glass helices
  d Stainless steel sponge

A

B

Figure 15.6 Columns for fractional distillation.

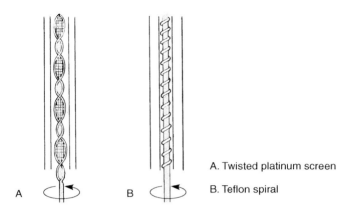

A. Twisted platinum screen

B. Teflon spiral

Figure 15.7 Bands for spinning-band columns.

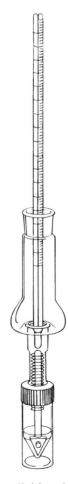

Figure 15.8 A commercially available microscale spinning-band column.

or 30 theoretical plates and can separate mixtures with a boiling-point difference of as little as 5–10°C.

Manufacturers of fractionating columns often offer them in a variety of lengths. Because the efficiency of a column is a function of its length, longer columns have more theoretical plates than shorter ones do. It is common to express efficiency of a column in a unit called **HETP,** the **H**eight of a column that is **E**quivalent to one **T**heoretical **P**late. HETP is usually expressed in units of cm/plate. When the height of the column (in centimeters) is divided by this value, the total number of theoretical plates is specified.

Fractionating columns must be insulated so that temperature equilibrium is maintained at all times. External temperature fluctuations will interfere with a good separation. Many fractionating columns are jacketed as a condenser is, but instead of water passing through the outer jacket, the jacket is evacuated and sealed. A vacuum jacket provides very good insulation of the inner column from the outside air temperature. In most student macroscale kits, the fractionating column is not evacuated but does have a jacket for insulation. This jacket, even though not evacuated, is usually sufficient for the demands of the introductory laboratory. The fractionating column looks very much like a water condenser; however, it has a larger diameter both for the inner tube and for the jacket. Be sure to take care to distinguish the larger-diameter fractionating column from the smaller-diameter water condenser.

15.6 FRACTIONAL DISTILLATION: METHODS AND PRACTICE

Many fractionating columns must be insulated so that temperature equilibrium is maintained at all times. Additional insulation will not be required for columns that have an outer jacket, but those that do not can benefit from being wrapped in insulation.

Cotton and aluminum foil (shiny side in) are often used for insulation. You can wrap the column with cotton and then use a wrapping of the aluminum foil to keep it in place. Another version of this method, which is especially effective, is to make an insulation blanket by placing a layer of cotton between two rectangles of aluminum foil, placed shiny side in. The sandwich is bound together with duct tape. This blanket, which is reusable, can be wrapped around the column and held in place with twist ties or tape.

The **reflux ratio** is defined as the ratio of the number of drops of distillate that return to the distillation flask compared to the number of drops of distillate collected. In an efficient column, the reflux ratio should equal or exceed the number of theoretical plates. A high reflux ratio ensures that the column will achieve temperature equilibrium and achieve its maximum efficiency. This ratio is not easy to determine; in fact, it is impossible to determine when using a Hickman head, and it should not concern a beginning student. In some cases, the **throughput,** or **rate of takeoff,** of a column may be specified. This is expressed as the number of milliliters of distillate that can be collected per unit of time, usually as mL/min.

Macroscale Apparatus. Figure 15.2 illustrates a fractional distillation assembly that can be used for larger-scale distillations. It has a glass-jacketed column that is packed with a stainless steel sponge. This apparatus would be common in situations where quantities of liquid in excess of 10 mL were to be distilled.

In a fractional distillation, the column should be clamped in a vertical position. The distilling flask would normally be heated by a heating mantle, which allows a precise adjustment of the temperature. A proper rate of distillation is extremely important. The distillation should be conducted as slowly as possible to allow as many vaporization–condensation cycles as possible to occur as the vapor passes through the column. However, the rate of distillation must be steady enough to produce a constant temperature reading at the thermometer. A rate that is too fast will cause the column to "flood" or "choke." In this instance, there is so much condensing liquid flowing downward in the column that the vapor cannot rise upward, and the column fills with liquid. Flooding can also occur if the column is not well insulated and has a large temperature difference from bottom to top. This situation can be remedied by employing one of the insulation methods that uses cotton or aluminum foil, as described in Section 15.5. It may also be necessary to insulate the distilling head at the top of the column. If the distilling head is cold, it will stop the progress of the distilling vapor. The distillation temperature can be monitored most accurately by using a partial immersion mercury thermometer (see Technique 13, Section 13.4, page 729.)

Microscale Apparatus. The apparatus shown in Figure 15.9 is the one you are most likely to use in the microscale laboratory. If your laboratory is one of the better equipped ones, you may have access to spinning-band columns like the one shown in Figure 15.8.

Part B.   Azeotropes

15.7 NONIDEAL SOLUTIONS: AZEOTROPES

Some mixtures of liquids, because of attractions or repulsions between the molecules, do not behave ideally; they do not follow Raoult's Law. There are two types of vapor–liquid composition diagrams that result from this nonideal behavior: **minimum-boiling-point** and **maximum-boiling-point** diagrams. The minimum or maximum points in these diagrams correspond to a constant-boiling mixture called an **azeotrope.** An azeotrope is a mixture with a fixed composition that cannot be altered by either simple or fractional distillation. An azeotrope behaves as if it were a pure compound, and it distills from the beginning to the end of its distillation at a constant temperature, giving a distillate of constant (azeotropic) composition. The vapor in equilibrium with an azeotropic liquid has the same composition as the azeotrope. Because of this, an azeotrope is represented as a *point* on a vapor–liquid composition diagram.

A.   Minimum-Boiling-Point Diagrams

A minimum-boiling-point azeotrope results from a slight incompatibility (repulsion) between the liquids being mixed. This incompatibility leads to a higher-than-expected combined vapor pressure from the solution. This higher combined vapor pressure brings about a lower boiling point for the mixture than is observed for the pure components. The most common two-component mixture that gives a minimum-boiling-point azeotrope is the ethanol–water system shown in Figure 15.10. The azeotrope at V_3 has a composition of 96% ethanol–4% water and a boiling point of 78.1°C. This boiling point is not much lower than

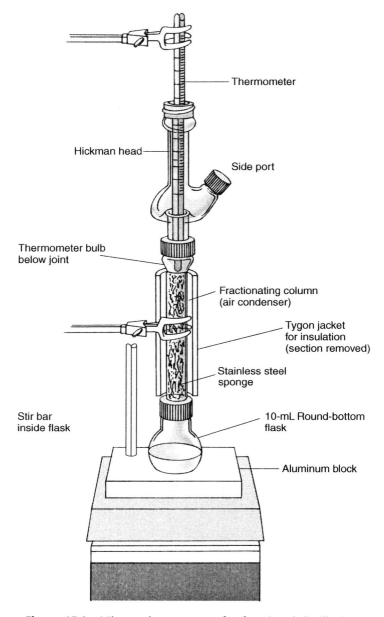

Figure 15.9 Microscale apparatus for fractional distillation.

that of pure ethanol (78.3°C), but it means that it is impossible to obtain pure ethanol from the distillation of any ethanol–water mixture that contains more than 4% water. Even with the best fractionating column, you cannot obtain 100% ethanol. The remaining 4% of water can be removed by adding benzene and removing a different azeotrope, the ternary benzene–water–ethanol azeotrope (bp 65°C). Once the water is removed, the excess benzene is removed as an ethanol–benzene azeotrope (bp 68°C). The resulting material is free of water and is called "absolute" ethanol.

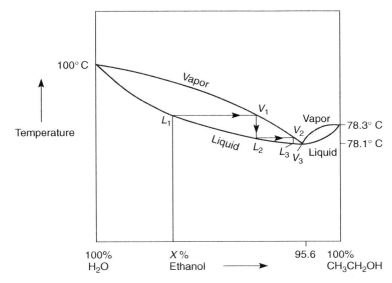

Figure 15.10 Ethanol–water minimum-boiling-point phase diagram.

The fractional distillation of an ethanol–water mixture of composition X can be described as follows. The mixture is heated (follow line XL_1) until it is observed to boil at L_1. The resulting vapor at V_1 will be richer in the lower-boiling component, ethanol, than the original mixture was.[1] The condensate at L_2 is vaporized to give V_2. The process continues, following the lines to the right, until the azeotrope is obtained at V_3. The liquid that distills is not pure ethanol, but it has the azeotropic composition of 96% ethanol and 4% water, and it distills at 78.1°C. The azeotrope, which is richer in ethanol than the original mixture was, continues to distill. As it distills, the percentage of water left behind in the distillation flask continues to increase. When all the ethanol has been distilled (as the azeotrope), pure water remains behind in the distillation flask, and it distills at 100°C.

If the azeotrope obtained by the preceding procedure is redistilled, it distills from the beginning to the end of the distillation at a constant temperature of 78.1°C as if it were a pure substance. There is no change in the composition of the vapor during the distillation.

Some common minimum-boiling-point azeotropes are given in Table 15.3. Numerous other azeotropes are formed in two- and three-component systems; such azeotropes are common. Water forms azeotropes with many substances; therefore, water must be carefully removed with **drying agents** whenever possible before compounds are distilled. Extensive azeotropic data are available in references such as the *CRC Handbook of Chemistry and Physics*.[2]

B. Maximum-Boiling-Point Diagrams

A maximum-boiling-point azeotrope results from a slight attraction between the component molecules. This attraction leads to lower combined vapor pressure than expected in

---

[1] Keep in mind that this distillate is not pure ethanol but is an ethanol–water mixture.

[2] More examples of azeotropes, with their compositions and boiling points, can be found in the *CRC Handbook of Chemistry and Physics;* also in L. H. Horsley, ed., *Advances in Chemistry Series,* No. 116, Azeotropic Data, III (Washington, DC: American Chemical Society, 1973).

TABLE 15.3   Common Minimum-Boiling-Point Azeotropes

Azeotrope	Composition (weight percentage)	Boiling Point (°C)
Ethanol–water	95.6% C_2H_5OH, 4.4% H_2O	78.17
Benzene–water	91.1% C_6H_6, 8.9% H_2O	69.4
Benzene–water–ethanol	74.1% C_6H_6, 7.4% H_2O, 18.5% C_2H_5OH	64.9
Methanol–carbon tetrachloride	20.6% CH_3OH, 79.4% CCl_4	55.7
Ethanol–benzene	32.4% C_2H_5OH, 67.6% C_6H_6	67.8
Methanol–toluene	72.4% CH_3OH, 27.6% $C_6H_5CH_3$	63.7
Methanol–benzene	39.5% CH_3OH, 60.5% C_6H_6	58.3
Cyclohexane–ethanol	69.5% C_6H_{12}, 30.5% C_2H_5OH	64.9
2-Propanol–water	87.8% $(CH_3)_2CHOH$, 12.2% H_2O	80.4
Butyl acetate–water	72.9% $CH_3COOC_4H_9$, 27.1% H_2O	90.7
Phenol–water	9.2% C_6H_5OH, 90.8% H_2O	99.5

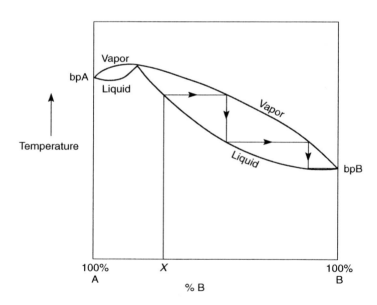

Figure 15.11 A maximum-boiling-point phase diagram.

the solution. The lower combined vapor pressures cause a higher boiling point than what would be characteristic for the components. A two-component maximum-boiling-point azeotrope is illustrated in Figure 15.11. Because the azeotrope has a higher boiling point than any of the components, it will be concentrated in the distillation flask as the distillate (pure B) is removed. The distillation of a solution of composition X would follow to the right along the lines in Figure 15.11. Once the composition of the material remaining in the flask has reached that of the azeotrope, the temperature will rise, and the azeotrope will be-

TABLE 15.4 Maximum-Boiling-Point Azeotropes

Azeotrope	Composition (weight percentage)	Boiling Point (°C)
Acetone–chloroform	20.0% CH_3COCH_3, 80.0% $CHCl_3$	64.7
Chloroform–methyl ethyl ketone	17.0% $CHCl_3$, 83.0% $CH_3COCH_2CH_3$	79.9
Hydrochloric acid	20.2% HCl, 79.8% H_2O	108.6
Acetic acid–dioxane	77.0% CH_3COCH, 23.0% $C_4H_8O_2$	119.5
Benzaldehyde–phenol	49.0% C_6H_5CHO, 51.0% C_6H_5OH	185.6

gin to distill. The azeotrope will continue to distill until all the material in the distillation flask has been exhausted.

Some maximum-boiling-point azeotropes are listed in Table 15.4. They are not nearly as common as minimum-boiling-point azeotropes.[3]

C. Generalizations

There are some generalizations that can be made about azeotropic behavior. They are presented here without explanation, but you should be able to verify them by thinking through each case using the phase diagrams given. (Note that pure A is always to the left of the azeotrope in these diagrams, and pure B is to the right of the azeotrope.)

Minimum-Boiling-Point Azeotropes

Initial Composition	Experimental Result
To left of azeotrope	Azeotrope distills first, pure A second
Azeotrope	Unseparable
To right of azeotrope	Azeotrope distills first, pure B second

Maximum-Boiling-Point Azeotropes

Initial Composition	Experimental Result
To left of azeotrope	Pure A distills first, azeotrope second
Azeotrope	Unseparable
To right of azeotrope	Pure B distills first, azeotrope second

[3]See footnote 2.

15.8 AZEOTROPIC DISTILLATION: APPLICATIONS

There are numerous examples of chemical reactions in which the amount of product is low because of an unfavorable equilibrium. An example is the direct acid-catalyzed esterification of a carboxylic acid with an alcohol:

$$R-\overset{\overset{\displaystyle O}{\|}}{C}-OH + R-O-H \xrightleftharpoons{H^+} R-\overset{\overset{\displaystyle O}{\|}}{C}-OR + H_2O$$

Because the equilibrium does not favor formation of the ester, it must be shifted to the right, in favor of the product, by using an excess of one of the starting materials. In most cases, the alcohol is the least expensive reagent and is the material used in excess. Isopentyl acetate (Experiment 12) and methyl salicylate (Experiment 13) are examples of esters prepared by using one of the starting materials in excess.

Another way of shifting the equilibrium to the right is to remove one of the products from the reaction mixture as it is formed. In the previous example, water can be removed as it is formed by **azeotropic distillation.** A common large-scale method is to use the Dean–Stark water separator shown in Figure 15.12A. In this technique, an inert solvent, commonly benzene or toluene, is added to the reaction mixture contained in the round-bottom flask. The sidearm of the water separator is also filled with this solvent. If benzene is used, as the mixture is heated under reflux, the benzene–water azeotrope (bp 69.4°C, Table 15.3) distills out of the flask.[4] When the vapor condenses, it enters the sidearm directly below the condenser, and water separates from the benzene–water condensate; benzene and water mix as vapors, but they are not miscible as cooled liquids. Once the water (lower phase) separates from the benzene (upper phase), liquid benzene overflows from the sidearm back into the flask. The cycle is repeated continuously until no more water forms in the sidearm. You may calculate the weight of water that should theoretically be produced and compare this value with the amount of water collected in the sidearm. Because the density of water is 1.0, the volume of water collected can be compared directly with the calculated amount, assuming 100% yield.

An improvised water separator, constructed from the components found in the traditional organic kit, is shown in Figure 15.12B. Although this requires the condenser to be placed in a nonvertical position, it works quite well.

At the microscale level, water separation can be achieved using a standard distillation assembly with a water condenser and a Hickman head (Figure 15.13). The side-ported variation of the Hickman head is the most convenient one to use for this purpose, but it is not essential. In this variation, you simply remove all the distillate (both solvent and water) several times during the course of the reaction. Use a Pasteur pipet to remove the distillate, as shown in Technique 14 (Figure 14.7, p. 743). Because both the solvent and water are re-

---

[4] Actually, with ethanol, a lower-boiling-point, three-component azeotrope distills at 64.9°C (see Table 15.3). It consists of benzene–water–ethanol. Because some ethanol is lost in the azeotropic distillation, a large excess of ethanol is used in esterification reactions. The excess also helps to shift the equilibrium to the right.

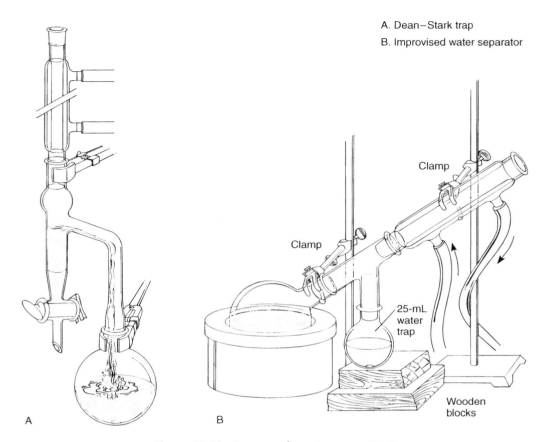

A. Dean–Stark trap

B. Improvised water separator

Clamp

Clamp

25-mL
water
trap

Wooden
blocks

A   B

Figure 15.12   Large-scale water separators.

moved in this procedure, it may be desirable to add more solvent from time to time, adding it through the condenser with a Pasteur pipet.

The most important consideration in using azeotropic distillation to prepare an ester (described on p. 760) is that the azeotrope containing water must have a **lower boiling point** than the alcohol used. With ethanol, the benzene–water azeotrope boils at a much lower temperature (69.4°C) than ethanol (78.3°C), and the technique previously described works well. With higher-boiling-point alcohols, azeotropic distillation works well because of the large boiling-point difference between the azeotrope and the alcohol.

With methanol (bp 65°C), however, the boiling point of the benzene–water azeotrope is actually *higher* by about 5°C, and methanol distills first. Thus, in esterifications involving methanol, a totally different approach must be taken. For example, you can mix the carboxylic acid, methanol, the acid catalyst, and *1,2-dichloroethane* in a conventional reflux apparatus (Technique 7, Figure 7.6, p. 628) without a water separator. During the reaction, water separates from the 1,2-dichloroethane because it is not miscible; however, the remainder of the components are soluble, so the reaction can continue. The equilibrium is shifted to the right by the "removal" of water from the reaction mixture.

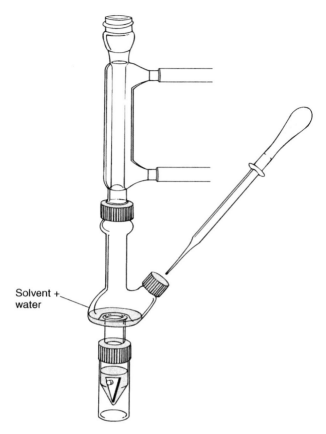

Figure 15.13 Microscale water separator (both layers are removed).

Azeotropic distillation is also used in other types of reactions, such as ketal or acetal formation, and in enamine formation.

$$\text{Acetal formation} \quad \underset{\substack{\\ }}{R-\overset{\displaystyle O}{\overset{\displaystyle \|}{C}}-H} + 2\,ROH \underset{}{\overset{H^+}{\rightleftharpoons}} \underset{\substack{|\\ OR}}{R-\overset{OR}{\underset{|}{C}}-H} + H_2O$$

Enamine formation

$$RCH_2-\underset{\underset{O}{\|}}{C}-CH_2R + \underset{\underset{H}{\overset{|}{N}}}{\bigcirc} \overset{H^+}{\rightleftharpoons} RCH{=}\underset{\underset{N}{|}}{C}-CH_2R + H_2O$$

PROBLEMS

1. In the accompanying chart are approximate vapor pressures for benzene and toluene at various temperatures.

Temp (°C)	mmHg	Temp (°C)	mmHg
Benzene 30	120	Toluene 30	37
40	180	40	60
50	270	50	95
60	390	60	140
70	550	70	200
80	760	80	290
90	1010	90	405
100	1340	100	560
		110	760

   a. What is the mole fraction of each component if 3.9 g of benzene C_6H_6 is dissolved in 4.6 g of toluene C_7H_8?
   b. Assuming that this mixture is ideal, that is, it follows Raoult's Law, what is the partial vapor pressure of benzene in this mixture at 50°C?
   c. Estimate to the nearest degree the temperature at which the vapor pressure of the solution equals 1 atm (bp of the solution).
   d. Calculate the composition of the vapor (mole fraction of each component) that is in equilibrium in the solution at the boiling point of this solution.
   e. Calculate the composition in weight percentage of the vapor that is in equilibrium with the solution.

2. Estimate how many theoretical plates are needed to separate a mixture that has a mole fraction of B equal to 0.70 (70% B) in Figure 15.3.

3. Two moles of sucrose are dissolved in 8 moles of water. Assume that the solution follows Raoult's Law and that the vapor pressure of sucrose is negligible. The boiling point of water is 100°C. The distillation is carried out at 1 atm (760 mmHg).
   a. Calculate the vapor pressure of the solution when the temperature reaches 100°C.
   b. What temperature would be observed during the entire distillation?
   c. What would be the composition of the distillate?
   d. If a thermometer were immersed below the surface of the liquid of the boiling flask, what temperature would be observed?

4. Explain why the boiling point of a two-component mixture rises slowly throughout a simple distillation when the boiling-point differences are not large.

5. Given the boiling points of several known mixtures of A and B (mole fractions are known) and the vapor pressures of A and B in the pure state (P_A^0 and P_B^0) at these same temperatures, how would you construct a boiling-point-composition phase diagram for A and B? Give a stepwise explanation.

6. Describe the behavior on distillation of a 98% ethanol solution through an efficient column. Refer to Figure 15.10.

7. Construct an approximate boiling-point-composition diagram for a benzene-methanol system. The mixture shows azeotropic behavior (see Table 15.3). Include on the graph the boiling points of pure benzene and pure methanol and the boiling point of the azeotrope. Describe the behavior for a mixture that is initially rich in benzene (90%) and then for a mixture that is initially rich in methanol (90%).

8. Construct an approximate boiling-point-composition diagram for an acetone–chloroform system, which forms a maximum-boiling-point azeotrope (Table 15.4). Describe the behavior on distillation of a mixture that is initially rich in acetone (90%), and then describe the behavior of a mixture that is initially rich in chloroform (90%).

9. Two components have boiling points of 130°C and 150°C. Estimate the number of theoretical plates needed to separate these substances in a fractional distillation.

10. A spinning-band column has an HETP of 0.25 in./plate. If the column has 12 theoretical plates, how long is it?

T E C H N I Q U E   1 9

Column Chromatography

The most modern and sophisticated methods of separating mixtures available to the organic chemist all involve **chromatography.** Chromatography is defined as the separation of a mixture of two or more different compounds or ions by distribution between two phases, one of which is stationary and the other of which is moving. Various types of chromatography are possible, depending on the nature of the two phases involved: **solid–liquid** (column, thin-layer, and paper), **liquid–liquid** (high-performance liquid), and **gas–liquid** (vapor-phase) chromatographic methods are common.

All chromatography works on much the same principle as solvent extraction (Technique 12). Basically, the methods depend on the differential solubilities or adsorptivities of the substances to be separated relative to the two phases between which they are to be partitioned. Here, column chromatography, a solid–liquid method, is considered. Thin-layer chromatography is examined in Technique 20; high-performance liquid chromatography is discussed in Technique 21; and gas chromatography, a gas–liquid method, is discussed in Technique 22.

19.1 ADSORBENTS

Column chromatography is a technique based on both adsorptivity and solubility. It is a solid–liquid phase-partitioning technique. The solid may be almost any material that does not dissolve in the associated liquid phase; the solids used most commonly are silica gel $SiO_2 \cdot xH_2O$, also called silicic acid, and alumina $Al_2O_3 \cdot xH_2O$. These compounds are used in their powdered or finely ground forms (usually 200–400 mesh).[1]

Most alumina used for chromatography is prepared from the impure ore bauxite $Al_2O_3 \cdot xH_2O + Fe_2O_3$. The bauxite is dissolved in hot sodium hydroxide and filtered to remove the insoluble iron oxides; the alumina in the ore forms the soluble amphoteric hydroxide $Al(OH)_4^-$. The hydroxide is precipitated by CO_2, which reduces the pH, as $Al(OH)_3$. When heated, the $Al(OH)_3$ loses water to form pure alumina Al_2O_3.

$$\text{Bauxite (crude)} \xrightarrow{\text{hot NaOH}} Al(OH)_4^- \text{ (aq)} + Fe_2O_3 \text{ (insoluble)}$$

$$Al(OH)_4^- \text{ (aq)} + CO_2 \longrightarrow Al(OH)_3 + HCO_3^-$$

$$2Al(OH)_3 \xrightarrow{\text{heat}} Al_2O_3 \text{ (s)} + 3H_2O$$

Alumina prepared in this way is called **basic alumina** because it still contains some hydroxides. Basic alumina cannot be used for chromatography of compounds that are base

---

[1] The term "mesh" refers to the number of openings per linear inch found in a screen. A large number refers to a fine screen (finer wires more closely spaced). When particles are sieved through a series of these screens, they are classified by the smallest mesh screen that they will pass through. Mesh 5 would represent a coarse gravel, and mesh 800 would be a fine powder.

sensitive. Therefore, it is washed with acid to neutralize the base, giving **acid-washed alumina.** This material is unsatisfactory unless it has been washed with enough water to remove *all* the acid; on being so washed, it becomes the best chromatographic material, called **neutral alumina.** If a compound is acid sensitive, either basic or neutral alumina must be used. You should be careful to ascertain what type of alumina is being used for chromatography. Silica gel is not available in any form other than that suitable for chromatography.

19.2 INTERACTIONS

If powdered or finely ground alumina (or silica gel) is added to a solution containing an organic compound, some of the organic compound will **adsorb** onto or adhere to the fine particles of alumina. Many kinds of intermolecular forces cause organic molecules to bind to alumina. These forces vary in strength according to their type. Nonpolar compounds bind to the alumina using only van der Waals forces. These are weak forces, and nonpolar molecules do not bind strongly unless they have extremely high molecular weights. The most important interactions are those typical of polar organic compounds. Either these forces are of the dipole–dipole type or they involve some direct interaction (coordination, hydrogen bonding, or salt formation). These types of interactions are illustrated in Figure 19.1, which for convenience shows only a portion of the alumina structure. Similar interactions occur with silica gel. The strengths of such interactions vary in the following approximate order:

Salt formation > coordination > hydrogen bonding > dipole–dipole > van der Waals

Strength of interaction varies among compounds. For instance, a strongly basic amine would bind more strongly than a weakly basic one (by coordination). In fact, strong bases and strong acids often interact so strongly that they **dissolve** alumina to some extent. You can use the following rule of thumb:

> The more polar the functional group, the stronger the bond to alumina (or silica gel).

A similar rule holds for solubility. Polar solvents dissolve polar compounds more effectively than nonpolar solvents do; nonpolar compounds are dissolved best by nonpolar solvents. Thus, the extent to which any given solvent can wash an adsorbed compound from alumina depends almost directly on the relative polarity of the solvent. For example, although a ketone adsorbed on alumina might not be removed by hexane, it might be removed completely by chloroform. For any adsorbed material, a kind of **distribution** equilibrium can be envisioned between the adsorbent material and the solvent. This is illustrated in Figure 19.2.

The distribution equilibrium is **dynamic,** with molecules constantly **adsorbing** from the solution and **desorbing** into it. The average number of molecules remaining adsorbed on the solid particles at equilibrium depends both on the particular molecule (RX) involved and the dissolving power of the solvent with which the adsorbent must compete.

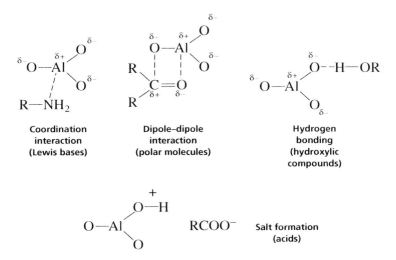

Figure 19.1 Possible interactions of organic compounds with alumina.

19.3 PRINCIPLE OF COLUMN CHROMATOGRAPHIC SEPARATION

The dynamic equilibrium mentioned previously and the variations in the extent to which different compounds adsorb on alumina or silica gel underlie a versatile and ingen-

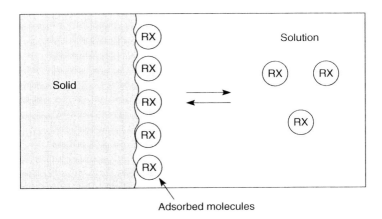

Figure 19.2 Dynamic adsorption equilibrium.

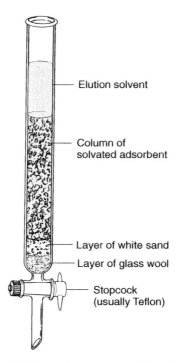

— Elution solvent

— Column of
solvated adsorbent

— Layer of white sand
— Layer of glass wool

— Stopcock
(usually Teflon)

Figure 19.3 A chromatographic column.

ious method for **separating** mixtures of organic compounds. In this method, the mixture of compounds to be separated is introduced onto the top of a cylindrical glass column (Figure 19.3) **packed** or filled with fine alumina particles (stationary solid phase). The adsorbent is continuously washed by a flow of solvent (moving phase) passing through the column.

Initially, the components of the mixture adsorb onto the alumina particles at the top of the column. The continuous flow of solvent through the column **elutes,** or washes, the solutes off the alumina and sweeps them down the column. The solutes (or materials to be separated) are called **eluates** or **elutants,** and the solvents are called **eluents.** As the solutes pass down the column to fresh alumina, new equilibria are established among the adsorbent, the solutes, and the solvent. The constant equilibration means that different compounds will move down at differing rates depending on their relative affinity for the adsorbent on the one hand, and for the solvent on the other. Because the number of alumina particles is large, because they are closely packed, and because fresh solvent is being added continuously, the number of equilibrations between adsorbent and solvent that the solutes experience is enormous.

As the components of the mixture are separated, they begin to form moving bands (or zones), with each band containing a single component. If the column is long enough and the other parameters (column diameter, adsorbent, solvent, and flow rate) are correctly chosen, the bands separate from one another, leaving gaps of pure solvent in between. As each band (solvent and solute) passes out from the bottom of the column, it can be collected before the next band arrives. If the parameters mentioned are poorly chosen, the various bands either overlap or coincide, in which case either a poor separation or no separation is the result. A successful chromatographic separation is illustrated in Figure 19.4.

19.4 PARAMETERS AFFECTING SEPARATION

The versatility of column chromatography results from the many factors that can be adjusted. These include

1. Adsorbent chosen
2. Polarity of the solvents chosen
3. Size of the column (both length and diameter) relative to the amount of material to be chromatographed
4. Rate of elution (or flow)

If the conditions are carefully chosen, almost any mixture can be separated. This technique has even been used to separate optical isomers. An optically active solid-phase adsorbent was used to separate the enantiomers.

Two fundamental choices for anyone attempting a chromatographic separation are the kind of adsorbent and the solvent system. In general, nonpolar compounds pass through the column faster than polar compounds, because they have a smaller affinity for the adsorbent. If the adsorbent chosen binds all the solute molecules (both polar and nonpolar) strongly, they will not move down the column. On the other hand, if too polar a solvent is chosen, all the solutes (polar and nonpolar) may simply be washed through the column, with no separation taking place. The adsorbent and the solvent should be chosen so that neither is favored excessively in the equilibrium competition for solute molecules.[2]

---

[2]Often, the chemist uses thin-layer chromatography (TLC), which is described in Technique 20, to arrive at the best choices of solvents and adsorbents for the best separation. The TLC experimentation can be performed quickly and with extremely small amounts (microgram quantities) of the mixture to be separated. This saves significant time and materials. Technique 20, Section 20.10, describes this use of TLC.

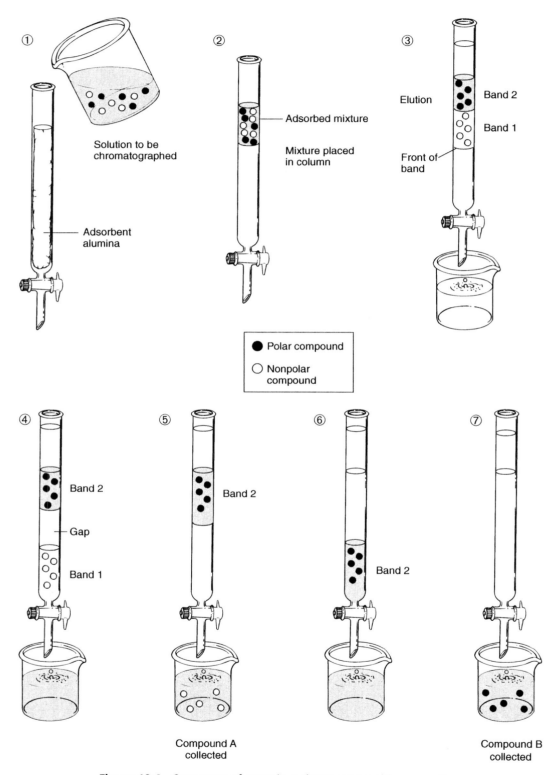

① Solution to be chromatographed

Adsorbent alumina

② Adsorbed mixture

Mixture placed in column

③ Elution

Band 2

Band 1

Front of band

● Polar compound
○ Nonpolar compound

④ Band 2

Gap

Band 1

⑤ Band 2

Compound A collected

⑥ Band 2

⑦ Compound B collected

Figure 19.4 Sequence of steps in a chromatographic separation.

226

TABLE 19.1   Solid Adsorbents for Column Chromatography

Paper	
Cellulose	
Starch	
Sugars	
Magnesium silicate	Increasing strength of
Calcium sulfate	binding interactions
Silicic acid	toward polar compounds
Florisil	
Magnesium oxide	
Aluminum oxide (alumina)[a]	
Activated charcoal (Norit)	

[a]Basic, acid washed, and neutral.

A. Adsorbents

In Table 19.1, various kinds of adsorbents (solid phases) used in column chromatography are listed. The choice of adsorbent often depends on the types of compounds to be separated. Cellulose, starch, and sugars are used for polyfunctional plant and animal materials (natural products) that are very sensitive to acid–base interactions. Magnesium silicate is often used for separating acetylated sugars, steroids, and essential oils. Silica gel and Florisil are relatively mild toward most compounds and are widely used for a variety of functional groups—hydrocarbons, alcohols, ketones, esters, acids, azo compounds, and amines. Alumina is the most widely used adsorbent and is obtained in the three forms mentioned in Section 19.1: acidic, basic, and neutral. The pH of acidic or acid-washed alumina is approximately 4. This adsorbent is particularly useful for separating acidic materials such as carboxylic acids and amino acids. Basic alumina has a pH of 10 and is useful in separating amines. Neutral alumina can be used to separate a variety of nonacidic and nonbasic materials.

The approximate strength of the various adsorbents listed in Table 19.1 is also given. The order is only approximate, and therefore it may vary. For instance, the strength, or separating abilities, of alumina and silica gel largely depends on the amount of water present. Water binds very tightly to either adsorbent, taking up sites on the particles that could otherwise be used for equilibration with solute molecules. If water is added to the adsorbent, it is said to have been **deactivated.** Anhydrous alumina or silica gel is said to be highly **activated.** High activity is usually avoided with these adsorbents. Use of the highly active forms of either alumina or silica gel, or of the acidic or basic forms of alumina, can often lead to molecular rearrangement or decomposition in certain types of solute compounds.

The chemist can select the degree of activity that is appropriate to carry out a particular separation. To accomplish this, highly activated alumina is mixed thoroughly with a precisely measured quantity of water. The water partially hydrates the alumina and thus reduces its activity. By carefully determining the amount of water required, the chemist can have available an entire spectrum of possible activities.

TABLE 19.2 Solvents (Eluents) for Chromatography

Petroleum ether	
Cyclohexane	
Carbon tetrachloride[a]	
Toluene	
Chloroform[a]	
Methylene chloride	Increasing polarity and
Diethyl ether	"solvent power" toward
Ethyl acetate	polar functional groups
Acetone	
Pyridine	
Ethanol	
Methanol	
Water	
Acetic acid	

[a]Suspected carcinogens.

TABLE 19.3 Elution Sequence for Compounds

Hydrocarbons	Fastest (will elute with nonpolar solvent)
Olefins	
Ethers	
Halocarbons	
Aromatics	
Ketones	Order of elution
Aldehydes	
Esters	
Alcohols	
Amines	
Acids, strong bases	Slowest (needs a polar solvent)

B. Solvents

In Table 19.2, some common chromatographic solvents are listed along with their relative ability to dissolve polar compounds. Sometimes a single solvent can be found that will separate all the components of a mixture. Sometimes a mixture of solvents can be found that will achieve separation. More often you must start elution with a nonpolar solvent to remove relatively nonpolar compounds from the column and then gradually increase the solvent polarity to force compounds of greater polarity to come down the column, or to elute. The approximate order in which various classes of compounds elute by this procedure is given in Table 19.3. In general, nonpolar compounds travel through the column faster (elute first), and polar compounds travel more slowly (elute last). However, molecular weight is also a factor in determining the order of elution. A nonpolar compound of high molecular weight travels more slowly than a nonpolar compound of low molecular weight, and it may even be passed by some polar compounds.

Solvent polarity functions in two ways in column chromatography. First, a polar solvent will better dissolve a polar compound and move it down the column faster. Therefore, as already mentioned, the polarity of the solvent is usually increased during column chromatography to wash down compounds of increasing polarity. Second, as the polarity of the solvent increases, the solvent itself will displace adsorbed molecules from the alumina or silica and take their place on the column. Because of this second effect, a polar solvent will move **all types of compounds,** both polar and nonpolar, down the column at a faster rate than a nonpolar solvent will.

When the polarity of the solvent has to be changed during a chromatographic separation, some precautions must be taken. Rapid changes from one solvent to another are to be avoided (especially when silica gel or alumina is involved). Usually, small percentages of a new solvent are mixed slowly into the one in use until the percentage reaches the desired level. If this is not done, the column packing often "cracks" as a result of the heat liberated when alumina or silica gel is mixed with a solvent. The solvent solvates the adsorbent, and the formation of a weak bond generates heat.

$$\text{Solvent} + \text{alumina} \rightarrow (\text{alumina} \cdot \text{solvent}) + \text{heat}$$

Often, enough heat is generated locally to evaporate the solvent. The formation of vapor creates bubbles, which forces a separation of the column packing; this is called **cracking.** A cracked column does not produce a good separation because it has discontinuities in the packing. The way in which a column is packed or filled is also very important in preventing cracking.

Certain solvents should be avoided with alumina or silica gel, especially with the acidic, basic, and highly active forms. For instance, with any of these adsorbents, acetone dimerizes via an aldol condensation to give diacetone alcohol. Mixtures of esters **trans-esterify** (exchange their alcoholic portions) when ethyl acetate or an alcohol is the eluent. Finally, the most active solvents (pyridine, methanol, water, and acetic acid) dissolve and elute some of the adsorbent itself. Generally, try to avoid solvents more polar than diethyl ether or methylene chloride in the eluent series (Table 19.2).

C. Column Size and Adsorbent Quantity

The column size and the amount of adsorbent must also be selected correctly to separate a given amount of sample well. As a rule of thumb, the amount of adsorbent should be 25 to 30 times, by weight, the amount of material to be separated by chromatography. Furthermore, the column should have a height-to-diameter ratio of about 8:1. Some typical relations of this sort are given in Table 19.4.

Note, as a caution, that the difficulty of the separation is also a factor in determining the size and length of the column to be used and the amount of adsorbent needed. Compounds that do not separate easily may require longer columns and more adsorbent than specified in Table 19.4. For easily separated compounds, a shorter column and less adsorbent may suffice.

TABLE 19.4 Size of Column and Amount of Adsorbent
for Typical Sample Sizes

Amount of Sample (g)	Amount of Adsorbent (g)	Column Diameter (mm)	Column Height (mm)
0.01	0.3	3.5	30
0.10	3.0	7.5	60
1.00	30.0	16.0	130
10.00	300.0	35.0	280

D. Flow Rate

The rate at which solvent flows through the column is also significant in the effectiveness of a separation. In general, the time the mixture to be separated remains on the column is directly proportional to the extent of equilibration between stationary and moving phases. Thus, similar compounds eventually separate if they remain on the column long enough. The time a material remains on the column depends on the flow rate of the solvent. If the flow is too slow, however, the dissolved substances in the mixture may diffuse faster than the rate at which they move down the column. Then the bands grow wider and more diffuse, and the separation becomes poor.

19.5 PACKING THE COLUMN: TYPICAL PROBLEMS

The most critical operation in column chromatography is packing (filling) the column with adsorbent. The **column packing** must be evenly packed and free of irregularities, air bubbles, and gaps. As a compound travels down the column, it moves in an advancing zone, or **band.** It is important that the leading edge, or **front,** of this band be horizontal, or perpendicular to the long axis of the column. If two bands are close together and do not have horizontal band fronts, it is impossible to collect one band while completely excluding the other. The leading edge of the second band begins to elute before the first band has finished eluting. This condition can be seen in Figure 19.5. There are two main reasons for this problem. First, if the top surface edge of the adsorbent packing is not level, nonhorizontal bands result. Second, bands may be nonhorizontal if the column is not held in an exactly vertical position in both planes (front to back and side to side). When preparing a column, you must watch both these factors carefully.

Another phenomenon, called **streaming** or **channeling,** occurs when part of the band front advances ahead of the major part of the band. Channeling occurs if there are any cracks or irregularities in the adsorbent surface or any irregularities caused by air bubbles in the packing. A part of the advancing front moves ahead of the rest of the band by flowing through the channel. Two examples of channeling are shown in Figure 19.6.

The methods outlined in Sections 19.6, 19.7, and 19.8 are used to avoid problems resulting from uneven packing and column irregularities. These procedures should be fol-

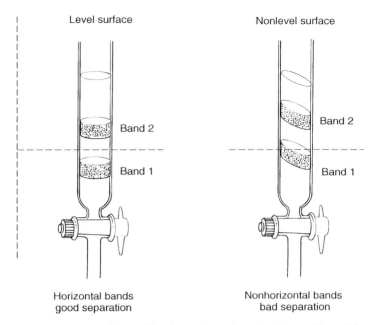

Figure 19.5 Comparison of horizontal and nonhorizontal band fronts.

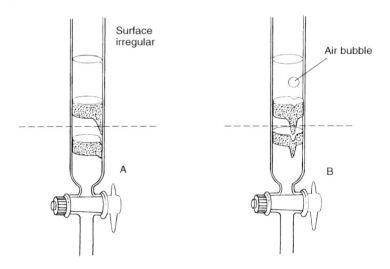

Figure 19.6 Channeling complications.

lowed carefully in preparing a chromatography column. Failure to pay close attention to the preparation of the column may affect the quality of the separation.

19.6 PACKING THE COLUMN: PREPARING THE SUPPORT BASE

Preparation of a column involves two distinct stages. In the first stage, a support base on which the packing will rest is prepared. This must be done so that the packing, a finely

231

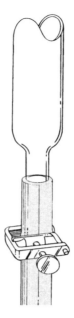

Figure 19.7 Tubing with screw clamp to regulate solvent flow on a chromatography column.

divided material, does not wash out of the bottom of the column. In the second stage, the column of adsorbent is deposited on top of the supporting base.

A. Macroscale Columns

For large-scale applications, a chromatography column is clamped upright (vertically). The column (Figure 19.3) is a piece of cylindrical glass tubing with a stopcock attached at one end. The stopcock usually has a Teflon plug, because stopcock grease (used on glass plugs) dissolves in many of the organic solvents used as eluents. Stopcock grease in the eluent will contaminate the eluates.

Instead of a stopcock, a piece of flexible tubing may be attached to the bottom of the column, with a screw clamp used to stop or regulate the flow (Figure 19.7). When a screw clamp is used, care must be taken that the tubing used is not dissolved by the solvents that will pass through the column during the experiment. Rubber, for instance, dissolves in chloroform, benzene, methylene chloride, toluene, or tetrahydrofuran (THF). Tygon tubing dissolves (actually, the plasticizer is removed) in many solvents, including benzene, methylene chloride, chloroform, ether, ethyl acetate, toluene, and THF. Polyethylene tubing is the best choice for use at the end of a column because it is inert with most solvents.

Next, the column is partially filled with a quantity of solvent, usually a nonpolar solvent such as hexane, and a support for the finely divided adsorbent is prepared in the following way. A loose plug of glass wool is tamped down into the bottom of the column with a long glass rod until all entrapped air is forced out as bubbles. Take care not to plug the column totally by tamping the glass wool too hard. A small layer of clean, white sand is formed on top of the glass wool by pouring sand into the column. The column is tapped to level the surface of the sand. Any sand adhering to the side of the column is washed down with a small quantity of solvent. The sand forms a base that supports the column of adsorbent and prevents it from washing through the stopcock. The column is packed in one of two ways: by the slurry method (Section 9.8) or by the dry pack method (Section 9.7).

B. Semi-microscale Columns

An alternative apparatus for macroscale column chromatography on a smaller scale is a commercial column, such as the one shown in Figure 19.8. This type of column is made of glass and has a solvent-resistant plastic stopcock at the bottom.[3] The stopcock assembly contains a filter disc to support the adsorbent column. An optional upper fitting, also made of solvent-resistant plastic, serves as a solvent reservoir. The column shown in Figure 19.8 is equipped with the solvent reservoir. This type of column is available in a variety of lengths, ranging from 100 mm to 300 mm. Because the column has a built-in filter disc, it is not necessary to prepare a support base before the adsorbent is added.

C. Microscale Columns

For microscale applications, a Pasteur pipet (5¾-inch) is used; it is clamped upright (vertically). To reduce the amount of solvent needed to fill the column, you may break off most of the tip of the pipet. A small ball of cotton is placed in the pipet and tamped into position using a glass rod or a piece of wire. Take care not to plug the column totally by tamping the cotton too hard. The correct position of the cotton is shown in Figure 19.9. A microscale chromatography column is packed by one of the dry pack methods described in Section 19.7.

19.7 PACKING THE COLUMN: DEPOSITING THE ADSORBENT—DRY PACK METHODS

A. Dry Pack Method 1

Macroscale Columns. In the first of the dry pack methods introduced here, the column is filled with solvent and allowed to drain *slowly*. The dry adsorbent is added, a little at a time, while the column is tapped gently with a pencil, finger, or glass rod.

A plug of cotton is placed at the base of the column, and an even layer of sand is formed on top (see p. 805). The column is filled about half-full with solvent, and the solid adsorbent is added carefully from a beaker while the solvent is allowed to flow slowly from the column. As the solid is added, the column is tapped as described for the slurry method (see p. 809) to ensure that the column is packed evenly. When the column has the desired length, no more adsorbent is added. This method produces an evenly packed column. Solvent should be cycled through this column (for macroscale applications) sev-

---

[3] Note to the instructor: With certain organic solvents, we have found that the "solvent-resistant" plastic stopcock may tend to dissolve! We recommend that instructors test their equipment with the solvent that they intend to use before the start of the laboratory class.

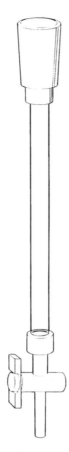

Figure 19.8 A commercial semi-microscale chromatography column. (The column shown is equipped with an optional solvent reservoir.)

eral times before each use. The same portion of solvent that has drained from the column during the packing is used to cycle through the column.

Semi-microscale Columns. The procedure to fill a commercial semi-microscale column is essentially the same as that used to fill a Pasteur pipet (see the following paragraph). The commercial column has the advantage that it is much easier to control the flow of solvent from the column during the filling process, because the stopcock can be adjusted appropriately. It is not necessary to use a cotton plug or to deposit a layer of sand before adding the adsorbent. The presence of the fritted disc at the base of the column prevents adsorbent from escaping from the column.

Microscale Columns. To fill a microscale column, fill the Pasteur pipet (with the cotton plug, prepared as described in Section 19.6) about half full with solvent. Using a microspatula, add the solid adsorbent slowly to the solvent in the column. As you add the solid, tap the column *gently* with a pencil, a finger, or a glass rod. The tapping promotes even settling and mixing and gives an evenly packed column free of air bubbles. As the adsorbent is added, solvent flows out of the Pasteur pipet. Because the adsorbent must not be allowed to dry during the packing process, you must use a means of controlling the solvent flow. If a piece of small-diameter plastic tubing is available, it can be fitted over the narrow

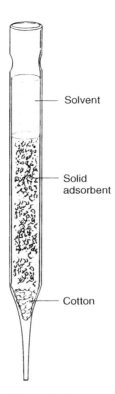

Figure 19.9 A microscale chromatography column.

tip of the Pasteur pipet. The flow rate can then be controlled using a screw clamp. A simple approach to controlling the flow rate is to use a finger over the top of the Pasteur pipet, much as you control the flow of liquid in a volumetric pipet. Continue adding the adsorbent slowly, with constant tapping, until the adsorbent has reached the desired level. As you pack the column, be careful not to let the column run dry. The final column should appear as shown in Figure 19.9.

B. Dry Pack Method 2

Macroscale Columns. Macroscale columns can also be packed by a dry pack method that is commonly used in the packing of microscale columns (see "Microscale Columns," following). In this method, the column is filled with dry adsorbent without any solvent. When the desired amount of adsorbent has been added, solvent is allowed to percolate through the column. The disadvantages described for the microscale method also apply to the macroscale method. This method is not recommended for use with silica gel or alumina because the combination leads to uneven packing, air bubbles, and cracking, especially if a solvent that has a highly exothermic heat of solvation is used.

Semi-microscale Columns. The dry pack method 2 for semi-microscale columns is similar to that described for Pasteur pipets (see next paragraph), except that the plug of cotton is not required. The flow rate of solvent through the column can be controlled using the stopcock, which is part of the column assembly (see Figure 19.8).

Microscale Columns.   An alternative dry pack method for microscale columns is to fill the Pasteur pipet with *dry* adsorbent, without any solvent. Position a plug of cotton in the bottom of the Pasteur pipet. The desired amount of adsorbent is added slowly, and the pipet is tapped constantly until the level of adsorbent has reached the desired height. Figure 19.9 can be used as a guide to judge the correct height of the column of adsorbent. When the column is packed, added solvent is allowed to percolate through the adsorbent until the entire column is moistened. The solvent is not added until just before the column is to be used.

This method is useful when the adsorbent is alumina, but it does not produce satisfactory results with silica gel. Even with alumina, poor separations can arise due to uneven packing, air bubbles, and cracking, especially if a solvent that has a highly exothermic heat of solvation is used.

19.8 PACKING THE COLUMN: DEPOSITING THE ADSORBENT—THE SLURRY METHOD

The slurry method is not recommended as a microscale method for use with Pasteur pipets. On a very small scale, it is too difficult to pack the column with the slurry without losing the solvent before the packing has been completed. Microscale columns should be packed by one of the dry pack methods, as described in Section 19.7.

In the slurry method, the adsorbent is packed into the column as a mixture of a solvent and an undissolved solid. The slurry is prepared in a separate container (Erlenmeyer flask) by adding the solid adsorbent, a little at a time, to a quantity of the solvent. This order of addition (adsorbent added to solvent) should be followed strictly, because the adsorbent solvates and liberates heat. If the solvent is added to the adsorbent, it may boil away almost as fast as it is added due to heat evolved. This will be especially true if ether or another low-boiling solvent is used. When this happens, the final mixture will be uneven and lumpy. Enough adsorbent is added to the solvent, and mixed by swirling the container, to form a thick, but flowing, slurry. The container should be swirled until the mixture is homogeneous and relatively free of entrapped air bubbles.

For a macroscale column, the procedure is as follows. When the slurry has been prepared, the column is filled about half full with solvent, and the stopcock is opened to allow solvent to drain slowly into a large beaker. The slurry is mixed by swirling and is then poured in portions into the top of the draining column (a wide-necked funnel may be useful here). Be sure to swirl the slurry thoroughly before each addition to the column. The column is tapped constantly and *gently* on the side during the pouring operation, with the fingers or with a pencil fitted with a rubber stopper. A short piece of large-diameter pressure tubing may also be used for tapping. The tapping promotes even settling and mixing and gives an evenly packed column free of air bubbles. Tapping is continued until all the material has settled, showing a well-defined level at the top of the column. Solvent from the collecting beaker may be readded to the slurry if it becomes too thick to be poured into the column at one time. In fact, the collected solvent should be cycled through the column several times to ensure that settling is complete and that the column is firmly packed. The downward flow of solvent tends to compact the adsorbent. Take care never to let the column "run dry" during packing. There should always be solvent on top of the absorbent column.

19.9 APPLYING THE SAMPLE TO THE COLUMN

The solvent (or solvent mixture) used to pack the column is normally the least polar elution solvent that can be used during chromatography. The compounds to be chromatographed are not highly soluble in the solvent. If they were, they would probably have a greater affinity for the solvent than for the adsorbent and would pass right through the column without equilibrating with the stationary phase.

The first elution solvent, however, is generally not a good solvent to use in preparing the sample to be placed on the column. Because the compounds are not highly soluble in nonpolar solvents, it takes a large amount of the initial solvent to dissolve the compounds, and it is difficult to get the mixture to form a narrow band on top of the column. A narrow band is ideal for an optimum separation of components. For the best separation, therefore, the compound is applied to the top of the column undiluted if it is a liquid, or in a *very small* amount of polar solvent if it is a solid. Water must not be used to dissolve the initial sample being chromatographed because it reacts with the column packing.

In adding the sample to the column, use the following procedure. Lower the solvent level to the top of the adsorbent column by draining the solvent from the column. Add the sample (either a pure liquid or a solution) to form a small layer on top of the adsorbent. A Pasteur pipet is convenient for adding the sample to the column. Take care not to disturb the surface of the adsorbent. This is best accomplished by touching the pipet to the inside of the glass column and slowly draining it to allow the sample to spread into a thin film, which slowly descends to cover the entire adsorbent surface. Drain the pipet close to the surface of the adsorbent. When all the sample has been added, drain this small layer of liquid into the column until the top surface of the column *just begins* to dry. Then add a small layer of the chromatographic solvent carefully with a Pasteur pipet, again being careful not to disturb the surface. Drain this small layer of solvent into the column until the top surface of the column just dries. Add another small layer of fresh solvent, if necessary, and repeat the process until it is clear that the sample is strongly adsorbed on the top of the column. If the sample is colored and the fresh layer of solvent acquires some of this color, the sample has not been properly adsorbed. Once the sample has been properly applied, you can protect the level surface of the adsorbent by carefully filling the top of the column with solvent and sprinkling clean, white sand into the column to form a small protective layer on top of the adsorbent. For microscale applications, this layer of sand is not required.

Separations are often better if the sample is allowed to stand a short time on the column before elution. This allows a true equilibrium to be established. In columns that stand for too long, however, the adsorbent often compacts or even swells, and the flow can become annoyingly slow. Diffusion of the sample to widen the bands also becomes a problem if a column is allowed to stand over an extended period. For small-scale chromatography using Pasteur pipets, there is no stopcock, and it is not possible to stop the flow. In this case, it is not necessary to allow the column to stand.

19.10 ELUTION TECHNIQUES

Solvents for analytical and preparative chromatography should be pure reagents. Commercial-grade solvents often contain small amounts of residue, which remain when the solvent is evaporated. For routine work and for relatively easy separations that take only small amounts of solvent, the residue usually presents few problems. For large-scale work, commercial-grade solvents may have to be redistilled before use. This is especially true for hydrocarbon solvents, which tend to have more residue than other solvent types.

Elution of the products is usually begun with a nonpolar solvent, such as hexane or petroleum ether. The polarity of the elution solvent can be increased gradually by adding successively greater percentages of ether or toluene (for instance, 1, 2, 5, 10, 15, 25, 50, or 100%) or some other solvent of greater solvent power (polarity) than hexane. The transition from one solvent to another should not be too rapid in most solvent changes. If the two solvents to be changed differ greatly in their heats of solvation in binding to the adsorbent, enough heat can be generated to crack the column. Ether is especially troublesome in this respect, as it has both a low boiling point and a relatively high heat of solvation. Most organic compounds can be separated on silica gel or alumina using hexane–ether or hexane–toluene combinations for elution, and following these by pure methylene chloride. Solvents of greater polarity are usually avoided for the various reasons mentioned previously. In microscale work, the usual procedure is to use only one solvent for the chromatography.

The flow of solvent through the column should not be too rapid, or the solutes will not have time to equilibrate with the adsorbent as they pass down the column. If the rate of flow is too low or stopped for a period, diffusion can become a problem—the solute band will diffuse, or spread out, in all directions. In either of these cases, separation will be poor. As a general rule (and only an approximate one), most macroscale columns are run with flow rates ranging from 5 to 50 drops of effluent per minute; a steady flow of solvent is usually avoided. Microscale columns made from Pasteur pipets do not have a means of controlling the solvent flow rate, but commercial microscale columns are equipped with stopcocks. The solvent flow rate in this type of column can be adjusted in a manner similar to that used with larger columns. To avoid diffusion of the bands, do not stop the column, and do not set it aside overnight.

In some cases, the chromatography may proceed too slowly; the rate of solvent flow can be accelerated by attaching a rubber dropper bulb to the top of the Pasteur pipet column and squeezing *gently*. The additional air pressure forces the solvent through the column more rapidly. If this technique is used, however, care must be taken to remove the rubber bulb from the column before releasing it. Otherwise, air may be drawn up through the bottom of the column, destroying the column packing.

19.11 RESERVOIRS

When large quantities of solvent are used in a chromatographic separation, it is often convenient to use a solvent reservoir to forestall having to add small portions of fresh solvent continually. The simplest type of reservoir, a feature of many columns, is created by fusing the top of the column to a round-bottom flask (Figure 19.10A). If the column has a standard-taper joint at its top, a reservoir can be created by joining a standard-taper separatory funnel to the column (Figure 19.10B). In this arrangement, the stopcock is left open, and no stopper is placed in the top of the separatory funnel. A third common arrangement is shown in Figure 19.10C. A separatory funnel is filled with solvent; its stopper is wetted with solvent and put *firmly* in place. The funnel is inserted into the empty filling space at the top of the chromatographic column, and the stopcock is opened. Solvent flows out of the funnel, filling the space at the top of the column until the solvent level is well above the

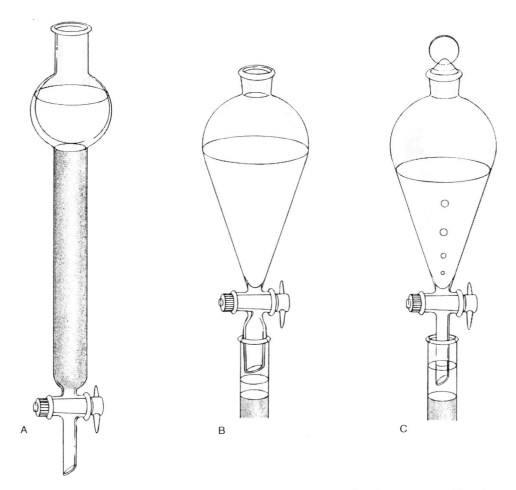

Figure 19.10 Various types of solvent-reservoir arrangements for chromatographic columns.

outlet of the separatory funnel. As solvent drains from the column, this arrangement automatically refills the space at the top of the column by allowing air to enter through the stem of the separatory funnel.

Some semi-microscale columns, such as that shown in Figure 19.8, are equipped with a solvent reservoir that fits onto the top of the column. It functions just as the reservoirs do that are described in this section.

For a microscale chromatography, the portion of the Pasteur pipet above the adsorbent is used as a reservoir of solvent. Fresh solvent, as needed, is added by means of another Pasteur pipet. When it is necessary to change solvent, the new solvent is also added in this manner.

19.12 MONITORING THE COLUMN

It is a lucky circumstance when the compounds to be separated are colored. The separation can then be followed visually and the various bands collected separately as they elute

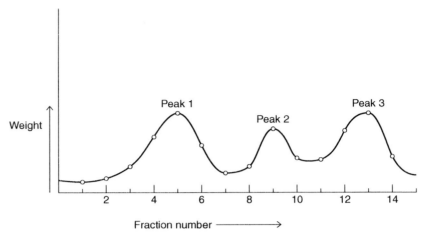

Figure 19.11 A typical elution graph.

from the column. For the majority of organic compounds, however, this lucky circumstance does not exist, and other methods must be used to determine the positions of the bands. The most common method of following a separation of colorless compounds is to collect *fractions* of constant volume in preweighed flasks or test tubes, to evaporate the solvent from each fraction, and to reweigh the container plus any residue. A plot of fraction number versus the weight of the residues after evaporation of solvent gives a plot similar to that in Figure 19.11. Clearly, fractions 2 through 7 (peak 1) may be combined as a single compound, and so can fractions 8 through 11 (peak 2) and 12 through 15 (peak 3). The size of the fractions collected (1, 10, 100, or 500 mL) depends on the size of the column and the ease of separation.

Another common method of monitoring the column is to mix an inorganic phosphor into the adsorbent used to pack the column. When the column is illuminated with an ultraviolet light, the adsorbent treated in this way fluoresces. However, many solutes have the ability to **quench** the fluorescence of the indicator phosphor. In areas in which solutes are present, the adsorbent does not fluoresce, and a dark band is visible. In this type of column, the separation can also be followed visually.

Thin-layer chromatography is often used to monitor a column. This method is described in Technique 20 (Section 20.10, p. 828). Several sophisticated instrumental and spectroscopic methods, which we shall not detail, can also monitor a chromatographic separation.

19.13 TAILING

When a single solvent is used for elution, an elution curve (weight versus fraction) such as that shown as a solid line in Figure 19.12 is often observed. An ideal elution curve is shown by dashed lines. In the nonideal curve, the compound is said to be **tailing.** Tailing can interfere with the beginning of a curve or a peak of a second component and lead to a poor separation. One way to avoid this is to increase the polarity of the solvent constantly while eluting. In this way, at the tail of the peak, where the

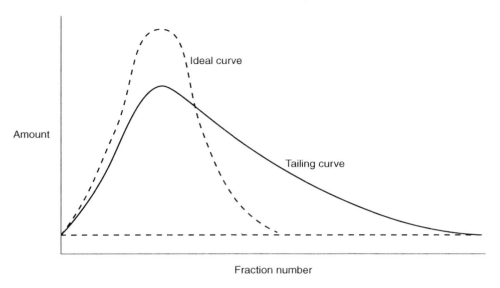

Figure 19.12 Elution curves: one ideal and one that "tails."

solvent polarity is increasing, the compound will move slightly faster than at the front and allow the tail to squeeze forward, forming a more nearly ideal band.

19.14 RECOVERING THE SEPARATED COMPOUNDS

In recovering each of the separated compounds of a chromatographic separation when they are solids, the various correct fractions are combined and evaporated. If the combined fractions contain sufficient material, they may be purified by recrystallization. If the compounds are liquids, the correct fractions are combined, and the solvent is evaporated. If sufficient material has been collected, liquid samples can be purified by distillation. The combination of chromatography–crystallization or chromatography–distillation usually yields very pure compounds. For microscale applications, the amount of sample collected is too small to allow a purification by crystallization or distillation. The samples that are obtained after the solvent has been evaporated are considered to be sufficiently pure, and no additional purification is attempted.

19.15 DECOLORIZATION BY COLUMN CHROMATOGRAPHY

A common outcome of organic reactions is the formation of a product that is contaminated by highly colored impurities. Very often, these impurities are highly polar, and they have a high molecular weight as well as being colored. The purification of the desired product requires that these impurities be removed. Section 11.7 of Technique 11 (pp. 693–694) details methods of decolorizing an organic product. In most cases, these methods involve the use of a form of activated charcoal, or Norit.

241

An alternative, which is applied conveniently in microscale experiments, is to remove the colored impurity by column chromatography. Because of the polarity of the impurities, the colored components are strongly adsorbed on the stationary phase of the column, and the less polar desired product passes through the column and is collected.

Microscale decolorization of a solution on a chromatography column requires that a column be prepared in a Pasteur pipet, using either alumina or silica gel as the adsorbent (Sections 19.6 and 19.7). The sample to be decolorized is diluted to the point where crystallization within the column will not take place, and it is then passed through the column in the usual manner. The desired compound is collected as it exits the column, and the excess solvent is removed by evaporation (Technique 7, Section 7.10, p. 639).

19.16 GEL CHROMATOGRAPHY

The stationary phase in gel chromatography consists of a cross-linked polymeric material. Molecules are separated according to their *size* by their ability to penetrate a sievelike structure. Molecules permeate the porous stationary phase as they move down the column. Small molecules penetrate the porous structure more easily than large ones. Thus, the large molecules move through the column faster than the smaller ones and elute first. The separation of molecules by gel chromatography is depicted in Figure 19.13. With adsorption chromatography using materials such as alumina or silica, the order is usually the reverse. Small

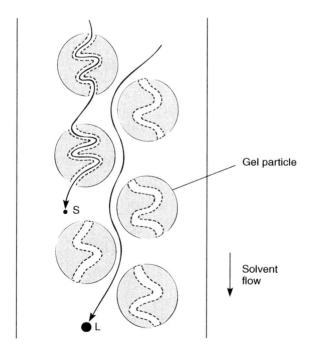

Figure 19.13 Gel chromatography. Comparison of the paths of large (L) and small (S) molecules through the column during the same interval of time.

molecules (of low molecular weight) pass through the column *faster* than large molecules (of high molecular weight) because large molecules are more strongly attracted to the polar stationary phase.

Equivalent terms used by chemists for the gel chromatography technique are **gel-filtration chromatography** (biochemistry term), **gel-permeation chromatography** (polymer chemistry term), and **molecular-sieve chromatography. Size-exclusion chromatography** is a general term for the technique, and it is perhaps the most descriptive term for what occurs on a molecular level.

Sephadex is one of the most popular materials for gel chromatography. It is widely used by biochemists for separating proteins, nucleic acids, enzymes, and carbohydrates. Most often, water or aqueous solutions of buffers are used as the moving phase. Chemically, Sephadex is a polymeric carbohydrate that has been cross linked. The degree of cross-linking determines the size of the "holes" in the polymer matrix. In addition, the hydroxyl groups on the polymer can adsorb water, which causes the material to swell. As it expands, "holes" are created in the matrix. Several different gels are available from manufacturers, each with its own set of characteristics. For example, a typical Sephadex gel, such as G-75, can separate molecules in the molecular weight (MW) range 3000 to 70,000. Assume a four-component mixture containing compounds with molecular weights of 10,000, 20,000, 50,000, and 100,000. The 100,000-MW compound would pass through the column first, because it cannot penetrate the polymer matrix. The 50,000-, 20,000-, and 10,000-MW compounds penetrate the matrix to varying degrees and would be separated. The molecules would elute in the order given (decreasing order of molecular weights). The gel separates on the basis of molecular size and configuration rather than molecular weight.

Sephadex LH-20 has been developed for nonaqueous solvents. Some of the hydroxyl groups have been alkylated, and thus the material can swell under both aqueous and nonaqueous conditions (it now has "organic" character). This material can be used with several organic solvents, such as alcohol, acetone, methylene chloride, and aromatic hydrocarbons.

Another type of gel is based on a polyacrylamide structure (Bio-Gel P and Poly-Sep AA). A portion of a polyacrylamide chain is shown here:

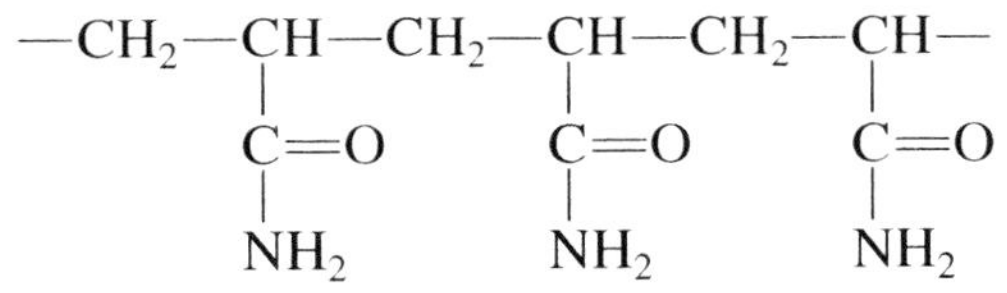

$$-CH_2-CH-CH_2-CH-CH_2-CH-$$
$$\quad\quad\quad | \quad\quad\quad\quad | \quad\quad\quad\quad |$$
$$\quad\quad C=O \quad\quad C=O \quad\quad C=O$$
$$\quad\quad\quad | \quad\quad\quad\quad | \quad\quad\quad\quad |$$
$$\quad\quad NH_2 \quad\quad NH_2 \quad\quad NH_2$$

Gels of this type can also be used in water and some polar organic solvents. They tend to be more stable than Sephadex, especially under acidic conditions. Polyacrylamides can be used for many biochemical applications involving macromolecules. For separating synthetic polymers, cross-linked polystyrene beads (copolymer of styrene and divinylbenzene) find common application. Again, the beads are swollen before use. Common organic solvents can be used to elute the polymers. As with other gels, the higher-molecular-weight compounds elute before the lower-molecular-weight compounds.

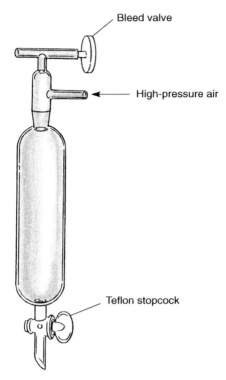

Bleed valve

High-pressure air

Teflon stopcock

Figure 19.14 Apparatus for flash chromatography.

19.17 FLASH CHROMATOGRAPHY

One of the drawbacks to column chromatography is that for large-scale preparative separations, the time required to complete a separation may be very long. Furthermore, the resolution that is possible for a particular experiment tends to deteriorate as the time for the experiment grows longer. This latter effect arises because the bands of compounds that move very slowly through a column tend to "tail."

A technique that can be useful in overcoming these problems has been developed. This technique, called **flash chromatography,** is actually a very simple modification of an ordinary column chromatography. In flash chromatography, the adsorbent is packed into a relatively short glass column, and air pressure is used to force the solvent through the adsorbent.

The apparatus used for flash chromatography is shown in Figure 19.14. The glass column is fitted with a Teflon stopcock at the bottom to control the flow rate of solvent. A plug of glass wool is placed in the bottom of the column to act as a support for the adsorbent. A layer of sand may also be added on top of the glass wool. The column is filled with adsorbent using the dry pack method. When the column has been filled, a fitting is attached to the top of the column, and the entire apparatus is connected to a source of high-pressure air or nitrogen. The fitting is designed so that the pressure applied to the top of the column can be adjusted precisely. The source of the high-pressure air is often a specially adapted air pump.

A typical column would use silica gel adsorbent (particle size = 40–63 μm) packed

244

to a height of 5 inches in a glass column of 20-mm diameter. The pressure applied to the column would be adjusted to achieve a solvent flow rate such that the solvent level in the column would decrease by about 2 inches/minute. This system would be appropriate to separate the components of a 250-mg sample.

The high-pressure air forces the solvent through the column of adsorbent at a rate that is much greater than what would be achieved if the solvent flowed through the column under the force of gravity. Because the solvent is made to flow faster, the time required for substances to pass through the column is reduced. By itself, simply applying air pressure to the column might reduce the clarity of the separation, because the components of the mixture would not have time to establish themselves into distinctly separate bands. However, in flash chromatography, you can use a much finer adsorbent than would be used in ordinary chromatography. With a much smaller particle size for the adsorbent, the surface area is increased, and the resolution possible thereby improves.

A simple variation on this idea does not use air pressure. Instead, the lower end of the column is inserted into a stopper, which is fitted into the top of a suction flask. Vacuum is applied to the system, and the vacuum acts to draw the solvent through the adsorbent column. The overall effect of this variation is similar to that obtained when air pressure is applied to the top of the column.

REFERENCES

Deyl, Z., Macek, K., and Janák, J. *Liquid Column Chromatography.* Amsterdam: Elsevier, 1975.

Heftmann, E. *Chromatography,* 3rd ed. New York: Van Nostrand Reinhold, 1975.

Jacobson, B. M. "An Inexpensive Way to Do Flash Chromatography." *Journal of Chemical Education, 65* (May 1988): 459.

Still, W. C., Kahn, M., and Mitra, A. "Rapid Chromatographic Technique for Preparative Separations with Moderate Resolution." *Journal of Organic Chemistry, 43* (1978): 2923.

PROBLEMS

1. A sample was placed on a chromatography column. Methylene chloride was used as the eluting solvent. All of the components eluted off the column, but no separation was observed. What must have been happening during this experiment? How would you change the experiment to overcome this problem?

2. You are about to purify an impure sample of naphthalene by column chromatography. What solvent should you use to elute the sample?

3. Consider a sample that is a mixture composed of biphenyl, benzoic acid, and benzyl alcohol. Predict the order of elution of the components in this mixture. Assume that the chromatography uses a silica column and the solvent system is based on cyclohexane, with an increasing proportion of methylene chloride added as a function of time.

4. An orange compound was added to the top of a chromatography column. Solvent was added immediately, and the entire volume of solvent in the solvent reservoir turned orange. No separation could be obtained from the chromatography experiment. What went wrong?

5. A yellow compound dissolved in methylene chloride is added to a chromatography column. The elution is begun using petroleum ether as the solvent. After 6 L of solvent had passed through the column, the yellow band still had not traveled down the column appreciably. What should be done to make this experiment work better?

6. You have 0.50 g of a mixture that you wish to purify by column chromatography. How much adsorbent should you use to pack the column? Estimate the appropriate column diameter and height.

7. In a particular sample, you wish to collect the component with the *highest* molecular weight as the *first* fraction. What chromatographic technique should you use?

8. A colored band shows an excessive amount of tailing as it passes through the column. What can you do to rectify this problem?

9. How would you monitor the progress of a column chromatography when the sample is colorless? Describe at least two methods.

T E C H N I Q U E   2 0

Thin-Layer Chromatography

Thin-layer chromatography (TLC) is a very important technique for the rapid separation and qualitative analysis of small amounts of material. It is ideally suited for the analysis of mixtures and reaction products in both macroscale and microscale experiments. The technique is closely related to column chromatography. In fact, TLC can be considered column chromatography *in reverse,* with the solvent ascending the adsorbent rather than descending. Because of this close relationship to column chromatography and because the principles governing the two techniques are similar, Technique 19, on column chromatography, should be read first.

20.1 PRINCIPLES OF THIN-LAYER CHROMATOGRAPHY

Like column chromatography, TLC is a solid–liquid partitioning technique. However, the moving liquid phase is not allowed to percolate down the adsorbent; it is caused to *ascend* a thin layer of adsorbent coated onto a backing support. The most typical backing is a plastic material, but other materials are also used. A thin layer of the adsorbent is spread onto the plate and allowed to dry. A coated and dried plate is called a **thin-layer plate** or a **thin-layer slide.** (Microscope slides were often used to prepare small thin-layer plates, thus the reference to *slide.*) When a thin-layer plate is placed upright in a vessel that contains a shallow layer of solvent, the solvent ascends the layer of adsorbent on the plate by capillary action.

In TLC, the sample is applied to the plate before the solvent is allowed to ascend the adsorbent layer. The sample is usually applied as a small spot near the base of the plate; this technique is often referred to as **spotting.** The plate is spotted by repeated applications of a sample solution from a small capillary pipet. When the filled pipet touches the plate, capillary action delivers its contents to the plate, and a small spot is formed.

As the solvent ascends the plate, the sample is partitioned between the moving liquid phase and the stationary solid phase. During this process, you are **developing,** or **running,** the thin-layer plate. In development, the various components in the applied mixture are separated. The separation is based on the many equilibrations the solutes experience between the moving and the stationary phases. (The nature of these equilibrations was thoroughly discussed in Technique 19, Sections 19.2 and 19.3, pp. 795–798.) As in column chromatography, the least polar substances advance faster than the most polar substances. A separation results from the differences in the rates at which the individual components of the mixture advance upward on the plate. When many substances are present in a mixture, each has its own characteristic solubility and adsorptivity properties, depending on the functional groups in its structure. In general, the stationary phase is strongly polar and strongly binds polar substances. The moving liquid phase is usually less polar than the adsorbent and most easily dissolves substances that are less polar or even nonpolar. Thus, the most polar substances travel slowly upward, or not at all, and nonpolar substances travel more rapidly if the solvent is sufficiently nonpolar.

When the thin-layer plate has been developed, it is removed from the developing tank and allowed to dry until it is free of solvent. If the mixture that was originally spotted on the plate was separated, there will be a vertical series of spots on the plate. Each spot corresponds to a separate component or compound from the original mixture. If the components of the mixture are colored substances, the various spots will be clearly visible after development. More often, however, the "spots" will not be visible because they correspond to colorless substances. If spots are not apparent, they can be made visible only if a **visualization method** is used. Often, spots can be seen when the thin-layer plate is held under ultraviolet light; the ultraviolet lamp is a common visualization method. Also common is the use of iodine vapor. The plates are placed in a chamber containing iodine crystals and left to stand for a short time. The iodine reacts with the various compounds adsorbed on the plate to give colored complexes that are clearly visible. Because iodine often changes the compounds by reaction, the components of the mixture cannot be recovered from the plate when the iodine method is used. (Other methods of visualization are discussed in Section 20.7.)

20.2 COMMERCIALLY PREPARED TLC PLATES

The most convenient type of TLC plate is prepared commercially and sold in a ready-to-use form. Many manufacturers supply glass plates precoated with a durable layer of silica gel or alumina. More conveniently, plates are also available that have either a flexible plastic backing or an aluminum backing. The most common types of commercial TLC plates are composed of plastic sheets that are coated with silica gel and polyacrylic acid, which serves as a binder. A fluorescent indicator may be mixed with the silica gel. Due to the presence of compounds in the sample, the indicator renders the spots visible under ultraviolet light (see Section 20.7). Although these plates are relatively expensive compared with plates prepared in the laboratory, they are far more convenient to use, and they provide more consistent results. The plates are manufactured quite uniformly. Because the plastic backing is flexible, an additional advantage is that the coating does not flake off the plates easily. The plastic sheets (usually 8 in. × 8 in. square) can also be cut with a pair of scissors or paper cutter to whatever size may be required.

If the package of commercially prepared TLC plates has been opened previously or if the plates have not been purchased recently, they should be dried before use. Dry the plates by placing them in an oven at 100°C for 30 minutes and store them in a desiccator until they are to be used.

20.3 PREPARATION OF THIN-LAYER SLIDES AND PLATES

Commercially prepared plates (Section 20.2) are the most convenient to use, and we recommend their use for most applications. If you must prepare your own slides or plates, this section provides directions for doing so. The two adsorbent materials used most often for TLC are alumina G (aluminum oxide) and silica gel G (silicic acid). The G designation stands for gypsum (calcium sulfate). Calcined gypsum $CaSO_4 \cdot \frac{1}{2}H_2O$ is better known as plaster of paris. When exposed to water or moisture, gypsum sets in a rigid mass $CaSO_4 \cdot 2H_2O$, which binds the adsorbent together and to the glass plates used as a backing support. In the adsorbents used for TLC, about 10–13% by weight of gypsum is added as a binder. The adsorbent materials are otherwise similar to those used in column chromatography; the adsorbents used in column chromatography have a larger particle size, however. The material for thin-layer work is a fine powder. The small particle size, along with the added gypsum, makes it impossible to use silica gel G or alumina G for column work. In a column, these adsorbents generally set so rigidly that solvent virtually stops flowing through the column.

For separations involving large amounts of material or for difficult separations, it may be necessary to use larger thin-layer plates. Under these circumstances, you may have to prepare your own plates. Plates with dimensions up to 200–250 cm^2 are common. With larger plates, it is desirable to have a somewhat durable coating, and a water slurry of the adsorbent should be used to prepare them. If silica gel is used, the slurry should be prepared in the ratio of about 1 g silica gel G to each 2 mL of water. The glass plate used for the thin-layer plate should be washed, dried, and placed on a sheet of newspaper. Place two strips of masking tape along two edges of the plate. Use more than one layer of masking tape if a thicker coating is desired on the plate. A slurry is prepared, shaken well, and poured along one of the untaped edges of the plate.

Caution: Avoid breathing silica dust or methylene chloride, prepare and use the slurry in a hood, and avoid getting methylene chloride or the slurry mixture on your skin. Perform the coating operation under a hood.

A heavy piece of glass rod, long enough to span the taped edges, is used to level and spread the slurry over the plate. While the rod is resting on the tape, it is pushed along the plate from the end at which the slurry was poured toward the opposite end of the plate. This is illustrated in Figure 20.1. After the slurry is spread, the masking tape strips are removed, and the plates are dried in a 110°C oven for about 1 hour. Plates of 200–250 cm^2 are easily prepared by this method. Larger plates present more difficulties. Many laboratories have a commercially manufactured spreading machine that makes the entire operation simpler.

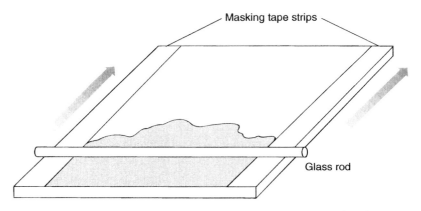

Masking tape strips

Glass rod

Figure 20.1   Preparing a large thin-layer chromatography plate.

20.4 SAMPLE APPLICATION: SPOTTING THE PLATES

A. Preparing a Micropipet

To apply the sample that is to be separated to the thin-layer plate, use a micropipet. A micropipet is easily made from a short length of thin-walled capillary tubing such as that used for melting-point determinations, but open at both ends. The capillary tubing is heated at its midpoint with a microburner and rotated until it is soft. When the tubing is soft, the heated portion of the tubing is drawn out until a constricted portion of tubing 4–5 cm long is formed. After cooling, the constricted portion of tubing is scored at its center with a file or scorer and broken. The two halves yield two capillary micropipets. Try to make a clean break without jagged or sharp edges. Figure 20.2 shows how to make such pipets.

B. Spotting the Plate

To apply a sample to the plate, begin by placing about 1 mg of a solid test substance or 1 drop of a liquid test substance in a small container such as a watch glass or a test tube. Dissolve the sample in a few drops of a volatile solvent. Acetone or methylene chloride is usually a suitable solvent. If a solution is to be tested, it can often be used directly (undiluted). The small capillary pipet, prepared as described, is filled by dipping the pulled end into the solution to be examined. Capillary action fills the pipet. Empty the pipet by touching it lightly to the thin-layer plate at a point about 1 cm from the bottom (Figure 20.3). The spot must be high enough so that it does not dissolve in the developing solvent. It is important to touch the plate very lightly and not to gouge a hole in the adsorbent. When the pipet touches the plate, the solution is transferred to the plate as a small spot. The pipet should be touched to the plate very briefly and then removed. If the pipet is held to the plate, its entire contents will be delivered to the plate. Only a small amount of material is needed. It is often helpful to blow gently on the plate as the sample is applied. This helps keep the spot small by evaporating the solvent before it can spread out on the plate. The smaller the spot formed, the better the separation obtainable. If needed, additional material can be applied to the plate by repeating the spotting procedure. You should repeat the procedure with several small amounts rather than apply one large amount. The solvent should be allowed to evaporate between ap-

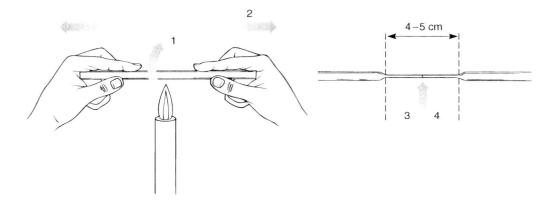

① Rotate in flame until soft.
② Remove from flame and pull.

③ Score lightly in center of pulled section.
④ Break in half to give two pipets.

Figure 20.2   The construction of two capillary micropipets.

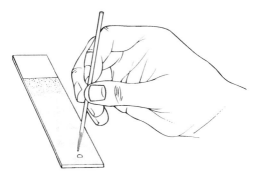

Figure 20.3   Spotting the thin-layer chromatography plate with a drawn capillary pipet.

plications. If the spot is not small (about 2 mm in diameter), a new plate should be prepared. The capillary pipet may be used several times if it is rinsed between uses. It is repeatedly dipped into a small portion of solvent to rinse it and touched to a paper towel to empty it.

As many as three different spots may be applied to a 1-inch-wide TLC plate. Each spot should be about 1 cm from the bottom of the plate, and all spots should be evenly spaced, with one spot in the center of the plate. Due to diffusion, spots often increase in diameter as the plate is developed. To keep spots containing different materials from merging and to avoid confusing the samples, do not place more than three spots on a single plate. Larger plates can accommodate many more samples.

20.5 DEVELOPING (RUNNING) TLC PLATES

A. Preparing a Development Chamber

A convenient development chamber for TLC plates can be made from a 4-oz wide-mouth jar. An alternative development chamber can be constructed from a beaker, using alu-

251

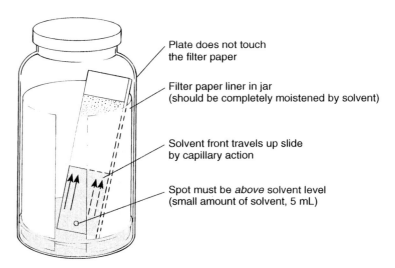

Plate does not touch
the filter paper

Filter paper liner in jar
(should be completely moistened by solvent)

Solvent front travels up slide
by capillary action

Spot must be *above* solvent level
(small amount of solvent, 5 mL)

Figure 20.4 A development chamber with a thin-layer chromatography plate undergoing development.

minum foil to cover the opening. The inside of the jar or beaker should be lined with a piece of filter paper, cut so that it does not quite extend around the inside of the jar. A small vertical opening (2–3 cm) should be left in the filter paper so the development can be observed. Before development, the filter paper inside the jar or beaker should be thoroughly moistened with the development solvent. The solvent-saturated liner helps to keep the chamber saturated with solvent vapors, thereby speeding the development. Once the liner is saturated, the level of solvent in the bottom of the development chamber is adjusted to a depth of about 5 mm, and the chamber is capped (or covered with aluminum foil) and set aside until it is to be used. A correctly prepared development chamber (with TLC plate in place) is shown in Figure 20.4.

B. Developing the TLC Plate

Once the spot has been applied to the thin-layer plate and the solvent has been selected (see Section 20.6), the plate is placed in the chamber for development. The plate must be placed in the chamber carefully so that no part of the plate touches the filter paper liner. In addition, the solvent level in the bottom of the chamber must not be above the spot that was applied to the plate, or the spotted material will dissolve in the pool of solvent instead of undergoing chromatography. Once the plate has been placed correctly, replace the cap on the developing chamber and wait for the solvent to advance up the plate by capillary action. This generally occurs rapidly, and you should watch carefully. As the solvent rises, the plate becomes visibly moist. When the solvent has advanced to within 5 mm of the end of the coated surface, the plate should be removed, and the position of the solvent front should be marked immediately by scoring the plate along the solvent line with a pencil. The solvent front must not be allowed to travel beyond the end of the coated surface. The plate should be removed before this happens. The solvent will not actually advance beyond the end of the plate, but spots allowed to stand on a completely moistened plate on which the solvent is not in motion expand by diffusion. Once the plate has dried, any visible spots should be outlined on the plate with a pencil. If no spots are apparent, a visualization method (Section 20.7) may be needed.

20.6 CHOOSING A SOLVENT FOR DEVELOPMENT

The development solvent used depends on the materials to be separated. You may have to try several solvents before a satisfactory separation is achieved. Because small TLC plates can be prepared and developed rapidly, an empirical choice is usually not hard to make. A solvent that causes all the spotted material to move with the solvent front is too polar. One that does not cause any of the material in the spot to move is not polar enough. As a guide to the relative polarity of solvents, consult Table 19.2 in Technique 19 (p. 801).

Methylene chloride and toluene are solvents of intermediate polarity and good choices for a wide variety of functional groups to be separated. For hydrocarbon materials, good first choices are hexane, petroleum ether (ligroin), or toluene. Hexane or petroleum ether with varying proportions of toluene or ether gives solvent mixtures of moderate polarity that are useful for many common functional groups. Polar materials may require ethyl acetate, acetone, or methanol.

A rapid way to determine a good solvent is to apply several sample spots to a single plate. The spots should be placed a minimum of 1 cm apart. A capillary pipet is filled with a solvent and gently touched to one of the spots. The solvent expands outward in a circle. The solvent front should be marked with a pencil. A different solvent is applied to each spot. As the solvents expand outward, the spots expand as concentric rings. From the appearance of the rings, you can judge approximately the suitability of the solvent. Several types of behavior experienced with this method of testing are shown in Figure 20.5.

20.7 VISUALIZATION METHODS

It is fortunate when the compounds separated by TLC are colored because the separation can be followed visually. More often than not, however, the compounds are colorless. In that case, some reagent or some method must be used to make the separated materials visible. Reagents that give rise to colored spots are called **visualization reagents.** Methods of viewing that make the spots apparent are **visualization methods.**

The most common method of visualization is by an ultraviolet (UV) lamp. Under UV

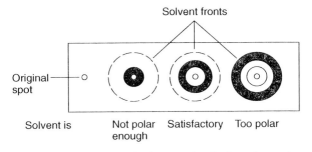

Figure 20.5 The concentric ring method of testing solvents.

light, compounds often look like bright spots on the plate. This often suggests the structure of the compound. Certain types of compounds shine very brightly under UV light because they fluoresce.

Plates can be purchased with a fluorescent indicator added to the adsorbent. A mixture of zinc and cadmium sulfides is often used. When treated in this way and held under UV light, the entire plate fluoresces. However, dark spots appear on the plate where the separated compounds are seen to quench this fluorescence.

Iodine is also used to visualize plates. Iodine reacts with many organic materials to form complexes that are either brown or yellow. In this visualization method, the developed and dried TLC plate is placed in a 4-oz wide-mouth, screw-cap jar along with a few crystals of iodine. The jar is capped and gently warmed on a steam bath or a hot plate at low heat. The jar fills with iodine vapors, and the spots begin to appear. When the spots are sufficiently intense, the plate is removed from the jar, and the spots are outlined with a pencil. The spots are not permanent. Their appearance results from the formation of complexes the iodine makes with the organic substances. As the iodine sublimes off the plate, the spots fade. Hence, they should be marked immediately. Nearly all compounds except saturated hydrocarbons and alkyl halides form complexes with iodine. The intensities of the spots do not accurately indicate the amount of material present, except in the crudest way.

In addition to the preceding methods, several chemical methods are available that either destroy or permanently alter the separated compounds through reaction. Many of these methods are specific for particular functional groups.

Alkyl halides can be visualized if a dilute solution of silver nitrate is sprayed on the plates. Silver halides are formed. These halides decompose if exposed to light, giving rise to dark spots (free silver) on the TLC plate.

Most organic functional groups can be made visible if they are charred with sulfuric acid. Concentrated sulfuric acid is sprayed on the plate, which is then heated in an oven at 110°C to complete the charring. Permanent spots are thus created.

Colored compounds can be prepared from colorless compounds by making derivatives before spotting them on the plate. An example of this is the preparation of 2,4-dinitrophenylhydrazones from aldehydes and ketones to produce yellow and orange compounds. You may also spray the 2,4-dinitrophenylhydrazine reagent on the plate after the ketones or aldehydes have separated. Red and yellow spots form where the compounds are located. Other examples of this method are the use of ferric chloride to visualize phenols and the use of bromocresol green to detect carboxylic acids. Chromium trioxide, potassium dichromate, and potassium permanganate can be used to visualize compounds that are easily oxidized. *p*-Dimethylaminobenzaldehyde easily detects amines. Ninhydrin reacts with amino acids to make them visible. Numerous other methods and reagents available from various supply outlets are specific for certain types of functional groups. These visualize only the class of compounds of interest.

20.8 PREPARATIVE PLATES

If you use large plates (Section 20.3), materials can be separated, and the separated components can be recovered individually from the plates. Plates used in this way are called **preparative plates.** For preparative plates, a thick layer of adsorbent is generally used. Instead of being applied as a spot or a series of spots, the mixture to be separated is applied as a line of material about 1 cm from the bottom of the plate. As the plate is developed, the separated materials form bands. After development, you can observe the separated bands, usually by UV light, and outline the zones in pencil. If the method of visualization is destructive, most of the plate is covered with paper to protect it, and the reagent is applied only at the extreme edge of the plate.

Once the zones have been identified, the adsorbent in those bands is scraped from the plate and extracted with solvent to remove the adsorbed material. Filtration removes the adsorbent, and evaporation of the solvent gives the recovered component from the mixture.

20.9 THE R_f VALUE

Thin-layer chromatography conditions include

1. Solvent system
2. Adsorbent
3. Thickness of the adsorbent layer
4. Relative amount of material spotted

Under an established set of such conditions, a given compound always travels a fixed distance relative to the distance the solvent front travels. This ratio of the distance the compound travels to the distance the solvent travels is called the R_f **value.** The symbol R_f stands for "retardation factor," or "ratio to front," and it is expressed as a decimal fraction:

$$R_f = \frac{\text{distance traveled by substance}}{\text{distance traveled by solvent front}}$$

When the conditions of measurement are completely specified, the R_f value is constant for any given compound, and it corresponds to a physical property of that compound.

The R_f value can be used to identify an unknown compound, but like any other identification based on a single piece of data, the R_f value is best confirmed with some additional data. Many compounds can have the same R_f value, just as many compounds have the same melting point.

It is not always possible, in measuring an R_f value, to duplicate exactly the conditions of measurement another researcher has used. Therefore, R_f values tend to be of more use to a single researcher in one laboratory than they are to researchers in different laboratories. The only exception to this occurs when two researchers use TLC plates from the same source, as in commercial plates, or know the exact details of how the plates were prepared. Nevertheless, the R_f value can be a useful guide. If exact values cannot be relied on, the relative values can provide another researcher with useful information about what to expect. Anyone using published R_f values will find it a good idea to check them by comparing them with standard substances whose identity and R_f values are known.

To calculate the R_f value for a given compound, measure the distance that the compound has traveled from the point at which it was originally spotted. For spots that are not too large, measure to the center of the migrated spot. For large spots, the measurement should be repeated on a new plate, using less material. For spots that show tailing, the measurement is made to the "center of gravity" of the spot. This first distance measurement is

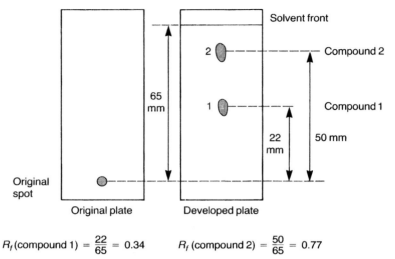

$$R_f(\text{compound 1}) = \frac{22}{65} = 0.34 \qquad R_f(\text{compound 2}) = \frac{50}{65} = 0.77$$

Figure 20.6 Sample calculation of R_f values.

then divided by the distance the solvent front has traveled from the same original spot. A sample calculation of the R_f values of two compounds is illustrated in Figure 20.6.

20.10 THIN-LAYER CHROMATOGRAPHY APPLIED IN ORGANIC CHEMISTRY

Thin-layer chromatography has several important uses in organic chemistry. It can be used in the following applications:

1. To establish that two compounds are identical
2. To determine the number of components in a mixture
3. To determine the appropriate solvent for a column-chromatographic separation
4. To monitor a column-chromatographic separation
5. To check the effectiveness of a separation achieved on a column, by crystallization or by extraction
6. To monitor the progress of a reaction

In all these applications, TLC has the advantage that only small amounts of material are necessary. Material is not wasted. With many of the visualization methods, less than a tenth of a microgram (10^{-7} g) of material can be detected. On the other hand, samples as large as a milligram may be used. With preparative plates that are large (about 9 inches on a side) and have a relatively thick coating of adsorbent ($> 500 \ \mu$m), it is often possible to separate from 0.2 g to 0.5 g of material at one time. The main disadvantage of TLC is that volatile materials cannot be used because they evaporate from the plates.

Thin-layer chromatography can establish that two compounds suspected to be identical are in fact identical. Simply spot both compounds side by side on a single plate and develop the plate. If both compounds travel the same distance on the plate (have the same R_f value), they are probably identical. If the spot positions are not the same, the compounds are definitely not identical. It is important to spot compounds *on the same plate*. This is especially important with slides and plates that you prepare yourself. Because plates vary widely from one sample to another, no two plates have exactly the same thickness of adsorbent. If you use commercial plates, this precaution is not necessary, although it is nevertheless strongly recommended.

Thin-layer chromatography can establish whether a sample is a single substance or a mixture. A single substance gives a single spot no matter which solvent is used to develop the plate. However, the number of components in a mixture can be established by trying various solvents on a mixture. A word of caution should be given. It may be difficult, in dealing with compounds of very similar properties, such as isomers, to find a solvent that will separate the mixture. Inability to achieve a separation is not absolute proof that a sample is a single pure substance. Many compounds can be separated only by *multiple developments* of the TLC slide with a fairly nonpolar solvent. In this method, you remove the plate after the first development and allow it to dry. After being dried, it is placed in the chamber again and developed once more. This effectively doubles the length of the slide. At times, several developments may be necessary.

When a mixture is to be separated, you can use TLC to choose the best solvent to separate it if column chromatography is contemplated. You can try various solvents on a plate coated with the same adsorbent as will be used in the column. The solvent that resolves the components best will probably work well on the column. These small-scale experiments are quick, use very little material, and save time that would be wasted by attempting to separate the entire mixture on the column. Similarly, TLC plates can *monitor* a column. A hypothetical situation is shown in Figure 20.7. A solvent was found that would separate the mixture into four components (A–D). A column was run using this solvent, and 11 fractions of 15 mL each were collected. Thin-layer analysis of the various fractions showed that fractions 1–3 contained component A; fractions 4–7, component B; fractions 8–9, component C; and fractions 10–11, component D. A small amount of cross-contamination was observed in fractions 3, 4, 7, and 9.

In another TLC example, a researcher found a product from a reaction to be a mix-

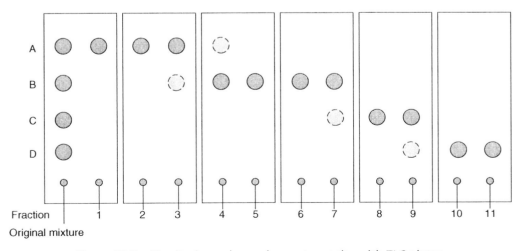

Figure 20.7 Monitoring column chromatography with TLC plates.

257

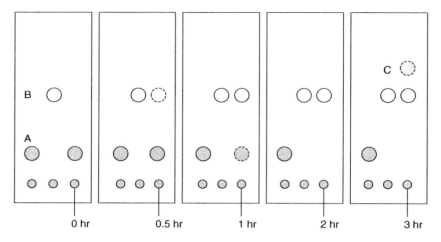

Figure 20.8 Monitoring a reaction with TLC plates.

ture. It gave two spots, A and B, on a TLC plate. After the product was crystallized, the crystals were found by TLC to be pure A, whereas the mother liquor was found to have a mixture of A and B. The crystallization was judged to have purified A satisfactorily.

Finally, it is often possible to monitor the progress of a reaction by TLC. At various points during a reaction, samples of the reaction mixture are taken and subjected to TLC analysis. An example is given in Figure 20.8. In this case, the desired reaction was the conversion of A to B. At the beginning of the reaction (0 hour), a TLC plate was prepared that was spotted with pure A, pure B, and the reaction mixture. Similar plates were prepared at 0.5, 1, 2, and 3 hours after the start of the reaction. The plates showed that the reaction was complete in 2 hours. When the reaction was run longer than 2 hours, a new compound, side product C, began to appear. Thus, the optimum reaction time was judged to be 2 hours.

20.11 PAPER CHROMATOGRAPHY

Paper chromatography is often considered to be related to thin-layer chromatography. The experimental techniques are somewhat like those of TLC, but the principles are more closely related to those of extraction. Paper chromatography is actually a liquid–liquid partitioning technique rather than a solid–liquid technique. For paper chromatography, a spot is placed near the bottom of a piece of high-grade filter paper (Whatman No. 1 is often used). Then the paper is placed in a developing chamber. The development solvent ascends the paper by capillary action and moves the components of the spotted mixture upward at differing rates. Although paper consists mainly of pure cellulose, the cellulose itself does not function as the stationary phase. Rather, the cellulose absorbs water from the atmosphere, especially from an atmosphere saturated with water vapor. Cellulose can absorb up to about 22% of water. It is this water adsorbed on the cellulose that functions as the stationary phase. To ensure that the cellulose is kept saturated with water, many development solvents used in paper chromatography contain water as a component. As the solvent ascends the paper, the compounds are partitioned between the stationary water phase and the moving solvent. Because the water phase is stationary, the components in a mixture that are most highly water soluble, or those that have the greatest hydrogen-bonding capacity, are the ones that are held back and move most slowly. Paper chromatography applies mostly to highly polar compounds or to compounds that are polyfunctional. The most common use of paper chromatography is for sugars, amino acids, and natural pigments. Because filter paper is manufactured consistently, R_f values can often be relied on in paper chromatographic work. However, R_f values are customarily measured from the leading edge (top) of the spot—not from its center, as is customary in TLC.

PROBLEMS

1. A student spots an unknown sample on a TLC plate and develops it in dichloromethane solvent. Only one spot, for which the R_f value is 0.95, is observed. Does this indicate that the unknown material is a pure compound? What can be done to verify the purity of the sample using thin-layer chromatography?

2. You and another student were each given an unknown compound. Both samples contained colorless material. You each used the same brand of commercially prepared TLC plate and developed the plates using the same solvent. Each of you obtained a single spot of $R_f = 0.75$. Were the two samples necessarily the same substances? How could you prove unambiguously that they were identical using TLC?

3. Each of the solvents given should effectively separate one of the following mixtures by TLC. Match the appropriate solvent with the mixture that you would expect to separate well with that solvent. Select your solvent from the following: hexane, methylene chloride, or acetone. You may need to look up the structures of the solvents and compounds in a handbook.

    a. 2-Phenylethanol and acetophenone

    b. Bromobenzene and *p*-xylene

    c. Benzoic acid, 2,4-dinitrobenzoic acid, and 2,4,6-trinitrobenzoic acid

4. Consider a sample that is a mixture composed of biphenyl, benzoic acid, and benzyl alcohol. The sample is spotted on a TLC plate and developed in a dichloromethane–cyclohexane solvent mixture. Predict the relative R_f values for the three components in the sample. (*Hint:* See Table 19.3.)

5. Consider the following errors that could be made when running TLC. Indicate what should be done to correct the error.

    a. A two-component mixture containing 1-octene and 1,4-dimethylbenzene gave only one spot with an R_f value of 0.95. The solvent used was acetone.

    b. A two-component mixture containing a dicarboxylic acid and a tricarboxylic acid gave only one spot with an R_f value of 0.05. The solvent used was hexane.

    c. When a TLC plate was developed, the solvent front ran off the top of the plate.

6. Calculate the R_f value of a spot that travels 5.7 cm, with a solvent front that travels 13 cm.

7. A student spots an unknown sample on a TLC plate and develops it in pentane solvent. Only one spot, for which the R_f value is 0.05, is observed. Is the unknown material a pure compound? What can be done to verify the purity of the sample using thin-layer chromatography?

8. A colorless unknown substance is spotted on a TLC plate and developed in the correct solvent. The spots do not appear when visualization with a UV lamp or iodine vapors is attempted. What could you do to visualize the spots if the compound is the following?

    a. An alkyl halide

    b. A ketone

    c. An amino acid

    d. A sugar

T E C H N I Q U E   2 1

High-Performance Liquid Chromatography (HPLC)

The separation that can be achieved is greater if the column packing used in column chromatography is made denser by using an adsorbent that has a smaller particle size. The solute molecules encounter a much larger surface area on which they can be adsorbed as they pass through the column packing. At the same time, the solvent spaces between the particles are reduced in size. As a result of this tight packing, equilibrium between the liquid and solid phases can be established very rapidly with a fairly short column, and the degree of separation is markedly improved. The disadvantage of making the column packing denser is that the solvent flow rate becomes very slow or even stops. Gravity is not strong enough to pull the solvent through a tightly packed column.

A recently developed technique can be applied to obtain much better separations with tightly packed columns. A pump forces the solvent through the column packing. As a result, solvent flow rate is increased, and the advantage of better separation is retained. This technique, called **high-performance liquid chromatography (HPLC),** is becoming widely applied to problems in which separations by ordinary column chromatography are unsatisfactory. Because the pump often provides pressures in excess of 1000 pounds per square inch (psi), this method is also known as **high-pressure liquid chromatography.** High pressures are not required, however, and satisfactory separations can be achieved with pressures as low as 100 psi.

The basic design of an HPLC instrument is shown in Figure 21.1. The instrument contains the following essential components:

1. Solvent reservoir
2. Solvent filter and degasser
3. Pump
4. Pressure gauge
5. Sample injection system
6. Column
7. Detector
8. Amplifier and electronic controls
9. Chart recorder

There may be other variations on this simple design. Some instruments have heated ovens to maintain the column at a specified temperature, fraction collectors, and microprocessor-controlled data-handling systems. Additional filters for the solvent and sample may also be included. You may find it interesting to compare this schematic diagram with Figure 22.2 in Technique 22 (p. 839) for a gas chromatography instrument. Many of the essential components are common to both types of instruments.

21.1 ADSORBENTS AND COLUMNS

The most important factor to consider when choosing a set of experimental conditions is the nature of the material packed into the column. You must also consider the size of

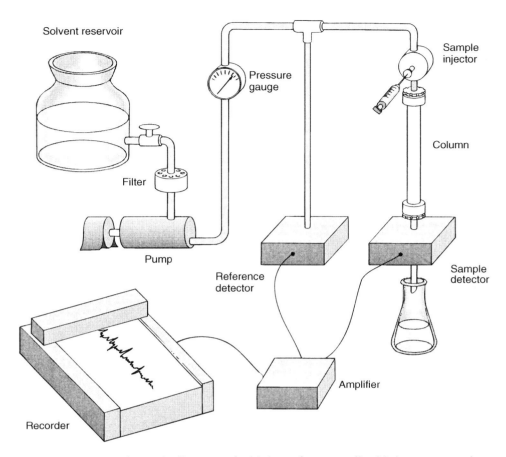

Figure 21.1   A schematic diagram of a high-performance liquid chromatograph.

the column that will be selected. The chromatography column is generally packed with silica or alumina adsorbents. However, the adsorbents used for HPLC have a much smaller particle size than those used in column chromatography. Typically, particle size ranges from 5 μm to 20 μm in diameter for HPLC and on the order of 100 μm for column chromatography.

The adsorbent is packed into a column that can withstand the elevated pressures typical of this type of experiment. Generally, the column is constructed of stainless steel, although some columns that are constructed of a rigid polymeric material ("PEEK"—Poly Ether Ether Ketone) are available commercially. A strong column is required to withstand the high pressures that may be used. The columns are fitted with stainless steel connectors, which ensure a pressure-tight fit between the column and the tubing that connects the column to the other components of the instrument.

Columns that fulfill a large number of specialized purposes are available. Here, we consider only the four most important types of columns:

1. Normal-phase chromatography
2. Reversed-phase chromatography

3. Ion-exchange chromatography

4. Size-exclusion chromatography

In most types of chromatography, the adsorbent is more polar than the mobile phase. For example, the solid packing material, which may be either silica or alumina, has a stronger affinity for polar molecules than does the solvent. As a result, the molecules in the sample adhere strongly to the solid phase, and their progress down the column is much slower than the rate at which solvent moves through the column. The time required for a substance to move through the column can be altered by changing the polarity of the solvent. In general, as the solvent becomes more polar, the faster substances move through the column. This type of behavior is known as **normal-phase chromatography.** In HPLC, you inject a sample onto a normal-phase column and elute it by varying the polarity of the solvent, much as you do with ordinary column chromatography. Disadvantages of normal-phase chromatography are that retention times tend to be long and bands have a tendency to "tail."

These disadvantages can be ameliorated by selecting a column in which the solid support is *less polar* than the moving solvent phase. This type of chromatography is known as **reversed-phase chromatography.** In this type of chromatography, the silica column packing is treated with alkylating agents. As a result, nonpolar alkyl groups are bonded to the silica surface, making the adsorbent nonpolar. The alkylating agents that are used most commonly can attach methyl ($—CH_3$), octyl ($—C_8H_{17}$), or octadecyl ($—C_{18}H_{37}$) groups to the silica surface. The latter variation, in which an 18-carbon chain is attached to the silica, is the most popular. This type of column is known as a **C_{18} column.** The bonded alkyl groups have an effect similar to what would be produced by an extremely thin organic solvent layer coating the surface of the silica particles. The interactions that take place between the substances dissolved in the solvent and the stationary phase thus become more like those observed in a liquid–liquid extraction. The solute particles distribute themselves between the two "solvents"—that is, between the moving solvent and the organic coating on the silica. The longer the chains of the alkyl groups that are bonded to the silica, the more effective the alkyl groups are as they interact with solute molecules.

Reversed-phase chromatography is widely used because the rate at which solute molecules exchange between moving phase and stationary phase is very rapid, which means that substances pass through the column relatively quickly. Furthermore, problems arising from the "tailing" of peaks are reduced. A disadvantage of this type of column, however, is that the chemically bonded solid phases tend to decompose. The organic groups are slowly hydrolyzed from the surface of the silica, which leaves a normal silica surface exposed. Thus, the chromatographic process that takes place on the column slowly shifts from a reversed-phase to a normal-phase separation mechanism.

Another type of solid support that is sometimes used in reversed-phase chromatography is organic polymer beads. These beads present a surface to the moving phase that is largely organic in nature.

For solutions of ions, select a column that is packed with an ion-exchange resin. This type of chromatography is known as **ion-exchange chromatography.** The ion-exchange resin that is chosen can be either an anion-exchange resin or a cation-exchange resin, depending upon the nature of the sample being examined.

A fourth type of column is known as a **size-exclusion column** or a **gel-filtration col-**

umn. The interaction that takes place on this type of column is similar to that described in Technique 19, Section 19.16, p. 815.

21.2 COLUMN DIMENSIONS

The dimensions of the column that you use depend upon the application. For analytical applications, a typical column is constructed of tubing that has an inside diameter of between 4 mm and 5 mm, although analytical columns with inside diameters of 1 mm or 2 mm are also available. A typical analytical column has a length of about 7.5 cm to 30 cm. This type of column is suitable for the separation of a 0.1-mg to 5-mg sample. With columns of smaller diameter, it is possible to perform an analysis with samples smaller than 1 *micro*gram.

High-performance liquid chromatography is an excellent analytical technique, but the separated compounds may also be isolated. The technique can be used for preparative experiments. Just as in column chromatography, the fractions can be collected into individual receiving containers as they pass through the column. The solvents can be evaporated from these fractions, allowing you to isolate separated components of the original mixture. Samples that range in size from 5 mg to 100 mg can be separated on a semipreparative, or **semiprep column.** The dimensions of a semiprep column are typically 8 mm inside diameter and 10 cm in length. A semiprep column is a practical choice when you wish to use the same column for both analytical and preparative separations. A semiprep column is small enough to provide reasonable sensitivity in analyses, but it is also capable of handling moderate-sized samples when you need to isolate the components of a mixture. Even larger samples can be separated using a **preparative column.** This type of column is useful when you wish to collect the components of a mixture and then use the pure samples for additional study (for example, for a subsequent chemical reaction or for spectroscopic analysis). A preparative column may be as large as 20 mm inside diameter and 30 cm in length. A preparative column can handle samples as large as 1 g per injection.

21.3 SOLVENTS

The choice of solvent used for an HPLC separation depends on the type of chromatographic process selected. For a normal-phase separation, the solvent is selected based on its polarity. The criteria described in Technique 19, Section 19.4B, p. 801, are used. A solvent of very low polarity might be pentane, petroleum ether, hexane, or carbon tetrachloride; a solvent of very high polarity might be water, acetic acid, methanol, or 1-propanol.

For a reversed-phase experiment, a less polar solvent causes solutes to migrate *faster.* For example, for a mixed methanol–water solvent, as the percentage of methanol in the solvent increases (solvent becomes less polar), the time required to elute the components of a mixture from a column decreases. The behavior of solvents as eluents in a reversed-phase chromatography would be the reverse of the order shown in Table 19.2 on p. 801.

If a single solvent (or solvent mixture) is used for the entire separation, the chromatogram is said to be **isochratic.** Special electronic devices are available with HPLC instruments that allow you to program changes in the solvent composition from the beginning to the end of the chromatography. These are called **gradient elution systems.** With gradient elution, the time required for a separation may be shortened considerably.

The need for pure solvents is especially acute with HPLC. The narrow bore of the column and the very small particle size of the column packing require that solvents be particularly pure and free of insoluble residue. In most cases, the solvents must be filtered through ultrafine filters and **degassed** (have dissolved gases removed) before they can be used.

The solvent gradient is chosen so that the eluting power of the solvent increases over the duration of the experiment. The result is that components of the mixture that tend to move very slowly through the column are caused to move faster as the eluting power of the solvent gradually increases. The instrument can be programmed to change the composition of the solvent following a linear gradient or a nonlinear gradient, depending on the specific requirements of the separation.

21.4 DETECTORS

A flow-through **detector** must be provided to determine when a substance has passed through the column. In most applications, the detector detects either the change in index of refraction of the liquid as its composition changes or the presence of solute by its absorption of ultraviolet or visible light. The signal generated by the detector is amplified and treated electronically in a manner similar to that found in gas chromatography (Technique 22, Section 22.6, p. 843).

A detector that responds to changes in the index of refraction of the solution may be considered the most universal of the HPLC detectors. The refractive index of the liquid passing through the detector changes slightly, but significantly, as the liquid changes from pure solvent to a liquid where the solvent contains some type of organic solute. This change in refractive index can be detected and compared to the refractive index of pure solvent. The difference in index values is then recorded as a peak on a chart. A disadvantage of this type of detector is that it must respond to very small changes in refractive index. As a result, the detector tends to be unstable and difficult to balance.

When the components of the mixture have some type of absorption in the ultraviolet or visible regions of the spectrum, a detector that is adjusted to detect absorption at a particular wavelength of light can be used. This type of detector is much more stable, and the readings tend to be more reliable. Unfortunately, many organic compounds do not absorb ultraviolet light, and this type of detector cannot be used.

21.5 PRESENTATION OF DATA

The data produced by an HPLC instrument appear in the form of a chart, where detector response is the vertical axis and time is represented on the horizontal axis. These are recorded on a continuously moving strip of chart paper, although they may also be observed in graphic form on a computer display. In virtually all respects, the form of the data is identical to that produced by a gas chromatograph; in fact, in many cases, the data-handling system for the two types of instruments is essentially identical. To understand how to analyze the data from an HPLC instrument, read Sections 22.11 and 22.12 in Technique 22.

REFERENCES

Bidlingmeyer, B. A. *Practical HPLC Methodology and Applications,* New York: Wiley, 1992.

Katz, E., editor. *Handbook of HPLC.* Volume 78 in Chromatographic Science Series, New York: M. Dekker, 1998.

Lough, W. J., and Wainer, I. W., editors. *High Performance Liquid Chromatography: Fundamental Principles and Practice.* London and New York: Blackie Academic & Professional, 1996.

Rubinson, K. A. "Liquid Chromatography." Chap. 14 in *Chemical Analysis.* Boston: Little, Brown and Co., 1987.

PROBLEMS

1. For a mixture of biphenyl, benzoic acid, and benzyl alcohol, predict the order of elution and describe any differences that you would expect for a normal-phase HPLC experiment (in hexane solvent) compared with a reversed-phase experiment (in tetrahydrofuran–water solvent).

2. How would the gradient elution program differ between normal-phase and reversed-phase chromatography?

TECHNIQUE 22

Gas Chromatography

Gas chromatography is one of the most useful instrumental tools for separating and analyzing organic compounds that can be vaporized without decomposition. Common uses include testing the purity of a substance and separating the components of a mixture. The relative amounts of the components in a mixture may also be determined. In some cases, gas chromatography can be used to identify a compound. In microscale work, it can also be used as a preparative method to isolate pure compounds from a small amount of a mixture.

Gas chromatography resembles column chromatography in principle, but it differs in three respects. First, the partitioning processes for the compounds to be separated are carried out between a **moving gas phase** and a **stationary liquid phase.** (Recall that in column chromatography, the moving phase is a liquid, and the stationary phase is a solid adsorbent.) Second, the temperature of the gas system can be controlled, because the column is contained in an insulated oven. And third, the concentration of any given compound in the gas phase is a function of its vapor pressure only. Because gas chromatography separates the components of a mixture primarily on the basis of their vapor pressures (or boiling points), this technique is also similar in principle to fractional distillation. In microscale work, it is sometimes used to separate and isolate compounds from a mixture; fractional distillation would normally be used with larger amounts of material.

Gas chromatography (GC) is also known as vapor-phase chromatography (VPC) and as gas–liquid partition chromatography (GLPC). All three names, as well as their indicated abbreviations, are often found in the literature of organic chemistry. In reference to the technique, the last term, GLPC, is the most strictly correct and is preferred by most authors.

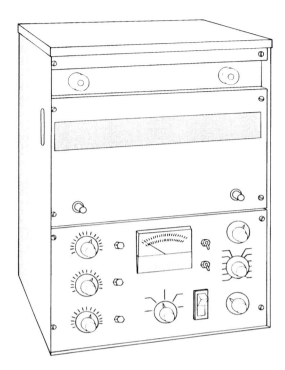

Figure 22.1 A gas chromatograph.

22.1 THE GAS CHROMATOGRAPH

The apparatus used to carry out a gas–liquid chromatographic separation is generally called a **gas chromatograph.** A typical student-model gas chromatograph, the GOW-MAC model 69-350, is illustrated in Figure 22.1. A schematic block diagram of a basic gas chromatograph is shown in Figure 22.2. The basic elements of the apparatus are apparent. The sample is injected into the chromatograph, and it is immediately vaporized in a heated injection chamber and introduced into a moving stream of gas, called the **carrier gas.** The vaporized sample is then swept into a column filled with particles coated with a liquid adsorbent. The column is contained in a temperature-controlled oven. As the sample passes through the column, it is subjected to many gas–liquid partitioning processes, and the components are separated. As each component leaves the column, its presence is detected by an electrical detector that generates a signal that is recorded on a strip chart recorder.

Many modern instruments are also equipped with a microprocessor, which can be programmed to change parameters, such as the temperature of the oven, while a mixture is being separated on a column. With this capability, it is possible to optimize the separation of components and to complete a run in a relatively short time.

22.2 THE COLUMN

The heart of the gas chromatograph is the packed column. This column is usually made of copper or stainless steel tubing, but sometimes glass is used. The most common di-

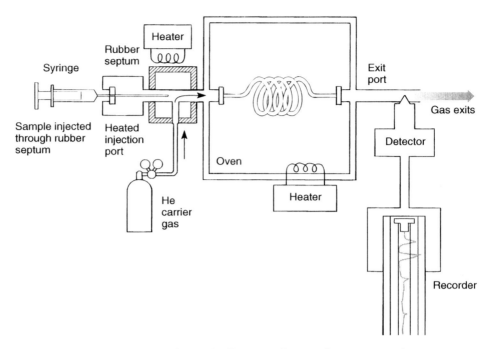

Figure 22.2 A schematic diagram of a gas chromatograph.

ameters of tubing are ⅛ inch (3 mm) and ¼ inch (6 mm). To construct a column, cut a piece of tubing to the desired length and attach the proper fittings on each of the two ends to connect to the apparatus. The most common length is 4–12 feet, but some columns may be up to 50 feet in length.

The tubing (column) is then packed with the **stationary phase.** The material chosen for the stationary phase is usually a liquid, a wax, or a low-melting solid. This material should be relatively nonvolatile; that is, it should have a low vapor pressure and a high boiling point. Liquids commonly used are high-boiling hydrocarbons, silicone oils, waxes, and polymeric esters, ethers, and amides. Some typical substances are listed in Table 22.1.

The liquid phase is usually coated onto a **support material.** A common support material is crushed firebrick. Many methods exist for coating the high-boiling liquid phase onto the support particles. The easiest is to dissolve the liquid (or low-melting wax or solid) in a volatile solvent such as methylene chloride (bp 40°C). The firebrick (or other support) is added to this solution, which is then slowly evaporated (rotary evaporator) so as to leave each particle of support material evenly coated. Other support materials are listed in Table 22.2.

In the final step, the liquid-phase-coated support material is packed into the tubing as evenly as possible. The tubing is bent or coiled so that it fits into the oven of the gas chromatograph with its two ends connected to the gas entrance and exit ports.

Selection of a liquid phase usually revolves about two factors. First, most liquid phases have an upper temperature limit above which they cannot be used. Above the specified limit of temperature, the liquid phase itself will begin to "bleed" off the column. Second, the materials to be separated must be considered. For polar samples, it is usually best to use a polar liquid phase; for nonpolar samples, a nonpolar liquid phase is indicated. The liquid phase performs best when the substances to be separated *dissolve* in it.

TABLE 22.1 Typical Liquid Phases

	Type	Composition	Maximum Temperature (°C)	Typical Use
Apiezons (L, M, N, etc.)	Hydrocarbon greases (varying MW)	Hydrocarbon mixtures	250–300	Hydrocarbons
SE-30	Methyl silicone rubber	Like silicone oil, but cross-linked	350	General applications
DC-200	Silicone oil (R = CH$_3$)	$R_3Si-O-[Si-O]_n-SiR_3$ (with R, R groups)	225	Aldehydes, ketones, halocarbons
DC-710	Silicone oil (R = CH$_3$) (R′ = C$_6$H$_5$)	$[R'-Si-O-R]_n$	300	General applications
Carbowaxes (400–20M)	Polyethylene glycols (varying chain lengths)	Polyether $HO-(CH_2CH_2-O)n-CH_2CH_2OH$	Up to 250	Alcohols, ethers, halocarbons
DEGS	Diethylene glycol succinate	Polyester $\left[CH_2CH_2-O-C(=O)-(CH_2)_2-C(=O)-O\right]_n$	200	General applications

Increasing polarity →

269

TABLE 22.2 Typical Solid Supports

Crushed firebrick	Chromosorb T
Nylon beads	(Teflon beads)
Glass beads	Chromosorb P
Silica	(pink diatomaceous earth,
Alumina	highly absorptive, pH 6–7)
Charcoal	Chromosorb W
Molecular sieves	(white diatomaceous earth,
	medium absorptivity, pH 8–10)
	Chromosorb G
	(like the above,
	low absorptivity, pH 8.5)

Most researchers today buy packed columns from commercial sources rather than pack their own. A wide variety of types and lengths is available.

Alternatives to packed columns are Golay or glass capillary columns of diameters 0.1–0.2 mm. With these columns, no solid support is required, and the liquid is coated directly on the inner walls of the tubing. Liquid phases commonly used in glass capillary columns are similar in composition to those used in packed columns. They include DB-1 (similar to SE-30), DB-17 (similar to DC-710), and DB-WAX (similar to Carbowax 20M). The length of a capillary column is usually very long, typically 50–100 feet. Because of the length and small diameter, there is increased interaction between the sample and the stationary phase. Gas chromatographs equipped with these small-diameter columns are able to separate components more effectively than instruments using larger packed columns.

22.3 PRINCIPLES OF SEPARATION

After a column is selected, packed, and installed, the **carrier gas** (usually helium, argon, or nitrogen) is allowed to flow through the column supporting the liquid phase. The mixture of compounds to be separated is introduced into the carrier gas stream, where its components are equilibrated (or partitioned) between the moving gas phase and the stationary liquid phase (Figure 22.3). The latter is held stationary because it is adsorbed onto the surfaces of the support material.

The sample is introduced into the gas chromatograph by a microliter syringe. It is injected as a liquid or as a solution through a rubber septum into a heated chamber, called the **injection port,** where it is vaporized and mixed with the carrier gas. As this mixture reaches the column, which is heated in a controlled oven, it begins to equilibrate between the liquid and gas phases. The length of time required for a sample to move through the column is a function of how much time the sample spends in the vapor phase and how much time it spends in the liquid phase. The more time the sample spends in the vapor phase, the faster it gets to the end of the column. In most separations, the components of a sample have similar solubilities in the liquid phase. Therefore, the time the different compounds spend in the vapor phase is primarily a function of the vapor pressure of the compounds, and the

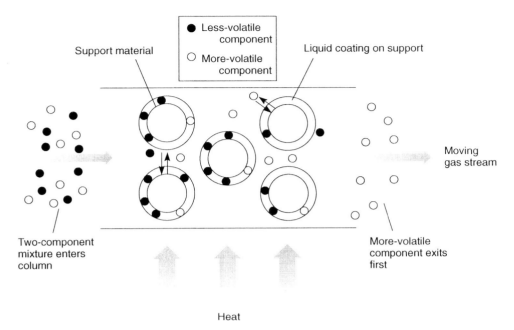

Less-volatile component

More-volatile component

Support material

Liquid coating on support

Moving gas stream

Two-component mixture enters column

More-volatile component exits first

Heat

Figure 22.3 The separation process.

more-volatile component arrives at the end of the column first, as illustrated in Figure 22.3. When the correct temperature of the oven and the correct liquid phase have been selected, the compounds in the injected mixture travel through the column at different rates and are separated.

22.4 FACTORS AFFECTING SEPARATION

Several factors determine the rate at which a given compound travels through a gas chromatograph. First, compounds with low boiling points will generally travel through the gas chromatograph faster than compounds with higher boiling points. The reason is that the column is heated, and low-boiling compounds always have higher vapor pressures than higher-boiling compounds. In general, therefore, for compounds with the same functional group, the higher the molecular weight, the longer the retention time. For most molecules, the boiling point increases as the molecular weight increases. If the column is heated to a temperature that is too high, however, the entire mixture to be separated is flushed through the column at the same rate as the carrier gas, and no equilibration takes place with the liquid phase. On the other hand, at too low a temperature, the mixture dissolves in the liquid phase and never revaporizes. Thus, it is retained on the column.

The second factor is the rate of flow of the carrier gas. The carrier gas must not move so rapidly that molecules of the sample in the vapor phase cannot equilibrate with those dissolved in the liquid phase. This may result in poor separation between components in the injected mixture. If the rate of flow is too slow, however, the bands broaden significantly, leading to poor resolution (see Section 22.8).

271

The third factor is the choice of liquid phase used in the column. The molecular weights, functional groups, and polarities of the component molecules in the mixture to be separated must be considered when a liquid phase is being chosen. A different type of material is generally used for hydrocarbons, for instance, than for esters. The materials to be separated should dissolve in the liquid. The useful temperature limit of the liquid phase selected must also be considered.

The fourth factor is the length of the column. Compounds that resemble one another closely, in general, require longer columns than dissimilar compounds. Many kinds of isomeric mixtures fit into the "difficult" category. The components of isomeric mixtures are so much alike that they travel through the column at very similar rates. You need a longer column, therefore, to take advantage of any differences that may exist.

22.5 ADVANTAGES OF GAS CHROMATOGRAPHY

All factors that have been mentioned must be adjusted by the chemist for any mixture to be separated. Considerable preliminary investigation is often required before a mixture can be separated successfully into its components by gas chromatography. Nevertheless, the advantages of the technique are many.

First, many mixtures can be separated by this technique when no other method is adequate. Second, as little as $1-10$ μL (1 $\mu L = 10^{-6}L$) of a mixture can be separated by this technique. This advantage is particularly important when working at the microscale level. Third, when gas chromatography is coupled with an electronic recording device (see following discussion), the amount of each component present in the separated mixture can be estimated quantitatively.

The range of compounds that can be separated by gas chromatography extends from gases, such as oxygen (bp $-183°C$) and nitrogen (bp $-196°C$), to organic compounds with boiling points over $400°C$. The only requirement for the compounds to be separated is that they have an appreciable vapor pressure at a temperature at which they can be separated and that they be thermally stable at this temperature.

22.6 MONITORING THE COLUMN (THE DETECTOR)

To follow the separation of the mixture injected into the gas chromatograph, it is necessary to use an electrical device called a **detector.** Two types of detectors in common use are the **thermal conductivity detector (TCD)** and the **flame-ionization detector (FID).**

The thermal conductivity detector is simply a hot wire placed in the gas stream at the column exit. The wire is heated by constant electrical voltage. When a steady stream of carrier gas passes over this wire, the rate at which it loses heat and its electrical conductance have constant values. When the composition of the vapor stream changes, the rate of heat flow from the wire, and hence its resistance, changes. Helium, which has a thermal conductivity higher than that of most organic substances, is a common carrier gas. Thus, when a substance elutes in the vapor stream, the thermal conductivity of the moving gases will be lower than with helium alone. The wire then heats up, and its resistance decreases.

A typical TCD operates by difference. Two detectors are used: one exposed to the ac-

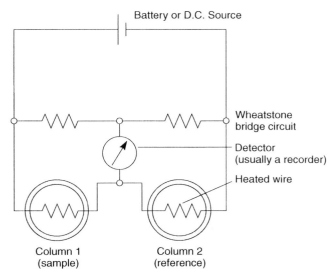

Figure 22.4 A typical thermal conductivity detector.

tual effluent gas and the other exposed to a reference flow of carrier gas only. To achieve this situation, a portion of the carrier gas stream is diverted before it enters the injection port. The diverted gas is routed through a reference column into which no sample has been admitted. The detectors mounted in the sample and reference columns are arranged to form the arms of a Wheatstone bridge circuit, as shown in Figure 22.4. As long as the carrier gas alone flows over both detectors, the circuit is in balance. However, when a sample elutes from the sample column, the bridge circuit becomes unbalanced, creating an electrical signal. This signal can be amplified and used to activate a strip chart recorder. The recorder is an instrument that plots, by means of a moving pen, the unbalanced bridge current versus time on a continuously moving roll of chart paper. This record of detector response (current) versus time is called a **chromatogram.** A typical gas chromatogram is illustrated in Figure 22.5. Deflections of the pen are called **peaks.**

When a sample is injected, some air (CO_2, H_2O, N_2, and O_2) is introduced along with the sample. The air travels through the column almost as rapidly as the carrier gas; as air passes the detector, it causes a small pen response, thereby giving a peak, called the **air peak.** At later times (t_1, t_2, t_3), the components also give rise to peaks on the chromatogram as they pass out of the column and past the detector.

In a flame-ionization detector, the effluent from the column is directed into a flame produced by the combustion of hydrogen, as illustrated in Figure 22.6. As organic compounds burn in the flame, ion fragments are produced and collect on the ring above the flame. The resulting electrical signal is amplified and sent to a recorder in a manner similar to that for a TCD, except that an FID does not produce an air peak. The main advantage of the FID is that it is more sensitive and can be used to analyze smaller quantities of sample. Also, because an FID does not respond to water, a gas chromatograph with this detector can be used to analyze aqueous solutions. Two disadvantages are that it is more difficult to operate and the detection process destroys the sample. Therefore, an FID gas chromatograph cannot be used to do preparative work.

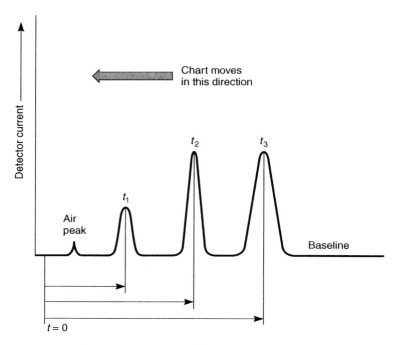

Figure 22.5 A typical gas chromatograph.

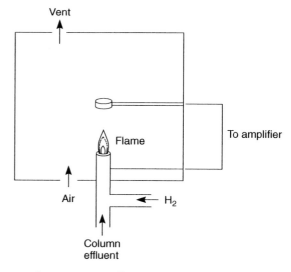

Figure 22.6 A flame-ionization detector.

22.7 RETENTION TIME

The period following injection that is required for a compound to pass through the column is called the **retention time** of that compound. For a given set of constant conditions (flow rate of carrier gas, column temperature, column length, liquid phase, injection port temperature, carrier), the retention time of any compound is always constant (much like the

R_f value in thin-layer chromatography, as described in Technique 20, Section 20.9, p. 827). The retention time is measured from the time of injection to the time of maximum pen deflection (detector current) for the component being observed. This value, when obtained under controlled conditions, can identify a compound by a direct comparison of it with values for known compounds determined under the same conditions. For easier measurement of retention times, most strip chart recorders are adjusted to move the paper at a rate that corresponds to time divisions calibrated on the chart paper. The retention times (t_1, t_2, t_3) are indicated in Figure 22.5 for the three peaks illustrated.

Most modern gas chromatographs are attached to a "data station," which uses a computer or a microprocessor to process the data. With these instruments, the chart often does not have divisions. Instead, the computer prints the retention time, usually to the nearest 0.01 minute, above each peak. A more complete discussion of the results obtained from a modern data station and how these data are treated may be found in Section 22.12.

22.8 POOR RESOLUTION AND TAILING

The peaks in Figure 22.5 are well **resolved.** That is, the peaks are separated from one another, and between each pair of adjacent peaks the tracing returns to the baseline. In Figure 22.7, the peaks overlap, and the resolution is not good. Poor resolution is often caused by using too much sample; by a column that is too short, has too high a temperature, or has too large a diameter; by a liquid phase that does not discriminate well between the two components; or, in short, by almost any wrongly adjusted parameter. When peaks are poorly resolved, it is more difficult to determine the relative amount of each component. Methods for determining the relative percentages of each component are given in Section 22.11.

Another desirable feature illustrated by the chromatogram in Figure 22.5 is that each peak is symmetrical. A common example of an unsymmetrical peak is one in which **tailing** has occurred, as shown in Figure 22.8. Tailing usually results from injecting too much sample into the gas chromatograph. Another cause of tailing occurs with polar compounds, such as alcohols and aldehydes. These compounds may be temporarily adsorbed on column walls or areas of the support material that are not adequately coated by the liquid phase. Therefore, they do not leave in a band, and tailing results.

22.9 QUALITATIVE ANALYSIS

A disadvantage of the gas chromatograph is that it gives no information about the identities of the substances it has separated. The little information it does provide is given

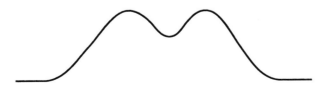

Figure 22.7 Poor resolution, or peaks overlap.

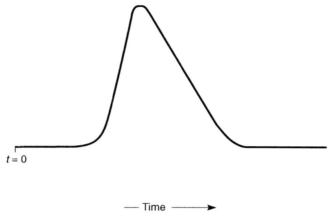

$t = 0$

— Time ——▶

Figure 22.8 Tailing.

by the retention time. It is hard to reproduce this quantity from day to day, however, and exact duplications of separations performed last month may be difficult to make this month. It is usually necessary to **calibrate** the column each time it is used. That is, you must run pure samples of all known and suspected components of a mixture individually, just before chromatographing the mixture, to obtain the retention time of each known compound. As an alternative, each suspected component can be added, one by one, to the unknown mixture while the operator looks to see which peak has its intensity increased relative to the unmodified mixture. Another solution is to collect the components individually as they emerge from the gas chromatograph. Each component can then be identified by other means, such as by infrared or nuclear magnetic resonance spectroscopy or by mass spectrometry.

22.10 COLLECTING THE SAMPLE

For gas chromatographs with a thermal conductivity detector, it is possible to collect samples that have passed through the column. One method uses a gas collection tube (see Figure 22.9), which is included in most microscale glassware kits. A collection tube is joined to the exit port of the column by inserting the ⚭ 5/5 inner joint into a metal adapter, which is connected to the exit port. When a sample is eluted from the column in the vapor state, it is cooled by the connecting adapter and the gas collection tube and condenses in the collection tube. The gas collection tube is removed from the adapter when the recorder indicates that the desired sample has completely passed through the column. After the first sample has been collected, the process can be repeated with another gas collection tube.

To isolate the liquid, insert the tapered joint of the collection tube into a 0.1-mL conical vial, which has a ⚭ 5/5 outer joint. Place the assembly into a test tube, as illustrated in Figure 22.10. During centrifugation, the sample is forced into the bottom of the conical vial. After disassembling the apparatus, the liquid can be removed from the vial with a syringe for a boiling-point determination or analysis by infrared spectroscopy. If a determination of the sample weight is desired, the empty conical vial and cap should be tared and reweighed after the liquid has been collected. It is advisable to dry the gas collection tube and the con-

276

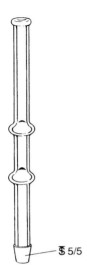

Figure 22.9 A gas chromatography collection tube.

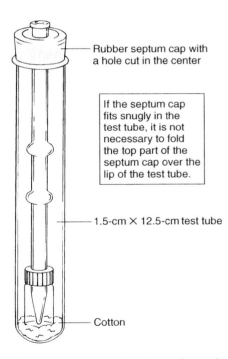

Rubber septum cap with
a hole cut in the center

If the septum cap
fits snugly in the
test tube, it is not
necessary to fold
the top part of the
septum cap over the
lip of the test tube.

1.5-cm × 12.5-cm test tube

Cotton

Figure 22.10 A gas chromatography collection tube and a 0.1-mL conical vial.

ical vial in an oven before use to prevent contamination by water or other solvents used in cleaning this glassware.

Another method for collecting samples is to connect a cooled trap to the exit port of the column. A simple trap, suitable for microscale work, is illustrated in Figure 22.11. Suitable coolants include ice water, liquid nitrogen, or dry ice–acetone. For instance, if the

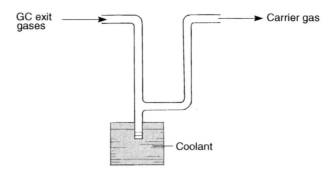

Figure 22.11 A collection trap.

coolant is liquid nitrogen (bp –196°C) and the carrier gas is helium (bp –269°C), compounds boiling above the temperature of liquid nitrogen generally are condensed or trapped in the small tube at the bottom of the U-shaped tube. The small tube is scored with a file just below the point at which it is connected to the larger tube, the tube is broken off, and the sample is removed for analysis. To collect each component of the mixture, you must change the trap after each sample is collected.

22.11 QUANTITATIVE ANALYSIS

The area under a gas chromatograph peak is proportional to the amount (moles) of compound eluted. Hence, the molar percentage composition of a mixture can be approximated by comparing relative peak areas. This method of analysis assumes that the detector is equally sensitive to all compounds eluted and that it gives a linear response with respect to amount. Nevertheless, it gives reasonably accurate results.

The simplest method of measuring the area of a peak is by geometric approximation, or triangulation. In this method, you multiply the height h of the peak above the baseline of the chromatogram by the width of the peak at half of its height $w_{1/2}$. This is illustrated in Figure 22.12. The baseline is approximated by drawing a line between the two sidearms of the peak. This method works well only if the peak is symmetrical. If the peak has tailed or is unsymmetrical, it is best to cut out the peaks with scissors and weigh the pieces of paper on an **analytical balance.** Because the weight per area of a piece of good chart paper is reasonably constant from place to place, the ratio of the areas is the same as the ratio of the weights. To obtain a percentage composition for the mixture, first add all the peak areas (weights). Then, to calculate the percentage of any component in the mixture, divide its individual area by the total area and multiply the result by 100. A sample calculation is illustrated in Figure 22.13. If peaks overlap (see Figure 22.7), either the gas chromatographic conditions must be readjusted to achieve better resolution of the peaks or the peak shape must be estimated.

There are various instrumental means, which are built into recorders, of detecting the amounts of each sample automatically. One method uses a separate pen that produces a trace that integrates the area under each peak. Another method employs an electronic device that automatically prints out the area under each peak and the percentage composition of the sample.

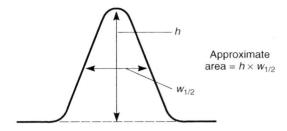

Figure 22.12 Triangulation of a peak.

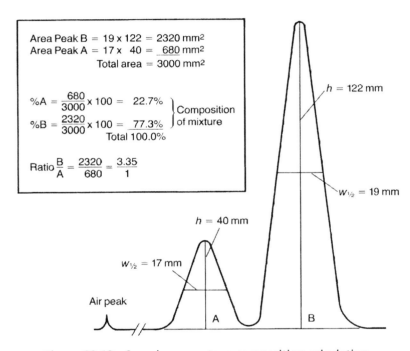

Area Peak B = 19 x 122 = 2320 mm²
Area Peak A = 17 x   40 =   680 mm²
                Total area = 3000 mm²

$\%A = \dfrac{680}{3000} \times 100 = 22.7\%$ ⎫ Composition
$\%B = \dfrac{2320}{3000} \times 100 = 77.3\%$ ⎬ of mixture
                Total 100.0%

$Ratio \dfrac{B}{A} = \dfrac{2320}{680} = \dfrac{3.35}{1}$

$h = 122$ mm

$w_{1/2} = 19$ mm

$h = 40$ mm

$w_{1/2} = 17$ mm

Air peak

A   B

Figure 22.13 Sample percentage composition calculation.

Most modern data stations (see Section 22.12) label the top of each peak with its retention time in minutes. When the trace is completed, the computer prints a table of all the peaks with their retention times, areas, and the percentage of the total area (sum of all the peaks) that each peak represents. Some caution should be used with these results because the computer often does not include smaller peaks and occasionally does not resolve narrow peaks that are so close together that they overlap. If the trace has several peaks and you would like the ratio of only two of them, you will have to determine their percentages yourself using only their two areas or instruct the instrument to integrate only these two peaks.

For many applications, one assumes that the detector is equally sensitive to all compounds eluted. Compounds with different functional groups or with widely varying molecular weights, however, produce different responses with both TCD and FID gas chromatographs. With a TCD, the responses are different because not all compounds have the same thermal conductivity. Different compounds analyzed with an FID gas chromatograph also give different responses because the detector response varies with the type of ions produced. For both types of detectors, it is possible to calculate a **response factor** for each compound in a mixture. Response factors are usually determined by making up an equimolar mixture of two compounds, one of which is considered to be the reference. The mixture is separated on a gas chromatograph, and the relative percentages are calculated using one of the methods described previously. From these percentages, you can determine a response factor for the compound being compared to the reference. If you do this for all the components in a mixture, you can then use these correction factors to make more accurate calculations of the relative percentages for the compounds in the mixture.

To illustrate how response factors are determined, consider the following example. An equimolar mixture of benzene, hexane, and ethyl acetate is prepared and analyzed using a flame-ionization gas chromatograph. The peak areas obtained are

Hexane	831158
Ethyl acetate	1449695
Benzene	966463

In most cases, benzene is taken as the standard, and its response factor is defined to be equal to 1.00. Calculation of the response factors for the other components of the test mixture proceeds as follows:

Hexane	831158/966463 = 0.86
Ethyl acetate	1449695/966463 = 1.50
Benzene	966463/966463 = 1.00 (by definition)

Notice that the response factors calculated in this example are molar response factors. It is necessary to correct these values by the relative molecular weights of each substance to obtain weight response factors.

When you use a flame-ionization gas chromatograph for quantitative analysis, it is first necessary to determine the response factors for each component of the mixture being analyzed, as just shown. For a quantitative analysis, it is likely that you will have to convert molar response factors into weight response factors. Next, the chromatography experiment using the unknown samples is performed. The observed peak areas for each component are corrected using the response factors in order to arrive at the correct weight percentage of each component in the sample. The application of response factors to correct the original results of a quantitative analysis will be illustrated in the following section.

22.12 TREATMENT OF DATA: CHROMATOGRAMS PRODUCED BY MODERN DATA STATIONS

A. Gas Chromatograms and Data Tables

Most modern gas chromatography instruments are equipped with computer-based data stations. Interfacing the instrument with a computer allows the operator to display and manipulate the results in whatever manner might be desired. The operator thus can view the output in a convenient form. The computer can both display the actual gas chromatogram and display the integration results. It can even display the result of two experiments simultaneously, making a comparison of parallel experiments convenient.

Figure 22.14 shows a gas chromatogram of a mixture of hexane, ethyl acetate, and benzene. The peaks corresponding to each peak can be seen; the peaks are labeled with their respective retention times:

	Retention Time (minutes)
Hexane	2.959
Ethyl acetate	3.160
Benzene	3.960

We can also see that there is a very small amount of an unspecified impurity, with a retention time of about 3.4 minutes.

Figure 22.15 shows part of the printed output that accompanies the gas chromatogram. It is this information that is used in the quantitative analysis of the mixture. According to the printout, the first peak has a retention time of 2.954 minutes (the difference between the retention times that appear as labels on the graph and those that appear in the data table are not significant). The computer has also determined the area under this peak (422373 counts). Finally, the computer has calculated the percentage of the first substance (hexane) by determining the total area of all the peaks in the chromatogram (1227054 counts) and dividing that into the area for the hexane peak. The result is displayed as 34.4217%. In a similar manner, the data table shows the retention times and peak areas for the other two peaks in the sample, along with a determination of the percentage of each substance in the mixture.

B. Application of Response Factors

If the detector responded with equal sensitivity to each of the components of the mixture, the data table shown in Figure 22.15 would contain the complete quantitative analysis of the sample. Unfortunately, as we have seen (Section 22.11), gas chromatography detectors respond more sensitively to some substances than they do to others. To correct for this discrepancy, it is necessary to apply corrections that are based on the **response factors** for each component of the mixture.

The method for determining the response factors was introduced in Section 22.11. In this section we will see how this information is applied in order to obtain a correct analysis. This example should serve to demonstrate the procedure for correcting raw gas chromatography results when response factors are known. According to the data table, the reported peak area for the first (hexane) peak is 422373 counts. The response factor for hexane was previously determined to be 0.86. The area of the hexane peak is thus corrected as follows:

$$422373/0.86 = 491000$$

Notice that the calculated result has been adjusted to reflect a reasonable number of significant figures.

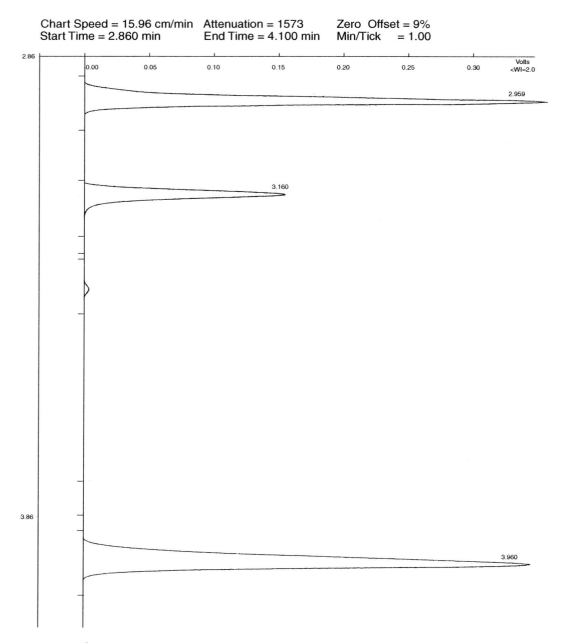

Chart Speed = 15.96 cm/min   Attenuation = 1573   Zero Offset = 9%
Start Time = 2.860 min   End Time = 4.100 min   Min/Tick = 1.00

Figure 22.14 A sample gas chromatogram obtained from a data station.

282

```
Run Mode        : Analysis
Peak Measurement: Peak Area
Calculation Type: Percent

                         Ret.   Time                    Width
Peak    Peak     Result  Time   Offset    Area    Sep.  1/2    Status
No.     Name     ()      (min)  (min)     (counts) Code (sec)  Codes
----  ---------- ------  -----  ------   ---------- ---- -----  ------
  1              34.4217 2.954  0.000     422373    BB   1.0
  2              16.6599 3.155  0.000     204426    BB   1.2
  3              48.9184 3.954  0.000     600255    BB   1.6
----  ---------- ======  -----  ======   ==========  ----  -----  ------
      Totals:    100.0000       0.000    1227054

Total Unidentified Counts :     1227054 counts

Detected Peaks: 8        Rejected Peaks: 5        Identified Peaks: 0

Multiplier: 1            Divisor: 1       Unidentified Peak Factor: 0

Baseline Offset: 1 microVolts

Noise (used): 28 microVolts — monitored before this run

Manual injection
```

★ ★

Figure 22.15   A data table to accompany the gas chromatogram shown in Figure 22.14.

The areas for the other peaks in the gas chromatogram are corrected in a similar manner:

Hexane	$422373/0.86 =$	491000
Ethyl acetate	$204426/1.50 =$	136000
Benzene	$600255/1.00 =$	600000
Total peak area		1227000

Using these corrected areas, the true percentages of each component can be easily determined:

		Composition
Hexane	491000/1227000	40.0%
Ethyl acetate	136000/1227000	11.1%
Benzene	600000/1227000	48.9%
Total		100.0%

C. Determination of Relative Percentages of Components in a Complex Mixture

In some circumstances, one may wish to determine the relative percentages of two components when the mixture being analyzed may be more complex and may contain more than two components. Examples of this situation might include the analysis of a reaction product where the laboratory worker might be interested in the relative percentages of two isomeric products when the sample might also contain peaks arising from the solvent, unreacted starting material, or some other product or impurity.

The example provided in Figures 22.14 and 22.15 can be used to illustrate the method of determining the relative percentages of some, but not all, of the components in the sample. Assume we are interested in the relative percentages of hexane and ethyl acetate in the sample but not in the percentage of benzene, which may be a solvent or an impurity. We know from the previous discussion that the *corrected* relative areas of the two peaks of interest are as follows:

	Relative Area
Hexane	491000
Ethyl acetate	136000
Total	627000

We can determine the relative percentages of the two components simply by dividing the area of each peak by the total area of the two peaks:

		Percentage
Hexane	491000/627000	78.3%
Ethyl acetate	136000/627000	21.7%
Total		100.0%

22.13 GAS CHROMATOGRAPHY–MASS SPECTROMETRY (GC–MS)

A recently developed variation on gas chromatography is **gas chromatography–mass spectrometry,** also known as **GC–MS.** In this technique, a gas chromatograph is coupled to a mass spectrometer (see Technique 28). In effect, the mass spectrometer acts as a detector. The gas stream emerging from the gas chromatograph is admitted through a valve into a tube, where it passes over the sample inlet system of the mass spectrometer. Some of the gas stream is thus admitted into the ionization chamber of the mass spectrometer.

The molecules in the gas stream are converted into ions in the ionization chamber, and thus the gas chromatogram is actually a plot of time versus **ion current,** a measure of the number of ions produced. At the same time that the molecules are converted into ions, they are also accelerated and passed through the **mass analyzer** of the instrument. The instrument, therefore, determines the mass spectrum of each fraction eluting from the gas chromatography column.

A drawback of this method involves the need for rapid scanning by the mass spectrometer. The instrument must determine the mass spectrum of each component in the mixture before the next component exits from the column so that the spectrum of one substance is not contaminated by the spectrum of the next fraction.

Because high-efficiency capillary columns are used in the gas chromatograph, in most cases compounds are completely separated before the gas stream is analyzed. The typical GC–MS instrument has the capability of obtaining at least one scan per second in the range of 10–300 amu. Even more scans are possible if a narrow range of masses is analyzed. Using capillary columns, however, requires the user to take particular care to ensure that the sample does not contain any particles that might obstruct the flow of gases through the column. For this reason, the sample is carefully filtered through a very fine filter before the sample is injected into the chromatograph.

With a GC–MS system, a mixture can be analyzed and results obtained that resemble very closely those shown in Figures 22.14 and 22.15. A library search on each component of the mixture can also be conducted. The data stations of most instruments contain a library of standard mass spectra in their computer memory. If the components are known compounds, they can be identified tentatively by a comparison of their mass spectrum with the spectra of compounds found in the computer library. In this way, a "hit list" can be generated that reports on the probability that the compound in the library matches the known substance. A typical printout from a GC–MS instrument will list probable compounds that fit the mass spectrum of the component, the names of the compounds, their CAS Nos. (see Technique 29, Section 29.11, p. 993), and a "quality" or "confidence" number. This last number provides an estimate of how closely the mass spectrum of the component matches the mass spectrum of the substance in the computer library.

A variation on the GC–MS technique includes coupling a Fourier-transform infrared spectrometer (FT–IR) to a gas chromatograph. The substances that elute from the gas chromatograph are detected by determining their infrared spectra rather than their mass spectra. A new technique that also resembles GC–MS is **high-performance liquid chromatography–mass spectrometry (HPLC–MS).** An HPLC instrument is coupled through a special interface to a mass spectrometer. The substances that elute from the HPLC column are detected by the mass spectrometer, and their mass spectra can be displayed, analyzed, and compared with standard spectra found in the computer library built into the instrument.

PROBLEMS

1. a. A sample consisting of 1-bromopropane and 1-chloropropane is injected into a gas chromatograph equipped with a nonpolar column. Which compound has the shorter retention time? Explain your answer.

   b. If the same sample were run several days later with the conditions as nearly the same as possible, would you expect the retention times to be identical to those obtained the first time? Explain.

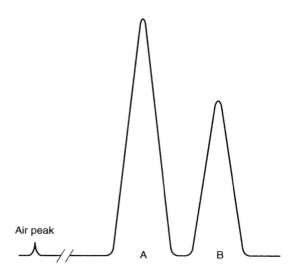

Air peak

A   B

Figure 22.16   A chromatogram for problem 2.

2. Using triangulation, calculate the percentage of each component in a mixture composed of two substances, A and B. The chromatogram is shown in Figure 22.16.

3. Make a photocopy of the chromatogram in Figure 22.16. Cut out the peaks and weigh them on an analytical balance. Use the weights to calculate the percentage of each component in the mixture. Compare your answer to what you calculated in problem 2.

4. What would happen to the retention time of a compound if the following changes were made?

    a.   Decrease the flow rate of the carrier gas

    b.   Increase the temperature of the column

    c.   Increase the length of the column

TECHNIQUE 25

Infrared Spectroscopy

Almost any compound having covalent bonds, whether organic or inorganic, will be found to absorb frequencies of electromagnetic radiation in the infrared region of the spectrum. The infrared region of the electromagnetic spectrum lies at wavelengths longer than those associated with visible light, which includes wavelengths from approximately 400 nm to 800 nm (1 nm = 10^{-9} m), but at wavelengths shorter than those associated with radio waves, which have wavelengths longer than 1 cm. For chemical purposes, we are interested in the *vibrational* portion of the infrared region. This portion includes radiations with wavelengths (λ) between 2.5 μm and 15 μm (1 μm = 10^{-6} m). The relation of the infrared region to other regions included in the electromagnetic spectrum is illustrated in Figure 25.1.

As with other types of energy absorption, molecules are excited to a higher energy state when they absorb infrared radiation. The absorption of the infrared radiation is, like other absorption processes, a quantized process. Only selected frequencies (energies) of infrared radiation are absorbed by a molecule. The absorption of infrared radiation corresponds to energy changes on the order of 8–40 kJ/mole (2–10 kcal/mole). Radiation in this energy range corresponds to the range encompassing the stretching and bending vibrational frequencies of the bonds in most covalent molecules. In the absorption process, those frequencies of infrared radiation that match the natural vibrational frequencies of the molecule in question are absorbed, and the energy absorbed increases the *amplitude* of the vibrational motions of the bonds in the molecule.

Most chemists refer to the radiation in the vibrational infrared region of the electromagnetic spectrum by units called **wavenumbers** ($\overline{\nu}$). Wavenumbers are expressed in reciprocal centimeters (cm^{-1}) and are easily computed by taking the reciprocal of the wavelength (λ) expressed in centimeters. This unit has the advantage, for those performing calculations, of being directly proportional to energy. Thus, the vibrational infrared region of the spectrum extends from about 4000 cm^{-1} to 650 cm^{-1} (or wavenumbers).

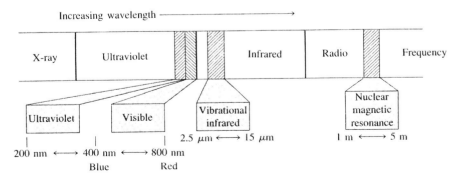

Figure 25.1 A portion of the electromagnetic spectrum showing the relation of vibrational infrared radiation to other types of radiation.

Wavelengths (μm) and wavenumbers (cm^{-1}) can be interconverted by the following relationships:

$$cm^{-1} = \frac{1}{(\mu m)} \times 10,000$$

$$\mu m = \frac{1}{(cm)^{-1}} \times 10,000$$

Part A.   Sample Preparation and Recording the Spectrum

25.1 INTRODUCTION

To determine the infrared spectrum of the compound, one must place the compound in a sample holder or cell. In infrared spectroscopy, this immediately poses a problem. Glass, quartz, and plastics absorb strongly throughout the infrared region of the spectrum (any compound with covalent bonds usually absorbs) and cannot be used to construct sample cells. Ionic substances must be used in cell construction. Metal halides (sodium chloride, potassium bromide, silver chloride) are commonly used for this purpose.

Sodium Chloride Cells.   Single crystals of sodium chloride are cut and polished to give plates that are transparent throughout the infrared region. These plates are then used to fabricate cells that can be used to hold *liquid* samples. Because sodium chloride is water soluble, samples must be *dry* before a spectrum can be obtained. In general, sodium chloride plates are preferred for most applications involving liquid samples. Potassium bromide plates may also be used in place of sodium chloride.

Silver Chloride Cells.   Cells may be constructed of silver chloride. These plates may be used for *liquid* samples that contain small amounts of water, because silver chloride is water insoluble. However, because water absorbs in the infrared region, as much water as possible should be removed, even when using silver chloride. Silver chloride plates must be stored in the dark. They darken when exposed to light, and they cannot be used with compounds that have an amino functional group. Amines react with silver chloride.

Solid Samples.   The easiest way to hold a *solid* sample in place is to dissolve the sample in a volatile organic solvent, place several drops of this solution on a salt plate, and allow the solvent to evaporate. This dry film method can be used only with modern FT-IR spectrometers. The other methods described here can be used with both FT-IR and dispersion spectrometers. A solid sample can also be held in place by making a potassium bromide pellet that contains a small amount of dispersed compound. A solid sample may also be suspended in mineral oil, which absorbs only in specific regions of the infrared spectrum. Another method is to dissolve the solid compound in an appropriate solvent and place the solution between two sodium chloride or silver chloride plates.

25.2 LIQUID SAMPLES—NaCl PLATES

The simplest method of preparing the sample, if it is a liquid, is to place a thin layer of the liquid between two sodium chloride plates that have been ground flat and polished. This is the method of choice when you need to determine the infrared spectrum of a pure liquid. A spectrum determined by this method is referred to as a **neat** spectrum. No solvent is used. The polished plates are expensive because they are cut from a large, single crystal of sodium chloride. Salt plates break easily, and they are water soluble.

Preparing the Sample.   Obtain two sodium chloride plates and a holder from the desiccator where they are stored. Moisture from fingers will mar and occlude the polished surfaces. Samples that contain water will destroy the plates.

> **Note:** The plates should be touched only on their edges. Be certain to use a sample that is dry or free from water.

Add 1 or 2 drops of the liquid to the surface of one plate, and then place the second plate on top.[1] The pressure of this second plate causes the liquid to spread out and form a thin capillary film between the two plates. As shown in Figure 25.2, set the plates between

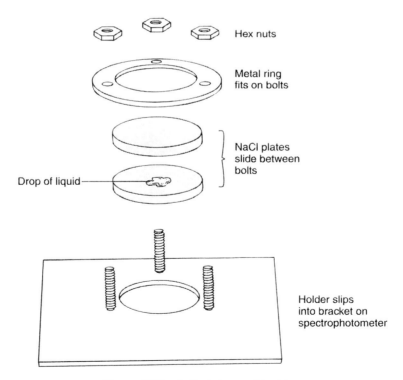

Figure 25.2   Salt plates and holder.

---

[1] Use a Pasteur pipet or a short length of microcapillary tubing. If you use the microcapillary tubing, it can be filled by touching it into the liquid sample. When you touch it (lightly) to the salt plate, it will empty. Be careful not to scratch the plate.

the bolts in a holder and place the metal ring carefully on the salt plates. Use the hex nuts to hold the salt plates in place.

> **Note:** Do not overtighten the nuts, or the salt plates will cleave or split.

Tighten the nuts firmly, but do not use any force to turn them. Spin them with the fingers until they stop; then turn them just another fraction of a full turn, and they will be tight enough. If the nuts have been tightened carefully, you should observe a *transparent film of sample* (a uniform wetting of the surface). If a thin film has not been obtained, either loosen one or more of the hex nuts and adjust them so that a uniform film is obtained or add more sample.

The thickness of the film obtained between the two plates is a function of two factors: (1) the amount of liquid placed on the first plate (1 drop, 2 drops, and so on) and (2) the pressure used to hold the plates together. If more than 1 or 2 drops of liquid have been used, the amount will probably be too much, and the resulting spectrum will show strong absorptions that are off the scale of the chart paper. Only enough liquid to wet both surfaces is needed.

If the sample has a very low viscosity, the capillary film may be too thin to produce a good spectrum. Another problem you may find is that the liquid is so volatile that the sample evaporates before the spectrum can be determined. In these cases, you may need to use the silver chloride plates discussed in Section 25.3 or a solution cell described in Section 25.6. Often, you can obtain a reasonable spectrum by assembling the cell quickly and running the spectrum before the sample runs out of the salt plates or evaporates.

Determining the Infrared Spectrum. Slide the holder into the slot in the sample beam of the spectrophotometer. Determine the spectrum according to the instructions provided by your instructor. In some cases, your instructor may ask you to calibrate your spectrum. If this is the case, refer to Section 25.8.

Cleaning and Storing the Salt Plates. Once the spectrum has been determined, demount the holder and rinse the salt plates with methylene chloride (or *dry* acetone). (Keep the plates away from water!) Use a soft tissue, moistened with the solvent, to wipe the plates. If some of your compound remains on the plates, you may observe a shiny surface. Continue to clean the plates with solvent until no more compound remains on the surfaces of the plates.

> **Caution:** Avoid direct contact with methylene chloride. Return the salt plates and holder to the desiccator for storage.

25.3 LIQUID SAMPLES—AgCl PLATES

The minicell shown in Figure 25.3 may also be used with liquids.[2] The cell assembly consists of a two-piece threaded body, an O-ring, and two silver chloride plates. The plates

---

[2] The Wilks Mini-Cell liquid sample holder is available from the Foxboro Company, 151 Woodward Avenue, South Norwalk, CT 06856. We recommend the AgCl cell windows with 0.10-mm depression rather than the 0.025-mm depression.

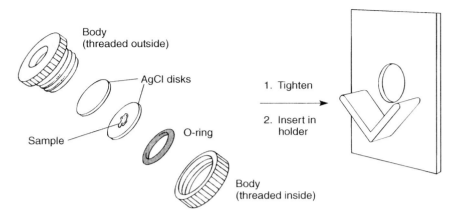

Figure 25.3 AgCl minicell liquid sample cell and V-mount holder.

are flat on one side, and there is a circular depression (0.025 mm or 0.10 mm deep) on the other side of the plate. An advantage of using silver chloride plates is that they may be used with wet samples or solutions. A disadvantage is that silver chloride darkens when exposed to light for extended periods. Silver chloride plates also scratch more easily than salt plates and react with amines.

Preparing the Sample.   Silver chloride plates should be handled in the same way as salt plates. Unfortunately, they are smaller and thinner (about like a contact lens) than salt plates, and care must be taken not to lose them! Remove them from the light-tight container with care. It is difficult to tell which side of the plate has the slight circular depression. Your instructor may have etched a letter on each plate to indicate which side is the flat one. To determine the infrared spectrum of a pure liquid (neat spectrum), select the flat side of each silver chloride plate. Insert the O-ring into the cell body as shown in Figure 25.3, place the plate into the cell body with the flat surface up, and add 1 drop or less of liquid to the plate.

Note: Do not use amines with AgCl plates.

Place the second plate on top of the first with the flat side down. The orientation of the silver chloride plates is shown in Figure 25.4A. This arrangement is used to obtain a capillary film of your sample. Screw the top of the minicell into the body of the cell so that the silver chloride plates are held firmly together. A tight seal forms because AgCl deforms under pressure.

Other combinations may be used with these plates. For example, you may vary the sample path length by using the orientations shown in Figures 25.4B and C. If you add your

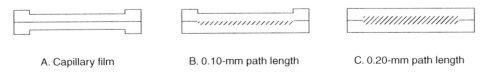

A. Capillary film   B. 0.10-mm path length   C. 0.20-mm path length

Figure 25.4 Path length variations for AgCl plates.

sample and the 0.10-mm depression of one plate and cover it with the flat side of the other one, you obtain a path length of 0.10 mm (Figure 25.4B). This arrangement is useful for analyzing volatile or low-viscosity liquids. Placement of the two plates with their depressions toward each other gives a path length of 0.20 mm (Figure 25.4C). This orientation may be used for a solution of a solid (or liquid) in carbon tetrachloride (Section 25.6B).

Determining the Spectrum. Slide the V-mount holder shown in Figure 25.3 into the slot on the infrared spectrophotometer. Set the cell assembly in the V-mount holder, and determine the infrared spectrum of the liquid.

Cleaning and Storing the AgCl Plates. Once the spectrum has been determined, the cell assembly holder should be demounted and the AgCl plates rinsed with methylene chloride or acetone. Do not use tissue to wipe the plates, as they scratch easily. AgCl plates are light sensitive. Store the plates in a light-tight container.

25.4 SOLID SAMPLES—DRY FILM

A simple method for determining the infrared spectrum of a solid sample is the **dry film** method. This method is easier than the other methods described here, it does not require any specialized equipment, and the spectra are excellent.[3] The disadvantage is that the dry film method can be used only with modern FT-IR spectrometers.

To use this method, place about 5 mg of your solid sample in a small, clean test tube. Add about 5 drops of methylene chloride (or diethyl ether or pentane), and stir the mixture to dissolve the solid. Using a Pasteur pipet (not a capillary tube), place several drops of the solution on the face of a salt plate. Allow the solvent to evaporate; a uniform deposit of your product will remain as a dry film coating the salt plate. Mount the salt plate on a V-shaped holder in the infrared beam. Note that only one salt plate is used; the second salt plate is not used to cover the first. Once the salt plate is positioned properly, you may determine the spectrum in the normal manner. With this method, it is *very important* that you clean your material off the salt plate. When you are finished, use methylene chloride or dry acetone to clean the salt plate.

25.5 SOLID SAMPLES—KBr PELLETS AND NUJOL MULLS

The methods described in this section can be used with both FT-IR and dispersion spectrometers.

A. KBr Pellets

One method of preparing a solid sample is to make a **potassium bromide (KBr) pellet.** When KBr is placed under pressure, it melts, flows, and seals the sample into a solid solution, or matrix. Because potassium bromide does not absorb in the infrared spectrum, a spectrum can be obtained on a sample without interference.

---

[3]P. L. Feist, *Journal of Chemical Education, 78* (2001): 351.

Preparing the Sample. Remove the agate mortar and pestle from the desiccator for use in preparing the sample. (Take care of them; they are expensive.) Grind 1 mg (0.001 g) of the solid sample for 1 minute in the agate mortar. At this point, the particle size will become so small that the surface of the solid appears shiny. Add 80 mg (0.080 g) of *powdered* potassium bromide and grind the mixture for about 30 seconds with the pestle. Scrape the mixture into the middle with a spatula and grind the mixture again for about 15 seconds. This grinding operation helps to mix the sample thoroughly with the KBr. You should work as rapidly as possible, because KBr absorbs water. The sample and KBr must be finely ground, or the mixture will scatter the infrared radiation excessively. Using your spatula, heap the mixture in the center of the mortar. Return the bottle of potassium bromide to the desiccator where it is stored when it is not in use.

The sample and potassium bromide should be weighed on an analytical balance the first few times that a pellet is prepared. After some experience, you can estimate these quantities quite accurately by eye.

Making a Pellet Using a KBr Handpress. Two methods are commonly used to prepare KBr pellets. The first method uses the handpress apparatus shown in Figure 25.5.[4]

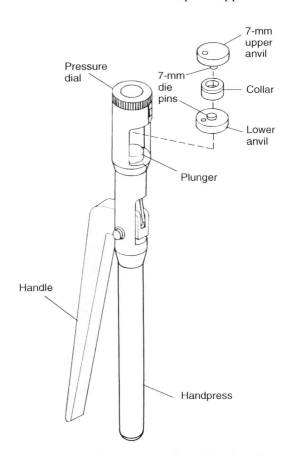

Figure 25.5 Making a KBr pellet with a handpress.

[4] KBr Quick Press unit is available from Wilmad Glass Company, Inc., Route 40 and Oak Road, Buena, NJ 08310.

Remove the die set from the storage container. Take extreme care to avoid scratching the polished surfaces of the die set. Place the anvil with the shorter die pin (lower anvil in Figure 25.5) on a bench. Slip the collar over the pin. Remove about one-fourth of your KBr mixture with a spatula and transfer it into the collar. The powder may not cover the head of the pin completely, but do not be concerned about this. Place the anvil with the longer die pin into the collar so that the die pin comes into contact with the sample. Never press the die set unless it contains a sample.

Lift the die set carefully by holding onto the lower anvil so that the collar stays in place. If you are careless with this operation, the collar may move enough to allow the powder to escape. Open the handle of the handpress slightly, tilt the press back a bit, and insert the die set into the press. Make sure that the die set is seated against the side wall of the chamber. Close the handle. It is imperative that the die set be seated against the side wall of the chamber so that the die is centered in the chamber. Pressing the die in an off-centered position can bend the anvil pins.

With the handle in the closed position, rotate the pressure dial so that the upper ram of the handpress just touches the upper anvil of the die assembly. Tilt the unit back so that the die set does not fall out of the handpress. Open the handle and rotate the pressure dial clockwise about one-half turn. Slowly compress the KBr mixture by closing the handle. The pressure should be no greater than that exerted by a very firm handshake. Do not apply excessive pressure, or the dies may be damaged. If in doubt, rotate the pressure dial counterclockwise to lower the pressure. If the handle closes too easily, open the handle, rotate the pressure dial clockwise, and compress the sample again. Compress the sample for about 60 seconds.

After this time, tilt the unit back so that the die set does not fall out of the handpress. Open the handle and carefully remove the die set from the unit. Turn the pressure dial counterclockwise about one full turn. Pull the die set apart and inspect the KBr pellet. Ideally, the pellet should appear clear like a piece of glass, but usually it will be translucent or somewhat opaque. There may be some cracks or holes in the pellet. The pellet will produce a good spectrum, even with imperfections, as long as light can travel through the pellet.

Making a Pellet with a KBr Minipress. The second method of preparing a pellet uses the minipress apparatus shown in Figure 25.6. Obtain a ground KBr mixture as described in "Preparing the Sample" and transfer a portion of the finely ground powder (usually not more than half) into a die that compresses it into a translucent pellet. As shown in Figure 25.6, the die consists of two stainless steel bolts and a threaded barrel. The bolts have their ends ground flat. To use this die, screw one of the bolts into the barrel, but not all the way; leave one or two turns. Carefully add the powder with a spatula into the open end of the partly assembled die and tap it lightly on the benchtop to give an even layer on the face of the bolt. While keeping the barrel upright, carefully screw the second bolt into the barrel until it is finger tight. Insert the head of the bottom bolt into the hexagonal hole in a plate bolted to the benchtop. This plate keeps the head of one bolt from turning. The top bolt is tightened with a torque wrench to compress the KBr mixture. Continue to turn the torque wrench until you hear a loud click (the ratchet mechanism makes softer clicks) or until you reach the appropriate torque value (20 ft-lb). If you tighten the bolt beyond this point, you may twist the head off one of the bolts. Leave the die under pressure for about 60 seconds; then reverse the ratchet on the torque wrench or pull the torque wrench in the opposite direction to open the assembly. When the two bolts are loose, hold the barrel horizontally and

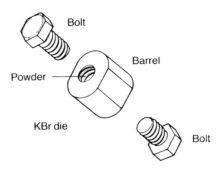

Figure 25.6   Making a KBr pellet with a minipress.

carefully remove the two bolts. You should observe a clear or translucent KBr pellet in the center of the barrel. Even if the pellet is not totally transparent, you should be able to obtain a satisfactory spectrum as long as light passes through the pellet.

Determining the Infrared Spectrum.   To obtain the spectrum, slide the holder appropriate for the type of die that you are using into the slot on the infrared spectrophotometer. Set the die containing the pellet in the holder so that the sample is centered in the optical path. Obtain the infrared spectrum. If you are using a double-beam instrument, you may be able to compensate (at least partially) for a marginal pellet by placing a wire screen or attenuator in the reference beam, thereby balancing the lowered transmittance of the pellet. An FT-IR instrument will automatically deal with the low intensity if you select the "autoscale" option.

Problems with an Unsatisfactory Pellet.   If the pellet is unsatisfactory (too cloudy to pass light), one of several things may have been wrong:

1. The KBr mixture may not have been ground finely enough, and the particle size may be too big. The large particle size creates too much light scattering.
2. The sample may not be dry.
3. Too much sample may have been used for the amount of KBr taken.
4. The pellet may be too thick; that is, too much of the powdered mixture was put into the die.
5. The KBr may have been "wet" or have acquired moisture from the air while the mixture was being ground in the mortar.
6. The sample may have a low melting point. Low-melting solids not only are difficult to dry but also melt under pressure. You may need to dissolve the compound in a solvent and run the spectrum in solution (Section 25.6).

Cleaning and Storing the Equipment.   After you have determined the spectrum, punch the pellet out of the die with a wooden applicator stick (a spatula should not be used as it may scratch the dies). Remember that the polished faces of the die set must not be scratched, or they become useless. Pull a piece of Kimwipe through the die unit to remove all the sample. Also wipe any surfaces with a Kimwipe. *Do not wash the dies with water.* Check with your instructor to see if there are additional instructions for cleaning the die set. Return the dies to the storage container. Wash the mortar and pestle with water, dry them carefully with paper towels, and return them to the desiccator. Return the KBr powder to its desiccator.

B. Nujol Mulls

If an adequate KBr pellet cannot be obtained or if the solid is insoluble in a suitable solvent, the spectrum of a solid may be determined as a **Nujol mull.** In this method, finely grind about 5 mg of the solid sample in an agate mortar with a pestle. Then add 1 or 2 drops of Nujol mineral oil (white) and grind the mixture to a very fine dispersion. The solid is not dissolved in the Nujol; it is actually a suspension. This mull is then placed between two salt plates using a rubber policeman. Mount the salt plates in the holder in the same way as for liquid samples (Section 25.2).

Nujol is a mixture of high-molecular-weight hydrocarbons. Hence, it has absorptions in the C—H stretch and CH_2 and CH_3 bending regions of the spectrum (Figure 25.7). Clearly, if Nujol is used, no information can be obtained in these portions of the spectrum. In interpreting the spectrum, you must ignore these Nujol peaks. It is important to label the spectrum immediately after it was determined, noting that it was determined as a Nujol mull. Otherwise, you might forget that the C—H peaks belong to Nujol and not to the dispersed solid.

25.6 SOLID SAMPLES—SOLUTION SPECTRA

A. Method A—Solution between Salt (NaCl) Plates

For substances that are soluble in carbon tetrachloride, a quick and easy method for determining the spectra of solids is available. Dissolve as much solid as possible in 0.1 mL of carbon tetrachloride. Place 1 or 2 drops of the solution between sodium chloride plates in precisely the same manner as used for pure liquids (Section 25.2). The spectrum is determined as described for pure liquids using salt plates (Section 25.2). You should work as

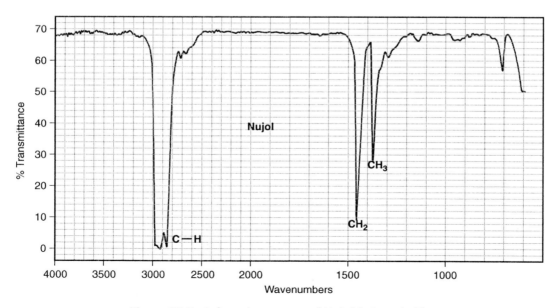

Figure 25.7 Infrared spectrum of Nujol (mineral oil).

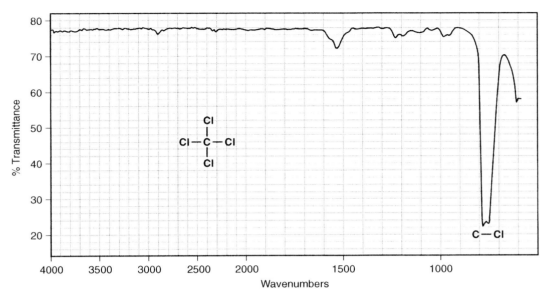

Figure 25.8 Infrared spectrum of carbon tetrachloride.

quickly as possible. If there is a delay, the solvent will evaporate from between the plates before the spectrum is recorded. Because the spectrum contains the absorptions of the solute superimposed on the absorptions of carbon tetrachloride, it is important to remember that any absorption that appears near 800 cm^{-1} may be due to the stretching of the C—Cl bond of the solvent. Information contained to the right of about 900 cm^{-1} is not usable in this method. There are no other interfering bands for this solvent (see Figure 25.8), and any other absorptions can be attributed to your sample. Chloroform solutions should not be studied by this method because the solvent has too many interfering absorptions (see Figure 25.9).

> **Caution:** Carbon tetrachloride is a hazardous solvent. Work under the hood!

Carbon tetrachloride, besides being toxic, is suspected of being a carcinogen. In spite of the health problems associated with its use, there is no suitable alternative solvent for infrared spectroscopy. Other solvents have too many interfering infrared absorption bands. Handle carbon tetrachloride very carefully to minimize the adverse health effects. The spectroscopic-grade carbon tetrachloride should be stored in a glass-stoppered bottle in a hood. A Pasteur pipet should be attached to the bottle, possibly by storing it in a test tube taped to the side of the bottle. All sample preparation should be conducted in a hood. Rubber or plastic gloves should be worn. The cells should also be cleaned in the hood. All carbon tetrachloride used in preparing samples should be disposed of in an appropriately marked waste container.

297

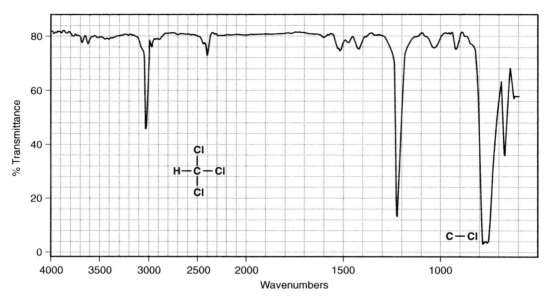

Figure 25.9 Infrared spectrum of chloroform.

B. Method B—AgCl Minicell

The AgCl minicell described in Section 25.3 may be used to determine the infrared spectrum of a solid dissolved in carbon tetrachloride. Prepare a 5–10% solution (5–10 mg in 0.1 mL) in carbon tetrachloride. If it is not possible to prepare a solution of this concentration because of low solubility, dissolve as much solid as possible in the solvent. Following the instructions given in Section 25.3, position the AgCl plates as shown in Figure 25.4C to obtain the maximum possible path length of 0.20 mm. When the cell is tightened firmly, the cell will not leak.

As indicated in method A, the spectrum will contain the absorptions of the dissolved solid superimposed on the absorptions of carbon tetrachloride. A strong absorption appears near 800 cm^{-1} for C—Cl stretch in the solvent. No useful information may be obtained for the sample to the right of about 900 cm^{-1}, but other bands that appear in the spectrum will belong to your sample. Read the safety material provided in method A. Carbon tetrachloride is toxic, and it should be used under a hood.

> **Note:** Care should be taken in cleaning the AgCl plates. Because AgCl plates scratch easily, they should not be wiped with tissue. Rinse them with methylene chloride and keep them in a dark place. Amines will destroy the plates.

C. Method C—Solution Cells (NaCl)

The spectra of solids may also be determined in a type of permanent sample cell called a **solution cell.** (The infrared spectra of liquids may also be determined in this cell.) The so-

298

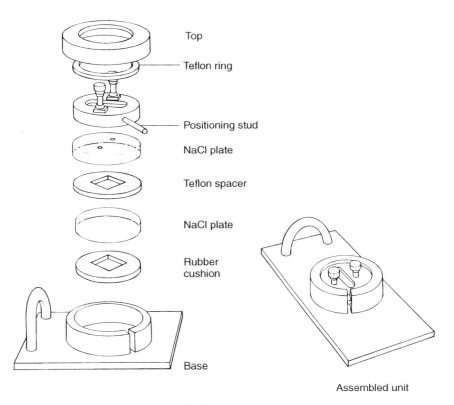

Figure 25.10 A solution cell.

lution cell, shown in Figure 25.10, is made from two salt plates, mounted with a Teflon spacer between them to control the thickness of the sample. The top sodium chloride plate has two holes drilled in it so that the sample can be introduced into the cavity between the two plates. These holes are extended through the face plate by two tubular extensions designed to hold Teflon plugs, which seal the internal chamber and prevent evaporation. The tubular extensions are tapered so that a syringe body (Luer lock without a needle) will fit snugly into them from the outside. The cells are thus filled from a syringe; usually, they are held upright and filled from the bottom entrance port.

These cells are very expensive, and you should try either method A or B before using solution cells. If you do need them, obtain your instructor's permission and receive instruction before using the cells. The cells are purchased in matched pairs, with identical path lengths. Dissolve a solid in a suitable solvent, usually carbon tetrachloride, and add the solution to one of the cells (**sample cell**) as described in the previous paragraph. The pure solvent, identical to that used to dissolve the solid, is placed in the other cell (**reference cell**). The spectrum of the solvent is subtracted from the spectrum of the solution (not always completely), and a spectrum of the solute is thus provided. For the solvent compensation to be as exact as possible and to avoid contamination of the reference cell, it is essential that one cell be used as a reference and that the other cell be used as a sample cell without ever being interchanged. After the spectrum is determined, it is important to clean the cells by flushing them with clean solvent. They should be dried by passing dry air through the cell.

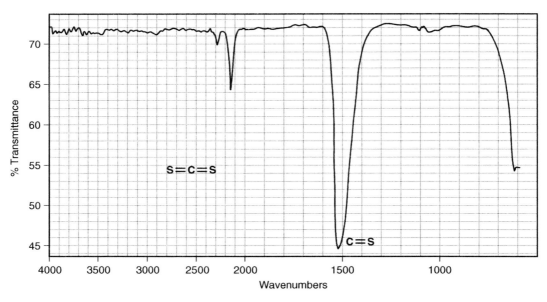

Figure 25.11 Infrared spectrum of carbon disulfide.

Solvents most often used in determining infrared spectra are carbon tetrachloride (Figure 25.8), chloroform (Figure 25.9), and carbon disulfide (Figure 25.11). A 5–10% solution of solid in one of these solvents usually gives a good spectrum. Carbon tetrachloride and chloroform are suspected carcinogens; however, because there are no suitable alternative solvents, these compounds must be used in infrared spectroscopy. The procedure outlined on page 883 for carbon tetrachloride should be followed. This procedure serves equally well for chloroform.

> **Note:** Before you use the solution cells, you must obtain the instructor's permission and instruction on how to fill and clean the cells.

25.7 RECORDING THE SPECTRUM

The instructor will describe how to operate the infrared spectrophotometer, because the controls vary considerably, depending on the manufacturer, model of the instrument, and type. For example, some instruments involve pushing only a few buttons, whereas others use a more complicated computer interface system.

In all cases, it is important that the sample, the solvent, the type of cell or method used, and any other pertinent information be written on the spectrum immediately after the determination. This information may be important, and it is easily forgotten if not recorded. You may also need to calibrate the instrument (Section 25.8).

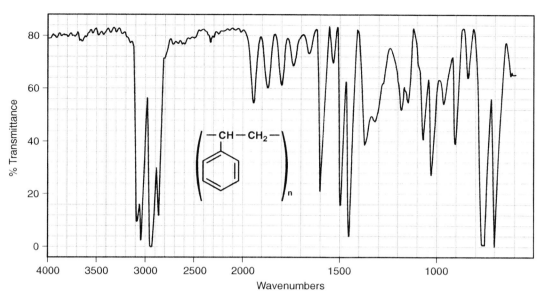

Figure 25.12 Infrared spectrum of polystyrene (thin film).

25.8 CALIBRATION

For some instruments, the frequency scale of the spectrum must be calibrated so that you know the position of each absorption peak precisely. You can recalibrate by recording a very small portion of the spectrum of polystyrene over the spectrum of your sample. The complete spectrum of polystyrene is shown in Figure 25.12. The most important of these peaks is at 1603 cm^{-1}; other useful peaks are at 2850 cm^{-1} and 906 cm^{-1}. After you record the spectrum of your sample, substitute a thin film of polystyrene for the sample cell and record the **tips** (not the entire spectrum) of the most important peaks over the sample spectrum.

It is always a good idea to calibrate a spectrum when the instrument uses chart paper with a preprinted scale. It is difficult to align the paper properly so that the scale matches the absorption lines precisely. You often need to know the precise values for certain functional groups (for example, the carbonyl group). Calibration is essential in these cases.

With computer-interfaced instruments, the instrument does not need to be calibrated. With this type of instrument, the spectrum and scale are printed on blank paper at the same time. The instrument has an internal calibration that ensures that the positions of the absorptions are known precisely and that they are placed at the proper positions on the scale. With this type of instrument, it is often possible to print a list of the locations of the major peaks as well as to obtain the complete spectrum of your compound.

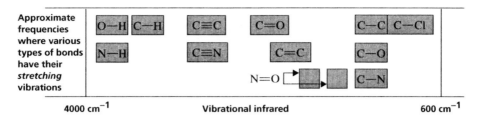

Figure 25.13 Approximate regions in which various common types of bonds absorb. (Bending, twisting, and other types of bond vibration have been omitted for clarity.)

Part B.   Infrared Spectroscopy

25.9 USES OF THE INFRARED SPECTRUM

Because every type of bond has a different natural frequency of vibration and because the same type of bond in two different compounds is in a slightly different environment, no two molecules of different structure have exactly the same infrared absorption pattern, or **infrared spectrum.** Although some of the frequencies absorbed in the two cases might be the same, in no case of two different molecules will their infrared spectra (the patterns of absorption) be identical. Thus, the infrared spectrum can be used to identify molecules much as a fingerprint can be used to identify people. Comparing the infrared spectra of two substances thought to be identical will establish whether or not they are in fact identical. If the infrared spectra of two substances coincide peak for peak (absorption for absorption), in most cases, the substances are identical.

A second and more important use of the infrared spectrum is that it gives structural information about a molecule. The absorptions of each type of bond (N—H, C—H, O—H, C—X, C=O, C—O, C—C, C=C, $C\equiv C$, $C\equiv N$, and so on) are regularly found only in certain small portions of the vibrational infrared region. A small range of absorption can be defined for each type of bond. Outside this range, absorptions will normally be due to some other type of bond. Thus, for instance, any absorption in the range $3000 \pm 150 \text{ cm}^{-1}$ will almost always be due to the presence of a CH bond in the molecule; an absorption in the range $1700 \pm 100 \text{ cm}^{-1}$ will normally be due to the presence of a C=O bond (carbonyl group) in the molecule. The same type of range applies to each type of bond. The way these are spread out over the vibrational infrared is illustrated schematically in Figure 25.13. It is a good idea to remember this general scheme for future convenience.

25.10 MODES OF VIBRATION

The simplest types, or **modes,** of vibrational motion in a molecule that are **infrared active,** that is, give rise to absorptions, are the stretching and bending modes.

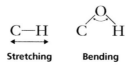

Other, more complex types of stretching and bending are also active, however. To introduce several words of terminology, the normal modes of vibration for a methylene group are shown below.

In any group of three or more atoms—at least two of which are identical—there are *two* modes of stretching or bending: the symmetric mode and asymmetric mode. Examples of such groupings are $-CH_3$, $-CH_2-$, $-NO_2$, $-NH_2$, and anhydrides $(CO)_2O$. For the anhydride, owing to asymmetric and symmetric modes of stretch, this functional group gives *two* absorptions in the $C=O$ region. A similar phenomenon is seen for amino groups, where primary amines usually have *two* absorptions in the NH stretch region, whereas secondary amines R_2NH have only one absorption peak. Amides show similar bands. There are two strong $N=O$ stretch peaks for a nitro group, which are caused by asymmetric and symmetric stretching modes.

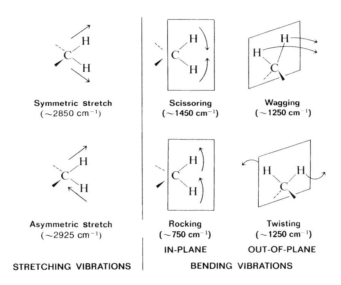

Symmetric Stretch
(~2850 cm⁻¹)

Scissoring
(~1450 cm⁻¹)

Wagging
(~1250 cm⁻¹)

Asymmetric Stretch
(~2925 cm⁻¹)

Rocking
(~750 cm⁻¹)

Twisting
(~1250 cm⁻¹)

IN-PLANE   OUT-OF-PLANE

STRETCHING VIBRATIONS   BENDING VIBRATIONS

25.11 WHAT TO LOOK FOR IN EXAMINING INFRARED SPECTRA

The instrument that determines the absorption spectrum for a compound is called an **infrared spectrophotometer.** The spectrophotometer determines the relative strengths and positions of all the absorptions in the infrared region and plots this information on a piece of paper. This plot of absorption intensity versus wavenumber or wavelength is referred to as the **infrared spectrum** of the compound. A typical infrared spectrum, that of methyl isopropyl ketone, is shown in Figure 25.14.

The strong absorption in the middle of the spectrum corresponds to $C=O$, the carbonyl group. Note that the $C=O$ peak is quite intense. In addition to the characteristic position of absorption, the **shape** and **intensity** of this peak are also unique to the $C=O$ bond. This is true for almost every type of absorption peak; both shape and intensity characteristics can be described, and these characteristics often make it possible to distinguish the peak

303

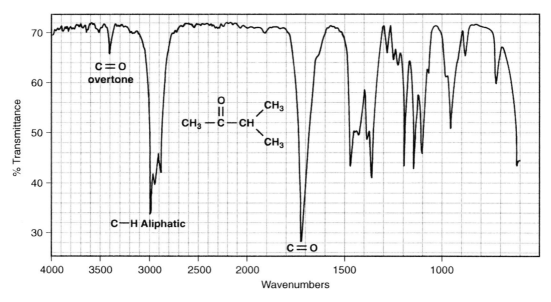

Figure 25.14 Infrared spectrum of methyl isopropyl ketone (neat liquid, salt plates).

in a confusing situation. For instance, to some extent both $C{=}O$ and $C{=}C$ bonds absorb in the same region of the infrared spectrum:

$$C{=}O \quad 1850\text{–}1630 \text{ cm}^{-1}$$
$$C{=}C \quad 1680\text{–}1620 \text{ cm}^{-1}$$

However, the $C{=}O$ bond is a strong absorber, whereas the $C{=}C$ bond generally absorbs only weakly. Hence, a trained observer would not normally interpret a strong peak at 1670 cm^{-1} to be a carbon–carbon double bond nor a weak absorption at this frequency to be due to a carbonyl group.

The shape of a peak often gives a clue to its identity as well. Thus, although the NH and OH regions of the infrared overlap,

$$OH \quad 3650\text{–}3200 \text{ cm}^{-1}$$
$$NH \quad 3500\text{–}3300 \text{ cm}^{-1}$$

NH usually gives a **sharp** absorption peak (absorbs a very narrow range of frequencies), and OH, when it is in the NH region, usually gives a **broad** absorption peak. Primary amines give *two* absorptions in this region, whereas alcohols give only one.

Therefore, while you are studying the sample spectra in the pages that follow, you should also notice shapes and intensities. They are as important as the frequency at which an absorption occurs, and you must train your eye to recognize these features. In the literature of organic chemistry, you will often find absorptions referred to as strong (s), medium (m), weak (w), broad, or sharp. The author is trying to convey some idea of what the peak looks like without actually drawing the spectrum. Although the intensity of an absorption often provides useful information about the identity of a peak, be aware that the relative intensities of all the peaks in the spectrum are dependent on the amount of sample that is used and the sensitivity setting of the instrument. Therefore, the *actual* intensity of a particular peak may vary from spectrum to spectrum, and you must pay attention to *relative* intensities.

25.12 CORRELATION CHARTS AND TABLES

To extract structural information from infrared spectra, you must know the frequencies or wavelengths at which various functional groups absorb. Infrared **correlation tables** present as much information as is known about where the various functional groups absorb. The books listed at the end of this chapter present extensive lists of correlation tables. Sometimes, the absorption information is given in a chart, called a **correlation chart.** A simplified correlation table is given in Table 25.1.

Although you may think assimilating the mass of data in Table 25.1 will be difficult, it is not if you make a modest start and then gradually increase your familiarity with the data. An ability to interpret the fine details of an infrared spectrum will follow. This is most easily accomplished by first establishing the broad visual patterns of Figure 25.13 firmly in mind. Then, as a second step, a "typical absorption value" can be memorized for each of the functional groups in this pattern. This value will be a single number that can be used as a pivot value for the memory. For instance, start with a simple aliphatic ketone as a model for all typical carbonyl compounds. The typical aliphatic ketone has carbonyl absorption of 1715 ± 10 cm^{-1}. Without worrying about the variation, memorize 1715 cm^{-1} as the base value for carbonyl absorption. Then learn the extent of the carbonyl range and the visual pattern of how the different kinds of carbonyl groups are arranged throughout this region. See, for instance, Figure 25.27 (page 902), which gives typical values for carbonyl compounds. Also learn how factors such as ring size (when the functional group is contained in a ring) and conjugation affect the base values (that is, in which direction the values are shifted). Learn the trends—always remembering the base value (1715 cm^{-1}). It might prove useful as a beginning to memorize the base values in Table 25.2 for this approach. Notice that there are only eight values.

25.13 ANALYZING A SPECTRUM (OR WHAT YOU CAN TELL AT A GLANCE)

In analyzing the spectrum of an unknown, concentrate first on establishing the presence (or absence) of a few major functional groups. The most conspicuous peaks are C=O, O—H, N—H, C—O, C=C, C≡C, C≡N, and NO$_2$. If they are present, they give immediate structural information. Do not try to analyze in detail the CH absorptions near 3000 cm^{-1}; almost all compounds have these absorptions. Do not worry about subtleties of the exact type of environment in which the functional group is found. A checklist of the important gross features follows:

1. Is a carbonyl group present?
   The C=O group gives rise to a strong absorption in the region 1820–1600 cm^{-1}. The peak is often the strongest in the spectrum and of medium width. You can't miss it.
2. If C=O is present, check the following types. (If it is absent, go to item 3.)
   Acids   Is O—H also present?

TABLE 25.1 A Simplified Correlation Table

	Type of Vibration		Frequency (cm⁻¹)	Intensity[a]
C—H	Alkanes	(stretch)	3000–2850	s
	—CH₃	(bend)	1450 and 1375	m
	—CH₂—	(bend)	1465	m
	Alkenes	(stretch)	3100–3000	m
		(bend)	1700–1000	s
	Aromatics	(stretch)	3150–3050	s
		(out-of-plane bend)	1000–700	s
	Alkyne	(stretch)	ca. 3300	s
	Aldehyde		2900–2800	w
			2800–2700	w
C—C	Alkane	Not interpretatively useful		
C=C	Alkene		1680–1600	m–w
	Aromatic		1600–1400	m–w
C≡C	Alkyne		2250–2100	m–w
C=O	Aldehyde		1740–1720	s
	Ketone (acyclic)		1725–1705	s
	Carboxylic acid		1725–1700	s
	Ester		1750–1730	s
	Amide		1700–1640	s
	Anhydride		ca. 1810	s
			ca. 1760	s
C—O	Alcohols, ethers, esters, carboxylic acids		1300–1000	s
O—H	Alcohol, phenols			
	Free		3650–3600	m
	H-Bonded		3400–3200	m
	Carboxylic acids		3300–2500	m
N—H	Primary and secondary amines		ca. 3500	m
C≡N	Nitriles		2260–2240	m
N=O	Nitro (R—NO₂)		1600–1500	s
			1400–1300	s
C—X	Fluoride		1400–1000	s
	Chloride		800–600	s
	Bromide, iodide		< 600	s

[a]s, strong; m, medium; w, weak.

TABLE 25.2 Base Values for Absorptions of Bonds

O—H	3400 cm⁻¹	C≡C	2150 cm⁻¹
N—H	3500 cm⁻¹	C=O	1715 cm⁻¹
C—H	3000 cm⁻¹	C=C	1650 cm⁻¹
C≡N	2250 cm⁻¹	C—O	1100 cm⁻¹

	Broad absorption near 3300–2500 cm^{-1} (usually overlaps C—H).
Amides	Is N—H also present?
	Medium absorption near 3500 cm^{-1}, sometimes a double peak, equivalent halves.
Esters	Is C—O also present?
	Medium intensity absorptions near 1300–1000 cm^{-1}.
Anhydrides	Have *two* C=O absorptions near 1810 and 1760 cm^{-1}.
Aldehydes	Is aldehyde C—H present?
	Two weak absorptions near 2850 cm^{-1} and 2750 cm^{-1} on the right side of C—H absorptions.
Ketones	The preceding five choices have been eliminated.

3. If C=O is absent

Alcohols	Check for O—H.
or Phenols	**Broad** absorption near 3600–3300 cm^{-1}.
	Confirm this by finding C—O near 1300–1000 cm^{-1}.
Amines	Check for N—H.
	Medium absorption(s) near 3500 cm^{-1}.
Ethers	Check for C—O (and absence of O—H) near 1300–1000 cm^{-1}.

4. Double bonds or aromatic rings or both

C=C is a **weak** absorption near 1650 cm^{-1}.

Medium to strong absorptions in the region 1650–1450 cm^{-1} often imply an aromatic ring.

Confirm the above by consulting the C—H region.

Aromatic and vinyl C—H occur to the left of 3000 cm^{-1} (aliphatic C—H occurs to the right of this value).

5. Triple bonds

C≡N is a medium, sharp absorption near 2250 cm^{-1}.

C≡C is a weak but sharp absorption near 2150 cm^{-1}.

Check also for acetylenic C—H near 3300 cm^{-1}.

6. Nitro groups   *Two* strong absorptions near 1600–1500 cm^{-1} and 1390–1300 cm^{-1}.

7. Hydrocarbons   None of the above is found.

Main absorptions are in the C—H region near 3000 cm^{-1}.

Very simple spectrum, only other absorptions are near 1450 cm^{-1} and 1375 cm^{-1}.

The beginning student should resist the idea of trying to assign or interpret *every* peak in the spectrum. You simply will not be able to do this. Concentrate first on learning the principal peaks and recognizing their presence or absence. This is best done by carefully studying the illustrative spectra in the section that follows.

Note: In describing the shifts of absorption peaks or their relative positions, we have used the phrases "to the left" and "to the right." This was done to simplify descriptions of peak positions. The meaning is clear, because all spectra are conventionally presented left to right from 4000 to 600 cm^{-1}.

25.14 SURVEY OF THE IMPORTANT FUNCTIONAL GROUPS

A. Alkanes

The spectrum is usually simple, with a few peaks.

C—H   Stretch occurs around 3000 cm^{-1}.
  1. In alkanes (except strained ring compounds), absorption always occurs to the right of 3000 cm^{-1}.
  2. If a compound has vinylic, aromatic, acetylenic, or cyclopropyl hydrogens, the CH absorption is to the left of 3000 cm^{-1}.

CH$_2$ Methylene groups have a characteristic absorption at approximately 1450 cm^{-1}.

CH$_3$ Methyl groups have a characteristic absorption at approximately 1375 cm^{-1}.

C—C   Stretch—not interpretatively useful—has many peaks.

The spectrum of decane is shown in Figure 25.15.

B. Alkenes

=C—H   Stretch occurs to the left of 3000 cm^{-1}.

=C—H   Out-of-plane (oop) bending occurs at 1000–650 cm^{-1}.
  The C—H out-of-plane absorptions often allow you to determine the type of substitution pattern on the double bond, according to the number of absorptions and their positions. The correlation chart in Figure 25.16 shows the positions of these bands.

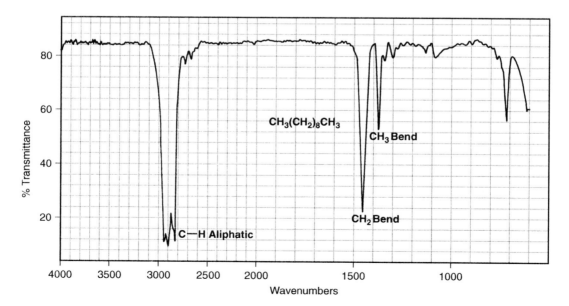

Figure 25.15   Infrared spectrum of decane (neat liquid, salt plates).

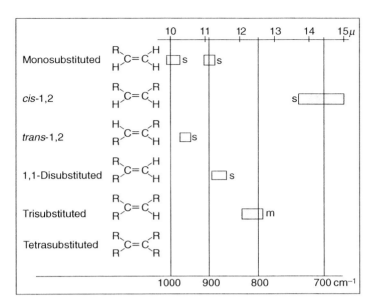

Figure 25.16 The C—H out-of-plane bending vibrations for substituted alkenes.

C=C   Stretch 1675–1600cm^{-1}, often weak.

Conjugation moves C=C stretch to the right.

Symmetrically substituted bonds, as in 2,3-dimethyl-2-butene, do not absorb in the infrared region (no dipole change). Highly substituted double bonds are often vanishingly weak in absorption.

The spectra of 4-methylcyclohexene and styrene are shown in Figures 25.17 and 25.18.

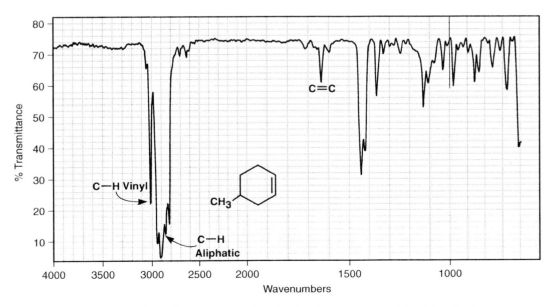

Figure 25.17 Infrared spectrum of 4-methylcyclohexene (neat liquid, salt plates).

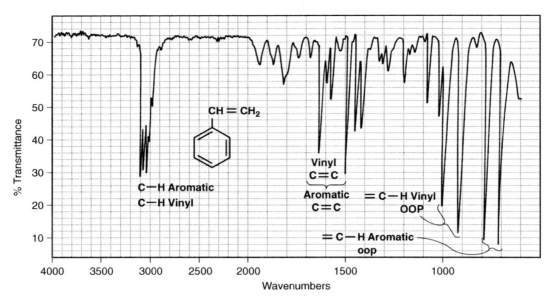

Figure 25.18 Infrared spectrum of styrene (neat liquid, salt plates).

C. Aromatic Rings

=C—H Stretch is always to the left of 3000 cm^{-1}.

=C—H Out-of-plane (oop) bending occurs at 900 to 690 cm^{-1}.

      The C—H out-of-plane absorptions often allow you to determine the type of ring substitution by their numbers, intensities, and positions. The correlation chart in Figure 25.19A indicates the positions of these bands.

      The patterns are generally reliable—they are most reliable for rings with alkyl substituents and least reliable for polar substituents.

    Ring Absorptions (C=C). There are often four sharp absorptions that occur in pairs at 1600 cm^{-1} and 1450 cm^{-1} and are characteristic of an aromatic ring. See, for example, the spectra of anisole (Figure 25.23), benzonitrile (Figure 25.26), and methyl benzoate (Figure 25.35).

    There are many weak combination and overtone absorptions that appear between 2000 cm^{-1} and 1667 cm^{-1}. The relative shapes and numbers of these peaks can be used to determine whether an aromatic ring is monosubstituted or di-, tri-, tetra-, penta-, or hexasubstituted. Positional isomers can also be distinguished. Because the absorptions are weak, these bands are best observed by using neat liquids or concentrated solutions. If the compound has a high-frequency carbonyl group, this absorption overlaps the weak overtone bands, so no useful information can be obtained from analyzing this region. The various patterns that are obtained in this region are shown in Figure 25.19B.

    The spectra of styrene and *o*-dichlorobenzene are shown in Figures 25.18 and 25.20.

D. Alkynes

≡C—H Stretch is usually near 3300 cm^{-1}, sharp peak.

C≡C Stretch is near 2150 cm^{-1}, sharp peak.

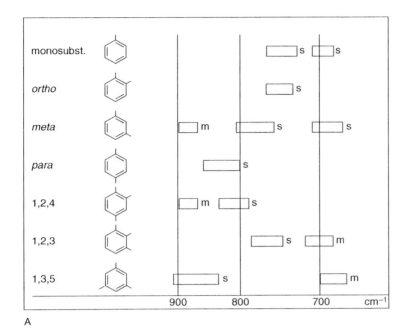
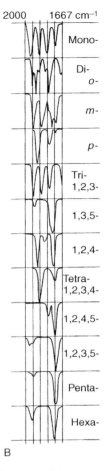

Figure 25.19 (A) The C—H out-of-plane bending vibrations for substituted benzenoid compounds. (B) The 2000–1667 cm-1 region for substituted benzenoid compounds. (From John R. Dyer, *Applications of Absorption Spectroscopy of Organic Compounds*, Englewood Cliffs, NJ: Prentice Hall, 1965.)

Conjugation moves C≡C stretch to the right.

Disubstituted or symmetrically substituted triple bonds give either no absorption or weak absorption.

E. Alcohols and Phenols

O—H   Stretch is a sharp peak at 3650–3600 cm^{-1} if no hydrogen bonding takes place. (This is usually observed only in dilute solutions.)

If there is hydrogen bonding (usual in neat or concentrated solutions), the absorption is *broad* and occurs more to the right at 3500–3200 cm^{-1}, sometimes overlapping C—H stretch absorptions.

C—O   Stretch is usually in the range of 1300–1000 cm^{-1}.

Phenols are like alcohols. The 2-naphthol shown in Figure 25.21 has some molecules hydrogen bonded and some free. The spectrum of

311

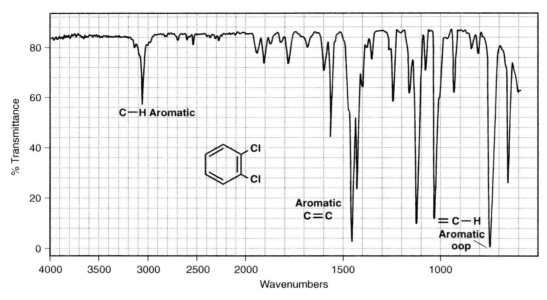

Figure 25.20 Infrared spectrum of *o*-dichlorobenzene (neat liquid, salt plates).

4-methylcyclohexanol is shown in Figure 25.22. This alcohol, which was determined neat, would also have had a free OH spike to the left of this hydrogen-bonded band if it had been determined in dilute solution.

F. Ethers

C—O   The most prominent band is due to C—O stretch at 1300–1000 cm^{-1}. Absence of C=O and O—H bands is required to be sure C—O stretch is not due to an alcohol or ester. Phenyl and vinyl ethers are found in the left portion of the range, aliphatic ethers in the right. (Conjugation with the oxygen moves the absorption to the left.)

The spectrum of anisole is shown in Figure 25.23.

G. Amines

N—H   Stretch occurs in the range of 3500–3300 cm^{-1}.
        Primary amines have *two* bands typically 30 cm^{-1} apart.
        Secondary amines have one band, often vanishingly weak.
        Tertiary amines have no NH stretch.
C—N   Stretch is weak and occurs in the range of 1350–1000 cm^{-1}.
N—H   Scissoring bending mode occurs in the range of 1640–1560 cm^{-1} (broad).
        An out-of-plane bending absorption can sometimes be observed at about 800 cm^{-1}.

The spectrum of *n*-butylamine is shown in Figure 25.24.

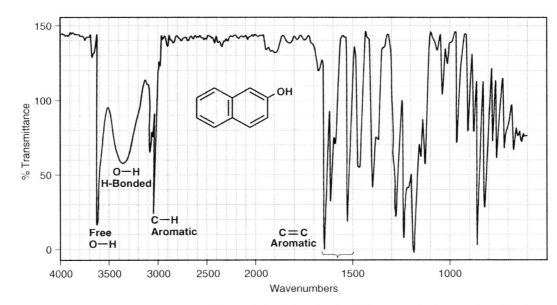

Figure 25.21 Infrared spectrum of 2-naphthol showing both free and hydrogen-bonded OH (CHCl$_3$ solution).

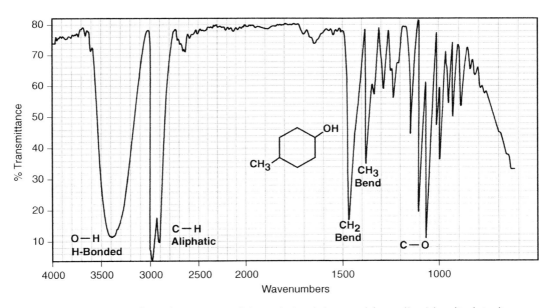

Figure 25.22 Infrared spectrum of 4-methylcyclohexanol (neat liquid, salt plates).

H. Nitro Compounds

N=O   Stretch is usually two strong bands at 1600–1500 cm^{-1} and 1390–1300 cm^{-1}.

The spectrum of nitrobenzene is shown in Figure 25.25.

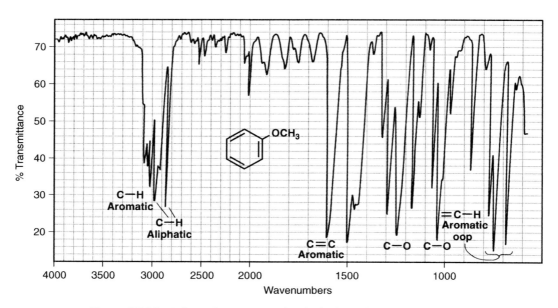

Figure 25.23 Infrared spectrum of anisole (neat liquid, salt plates).

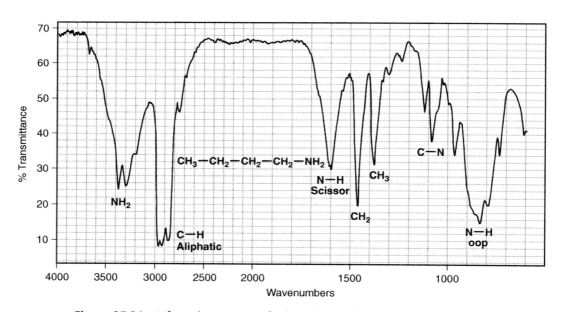

Figure 25.24 Infrared spectrum of *n*-butylamine (neat liquid, salt plates).

I. Nitriles

C≡N   Stretch is a sharp absorption near 2250 cm^{-1}.
Conjugation with double bonds or aromatic rings moves the absorption to the right.

The spectrum of benzonitrile is shown in Figure 25.26.

314

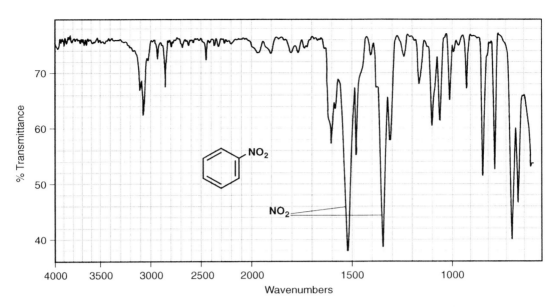

Figure 25.25 Infrared spectrum of nitrobenzene (neat liquid, salt plates).

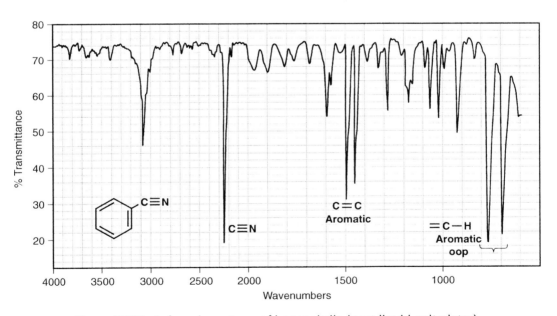

Figure 25.26 Infrared spectrum of benzonitrile (neat liquid, salt plates).

J. Carbonyl Compounds

The carbonyl group is one of the most strongly absorbing groups in the infrared region of the spectrum. This is mainly due to its large dipole moment. It absorbs in a variety of compounds (aldehydes, ketones, acids, esters, amides, anhydrides, and so on) in the range of 1850–1650 cm^{-1}. In Figure 25.27, the normal values for the various types of carbonyl groups are compared. In the sections that follow, each type is examined separately.

315

1810	1760	1735	1725	1715	1710	1690	cm⁻¹
Anhydride (Band 1)		Esters		Ketones		Amides	
	Anhydride (Band 2)		Aldehydes		Carboxylic acids		

Figure 25.27   Normal values (± 10 cm^{-1}) for various types of carbonyl groups.

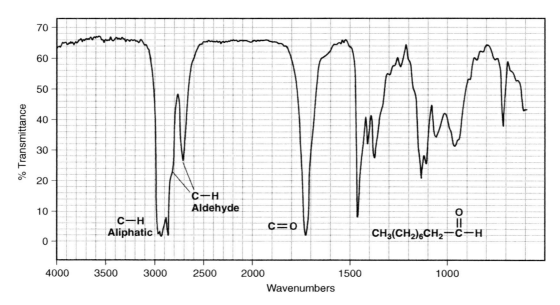

Figure 25.28   Infrared spectrum of nonanal (neat liquid, salt plates).

K. Aldehydes

C=O   Stretch at approximately 1725 cm^{-1} is normal.
Aldehydes *seldom* absorb to the left of this value.
Conjugation moves the absorption to the right.

C—H   Stretch, aldehyde hydrogen (—CHO), consists of *weak* bands at about
2750 cm^{-1} and 2850 cm^{-1}. Note that the CH stretch in alkyl chains does
not usually extend this far to the right.

The spectrum of an unconjugated aldehyde, nonanal, is shown in Figure 25.28, and the conjugated aldehyde, benzaldehyde, is shown in Figure 25.29.

L. Ketones

C=O   Stretch at approximately at 1715 cm^{-1} is normal.
Conjugation moves the absorption to the right.
Ring strain moves the absorption to the left in cyclic ketones. (See Figure 25.30.)

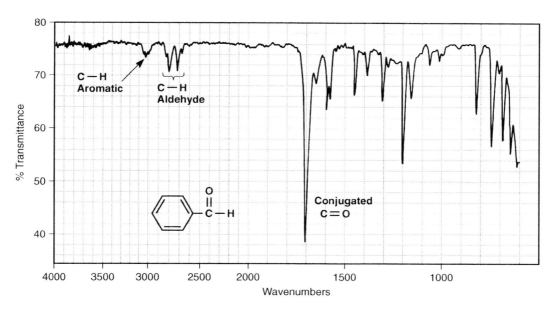

Figure 25.29 Infrared spectrum of benzaldehyde (neat liquid, salt plates).

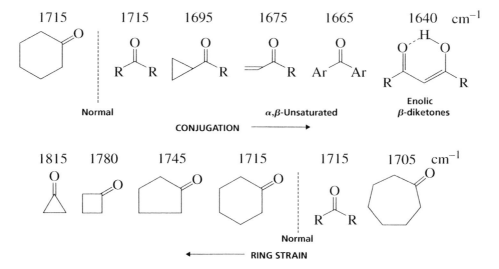

Figure 25.30 Effects of conjugation and ring strain on carbonyl frequencies in ketones.

The spectra of methyl isopropyl ketone and mesityl oxide are shown in Figures 25.14 and 25.31. The spectrum of camphor, shown in Figure 25.32, has a carbonyl group that has been shifted to a higher frequency because of ring strain (1745 cm^{-1}).

M. Acids

O—H   Stretch, usually *very broad* (strongly hydrogen bonded) at 3300–2500 cm^{-1}, often interferes with C—H absorptions.

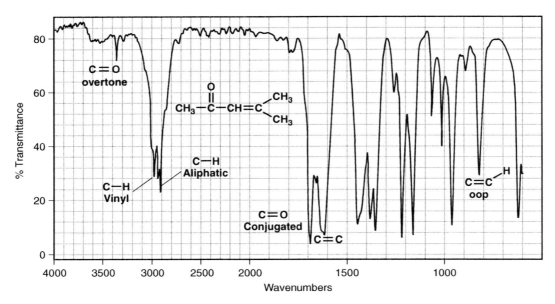

Figure 25.31 Infrared spectrum of mesityl oxide (neat liquid, salt plates).

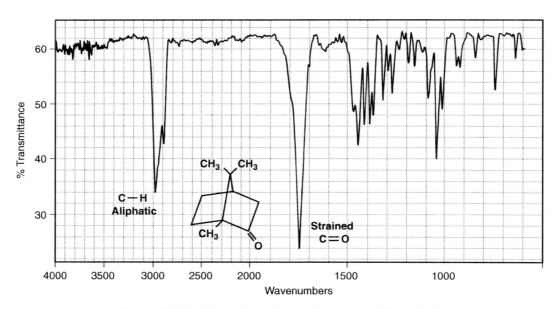

Figure 25.32 Infrared spectrum of camphor (KBr pellet).

C=O   Stretch, broad, 1730–1700 cm^{-1}.
       Conjugation moves the absorption to the right.
C—O   Stretch, in the range of 1320–1210 cm^{-1}, is strong.

The spectrum of benzoic acid is shown in Figure 25.33.

318

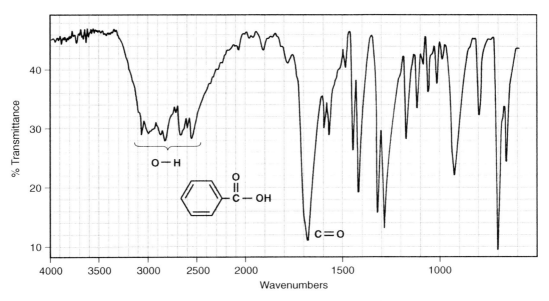

Figure 25.33 Infrared spectrum of benzoic acid (KBr pellet).

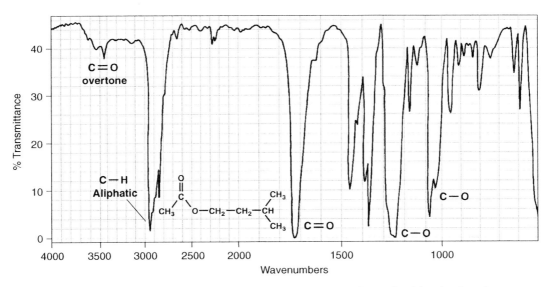

Figure 25.34 Infrared spectrum of isopentyl acetate (neat liquid, salt plates).

N. Esters (R—C(=O)—OR′)

C=O   Stretch occurs at about 1735 cm^{-1} in normal esters.

1. Conjugation in the R part moves the absorption to the right.
2. Conjugation with the O in the R′ part moves the absorption to the left.
3. Ring strain (lactones) moves the absorption to the left.

319

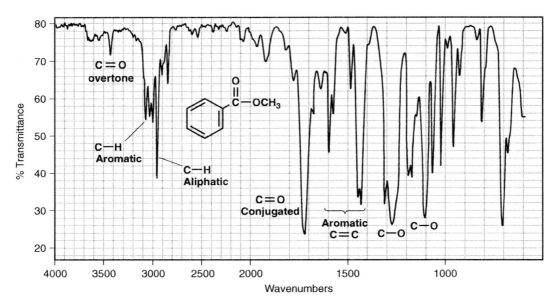

Figure 25.35 Infrared spectrum of methyl benzoate (neat liquid, salt plates).

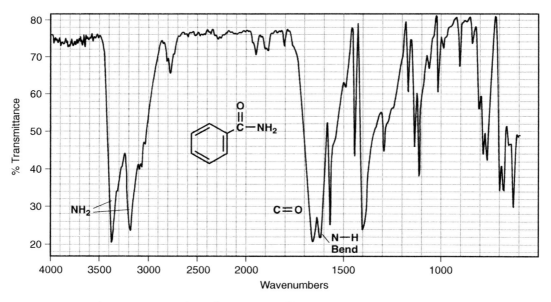

Figure 25.36 Infrared spectrum of benzamide (solid phase, KBr).

C—O   Stretch, two bands or more, one stronger than the others, is in the range of 1300–1000 cm^{-1}.

The spectrum of an unconjugated ester, isopentyl acetate, is shown in Figure 25.34 (C=O appears at 1740 cm^{-1}). A conjugated ester, methyl benzoate, is shown in Figure 25.35 (C=O appears at 1720 cm^{-1}).

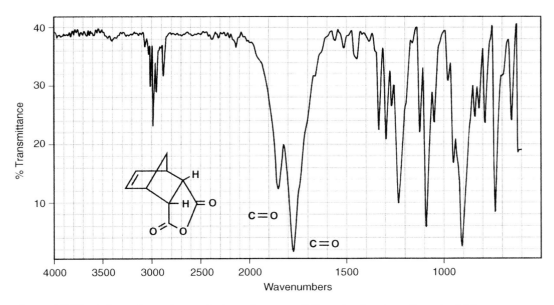

Figure 25.37 Infrared spectrum of *cis*-norbornene-5,6-*endo*-dicarboxylic anhydride (KBr pellet).

O. Amides

C=O   Stretch is at approximately 1670–1640 cm^{-1}.
        Conjugation and ring size (lactams) have the usual effects.
N—H   Stretch (if monosubstituted or unsubstituted) is at 3500–3100 cm^{-1}.
        Unsubstituted amides have two bands (—NH$_2$) in this region.
N—H   Bending around 1640–1550 cm^{-1}.

The spectrum of benzamide is shown in Figure 25.36.

P. Anhydrides

C=O   Stretch always has *two* bands: 1830–1800 cm^{-1} and 1775–1740 cm^{-1}.
        Unsaturation moves the absorptions to the right.
        Ring strain (cyclic anhydrides) moves the absorptions to the left.
C—O   Stretch is at 1300–900 cm^{-1}. The spectrum of *cis*-norbornene-5,6-*endo*-dicarboxylic anhydride is shown in Figure 25.37.

Q. Halides

It is often difficult to determine either the presence or the absence of a halide in a compound by infrared spectroscopy. The absorption bands cannot be relied on, especially if the spectrum is being determined with the compound dissolved in CCl$_4$ or CHCl$_3$ solution.

C—F   Stretch, 1350–960 cm^{-1}.
C—Cl   Stretch, 850–500 cm^{-1}.

321

C—Br   Stretch, to the right of 667 cm^{-1}.
C—I   Stretch, to the right of 667 cm^{-1}.

The spectra of the solvents, carbon tetrachloride and chloroform, are shown in Figures 25.8 and 25.9, respectively.

REFERENCES

Bellamy, L. J. *The Infra-red Spectra of Complex Molecules,* 3rd ed. New York: Methuen, 1975.

Colthup, N. B., Daly, L. H., and Wiberly, S. E. *Introduction to Infrared and Raman Spectroscopy,* 3rd ed. San Diego, CA: Academic Press, 1990.

Dyer, J. R. *Applications of Absorption Spectroscopy of Organic Compounds.* Englewood Cliffs, NJ: Prentice-Hall, 1965.

Lin-Vien, D., Colthup, N. B., Fateley, W. G., and Grasselli, J. G. *Infrared and Raman Characteristic Frequencies of Organic Molecules.* San Diego, CA: Academic Press, 1991.

Nakanishi, K., and Soloman, P. H. *Infrared Absorption Spectroscopy,* 2nd ed. San Francisco: Holden-Day, 1977.

Pavia, D. L., Lampman, G. M., and Kriz, G. S. *Introduction to Spectroscopy: A Guide for Students of Organic Chemistry,* 3rd ed. Philadelphia: Saunders, 2001.

Silverstein, R. M., and Webster, F. X. *Spectrometric Identification of Organic Compounds,* 6th ed., New York: John Wiley & Sons, 1998.

PROBLEMS

1. Comment on the suitability of running the infrared spectrum under each of the following conditions. If there is a problem with the conditions given, provide a suitable alternative method.

  a. A neat spectrum of liquid with a boiling point of 150°C is determined using salt plates.
  b. A neat spectrum of a liquid with a boiling point of 35°C is determined using salt plates.
  c. A KBr pellet is prepared with a compound that melts at 200°C.
  d. A KBr pellet is prepared with a compound that melts at 30°C.
  e. A solid aliphatic hydrocarbon compound is determined as a Nujol mull.
  f. Silver chloride plates are used to determine the spectrum of aniline.
  g. Sodium chloride plates are selected to run the spectrum of a compound that contains some water.

2. Indicate how you could distinguish between the following pairs of compounds by using infrared spectroscopy.

a. $CH_3CH_2CH_2\overset{\displaystyle O}{\overset{\displaystyle \|}{C}}\!-\!H$ 　　　　　　$CH_3CH_2\overset{\displaystyle O}{\overset{\displaystyle \|}{C}}CH_3$

b. 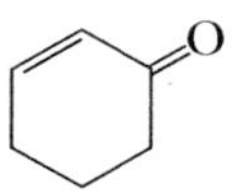 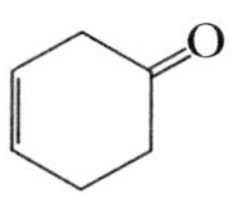 　　　　　　

c. $CH_3CH_2\overset{\displaystyle H}{\overset{\displaystyle |}{N}}CH_2CH_3$ 　　　　　　$CH_3CH_2CH_2CH_2NH_2$

d. $CH_3CH_2\overset{\displaystyle O}{\overset{\|}{C}}OCH_2CH_3$ $CH_3CH_2\overset{\displaystyle O}{\overset{\|}{C}}CH_2OCH_3$

e. $CH_3CH_2\overset{\displaystyle O}{\overset{\|}{C}}OH$ $CH_3CH_2CH_2OH$

f.

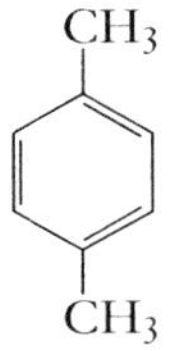

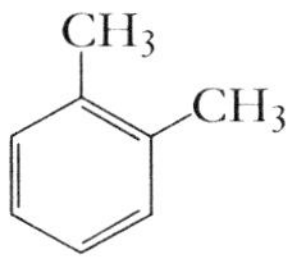

g. $CH_3CH_2CH{=}CH_2$ $CH_3CH{=}CHCH_3$ (trans)

h. $CH_3CH_2CH_2C{\equiv}CH$ $CH_3CH_2CH_2CH{=}CH_2$

i.

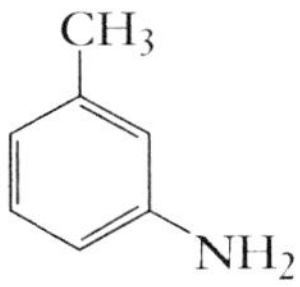

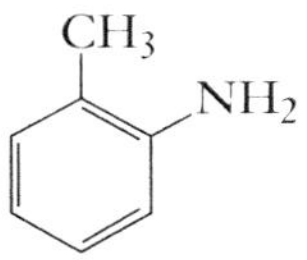

j. $CH_3CH_2CH_2CH_2\overset{\displaystyle O}{\overset{\|}{C}}{-}OH$ $CH_3CH_2CH_2\overset{\displaystyle O}{\overset{\|}{C}}OCH_3$

k. $CH_3CH_2CH_2CH_2CH_3$ $CH_2{=}CHCH_2CH_2CH_2CH_3$

l. $CH_3CH_2CH_2CH_2C{\equiv}CH$ $CH_3CH_2CH_2C{\equiv}CCH_3$

T E C H N I Q U E   2 9

Guide to the Chemical Literature

Often, you may need to go beyond the information contained in the typical organic chemistry textbook and to use reference material in the library. At first glance, using library materials may seem formidable because of the numerous sources the library contains. If, however, you adopt a systematic approach, the task can prove rather useful. This description of various popular sources and an outline of logical steps to follow in the typical literature search should be helpful.

29.1 LOCATING PHYSICAL CONSTANTS: HANDBOOKS

To find information on routine physical constants, such as melting points, boiling points, indices of refraction, and densities, you should first consider a handbook. Examples of suitable handbooks are

Aldrich Handbook of Fine Chemicals. Milwaukee, WI: Sigma-Aldrich, 2003–2004.
Budavari, S., ed. *The Merck Index,* 12th ed. Whitehouse Station, NJ: Merck, 1996.
Dean, J. A., ed. *Lange's Handbook of Chemistry,* 14th ed. New York: McGraw-Hill, 1992.
Lide, D. R., ed. *CRC Handbook of Chemistry and Physics,* 80th ed. Boca Raton, FL: CRC Press, 1999.

Each of these references is discussed in detail in Technique 4. The *CRC Handbook* is the reference consulted most often because the book is so widely available. There are, however, distinct advantages to using the other handbooks. The *CRC Handbook* uses the *Chemical Abstracts* system of nomenclature that requires you to identify the parent name; 3-methyl-1-butanol is listed as 1-butanol, 3-methyl.

The Merck Index has fewer compounds listed, but for the ones listed, there is far more information provided. If the compound is a medicinal or natural product, this is the reference of choice. This handbook contains literature references on the isolation and synthesis of a compound, along with certain properties of medicinal interest, such as toxicity. *Lange's Handbook* and the *Aldrich Handbook* list compounds in alphabetical order; 3-methyl-1-butanol is listed as 3-methyl-1-butanol.

A more complete handbook that is usually housed in the library is

Buckingham, J., ed. *Dictionary of Organic Compounds.* New York: Chapman & Hall/Methuen, 1982–1992.

This is a revised version of an earlier four-volume handbook edited by I. M. Heilbron and H. M. Bunbury. In its present form, it consists of seven volumes with 10 supplements.

29.2 GENERAL SYNTHETIC METHODS

Many standard introductory textbooks in organic chemistry provide tables that summarize most of the common reactions, including side reactions, for a given class of compounds. These books also describe alternative methods of preparing compounds.

Brown, W. H., and Foote, C. *Organic Chemistry,* 3rd ed. Pacific Grove, CA: Brooks/Cole, 2002.

Carey, F. A. *Organic Chemistry,* 5th ed. New York: McGraw-Hill, 2003.

Ege, S. *Organic Chemistry,* 5th ed. Boston: Houghton-Mifflin, 2004.

Fessenden, R. J., and Fessenden, J. S. *Organic Chemistry,* 6th ed. Pacific Grove, CA: Brooks/Cole, 1998.

Fox, M. A., and Whitesell, J. K. *Organic Chemistry,* 2nd ed. Boston: Jones & Bartlett, 1997.

Hornback, Joe, *Organic Chemistry.* Pacific Grove, CA: Brooks/Cole, 1998.

Jones, M., Jr. *Organic Chemistry,* 3rd ed. New York: W. W. Norton, 2003.

Loudon, G. M. *Organic Chemistry,* 4th ed. Menlo Park, CA: Benjamin/Cummings, 2004.

McMurry, J. *Organic Chemistry,* 6th ed. Pacific Grove, CA: Brooks/Cole, 2004.

Morrison, R. T., and Boyd, R. N. *Organic Chemistry,* 7th ed. Englewood Cliffs, NJ: Prentice-Hall, 1999.

Smith, M. B., and March, J. *Advanced Organic Chemistry,* 5th ed. New York: John Wiley & Sons, 2001.

Solomons, T. W. G., and Fryhle, C. *Organic Chemistry,* 8th ed. New York: John Wiley & Sons, 2003.

Streitwieser, A., Heathcock, C. H., and Kosower, E. M. *Introduction to Organic Chemistry,* 4th ed. New York: Prentice-Hall, 1992.

Vollhardt, K. P. C., and Schore, N. E. *Organic Chemistry,* 4th ed. New York: W. H. Freeman, 2003.

Wade, L. G., Jr. *Organic Chemistry,* 5th ed. Englewood Cliffs, NJ: Prentice-Hall, 2003.

29.3 SEARCHING THE CHEMICAL LITERATURE

If the information you are seeking is not available in any of the handbooks mentioned in Section 29.1 or if you are searching for more detailed information than they can provide, then a proper literature search is in order. Although an examination of standard textbooks can provide some help, you often must use all the resources of the library, including journals, reference collections, and abstracts. The following sections outline how the various types of sources should be used and what sort of information can be obtained from them.

The methods discussed for searching the literature use mainly printed materials. Modern search methods also make use of computerized databases and are discussed in Section 29.11. These are vast collections of data and bibliographic materials that can be scanned very rapidly from remote computer terminals. Although computerized searching is widely available, its use may not be readily accessible to undergraduate students. The following references provide excellent introductions to the literature of organic chemistry:

Carr, C. "Teaching and Using Chemical Information." *Journal of Chemical Education, 70* (September 1993): 719.

Maizell, R. E. *How to Find Chemical Information,* 3rd ed. New York: John Wiley & Sons, 1998.

Smith, M. B., and March, J. *Advanced Organic Chemistry,* 5th ed. New York: John Wiley & Sons, 2001.

Somerville, A. N. "Information Sources for Organic Chemistry, 1: Searching by Name Reaction and Reaction Type." *Journal of Chemical Education, 68* (July 1991): 553.

Somerville, A. N. "Information Sources for Organic Chemistry, 2: Searching by Functional Group." *Journal of Chemical Education, 68* (October 1991): 842.

Somerville, A. N. "Information Sources for Organic Chemistry, 3: Searching by Reagent." *Journal of Chemical Education, 69* (May 1992): 379.

Wiggins, G. *Chemical Information Sources.* New York: McGraw-Hill, 1991. Integrates printed materials and computer sources of information.

29.4 COLLECTIONS OF SPECTRA

Collections of infrared, nuclear magnetic resonance, and mass spectra can be found in the following catalogues of spectra:

Cornu, A., and Massot, R. *Compilation of Mass Spectral Data,* 2nd ed. London: Heyden and Sons, 1975.

High-Resolution NMR Spectra Catalog. Palo Alto, CA: Varian Associates. Vol. 1, 1962; Vol. 2, 1963.

Johnson, L. F., and Jankowski, W. C. *Carbon-13 NMR Spectra.* New York: John Wiley & Sons, 1972.

Pouchert, C. J. *Aldrich Library of Infrared Spectra,* 3rd ed. Milwaukee: Aldrich Chemical Co., 1981.

Pouchert, C. J. *Aldrich Library of FT-IR Spectra,* 2nd ed. Milwaukee: Aldrich Chemical Co., 1997.

Pouchert, C. J. *Aldrich Library of NMR Spectra,* 2nd ed. Milwaukee: Aldrich Chemical Co., 1983.

Pouchert, C. J., and Behnke, J. *Aldrich Library of ^{13}C and ^{1}H FT NMR Spectra.* Milwaukee: Aldrich Chemical Co., 1993.

Sadtler Standard Spectra. Philadelphia: Sadtler Research Laboratories. Continuing collection.

Stenhagen, E., Abrahamsson, S., and McLafferty, F. W. *Registry of Mass Spectral Data,* 4 vols. New York: Wiley-Interscience, 1974.

The American Petroleum Institute has also published collections of infrared, nuclear magnetic resonance, and mass spectra.

29.5 ADVANCED TEXTBOOKS

Much information about synthetic methods, reaction mechanisms, and reactions of organic compounds is available in any of the many current advanced textbooks in organic chemistry. Examples of such books are

Carey, F. A., and Sundberg, R. J. *Advanced Organic Chemistry. Part A. Structure and Mechanisms; Part B. Reactions and Synthesis,* 4th ed. New York: Kluwer Academic, 2001.

Carruthers, W. *Some Modern Methods of Organic Synthesis,* 3rd ed. Cambridge, UK: Cambridge University Press, 1986.

Corey, E. J., and Cheng, Xue-Min. *The Logic of Chemical Synthesis.* New York: John Wiley & Sons, 1989.

Fieser, L. F., and Fieser, M. *Advanced Organic Chemistry.* New York: Reinhold, 1961.

Finar, I. L. *Organic Chemistry,* 6th ed. London: Longman Group, 1986.

House, H. O. *Modern Synthetic Reactions,* 2nd ed. Menlo Park, CA: W. H. Benjamin, 1972.

Noller, C. R. *Chemistry of Organic Compounds,* 3rd ed. Philadelphia: W. B. Saunders, 1965.

Smith, M. B. *Organic Synthesis,* 2nd ed. New York: McGraw-Hill, 2002.

Smith, M. B., and March, J. *Advanced Organic Chemistry,* 5th ed. New York: John Wiley & Sons, 2001.

Stowell, J. C. *Intermediate Organic Chemistry,* 2nd ed. New York: John Wiley & Sons, 1993.

Warren, S. *Organic Synthesis: The Disconnection Approach.* New York: John Wiley & Sons, 1982.

These books often contain references to original papers in the literature for students wanting to follow the subject further. Consequently you obtain not only a review of the subject from such a textbook but also a key reference that is helpful toward a more extensive literature search. The textbook by Smith and March is particularly useful for this purpose.

29.6 SPECIFIC SYNTHETIC METHODS

Anyone interested in locating information about a particular method of synthesizing a compound should first consult one of the many general textbooks on the subject. Useful ones are

Anand, N., Bindra, J. S., and Ranganathan, S. *Art in Organic Synthesis,* 2nd ed. New York: John Wiley & Sons, 1988.

Barton, D., and Ollis, W. D., eds. *Comprehensive Organic Chemistry,* 6 vols. Oxford: Pergamon Press, 1979.

Buehler, C. A., and Pearson, D. E. *Survey of Organic Syntheses.* New York: Wiley-Interscience, 1970, 2 vols., 1977.

Carey, F. A., and Sundberg, R. J. *Advanced Organic Chemistry. Part B. Reactions and Synthesis,* 4th ed. New York: Kluwer, 2000.

Compendium of Organic Synthetic Methods. New York: Wiley-Interscience, 1971–2002. This is a continuing series, now in 10 volumes.

Fieser, L. F., and Fieser, M. *Reagents for Organic Synthesis.* New York: Wiley-Interscience, 1967–1999. This is a continuing series, now in 21 volumes.

Greene, T. W., and Wuts, P. G. M. *Protective Groups in Organic Synthesis,* 3rd ed. New York: John Wiley & Sons, 1999.

House, H. O. *Modern Synthetic Reactions,* 2nd ed. Menlo Park, CA: W. H. Benjamin, 1972.

Larock, R. C. *Comprehensive Organic Transformations,* 2nd ed. New York: Wiley-VCH, 1999.

Mundy, B. P., and Ellerd, M. G. *Name Reactions and Reagents in Organic Synthesis.* New York: John Wiley & Sons, 1988.

Patai, S., ed. *The Chemistry of the Functional Groups.* London: Interscience, 1964–present. This series consists of many volumes, each one specializing in a particular functional group.

Smith, M. B., and March, J. *Advanced Organic Chemistry,* 5th ed. New York: John Wiley & Sons, 2001.

Trost, B. M., and Fleming, I. *Comprehensive Organic Synthesis.* Amsterdam: Pergamon/Elsevier Science, 1992. This series consist of 9 volumes plus supplements.

Vogel, A. I. *Vogel's Textbook of Practical Organic Chemistry, including Qualitative Organic Analysis,* 5th ed. London: Longman Group, 1989. Revised by members of the School of Chemistry, Thames Polytechnic.

Wagner, R. B., and Zook, H. D. *Synthetic Organic Chemistry.* New York: John Wiley & Sons, 1956.

More specific information, including actual reaction conditions, exists in collections specializing in organic synthetic methods. The most important of these are

Organic Syntheses. New York: John Wiley & Sons, 1921–present. Published annually.
Organic Syntheses, Collective Volumes. New York: John Wiley & Sons, 1941–1993.
Vol. 1, 1941, Annual Volumes 1–9
Vol. 2, 1943, Annual Volumes 10–19
Vol. 3, 1955, Annual Volumes 20–29
Vol. 4, 1963, Annual Volumes 30–39

Vol. 5, 1973, Annual Volumes 40–49
Vol. 6, 1988, Annual Volumes 50–59
Vol. 7, 1990, Annual Volumes 60–64
Vol. 8, 1993, Annual Volumes 65–69
Vol. 9, 1998, Annual Volumes 70–74

It is much more convenient to use the collective volumes where the earlier annual volumes of *Organic Syntheses* are combined in groups of 9 or 10 in the first six collective volumes (Volumes 1–6), and then in groups of 5 for the next three volumes (Volumes 7, 8, and 9). Useful indices are included at the end of each of the collective volumes that classify methods according to the type of reaction, type of compound prepared, formula of compound prepared, preparation or purification of solvents and reagents, and use of various types of specialized apparatus.

The main advantage of using one of the *Organic Syntheses* procedures is that they have been tested to make sure that they work as written. Often, an organic chemist will adapt one of these tested procedures to the preparation of another compound. One of the features of the advanced organic textbook by Smith and March is that it includes references to specific preparative methods contained in *Organic Syntheses.*

More advanced material on organic chemical reactions and synthetic methods may be found in any one of a number of annual publications that review the original literature and summarize it. Examples include

Advances in Organic Chemistry: Methods and Results. New York: John Wiley & Sons, 1960–present.
Annual Reports in Organic Synthesis. Orlando, FL: Academic Press, 1985–1995.
Annual Reports of the Chemical Society, Section B. London: Chemical Society, 1905–present. Specifically, the section "Synthetic Methods."
Organic Reactions. New York: John Wiley & Sons, 1942–present.
Progress in Organic Chemistry. New York: John Wiley & Sons, 1952–1973.

Each of these publications contains a great many citations to the appropriate articles in the original literature.

29.7 ADVANCED LABORATORY TECHNIQUES

The student who is interested in reading about techniques more advanced than those described in this textbook, or in more complete descriptions of techniques, should consult one of the advanced textbooks specializing in organic laboratory techniques. Besides focusing on apparatus construction and the performance of complex reactions, these books provide advice on purifying reagents and solvents. Useful sources of information on organic laboratory techniques include

Bates, R. B., and Schaefer, J. P. *Research Techniques in Organic Chemistry.* Englewood Cliffs, NJ: Prentice-Hall, 1971.
Krubsack, A. J. *Experimental Organic Chemistry.* Boston: Allyn & Bacon, 1973.
Leonard, J., Lygo, B., and Procter, G. *Advanced Practical Organic Chemistry,* 2nd ed. London: Chapman & Hall, 1995.

Monson, R. S. *Advanced Organic Synthesis: Methods and Techniques.* New York: Academic Press, 1971.

Techniques of Chemistry. New York: John Wiley & Sons, 1970–present. Currently 23 volumes. The successor to *Technique of Organic Chemistry,* this series covers experimental methods of chemistry, such as purification of solvents, spectral methods, and kinetic methods.

Weissberger, A., et al., eds. *Technique of Organic Chemistry,* 3rd ed, 14 vol. New York: Wiley-Interscience, 1959–1969.

Wiberg, K. B. *Laboratory Technique in Organic Chemistry.* New York: McGraw-Hill, 1960.

Numerous works and some general textbooks specialize in particular techniques. The preceding list is representative only of the most common books in this category. The following books deal specifically with microscale and semi-microscale techniques.

Cheronis, N. D. "Micro and Semimicro Methods." In A. Weissberger, ed., *Technique of Organic Chemistry,* Vol. 6. New York: Wiley-Interscience, 1954.

Cheronis, N. D., and Ma, T. S. *Organic Functional Group Analysis by Micro and Semimicro Methods.* New York: Wiley-Interscience, 1964.

Ma, T. S., and Horak, V. *Microscale Manipulations in Chemistry.* New York: Wiley-Interscience, 1976.

29.8 REACTION MECHANISMS

As with the case of locating information on synthetic methods, you can obtain a great deal of information about reaction mechanisms by consulting one of the common textbooks on physical organic chemistry. The textbooks listed here provide a general description of mechanisms, but they do not contain specific literature citations. Very general textbooks include

Bruckner, R. *Advanced Organic Chemistry: Reaction Mechanisms.* New York: Academic Press, 2001.

Miller, A., and Solomon, P. *Writing Reaction Mechanisms in Organic Chemistry,* 2nd ed. San Diego, CA: Academic Press, 1999.

Sykes, P. *A Primer to Mechanisms in Organic Chemistry.* Menlo Park, CA: Benjamin/Cummings, 1995.

More advanced textbooks include

Carey, F. A., and Sundberg, R. J. *Advanced Organic Chemistry. Part A. Structure and Mechanisms,* 4th ed. New York: Kluwer, 2000.

Hammett, L. P. *Physical Organic Chemistry: Reaction Rates, Equilibria, and Mechanisms,* 2nd ed. New York: McGraw-Hill, 1970.

Hine, J. *Physical Organic Chemistry,* 2nd ed. New York: McGraw-Hill, 1962.

Ingold, C. K. *Structure and Mechanism in Organic Chemistry,* 2nd ed. Ithaca, NY: Cornell University Press, 1969.

Isaacs, N. S. *Physical Organic Chemistry,* 2nd ed. New York: John Wiley & Sons, 1995.

Jones, R. A. Y. *Physical and Mechanistic Organic Chemistry,* 2nd ed. Cambridge: Cambridge University Press, 1984.

Lowry, T. H., and Richardson, K. S. *Mechanism and Theory in Organic Chemistry,* 3rd ed. New York: Harper & Row, 1987.

Moore, J. W., and Pearson, R. G. *Kinetics and Mechanism,* 3rd ed. New York: John Wiley & Sons, 1981.

Smith, M. B., and March, J. *Advanced Organic Chemistry,* 5th ed. New York: John Wiley & Sons, 2001.

These books include extensive bibliographies that permit the reader to delve more deeply into the subject.

Most libraries also subscribe to annual series of publications that specialize in articles dealing with reaction mechanisms. Among these are

Advances in Physical Organic Chemistry. London: Academic Press, 1963–present.

Annual Reports of the Chemical Society. Section B. London: Chemical Society, 1905–present. Specifically, the section "Reaction Mechanisms."

Organic Reaction Mechanisms. Chichester: John Wiley & Sons, 1965–present.

Progress in Physical Organic Chemistry. New York: Interscience, 1963–present.

These publications provide the reader with citations from the original literature that can be very useful in an extensive literature search.

29.9 ORGANIC QUALITATIVE ANALYSIS

Many laboratory manuals provide basic procedures for identifying organic compounds through a series of chemical tests and reactions. Occasionally, you might require a more complete description of analytical methods or a more complete set of tables of derivatives. Textbooks specializing in organic qualitative analysis should fill this need. Examples of sources for such information include

Cheronis, N. D., and Entriken, J. B. *Identification of Organic Compounds: A Student's Text Using Semimicro Techniques.* New York: Interscience, 1963.

Pasto, D. J., and Johnson, C. R. *Laboratory Text for Organic Chemistry: A Source Book of Chemical and Physical Techniques.* Englewood Cliffs, NJ: Prentice-Hall, 1979.

Rappoport, Z. ed. *Handbook of Tables for Organic Compound Identification,* 3rd ed. Boca Raton, FL: CRC Press, 1967.

Shriner, R. L., Hermann, C. K. F., Merrill, T. C., Curtin, D. Y., and Fuson, R. C. *The Systematic Identification of Organic Compounds,* 7th ed. New York: John Wiley & Sons, 1998.

Vogel, A. I. *Elementary Practical Organic Chemistry. Part 2. Qualitative Organic Analysis,* 2nd ed. New York: John Wiley & Sons, 1966.

Vogel, A. I. *Vogel's Textbook of Practical Organic Chemistry, including Qualitative Organic Analysis,* 5th ed. London: Longman Group, 1989. Revised by members of the School of Chemistry, Thames Polytechnic.

29.10 *BEILSTEIN* AND *CHEMICAL ABSTRACTS*

One of the most useful sources of information about the physical properties, synthesis, and reactions of organic compounds is *Beilsteins Handbuch der Organischen Chemie.* This is a monumental work, initially edited by Friedrich Konrad Beilstein and updated through several revisions by the Beilstein Institute in Frankfurt am Main, Germany. The original edition (the *Hauptwerk,* abbreviated H) was published in 1918 and covers completely the literature to 1909. Five supplementary series (*Ergänzungswerken*) have been published since that time. The first supplement (*Erstes Ergänzungswerk,* abbreviated E I) covers the literature from 1910 to 1919; the second supplement (*Zweites Ergänzungswerk,* E II) covers 1920–1929; the third supplement (*Drittes Ergänzungswerk,* E III) covers 1930–1949; the fourth supplement (*Viertes Ergänzungswerk,* E IV) covers 1950–1959; and the fifth supplement (in English) covers 1960–1979. Volumes 17–27 of supplementary series III and IV, covering heterocyclic compounds, are combined in a joint issue, E III/IV. Supplementary series III, IV, and V are not complete, so the coverage of *Handbuch der Organischen Chemie* can be considered complete to 1929, with partial coverage to 1979.

Beilsteins Handbuch der Organischen Chemie, usually referred to simply as *Beilstein,* also contains two types of cumulative indices. The first of these is a name index (*Sachregister*), and the second is a formula index (*Formelregister*). These indices are particularly useful for a person wishing to locate a compound in *Beilstein.*

The principal difficulty in using *Beilstein* is that it is written in German through the fourth supplement. The fifth supplement is in English. Although some reading knowledge of German is useful, you can obtain information from the work by learning a few key phrases. For example, *Bildung* is "formation" or "structure." *Darst* or *Darstellung* is "preparation," K_P or *Siedepunkt* is "boiling point," and *F* or *Schmelzpunkt* is "melting point." Furthermore, the names of some compounds in German are not cognates of the English names. Some examples are *Apfelsäure* for "malic acid" (*säure* means "acid"), *Harnstoff* for "urea," *Jod* for "iodine," and *Zimtsäure* for "cinnamic acid." If you have access to a German–English dictionary for chemists, many of these difficulties can be overcome. The best such dictionary is

Patterson, A. M. *German–English Dictionary for Chemists,* 4th ed. New York: John Wiley & Sons, 1991.

Beilstein is organized according to a very sophisticated and complicated system. However, most students do not wish to become experts on *Beilstein* to this extent. A simpler, though slightly less reliable, method is to look for the compound in the formula index that accompanies the second supplement. By looking under the molecular formula, you will find the names of compounds that have that formula. After that name will be a series of numbers that indicate the pages and volume in which that compound is listed. Suppose, as an example, that you are searching for information on *p*-nitroaniline. This compound has the molecular formula $C_6H_6N_2O_2$. Searching for this formula in the formula index to the second supplement, you find

4-Nitro-anilin **12** 711, **I** 349, **II** 383

This information tells you that *p*-nitroaniline is listed in the main edition, *Hauptwerk,* in Volume 12, p. 711. Locate this particular volume, which is devoted to isocyclic monoamines, turn to page 711 to find the beginning of the section on *p*-nitroaniline. At the left side of the top of this page is "Syst. No. 1671." This is the system number given to compounds in this part of Volume 12. The system number is useful, as it can help you find entries for this compound in subsequent supplements. The organization of *Beilstein* is such that all entries on *p*-nitroaniline in each of the supplements will be found in Volume 12. The entry in the formula index also indicates that material on this compound may be found in the first supplement on page 349 and in the second supplement on page 383. On page 349 of Volume 12 of the first supplement, there is a heading, "XII, 710–712," and on the left is "Syst. No. 1671." Material on *p*-nitroaniline is found in each supplement on a page that is headed with the volume and page of the *Hauptwerk* in which the same compound is found. On page 383 of Volume 12 of the second supplement, the heading in the center of the top of the page is "H12, 710–712." On the left, you find "Syst. No. 1671." Again, because *p*-nitroaniline appeared in Volume 12, page 711, of the main edition, you can locate it by searching through Volume 12 of any supplement until you find a page with the heading corresponding to Volume 12, page 711.

Because the third and fourth supplements are not complete, there is no comprehensive formula index for these supplements. However, you can still find material on *p*-nitroaniline by using the system number and the volume and page in the main work. In the third supplement, because the amount of information available has grown so much since the early days of Beilstein's work, Volume 12 has now expanded so that it is found in several bound parts. However, you select the part that includes system number 1671. In this part of Volume 12, you look through the pages until you find a page headed "Syst. No. 1671/H711." The information on *p*-nitroaniline is found on this page (page 1580). If Volume 12 of the fourth supplement were available, you would go on in the same way to locate more recent data on *p*-nitroaniline. This example is meant to illustrate how you can locate information on particular compounds without having to learn the *Beilstein* system of classification. You might do well to test your ability at finding compounds in *Beilstein* as we have described here.

Guidebooks to using *Beilstein,* which include a description of the *Beilstein* system, are recommended for anyone who wants to work extensively with *Beilstein.* Among such sources are

Heller, S. R. *The Beilstein System: Strategies for Effective Searching.* New York: Oxford University Press, 1997.
How to Use Beilstein. Beilstein Institute, Frankfurt am Main. Berlin: Springer-Verlag.
Huntress, E. H. *A Brief Introduction to the Use of* Beilsteins Handbuch der Organischen Chemie, 2nd ed. New York: John Wiley & Sons, 1938.
Weissbach, O. *The Beilstein Guide: A Manual for the Use of* Beilsteins Handbuch der Organischen Chemie. New York: Springer-Verlag, 1976.

Beilstein reference numbers are listed in such handbooks as *CRC Handbook of Chemistry and Physics* and *Lange's Handbook of Chemistry.* Additionally, *Beilstein* numbers are included in the *Aldrich Handbook of Fine Chemicals,* issued by the Aldrich Chemical Company. If the compound you are seeking is listed in one of these handbooks, you will find that using *Beilstein* is simplified.

Another very useful publication for finding references for research on a particular topic is *Chemical Abstracts,* published by the Chemical Abstracts Service of the American Chemical Society. *Chemical Abstracts* contains abstracts of articles appearing in more than 10,000 journals from virtually every country conducting scientific research. These abstracts list the authors, the journal in which the article appeared, the title of the paper, and a short summary of the contents of the article. Abstracts of articles that appeared originally in a foreign language are provided in English, with a notation indicating the original language.

To use *Chemical Abstracts,* you must know how to use the various indices that accompany it. At the end of each volume, there appears a set of indices, including a formula index, a general subject index, a chemical substances index, an author index, and a patent index. The listings in each index refer the reader to the appropriate abstract according to the number assigned to it. There are also collective indices that combine all the indexed material appearing in a 5-year period (10-year period before 1956). In the collective indices, the listings include the volume number as well as the abstract number.

For material after 1929, *Chemical Abstracts* provides the most complete coverage of the literature. For material before 1929, use *Beilstein* before consulting *Chemical Abstracts. Chemical Abstracts* has the advantage that it is written entirely in English. Nevertheless, most students perform a literature search to find a relatively simple compound. Finding the desired entry for a simple compound is much easier in *Beilstein* than in *Chemical Abstracts.* For simple compounds, the indices in *Chemical Abstracts* are likely to contain very many entries. To locate the desired information, you must comb through this multitude of listings—potentially a very time-consuming task.

The opening pages of each index in *Chemical Abstracts* contain a brief set of instructions on using that index. If you want a more complete guide to *Chemical Abstracts,* consult a textbook designed to familiarize you with these abstracts and indices. Two such books are

CAS Printed Access Tools: A Workbook. Washington, DC: Chemical Abstracts Service, American Chemical Society, 1977.
How to Search Printed CA. Washington, DC: Chemical Abstracts Service, American Chemical Society, 1989.

Chemical Abstracts Service maintains a computerized database that permits users to search through *Chemical Abstracts* very rapidly and thoroughly. This service, which is called *CA Online,* is described in Section 29.11. *Beilstein* is also available for online searching by computer.

29.11 COMPUTER ONLINE SEARCHING

You can search a number of chemistry databases online by using a computer and modem or a direct Internet connection. Many academic and industrial libraries can access these databases through their computers. One organization that maintains a large number of databases is the Scientific and Technical Information Network (STN International). The fee charged to the library for this service depends on the total time used in making the search, the type of information being asked for, the time of day when the search is being conducted, and the type of database being searched.

The Chemical Abstracts Service database (*CA Online*) is one of many databases available on STN. It is particularly useful to chemists. Unfortunately, this database extends back only to about 1967, although some earlier references are available. Searches for references earlier than 1967 must be made with printed abstracts (Section 29.10). Searching online is much faster than searching in the printed abstracts. In addition, you can tailor the search in a number of ways by using keywords and the Chemical Abstracts Service Registry Number (CAS Number) as part of the search routine. The CAS Number is a specific number assigned to every compound listed in the *Chemical Abstracts* database. The CAS Number is used as a key in an online search to locate information about the compound. For the more common organic compounds, you can easily obtain CAS Numbers from the catalogs of most of the companies that supply chemicals. Another advantage of performing an online search is that the *Chemical Abstracts* files are updated much more quickly than the printed versions of abstracts. This means that your search is more likely to reveal the most current information available.

Other useful databases available from STN include *Beilstein* and *CASREACTS.* As described in Section 29.10, *Beilstein* is very useful to organic chemists. Currently, there are over 3.5 million compounds listed in the database. You can use the CAS Numbers to help in a search that has the potential of going back to 1830. *CASREACTS* is a chemical reactions database derived from over 100 journals covered by *Chemical Abstracts,* starting in 1985. With this database, you can specify a starting material and a product using the CAS Numbers. Further information on *CA Online, Beilstein, CASREACTS,* and other databases can be obtained from the following references:

Smith, M. B., and March, J. *Advanced Organic Chemistry,* 5th ed. New York: John Wiley & Sons, 2001.
Somerville, A. N. "Information Sources for Organic Chemistry, 2: Searching by Functional Group." *Journal of Chemical Education, 68* (October 1991): 842.
Somerville, A. N. "Subject Searching of Chemical Abstracts Online." *Journal of Chemical Education, 70* (March 1993): 200.
Wiggins, G. *Chemical Information Sources.* New York: McGraw-Hill, 1990. Integrates printed materials and computer sources of information.

29.12 SCIENTIFIC JOURNALS

Ultimately, someone wanting information about a particular area of research will be required to read articles from the scientific journals. These journals are of two basic types: review journals and primary scientific journals. Journals that specialize in review articles summarize all the work that bears on the particular topic. These articles may focus on the contributions of one particular researcher but often consider the contributions of many researchers to the subject. These articles also contain extensive bibliographies, which refer you to the original research articles. Among the important journals devoted, at least partly, to review articles are

Accounts of Chemical Research
Angewandte Chemie (International Edition, in English)
Chemical Reviews
Chemical Society Reviews (formerly known as *Quarterly Reviews*)
Nature
Science

The details of the research of interest appear in the primary scientific journals. Although there are thousands of journals published in the world, a few important journals specializing in articles dealing with organic chemistry include

Canadian Journal of Chemistry
European Journal of Organic Chemistry (formerly known as *Chemische Berichte*)
Journal of Organic Chemistry
Journal of the American Chemical Society
Journal of the Chemical Society, Chemical Communications

Journal of the Chemical Society, Perkin Transactions (Parts I and II)
Journal of Organometallic Chemistry
Organic Letters
Organometallics
Synlett
Synthesis
Tetrahedron
Tetrahedron Letters

29.13 TOPICS OF CURRENT INTEREST

The following journals and magazines are good sources for topics of educational and current interest. They specialize in news articles and focus on current events in chemistry or in science in general. Articles in these journals (magazines) can be useful in keeping you abreast of developments in science that are not part of your normal specialized scientific reading.

American Scientist
Chemical and Engineering News
Chemistry and Industry
Chemistry in Britain
Chemtech
Discover
Journal of Chemical Education
Nature
Omni
Science
Scientific American

Other sources for topics of current interest include the following:

Encyclopedia of Chemical Technology, 4th ed., 25 vols. plus index and supplements, 1992. Also called *Kirk-Othmer Encyclopedia of Chemical Technology.*
McGraw-Hill Encyclopedia of Science and Technology, 20 volumes and supplements, 1997.

29.14 HOW TO CONDUCT A LITERATURE SEARCH

The easiest method to follow in searching the literature is to begin with secondary sources and then go to the primary sources. In other words, you would try to locate material in a textbook, *Beilstein,* or *Chemical Abstracts.* From the results of that search, you would then consult one of the primary scientific journals.

A literature search that ultimately requires you to read one or more papers in the scientific journals is best conducted if you can identify a particular paper central to the study. Often, you can obtain this reference from a textbook or a review article on the subject. If this is not available, a search through *Beilstein* is required. A search through one of the handbooks that provides *Beilstein* reference numbers (see Section 29.10) may be helpful. Searching through *Chemical Abstracts* would be considered the next logical step. From these sources, you should be able to identify citations from the original literature on the subject.

Additional citations may be found in the references cited in the journal article. In this way, the background leading to the research can be examined. It is also possible to conduct a search forward in time from the date of the journal article through the *Science Citation Index*. This publication provides the service of listing articles and the papers in which these articles were cited. Although the *Science Citation Index* consists of several types of indices, the *Citation Index* is most useful for the purposes described here. A person who knows of a particular key reference on a subject can examine the *Science Citation Index* to obtain a list of papers that have used that seminal reference in support of the work described. The *Citation Index* lists papers by their senior author, journal, volume, page, and date, followed by citations of papers that have referred to that article, author, journal, volume, page, and date of each. The *Citation Index* is published in annual volumes, with quarterly supplements issued during the current year. Each volume contains a complete list of the citations of the key articles made during that year. A disadvantage is that *Science Citation Index* has been available only since 1961. An additional disadvantage is that you may miss journal articles on the subject of interest if *Citation Index* failed to cite that particular key reference in its bibliographies—a reasonably likely possibility.

You can, of course, conduct a literature search by a "brute force" method, by beginning the search with *Beilstein* or even with the indices in *Chemical Abstracts*. However, the task can be made much easier by performing a computer search (Section 29.11) or by starting with a book or an article of general and broad coverage, which can provide a few citations for starting points in the search.

The following guides to using the chemical literature are provided for the reader who is interested in going further into this subject.

Bottle, R. T., and Rowland, J. F. B., eds. *Information Sources in Chemistry,* 4th ed. New York: Bowker-Saur, 1992.

Maizell, R. E. *How to Find Chemical Information: A Guide for Practicing Chemists, Educators, and Students,* 3rd ed. New York: John Wiley & Sons, 1998.

Mellon, M. G. *Chemical Publications,* 5th ed. New York: McGraw-Hill, 1982.

Wiggins, G. *Chemical Information Sources.* New York: McGraw-Hill, 1991. Integrates printed materials and computer sources of information.

PROBLEMS

1. Find the following compounds in the formula index for the *Second Supplement of Beilstein* (Section 29.10). (1) List the page numbers from the main work and the supplements (first and second). (2) Using these page numbers, look up the system number (Syst. No.) and the main work number (*Hauptwerk* number, H) for each compound in the main work and the first and second supplements. In some cases, a compound may not be found in all three places. (3) Now use the system number and main work number to find each of these compounds in the third and fourth supplements. List the page numbers where these compounds are found.

   a. 2,5-hexanedione (acetonylacetone)

   b. 3-nitroacetophenone

   c. 4-*tert*-butylcyclohexanone

   d. 4-phenylbutanoic acid (4-phenylbutyric acid, γ-phenylbuttersäure)

2. Using the *Science Citation Index* (Section 29.14), list five research papers by complete title and journal citation for each of the following chemists who have been awarded the Nobel Prize. Use the *Five-Year Cumulative Source Index* for the years 1980–1984 as your source.

    a. H. C. Brown

    b. R. B. Woodward

    c. D. J. Cram

    d. G. Olah

3. The reference book by Smith and March is listed in Section 29.2. Using Appendix 2 in this book, give two methods for preparing the following functional groups. You will need to provide equations.

    a. carboxylic acids

    b. aldehydes

    c. esters (carboxylic esters)

4. *Organic Syntheses* is described in Section 29.6. There are currently nine collective volumes in the series, each with its own index. Find the compounds listed below and provide the equations for preparing each compound.

    a. 2-methylcyclopentane-1,3-dione

    b. *cis*-Δ^4-tetrahydrophthalic anhydride (listed as tetrahydrophthalic anhydride)

5. Provide four ways that may be used to oxidize an alcohol to an aldehyde. Give complete literature references for each method, as well as equations. Use the *Compendium of Organic Synthetic Methods* or *Survey of Organic Syntheses* by Buehler and Pearson (Section 29.6).

Appendix A: The Twelve Principles of Green Chemistry

This text approaches the development of green chemical processes by considering a generic chemical equation and the ways in which one may reduce the hazards and environmental impacts arising from each component of this equation (Chapter 5). Anastas and Warner have formulated twelve fundamental principles of green chemistry, and these principles, as put forth in P. T. Anastas and J. C. Warner, "Green Chemistry: Theory and Practice;" Oxford University Press: Oxford, UK (1998), are reproduced below. Although we have not organized the discussions of this text around these principles, the concepts contained within each should sound familiar to you.

1. It is better to prevent waste than to treat or clean up waste after it is formed.

2. Synthetic methods should be designed to maximize the incorporation of all materials used in the process into the final product.

3. Wherever practicable, synthetic methodologies should be designed to use and generate substances that possess little or no toxicity to human health and the environment.

4. Chemical products should be designed to preserve efficacy of function while reducing toxicity.

5. The use of auxiliary substances (e.g. solvents, separation agents, etc.) should be made unnecessary wherever possible and innocuous when used.

6. Energy requirements should be recognized for their environmental and economic impacts and should be minimized. Synthetic methods should be conducted at ambient temperature and pressure.

7. A raw material or feedstock should be renewable rather than depleting wherever technically and economically practicable.

8. Unnecessary derivatization (blocking group, protection/deprotection, temporary modification of physical/chemical processes) should be avoided whenever possible.

9. Catalytic reagents (as selective as possible) are superior to stoichiometric reagents.

10. Chemical products should be designed so that at the end of their function they do not persist in the environment and break down into innocuous degradation products.

11. Analytical methodologies need to be further developed to allow for real-time, in-process monitoring and control prior to the formation of hazardous substances.

12. Substances and the form of a substance used in a chemical process should be chosen so as to minimize the potential for chemical accidents, including releases, explosions, and fires.

EXPERIMENT 8
MICROWAVE SYNTHESIS OF 5,10,15,20-TETRAPHENYLPORPHYRIN

Chemical Concepts

Electrophilic aromatic substitution; visible spectroscopy; column chromatography; thin-layer chromatography.

Green Lessons

Solvent-free reactions; solid-supported synthesis; microwave heating of reaction mixtures; safer solvents (for chromatography).

Estimated Lab Time

2.5 hours

Introduction

The preceding experiment introduced the chemistry of porphyrins and related compounds and discussed some of the chemistry involved in their synthesis. In this experiment you will explore an alternative solvent-free synthesis of 5,10,15,20-tetraphenylporphyrin from benzaldehyde and pyrrole. Instead of a gas-phase reaction at high temperature, you will use microwave irradiation to heat the reactants. In this case, the liquid reactants are adsorbed on a solid support, silica gel, which may act as a Lewis acid catalyst to facilitate the reaction. As in the preceding experiment, the reaction presumably forms a porphyrinogen, which is then oxidized to the porphyrin product by atmospheric oxygen.

Isolation and purification of the tetraphenylporphyrin product is effected by removal of the crude product from the silica, followed by column chromatography. As in the gas-phase synthesis procedure, this chromatography utilizes a safer solvent (a mixture of hexanes and ethyl acetate) than the halogenated solvents traditionally employed. This experiment, which clearly complements the preceding gas-phase synthesis, illustrates a number of other green chemical issues, including the avoidance of solvent usage, the use of solid-supported reactions, and the use of alternative energy sources (here, microwave energy) to effect chemical reactions.

Pre-Lab Preparation

1. Study the technique sections in your lab manual regarding column chromatography, TLC, visible spectroscopy, and use of the rotary evaporator.

2. Carry out pre-lab preparations as described in Chapter 11, section 11.6A, or as called for by your instructor.

Experimental Procedure

> SAFETY PRECAUTIONS: Ethyl acetate, hexanes, and acetone are flammable; avoid exposure to open flames. Avoid inhalation of silica gel particles or fumes of benzaldehyde or pyrrole. Pyrrole and benzaldehyde can be irritating to the skin – avoid contact. When the reaction vessel is removed from the microwave oven, it will be very hot – take care to avoid thermal burns.

Reaction

1. Mix 0.43 mL of benzaldehyde and 0.3 mL of pyrrole in a 25 mL Erlenmeyer flask. Once the reactants are thoroughly mixed, add 0.63 g of silica gel, stopper the flask, and mix well until the silica gel is evenly and completely covered with the reactant mixture.

2. Place the flask containing the reaction mixture in the microwave oven (a standard 1000 W model), cover with a Pyrex watch glass, and heat for a total of 10 minutes in five 2-minute intervals.

3. Once the reaction is complete, allow the mixture to cool to room temperature, then add approximately 15 mL of ethyl acetate. Filter the solution to remove the silica gel, then remove the ethyl acetate using a rotary evaporator. Extract the residue with 1 mL of CH_2Cl_2 to prepare for chromatography.

Isolation and Characterization

4. Carry out thin layer chromatographic analysis of your crude reaction mixture, column chromatography to separate the tetraphenylporphyrin, and UV/visible spectroscopic analysis to estimate the yield of your product as described in the preceding experiment. If you plan to carry out the following experiment in this text – the metallation of 5,10,15,20-tetraphenylporphyrin – save the first three drops of porphyrin-containing solution eluted from your column chromatography.

5. This procedure provides tetraphenylporphyrin of approximately 85% purity, as determined by ^{1}H NMR integration. The major impurity can be seen in the ^{1}H NMR spectrum as a broad multiplet near 7.3 ppm. The impurity does not affect the UV/visible spectrum of the porphyrin, and the product is of satisfactory purity for use in the following experiment.

Post-Lab Questions and Exercises

1. To the best of your ability based on your spectroscopic analysis, report the mass and percent of theoretical yield of the product.

2. Describe your TLC results for the reaction mixture. What were the R_f values for the spot(s)?

3. Describe what happened during column chromatography. What bands did you see elute, in what order?

4. Attach your UV/visible spectra. Be sure to indicate which fraction from the column chromatography you used to obtain these spectra. Label the absorbance and wavelength of each peak in the spectrum.

5. Compare the "greenness" of this procedure with a more conventional synthesis in hot propanoic acid.

6. Assuming that this procedure affords a 5% yield, how much pyrrole, benzaldehyde and silica gel would you need to prepare 100 mg of tetraphenylporphyrin?

7. Most organic compounds display proton NMR resonances in the range of 0 – 10 ppm. In addition to a number of peaks in this "normal" region, the proton NMR spectrum of tetraphenylporphyrin

displays a resonance at –2.7 ppm (i.e., 2.7 ppm *upfield* from tetramethylsilane). Suggest which protons are responsible for this unusual resonance and explain why it appears so far upfield.

Experiment Development Notes

This experiment was developed, with extensive modification for use in the organic teaching lab [50], based upon the original report from Petit, *et al.* [52]. Although this preparation offers a number of advantages over traditional methods, there is room for further improvements, some of which could form the basis of student inquiry-driven investigation. Development of alternative chromatographic procedures that could reduce solvent usage during chromatography is desirable. (Although one of the primary goals of this experiment is to provide experience with column chromatography, eliminating the chromatography step is a possible option if this experience is not deemed necessary.)

Use of more benign benzaldehyde derivatives in place of benzaldehyde itself would also be desirable. This actually suggests an interesting possible extension of the experiment to the use of *ortho*-substituted benzaldehyde derivatives. The resulting *ortho*-substituted tetraphenylporphyrins will display interesting TLC and ^{1}H NMR spectral behavior due to restricted rotation (atropisomerism) [53]. This provides a platform for the discussion of more advanced topics in spectroscopy, such as the observation of temperature dependent phenomena and measurement of rates of interconversion by line broadening methods. Finally, the porphyrin product can also be used to construct a functioning solar cells according to a procedure published in the recent literature [54]. We hope to include this experiment in the next edition of this text.

52.   A. Petit, A. Loupy, P. Maillard, and M. Momenteau *Synth. Commun.* **1992**, *22*, 1137.
53.   R. F. Beeston, S. E. Stitzel, and M. A. Rhea, *J. Chem. Ed.* **1997**, *74*, 1468.
54.   E. N. Durantini and L. Otero, *Chem. Educator* **1999**, *4*, 144.

ESSAY

Analgesics

Acylated aromatic amines (those having an acyl group, $R\overset{\overset{\displaystyle O}{\|}}{-C}-$, substituted on nitrogen) are important in over-the-counter headache remedies. Over-the-counter drugs are those you may buy without a prescription. Acetanilide, phenacetin, and acetaminophen are mild analgesics (relieve pain) and antipyretics (reduce fever) and are important, along with aspirin, in many nonprescription drugs.

Acetanilide   Phenacetin   Acetaminophen

The discovery that acetanilide was an effective antipyretic came about by accident in 1886. Two doctors, Cahn and Hepp, had been testing naphthalene as a possible **vermifuge** (an agent that expels worms). Their early results on simple worm cases were very discouraging, so Dr. Hepp decided to test the compound on a patient with a larger variety of complaints, including worms—a sort of shotgun approach. A short time later, Dr. Hepp excitedly reported to his colleague, Dr. Cahn, that naphthalene had miraculous fever-reducing properties.

In trying to verify this observation, the doctors discovered that the bottle they thought contained naphthalene had apparently been mislabeled. In fact, the bottle brought to them by their assistant had a label so faint as to be illegible. They were sure that the sample was not naphthalene, because it had no odor. Naphthalene has a strong odor reminiscent of mothballs. So close to an important discovery, the doctors were nevertheless stymied; they appealed to a cousin of Hepp, who was a chemist in a nearby dye factory, to help them identify the unknown compound. This compound turned out to be acetanilide, a compound

Naphthalene

with a structure not at all like that of naphthalene. Certainly, Hepp's unscientific and risky approach would be frowned on by doctors today; and to be sure, the Food and Drug Administration (FDA) would never allow human testing before extensive animal testing (consumer protection has progressed). Nevertheless, Cahn and Hepp made an important discovery.

In another instance of serendipity, the publication of Cahn and Hepp, describing their experiments with acetanilide, caught the attention of Carl Duisberg, director of research at the Bayer Company in Germany. Duisberg was confronted with the problem of profitably getting rid of nearly 50 tons of p-aminophenol, a by-product of the synthesis of one of Bayer's other commercial products. He immediately saw the possibility of converting p-aminophenol to a compound similar in structure to acetanilide by putting an acyl group on the nitrogen. It was then believed, however, that all compounds having a hydroxyl group on a benzene ring (that is, phenols) were toxic. Duisberg devised a scheme of structural modification of p-aminophenol to synthesize the compound phenacetin. The reaction scheme is shown here.

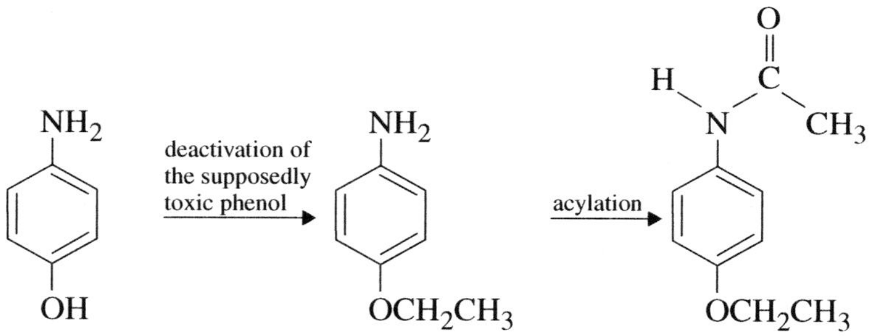

p-Aminophenol   Phenacetin

Phenacetin turned out to be a highly effective analgesic and antipyretic. A common form of combination pain reliever, called an APC tablet, was once available. An APC tablet contained **A**spirin, **P**henacetin, and **C**affeine (hence, **APC**). Phenacetin is no longer used in commercial pain-relief preparations. It was later found that not all aromatic hydroxyl groups lead to toxic compounds, and today the compound acetaminophen is very widely used as an analgesic in place of phenacetin.

Another analgesic, structurally similar to aspirin, that has found some application is **salicylamide.** Salicylamide is found as an ingredient in some pain-relief preparations, although its use is declining.

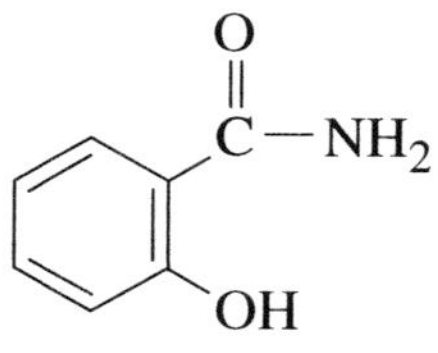

Salicylamide

On continued or excessive use, acetanilide can cause a serious blood disorder called **methemoglobinemia.** In this disorder, the central iron atom in hemoglobin is converted from Fe(II) to Fe(III) to give methemoglobin. Methemoglobin will not function as an oxygen carrier in the bloodstream. The result is a type of anemia (deficiency of hemoglobin or lack of red blood cells). Phenacetin and acetaminophen cause the same disorder, but to a much lesser degree. Because they are also more effective as antipyretic and analgesic drugs than acetanilide, they are preferred remedies. Acetaminophen is marketed under a variety of trade names, including Tylenol, Datril, and Panadol, and is often successfully used by people who are allergic to aspirin.

Heme portion of blood-oxygen carrier, hemoglobin.

More recently, a new drug has appeared in over-the-counter preparations. This drug is **ibuprofen,** which is marketed as a prescription drug in the United States under the name Motrin. Ibuprofen was first developed in England in 1964. United States marketing rights were obtained in 1974. Ibuprofen is now sold without prescription under brand names, which include Advil, Motrin, and Nuprin. Ibuprofen is principally an anti-inflammatory drug, but it is also effective as an analgesic and an antipyretic. It is particularly effective in treating the symptoms of rheumatoid arthritis and menstrual cramps. Ibuprofen appears to control the production of prostaglandins, which parallels the mode of action of aspirin. An important advantage of ibuprofen is that it is a very powerful pain reliever. One 200-mg tablet is as effective as two tablets (650 mg) of aspirin. Furthermore, ibuprofen has a more advantageous dose–response curve, which means that taking two tablets of this drug is approximately twice as effective as one tablet for certain types of pain. Aspirin and acetaminophen reach their maximum effective dose at two tablets. Little additional relief is gained at doses above that level. Ibuprofen, however, continues to increase its effectiveness up to the 400-mg level (the equivalent of four tablets of aspirin or acetaminophen). Ibuprofen is a relatively safe drug, but its use should be avoided in cases of aspirin allergy, kidney problems, ulcers, asthma, hypertension, or heart disease.

Ibuprofen

The Food and Drug Administration has also approved two other drugs with similar structures to ibuprofen for over-the-counter use as pain relievers. These new drugs are known by their generic names, **naproxen** and **ketoprofen.** Naproxen is often administered in the form of its sodium salt. Naproxen and ketoprofen can be used to alleviate the pain of

Analgesics and Caffeine in Some Common Preparations

	Aspirin	Acetaminophen	Caffeine
Aspirin*	0.325 g	—	—
Anacin	0.400 g	—	0.032 g
Bufferin	0.325 g	—	—
Cope	0.421 g	—	0.032 g
Excedrin (Extra-Strength)	0.250 g	0.250 g	0.065 g
Tylenol	—	0.325 g	—
B. C. Tablets	0.325 g	—	0.016 g
Advil	—	—	—
Aleve	—	—	—
Orudis	—	—	—

Note: Nonanalgesic ingredients (e.g., buffers) are not listed.

*5-grain tablet (1 grain = 0.0648 g).

headaches, toothaches, muscle aches, backaches, arthritis, and menstrual cramps, and they can also be used to reduce fever. They appear to have a longer duration of action than the older analgesics.

Naproxen   Ketoprofen

REFERENCES

Barr, W. H., and Penna, R. P. "O-T-C Internal Analgesics." In G. B. Griffenhagen, ed., *Handbook of Non-Prescription Drugs,* 7th ed. Washington, DC: American Pharmaceutical Association, 1982.

Bugg, C. E., Carson, W. M., and Montgomery, J. A. "Drugs by Design." *Scientific American,* 269 (December 1993): 92.

Flower, R. J., Moncada, S., and Vane, J. R. "Analgesic-Antipyretics and Anti-inflammatory Agents; Drugs Employed in the Treatment of Gout." In A. G. Gilman, L. S. Goodman, T. W. Rall, and F. Murad, *The Pharmacological Basis of Therapeutics,* 7th ed. New York: Macmillan, 1985.

Hansch, C. "Drug Research or the Luck of the Draw." *Journal of Chemical Education,* 51 (1974): 360.

"The New Pain Relievers." *Consumer Reports,* 49 (November 1984): 636–638.

Ray, O. S. "Internal Analgesics." *Drugs, Society, and Human Behavior,* 2nd ed. St. Louis: C. V. Mosby, 1978.

Salicylamide	Ibuprofen	Ketoprofen	Naproxen
—	—	—	—
—	—	—	—
—	—	—	—
—	—	—	—
—	—	—	—
—	—	—	—
0.095 g	—	—	—
—	0.200 g	—	—
—	—	—	0.220 g
—	—	0.0125 g	—

Senozan, N. M. "Methemoglobinemia: An Illness Caused by the Ferric State." *Journal of Chemical Education,* 62 (March 1985): 181.

EXPERIMENT 8

Acetanilide

Crystallization
Gravity filtration
Vacuum filtration
Decolorization
Preparation of an amide

An amine can be treated with an acid anhydride to form an amide. In this experiment, aniline, the amine, is reacted with acetic anhydride to form acetanilide, the amide, and acetic acid. Crude acetanilide contains a colored impurity that is removed by decolorization with charcoal. Acetanilide is purified further by crystallization from hot water.

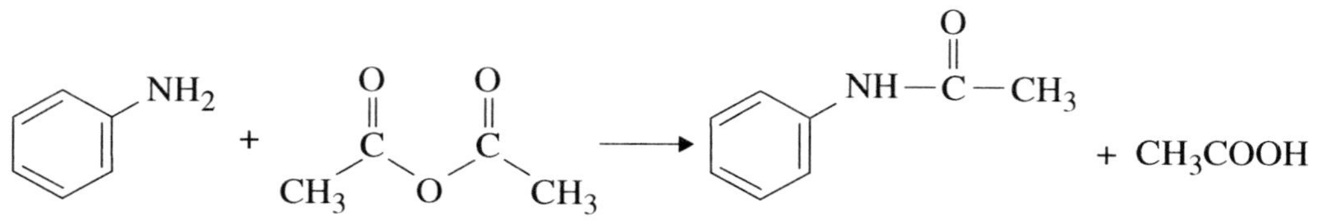

Aniline   Acetic anhydride   Acetanilide   Acetic acid

Amines can be acylated in several ways. Among these are the use of acetic anhydride, acetyl chloride, or glacial acetic acid. The procedure with glacial acetic acid is of commercial interest because it is economical. It requires long heating, however. Acetyl chloride is unsatisfactory for several reasons. Principally, it reacts vigorously, liberating HCl; this converts half of the amine to its hydrochloride salt, rendering it incapable of participating in the reaction. Acetic anhydride is preferred for a laboratory synthesis and is used in this experiment. Its rate of hydrolysis (reaction with water) is low enough to allow the acetylation of amines to be carried out in aqueous solutions. The procedure gives a product of high purity and in good yield, but it is not suitable for use with deactivated amines (weak bases) such as *ortho*- and *para*-nitroanilines.

Acetylation is often used to "protect" a primary or a secondary amine functional group. Acylated amines are less susceptible to oxidation, less reactive in aromatic substitution reactions (Experiments 42 and 46), and less prone to participate in many of the typical reactions of free amines, because they are less basic. The amino group can be regenerated readily by hydrolysis in acid or base (Experiment 46).

Required Reading

Review: Techniques 5 and 6
          Technique 7   Reaction Methods, Section 7.4
          Technique 8   Filtration, Sections 8.1–8.5
          Technique 9   Physical Constants of Solids: The Melting Point

350

New: Technique 11   Crystallization: Purification of Solids
               Essay   Analgesics

Special Instructions

Acetic anhydride can cause irritation of tissue, especially in nasal passages. Avoid breathing the vapor and avoid contact with skin and eyes. Aniline is a toxic substance, and it can be absorbed through the skin. Care should be exercised in handling it. You should be careful not to stop the experiment at any place where solid has not been filtered from the solution.

Suggested Waste Disposal

Aqueous solutions obtained from filtration operations should be poured into the container designated for aqueous wastes.

Notes to the Instructor

Aniline acquires a black color upon standing due to air oxidation. Because charcoal is very effective in decolorizing the crude acetanilide, it is recommended that students use impure aniline in this experiment. When very dark aniline is used, students can see just how effective charcoal can be in purifying organic compounds.

Procedure

Reaction Mixture. Weigh 2.0 g of aniline into a 125-mL Erlenmeyer flask. To avoid spills or contact with the skin, use a Pasteur pipet to transfer the aniline to the flask. Add 15 mL of water to the flask. Next, swirl the flask gently while slowly adding 2.5 mL of acetic anhydride (density 1.08 g/mL). Note in your laboratory notebook any changes that might occur during this reaction.

Once the crude acetanilide precipitates during this reaction, it must be crystallized. This crystallization will be accomplished in the same flask as the original reaction. Add 50 mL of water, along with a boiling stone, to the flask. Heat the mixture on a hot plate until all the solid and oily materials have dissolved. After removing the flask from the hot plate, pour about 1 mL of the hot solution into a small beaker and allow this material to cool.

Caution: The Erlenmeyer flask will be hot, so it is advisable to handle it with a paper towel. Do not use a test tube clamp or crucible tongs to remove the flask.

Decolorization. Add a small amount of activated charcoal, or Norit, to the Erlenmeyer flask and bring the mixture to a boil again. About one spatulaful should be enough charcoal. It is important *not* to add the charcoal to the solution while it is boiling vigorously, or violent frothing is likely. Swirl the mixture and allow it to boil gently for a few minutes.

Gravity Filtration. While the solution is boiling, assemble an apparatus for gravity filtration, equipped with a funnel (stemless, if possible) and fluted filter paper in a 125- or 250-mL Erlenmeyer flask (see Technique 8, Section 8.1, p. 645). Also prepare about 25 mL of boiling water, which will be needed as a washing solvent in the steps that follow.

Warm the funnel by pouring about 10 mL of the boiling water through it. Discard this warming water, put in the fluted filter paper (Figure 8.3, p. 648), and then filter the acetanilide–charcoal mixture as quickly as possible, but in small portions, through the fluted filter. Keep the solution warm on the hot plate until the solution is poured into the funnel. While pouring the solution through the filter, keep the collection flask warmed on the hot plate. The purpose of keeping these flasks on the hot plate is to allow the water vapor to warm the funnel stem and to reduce the likelihood that crystals will form in the funnel, clogging it. If all goes well, the charcoal remains behind on the fluted filter paper, and the aqueous solution containing acetanilide passes through the filter. If crystallization should begin in the funnel, add some hot water to the funnel to dissolve the crystals. Rinse the flask and the solid materials on the fluted filter paper with a little hot water and set the flask containing the filtrate aside to cool slowly to room temperature.

Crystallization and Vacuum Filtration. To complete the crystallization, place the flask in an ice bath for about 15 minutes. Using the instructions given in Section 8.3, page 651, prepare a Büchner funnel with filter paper. Collect the crystals by vacuum filtration and dry them as completely as possible by allowing air to be drawn through them while they remain on the Büchner funnel. Complete the drying by spreading the crystals on a watch glass, covering them with an inverted beaker, and allowing them to dry until the next laboratory period.

Collect the crystals that were not treated with charcoal in a Hirsch funnel or small Büchner funnel and compare the color of these crystals with the color of the crystals that were treated with charcoal. Record the results of the comparison in your laboratory notebook.

Record the weight of the pure crystallized product and calculate the percentage yield. Determine the melting point of both the pure and the impure samples of dried acetanilide. Place each sample of crystals in a separate, labeled vial and submit both samples to the instructor with your laboratory report.

QUESTIONS

1. Aniline is basic, and acetanilide is not basic. Explain this difference.

2. If 10 g of aniline are allowed to react with excess acetic anhydride, what is the theoretical yield of acetanilide in moles? in grams?

3. Give equations for the reactions of aniline with acetyl chloride and with acetic acid, to give acetanilide.

4. In the introduction to this experiment, the hydrolysis of acetic anhydride is mentioned as a competing reaction. Write an equation for this reaction.

5. During the crystallization of acetanilide, why was the mixture cooled in an ice bath?

6. Give two reasons why the crude product in most reactions is not pure.

Aspirin

Aspirin is one of the most popular cure-alls of modern life. Even though its curious history began more than 200 years ago, we still have much to learn about this enigmatic remedy. No one yet knows exactly how or why it works, yet more than 15 billion aspirin tablets are consumed each year in the United States.

The history of aspirin began on June 2, 1763, when Edward Stone, a clergyman, read a paper to the Royal Society of London entitled "An Account of the Success of the Bark of the Willow in the Cure of Agues." By *ague,* Stone was referring to what we now call malaria, but his use of the word *cure* was optimistic; what his extract of willow bark actually did was to reduce the feverish symptoms of the disease. Almost a century later, a Scottish physician was to find that extracts of willow bark would also alleviate the symptoms of acute rheumatism. This extract was ultimately found to be a powerful **analgesic** (pain reliever), **antipyretic** (fever reducer), and **anti-inflammatory** (reduces swelling) drug.

Soon thereafter, organic chemists working with willow bark extract and flowers of the meadowsweet plant (which gave a similar compound) isolated and identified the active ingredient as salicylic acid (from *salix,* the Latin name for the willow tree). The substance could then be chemically produced in large quantities for medical use. It soon became apparent that using salicylic acid as a remedy was severely limited by its acidic properties. The substance irritated the mucous membranes lining the mouth, gullet, and stomach. The first attempts at circumventing this problem by using the less acidic sodium salt (sodium salicylate) were only partially successful. This substance was less irritating but had such an objectionable sweetish taste that most people could not be induced to take it. The breakthrough came at the turn of the century (1893) when Felix Hofmann, a chemist for the German firm of Bayer, devised a practical route for synthesizing acetylsalicylic acid, which was found to have all the same medicinal properties without the highly objectionable taste or the high degree of mucosal-membrane irritation. Bayer called its new product "aspirin," a name derived from *a-* for acetyl, and the root *-spir,* from the Latin name for the meadowsweet plant, *spirea.*

Salicylic acid — Sodium salicylate — Acetylsalicylic acid (aspirin)

The history of aspirin is typical of many of the medicinal substances in current use. Many began as crude plant extracts or folk remedies whose active ingredients were isolated, and their structure was determined by chemists, who then improved on the original.

In the last few years, the mode of action of aspirin has just begun to be explained. A whole new class of compounds called **prostaglandins** has been found to be involved in the body's immune responses. Their synthesis is provoked by interference with the body's normal functioning by foreign substances or unaccustomed stimuli.

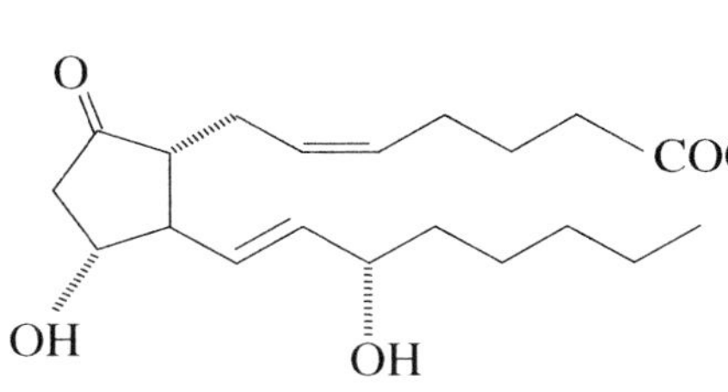

Prostaglandin E₂   Prostaglandin F₂ₐ

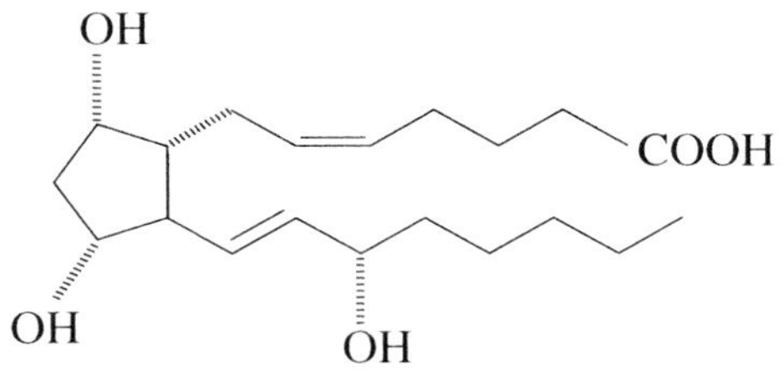

These substances are involved in a wide variety of physiological processes and are thought to be responsible for evoking pain, fever, and local inflammation. Aspirin has recently been shown to prevent bodily synthesis of prostaglandins and thus to alleviate the symptomatic portion (fever, pain, inflammation, menstrual cramps) of the body's immune responses (that is, the ones that let you know something is wrong). One report suggests that aspirin may inactivate one of the enzymes responsible for the synthesis of prostaglandins. The natural precursor for prostaglandin synthesis is **arachidonic acid.** This substance is converted to a peroxide intermediate by an enzyme called **cyclo-oxygenase,** or prostaglandin synthase. This intermediate is converted further to prostaglandin. The apparent role of aspirin is to attach an acetyl group to the active site of cyclo-oxygenase, thus rendering it unable to convert arachidonic acid to the peroxide intermediate. In this way, prostaglandin synthesis is blocked.

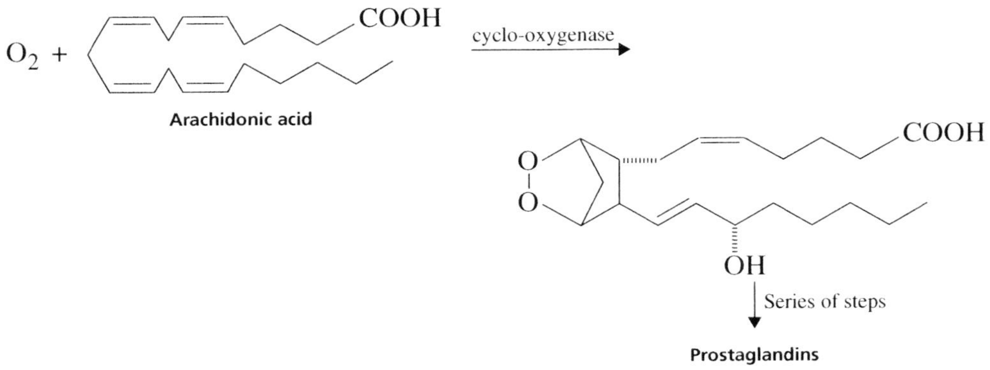

Arachidonic acid

Prostaglandins

Aspirin tablets (5-grain size) are usually compounded of about 0.32 g of acetylsalicylic acid pressed together with a small amount of starch, which binds the ingredients. Buffered aspirin usually contains a basic buffering agent to reduce the acidic irritation of mucous membranes in the stomach because the acetylated product is not totally free of this irritating effect. Bufferin contains 0.325 g of aspirin, together with calcium carbonate, magnesium oxide, and magnesium carbonate as buffering agents. Combination pain relievers usually contain aspirin, acetaminophen, and caffeine. Extra-Strength Excedrin, for instance, contains 0.250 g aspirin, 0.250 g acetaminophen, and 0.065 g caffeine.

REFERENCES

"Aspirin Cuts Deaths after Heart Attacks." *New Scientist,* 118 (April 7, 1988): 22.

Collier, H. O. J. "Aspirin." *Scientific American,* 209 (November 1963): 96.

Collier, H. O. J. "Prostaglandins and Aspirin." *Nature,* 232 (July 2, 1971): 17.

Disla, E., Rhim, H. R., Reddy, A., and Taranta, A. "Aspirin on Trial as HIV Treatment." *Nature,* 366 (November 18, 1993): 198.

Kingman, S. "Will an Aspirin a Day Keep the Doctor Away?" *New Scientist,* 117 (February 11, 1988): 26.

Kolata, G. "Study of Reye's–Aspirin Link Raises Concerns." *Science,* 227 (January 25, 1985): 391.

Macilwain, C. "Aspirin on Trial as HIV Treatment." *Nature,* 364 (July 29, 1993): 369.

Nelson, N. A., Kelly, R. C., and Johnson, R. A. "Prostaglandins and the Arachidonic Acid Cascade." *Chemical and Engineering News* (August 16, 1982): 30.

Pike, J. E. "Prostaglandins." *Scientific American,* 225 (November 1971): 84.

Roth, G. J., Stanford, N., and Majerus, P. W. "Acetylation of Prostaglandin Synthase by Aspirin." *Proceedings of the National Academy of Science of the U.S.A.,* 72 (1975): 3073.

Street, K. W. "Method Development for Analysis of Aspirin Tablets." *Journal of Chemical Education,* 65 (October 1988): 914.

Vane, J. R. "Inhibition of Prostaglandin Synthesis as a Mechanism of Action for Aspirin-Like Drugs." *Nature–New Biology,* 231 (June 23, 1971): 232.

Weissmann, G. "Aspirin." *Scientific American,* 264 (January 1991): 84.

Acetylsalicylic Acid

Crystallization

Vacuum filtration

Melting point

Esterification

Aspirin (acetylsalicylic acid) can be prepared by the reaction between salicylic acid and acetic anhydride:

| Salicylic acid | Acetic anhydride | Acetylsalicylic acid | Acetic acid |

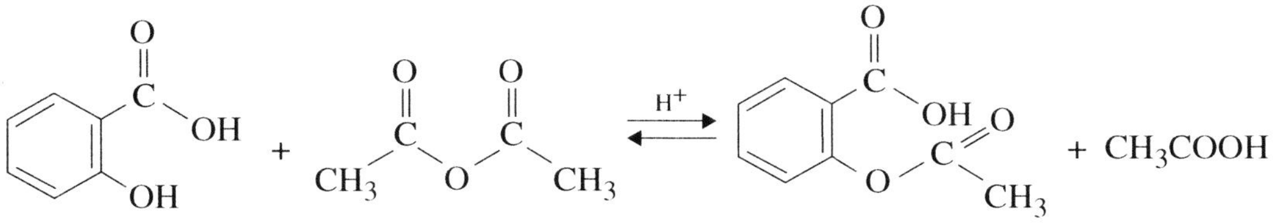

In this reaction, the **hydroxyl group** (—OH) on the benzene ring in salicylic acid reacts with acetic anhydride to form an **ester** functional group. Thus, the formation of acetylsalicylic acid is referred to as an **esterification** reaction. This reaction requires the presence of an acid catalyst, indicated by the H^+ above the equilibrium arrows.

When the reaction is complete, some unreacted salicylic acid and acetic anhydride will be present, along with acetylsalicylic acid, acetic acid, and the catalyst. The technique used to purify the acetylsalicylic acid from the other substances is called **crystallization.** This technique, which was introduced in Experiment 3, will be studied in more detail in Experiment 10. The basic principle is quite simple. At the end of this reaction, the reaction mixture will be hot, and all substances will be in solution. As the solution is allowed to cool, the solubility of acetylsalicylic acid will decrease, and it will gradually come out of solution, or crystallize. Because the other substances are either liquids at room temperature or are present in much smaller amounts, the crystals formed will be composed mainly of acetylsalicylic acid. Thus, a separation of acetylsalicylic acid from the other materials will have been accomplished. The purification process is facilitated by the addition of water after the crystals have formed. The water decreases the solubility of acetylsalicylic acid and dissolves some of the impurities.

The most likely impurity in the final product is salicylic acid itself, which can arise from incomplete reaction of the starting materials or from **hydrolysis** (reaction with water) of the product during the isolation steps. The hydrolysis reaction of acetylsalicylic acid produces salicylic acid. Salicylic acid and other compounds that contain a hydroxyl group on the benzene ring are referred to as **phenols.** Phenols form a highly colored complex with ferric chloride (Fe^{3+} ion). Aspirin is not a phenol, because it does not possess a hydroxyl group directly attached to the ring. Because aspirin will not give the color reaction with ferric chloride, the presence of salicylic acid in the final product is easily detected. The purity of your product will also be determined by obtaining the melting point.

REQUIRED READING

Review: Introduction to Microscale Laboratory (pp. 2–13)

    Technique 8   Filtration, Sections 8.1–8.6

    Technique 9   Physical Constants, Melting Points

New: Technique 5   Measurement of Volume and Weight

    Technique 6   Heating and Cooling Methods

    Technique 7   Reaction Methods, Sections 7.1–7.4

    Essay   Aspirin

SPECIAL INSTRUCTIONS

This experiment involves concentrated phosphoric acid, which is highly corrosive. It will cause burns if it is spilled on the skin. Exercise care in handling it. The acetylsalicylic acid crystals should be allowed to air-dry overnight after filtration on the Hirsch funnel.

SUGGESTED WASTE DISPOSAL

Dispose of the aqueous filtrate in the container for aqueous waste.

PROCEDURE

Preparation of Acetylsalicylic Acid (Aspirin)

Prepare a hot water bath using a 250-mL beaker and a hot plate. Use about 100 mL of water and adjust the temperature to about 50°C. Weigh 0.210 g of salicylic acid (*MW* = 138.1) and place this in a **dry** 5-mL conical vial. It is not necessary for you to weigh exactly 0.210 g of salicylic acid. Try to obtain a weight within about 0.005 g of the indicated weight without spending excessive time at the balance. Record the actual weight in your notebook, and use this weight in any subsequent calculations. Using an automatic pipet or a dispensing pump, add 0.480 mL of acetic anhydride (*MW* = 102.1, *d* = 1.08 g/mL), followed by exactly one drop of concentrated phosphoric acid from a Pasteur pipet.

CAUTION

Concentrated phosphoric acid is highly corrosive. You must handle it with great care.

Add a magnetic spin vane (Fig. 7.8a, p. 607) and attach an air condenser to the vial. Clamp this assembly so that the vial is partially submerged in the hot water bath (Fig. 6.6, p. 594). Stir the mixture with the spin vane until the salicylic acid dissolves. (If the spin vane becomes stuck in the solid salicylic acid, insert a microspatula through the air condenser into the conical vial and gently push the spin vane until it begins spinning.) Heat the mixture for 8–10 minutes after the solid dissolves to complete the reaction.

Crystallization of Acetylsalicylic Acid

Remove the vial from the water bath and allow it to cool. After the vial has cooled enough for you to handle it, detach the air condenser and remove the spin vane with forceps or a magnetic stirring bar. (If you use forceps, be sure to clean them.) Place the conical vial in a small beaker and allow the vial to cool to room temperature, during which time the acetylsalicylic acid should begin to crystallize from the reaction mixture. If it does not crystallize, scratch the walls of the vial with a glass rod (not fire-polished) and cool the mixture slightly in an ice-water bath (Technique 11, Section 11.3C, p. 655) until crystallization has occurred. (Scratching the inside walls of the container often helps to initiate crystallization.) After crystal formation is complete (usually when the product appears as a solid mass), add 3.0 mL of water (measured with a 10-mL graduated cylinder) and stir thoroughly with a microspatula.

Vacuum Filtration

Set up a Hirsch funnel for vacuum filtration (see Technique 8, Section 8.3, and Fig. 8.5, p. 622). Moisten the filter paper with a few drops of water and turn on the vacuum (or aspirator) to the fullest extent. Transfer the mixture in the conical vial to the Hirsch funnel. When you have removed as much product as possible from the vial, add about 1 mL of cold water to the vial using a calibrated Pasteur pipet (p. 11). Stir the mixture and transfer the remaining crystals and water to the Hirsch funnel. When all the crystals have been collected in the funnel, rinse them with several 0.5-mL portions of cold water. Continue drawing air through the crystals on the Hirsch funnel by suction until the crystals are nearly dry (5–10 minutes). Remove the crystals for air-drying on a watch glass or clay plate. It is convenient to hold the filter paper disc with forceps while *gently* scraping the crystals off the filter paper with a microspatula. If the paper is scraped too hard, small pieces of paper will be removed along with the crystals. To dry the crystals completely, you must set the crystals aside overnight. Weigh the dry product and calculate the percentage yield of acetylsalicylic acid (*MW* = 180.2).

Test for Purity

Ferric Chloride Test

You can perform this test on a sample of your product that is not completely dry. To determine if there is any salicylic acid remaining in your product, carry out the following procedure. Obtain three small test tubes. Add 0.5 mL of water to each test tube. Dissolve a small amount of salicylic acid in the first tube. Add a similar amount of your product to the second tube. The third test tube, which contains only solvent, will serve as the control. Add one drop of 1% ferric chloride solution to each tube and note the color after shaking. Formation of an iron–phenol complex with Fe(III) gives a definite color ranging from red to violet, depending on the particular phenol present.

Melting Point

As an additional test for purity, determine the melting point of your product (see Technique 9, Sections 9.5–9.8, pp. 631–636). The melting point must be obtained with a completely dried sample. Pure aspirin has a melting point of 135–136°C.

Place your product in a small vial, label it properly (p. 565), and submit it to your instructor.

Aspirin Tablets

Aspirin tablets are acetylsalicylic acid pressed together with a small amount of inert binding material. Common binding substances include starch, methylcellulose, and microcrystalline cellulose. You can test for the presence of starch by boiling approximately one-fourth of an aspirin tablet with 2 mL of water. Cool the liquid and add a drop of iodine solution. If starch is present, it will form a complex with the iodine. The starch–iodine complex is deep blue–violet. Repeat this test with a commercial aspirin tablet and with the acetylsalicylic acid prepared in this experiment.

QUESTIONS

1. What is the purpose of the concentrated phosphoric acid used in the first step? *acid catalyst*

2. What would happen if the phosphoric acid were left out? *slow, activ barrier not overcome*

3. If you used 250 mg of salicylic acid and excess acetic anhydride in the preceding synthesis of aspirin, what would be the theoretical yield of acetylsalicylic acid in moles? In milligrams?

4. What is the equation for the <u>decomposition reaction</u> that can occur with aspirin in water?

5. Most aspirin tablets contain five grains of acetylsalicylic acid. How many milligrams is this? (*Hint:* See the essay "Aspirin.")

6. A student performed the reaction in this experiment using a water bath at 90°C instead of 50°C. The final product was tested for the presence of phenols with ferric chloride. This test was negative (no color observed); however, the melting point of the dry product was 122–125°C. Explain these results as completely as possible. *dif prod...*

7. If the aspirin crystals were not completely dried before the melting point was determined, what effect would this have on the observed melting point? *water, solvent in it: lower MP*

MW: daltons
 # grams / mol

3.

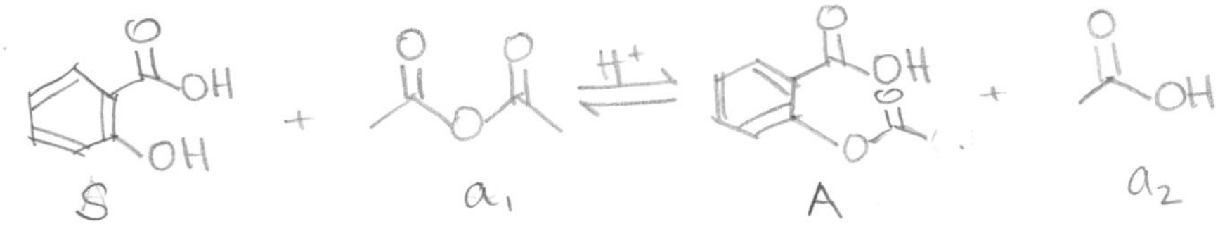

$$.250\,g\;S \times \frac{1\,mol\;S}{138.1\,g} \times \frac{1\,mol\;A}{1\,mol\;S} \times \frac{180.2\,g}{1\,mol\;A} = .326\,g\;A = 326\,mg$$

4. decomp: hydrolysis

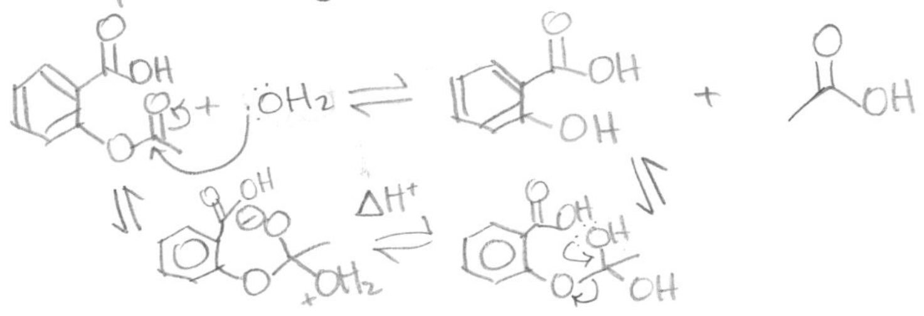

ESSAY

Fireflies and Photochemistry

The production of light as a result of a chemical reaction is called **chemilumines-cence.** A chemiluminescent reaction generally produces one of the product molecules in an electronically excited state. The excited state emits a photon, and light is produced. If a reaction that produces light is biochemical, occurring in a living organism, the phenomenon is called **bioluminescence.**

The light produced by fireflies and other bioluminescent organisms has fascinated observers for many years. Many different organisms have developed the ability to emit light. They include bacteria, fungi, protozoans, hydras, marine worms, sponges, corals, jellyfish, crustaceans, clams, snails, squids, fish, and insects. Curiously, among the higher forms of life, only fish are included on the list. Amphibians, reptiles, birds, mammals, and the higher plants are excluded. Among the marine species, none is a freshwater organism. The excellent *Scientific American* article by McElroy and Seliger (see References) delineates the natural history, characteristics, and habits of many bioluminescent organisms.

The first significant studies of a bioluminescent organism were performed by the French physiologist Raphael Dubois in 1887. He studied the mollusk *Pholas dactylis,* a bioluminescent clam indigenous to the Mediterranean Sea. Dubois found that a cold-water extract of the clam was able to emit light for several minutes following the extraction. When the light emission ceased, it could be restored, he found, by a material extracted from the clam by hot water. A hot-water extract of the clam alone did not produce the luminescence. Reasoning carefully, Dubois concluded that there was an enzyme in the cold-water extract that was destroyed in hot water. The luminescent compound, however, could be extracted without destruction in either hot or cold water. He called the luminescent material **luciferin,** and the enzyme that induced it to emit light, **luciferase;** both names were derived from *Lucifer,* a Latin name meaning "bearer of light." Today the luminescent materials from all organisms are called *luciferins,* and the associated enzymes are called *luciferases.*

The most extensively studied bioluminescent organism is the firefly. Fireflies are found in many parts of the world and probably represent the most familiar example of bioluminescence. In such areas, on a typical summer evening, fireflies, or "lightning bugs," can frequently be seen to emit flashes of light as they cavort over the lawn or in the garden. It is now universally accepted that the luminescence of fireflies is a mating device. The male firefly flies about 2 feet above the ground and emits flashes of light at regular intervals. The female, who remains stationary on the ground, waits a characteristic interval and then flashes a response. In return, the male reorients his direction of flight toward her and flashes a signal once again. The entire cycle is rarely repeated more than 5 to 10 times before the male reaches the female. Fireflies of different species can recognize one another by their flash patterns, which vary in number, rate, and duration among species.

Although the total structure of the luciferase enzyme of the American firefly *Photinus pyralis* is unknown, the structure of the luciferin has been established. In spite of a large amount of experimental work, however, the complete nature of the chemical reactions that produce the light is still subject to some controversy. It is possible, nevertheless, to outline the most salient details of the reaction.

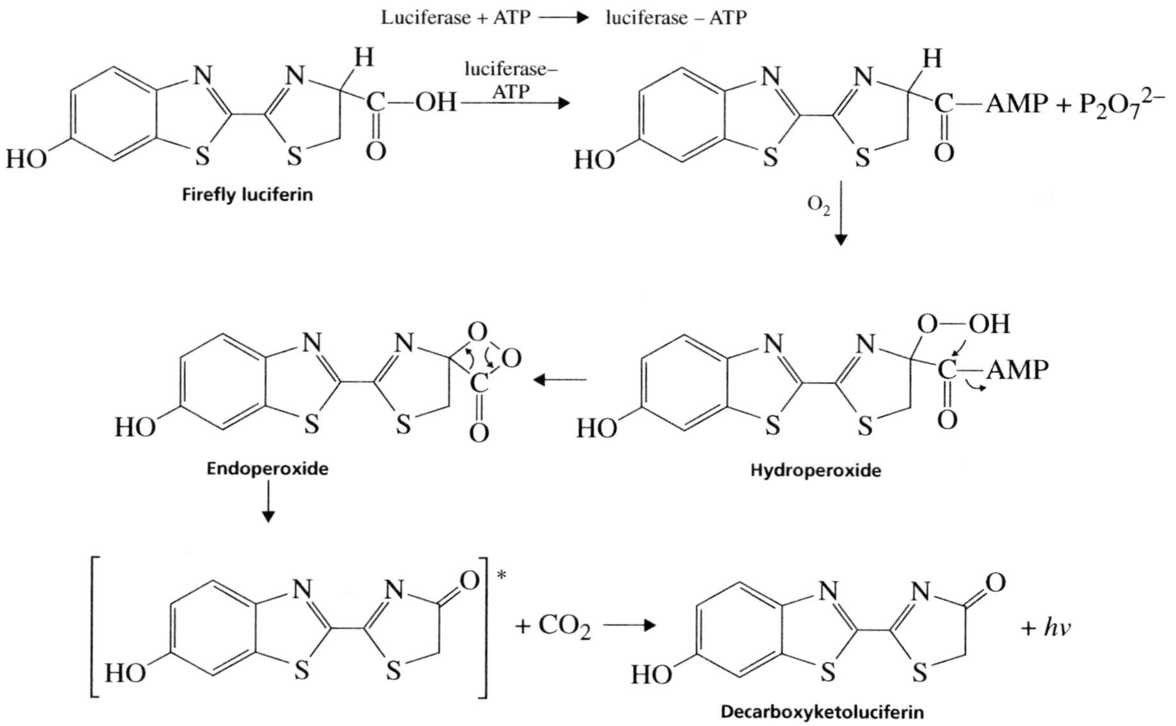

$$\text{Luciferase} + \text{ATP} \longrightarrow \text{luciferase} - \text{ATP}$$

Firefly luciferin

Endoperoxide **Hydroperoxide**

Decarboxyketoluciferin

Besides the luciferin and the luciferase, other substances—magnesium(II), ATP (adenosine triphosphate), and molecular oxygen—are needed to produce the luminescence. In the postulated first step of the reaction, the luciferase complexes with an ATP molecule. In the second step, the luciferin binds to the luciferase and reacts with the already bound ATP molecule to become "primed." In this reaction, pyrophosphate ion is expelled, and AMP (adenosine monophosphate) becomes attached to the carboxyl group of the luciferin. In the third step, the luciferin–AMP complex is oxidized by molecular oxygen to form a hydroperoxide; this cyclizes with the carboxyl group, expelling AMP and forming the cyclic endoperoxide. This reaction would be difficult if the carboxyl group of the luciferin had not been primed with ATP. The endoperoxide is unstable and readily decarboxylates, producing decarboxyketoluciferin in an *electronically excited state,* which is deactivated by the emission of a photon (fluorescence). Thus, it is the cleavage of the four-membered-ring endoperoxide that leads to the electronically excited molecule and hence the bioluminescence.

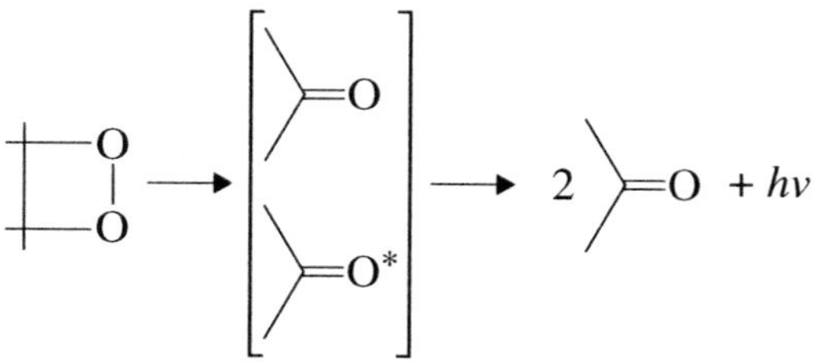

That one of the two carbonyl groups, either that of the decarboxyketoluciferin or that of the carbon dioxide, should be formed in an excited state can be readily predicted from the orbital symmetry conservation principles of Woodward and Hoffmann. This reaction is formally like the decomposition of a cyclobutane ring and yields two ethylene molecules. In analyzing the forward course of that reaction, that is, 2 ethylene $\rightarrow$ cyclobutane, one can easily show that the reaction, which involves four π electrons, is forbidden for two ground-state ethylenes but allowed for only one ethylene in the ground state and the other in an excited state. This suggests that, in the reverse process, one of the ethylene molecules should be formed in an excited state. Extending these arguments to the endoperoxide also suggests that one of the two carbonyl groups should be formed in its excited state.

The emitting molecule, decarboxyketoluciferin, has been isolated and synthesized. When it is excited photochemically by photon absorption in basic solution (pH $>$ 7.5–8.0), it fluoresces, giving a fluorescence emission spectrum that is identical to the emission spectrum produced by the interaction of firefly luciferin and firefly luciferase. The emitting form of decarboxyketoluciferin has thus been identified as the **enol dianion.** In neutral or acidic solution, the emission spectrum of decarboxyketoluciferin does not match the emission spectrum of the bioluminescent system.

The exact function of the enzyme firefly luciferase is not yet known, but it is clear that all these reactions occur while luciferin is bound to the enzyme as a substrate. Also, because the enzyme undoubtedly has several basic groups ($-COO^-$, $-NH_2$, and so on), the buffering action of those groups would easily explain why the enol dianion is also the emitting form of decarboxyketoluciferin in the biological system.

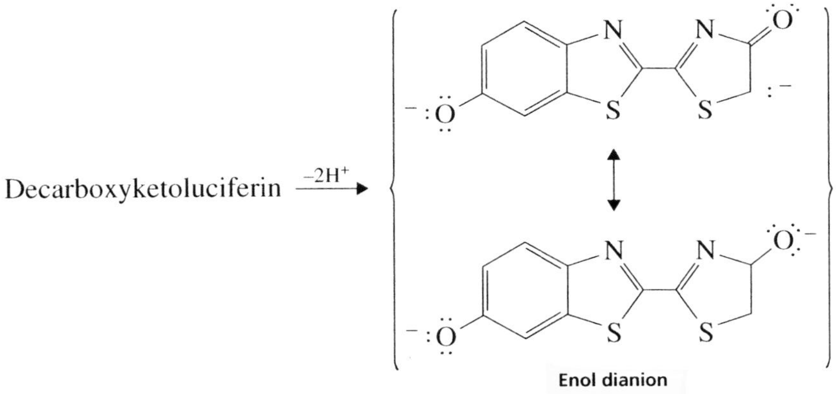

Enol dianion

Most chemiluminescent and bioluminescent reactions require oxygen. Likewise, most produce an electronically excited emitting species through the decomposition of a **peroxide** of one sort or another. In the experiment that follows, a **chemiluminescent** reaction that involves the decomposition of a peroxide intermediate is described.

REFERENCES

Clayton, R. K. "The Luminescence of Fireflies and Other Living Things." Chap. 6 in *Light and Living Matter.* Vol. 2: *The Biological Part.* New York: McGraw-Hill, 1971.

Fox, J. L. "Theory May Explain Firefly Luminescence." *Chemical and Engineering News, 56* (March 6, 1978): 17.

Harvey, E. N. *Bioluminescence.* New York: Academic Press, 1952.

Hastings, J. W. "Bioluminescence." *Annual Review of Biochemistry, 37* (1968): 597.

McCapra, F. "Chemical Mechanisms in Bioluminescence." *Accounts of Chemical Research, 9* (1976): 201.

McElroy, W. D., and Seliger, H. H. "Biological Luminescence." *Scientific American, 207* (December 1962): 76.

McElroy, W. D., Seliger, H. H., and White, E. H. "Mechanism of Bioluminescence, Chemiluminescence and Enzyme Function in the Oxidation of Firefly Luciferin." *Photochemistry and Photobiology, 10* (1969): 153.

Seliger, H. H., and McElroy, W. D. *Light: Physical and Biological Action.* New York: Academic Press, 1965.

EXPERIMENT 51

Luminol

Chemiluminescence
Energy transfer
Reduction of a nitro group
Amide formation

In this experiment, the chemiluminescent compound **luminol,** or **5-amino-phthalhydrazide,** will be synthesized from 3-nitrophthalic acid.

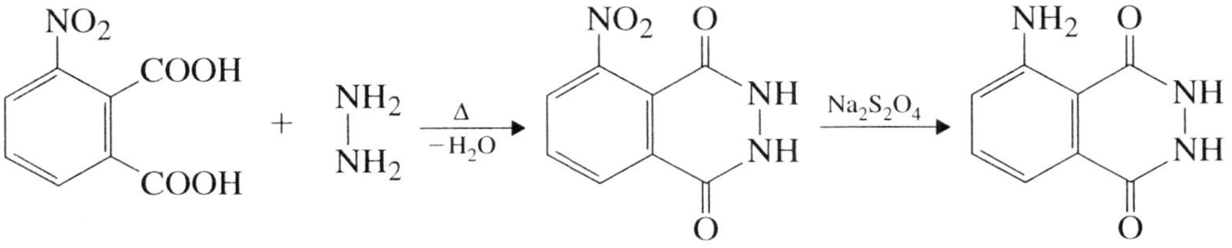

3-Nitrophthalic acid   Hydrazine   5-Nitrophthalhydrazide   Luminol

The first step of the synthesis is the simple formation of a cyclic diamide, 5-nitrophthalhydrazide, by reaction of 3-nitrophthalic acid with hydrazine. Reduction of the nitro group with sodium dithionite affords luminol.

In neutral solution, luminol exists largely as a dipolar anion (zwitterion). This dipolar ion exhibits a weak blue fluorescence after being exposed to light. However, in alkaline solution, luminol is converted to its dianion, which may be oxidized by molecular oxygen to give an intermediate that is chemiluminescent. The reaction is thought to have the following sequence:

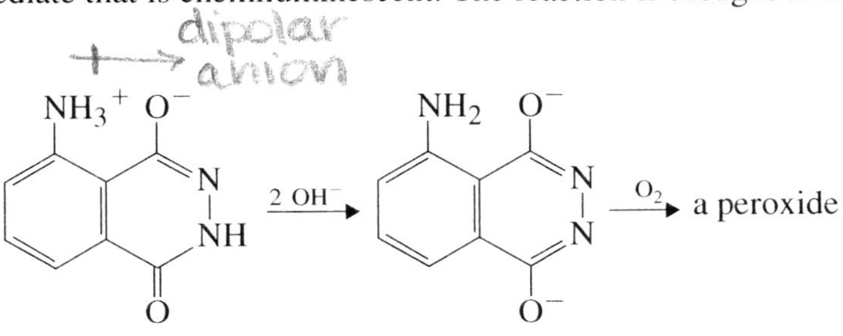

Luminol   Dianion

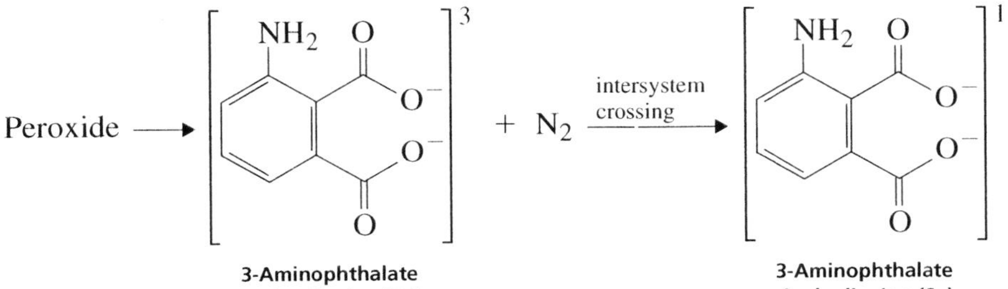

3-Aminophthalate
triplet dianion (T$_1$)   3-Aminophthalate
single dianion (S$_1$)

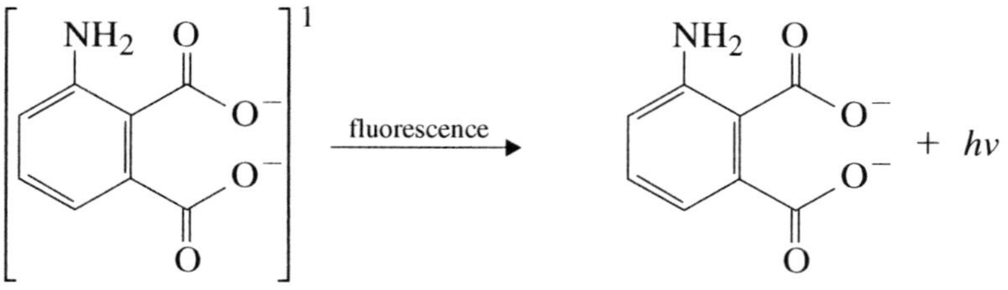

$$\text{S}_1 \xrightarrow{\text{fluorescence}} \text{3-Aminophthalate ground-state dianion, S}_0 + h\nu$$

The dianion of luminol undergoes a reaction with molecular oxygen to form a peroxide of unknown structure. This peroxide is unstable and decomposes with the evolution of nitrogen gas, producing the 3-aminophthalate dianion in an electronically excited state. The excited dianion emits a photon that is visible as light. One very attractive hypothesis for the structure of the peroxide postulates a cyclic endoperoxide that decomposes by the following mechanism:

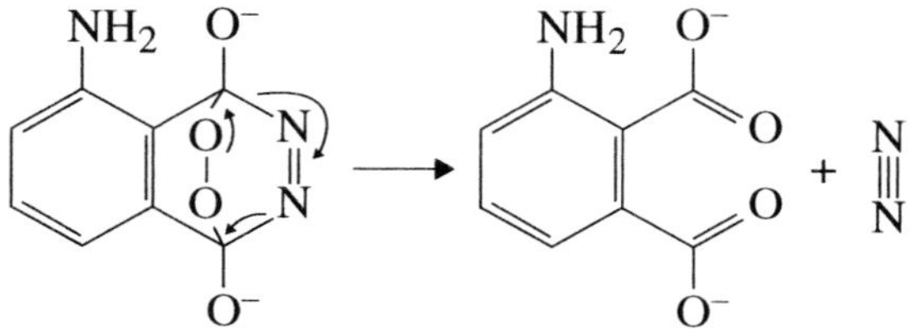

Certain experimental facts argue against this intermediate, however. For instance, certain acyclic hydrazides that cannot form a similar intermediate have also been found to be chemiluminescent.

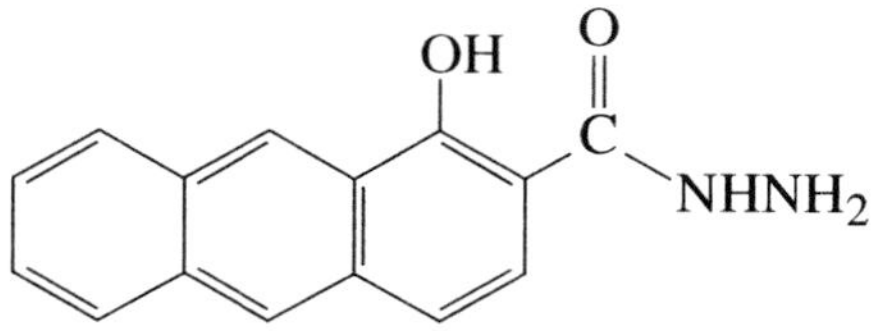

**1-Hydroxy-2-anthroic acid
hydrazide (chemiluminescent)**

Although the nature of the peroxide is still debatable, the remainder of the reaction is well understood. The chemical products of the reaction have been shown to be the 3-aminophthalate dianion and molecular nitrogen. The intermediate that emits light has been identified definitely as the *excited-state singlet* of the 3-aminophthalate dianion.[1] Thus, the fluorescence emission spectrum of the 3-aminophthalate dianion (produced by photon absorption) is identical to the spectrum of the light emitted from the chemiluminescent reaction. However, for numerous complicated reasons, it is believed that the 3-aminophthalate

---

[1] The terms *singlet, triplet, intersystem crossing, energy transfer,* and *quenching* are explained in Experiment 50.

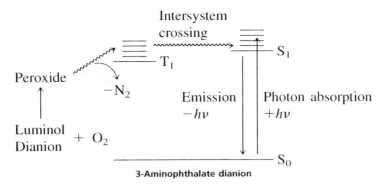

Fluorescence emission spectrum of the 3-aminophthalate dianion.

dianion is formed first as a vibrationally excited triplet state molecule, which makes the intersystem crossing to the singlet state before emission of a photon.

The excited state of the 3-aminophthalate dianion may be quenched by suitable acceptor molecules, or the energy (about 50–80 Kcal/mol) may be transferred to give emission from the acceptor molecules. Several such experiments are described in the following procedure.

The system chosen for the chemiluminescence studies of luminol in this experiment uses dimethylsulfoxide $(CH_3)_2SO$ as the solvent, potassium hydroxide as the base required for the formation of the dianion of luminol, and molecular oxygen. Several alternative systems have been used, substituting hydrogen peroxide and an oxidizing agent for molecular oxygen. An aqueous system using potassium ferricyanide and hydrogen peroxide is an alternative system used frequently.

References

Rahaut, M. M. "Chemiluminescence from Concerted Peroxide Decomposition Reactions." *Accounts of Chemical Research, 2* (1969): 80.

White, E. H., and Roswell, D. F. "The Chemiluminescence of Organic Hydrazides." *Accounts of Chemical Research, 3* (1970): 54.

Required Reading

Review:	Technique 7	Reaction Methods, Section 7.9
New:	Essay	Fireflies and Photochemistry

Special Instructions

This entire experiment can be completed in about 1 hour. When you are working with hydrazine, you should remember that it is toxic and should not be spilled on the skin. It is also a suspected carcinogen. Dimethylsulfoxide may also be toxic; avoid breathing the vapors or spilling it on your skin.

A darkened room is required to observe adequately the chemiluminescence of luminol. A darkened hood that has had its window covered with butcher paper or aluminum foil also works well. Other fluorescent dyes besides those mentioned (for instance, 9,10-diphenylanthracene) can also be used for the energy-transfer experiments. The dyes selected may depend on what is immediately available. The instructor may have each student use one dye for the energy-transfer experiments, with one student making a comparison experiment without a dye.

Suggested Waste Disposal

Dispose of the filtrate from the vacuum filtration of 5-nitrophthalhydrazide in the container designated for nonhalogenated organic solvents. The filtrate from the vacuum filtration of 5-aminophthalhydrazide may be diluted with water and poured into the waste container designated for aqueous waste. The mixture containing potassium hydroxide, dimethylsulfoxide, and luminol should be placed in the special container designated for this material.

Procedure

PART A.   3-NITROPHTHALHYDRAZIDE   *reactants—→intermed.*

Place 0.60 g of 3-nitrophthalic acid and 0.8 mL of a 10% aqueous solution of hydrazine (use gloves) in a small (15-mm × 125-mm) sidearm test tube.[2] At the same time, heat 8 mL of water in a beaker on a hot plate to about 80°C. Heat the test tube over a microburner until the solid dissolves. Add 1.6 mL of triethylene glycol and clamp the test tube in an upright position on a ring stand. Place a thermometer (do not seal the system) and a boiling stone in the test tube and attach a piece of pressure tubing to the sidearm. Connect this tubing to an aspirator (use a trap). The thermometer bulb should be in the liquid as much as possible. Heat the solution with a microburner until the liquid boils vigorously and the refluxing water vapor is drawn away by the aspirator vacuum (the temperature will rise to about 120°C). Continue heating and allow the temperature to increase rapidly until it rises just above 200°C. This heating requires 2–3 minutes, and you must watch the temperature closely to avoid heating the mixture well above 200°C. Remove the burner briefly when this temperature has been achieved and then resume gentle heating to maintain a fairly constant temperature of 220–230°C for about 3 minutes. Allow the test tube to cool to about 100°C, add the 8 mL of hot water that was prepared previously, and cool the test tube to

---

[2] A 10% aqueous solution of hydrazine can be prepared by diluting 15.6 g of a commercial 64% hydrazine solution to a volume of 100 mL using water.

room temperature by allowing tap water to flow over the outside of the test tube. Collect the brown crystals of 5-nitrophthalhydrazide by vacuum filtration, using a small Hirsch funnel. It is not necessary to dry the product before you go on with the next reaction step.

PART B. LUMINOL (5-AMINOPHTHALHYDRAZIDE)

Transfer the moist 5-nitrophthalhydrazide to a 20-mm × 150-mm test tube. Add 2.6 mL of a 10% sodium hydroxide solution and agitate the mixture until the hydrazide dissolves. Add 1.6 g of sodium dithionite dihydrate (sodium hydrosulfite dihydrate, $Na_2S_2O_4 \cdot 2 H_2O$). Using a Pasteur pipet, add 2–4 mL of water to wash the solid from the walls of the test tube. Add a boiling stone to the test tube. Heat the test tube until the solution boils. Agitate the solution and maintain the boiling, continuing the agitation for at least 5 minutes. Add 1.0 mL of glacial acetic acid and cool the test tube to room temperature by allowing tap water to flow over the outside of it. Agitate the mixture during the cooling step. Collect the light yellow or gold crystals of luminol by vacuum filtration, using a small Hirsch funnel. Save a small sample of this product, allow it to dry overnight, and determine its melting point (mp 319–320°C). The remainder of the luminol may be used without drying for the chemiluminescence experiments. When drying the luminol, it is best to use a vacuum desiccator charged with calcium sulfate drying agent.

PART C. CHEMILUMINESCENCE EXPERIMENTS

Caution: Be careful not to allow any of the mixture to touch your skin while shaking the flask. Hold the stopper securely.

Cover the bottom of a 10-mL Erlenmeyer flask with a layer of potassium hydroxide pellets. Add enough dimethylsulfoxide to cover the pellets. Add about 0.025 g of the moist luminol to the flask, stopper it, and shake it vigorously to mix air into the solution.[3] In a dark room, a faint glow of bluish white light will be visible. The intensity of the glow will increase with continued shaking of the flask and occasional removal of the stopper to admit more air.

To observe energy transfer to a fluorescent dye, dissolve 1 or 2 crystals of the indicator dye in about 0.25 mL of water. Add the dye solution to the dimethylsulfoxide solution of luminol, stopper the flask, and shake the mixture vigorously. Observe the intensity and the color of the light produced.

A table of some dyes and the colors produced when they are mixed with luminol follows. Other dyes not included on this list may also be tested in this experiment.

---

[3] An alternative method for demonstrating chemiluminescence, using potassium ferricyanide and hydrogen peroxide as oxidizing agents, is described in E. H. Huntress, L. N. Stanley, and A. S. Parker, *Journal of Chemical Education, 11* (1934): 142.

Fluorescent Dye	Color
No dye	Faint bluish white
2,6-Dichloroindophenol	Blue
9-Aminoacridine	Blue green
Eosin	Salmon pink
Fluorescein	Yellow green
Dichlorofluorescein	Yellow orange
Rhodamine B	Green
Phenolphthalein	Purple

EXPERIMENT 24

4-Methylcyclohexene

Preparation of an alkene
Dehydration of an alcohol
Distillation
Bromine and permanganate tests for unsaturation

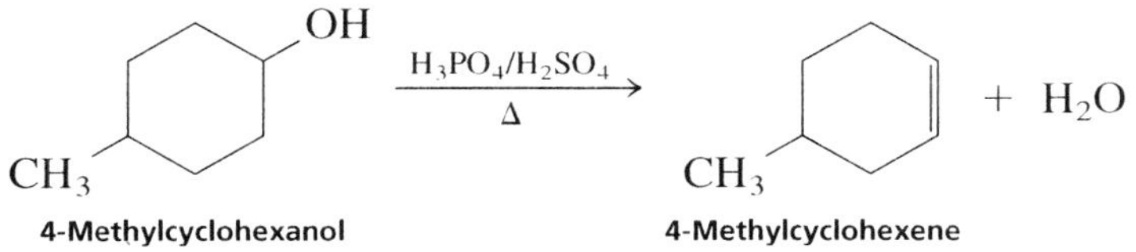

$$\text{4-Methylcyclohexanol} \xrightarrow[\Delta]{H_3PO_4/H_2SO_4} \text{4-Methylcyclohexene} + H_2O$$

Alcohol dehydration is an <u>acid-catalyzed reaction</u> performed by strong, concentrated mineral acids such as sulfuric and phosphoric acids. The acid protonates the alcoholic hydroxyl group, permitting it to dissociate as water. Loss of a proton from the intermediate (elimination) brings about an alkene. Because sulfuric acid often causes extensive <u>charring</u> in this reaction, phosphoric acid, which is comparatively free of this problem, is a better choice. In order to make the reaction proceed faster, however, you will also use a <u>minimal amount of sulfuric acid</u>.

The equilibrium that attends this reaction will be shifted in favor of the product by distilling it from the reaction mixture as it is formed. The <u>4-methylcyclohexene</u> (bp 101–102°C) will codistill with the water that is also formed. By continuously removing the products, you can obtain a high yield of 4-methylcyclohexene. Because the starting material, 4-methylcyclohexanol, also has a somewhat low boiling point (bp 171–173°C), the distillation must be done carefully so that the alcohol does not also distill.

Unavoidably, <u>a small amount of phosphoric acid codistills with the product</u>. It is removed by washing the distillate mixture with a <u>saturated sodium chloride solution</u>. This step also <u>partially removes the water</u> from the 4-methylcyclohexene layer; the drying process will be completed by allowing the product to stand over anhydrous sodium sulfate.

Compounds containing double bonds react with a bromine solution <u>(red)</u> to <u>decolorize</u> it. Similarly, they react with a solution of <u>potassium permanganate (purple)</u> to discharge its color and produce a <u>brown precipitate (MnO₂)</u>. These reactions are often used as qualitative tests to determine the presence of a double bond in an organic molecule (see Experiment 55). Both tests will be performed on the 4-methylcyclohexene formed in this experiment.

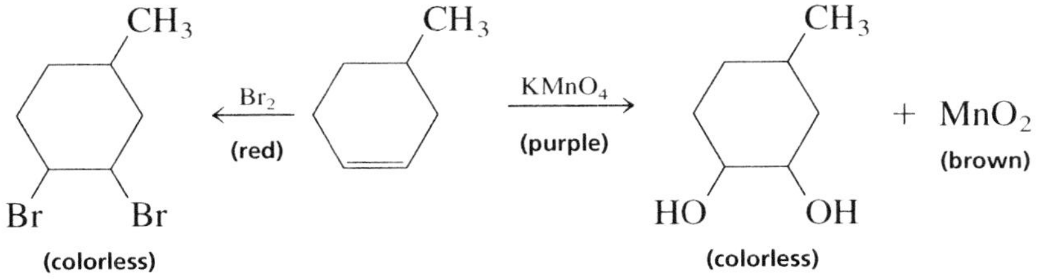

$$\underset{\text{(colorless)}}{\overset{CH_3}{\text{Br}\quad\text{Br}}} \xleftarrow[\text{(red)}]{Br_2} \overset{CH_3}{\bigcirc} \xrightarrow[\text{(purple)}]{KMnO_4} \underset{\text{(colorless)}}{\overset{CH_3}{\text{HO}\quad\text{OH}}} + \underset{\text{(brown)}}{MnO_2}$$

Review: Techniques 5 and 6
Technique 12   Extractions, Separations, and Drying Agents,
Sections 12.7, 12.8, and 12.9

New: Technique 14   Simple Distillation

If performing the optional infrared spectroscopy, also read
Technique 25   Infrared Spectroscopy

Special Instructions

Phosphoric and sulfuric acids are very corrosive. Do not allow either acid to touch your skin.

Suggested Waste Disposal

Dispose of aqueous wastes by pouring them into the container designated for aqueous wastes. Residues that remain after the first distillation may also be placed in the aqueous waste container. Discard the solutions that remain after the bromine test for unsaturation in an organic waste container designated for the disposal of *halogenated* wastes. The solutions that remain after the potassium permanganate test should be discarded into a waste container specifically marked for the disposal of potassium permanganate waste.

Procedure

Apparatus Assembly.   Place 7.5 mL of 4-methylcyclohexanol (*MW* = 114.2) in a tared 50-mL round-bottom flask and reweigh the flask to determine an accurate weight for the alcohol. Add 2.0 mL of 85% phosphoric acid and 30 drops (0.40 mL) of concentrated sulfuric acid to the flask. Mix the liquids thoroughly using a glass stirring rod and add a boiling stone. Assemble a distillation apparatus as shown in Technique 14, Figure 14.1, p. 734 (omit the condenser), using a 25-mL flask as a receiver. Immerse the receiving flask in an ice-water bath to minimize the possibility that 4-methylcyclohexene vapors will escape into the laboratory.

Dehydration.   Start circulating the cooling water in the condenser and heat the mixture with a heating mantle until the product begins to distill and collect in the receiver. The heating should be regulated so that the distillation requires about 30 minutes. Too rapid distillation leads to incomplete reaction and isolation of the starting material, 4-methylcyclohexanol. Continue the distillation until no more liquid is collected. The distillate contains 4-methylcyclohexene as well as water.

Isolation and Drying of the Product.   Transfer the distillate to a centrifuge tube with the aid of 1 or 2 mL of saturated sodium chloride solution. Allow the layers to

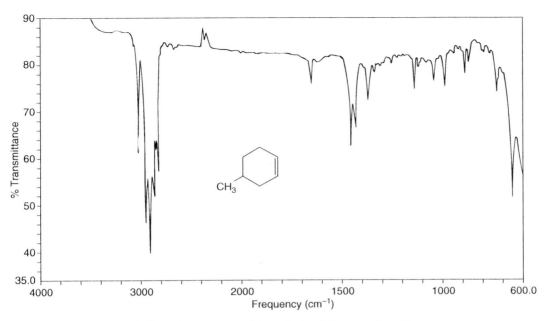

Infrared spectrum of 4-methylcyclohexene (neat).

separate and remove the bottom aqueous layer with a Pasteur pipet (discard it). Using a dry Pasteur pipet, transfer the organic layer remaining in the centrifuge tube to an Erlenmeyer flask containing a small amount of granular anhydrous sodium sulfate. Place a stopper in the flask and set it aside for 10–15 minutes to remove the last traces of water. During this time, wash and dry the distillation apparatus, using small amounts of acetone and an air stream to aid the drying process.

Distillation. Transfer as much of the dried liquid as possible to the clean, dry 50-mL round-bottom flask, being careful to leave as much of the solid drying agent behind as possible. Add a boiling stone to the flask and assemble the distillation apparatus as before, using a *preweighed* 25-mL receiving flask. Because 4-methylcyclohexene is so volatile, you will recover more product if you cool the receiver in an ice-water bath. Using a heating mantle, distill the 4-methylcyclohexene, collecting the material that boils over the range 100–105°C. Record your observed boiling-point range in your notebook. There will be little or no forerun, and very little liquid will remain in the distilling flask at the end of the distillation. Reweigh the receiving flask to determine how much 4-methylcyclohexene you prepared. Calculate the percentage yield of 4-methylcyclohexene ($MW = 96.2$).

Spectroscopy. At the instructor's option, obtain the infrared spectrum of 4-methylcyclohexene (Technique 25, Section 25.2, p. 875, or 25.3, p. 876). Because 4-methylcyclohexene is so volatile, you must work quickly to obtain a good spectrum using sodium chloride plates. Compare the spectrum with the one shown in this experiment. After performing the following tests, submit your sample, along with the report, to the instructor.[1]

---

[1] The product of the distillation may also be analyzed by gas chromatography. We have found that when using gas chromatography–mass spectrometry to analyze the products of this reaction, it is possible to observe the presence of isomeric methylcyclohexenes. These isomers arise from rearrangement reactions that occur during the dehydration.

UNSATURATION TESTS

Place 4–5 drops of 4-methylcyclohexanol in each of two small test tubes. In each of another pair of small test tubes, place 4–5 drops of the 4-methylcyclohexene you prepared. Do not confuse the test tubes. Take one test tube from each group and add a solution of bromine in carbon tetrachloride or methylene chloride, drop by drop, to the contents of the test tube until the red color is no longer discharged. Record the result in each case, including the number of drops required. Test the remaining two test tubes in a similar fashion with a solution of potassium permanganate. Because aqueous potassium permanganate is not miscible with organic compounds, you will have to add about 0.3 mL of 1,2-dimethoxyethane to each test tube before making the test. Record your results and explain them.

QUESTIONS

1. Outline a mechanism for the dehydration of 4-methylcyclohexanol catalyzed by phosphoric acid.
2. What major alkene product is produced by the dehydration of the following alcohols?
   a. Cyclohexanol
   b. 1-Methylcyclohexanol
   c. 2-Methylcyclohexanol
   d. 2,2-Dimethylcyclohexanol
   e. 1,2-Cyclohexanediol (*Hint:* Consider keto-enol tautomerism.)
3. Compare and interpret the infrared spectra of 4-methylcyclohexene and 4-methylcyclohexanol.
4. Identify the C — H out-of-plane bending vibrations in the infrared spectrum of 4-methylcyclohexene. What structural information can be obtained from these bands?
5. In this experiment, 1–2 mL of saturated sodium chloride is used to transfer the crude product after the initial distillation. Why is saturated sodium chloride, rather than pure water, used for this procedure?

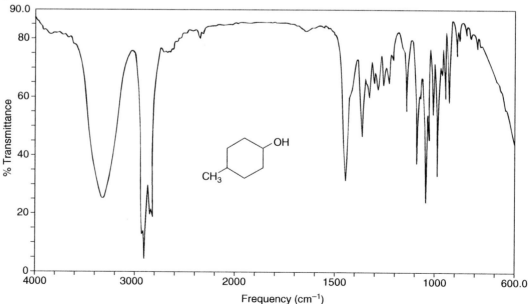

Infrared spectrum of 4-methylcyclohexanol (neat).

374

ESSAY

Identification of Drugs

Frequently, a chemist is called on to identify a particular unknown substance. If there is no prior information to work from, this can be a formidable task. There are several million known compounds, both inorganic and organic. For a completely unknown substance, the chemist must often use every available method. If the unknown substance is a mixture, then the mixture must be separated into its components and each component identified separately. A pure compound can often be identified from its physical properties (melting point, boiling point, density, refractive index, and so on) and a knowledge of its functional groups. These can be identified by the reactions that the compound is observed to undergo or by spectroscopy (infrared, ultraviolet, nuclear magnetic resonance, and mass spectroscopy). The techniques necessary for this type of identification are introduced in a later section.

A somewhat simpler situation often arises in drug identification. The scope of drug identification is more limited, and the chemist working in a hospital trying to identify the source of a drug overdose or the law enforcement officer trying to identify a suspected illicit drug or a poison usually has some prior clues to work from. So does the medicinal chemist working for a pharmaceutical manufacturer who might be trying to discover why a competitor's product may be better.

Consider a drug overdose case as an example. The patient is brought into the emergency ward of a hospital. This person may be in a coma or a hyperexcited state, have an allergic rash, or clearly be hallucinating. These physiological symptoms are themselves a clue to the nature of the drug. Samples of the drug may be found in the patient's possession. Correct medical treatment may require a rapid and accurate identification of a drug powder or capsule. If the patient is conscious, the necessary information can be elicited orally; if not, the drug must be examined. If the drug is a tablet or a capsule, the process is often simple, because many drugs are coded by a manufacturer's trademark or logo, by shape (round, oval, bullet shape), by formulation (tablet, gelatin capsule, time-release microcapsules), and by color. Some drugs bear an imprinted number or code.

It is more difficult to identify a powder, but under some circumstances such identification may be easy. Plant drugs are often easily identified because they contain microscopic bits and pieces of the plant from which they are obtained. This cellular debris is often characteristic for certain types of drugs, and they can be identified on this basis alone. A microscope is all that is needed. Sometimes chemical color tests can be used as confirmation. Certain drugs give rise to characteristic colors when treated with special reagents. Other drugs form crystalline precipitates of characteristic color and crystal structure when treated with appropriate reagents.

If the drug itself is not available and the patient is unconscious (or dead), identification may be more difficult. It may be necessary to pump the stomach or bladder contents of the patient (or corpse) or to obtain a blood sample and work on these. These samples of stomach fluid, urine, or blood would be extracted with an appropriate organic solvent, and the extract would be analyzed.

Often the final identification of a drug, as an extract of urine, serum, or stomach fluid, hinges on some type of **chromatography.** Thin-layer chromatography (TLC) is often used.

Under specified conditions, many drug substances can be identified by their R_f values and by the colors that their TLC spots turn when treated with various reagents or when they are observed under certain visualization methods. In the experiment that follows, TLC is applied to the analysis of an unknown analgesic drug.

REFERENCES

Keller, E. "Origin of Modern Criminology." *Chemistry, 42* (1969): 8.

Keller, E. "Forensic Toxicology: Poison Detection and Homicide." *Chemistry, 43* (1970): 14.

Lieu, V. T. "Analysis of APC Tablets." *Journal of Chemical Education, 48* (1971): 478.

Neman, R. L. "Thin Layer Chromatography of Drugs." *Journal of Chemical Education, 49* (1972): 834.

Rodgers, S. S. "Some Analytical Methods Used in Crime Laboratories." *Chemistry, 42* (1969): 29.

Tietz, N. W. *Fundamentals of Clinical Chemistry.* Philadelphia: W. B. Saunders, 1970.

Walls, H. J. *Forensic Science.* New York: Praeger, 1968.

A collection of articles on forensic chemistry can be found in

Berry, K., and Outlaw, H. E., eds. "Forensic Chemistry—A Symposium Collection." *Journal of Chemical Education, 62* (December 1985): 1043–1065.

EXPERIMENT 10

TLC Analysis of Analgesic Drugs

Thin-layer chromatography

In this experiment, thin-layer chromatography (TLC) will be used to determine the composition of various over-the-counter analgesics. If the instructor chooses, you may also be required to identify the components and actual identity (trade name) of an unknown analgesic. You will be given either two or three commercially prepared TLC plates with a flexible backing and a silica gel coating with a fluorescent indicator. On the first TLC plate, a reference plate, you will spot five standard compounds often used in analgesic formulations. In addition, a standard reference mixture containing four of these same compounds will be spotted. Ibuprofen is omitted from this standard mixture because it would overlap with salicylamide after the plate is developed. If your instructor wishes, you will spot five additional reference substances on a second reference plate, including the newest analgesic drugs. On the final plate (the sample plate) you will spot several commercial analgesic preparations in order to determine their composition. At your instructor's option, one or more of these may be an unknown.

The standard compounds will all be available as solutions of 1 g of each dissolved in 20 mL of a 50:50 mixture of methylene chloride and ethanol. The purpose of the first reference plate is to determine the order of elution (R_f values) of the known substances and to index the standard reference mixture. On the second reference plate (optional), several of

Reference Plate 1		Reference Plate 2 (optional)		Sample Plate
Acetaminophen	(Ac)	Aspirin	(Asp)	Five commercial preparations (or unknowns) plus the reference mixture
Aspirin	(Asp)	Ibuprofen	(Ibu)	
Caffeine	(Cf)	Ketoprofen	(Kpf)	
Ibuprofen	(Ibu)	Naproxen sodium	(Nap)	
Salicylamide	(Sal)	Salicylamide	(Sal)	
Reference mixture 1	(Ref-1)	Reference mixture 2	(Ref-2)	

the substances have similar R_f values, but you will note a different behavior for each spot with the visualization methods. On the sample plate, the standard reference mixture will be spotted, along with several solutions that you will prepare from commercial analgesic tablets. These tablets will each be crushed and dissolved in a 50:50 methylene chloride–ethanol mixture for spotting.

Two methods of visualization will be used to observe the positions of the spots on the developed TLC plates. First, the plates will be observed while under illumination from a short-wavelength ultraviolet (UV) lamp. This is done best in a darkened room or in a fume hood that has been darkened by taping butcher paper or aluminum foil over the lowered glass cover. Under these conditions, some of the spots will appear as dark areas on the plate, while others will fluoresce brightly. This difference in appearance under UV illumination will help to distinguish the substances from one another. You will find it convenient to outline very lightly in *pencil* the spots observed and to place a small **x** inside those spots that fluoresce. For a second means of visualization, iodine vapor will be used. Not all the spots will become visible when treated with iodine, but some will develop yellow, tan, or deep brown colors. The differences in the behaviors of the various spots with iodine can be used to further differentiate among them.

It is possible to use several developing solvents for this experiment, but ethyl acetate with 0.5% glacial acetic acid added is preferred. The small amount of glacial acetic acid supplies protons and suppresses ionization of aspirin, ibuprofen, naproxen sodium, and ketoprofen, allowing them to travel upward on the plates in their protonated form. Without the acid, these compounds do not move.

In some analgesics, you may find ingredients besides the five mentioned previously. Some include an antihistamine and some, a mild sedative. For instance, Midol contains N-cinnamylephedrine (cinnamedrine), an antihistamine, and Excedrin PM contains the sedative methapyrilene hydrochloride. Cope contains the related sedative methapyrilene fumarate. Some tablets may be colored with a chemical dye.

Required Reading

Review:	Essay	Analgesics
New:	Technique 19	Column Chromatography, Sections 19.1–19.3
	Technique 20	Thin-Layer Chromatography
	Essay	Identification of Drugs

Special Instructions

You must examine the developed plates under ultraviolet light first. After comparisons of *all* plates have been made with UV light, iodine vapor can be used. The iodine permanently affects some of the spots, making it impossible to go back and repeat the UV visualization. Take special care to notice those substances that have similar R_f values; these spots each have a different appearance when viewed under UV illumination or a different staining color with iodine, allowing you to distinguish among them.

Aspirin presents some special problems because it is present in a large amount in many of the analgesics and because it hydrolyzes easily. For these reasons, the aspirin spots often show excessive tailing.

Suggested Waste Disposal

Dispose of all development solvent in the container for nonhalogenated organic solvents. Dispose of the ethanol–methylene chloride mixture in the container for halogenated organic solvents. The micropipets used for spotting the solution should be placed in a special container labeled for that purpose. The TLC plates should be stapled in your lab notebook.

Notes to the Instructor

If you wish, students may work in pairs on this experiment, each one preparing one of the two reference plates and then cooperating on the third plate. Alternatively, especially if students are to work alone, you may wish to omit plate 2 and forgo identifying the two newest analgesics (ketoprofen and naproxen sodium).

Perform the thin-layer chromatography with flexible Silica Gel 60 F-254 plates (EM Science, No. 5554-7). If the TLC plates have not been purchased recently, you should place them in an oven at 100°C for 30 minutes and store them in a desiccator until used. If you use different thin-layer plates, try out the experiment before using them with a class. Other plates may not resolve all five substances.

Ibuprofen and salicylamide have approximately the same R_f value, but they show up differently under the detection methods. For reasons that are not yet clear, ibuprofen sometimes gives two or even three spots. Naproxen sodium and ketoprofen have approximately the same R_f as aspirin. Once again, however, they show up differently under the detection methods. Fortunately, none of the new drugs appears in combination, either together, or with aspirin or ibuprofen, in any current commercial product.

Procedure

Initial Preparations. You will need at least 12 capillary micropipets (18 if both reference plates are prepared) to spot the plates. The preparation of these pipets is described and illustrated in Technique 20, Section 20.4, page 822. A common error is to pull the center section out too far when making these pipets, with the result that too little sample is applied to the plate. If this happens, you won't see *any* spots. Follow the directions carefully.

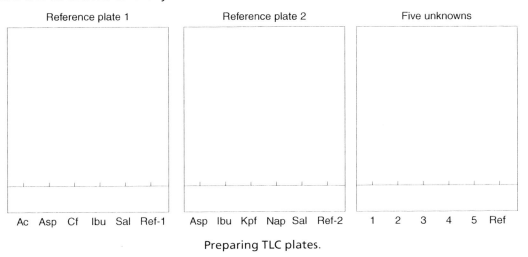

Preparing TLC plates.

379

After preparing the micropipets, obtain two (or three) 10-cm × 6.6-cm TLC plates (EM Science Silica Gel 60 F-254, No. 5554-7) from your instructor. These plates have a flexible backing, but they should not be bent excessively. Handle them carefully or the adsorbent may flake off. Also, you should handle them only by the edges; the surface should not be touched. Using a lead pencil (not a pen), *lightly* draw a line across the plates (short dimension) about l cm from the bottom. Using a centimeter ruler, move its index about 0.6 cm in from the edge of the plate and lightly mark off six 1-cm intervals on the line (see figure). These are the points at which the samples will be spotted. If you are preparing two reference plates, it would be a good idea to mark a small number **1** or **2** in the upper right-hand corner of each plate to allow easy identification.

Spotting the First Reference Plate.   On the first plate (marked 1), starting from left to right, spot acetaminophen, then aspirin, caffeine, ibuprofen, and salicylamide. This order is alphabetic and will avoid any further memory problems or confusion. Solutions of these compounds will be found in small bottles on the side shelf. The standard reference mixture (Ref-1), also found on the side shelf, is spotted in the last position. The correct method of spotting a TLC plate is described in Technique 20, Section 20.4, page 822. It is important that the spots be made as small as possible, but not too small. With too much sample, the spots will tail and will overlap one another after development. With too little sample, no spots will be observed after development. The optimum applied spot should be about 1–2 mm (1/16 in.) in diameter. If scrap pieces of the TLC plates are available, it would be a good idea to practice spotting on these before preparing the actual sample plates.

Spotting the Second Reference Plate (Optional).   On the second plate (marked 2), starting from left to right, spot aspirin, ibuprofen, ketoprofen, naproxen sodium, salicylamide, and the reference mixture (Ref-2). Follow the same procedure and take the precautions noted above for the first plate.

Preparing the Development Chamber.   When the reference plate (or plates) has been spotted, obtain a 16-oz wide-mouth, screw-cap jar (or other suitable container) for use as a development chamber. The preparation of a development chamber is described in Technique 20, Section 20.5, page 823. Because the backing on the TLC plates is very thin, if they touch the filter paper liner of the development chamber *at any point,* solvent will begin to diffuse onto the absorbent surface at that point. To avoid this, you may either omit the liner or make the following modification.

If you wish to use a liner, use a very narrow strip of filter paper (approximately 5 cm wide). Fold it into an L shape that is long enough to traverse the bottom of the jar and extend up the side to the top of the jar. TLC plates placed in the jar for development should *straddle* this liner strip but not touch it.

When the development chamber has been prepared, obtain a small amount of the development solvent (0.5% glacial acetic acid in ethyl acetate). Your instructor should prepare this mixture; it contains such a small amount of acetic acid that small individual portions are difficult to prepare. Fill the chamber with the development solvent to a depth of about 0.5–0.7 cm. If you are using a liner, be sure it is saturated with the solvent. Recall that the solvent level must not be above the spots on the plate or the samples will dissolve off the plate into the reservoir instead of developing.

Development of the Reference TLC Plates.   Place the spotted plate (or plates) in the chamber (straddling the liner if one is present) and allow the spots to develop. If you are doing two reference plates, both plates may be placed in the same development jar. Be sure the plates are placed in the developing jar so that their bottom edge is parallel to the bottom of the jar (straight, not tilted); if not, the solvent front will not advance evenly, increasing the difficulty of making good comparisons. The plates should face each other and slant or lean back in opposite directions. When the solvent has risen to a level about 0.5 cm from the top of the plate, remove each plate from the chamber (in the hood) and, using a lead pencil, mark the position of the solvent front. Set the plate on a piece of paper towel to dry. It may be helpful to place a small object under one end to allow optimum air flow around the drying plate.

UV Visualization of the Reference Plates. When the plates are dry, observe them under a short-wavelength UV lamp, preferably in a darkened hood or a darkened room. Lightly outline all of the observed spots with a pencil. Carefully notice any differences in behavior between the spotted substances, especially those on plate 2. Several compounds have similar R_f values, but the spots have a different appearance under UV illumination or iodine staining. Currently, there are no commercial analgesic preparations containing any compounds that have the same R_f values, but you will need to be able to distinguish them from one another to identify which one is present. Before proceeding, make a sketch of the plates in your notebook and note the differences in appearance that you observed. Using a ruler marked in millimeters, measure the distance that each spot has traveled relative to the solvent front. Calculate R_f values for each spot (Technique 20, Section 20.9, p. 827).

Analysis of Commercial Analgesics or Unknowns (Sample Plate). Next, obtain half a tablet of each of the analgesics to be analyzed on the final TLC plate. If you were issued an unknown, you may analyze four other analgesics of your choice; if not, you may analyze five. The experiment will be most interesting if you make your choices in a way that gives a wide spectrum of results. Try to pick at least one analgesic each containing aspirin, acetaminophen, ibuprofen, a newer analgesic, and, if available, salicylamide. If you have a favorite analgesic, you may wish to include it among your samples. Take each analgesic half-tablet, place it on a smooth piece of notebook paper, and crush it well with a spatula. Transfer each crushed half-tablet to a labeled test tube or a small Erlenmeyer flask. Using a graduated cylinder, mix 15 mL of absolute ethanol and 15 mL of methylene chloride. Mix the solution well. Add 5 mL of this solvent to each of the crushed half-tablets and then heat each of them *gently* for a few minutes on a steam bath or sand bath at about 100°C. Not all the tablet will dissolve, because the analgesics usually contain an insoluble binder. In addition, many of them contain inorganic buffering agents or coatings that are insoluble in this solvent mixture. After heating the samples, allow them to settle and then spot the clear liquid extracts on the sample plate. At the sixth position, spot the standard reference solution (Ref-1 or Ref-2). Develop the plate in 0.5% glacial acetic acid–ethyl acetate as before. Observe the plate under UV illumination and mark the visible spots as you did for the first plate. Sketch the plate in your notebook and record your conclusions about the contents of each tablet. This can be done by directly comparing your plate to the reference plate(s)—they can all be placed under the UV light at the same time. If you were issued an unknown, try to determine its identity (trade name).

Iodine Analysis. Do not perform this step until UV comparisons of all the plates are complete. When ready, place the plates in a jar containing a few iodine crystals, cap the jar, and warm it gently on a steam bath or warm hot plate until the spots begin to appear. Notice which spots become visible and note their relative colors. You can directly compare colors of the reference spots to those on the unknown plate(s). Remove the plates from the jar and record your observations in your notebook.

QUESTIONS

1. What happens if the spots are made too large when preparing a TLC plate for development?
2. What happens if the spots are made too small when preparing a TLC plate for development?
3. Why must the spots be above the level of the development solvent in the developing chamber?
4. What would happen if the spotting line and positions were marked on the plate with a ball-point pen?
5. Is it possible to distinguish two spots that have the same R_f value but represent different compounds? Give two different methods.
6. Name some advantages of using acetaminophen (Tylenol) instead of aspirin as an analgesic.

ESSAY

The Chemistry of Vision

An interesting and challenging topic for chemists to investigate is how the eye functions. What chemistry is involved in detection of light and transmission of that information to the brain? The first definitive studies on how the eye functions were begun in 1877 by Franz Boll. Boll demonstrated that the red color of the retina of a frog's eye could be bleached yellow by strong light. If the frog was then kept in the dark, the red color of the retina slowly returned. Boll recognized that a bleachable substance had to be connected somehow with the ability of the frog to perceive light.

Most of what is now known about the chemistry of vision is the result of the elegant work of George Wald, Harvard University; his studies, which began in 1933, ultimately resulted in his receiving the Nobel Prize in biology. Wald identified the sequence of chemical events during which light is converted into some form of electrical information that can be transmitted to the brain. Here is a brief outline of that process.

The retina of the eye is made up of two types of photoreceptor cells: **rods** and **cones.** The rods are responsible for vision in dim light, and the cones are responsible for color vision in bright light. The same principles apply to the chemical functioning of the rods and the cones; however, the details of functioning are less well understood for the cones than for the rods.

Each rod contains several million molecules of **rhodopsin.** Rhodospin is a complex of a protein, **opsin,** and a molecule derived from Vitamin A, 11-*cis*-retinal (sometimes called **retinene**). Very little is known about the structure of opsin. The structure of 11-*cis*-retinal is shown here.

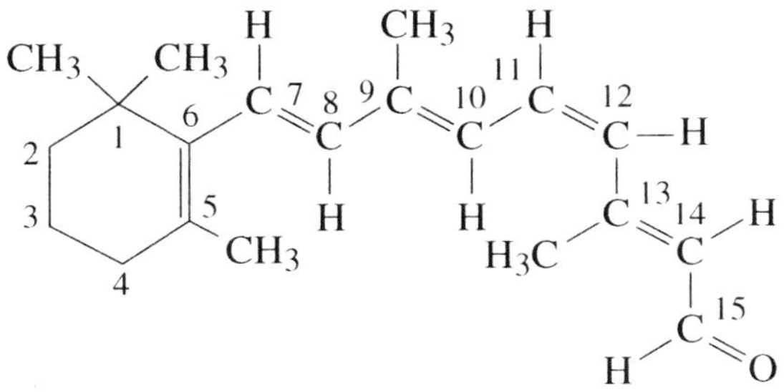

11-*cis*-retinal

The detection of light involves the initial conversion of 11-*cis*-retinal to its all-*trans* isomer. This is the only obvious role of light in this process. The high energy of a quantum of visible light promotes the fission of the π bond between carbons 11 and 12. When the π bond breaks, free rotation about the σ bond in the resulting radical is possible. When the π bond re-forms after such rotation, all-*trans*-retinal results. All-*trans*-retinal is more stable than 11-*cis*-retinal, which is the reason the isomerization proceeds spontaneously in the direction shown.

The two molecules have different shapes due to their different structures. The 11-*cis*-retinal has a fairly curved shape, and the parts of the molecule on either side of the *cis* double bond tend to lie in different planes. Because proteins have very complex and specific three-dimensional shapes (tertiary structures), 11-*cis*-retinal associates with the protein opsin in a particular manner. All-*trans*-retinal has an elongated shape, and the entire molecule tends to lie in a single plane. This different shape for the molecule, compared with that for the 11-*cis* isomer, means that all-*trans*-retinal will have a different association with the protein opsin.

In fact, all-*trans*-retinal associates very weakly with opsin because its shape does not fit the protein. Consequently, the next step after the isomerization of retinal is the dissociation of all-*trans*-retinal from opsin. The opsin protein undergoes a simultaneous change in conformation as the all-*trans*-retinal dissociates.

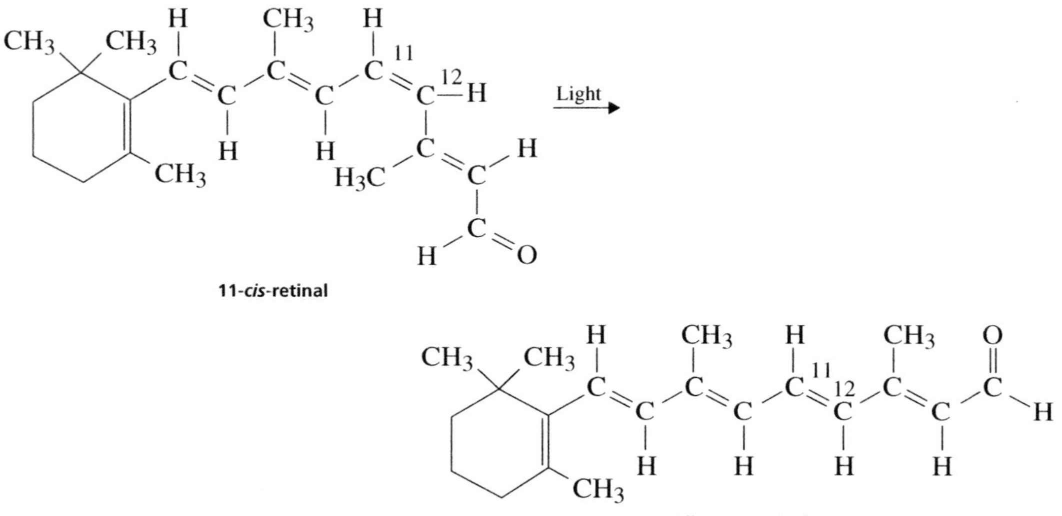

11-*cis*-retinal

All-*trans*-retinal

At some time after the 11-*cis*-retinal–opsin complex receives a photon, a message is received by the brain. It was originally thought that either the isomerization of 11-*cis*-retinal to all-*trans*-retinal or the conformational change of the opsin protein was an event that generated the electrical message sent to the brain. Current research, however, indicates that both these events occur too slowly relative to the speed with which the brain receives the message. Current hypotheses invoke involved quantum mechanical explanations, which hold it significant that the chromophores (light-absorbing groups) are arranged in a very precise geometrical pattern in the rods and cones, allowing the signal to be transmitted rapidly through space. The main physical and chemical events Wald discovered are illustrated in the figure for easy visualization. The question of how the electrical signal is transmitted still remains unsolved.

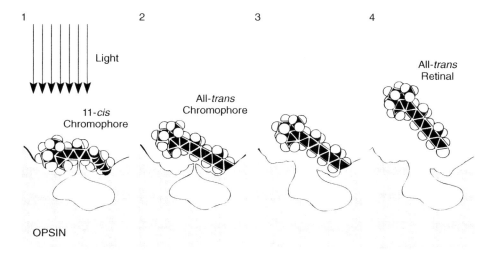

Wald was also able to explain the sequence of events by which the rhodopsin molecules are regenerated. After dissociation of all-*trans*-retinal from the protein, the following enzyme-mediated changes occur. All-*trans*-retinal is reduced to the alcohol all-*trans*-retinol, also called all-*trans*-Vitamin A.

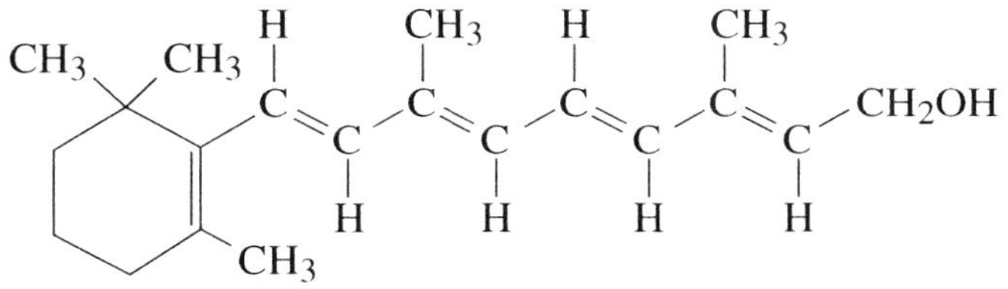

$$CH_3 \quad CH_3 \qquad \overset{H}{\underset{H}{C}} \quad \overset{CH_3}{C} \quad \overset{H}{\underset{H}{C}} \quad \overset{CH_3}{C}$$

All-*trans*-Vitamin A

All-*trans*-Vitamin A is then isomerized to its 11-*cis*-Vitamin A isomer. Following the isomerization, the 11-*cis*-Vitamin A is oxidized back to 11-*cis*-retinal, which forthwith recombines with the opsin protein to form rhodopsin. The regenerated rhodopsin is then ready to begin the cycle anew, as illustrated in the accompanying diagram.

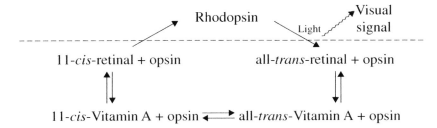

By this process, as little light as 10^{-14} of the number of protons emitted from a typical flashlight bulb can be detected. The conversion of light into isomerized retinal exhibits an ex-

385

traordinarily high quantum efficiency. Virtually every quantum of light absorbed by a molecule of rhodopsin causes the isomerization of 11-*cis*-retinal to all-*trans*-retinal.

As you can see from the reaction scheme, the retinal derives from Vitamin A, which merely requires the oxidation of a —CH$_2$OH group to a —CHO group to be converted to retinal. The precursor in the diet that is transformed to Vitamin A is β-carotene. The β-carotene is the yellow pigment of carrots and is an example of a family of long-chain polyenes called **carotenoids.**

β-Carotene

In 1907, Willstätter established the structure of carotene, but it was not known until 1931–1933 that there were actually three isomers of carotene. The α-carotene differs from β-carotene in that the α isomer has a double bond between C$_4$ and C$_5$ rather than between C$_5$ and C$_6$, as in the β isomer. The γ isomer has only one ring, identical to the ring in the β isomer, whereas the other ring is opened in the γ form between C$_1$′ and C$_6$′. The β isomer is by far the most common of the three.

The substance β-carotene is converted to Vitamin A in the liver. Theoretically, one molecule of β-carotene should give rise to two molecules of the vitamin by cleavage of the C$_{15}$–C$_{15}$′, double bond, but actually only one molecule of Vitamin A is produced from each molecule of the carotene. The Vitamin A thus produced is converted to 11-*cis*-retinal within the eye.

Along with the problem of how the electrical signal is transmitted, color perception is also currently under study. In the human eye there are three kinds of cone cells, which absorb light at 440, 535, and 575 nm, respectively. These cells discriminate among the primary colors. When combinations of them are stimulated, full color vision is the message received in the brain.

Because all these cone cells use 11-*cis*-retinal as a substrate-trigger, it has long been suspected that there must be three different opsin proteins. Recent work has begun to establish how the opsins vary the spectral sensitivity of the cone cells, even though all of them have the same kind of light-absorbing chromophore.

Retinal is an aldehyde, and it binds to the terminal amino group of a lysine residue in the opsin protein to form a Schiff base, or imine linkage (C=N—). This imine linkage is believed to be protonated (with a plus charge) and to be stabilized by being located near a negatively charged amino acid residue of the protein chain. A second negatively charged group is thought to be located near the 11-*cis* double bond. Researchers have recently shown, from synthetic models that use a simpler protein than opsin itself, that forcing these negatively charged groups to be located at different distances from the imine linkage causes the absorption maximum of the 11-*cis*-retinal chromophore to be varied over a wide enough range to explain color vision.

Rhodopsin.

Whether there are actually <u>three different opsin proteins</u>, or whether there are just <u>three different conformations</u> of the same protein in the three types of cone cells, will not be known until further work is completed on the structure of the opsin or opsins.

REFERENCES

Borman, S. "New Light Shed on Mechanism of Human Color Vision." *Chemical and Engineering News* (April 6, 1992): 27.

Fox, J. L. "Chemical Model for Color Vision Resolved." *Chemical and Engineering News, 57* (46) (November 12, 1979): 25. A review of articles by Honig and Nakanishi in the *Journal of the American Chemical Society, 101* (1979): 7082, 7084, 7086.

Hubbard, R., and Kropf, A. "Molecular Isomers in Vision." *Scientific American, 216* (June 1967): 64.

Hubbard, R., and Wald, G. "Pauling and Carotenoid Stereochemistry." In A. Rich and N. Davidson, eds., *Structural Chemistry and Molecular Biology.* San Francisco: W. H. Freeman, 1968.

MacNichol, E. F., Jr. "Three Pigment Color Vision." *Scientific American, 211* (December 1964): 48.

"Model Mechanism May Detail Chemistry of Vision." *Chemical and Engineering News* (January 7, 1985): 40.

Rushton, W. A. H. "Visual Pigments in Man." *Scientific American, 207* (November 1962): 120.

Wald, G. "Life and Light." *Scientific American, 201* (October 1959): 92.

Zurer, P. S. "The Chemistry of Vision." *Chemical and Engineering News, 61* (November 28, 1983): 24.

EXPERIMENT 16

Isolation of Chlorophyll and Carotenoid Pigments from Spinach

Isolation of a natural product
Extraction
Column chromatography
Thin-layer chromatography

Photosynthesis in plants takes place in organelles called **chloroplasts.** Chloroplasts contain a number of colored compounds (pigments) that fall into two categories: **chlorophylls** and **carotenoids.**

Carotenoids are yellow pigments that are also involved in the photosynthetic process. The structures of **α-** and **β-carotene** are given in the essay preceding this experiment. In addition, chloroplasts also contain several oxygen-containing derivatives of carotenes, called **xanthophylls.**

In this experiment, you will extract the chlorophyll and carotenoid pigments from spinach leaves using acetone as the solvent. The pigments will be separated by column chroma-

Chlorophyll a

$$Phytyl = -CH_2-CH=\overset{\overset{\displaystyle CH_3}{|}}{C}-CH_2-(CH_2-CH_2-\overset{\overset{\displaystyle CH_3}{|}}{C}H-CH_2)_2-CH_2-CH_2-\overset{\overset{\displaystyle CH_3}{|}}{C}H-CH_3$$

tography using alumina as the adsorbent. Increasingly more polar solvents will be used to elute the various components from the column. The colored fractions collected will then be analyzed using thin-layer chromatography. It should be possible for you to identify most of the pigments already discussed on your thin-layer plate after development.

In this experiment, you will extract the chlorophyll and carotenoid pigments from spinach leaves using acetone as the solvent. The pigments will be separated by column chromatography using alumina as the adsorbent. Increasingly more polar solvents will be used to elute the various components from the column. The colored fractions collected will then be analyzed using thin-layer chromatography. It should be possible for you to identify most of the pigments already discussed on your thin-layer plate after development.

Chlorophylls are the green pigments that act as the principal photoreceptor molecules of plants. They are capable of absorbing certain wavelengths of visible light that are then converted by plants into chemical energy. Two different forms of these pigments found in plants are **chlorophyll *a*** and **chlorophyll *b*.** The two forms are identical, except that the methyl group that is shaded in the structural formula of chlorophyll *a* is replaced by a —CHO group in chlorophyll *b*. **Pheophytin *a*** and **pheophytin *b*** are identical to chlorophyll *a* and chlorophyll *b*, respectively, except that in each case the magnesium ion Mg^{2+} has been replaced by two hydrogen ions $2H^+$.

Required Reading

Review:	Techniques 5 and 6	
	Technique 7	Reaction Methods, Section 7.10
	Technique 12	Extractions, Separations, and Drying Agents, Sections 12.7 and 12.9
	Technique 20	Thin-Layer Chromatography
New:	Technique 19	Column Chromatography
	Essay	The Chemistry of Vision

Special Instructions

Hexane and acetone are both highly flammable. Avoid the use of flames while working with these solvents. Perform the thin-layer chromatography in the hood. The procedure calls for a centrifuge tube with a tight-fitting cap. If this is not available, you can use a vortex mixer for mixing the liquids. Another alternative is to use a cork to stopper the tube; however, the cork will absorb some liquid.

Fresh spinach is preferable to frozen spinach. Because of handling, frozen spinach contains additional pigments that are difficult to identify. Because the pigments are light-sensitive and can undergo air oxidation, you should work quickly. Samples should be stored in closed containers and kept in the dark when possible. The column chromatography procedure takes less than 15 minutes to perform and cannot be stopped until it is completed. It is very important, therefore, that you have all the materials needed for this part of the experiment prepared in advance and that you are thoroughly familiar with the procedure before running the column. If you need to prepare the 70% hexane–30% acetone solvent mixture, be sure to mix it thoroughly before using.

Suggested Waste Disposal

Dispose of all organic solvents in the container for nonhalogenated organic solvents. Place the alumina in the container designated for wet alumina.

The column chromatography should be performed with activated alumina from EM Science (No. AX0612-1). The particle sizes are 80–200 mesh, and the material is Type F-20. Dry the alumina overnight in an oven at 110°C and store it in a tightly sealed bottle. Alumina more than several years old may need to be dried for a longer time at a higher temperature. Depending on how dry the alumina is, solvents of different polarity will be required to elute the components from the column.

For thin-layer chromatography, use flexible silica gel plates from Whatman with a fluorescent indicator (No. 4410 222). If the TLC plates have not been purchased recently, place them in an oven at 100°C for 30 minutes and store them in a desiccator until used.

If you use different alumina or different thin-layer plates, try out the experiment before using it in class. Materials other than those specified here may give different results than indicated in this experiment.

Procedure

PART A. EXTRACTION OF THE PIGMENTS

Weigh about 0.5 g of fresh (or 0.25 g of frozen) spinach leaves (avoid using stems or thick veins). Fresh spinach is preferable, if available. If you must use frozen spinach, dry the thawed leaves by pressing them between several layers of paper towels. Cut or tear the spinach leaves into small pieces and place them in a mortar along with 1.0 mL of cold acetone. Grind with a pestle until the spinach leaves have been broken into particles too small to be seen clearly. If too much acetone has evaporated, you may need to add an additional portion of acetone (0.5–1.0 mL) to perform the following step. Using a Pasteur pipet, transfer the mixture to a centrifuge tube. Rinse the mortar and pestle with 1.0 mL of cold acetone and transfer the remaining mixture to the centrifuge tube. Centrifuge the mixture (be sure to balance the centrifuge). Using a Pasteur pipet, transfer the liquid to a centrifuge tube with a tight-fitting cap (see "Special Instructions" if one is not available).

Add 2.0 mL of hexane to the tube, cap the tube, and shake the mixture thoroughly. Then add 2.0 mL of water and shake thoroughly with occasional venting. Centrifuge the mixture to break the emulsion, which usually appears as a cloudy, green layer in the middle of the mixture. Remove the bottom aqueous layer with a Pasteur pipet. Using a Pasteur pipet, prepare a column containing anhydrous sodium sulfate to dry the remaining hexane layer, which contains the dissolved pigments. Place a plug of cotton into a Pasteur pipet (5¾-inch) and tamp it into position using a glass rod. The correct position of the cotton is shown in the figure. Add about 0.5 g of powdered or granular anhydrous sodium sulfate and tap the column with your finger to pack the material.

Clamp the column in a vertical position and place a dry test tube (13-mm × 100-mm) under the bottom of the column. Label this test tube with an "**E**" for "extract" so that you don't confuse it with the test tubes you will be working with later in this experiment. With a Pasteur pipet, transfer the hexane layer to the column.

When all the solution has drained, add 0.5 mL of hexane to the column to extract all the pigments from the drying agent. Evaporate the solvent by placing the test tube in a warm water bath (40–60°C) and directing a stream of nitrogen gas (or dry air) into the tube. Dissolve the residue in 0.5 mL of hexane. Stopper the test tube and place it in your drawer until you are ready to run the alumina chromatography column.

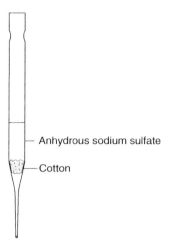

Column for drying extract.

PART B. COLUMN CHROMATOGRAPHY

Introduction.   The pigments are separated on a column packed with alumina. Although there are many different components in your sample, they usually separate into two main bands on the column. The first band to pass through the column is yellow and consists of the carotenes. This band may be less than 1 mm wide, and it may pass through the column very rapidly. It is easy to miss seeing the band as it passes through the alumina. The second band consists of all the other pigments discussed in the introduction to this experiment. Although it consists of both green and yellow pigments, it appears as a green band on the column. The green band spreads out on the column more than the yellow band, and it moves more slowly. Occasionally, the yellow and green components in this band will separate as the band moves down the column. If this begins to occur, you should change to a solvent of higher polarity so that the components come out as one band. As the samples elute from the column, collect the yellow band (carotenes) in one test tube and the green band in another test tube.

Because the moisture content of the alumina is difficult to control, different samples of alumina may have different activities. The activity of the alumina is an important factor in determining the polarity of the solvent required to elute each band of pigments. Several solvents with a range of polarities are used in this experiment. The solvents and their relative polarities follow:

$$\left[\begin{array}{l} \text{Hexane} \\ \text{70\% hexane–30\% acetone} \\ \text{Acetone} \\ \text{80\% acetone–20\% methanol} \end{array}\right. \quad \begin{array}{l} \text{increasing} \\ \text{polarity} \end{array} \downarrow$$

A solvent of lower polarity elutes the yellow band; a solvent of higher polarity is required to elute the green band. In this procedure, you first try to elute the yellow band with hexane. If the yellow band does not move with hexane, you then add the next more polar solvent. Continue this process until you find a solvent that moves the yellow band. When you find the appropriate solvent, continue using it until the yellow band is eluted from the column. When the yellow band is eluted, change to the next more polar solvent. When you find a solvent that moves the green band, continue using it until the green band is eluted. Remember that occasionally a second yellow band will begin to move down the column before the green band moves. This yellow band will be much wider than the first one. If this occurs, change to a more polar solvent. This should bring all the components in the green band down at the same time.

Advance Preparation. Before running the column, assemble the following glassware and liquids. Obtain five dry test tubes (16-mm × 100-mm) and number them 1 through 5. Prepare two dry Pasteur pipets with bulbs attached. Calibrate one of them to deliver a volume of about 0.25 mL (Technique 5, Section 5.4, p. 607). Place 10.0 mL of hexane, 6.0 mL of 70% hexane–30% acetone solution (by volume), 6.0 mL of acetone, and 6.0 mL of 80% acetone–20% methanol (by volume) into four separate containers. Clearly label each container. _weigh 0.25 g H₂O... 56_

Prepare a chromatography column packed with alumina. Place a *loose* plug of cotton in a Pasteur pipet (5¾-inch) and push it *gently* into position using a glass rod (see figure on p. 127 for the correct position of the cotton). Add 1.25 g of alumina (EM Science, No. AX0612-1) to the pipet while tapping the column gently with your finger. When all the alumina has been added, tap the column with your finger for several seconds to ensure that the alumina is tightly packed. Clamp the column in a vertical position so that the bottom of the column is just above the height of the test tubes you will be using to collect the fractions. Place test tube 1 under the column.

> **Note:** Read the following procedure on running the column. The chromatography procedure takes less than 15 minutes, and you cannot stop until all the material is eluted from the column. You must have a good understanding of the whole procedure before running the column.

Running the Column. Using a Pasteur pipet, slowly add about 3.0 mL of hexane to the column. The column must be completely moistened by the solvent. Drain the excess hexane until the level of hexane reaches the top of the alumina. Once you have added hexane to the alumina, the top of the column must not be allowed to run dry. If necessary, add more hexane.

> **Note:** It is essential that the liquid level not be allowed to drain below the surface of the alumina at any point during the procedure.

When the level of the hexane reaches the top of the alumina, add about half (0.25 mL) of the dissolved pigments to the column. Leave the remainder in the test tube for the thin-layer chromatography procedure. (Put a stopper on the tube and place it back in your drawer). Continue collecting the eluent in test tube 1. Just as the pigment solution penetrates the column, add 1 mL of hexane and drain until the surface of the liquid has reached the alumina.

Add about 4 mL of hexane. If the yellow band begins to separate from the green band, continue to add hexane until the yellow band passes through the column. If the yellow band does not separate from the green band, change to the next more polar solvent (70% hexane–30% acetone). When changing solvents, do not add the new solvent until the last solvent has nearly penetrated the alumina. When the appropriate solvent is found, add this solvent until the yellow band passes through the column. Just before the yellow band reaches the bottom of the column, place test tube 2 under the column. When the eluent becomes colorless again (the total volume of the yellow material should be less than 2 mL), place test tube 3 under the column.

Add several mL of the next more polar solvent when the level of the last solvent is almost at the top of the alumina. If the green band moves down the column, continue to add this solvent until the green band is eluted from the column. If the green band does not move or if a diffuse yellow band begins to move, change to the next more polar solvent. Change solvents again if necessary. Collect the green band in test tube 4. When there is little or no green color in the eluent, place test tube 5 under the column and stop the procedure.

Using a warm water bath (40–60°C) and a stream of nitrogen gas, evaporate the solvent from the tube containing the yellow band (tube 2), the tube containing the green band (tube 4), and the tube containing the original pigment solution (tube E). As soon as all the solvent has evaporated from each of the tubes, remove them from the water bath. Do not allow any of the tubes to remain in the water bath after the solvent has evaporated. Stopper the tubes and place them in your drawer.

PART C.   THIN-LAYER CHROMATOGRAPHY

Preparing the TLC Plate.   Technique 20 describes the procedures for thin-layer chromatography. Use a 10-cm × 3.3-cm TLC plate (Whatman Silica Gel Plates No. 4410 222). These plates have a flexible backing but should not be bent excessively. Handle them carefully, or the adsorbent may flake off them. Also, you should handle them only by the edges; the surface should not be touched. Using a lead pencil (not a pen), *lightly* draw a line across the plate (short dimension) about 1 cm from the bottom (see figure). Using a centimeter ruler, move its index about 0.6 cm in from the edge of the plate and lightly mark off three 1-cm intervals on the line. These are the points at which the samples will be spotted.

Prepare three micropipets to spot the plate. The preparation of these pipets is described and illustrated in Technique 20, Section 20.4, page 822. Prepare a TLC development chamber with 70% hexane–30% acetone (see Technique 20, Section 20.5, p. 823). A beaker covered with aluminum foil or a wide-mouth, screw-cap bottle is a suitable container to use (see Figure 20.4, p. 824). The backing on the TLC plates is very thin, so if they touch the filter paper liner of the development chamber *at any point,* solvent will begin to diffuse onto the absorbent surface at that point. To avoid this, be sure that the filter paper liner does not go completely around the inside of the container. A space about 2 inches wide must be provided.

Using a Pasteur pipet, add two drops of 70% hexane–30% acetone to each of the three test tubes containing dried pigments. Swirl the tubes so that the drops of solvent dissolve as much of the pigments as possible. The TLC plate should be spotted with three samples: the extract, the yellow band from the column, and the green band. For each of the three samples, use a different micropipet to spot the sample on the plate. The correct method of spotting a TLC plate is described in Technique 20, Section 20.4, page 822. Take up part of the sample in the pipet (don't use a bulb; capillary action will draw up the liquid). For the extract (tube E) and the green band (tube 4), touch the plate once *lightly* and let the solvent evaporate. The spot should be no longer than 2 mm in diameter and should be a fairly dark green. For the yellow band (tube 2), repeat the spotting technique 5–10 times, until the spot is a definite yellow color. Allow the solvent to evaporate completely between successive applications and spot the plate in exactly the same position each time. Save the samples in case you need to repeat the TLC.

Developing the TLC Plate. Place the TLC plate in the development chamber, making sure that the plate does not come in contact with the filter paper liner. Remove the plate when the solvent front is 1–2 cm from the top of the plate. Using a lead pencil, mark the position of the solvent front. As soon as the plates have dried,

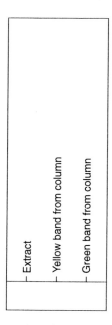

Preparing the TLC plate.

outline the spots with a pencil and indicate the colors. This is important to do soon after the plates have dried, because some of the pigments will change color when exposed to the air.

Analysis of the Results. In the crude extract, you should be able to see the following components (in order of decreasing R_f values):

Carotenes (1 spot) (yellow orange)

Pheophytin *a* (gray, may be nearly as intense as chlorophyll *b*)

Pheophytin *b* (gray, may not be visible)

Chlorophyll *a* (blue green, more intense than chlorophyll *b*)

Chlorophyll *b* (green)

Xanthophylls (possibly 3 spots: yellow)

Depending on the spinach sample, the conditions of the experiment, and the amount of sample spotted on the TLC plate, you may observe other pigments. These additional components can result from air oxidation, hydrolysis, or other chemical reactions involving the pigments discussed in this experiment. It is very common to observe other pigments in samples of frozen spinach. It is also common to observe components in the green band that were not present in the extract.

Identify as many of the spots in your samples as possible. Determine which pigments were present in the yellow band and in the green band. Draw a picture of the TLC plate in your notebook. Label each spot with its color and its identity, where possible. Calculate the R_f values for each spot produced by chromatography of the extract (see Technique 20, Section 20.9, p. 827). At the instructor's option, submit the TLC plate with your report.

255
→ larger, pos charge of Mg²⁺/H⁺
and polarity:
retained in solvent??

QUESTIONS

1. Why are the chlorophylls less mobile on column chromatography, and why do they have lower R_f values than the carotenes?

2. Propose structural formulas for pheophytin *a* and pheophytin *b*.

3. What would happen to the R_f values of the pigments if you were to increase the relative concentration of acetone in the developing solvent?

4. Using your results as a guide, comment on the purity of the material in the green and yellow bands.

ESSAY

Esters—Flavors and Fragrances

Esters are a class of compounds widely distributed in nature. They have the general formula

$$R - \overset{\displaystyle O}{\underset{\displaystyle \|}{C}} - OR'$$

The simple esters tend to have pleasant odors. In many cases, although not exclusively so, the characteristic flavors and fragrances of flowers and fruits are due to compounds with the ester functional group. An exception is the case of the essential oils. The **organoleptic** qualities (odors and flavors) of fruits and flowers may often be due to a single ester, but more often, the flavor or the aroma is due to a complex mixture in which a single ester predominates. Some common flavor principles are listed in Table One. Food and beverage manufacturers are thoroughly familiar with these esters and often use them as additives to spruce up the flavor or odor of a dessert or beverage. Many times, such flavors or odors do not even have a natural basis, as is the case with the "juicy fruit" principle, isopentenyl acetate. An instant pudding that has the flavor of rum may never have seen its alcoholic namesake—this flavor can be duplicated by the proper admixture, along with other minor components, of ethyl formate and isobutyl propionate. The natural flavor and odor are not exactly duplicated, but most people can be fooled. Often, only a trained person with a high degree of gustatory perception, a professional taster, can tell the difference.

A single compound is rarely used in good-quality imitation flavoring agents. A formula for an imitation pineapple flavor that might fool an expert is listed in Table Two. The formula includes 10 esters and carboxylic acids that can easily be synthesized in the laboratory. The remaining seven oils are isolated from natural sources.

Flavor is a combination of taste, sensation, and odor transmitted by receptors in the mouth (taste buds) and nose (olfactory receptors). The stereochemical theory of odor is discussed in the essay that precedes Experiment 15. The four basic tastes (sweet, sour, salty, and bitter) are perceived in specific areas of the tongue. The sides of the tongue perceive sour and salty tastes, the tip is most sensitive to sweet tastes, and the back of the tongue detects bitter tastes. The perception of flavor, however, is not so simple. If it were, it would require only the formulation of various combinations of four basic substances—a bitter substance (a base), a sour substance (an acid), a salty substance (sodium chloride), and a sweet substance (sugar)—to duplicate any flavor! In fact, we cannot duplicate flavors in this way. The human possesses 9,000 taste buds. The combined response of these taste buds is what allows perception of a particular flavor.

Although the "fruity" tastes and odors of esters are pleasant, they are seldom used in perfumes or scents that are applied to the body. The reason for this is chemical. The ester group is not as stable under perspiration as the ingredients of the more expensive essential-oil perfumes. The latter are usually hydrocarbons (terpenes), ketones, and ethers extracted from natural sources. Esters, however, are used only for the cheapest toilet waters, because

TABLE ONE Ester Flavors and Fragrances

Isoamyl acetate
(banana)
(alarm pheromone of honeybee)

$$CH_3 \overset{\overset{\displaystyle O}{\|}}{\underset{}{C}} OCH_2CH_2CH \overset{CH_3}{\underset{CH_3}{<}}$$

Ethyl butyrate
(pineapple)

$$CH_3CH_2CH_2 \overset{\overset{\displaystyle O}{\|}}{\underset{}{C}} OCH_2CH_3$$

Isobutyl propionate
(rum)

$$CH_3CH_2 \overset{\overset{\displaystyle O}{\|}}{\underset{}{C}} OCH_2CH \overset{CH_3}{\underset{CH_3}{<}}$$

Octyl acetate
(oranges)

$$CH_3 \overset{\overset{\displaystyle O}{\|}}{\underset{}{C}} O-CH_2(CH_2)_6CH_3$$

Methyl anthranilate
(grape)

$$NH_2 \quad \overset{\overset{\displaystyle O}{\|}}{\underset{}{C}} OCH_3$$

Isopentenyl acetate
("Juicy Fruit")

$$CH_3 \overset{\overset{\displaystyle O}{\|}}{\underset{}{C}} O-CH_2CH=C \overset{CH_3}{\underset{CH_3}{<}}$$

Benzyl acetate
(peach)

$$CH_3 \overset{\overset{\displaystyle O}{\|}}{\underset{}{C}} O-CH_2 \bigcirc$$

n-Propyl acetate
(pear)

$$CH_3 \overset{\overset{\displaystyle O}{\|}}{\underset{}{C}} O-CH_2CH_2CH_3$$

Methyl butyrate
(apple)

$$CH_3CH_2CH_2 \overset{\overset{\displaystyle O}{\|}}{\underset{}{C}} OCH_3$$

Ethyl phenylacetate
(honey)

$$\bigcirc -CH_2 \overset{\overset{\displaystyle O}{\|}}{\underset{}{C}} -OCH_2CH_3$$

on contact with sweat they undergo hydrolysis, giving organic acids. These acids, unlike their precursor esters, generally do not have a pleasant odor.

Butyric acid, for instance, has a strong odor like that of rancid butter (of which it is an ingredient) and is a component of what we normally call body odor. It is this substance that makes foul-smelling humans so easy for an animal to detect when downwind of them. It is also of great help to the bloodhound, which is trained to follow small traces of this odor.

TABLE TWO Artificial Pineapple Flavor

Pure Compounds	%	Essential Oils	%
Allyl caproate	5	Oil of sweet birch	1
Isoamyl acetate	3	Oil of spruce	2
Isoamyl isovalerate	3	Balsam Peru	4
Ethyl acetate	15	Volatile mustard oil	1
Ethyl butyrate	22	Oil cognac	5
Terpinyl propionate	3	Concentrated orange oil	4
Ethyl crotonate	5	Distilled oil of lime	2
Caproic acid	8		19
Butyric acid	12		
Acetic acid	5		
	81		

$$R-\overset{\overset{\displaystyle O}{\|}}{C}-OR' + H_2O \longrightarrow R-\overset{\overset{\displaystyle O}{\|}}{C}-OH + R'OH$$

Ethyl butyrate and methyl butyrate, however, which are the *esters* of butyric acid, smell like pineapple and apple, respectively.

A sweet, fruity odor also has the disadvantage of possibly attracting fruit flies and other insects in search of food. Isoamyl acetate, the familiar solvent called banana oil, is particularly interesting. It is identical to a component of the alarm **pheromone** of the honey-bee. Pheromone is the name applied to a chemical secreted by an organism that evokes a specific response in another member of the same species. This kind of communication is common among insects who otherwise lack means of intercourse. When a honeybee worker stings an intruder, an alarm pheromone, composed partly of isoamyl acetate, is secreted along with the sting venom. This chemical causes aggressive attack on the intruder by other bees, who swarm after the intruder. Obviously, it wouldn't be wise to wear a perfume compounded of isoamyl acetate near a beehive. Pheromones are discussed in more detail in the essay preceding Experiment 45.

REFERENCES

Bauer, K., and Garbe, D. *Common Fragrance and Flavor Materials.* Weinheim: VCH Publishers, 1985.

The Givaudan Index. New York: Givaudan-Delawanna, 1949. (Gives specifications of synthetics and isolates for perfumery.)

Gould, R. F., ed. *Flavor Chemistry, Advances in Chemistry,* No. 56. Washington, DC: American Chemical Society, 1966.

Layman, P. L. "Flavors and Fragrances Industry Taking on New Look." *Chemical and Engineering News* (July 20, 1987): 35.

Moyler, D. "Natural Ingredients for Flavours and Fragrances." *Chemistry and Industry* (January 7, 1991): 11.

Rasmussen, P. W. "Qualitative Analysis by Gas Chromatography—G.C. versus the Nose in Formulation of Artificial Fruit Flavors." *Journal of Chemical Education,* 61 (January 1984): 62.

Shreve, R. N., and Brink, J. *Chemical Process Industries,* 4th ed. New York: McGraw-Hill, 1977.

Welsh, F. W., and Williams, R. E. "Lipase Mediated Production of Flavor and Fragrance Esters from Fusel Oil." *Journal of Food Science, 54* (November/December 1989): 1565.

EXPERIMENT 12

Isopentyl Acetate (Banana Oil)

Esterification
Heating under reflux
Separatory funnel
Extraction
Simple distillation

In this experiment, you will prepare an ester, isopentyl acetate. This ester is often referred to as banana oil, because it has the familiar odor of this fruit.

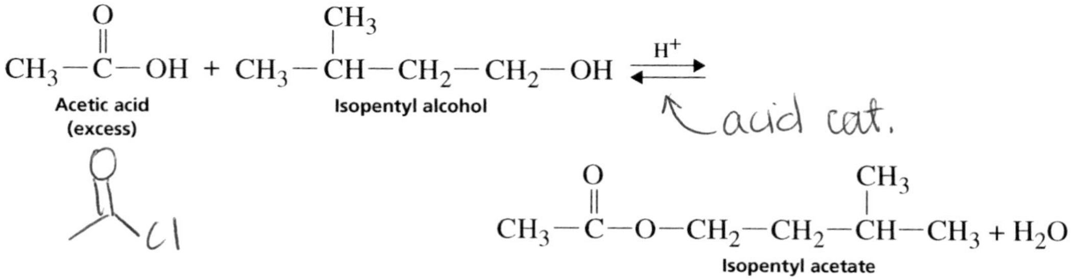

$$CH_3-\underset{\underset{O}{\|}}{C}-OH + CH_3-\underset{\underset{CH_3}{|}}{CH}-CH_2-CH_2-OH \; \overset{H^+}{\rightleftharpoons}$$

Acetic acid
(excess)

(handwritten: ~ acid cat.)

$$CH_3-\underset{\underset{O}{\|}}{C}-O-CH_2-CH_2-\underset{\underset{CH_3}{|}}{CH}-CH_3 + H_2O$$

Isopentyl acetate

Isopentyl acetate is prepared by the direct esterification of acetic acid with isopentyl alcohol. Because the equilibrium does not favor the formation of the ester, it must be shifted to the right, in favor of the product, by using an excess of one of the starting materials. Acetic acid is used in excess because it is less expensive than isopentyl alcohol and more easily removed from the reaction mixture.

In the isolation procedure, much of the excess acetic acid and the remaining isopentyl alcohol are removed by extraction with sodium bicarbonate and water. After drying with anhydrous sodium sulfate, the ester is purified by distillation. The purity of the liquid product is analyzed by determining the infrared spectrum.

Required Reading

Review: Techniques 5 and 6

New: Technique 7   Reaction Methods
               Technique 12   Extractions, Separations, and Drying Agents
               Technique 13   Physical Constants of Liquids, Part A.
                                        Boiling Points and Thermometer Correction
               Technique 14   Simple Distillation
               Essay   Esters—Flavors and Fragrances

If performing the optional infrared spectroscopy, also read

Technique 25, pages 874–887

Special Instructions

Be careful when dispensing sulfuric and glacial acetic acids. They are very corrosive and will attack your skin if you make contact with them. If you get one of these acids on your skin, wash the affected area with copious quantities of running water for 10–15 minutes.

Because a 1-hour reflux is required, you should start the experiment at the very beginning of the laboratory period. During the reflux period, you may perform other experimental work.

Suggested Waste Disposal

Any aqueous solutions should be placed in a container specially designated for dilute aqueous waste. Place any excess ester in the nonhalogenated organic waste container.

Notes to the Instructor

This experiment has been carried out successfully using Dowex 50X2-100 ion exchange resin instead of the sulfuric acid.

Procedure

Apparatus. Assemble a reflux apparatus, using a 25-mL round-bottom flask and a water-cooled condenser (refer to Technique 7, Fig. 7.6, p. 628). Use a heating mantle to heat. In order to control vapors, place a drying tube packed with calcium chloride on top of the condenser.

Reaction Mixture. Weigh (tare) an empty 10-mL graduated cylinder and record its weight. Place approximately 5.0 mL of isopentyl alcohol in the graduated cylinder and reweigh it to determine the weight of alcohol. Disconnect the round-bottom flask from the reflux apparatus and transfer the alcohol into it. Do not clean or wash the graduated cylinder. Using the same graduated cylinder, measure approximately 7.0 mL of glacial acetic acid ($MW = 60.1$, $d = 1.06$ g/mL) and add it to the alcohol already in the flask. Using a calibrated Pasteur pipet, add 1 mL of concentrated sulfuric acid, mixing *immediately* (swirl), to the reaction mixture contained in the flask. Add a corundum boiling stone and reconnect the flask. Do not use a calcium carbonate (marble) boiling stone because it will dissolve in the acidic medium.

Reflux. Start water circulating in the condenser and bring the mixture to a boil. Continue heating under reflux for 60–75 minutes. Then disconnect or remove the heating source and allow the mixture to cool to room temperature.

Extractions. Disassemble the apparatus and transfer the reaction mixture to a separatory funnel (125-mL) placed in a ring that is attached to a ring stand. Be sure that the stopcock is closed and, using a funnel, pour the mixture into the top of the separatory funnel. Also be careful to avoid transferring the boiling stone, or you will need to remove it after the transfer. Add 10 mL of water, stopper the funnel, and mix the phases by careful shaking and venting (Technique 12, Section 12.4, and Fig. 12.6, pp. 704 and 705). Allow the phases to separate and then unstopper the funnel and drain the lower aqueous layer through the stopcock into a beaker or other suitable container. Next, extract the organic layer with 5 mL of 5% aqueous sodium bicarbonate just as you did previously with water. Extract the organic layer once again, this time with 5 mL of saturated aqueous sodium chloride.

Drying. Transfer the crude ester to a clean, dry 25-mL Erlenmeyer flask and add approximately 1.0 g of anhydrous granular sodium sulfate. Cork the mixture and allow it to stand for 10–15 minutes while you prepare the apparatus for distillation. If the mixture does not appear dry (the drying agent clumps and does not "flow," the solution is cloudy, or drops of water are obvious), transfer the ester to a new clean, dry 25-mL Erlenmeyer flask and add a new 0.5-g portion of anhydrous sodium sulfate to complete the drying.

Distillation. Assemble a distillation apparatus using your smallest round-bottom flask to distill from (Technique 14, Fig. 14.1, p. 734). Use a heating mantle to heat. Preweigh (tare) and use another small round-bottom flask, or an Erlenmeyer flask, to collect the product. Immerse the collection flask in a beaker of ice to ensure condensation and to reduce odors. You should look up the boiling point of your expected product in a handbook so you will know what to expect. Continue distillation until only one or two drops of liquid remain in the distilling flask. Record the observed boiling point range in your notebook.

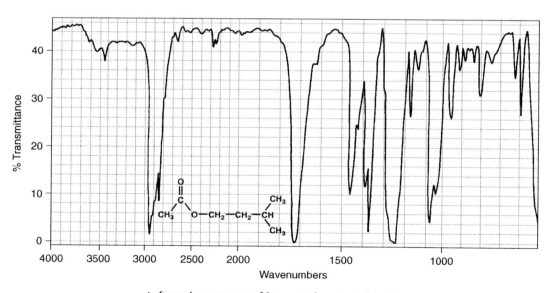

Infrared spectrum of isopentyl acetate (neat).

Yield Determination. Weigh the product and calculate the <u>percentage yield</u> of the ester. At the option of your instructor, determine the <u>boiling point</u> using one of the methods described in Technique 13, Sections 13.2 and 13.3, pages 724 and 727.

Spectroscopy. At your instructor's option, obtain an infrared spectrum using salt plates (Technique 25, Section 25.2, p. 875). Compare your spectrum with the one reproduced in the text. Interpret the spectrum and include it in your report to the instructor. You may also be required to determine and interpret the proton and carbon-13 NMR spectra (Technique 26, Part A, pp. 911–916, and Technique 27, Section 27.1, p. 947). Submit your sample in a properly labeled vial with your report.

QUESTIONS

1. One method of favoring the formation of an ester is to add excess acetic acid. Suggest another method, involving the right-hand side of the equation, that will favor the formation of the ester.

2. Why is the mixture extracted with sodium bicarbonate? Give an equation and explain its relevance.

3. Why are gas bubbles observed when the sodium bicarbonate is added?

4. Which starting material is the limiting reagent in this procedure? Which reagent is used in excess? How great is the molar excess (how many times greater)?

5. Outline a separation scheme for isolating pure isopentyl acetate from the reaction mixture.

6. Interpret the principal absorption bands in the infrared spectrum of isopentyl acetate or, if you did not determine the infrared spectrum of your ester, do this for the spectrum of isopentyl acetate shown in the previous figure. (Technique 25 may be of some help.)

7. Write a mechanism for the acid-catalyzed esterification of acetic acid with isopentyl alcohol.

8. Why is glacial acetic acid designated as "glacial"? (*Hint:* Consult a handbook of physical properties.)

EXPERIMENT 57

A Separation and Purification Scheme

Extraction
Crystallization
Devising a procedure
Critical thinking application

There are many organic experiments in which the components of a mixture must be separated, isolated, and purified. Although detailed procedures are usually given for carrying this out, devising your own scheme can help you understand these techniques more thoroughly. In this experiment, you will devise a separation and purification scheme for a three-component mixture that will be assigned to you. The mixture will contain a neutral organic compound and either an organic acid or base in nearly equal amounts. The third component, also a neutral compound, will be present in a much smaller amount. Your goal will be to isolate in pure form *two* of the three compounds. The components of your mixture may be separated and purified by a combination of acid–base extractions and crystallizations. You will be told the composition of your mixture well in advance of the laboratory period so that you will have time to write a procedure for this experiment.

This experiment can be performed at two different scales. In Experiment 57A, the procedure calls for 1.0 g of the assigned mixture, and the extraction procedures are carried out with a separatory funnel. In Experiment 57B, the extraction procedures are performed with a centrifuge tube using 0.5 g of the assigned mixture. Your instructor will tell you which procedure to follow.

Required Reading

Review: Technique 11   Crystallization: Purification of Solids
         Technique 12   Extractions, Separations, and Drying Agents

Suggested Waste Disposal

Dispose of all filtrates that may contain 1,4-dibromobenzene or methylene chloride into the container designated for halogenated organic wastes. All other filtrates may be disposed of into the container for nonhalogenated organic wastes.

Notes to the Instructor

Students must be told the composition of their mixture well in advance of the laboratory period so that they have enough time to devise a procedure. It is advisable to require

Experiment 57 is based on a similar experiment developed by James Patterson, University of Washington, Seattle.

that students turn in a copy of their procedure at the beginning of the lab period. You may wish to allow enough time for students to repeat the experiment if their procedure doesn't work the first time or if they want to improve on their percentage recovery and purity. If you allow enough time for students to perform this experiment just once, it will be helpful to put out pure samples of the compounds in the mixtures so students can try out different solvents to determine a good solvent for crystallizing each compound.

EXPERIMENT 57A

Extractions with a Separatory Funnel

Procedure

Advanced Preparation. Each student will be assigned a mixture of three compounds.[1] Before coming to the laboratory, you must work out a detailed procedure that can be used to separate, isolate, and purify *two* of the compounds in your mixture. You may not be able to specify all the reagents or the volumes required ahead of time, but the procedure should be as complete as possible. It will be helpful to consult the following experiments and techniques:

Experiment 1, "Solubility," Part D, pp. 11–12

Experiment 3, "Extraction," Part D, pp. 32–34

Technique 10, Section 10.2B, p. 673

Technique 12, Section 12.11, pp. 717–720

The following reagents will be available: 1 M NaOH, 6 M NaOH, 1 M HCl, 6 M HCl, 1 M NaHCO$_3$, saturated sodium chloride, diethyl ether, 95% ethanol, methanol, isopropyl alcohol, acetone, hexane, toluene, methylene chloride, and anhydrous sodium sulfate. Other solvents that can be used for crystallization may also be available.

Separation. The first step in your procedure should be to dissolve about 1.0 g (record exact weight) of the mixture in the minimum amount of diethyl ether or methylene chloride. If more than about 10 mL of a solvent is required, you should use the other solvent. Most of the compounds in the mixtures are more soluble in methylene chloride than diethyl ether; however, you may need to determine the appropriate solvent by experimentation. Once you have selected a solvent, this same solvent should be used throughout the procedure when an organic solvent is required. If you use diethyl ether, you must use two steps to dry the organic layer. First, the organic layer must be mixed with saturated sodium chloride (see p. 717), and then the liquid is dried over anhydrous sodium sulfate. For all extraction procedures in this experiment, you should use a separatory funnel.

---

[1] Your mixture may be one of the following: (1) 50% benzoic acid, 40% benzoin, 10% 1,4-dibromobenzene; (2) 50% fluorene, 40% o-toluic acid, 10% 1,4-dibromobenzene; (3) 50% phenanthrene, 40% methyl 4-aminobenzoate, 10% 1,4-dibromobenzene; or (4) 50% 4-aminoacetophenone, 40% 1,2,4,5-tetrachlorobenzene, 10% 1,4-dibromobenzene. Other mixtures are given in the Instructor's Manual along with some suggestions about these mixtures.

Purification. To improve the purity of your final samples, you should include a backwashing step at the appropriate place in your procedure. See Section 12.11, page 717, for a discussion of this technique. Crystallization will be required to purify both of the compounds you isolate. To find an appropriate solvent, you should consult a handbook. You can also use the procedure in Section 11.6, page 691, to determine a good solvent experimentally. Your procedure should include at least one method for determining if you have obtained both compounds in a pure form. Hand in each compound in a labeled vial.

When performing the laboratory work, you should strive to obtain a high recovery of both compounds in a highly pure form. If your procedure fails, modify it and repeat the experiment.

REPORT

Write out a complete procedure by which you separated and isolated pure samples of two of the compounds in your mixture. Describe how you determined that your procedure was successful and give any data or results used for this purpose. Calculate the percentage recovery for both compounds.

EXPERIMENT 57B

Extractions with a Screw-Cap Centrifuge Tube

Procedure

Follow the procedure given in Experiment 57A, except for the following changes in the "Separation" and "Purification" sections. Dissolve about 0.5 g of the assigned mixture in the minimum amount of diethyl ether or methylene chloride.[2] If more than about 4 mL of a solvent is required, you should use the other solvent. For all extraction procedures in this experiment, you should use a screw-cap centrifuge tube.

---

[2] See footnote 1, page 522.

The Diels-Alder Reaction: Preparation of 4-Cyclohexene-cis-1,2-dicarboxylic Anhydride

BACKGROUND

One of the most useful methods available to the organic chemist for the synthesis of six-membered rings involves the reaction between a 1,3-diene and an alkene (*dienophile*). This ring-forming process is an example of a *cycloaddition* reaction and is called the Diels-Alder reaction. In this experiment we will carry out a Diels-Alder [4 + 2] cycloaddition reaction between butadiene and maleic anhydride to prepare 4-cyclohexene-*cis*-1,2-dicarboxylic anhydride:

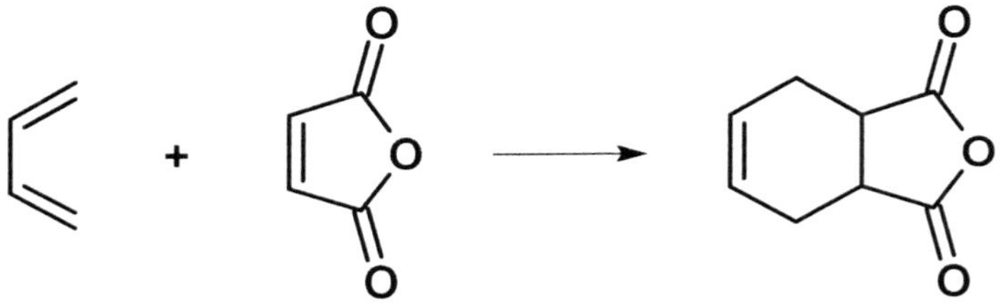

1,3-Butadiene is a gas a room temperature (bp -4.4°C). In this experiment, 1,3-butadiene will be generated *in situ* by the thermal decomposition of 3-sulfolene (a retro chelotropic reaction) and will then react with the dienophile (maleic anhydride) that is present:

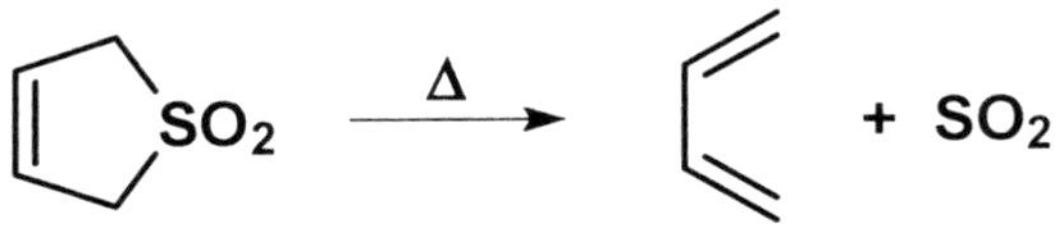

PROCEDURE

CAUTION: Be certain that all joints in the apparatus are tight and well lubricated before the reaction mixture is heated. The organic solvents used are flammable. Sulfur dioxide that is evolved is toxic and ill-smelling. Be sure the gas trap is functioning properly before heating the reaction mixture in order to avoid releasing gaseous SO$_2$ into the laboratory.

Place 10.0 g (0.085 mol) of 3-sulfolene, 6.0 g (0.061 mol) of finely pulverized maleic anhydride (*CAUTION: Corrosive! Toxic!*) (crush the maleic anhydride with a mortar and pestle just before use), 4 mL anhydrous xylene (*CAUTION: Flammable!*), and 3 boiling chips in a 100-mL round-bottomed flask equipped with a water-cooled reflux condenser. Fit the condenser with a gas trap connected to a water aspirator (**Fig. 13**). Warm the flask gently to effect solution, then heat the mixture to a gentle reflux, and continue refluxing for an additional 30 min.

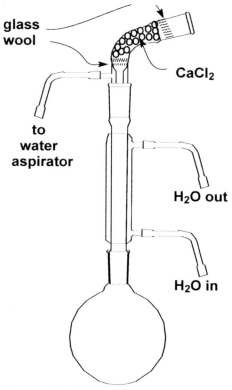

Figure 13. Reflux apparatus with SO$_2$ gas trap.

Cool the reaction mixture. Replace the gas trap with a CaCl$_2$ drying tube. Add an additional 30 mL of anhydrous xylene and about 1 g of activated charcoal (*CAUTION: Very messy!*), and heat the mixture with stirring for about 5 min. Filter the hot solution using a fluted filter paper and a short-stemmed funnel. Cool the filtrate in an ice bath and allow the product to crystallize. Collect the product by suction filtration, rinse with a small amount of ice-cold toluene, and then with petroleum ether (3 X) (*CAUTION: Flammable solvents!*). Allow the crystals to air dry, record the mass, and determine the melting point of your product. The literature melting point is 103-104°C.

Waste Disposal. Sulfolene, maleic anhydride, calcium chloride, and filter papers are discarded in the "Solid Chemical Waste" tub. Organic solvents (xylene, toluene, petroleum ether) and filtrates are discarded in the "Non-Chlorinated Solvent Waste" jug.

Turn in your Diels-Alder adduct in a properly labeled vial along with your report.
[100 points for your product; 200 points for your report]

REFERENCES

Roberts, R.M.; Gilbert, J.C.; Rodewald, L.B.; Wingrove, A.S. *Modern Experimental Organic Chemistry*, 4th Ed.; Saunders: Philadelphia, 1985; pp 384-405.

Sample, T. E.; Hatch, L. F. 3-Sulfolene: A Butadiene Source for a Diels-Alder Synthesis: An Undergraduate Laboratory Experiment. *J. Chem. Educ.* **1968**, *45*, 55.

THE DIELS-ALDER REACTION

Pre-Laboratory Questions/Exercises

Name _____   **Sec. No.** _____

1. What problems might arise if the solvent were not anhydrous?

2. Sketch the highest occupied molecular orbital (HOMO) of butadiene, sketch the lowest unoccupied molecular orbital (LUMO) of ethylene, and show that these orbitals have the correct symmetry for cycloaddition.

3. In the reaction between a 1,3-cyclopentadiene and maleic anhydride, why is the major product the more sterically hindered *endo* cycloadduct rather than the *exo*?

4. Draw the structures for the products of each of the following Diels-Alder reactions:

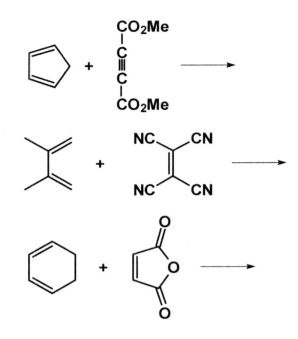

5. Show how you would prepare each of the following compounds using a Diels-Alder reaction:

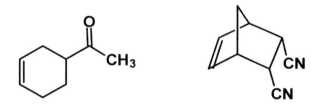

Isolation of Eugenol from Cloves

BACKGROUND

The main constituent in the essential oil of cloves is eugenol (4-allyl-2-methoxyphenol). Eugenol acetate, β-caryophyllene, and other compounds are found in small amounts.

Eugenol   **Eugenol acetate**   **β-Caryophyllene**

PROCEDURE

Hydrodistillation of Cloves (**read about Steam Distillation in FF&F, pp 107-110**). Place about 50 g whole cloves (weigh out to the nearest 0.01 g) and 150 mL water in a 500-mL round-bottom flask and assemble the apparatus for a direct steam distillation (flask fitted with Claisen adapter, 125-mL addition funnel with water, distillation head, condenser, and receiver; **see Fig. 10**). Heat the mixture with a heating mantle hot enough so that distillation occurs as rapidly as possible (as fast as the distillate will condense, or as quickly as possible without excessive bumping). After distillation begins, add water from the dropping funnel to maintain the original volume of liquid in the flask. Continue distilling until no further drops of oil can be seen coming over with the water. At least 75 mL of liquid should be collected.

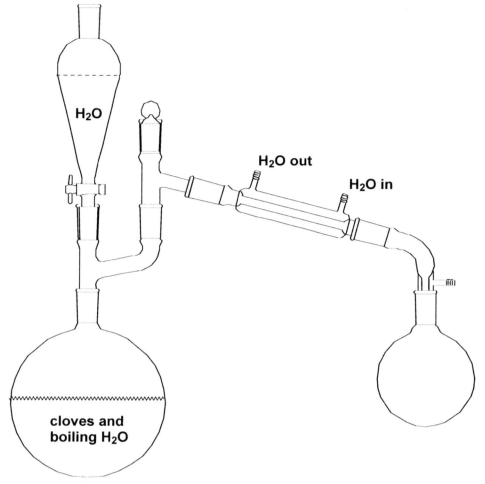

Figure 10. Hydrodistillation apparatus.

Extraction of the Essential Oil (read about Extraction in FF&F, pp 49-61). Dissolve approximately 6 g sodium chloride in the distillate and agitate to dissolve the salt. Pour the distillate into a separatory funnel and extract it three times with 25-mL portions of dichloromethane, and periodically releasing any internal pressure (**see Fig. 11**). (*CAUTION: Dichloromethane is toxic! Do not breathe it excessively or spill it on yourself!*)

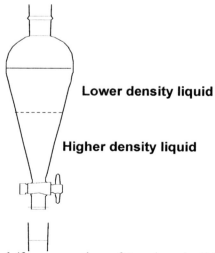

Lower density liquid

Higher density liquid

Figure 11. Separatory funnel (for separation of two immiscible liquids).

Combine the dichloromethane extracts (the aqueous layer can be discarded) and add just enough anhydrous calcium chloride so that the drying agent no longer clumps together. Swirl the flask for about one minute to complete the drying process and then decant the solvents into a dry graduated cylinder.

Measure the volume of the dichloromethane extract, place exactly one-fifth of the solution into a tared (pre-weighed) Erlenmeyer flask, add a boiling chip, and evaporate off the dichloromethane in a hood (carefully use a hot plate to remove much of the solvent and finish using a heat gun (hair dryer). The residue of crude clove oil will be used in the thin-layer chromatography analysis. From its mass the total yield of crude clove oil can be calculated.

Isolation of Eugenol. Transfer the remaining four-fifths of the dichloromethane extract back to the separatory funnel and extract with three 25-mL portions of 5% NaOH solution. **Eugenol is a phenol and is slightly acidic; it can be deprotonated by NaOH, converting it into the corresponding water-soluble sodium salt. The other components are not acidic, are not deprotonated, and therefore, remain soluble in dichloromethane.** Combine the basic aqueous layers and wash once with one 25-mL portion of dichloromethane. Combine the dichloromethane extracts and dry over $CaCl_2$. Decant the solution into a tared Erlenmeyer flask, and evaporate the solvent. The residue should consist mostly of eugenol acetate (acetyleugenol) with small amounts of caryophyllene and other steam-volatile neutral compounds from cloves.

Transfer the aqueous basic layer to a 250-mL beaker and *slowly* acidify the aqueous layer to pH 1 with 5% HCl solution. **Acidification serves to re-protonate the eugenol, making it insoluble in water but soluble in dichloromethane.** After acidification, transfer the solution back to the separatory funnel and extract the aqueous layer with three 25-mL portions of dichloromethane. Discard the aqueous wash. Wash the combined organic layers with one 25-mL portion of water, followed by one 25-mL portion of saturated NaCl solution. Dry the organic layer over a small amount of calcium chloride. Decant the dichloromethane solution from the drying agent into a pre-weighed Erlenmeyer flask and carefully evaporate the solvent. Determine the mass of eugenol. Determine the percentage yields of essential oil, eugenol, and eugenol acetate based upon the original weight of cloves used.

Thin-Layer Chromatographic Analysis (**read about Thin-Layer Chromatography in FF&F, pp 133-138**). Analyze your products by thin-layer chromatography. Use plastic sheets precoated with silica gel for TLC. One piece, 3 cm X 10 cm, should suffice. Spot crude clove oil, eugenol, and eugenol acetate side by side about 5 mm from one end of the plate (see Fig. 12). The spots should be very small. Immerse the end of the plate in a dichloromethane-hexane mixture (1:2) about 3 mm deep in a developing jar. Allow the solvent to elute to about 5 mm from the end of the plate. After running the chromatogram, evaporate off the solvent and observe the spots by developing in an iodine chamber. Report the R_f values of eugenol and eugenol acetate (R_f = distance spot traveled/distance solvent front).

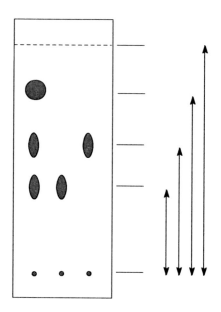

Figure 12. Thin-layer chromatographic (TLC) plate.

Waste Disposal. Used cloves can be discarded in the trash can. Dichloromethane should be discarded in the "Chlorinated Solvent Waste" jug. Used TLC plates are discarded in the "Solid Chemical Waste" tub.

Turn in your isolated eugenol in a properly labeled vial along with your report.
[100 points for your product; 300 points for your report]

REFERENCES

Eaton, D.C. *Laboratory Investigations in Organic Chemistry*; McGraw-Hill: New York, 1989; pp 213-236.

Ntamila, M.S.; Hassanali, A. Isolation of Oil of Clove and Separation of Eugenol and Acetyl Eugenol. An Instructive Experiment for Beginning Chemistry Undergraduates. *J. Chem. Educ.* **1976**, *53*, 263.

Flair, M.N.; Setzer, W.N. An Olfactory Indicator for Acid-Base Titrations: A Laboratory Technique for the Visually Impaired. *J. Chem. Educ.* **1990**, 67, 795-796.

ISOLATION OF EUGENOL FROM CLOVES

Pre-Laboratory Questions/Exercises

Name _____   Sec. No. _____

1. Construct a flow chart for the separation of eugenol from eugenol acetate and caryophyllene.

2. Extra Strength Excedrin® contains aspirin, acetaminophen, and caffeine. How would you separate this mixture? Hint: What are the acid-base properties of the compounds?

Aspirin   **Acetaminophen**   **Caffeine**

3. Calculate the R_f values for the following compounds:

   a) Spot 35 mm; solvent front 90 mm

   b) Spot 55 mm; solvent front 85 mm

c) Spot 14 cm; solvent front 18 cm

4. Eugenol has been used as an acid-base indicator for blind people (see Flair, M.N.; Setzer, W.N. An Olfactory Indicator for Acid-Base Titrations: A Laboratory Technique for the Visually Impaired. *J. Chem. Educ.* **1990**, 67, 795-796.). Explain how this works.

Synthesis of *trans*-9-(2-Phenylethenyl) anthracene: A Wittig Reaction

prepared by **William M. Loffredo**, East Stroudsburg University

PURPOSE OF THE EXPERIMENT

Synthesize *trans*-9-(2-phenylethenyl)anthracene using a Wittig reaction. Characterize the product by melting point, thin-layer chromatography, infrared spectroscopy, and nuclear magnetic resonance spectroscopy.

EXPERIMENTAL OPTIONS

Semi-Microscale Wittig Synthesis
Microscale Wittig Synthesis
Characterizing the Product

BACKGROUND REQUIRED

You should be familiar with techniques for drying organic solvents and measuring melting points. You should be familiar with the techniques for extraction, distillation, recrystallization, and vacuum filtration. You should know how to speed the evaporation of microscale quantities of solvent using air or nitrogen. You should be familiar with thin-layer chromatography (TLC), infrared spectroscopy (IR), and nuclear magnetic resonance spectroscopy (NMR).

BACKGROUND INFORMATION

Chemical reactions involving organic molecules can be classified into three very broad categories: molecular rearrangement, elimination, and addition. Although alkenes are commonly formed from *elimination* reactions, such as dehydration of alcohols and dehydrohalogenation of alkyl halides, these reactions usually result in a mixture of structural isomers. The Wittig reaction is often preferred as a method of synthesizing alkenes because of its high level of **regioselectivity**, which is the tendency of a reaction to form predominantly one isomer from a single reactant. The Wittig reaction allows the chemist to choose the precise location of the newly formed bond.

The Wittig reaction is an *addition* reaction. It generates an alkene from the reaction of a carbonyl compound with a carbon-containing phosphorus reagent known as an ylide, which is made from a phosphonium halide. The phosphonium halide is generated from the nucleophilic substitution reaction of a primary or secondary alkyl halide and triphenylphosphine, Ph_3P. Ph_3P is a good nucleophile and a relatively weak base. Therefore, the potentially competing elimination reaction does not occur. The substitution products are phosphonium salts, as shown in Equations 1 and 2.

$$RCH_2X \quad + \quad Ph_3P \quad \longrightarrow \quad RCH_2\overset{+}{P}Ph_3 \quad X^- \qquad \text{(Eq. 1)}$$

1° alkyl halide

$$R_2CHX \quad + \quad Ph_3P \quad \longrightarrow \quad R_2CH\overset{+}{P}Ph_3 \quad X^- \qquad \text{(Eq. 2)}$$

2° alkyl halide

The phosphonium salt must have phosphorus attached to a carbon containing at least one hydrogen atom. This hydrogen atom is moderately acidic and can be extracted in the presence of a strong base. Typically, alkyl lithium compounds or metal hydrides are used as the strong base. In this experiment, however, a concentrated solution of aqueous sodium hydroxide will be used.

The product resulting from the reaction of the phosphonium halide with a strong base is called an **ylide**. An ylide is a neutral molecule, which, among its atoms, has two adjacent atoms that have opposite charges. The two charged atoms are the phosphorus from the phosphine and the carbon from the alkyl halide, as shown in Equation 3.

$$RCH_2\overset{+}{P}Ph_3 \quad X^- \quad \xrightarrow{\text{base}} \quad R\overset{-}{C}H\overset{+}{P}Ph_3 \qquad \text{(Eq. 3)}$$

ylide

This carbon group attached to the phosphorus has carbanionic character and acts as a nucleophile toward carbonyl groups. The general mechanism of the reaction is shown in Equation 4.

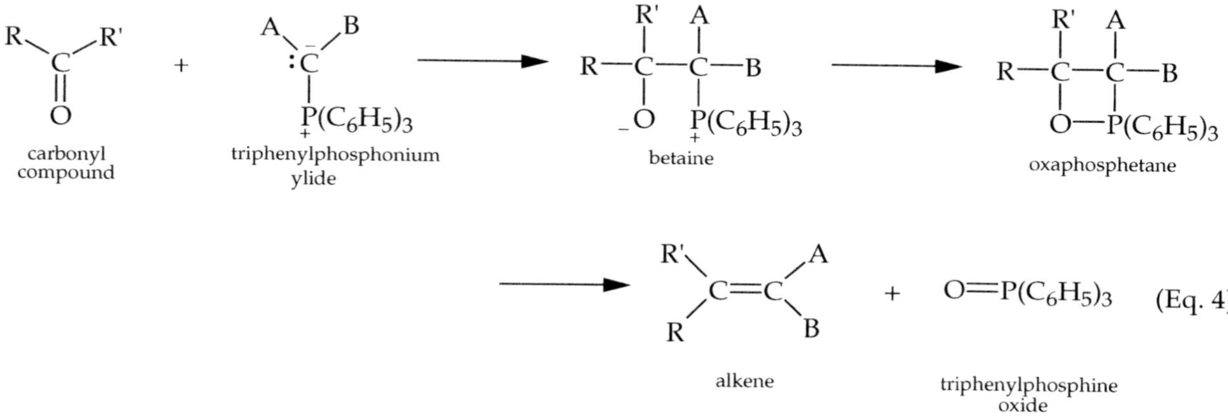

carbonyl compound   triphenylphosphonium ylide   betaine   oxaphosphetane

alkene   triphenylphosphine oxide   (Eq. 4)

The mechanism is still under investigation. The controversy lies in whether the oxaphosphetane intermediate is formed by a one-step concerted process or by a two-step process. Formation of the oxaphosphetane through a two-step process involves the initial formation of a dipolar intermediate known as a betaine. The betaine then reacts to form the oxaphosphetane. The oxaphosphetane is stable at $-78\,°C$, but at room temperature, it decomposes to yield the alkene and triphenyl-phosphine oxide. The driving force for the decomposition of the oxa-phosphetane is thought to be the formation of the strong phosphorus–oxygen bond of the phosphine oxide, a bond strength estimated to be at least 540 kJ/mol.

The Wittig reaction forms the carbon–carbon double bond between the carbonyl carbon and the carbon adjacent to the phosphorus atom in the ylide. For example, consider the formation of methylenecyclohexane.

The Wittig reaction could be conducted with formaldehyde and bromocyclohexane or with bromomethane and cyclohexanone, as shown in Equation 5.

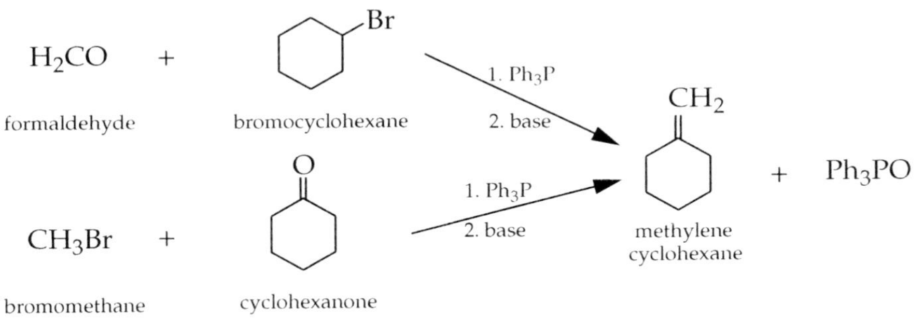

H_2CO +

formaldehyde   bromocyclohexane

CH_3Br +

bromomethane   cyclohexanone

1. Ph_3P
2. base

1. Ph_3P
2. base

methylene cyclohexane

+ Ph_3PO (Eq. 5)

The synthetic route chosen will depend on the availability of the possible starting materials.

In this experiment, the alkene *trans*-9-(2-phenylethenyl)anthracene will be synthesized from 9-anthraldehyde and the ylide derived from triphenylbenzylphosphonium chloride. The ylide formation and the subsequent reaction are shown in Equation 6.

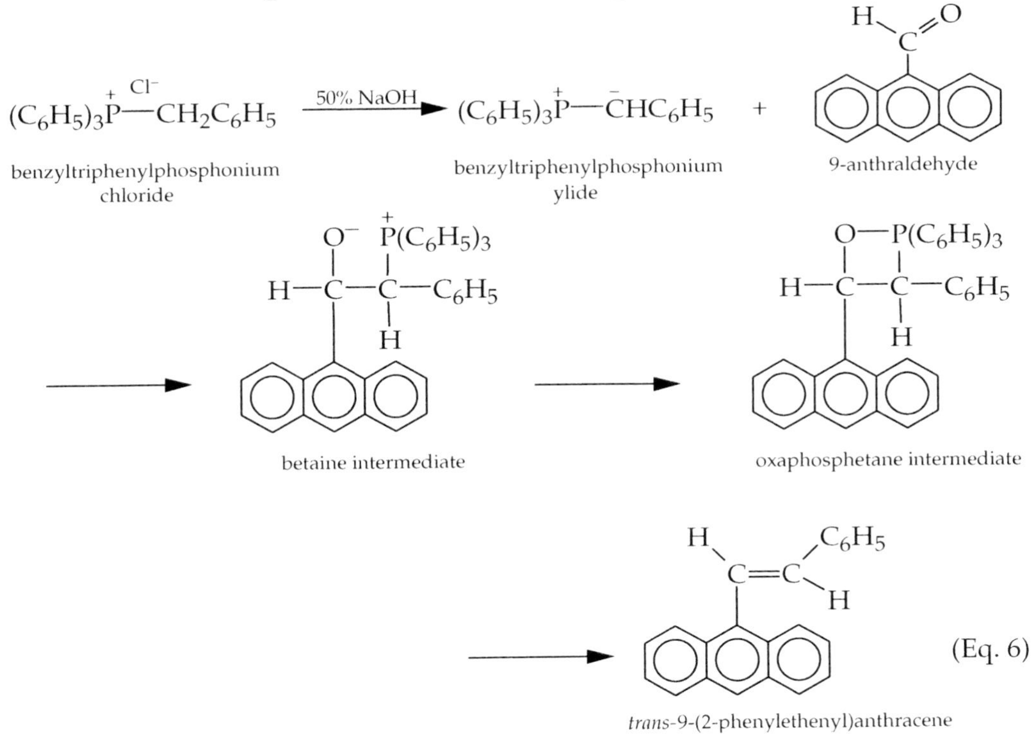

$(C_6H_5)_3\overset{+}{P}$—$CH_2C_6H_5$ $\xrightarrow{\text{50\% NaOH}}$ $(C_6H_5)_3\overset{+}{P}$—$\overset{-}{C}HC_6H_5$ +

benzyltriphenylphosphonium chloride

benzyltriphenylphosphonium ylide

9-anthraldehyde

betaine intermediate

oxaphosphetane intermediate

(Eq. 6)

trans-9-(2-phenylethenyl)anthracene

Semi-Microscale Wittig Synthesis

Equipment

50-mL beaker
2 beakers, 100-mL
250-mL beaker*
boiling chip

Büchner funnel, with adapter
condenser, with tubing
distilling head
25-mL Erlenmeyer flask

250-mL filter flask,
   with vacuum tubing
filter paper
10-mL graduated cylinder
hot plate
magnetic stir bar
magnetic stirrer
medicine dropper
*for ice bath and for hot-water bath

microspatula
product vial
25-mL round-bottom flask
125-mL separatory funnel
2 support stands
2 utility clamps
watch glass

Reagents and Properties

substance	quantity	molar mass (g/mol)	bp (°C)	mp (°C)	d (g/mL)
9-anthraldehyde	0.520 g	206.24		104–105	
benzyltriphenyl-phosphonium chloride	0.980 g	388.88			
calcium chloride, anhydrous	1 g	110.99			
dichloromethane	18 mL	84.93	40		1.325
trans-9-(2-phenyl-ethenyl)anthracene*		280.4		130–132	
2-propanol	20 mL	60.10	82		0.785
50% sodium hydroxide	1.3 mL				

*product

Preview

- Dissolve benzyltriphenylphosphonium chloride and 9-anthraldehyde in dichloromethane

- Add 50% aqueous sodium hydroxide

- Stir the reaction mixture vigorously for 30 min

- Use a separatory funnel to separate the dichloromethane layer from the aqueous layer

- Extract the aqueous layer with additional dichloromethane

- Dry the combined dichloromethane layers over anhydrous calcium chloride

- Remove the solvent from the crude product

- Recrystallize the crude product from 2-propanol

- Dry and weigh the product

PROCEDURE **Chemical Alert**

9-anthraldehyde—*irritant*

benzyltriphenylphosphonium chloride—*irritant and hygroscopic*

anhydrous calcium chloride—*irritant and hygroscopic*

dichloromethane—*toxic and irritant*

420

2-propanol—*flammable and irritant*

50% sodium hydroxide—*corrosive and toxic*

Caution: Wear departmentally approved safety goggles at all times while in the chemistry laboratory.

1. Using a Wittig Reagent to Synthesize *trans*-9-(2-Phenylethenyl)anthracene

Caution: Benzyltriphenylphosphonium chloride and 9-anthraldehyde are irritating. Dichloromethane is toxic and irritating. Use a ***fume hood***.

50% Sodium hydroxide (NaOH) is corrosive and toxic. Wear gloves when using this solution. Prevent eye, skin, and clothing contact. Avoid inhaling and ingesting these compounds.

Weigh 0.980 g of benzyltriphenylphosphonium chloride and 0.520 g of 9-anthraldehyde. Place them into a 25-mL Erlenmeyer flask. Add 3 mL of dichloromethane. Place the flask on top of a magnetic stirrer and add a stir bar.

While the mixture is vigorously stirring, add 1.3 mL of 50% aqueous sodium hydroxide at a rate of 1 drop every 7 s. Vigorously stir the reaction mixture for an additional 30 min.

2. Isolating *trans*-9-(2-Phenylethenyl)anthracene

Caution: 2-Propanol is flammable and irritating. Keep away from flames or other heat sources. Anhydrous calcium chloride ($CaCl_2$) is irritating and hygroscopic. Prevent eye, skin, and clothing contact. Avoid inhaling and ingesting these compounds.

Transfer the reaction mixture from the Erlenmeyer flask to a 125-mL separatory funnel. Rinse the reaction flask with 10 mL of dichloromethane and transfer the rinse to the separatory funnel. Then rinse the reaction flask with 10 mL of distilled or deionized water and transfer the rinse to the separatory funnel.

Shake and vent the contents in the funnel. Allow the layers to separate. Drain the organic layer from the funnel into a 100-mL beaker labeled, "Organic Layer".

Add an additional 5 mL of dichloromethane to the aqueous layer in the funnel. Shake and vent the contents in the funnel. Drain the organic layer into the beaker containing the initial organic layer.

Dry the combined organic layers by adding up to 1 g of anhydrous $CaCl_2$ to the beaker. Cover the beaker with a watch glass and allow the solution to dry for 10 min. Decant the organic layer from the drying agent into a dry 25-mL round-bottom flask.

3. Removing the Dichloromethane [NOTE 1]

Using a Rotary Evaporator

Use a rotary evaporator to collect the dichloromethane from the product, as directed by your laboratory instructor.

Using Distillation

Set up a simple distillation apparatus in the ***fume hood***. Use the 25-mL round-bottom flask containing your product as the distilling flask. Add a boiling chip. Use a hot-water bath to distill the dichloromethane from the product. Collect the dichloromethane in a 50-mL beaker.

NOTE 1: Use the separation method designated by your laboratory instructor.

| 4. **Purifying** *trans*-9-(2-Phenylethenyl) anthracene | Add 20 mL of 2-propanol to a 100-mL beaker. Heat the 2-propanol to boiling using a hot plate or electric flask heater. Recrystallize the crude product from 2-propanol. Allow the flask to cool to room temperature. Then place the solution in an ice-water bath for 5–10 min. |

Collect the product by vacuum filtration using a Büchner funnel. Continue the suction for 5 min to dry the product. Weigh the product and place it into a labeled product vial.

Proceed to the Characterizing the Product Section later in this experiment. Use the procedures designated by your laboratory instructor.

5. **Cleaning Up**   Use the labeled collection containers as directed by your laboratory instructor. Clean your glassware with soap or detergent.

Caution: Wash your hands with soap or detergent before leaving the laboratory.

Microscale Wittig Synthesis

Equipment

2 beakers, 10-mL	hot plate
250-mL beaker*	magnetic stir bar
10-mL centrifuge tube, with screw cap	magnetic stirrer
	medicine dropper
5-mL conical vial	microspatula
25-mL Erlenmeyer flask	2 Pasteur pipets, with latex bulb
25-mL filter flask, with vacuum tubing	1-mL pipet[†]
	product vial
filter paper	support stand
10-mL graduated cylinder	utility clamp
Hirsch funnel, with adapter	watch glass

*for ice bath and for hot-water bath
[†]or adjustable micropipet

Reagents and Properties

substance	quantity	molar mass (g/mol)	bp (°C)	mp (°C)	d (g/mL)
9-anthraldehyde	0.110 g	206.24		104–105	
benzyltriphenyl-phosphonium chloride	0.210 g	388.88			
calcium chloride, anhydrous	0.3 g	110.99			
dichloromethane	3.1 mL	84.93	40		1.325
trans-9-(2-phenyl-ethenyl)anthracene*		280.4		130–132	
2-propanol	5 mL	60.10	82		0.785
50% sodium hydroxide	0.26 mL				

*product

- Dissolve benzyltriphenylphosphonium chloride and 9-anthraldehyde in dichloromethane
- Add 50% aqueous sodium hydroxide
- Stir the reaction mixture vigorously for 30 min
- Separate the dichloromethane layer from the aqueous layer in a centrifuge tube
- Extract the aqueous layer with additional dichloromethane
- Dry the combined dicloromethane layers over anhydrous calcium chloride
- Remove the solvent from the crude product
- Recrystallize the crude product from 2-propanol
- Dry and weigh the product

PROCEDURE   ## Chemical Alert

9-anthraldehyde—*irritant*

benzyltriphenylphosphonium chloride—*irritant and hygroscopic*

anhydrous calcium chloride—*irritant and hygroscopic*

dichloromethane—*toxic and irritant*

2-propanol—*flammable and irritant*

50% sodium hydroxide—*corrosive and toxic*

Caution: Wear departmentally approved safety goggles at all times while in the chemistry laboratory.

1. Using a Wittig Reagent to Synthesize *trans*-9-(2-Phenylethenyl)anthracene

Caution: Benzyltriphenylphosphonium chloride and 9-anthraldehyde are irritating. Dichloromethane is toxic and irritating. Use a *fume hood*. Prevent eye, skin, and clothing contact. Avoid inhaling and ingesting these compounds.

50% Sodium hydroxide (NaOH) is corrosive and toxic. Wear gloves when using this solution. Prevent eye, skin, and clothing contact. Avoid inhaling and ingesting this compound.

Weigh 0.210 g of benzyltriphenylphosphonium chloride and 0.110 g of 9-anthraldehyde. Place them into a 5-mL conical vial. Add 0.6 mL of dichloromethane. Place the vial on top of a magnetic stirrer and add a stir bar. Clamp the vial in place for added stability.

While the mixture is vigorously stirring, add 0.26 mL of 50% aqueous sodium hydroxide at a rate of 1 drop every 7 s. Vigorously stir the reaction mixture for an additional 30 min.

2. Isolation and Purification of *trans*-9-(2-Phenylethenyl) anthracene

Transfer the reaction mixture from the vial to a 10-mL centrifuge tube. Rinse the reaction vial with 1.5 mL of dichloromethane and transfer the rinse to the centrifuge tube. Then rinse the reaction vial with 1.5 mL of distilled or deionized water and add the rinse to the centrifuge tube.

Screw the cap onto the centrifuge tube and shake it vigorously, venting the tube periodically. Allow the layers to separate. Using a Pasteur pipet, transfer the organic layer from the centrifuge tube to a 10-mL beaker labeled, "Organic Layer".

Add an additional 1 mL of dichloromethane to the aqueous layer in the centrifuge tube. Shake and vent the contents in the tube. Transfer the organic layer to the beaker containing the initial organic layer.

Dry the combined organic layers by adding up to 0.3 g of anhydrous $CaCl_2$ to the beaker. Cover the beaker with a watch glass and allow the solution to dry for 10 min.

Decant the organic layer from the drying agent into a dry 10-mL beaker. Use a steam bath or a hot-water bath in a *fume hood* to carefully evaporate the dichloromethane from the crude product. Do not overheat the beaker and melt the crude product. Use a *gentle* stream of air or nitrogen to speed the evaporation process.

Add 5 mL of 2-propanol to a 25-mL Erlenmeyer flask. Heat the 2-propanol to boiling, using a hot plate or electric flask heater. Recrystallize the crude product from hot 2-propanol. Allow the flask to cool to room temperature. Then place the solution in an ice-water bath for 5–10 min.

Collect the product by vacuum filtration using a Hirsch funnel. Continue the suction for 5 min to dry the product. Weigh the product and place it into a labeled product vial.

Proceed to the Characterizing the Product Section. Use the procedures designated by your laboratory instructor.

3. **Cleaning Up**   Use the labeled collection containers as directed by your laboratory instructor. Clean your glassware with soap or detergent.

Caution: Wash your hands with soap or detergent before leaving the laboratory.

Characterizing the Product

Equipment

Melting Point

melting point capillary tubes

Thin-Layer Chromatography

1.0-mL conical vial
12-cm filter paper,
    cut to fit the developing chamber
10-mL graduated cylinder
microburner
open-ended capillary tubes
*or 400-mL beakers, with aluminum foil covers

pencil
0.1-mL transfer pipet
ruler
2 screw-cap jars, 4-oz*
2 × 9-cm silica gel TLC plate,
    with fluorescent indicator

Infrared Analysis

KBr pellet press*
NaCl or AgCl plates, with sample holder†
*for KBr pellets
†for mull

NMR Analysis

3.0-mL conical vial
Pasteur pipet, with latex bulb

NMR sample tube

Reagents and Properties

substance	quantity	molar mass (g/mol)	bp (°C)	mp (°C)
9-anthraldehyde		206.24		104–105
deutero-chloroform	1 mL	120.39	60.9	
potassium bromide	100 mg			
toluene	10 mL	92.14	110.6	

Preview

- Measure the melting point of the product
- Prepare a thin-layer chromatogram and measure the product R_f
- Analyze the product using infrared spectroscopy
- Analyze the product using nuclear magnetic resonance spectroscopy

PROCEDURE   *Chemical Alert*

9-anthraldehyde—*irritant*

deutero-chloroform—*toxic and suspected carcinogen*

toluene—*flammable and toxic*

Caution: Wear departmentally approved safety goggles at all times while in the chemistry laboratory.

1. Measuring Melting Point   Take a melting point of the product. Heat the melting point tube quickly to 110 °C, then slow the heating rate to 2 °C per min. Observe and record the temperature range over which the solid melts.

2. Using Thin-Layer Chromatography   *Caution:*   Toluene is flammable and toxic. Do not use toluene near flames or other heat sources. *Use toluene only when all students have prepared their micropipets and all flames have been extinguished.* Use a *fume hood.* Prevent eye, skin, and clothing contact. Avoid inhaling vapors and ingesting toluene.

Prepare micropipets for spotting the TLC plate by drawing out open-ended capillary tubes.

Prepare a developing chamber using approximately 10 mL of toluene as the eluent.

Place 0.1-mL of toluene in a 1.0-mL conical vial. Add 1–2 mg of your product and mix to dissolve.

Using a *pencil*, lightly draw a line across the bottom of a TLC plate, 1 cm above the bottom. Carefully make two light hash marks on the line and label them as "starting material" and "product".

Caution: 9-Anthraldehyde is irritating. Prevent eye, skin, and clothing contact.

Spot 9-anthraldehyde, using the solution provided by your laboratory instructor, and the product, using the solution you prepared, on the plate. Place the plate into the developing chamber.

Develop the plate until the eluent front is approximately 1 cm from the top. Then remove the chromatogram from the chamber and *immediately* mark the eluent front with a pencil.

Caution: Ultraviolet radiation can cause severe damage to the eyes. Wear goggles. Do not look directly into the lamp.

Allow the eluent to evaporate under the *fume hood*. Examine the chromatogram under the UV lamp and lightly circle the spots using a pencil.

Using a ruler, measure the distance to the eluent front and to the center of each spot. Record the values.

3. **Using Infrared Spectroscopy** *Caution:* Potassium bromide (KBr) is irritating. Prevent eye, skin, and clothing contact. Avoid inhaling dust.

Prepare the sample for IR analysis following the instructions of your laboratory instructor. Obtain an IR spectrum of your sample.

4. **Using Nuclear Magnetic Resonance Spectroscopy** *Caution:* *deutero*-Chloroform (*d*-chloroform) is toxic and a suspected carcinogen. Use gloves. Use a *fume hood*. Prevent eye, skin, and clothing contact. Avoid inhaling vapors and ingesting the compound.

Obtain an NMR sample tube from your laboratory instructor. In a dry vial, place approximately 10 mg of product and 1 mL of *d*-chloroform. Swirl the vial until all of the solid has dissolved. Use a Pasteur pipet to transfer at least 0.600 mL of the solution to the NMR tube and cap the tube.

Follow the instructions of your laboratory instructor to obtain an NMR spectrum of your sample.

5. **Cleaning Up** Use the labeled collection containers as directed by your laboratory instructor. Clean your glassware with soap or detergent.

Caution: Wash your hands with soap or detergent before leaving the laboratory.

Post-Laboratory Questions

1. Calculate the percent yield of product you obtained from this reaction.
2. Calculate R_fs for each spot on your chromatogram.
3. Using your melting point data and thin-layer chromatogram, what evidence allows you to conclude that your product is *trans*-9-(2-phenylethenyl)anthracene?
4. Compare the IR spectra for 9-anthraldehyde and that of your product. What evidence allows you to conclude that your product is *trans*-9-(2-phenylethenyl) anthracene?
5. Using your IR and NMR spectra, what evidence supports the synthesis of the *trans* isomer rather than the *cis* isomer?

SYNT 721/Synthesis of trans-9-(2-Phenylethenyl)anthracene: A Wittig Reaction

Pre-Laboratory Assignment

1. What safety precautions must be observed when using
   (a) dichloromethane?

   (b) 50% aqueous sodium hydroxide?

   (c) toluene?

2. Briefly explain the advantage of a Wittig synthesis over the more common dehydrohalogenation reaction.

427

3. Using the data in the Reagents and Properties table,
    (a) identify which reactant is the limiting reagent in the reaction;

    (b) calculate the theoretical yield, in grams, of *trans*-9-(2-phenylethenyl)anthracene. Show your calculation here and in your laboratory notebook.

4. What combination of carbonyl compound and phosphorus ylide could you use to prepare the following alkenes?
    (a) $CH_3CH_2CH(CH_3)CH=CHCH_3$

    (b) $(CH_3)_2C=CHC_6H_5$

ISBN 0-87540-721-8

428

1,4-Diphenyl-1,3-butadiene

Wittig reaction
Working with sodium ethoxide
Thin-layer chromatography
UV/NMR spectroscopy
Solventless Wittig reactions

The Wittig reaction is often used to form alkenes from carbonyl compounds. In this experiment, the isomeric dienes *cis,trans-*, and *trans,trans-*1,4-diphenyl-1,3-butadiene will be formed from cinnamaldehyde and benzyltriphenylphosphonium chloride.

Two procedures are provided for preparing *trans,trans-*1,4-diphenyl-1,3-butadiene. In Experiment 44B, the reaction uses sodium ethoxide in ethanol solvent as the base, whereas in Experiment 44C, a green chemistry alternative is provided whereby potassium phosphate is employed as the base that is conducted without any solvent. The mechanism of the Wittig reaction in the presence of either sodium ethoxide or potassium phosphate is essentially identical. Sodium ethoxide is shown as the base in the mechanism that follows. In Experiment 44A, an optional procedure is provided for preparing one of the starting materials for the Wittig reaction.

The reaction is carried out in two steps. First, the phosphonium salt is formed by the reaction of triphenylphosphine with benzyl chloride in Experiment 44A. The reaction is a simple nucleophilic displacement of chloride ion by triphenylphosphine. The salt that is formed is called the "Wittig reagent" or "Wittig salt."

Benzyltriphenylphosphonium chloride
"Wittig salt"

When treated with base, the Wittig salt forms an **ylide.** An ylide is a species having adjacent atoms oppositely charged. The ylide is stabilized due to the ability of phosphorus to accept more than eight electrons in its valence shell. Phosphorus uses its 3d orbitals to form the overlap with the

2p orbital of carbon that is necessary for resonance stabilization. Resonance stabilizes the carbanion.

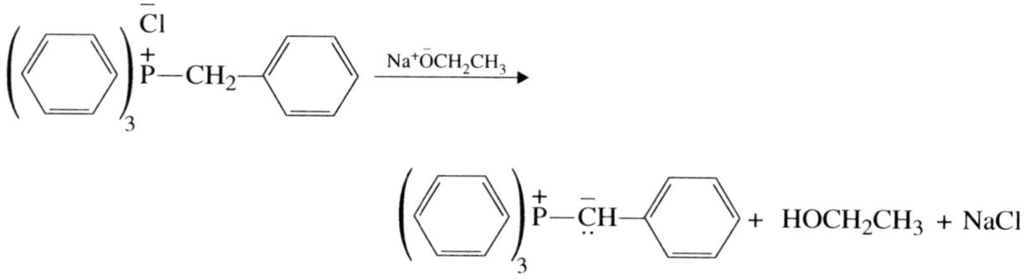

An ylide

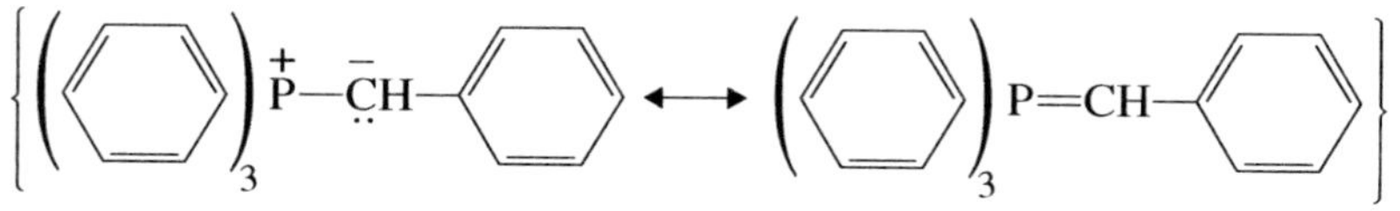

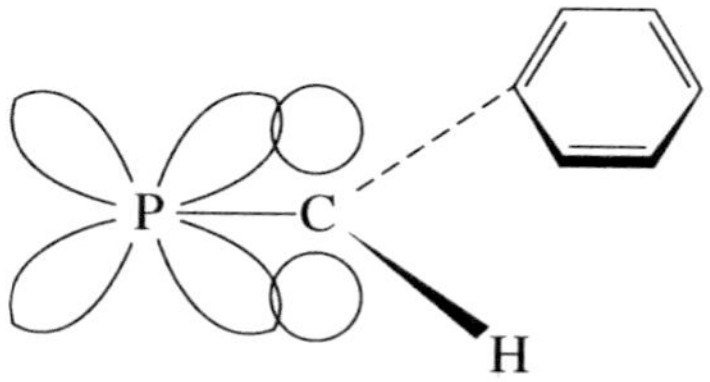

The ylide is a carbanion that acts as a nucleophile, and it adds to the carbonyl group in the first step of the mechanism. Following the initial nucleophilic addition, a remarkable sequence of events occurs, as outlined in the following mechanism:

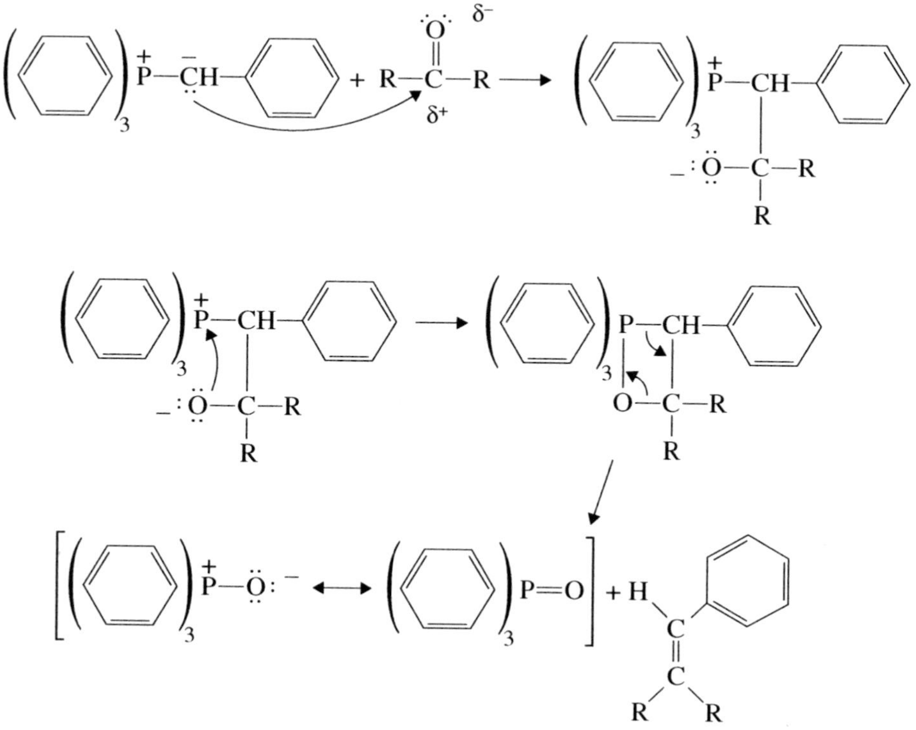

Triphenylphosphine oxide

An alkene

430

The addition intermediate, formed from the ylide and the carbonyl compound, cyclizes to form a four-membered-ring intermediate. This new intermediate is unstable and fragments into an alkene and triphenylphosphine oxide. Notice that the ring breaks open differently from the way it was formed. The driving force for this ring-opening process is the formation of a very stable substance, triphenylphosphine oxide. A large decrease in potential energy is achieved on the formation of this thermodynamically stable compound.

In this experiment, cinnamaldehyde is used as the carbonyl compound and yields mainly the *trans,trans*-1,4-diphenyl-1,3-butadiene, which is obtained as a solid. The *cis,trans* isomer is formed in smaller amounts, but it is a liquid that is not isolated in this experiment. The *trans,trans* isomer is the more stable isomer and is formed preferentially.

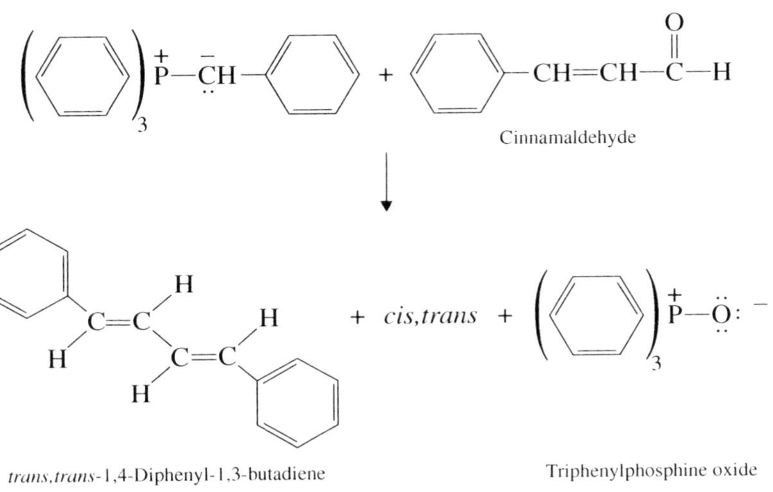

Cinnamaldehyde

trans,trans-1,4-Diphenyl-1,3-butadiene   Triphenylphosphine oxide

---

REQUIRED READING

Review: Technique 8   Section 8.3
Technique 20

SPECIAL INSTRUCTIONS

Your instructor may ask you to prepare 1,4-diphenyl-1,3-butadiene starting with commercially available benzyltriphenylphosphonium chloride. If so, start with Experiment 44B or 44C. The sodium ethoxide solution used in Experiment 44B must be kept tightly stoppered when not in use because it reacts readily with atmospheric water. Fresh cinnamaldehyde must be used in this experiment. Old cinnamaldehyde should be checked by infrared spectroscopy to be certain that it does not contain any cinnamic acid.

If your instructor asks you to prepare benzyltriphenylphosphonium chloride in Experiment 44A, you can conduct another experiment concurrently during the 1.5-hour reflux period. Triphenylphosphine is rather toxic. Be careful not to inhale the dust. Benzyl chloride is a skin irritant and a lachrymator. It should be handled in the hood with care.

SUGGESTED WASTE DISPOSAL

If you conducted Experiment 44A, place the wastes in the nonhalogenated waste container. For Experiment 44B and 44C, dispose of organic wastes in the nonhalogenated waste container. Place the aqueous waste into the bottle designated for aqueous wastes.

EXPERIMENT 44A (OPTIONAL)

Benzyltriphenylphosphonium Chloride (Wittig Salt)

Place 0.550 g of triphenylphosphine ($MW = 262.3$) into a 5-mL conical vial. In a hood, transfer 0.36 mL of benzyl chloride ($MW = 126.6$, $d = 1.10$ g/mL) to the vial and add 2.0 mL of xylenes (mixture of o-, m-, and p-isomers).

CAUTION

Benzyl chloride is a lachrymator, a tear-producing substance.

Add a magnetic spin vane to the conical vial and attach a water-cooled condenser. Boil the mixture using an aluminum block at about 165°C for at least 1.5 hours. An increased yield may be expected when the mixture is heated longer. In fact, you may begin heating the mixture before the temperature has reached the values given, but do not include this time in the 1.5-hour reaction period. The solution will be homogeneous at first, and then the Wittig salt will begin to precipitate. Maintain the stirring during the entire heating period or bumping may occur. Remove the apparatus from the aluminum block and allow it to cool for a few minutes. Remove the vial and cool it thoroughly in an ice bath for about 5 minutes.

Collect the Wittig salt by vacuum filtration using a Hirsch funnel. Use three 1-mL portions of cold petroleum ether (bp 60–90°C) to aid the transfer and to wash the crystals free of the xylene solvent. Dry the crystals, weigh them, and calculate the percentage yield of the Wittig salt. At the option of the instructor, obtain the proton NMR spectrum of the salt in CDCl$_3$. The methylene group appears as a doublet (J = 14 Hz) at 5.5 ppm because of ^{1}H-^{31}P coupling.

EXPERIMENT 44B

Preparation of 1,4-Diphenyl-1,3-Butadiene Using Sodium Ethoxide to Generate the Ylide

In the following operations, cap the 5-mL conical vial whenever possible to avoid contact with moisture from the atmosphere. If you prepared your own benzyltriphenylphosphonium chloride in Experiment 44A, you may need to supplement your yield in this part of the experiment.

Preparation of the Ylide

Place 0.480 g of benzyltriphenylphosphonium chloride (MW = 388.9) in a *dry* 5-mL conical vial. Add a magnetic spin vane. Transfer 2.0 mL of absolute (anhydrous) ethanol to the vial and stir the mixture to dissolve the phosphonium salt (Wittig salt). Add 0.75 mL of sodium ethoxide solution[1] to the vial using a *dry* pipet while stirring continuously. Cap the vial and stir this mixture for 15 minutes. During this period, the cloudy solution acquires the characteristic yellow color of the ylide.

Reaction of the Ylide with Cinnamaldehyde

Measure 0.15 mL of *pure* cinnamaldehyde (MW = 132.2, d = 1.11 g/mL) and place it in another small conical vial. Add 0.50 mL of absolute ethanol to the cinnamaldehyde. Cap the vial until it is needed. After the 15-minute period, use a Pasteur pipet to mix the cinnamaldehyde with the ethanol and add this solution to the ylide in the reaction vial. A color change should be observed as the ylide reacts with the aldehyde and the product precipitates. Stir the mixture for 10 minutes.

Separation of the Isomers of 1,4-Diphenyl-1,3-Butadiene

Cool the vial thoroughly in an ice-water bath (10 min), stir the mixture with a spatula, and transfer the material from the vial to a Hirsch funnel under vacuum. Use two 1-mL portions of ice-cold absolute ethanol to aid the transfer and to rinse the product. Dry the crystalline *trans,trans*-1,4-diphenyl-1,3-butadiene by drawing air through the solid. The product has a small amount of sodium chloride that is removed as described in the next paragraph. The cloudy material in the filter flask contains triphenylphosphine oxide, the *cis,trans*-isomer, and some *trans,trans* product. Pour the filtrate into a beaker and save it for the thin-layer chromatography experiment described in the next section.

Remove the *trans,trans*-1,4-diphenyl-1,3-butadiene from the filter paper, place the solid in a 10-mL beaker, and add 3 mL of water. Stir the mixture and filter it on a Hirsch funnel, under vacuum, to collect the nearly colorless crystalline *trans,trans* product. Use about 1 mL of water to aid the transfer. Allow the solid to dry thoroughly.

Thin-Layer Chromatography

Use thin-layer chromatography to analyze the filtrate that you saved in the previous section. This mixture must be analyzed as soon as possible so that the *cis,trans* isomer will not be photochemically converted to the *trans,trans* compound. Use a 2 × 8-cm silica gel TLC plate that has a fluorescent indicator

---

[1] This reagent is prepared in advance by the instructor. Carefully dry a 250-mL Erlenmeyer flask and insert a drying tube filled with calcium chloride into a one-hole rubber stopper. Obtain a large piece of sodium, clean it by cutting off the oxidized surface, weigh out a 2.30-g piece, cut it into 20 smaller pieces, and store it under xylene. Using tweezers, remove each piece, wipe off the xylene, and add the sodium slowly over a period of about 30 minutes to 40 mL of absolute (anhydrous) ethanol in the 250-mL Erlenmeyer flask. After the addition of each piece, replace the stopper. The ethanol will warm as the sodium reacts, but do not cool the flask. After the sodium has been added, warm the solution and shake it *gently* until all the sodium reacts. Cool the sodium ethoxide solution to room temperature. This reagent may be prepared in advance of the laboratory period, but it must be stored in a refrigerator between laboratory periods. When it is stored in a refrigerator, it may be kept for about 3 days. Before using this reagent, bring it to room temperature and swirl it gently in order to redissolve any precipitated sodium ethoxide. Keep the flask stoppered between each use.

(Eastman Chromatogram Sheet, No. EK 1224294). At one position on the TLC plate, spot the filtrate, as is, without dilution. Dissolve a few crystals of the *trans,trans*-1,4-diphenyl-1,3-butadiene in a few drops of acetone and spot it at another position on the plate. Use hexane as a solvent to develop (run) the plate.

Visualize the spots with a UV lamp using both the long and short wavelength settings. The order of increasing R_f values is as follows: triphenylphosphine oxide, *trans,trans*-diene, and *cis,trans*-diene. It is easy to identify the spot for the *trans,trans* isomer because it fluoresces brilliantly. What conclusion can you make about the contents of the filtrate and the purity of the *trans,trans* product? Report the results that you obtain, including R_f values and the appearance of the spots under illumination. Discard the filtrate in the container designated for nonhalogenated waste.

Yield Calculation and Melting-Point Determination

When the *trans,trans*-1,4-diphenyl-1,3-butadiene is dry, determine the melting point (literature, 151°C). Weigh the solid and determine the percentage yield. If the melting point is below 145°C, recrystallize a portion of the compound from hot 95% ethanol (20 mg/1.3 mL ethanol) in a Craig tube. Redetermine the melting point.

Preparation of 1,4-Diphenyl-1,3-Butadiene Using Potassium Phosphate to Generate the Ylide

Experiment 44C provides an alternative green chemistry method for preparing 1,4-diphenyl-1,3-butadiene by the Wittig reaction. No solvent is used in this experiment. Instead, the starting materials are ground together with potassium phosphate in a mortar and pestle. This experiment will demonstrate to students a more environmentally friendly method for carrying out a reaction that might be performed on a larger scale in industry.

The reaction will be accomplished by grinding cinnamaldehyde with benzyltriphenylphosphonium chloride and potassium phosphate (tribasic, K_3PO_4). This is done using a mortar and pestle. TLC will be used to analyze the crystallized *trans,trans*-1,4-diphenyl-1,3-butadiene product, as well as the filtrate from the crystallization procedure that contains both the *cis,trans* and *trans,trans*-1,4-diphenyl-1,3,-butadiene isomers.

Reaction

Using an analytical balance, weigh out 309 mg of benzyltriphenylphosphonium chloride and 656 mg of potassium phosphate (tribasic, K_3PO_4) and place the solids into a clean and dry 6-cm (inside diameter) porcelain mortar with a pour lip. Using an automatic pipet, measure and add 100 μL of cinnamaldehyde to the mixture in the mortar. Grind the mixture together for a total of 20 minutes. It is much easier to use a pestle that is long enough to grip securely in your hand, thus saving one's fingers from getting sore or tired. At the beginning of the grinding operation, the mixture will act like putty and will have a definite yellow color. After a few minutes of grinding, the mixture starts to turn into a thick paste that adheres to the inside of the mortar and the edges of the pestle. Bend the end of a spatula as shown in the figure. This bent spatula is useful for scraping the material off of the inside of the mortar and pestle and directing the mass into the center of the mortar. Repeat the scraping operation after every 1 to 2 minutes of grinding. Include that time in the total of 20 minutes of grinding time.

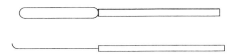

Isolation of Crude 1,4-Diphenyl-1,3-Butadiene

After 20 minutes, add a few milliliters of deionized water to the material in the mortar. Scrape the mortar and pestle a final time to loosen all of the product from the mortar. Pour the mixture into a Hirsch funnel inserted into a filter flask under vacuum. Use a squirt bottle with deionized water to transfer any remaining off-white product into the Hirsch funnel. Discard the filtrate that contains potassium phosphate and some triphenylphosphine oxide. The off-white solid consists of mainly of the *trans,trans* isomer, but some of the *cis,trans* isomer will be present, as well.

Crystallization

Purify the off-white solid by crystallization from absolute ethanol in a small test tube using the standard technique of adding hot solvent until the solid dissolves. A small amount of impurity might not dissolve. If this is the case, use a Pasteur pipet to *rapidly* remove the hot solution away from the impurity and transfer the hot solution to another test tube. Cork the test tube and place it in a warm 25-mL Erlenmeyer flask. Allow the solution to cool slowly. Once the test tube has cooled and crystals have formed, place the test tube in an ice bath for at least 10 minutes to complete the crystallization process. Place 2 mL of absolute ethanol in another test tube and cool the solvent in the ice bath (this solvent will be used to aid the transfer of the product). Loosen the crystals in the test tube with a microspatula and pour the contents of the test tube into a Hirsch funnel under vacuum. Remove the remaining crystals from the test tube using the chilled ethanol and a spatula. Dry the colorless crystalline (plates) of *trans,trans*-1,4-diphenyl-1,3-butadiene on the Hirsch funnel for about 5 minutes to completely dry them. Save the filtrate from the crystallization for analysis by thin-layer chromatography. The *cis,trans*-1,4-diphenyl-1,3-butadiene, which is also formed in the Wittig reaction, is a liquid, and crystallization effectively removes the isomer from the solid *trans,trans* product.

Yield Calculation and Melting Point Determination

Weigh the purified *trans,trans* product and calculate the percentage yield. Determine the melting point of the product (literature, 151°C).

Thin-Layer Chromatography

Following the procedure in Experiment 44B, analyze the filtrate from the crystallization and the purified solid product by thin-layer chromatography. Develop the plate with hexane. This solvent will separate the *cis,trans*-diene from the *trans,trans* isomer. The order of increasing R_f values is as follows: triphenylphosphine oxide, *trans,trans*-diene, and *cis-trans*-diene. Triphenylphosphine oxide is so polar that the R_f value will be nearly zero. After developing the plate in hexane, as indicated in Experiment 44B, use the short and long wavelength settings with a UV lamp to visualize the spots. Calculate the R_f values and record them in your notebook.

Spectroscopy (Optional)

Prepare an NMR sample by dissolving at least 20 mg of crystallized product in about 1 ml of $CDCl_3$ in a small test tube. Transfer the solution to an NMR tube and add more solvent until the level of the solution is about 50 mm in the tube. Run the proton and carbon NMR spectra on the sample. At 300 MHz, the proton spectrum shows multiplets at 6.68 ppm and 6.95 ppm for the vinyl protons and 7.24 ppm (triplet, 2 H), 7.34 ppm (triplet, 4 H), and 7.44 ppm (doublet, 4 H) for the aromatic protons. The carbon spectrum shows peaks at 125.4, 126.6, 127.7, 128.3, 131.8, and 136.4 ppm. To determine the UV spectrum of the product, dissolve a 10-mg sample in 100 mL of hexane in a volumetric flask. Remove 10 mL of this solution and dilute it to 100 mL in another volumetric flask. This concentration should be adequate for analysis. The *trans,trans* isomer absorbs at 328 nm and possesses fine structure, whereas the *cis,trans* isomer absorbs at 313 nm and has a smooth curve.[2] See if your spectrum is consistent with these observations. Submit the spectral data with your laboratory report.

QUESTIONS

1. There is an additional isomer of 1,4-diphenyl-1,3-butadiene (mp 70°C), which has not been shown in this experiment. Draw the structure and name it. Why is it not produced in this experiment? (*Hint:* The cinnamaldehyde has *trans* stereochemistry).

2. Why should the *trans,trans* isomer be the thermodynamically most stable one?

3. A lower yield of phosphonium salt is obtained in refluxing benzene than in xylene (Experiment 44A). Look up the boiling points for these solvents, and explain why the difference in boiling points might influence the yield.

4. Outline a synthesis for *cis* and *trans* stilbene (the 1,2-diphenylethenes) using the Wittig reaction.

5. The sex attractant of the female housefly (*Musca domestica*) is called **muscalure,** and its structure follows. Outline a synthesis of muscalure, using the Wittig reaction. Will your synthesis lead to the required *cis* isomer?

$$CH_3(CH_2)_7 \diagdown \diagup (CH_2)_{12}CH_3$$
$$C=C$$
$$H \diagup \diagdown H$$

Muscalure

[2] The comparative study of the stereoisometric 1,4-diphenyl-1,3-butadienes has been published: Pinkard, J. H., Wille, B., and Zechmeister, L. *Journal of the American Chemical Society, 70* (1948): 1938.

Essential Oils: Extraction of Oil of Cloves by Steam Distillation and Liquid Carbon Dioxide

Isolation of a natural product

Steam distillation

Green chemistry

Essential oils are volatile compounds responsible for the aromas commonly associated with many plants (see essay "Terpenes and Phenylpropanoids"). The chief constituent of the essential oil from cloves is aromatic and volatile with steam. In this experiment, you will isolate the main component derived from this spice by steam distillation. Steam distillation provides a means of isolating natural products, such as essential oils, without the risk of decomposing them thermally. Identification and characterization of this essential oil will be accomplished by infrared spectroscopy. Experiment 14C provides a Green Chemistry option in which the instructor may demonstrate the extraction of the oil with liquid CO_2.

Oil of cloves (from *Eugenia caryophyllata*) is rich in **eugenol** (4-allyl-2-methoxyphenol). Caryophyllene is present in small amounts, along with other terpenes. Eugenol (bp 250°C) is a phenol, or an aromatic hydroxy compound.

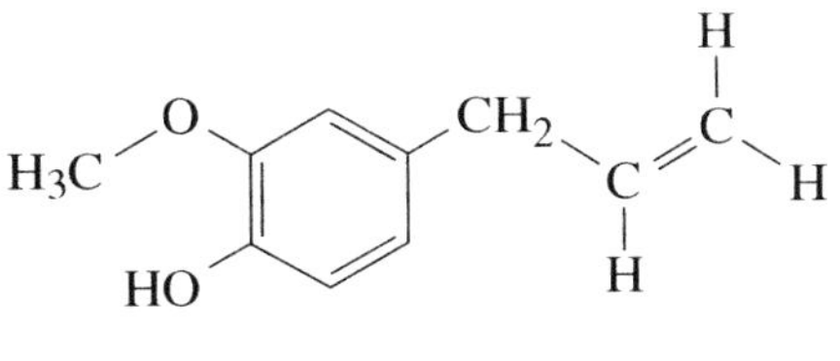

Eugenol 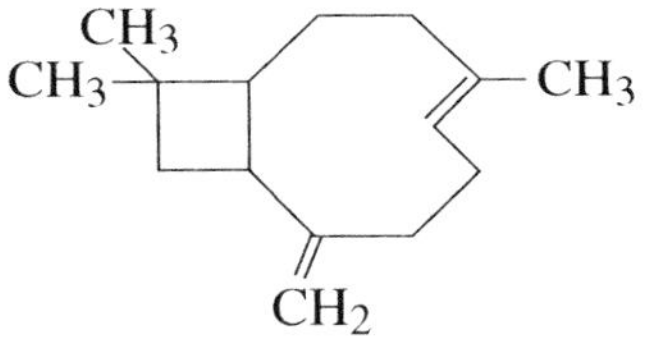   Caryophyllene

---

REQUIRED READING

Review: Techniques 5 and 6

Technique 7   Reaction Methods, Section 7.10

Technique 12   Extractions, Separations and Drying Agents, Sections 12.4 and 12.9

Technique 25   Infrared Spectroscopy

New: Technique 18   Steam Distillation

Essay   Terpenes and Phenylpropanoids

If performing the optional proton NMR analysis, also read

Technique 26   Nuclear Magnetic Resonance Spectroscopy

SPECIAL INSTRUCTIONS

Be careful when handling methylene chloride. It is a toxic solvent, and you should not breathe it excessively or spill it on yourself. To complete the distillation in a reasonable time, boil the mixture as rapidly as possible without allowing the boiling mixture to rise above the neck of the Hickman head. This requires that you work with careful attention during the distillation procedure. The distillation requires 1–2 hours.

SUGGESTED WASTE DISPOSAL

You must dispose of methylene chloride in a waste container marked for the disposal of halogenated organic waste. Any residue from the ground cloves can be disposed of in an ordinary trash can. Any aqueous solutions should be placed in the container specially designated for aqueous wastes.

EXPERIMENT 14A

Oil of Cloves (Microscale Procedure)

PROCEDURE

Assemble a steam distillation apparatus, as shown in Figure 18.3, page 753. Be sure to include the water condenser, as shown in the illustration. Use a 20- or 25-mL round-bottom flask as a distillation flask and either an aluminum block or a sand bath to heat the distillation flask. If you use a sand bath, you may need to cover the sand bath and distillation flask with aluminum foil.

Weight approximately 1.0 g of ground cloves or clove buds onto a weighing paper and record the exact weight. If your spice is already ground, you may proceed without grinding it; if you use clove buds, cut the buds into small pieces. Mix the spice with 12–15 mL of water in the round-bottom distillation flask, add a magnetic stirring bar, and attach the flask to the distillation apparatus. Allow the spice to soak in the water for about 15 minutes before beginning the heating. Be sure that all the spice is thoroughly wetted. Swirl the flask gently, if needed.

Steam Distillation

Turn on the cooling water in the condenser, begin stirring the mixture in the distillation flask, and begin heating the mixture to provide a steady rate of distillation. The temperature for the heating device should be about 130°C. If you approach the boiling point too quickly, you may have difficulty with frothing or bump-over. You need to find the amount of heating that provides a steady rate of distillation but avoids frothing or bumping. A good rate of distillation would be to have one drop of liquid collected every 2–5 seconds.

438

As the distillation proceeds, use a Pasteur pipet (5¾-inch) to transfer the distillate from the reservoir of the Hickman head to a 15-mL screw-cap centrifuge tube. If you are using a Hickman head with a side port, you can easily remove the distillate by opening the side port and withdrawing the liquid. If your Hickman head does not have a side port, you need to remove the condenser from the top of the distillation apparatus to remove the distillate. In this case, the transferring operation is best accomplished if the Pasteur pipet is bent slightly at the end. Continue distillation until 5–8 mL of distillate has been collected.

Normally in a steam distillation, the distillate is somewhat cloudy owing to separation of the essential oil as the vapors cool. You may not notice this, but you will still obtain satisfactory results.

Extraction of the Essential Oil

Collect all the distillate in a 15-mL screw-cap centrifuge tube. Using a calibrated Pasteur pipet (p. 11), add 2.0 mL of methylene chloride (dichloromethane) to extract the distillate. Cap the tube securely and shake it vigorously with frequent venting. Allow the layers to separate. Using a Pasteur pipet, transfer the lower methylene chloride layer to a clean, dry, 5-mL conical vial. Repeat this extraction procedure two more times with fresh 1.0-mL portions of methylene chloride and combine all the methylene chloride extracts in the same 5-mL conical vial that you used for the first extraction. If there are drops of water in the vial, it will be necessary to transfer the methylene chloride solution with a dry Pasteur pipet to another dry conical vial.

Drying

Dry the methylene chloride solution by adding granular anhydrous sodium sulfate to the conical vial (see Technique 12, Section 12.9, p. 680). Let the solution stand for 10–15 minutes with occasional stirring.

Evaporation

While the organic solution is being dried, clean and dry a 5-mL conical vial and weigh (tare) it accurately. With a clean, dry Pasteur pipet, transfer the dried organic layer to the tared vial, leaving the drying agent behind. Use small amounts of methylene chloride to rinse the solution completely into the tared vial. Be careful to keep any of the sodium sulfate from being transferred. Working in a hood, evaporate the methylene chloride from the solution by using a gentle stream of dry air or nitrogen while heating the vial in a warm water bath (temperature about 40°C). (See Technique 7, Section 7.10, p. 611). It is important that the stream of air or nitrogen be gentle or you will force your solution out of the conical vial. In addition, be careful not to overheat the sample. Be careful not to continue the evaporation beyond the point where all the methylene chloride has evaporated. Your product is a volatile oil (i.e., a liquid), and if you continue to heat and evaporate the liquid beyond the point where the solvent has been removed, you will likely lose your sample.

Yield Determination

When the solvent has been removed, weigh the conical vial. Calculate the weight percentage recovery (see p. 565) of the oil from the original amount of spice used. See page 115 for a spectral analysis.

Oil of Cloves (Semimicroscale Procedure)

PROCEDURE

Apparatus

Assemble a semimicroscale distillation apparatus, as shown in Figure 14.10, page 713. Use a 20- or 25-mL round-bottom flask as the distillation flask and either an aluminum block or a sand bath to heat the distillation flask. If you use a sand bath, you may need to cover the sand bath and distillation flask with aluminum foil.

Preparation

Use the amounts of cloves and water described in Experiment 14A, page 113.

Steam Distillation

Proceed with the distillation as described in Experiment 14A. Note, however, that you will not have to remove distillate during the course of the distillation. Continue with the extraction, drying, evaporation, and yield determination, as described on pages 113–114.

Spectroscopy (Experiment 14A and 14B)

Infrared Spectrum

Obtain the infrared spectrum of the oil as a pure liquid sample (Technique 25, Section 25.2, p. 834). Small amounts of water will damage the salt plates that are used as cells in infrared spectroscopy.

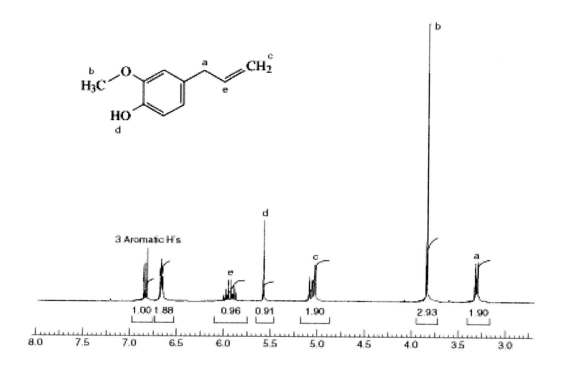

It may be necessary to use a capillary tube to transfer a sufficient amount of liquid to the salt plates. If the amount of liquid is too small to transfer, add one or two drops of methylene chloride to aid in the transfer. Gently blow on the plate to evaporate the solvent. Include the infrared spectrum in your laboratory report, along with an interpretation of the principal absorption peaks.

NMR Spectrum

At the instructor's option, determine the nuclear magnetic resonance spectrum of the oil (Technique 26, Section 26.1, p. 870).

QUESTIONS

1. Why is eugenol steam-distilled rather than purified by simple distillation?

2. A natural product (MW = 150) distills with steam at a boiling temperature of 99°C at atmospheric pressure. The vapor pressure of water at 99°C is 733 mm Hg.

   (a) Calculate the weight of the natural product that codistills with each gram of water at 99°C.

   (b) How much water must be removed by steam distillation to recover this natural product from 0.5 g of a spice that contains 10% of the desired substance?

3. In a steam distillation, the amount of water actually distilled is usually greater than the amount calculated, assuming that both water and organic substance exert the same vapor pressure when they are mixed that they exert when each is pure. Why does one recover more water in the steam distillation than was calculated? (*Hint:* Are the organic compound and water truly immiscible?)

4. Explain how caryophyllene fits the isoprene rule (see essay, "Terpenes and Phenyl-propanoids," p. 106).

EXPERIMENT 14C

Extraction of Oil of Cloves with Liquid Carbon Dioxide—A Demonstration

This experiment should be performed only by the instructor. Liquid CO_2, produced from crushed dry ice, is used to extract the essential oil eugenol from clove spice. After the isolation of eugenol, you will determine its infrared spectrum and assign the major peaks observed in the spectrum to structural features present in the molecule. Mass spectrometry and proton NMR may also be used to determine the structure and purity of the eugenol obtained.

REQUIRED READING

Review:	Technique 8	Section 8.1B, Fluted Filters
New:	Essay	Green Chemistry
	Technique 25	Infrared Spectroscopy

| Technique 26 | Nuclear Magnetic Resonance Spectroscopy (Optional) |
| Technique 28 | Mass Spectrometry (Optional) |

SPECIAL INSTRUCTIONS AND NOTES TO THE INSTRUCTOR

It is recommended that you begin with clove buds and finely grind them to a powder in a mortar and pestle to improve yield. Crush the dry ice with a hammer and store in a Styrofoam container or use immediately.

Special care needs to be taken as to the type of filter paper used in this experiment. It is recommended that fastest filter paper be available to increase yield. Whatman #4 (11 cm) filter paper may be used, but paper used in "Mr Coffee" type coffeemakers works even better as long as it is a low-quality basket-type filter paper. The basket-type filter paper should be cut to 11 cm in diameter.[1] Do not use the coffee filters that have been sealed on the edges to resemble a cone.

Use a **new** 50-mL plastic centrifuge tube made of durable polypropylene provided by VWR (catalog number 20171-029). The centrifuge tubes may be reused for up to 5 times, but then they must be replaced because they will not hold the pressure required for the carbon dioxide to be maintained in the liquid state. Unused centrifuge tubes and lids will assure you that a satisfactory seal will be maintained so that you will be able to attain the pressure required to form liquid CO_2.

SAFETY PRECAUTIONS

This demonstration must be performed with a new centrifuge tube in a hood, with the safety glass pulled down. The 1000-mL graduated cylinder must be made of plastic. Special care is required when the tube is in the water bath, because the centrifuge tube could explode or the lid could fly off due to the high pressure created in the tube during the extraction. See the Instructor's Manual for additional safety discussion. Use only the equipment and methods described here. **Do not under any circumstances use glass products or other plastic centrifuge tubes than the one specified here.**

SUGGESTED WASTE DISPOSAL

Solid waste from the spice should be disposed of in a garbage can.

PROCEDURE

Apparatus

Obtain a 50-mL *plastic* centrifuge tube and cap. **Perform this experiment in a hood, with the safety glass pulled down.**

CAUTION

Do not under any circumstances use glass centrifuge tubes as a substitute.

---

[1] Costco sells bulk basket-type coffee filters designed for 8–12 cups. This type of filter fits Mr. Coffee machines. The best paper is thin so that you can see light through the paper.

Coil a 15-cm piece of copper wire twice at one end so that it will fit inside the centrifuge tube. The wire should be long enough so that you will have a "handle" that can be used to lower the spice into the tube and will allow you to easily remove the filter cone after the extraction. The coil prevents the filter paper cone containing the spice from falling to the bottom of the tube into the extracted oil (see figures).

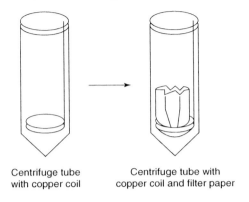

Centrifuge tube
with copper coil

Centrifuge tube with
copper coil and filter paper

Preparing the Spice

Grind about 2.0 g of clove buds to a fine powder in a mortar and pestle. Flute an 11-cm piece of filter paper by the procedure shown in Figure 8.3, page 619 (see "Special Instructions" and "Notes to the Instructor" for the type of paper required). Adjust the filter paper so that it will fit into the centrifuge tube and into the copper coil, but make sure that the tip of the filter paper doesn't project down too far into the tapered end of the centrifuge tube (see figure). It is critical that the filter paper does not touch the bottom of the centrifuge tube. Now transfer the powdered cloves to the preweighed fluted filter paper and record the exact weight of spice.

Extraction

Fill a 1000-mL **plastic** graduated cylinder two-thirds full with hot tap water (40–45°C) and place it in a hood. It is best to use a clear graduated cylinder so that you can observe the extraction as it occurs **but it must be made of plastic.** Working as quickly as possible, place some crushed dry ice *only* in the *tapered part* of the centrifuge tube at the bottom. Insert the fluted filter paper cone containing the ground spice into the copper coil and gently push the coil into the tube, sliding it down to the level of the dry ice. You will need to push the filter cone down into the tube with your index finger as you push the copper coil into the tube. Fill the remainder of the tube with the finely crushed dry ice, tapping the bottom of the tube on the counter and adding more dry ice until the tube is full. Then cap the centrifuge tube as tightly as you can. All of these operations must be carried out as quickly as possible. Proceed to the next step *immediately* after sealing the centrifuge tube.

CAUTION

Do not leave the centrifuge tube out in the open once you have twisted the cap onto the centrifuge tube. Immediately place it into the warm water in the hood.

Quickly lower the capped centrifuge tube, tapered end first, into the graduated cylinder containing warm water in a hood. Pull the hood safety glass down as soon as you place the centrifuge tube into the warm water. The dry ice should liquefy after a minute and remain in the liquid state for about 9 minutes. If the dry ice has not entered the liquid state after about 2 minutes, it is likely that the centrifuge tube leaked from around the cap and did not have an opportunity to build up sufficient pressure. You should replace the cap and tube and try again. Also, if you wait too long before sealing the centrifuge tube, the dry ice can fail to liquefy.

After about 9 minutes, all the liquid CO_2 should have vaporized, and the gas will have escaped from around the cap on the centrifuge tube. Take the centrifuge tube out of the graduated cylinder and remove the cap. Lift the filter cone out of the centrifuge tube using the wire handle on the copper coil. Dispose of the waste spice in a trash can. Remove the clove oil from the bottom of the centrifuge tube with a Pasteur pipet and transfer the clove oil to a small preweighed sample vial. Reweigh the vial to determine the weight of eugenol obtained from the extraction. Calculate the weight percentage recovery of the eugenol from the original weight of spice used.

Spectroscopy

Infrared Spectroscopy

Determine the infrared spectrum of the oil as a neat liquid sample. (Technique 25, Section 25.2) and provide copies for all students. Include the infrared spectrum with your laboratory report, along with an interpretation of the principal peaks.[2]

Nuclear Magnetic Resonance Spectroscopy (Optional)

At the instructor's option, determine the proton NMR spectrum of the eugenol. Assign the peaks in the spectrum to the structure of eugenol.

Mass Spectrometry (Optional)

At the instructor's option, determine the mass spectrum of the eugenol sample (Technique 28). Try to assign as many of the fragments in the spectrum as possible.

REPORT

Attach your infrared spectrum to your report and label the major peaks with the type of bond or group of atoms that is responsible for the absorption. If you have obtained the proton NMR spectrum of the sample, include the spectrum with your report. Be sure to interpret your spectrum fully. If you determined a mass spectrum, identify the important fragment ion peaks. Be sure to also include the weight percentage recovery calculation.

REFERENCE

McKenzie, L. C., Thompson, J. E., Sullivan, R., and Hutchison, J. E. "Green Chemical Processing in the Teaching Laboratory: A Convenient Liquid CO_2 Extraction of Natural Products." *Green Chemistry, 6* (2004): 355–358.

---

[2] Extraction of eugenol with liquid CO_2 yields an extra peak at 1764 cm^{-1} that is attributed to eugenol acetate, a by-product of the extraction; GC-MS will be useful as an optional experiment in identifying the impurity.

EXPERIMENT 1

SOLVENTLESS REACTIONS:

THE ALDOL REACTION

Chemical Concepts

Carbonyl chemistry; the aldol reaction; melting points of solids and mixtures; recrystallization.

Green Lessons

Solventless reactions between solids; atom economy.

Estimated Lab Time

1 – 2 hours

Introduction

The aldol condensation represents a powerful general method for the construction of carbon-carbon bonds, one of the central themes of synthetic organic chemistry. In the base-catalyzed aldol condensation reaction, deprotonation alpha (adjacent) to a carbonyl group affords a resonance-stabilized anion called an enolate, which then carries out nucleophilic attack at the carbonyl group of another molecule of the reactant. (Analogous acid-catalyzed reactions are also well-known.) The product, a beta-hydroxy carbonyl compound, often undergoes facile elimination of water (dehydration), affording an alpha, beta-unsaturated carbonyl compound as the final product.

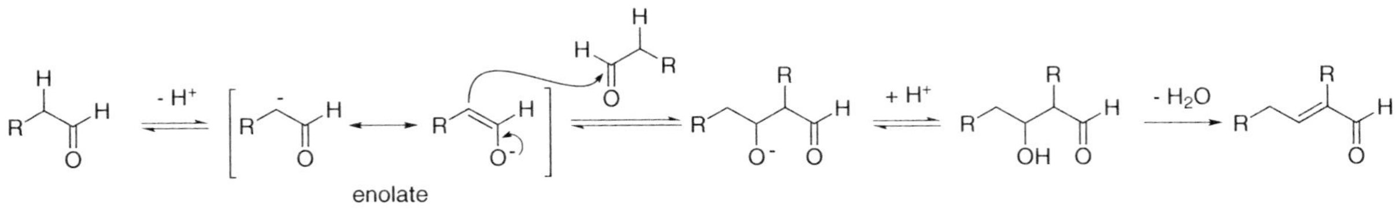

Mechanism of the base-catalyzed aldol condensation

Aldol condensation reactions between two different carbonyl compounds can lead to complex product mixtures, due to the possibility of enolate formation from either reactant and to the possibility of competing "homo" coupling rather than the desired "cross" coupling.

445

"Crossed" aldol condensation can afford complex mixtures

If, however, only one of the carbonyl compounds has alpha hydrogens available for deprotonation and enolate formation, the "crossed" aldol reaction can provide synthetically useful yields of products. Thus, for example, benzaldehyde cannot be converted to an enolate, yet reacts readily with enolates of other carbonyl compounds, including acetone.

A successful "crossed" aldol condensation

Homo coupling of acetone (or other ketones) is generally not a problem in such reactions, as the aldol condensation of ketones is generally not a very efficient reaction. (More specifically, each step of the aldol condensation is reversible under the reaction conditions – at least until the dehydration step – and thus equilibrium is established. With aldehydes, equilibrium favors the aldol product, but with ketones, primarily for steric reasons, very little aldol condensation product is present at equilibrium.)

In this experiment, you will explore the aldol condensation reaction of 3,4-dimethoxybenzaldehyde and 1-indanone.

3,4-dimethoxy-
benzaldehyde   1-indanone

446

In contrast to typical experimental procedures for aldol condensation reactions, this reaction will be carried out without solvent. Ongoing research is revealing a number of reactions that proceed nicely in the absence of solvent, representing the best possible solution to choice of a benign solvent. Although these reactions are frequently referred to as "solid-state" reactions, it has been noted [41] that in many cases, mixture of the solid reactants results in melting, so that the reactions actually occur in the liquid, albeit solvent-free state. This melting phenomenon is interesting and actually represents one of the key points of this experiment. You have learned that impurities lead to lower melting points. Here, you will experience this in a vivid way – as you mix the two solid reactants, they will melt. In addition to providing a memorable demonstration of the impact of impurities on melting points and illustrating the possibility of carrying out organic reactions in the absence of solvents, this experiment highlights another key green concept – the design of efficient, atom-economical reactions. The aldol condensation, if effected without dehydration, has an atom economy of 100% and requires only a catalytic amount of acid or base, and even with dehydration, the atom economy remains quite high.

Pre-Lab Preparation

1. Study the technique sections in your lab manual regarding melting points and recrystallization.
2. Carry out pre-lab preparations as described in Chapter 11, section 11.6A, or as called for by your instructor.

Experimental Procedure

SAFETY PRECAUTIONS: Use care to avoid contact with solid sodium hydroxide or the reaction mixture.

41.   G. Rothenberg, A. P. Downie, C. L. Raston, and J. L. Scott, "Understanding Solid/Solid Organic Reactions," *J. Am. Chem. Soc.* **2001**, *123*, 8701-8708.

Reaction

1. Place 0.25 g of 3,4-dimethoxybenzaldehyde and 0.20 g of 1-indanone in a test tube. Using a metal spatula, scrape and crush the two solids together until they become a brown oil. Use care to avoid breaking the test tube.

2. Add 0.05 g of finely ground (using a mortar and pestle) solid NaOH to the reaction mixture and continue scraping until the mixture becomes solid.

Workup and purification

3. Allow the mixture to stand for 15 minutes, then add about 2 mL of 10% aqueous HCl solution. Scrape well in order to dislodge the product from the walls of the test tube. Check the pH of the solution to make sure it is acidic.

4. Isolate the solid product by vacuum filtration, continuing to pull air through the solid to facilitate drying. Determine the mass of the crude product.

5. Recrystallize the product from 90% ethanol/10% water, using the hot solvent first to rinse any remaining product from the test tube. You should not require more than 20 mL of solvent to effect this recrystallization.

Characterization

6. Determine the mass and melting point of the recrystallized product. (A typical melting point range is 178 – 181 C.)

Post-Lab Questions and Exercises

1. Describe the physical properties (color and state) of your crude product. Report the mass and percent of theoretical yield of the crude product.

2. Report the color and melting point range of your recrystallized product. Report the mass and percent of theoretical yield of the recrystallized product.

3. Calculate the atom economy for the reaction.

4. Perform an economic analysis for the preparation of your product.

Experiment Development Notes

This experiment was adapted from the primary literature. Any number of solventless aldol reactions are possible [41], and it may be attractive to allow students some latitude in choosing their reactants, taking care to avoid unexpectedly hazardous reagents or products. The reactants reported here were chosen deliberately to highlight the melting point depression phenomenon; other pairs of reagents may or may not visibly melt upon mixing.